eighteenth
EDITION

# THE HARRIET LANE HANDBOOK

*A Manual for Pediatric House Officers*

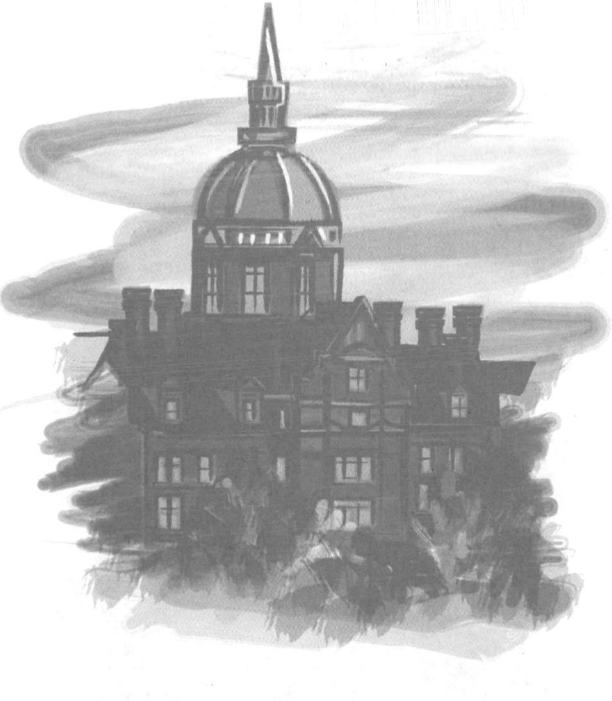

## RESUSCITATION MEDICATIONS

| Medication / Indication | Dose |
|---|---|
| **Adenosine**<br>• Supraventricular tachycardia | **0.1 mg/kg IV/IO RAPID BOLUS**<br>May repeat at 0.2 mg/kg IV/IO after 2 min.<br>Max first dose 6 mg, max subsequent dose 12 mg. |
| **Amiodarone**<br>• Ventricular tachycardia<br>• Ventricular fibrillation | **5 mg/kg IV/IO**<br>Push if no pulse.<br>Give over 15–20 min if pulse.<br>Monitor for hypotension. |
| **Atropine**<br>• Bradycardia (increased vagal tone)<br>• Primary AV block | **0.02 mg/kg IV/IO, 0.04–0.06 mg/kg ETT**<br>Min dose 0.1 mg<br>Max dose 0.5 mg (child), 1 mg (adolescent).<br>Repeat q5min to max dose of 1 mg (child), 2 mg (adol). |
| **Calcium chloride (10%)**<br>• Hypocalcemia | **20 mg/kg IV/IO (0.2 mL/kg)** |
| **Dextrose**<br>**(0.5–1 g/kg)** | **5–10 mL/kg 10% dextrose for <2 mo**<br>**2–4 mL/kg 25% dextrose for 2 mo–2 yr**<br>**1–2 mL/kg 50% dextrose for >2 yr** |
| **Epinephrine**<br>• Bradycardia<br>• Asystole<br>• Pulseless arrest | **0.01 mg/kg of 1 : 10,000 IV/IO ETT for <28 days old**<br>Repeat q3–5 min.<br>**0.1 mg/kg of 1 : 1000 ETT for >28 days old**<br>Dilute ETT dose to 2–5 mL with NS, follow with several positive-pressure ventilations.<br>**High-dose: 0.1 mg/kg 1 : 1000 IV/IO for anaphylaxis, beta blocker OD** |
| **Insulin**<br>• Hyperkalemia | **0.1 units/kg IV/IO with 0.5 g/kg of dextrose** |
| **Magnesium sulfate**<br>• Torsades de pointes<br>• Hypomagnesemia | **25–50 mg/kg IV/IO**<br>Push if no pulse.<br>Give over 15–20 min if pulse.<br>Monitor for hypotension/bradycardia. |
| **Nalaxone**<br>• Opioid overdose<br>• Coma | **<5 yr or <20 kg: 0.1 mg/kg IV/IO/IM/SC**<br>**>5 yr or >20 kg: 2 mg IV/IO/IM/SC**<br>ETT dose 2–3 times IV dose. |
| **Sodium bicarbonate**<br>• Metabolic acidosis<br>• Hyperkalemia<br>• Tricyclic antidepressant OD | **1 mEq/kg IV/IO**<br>Neonate: 0.5 mEq/kg IV/IO<br>Dilute 1 : 1 with sterile water for <10 kg. |
| **Vasopressin** | 0.5 units/kg/dose IV/IO |

ETT Meds ("LANE": lidocaine, atropine, naloxone, epinephrine)—dilute meds to 3–5 mL with NS, follow with positive-pressure ventilation.

## GLASCOW COMA SCALE

| Activity | Score | Child/Adult | Score | Infant |
|---|---|---|---|---|
| **Eye Opening** | 4 | Spontaneous | 4 | Spontaneous |
| | 3 | To speech | 3 | To speech/sound |
| | 2 | To pain | 2 | To pain |
| | 1 | None | 1 | None |
| **Verbal** | 5 | Oriented | 5 | Coos/babbles |
| | 4 | Confused | 4 | Irritable cry |
| | 3 | Inappropriate | 3 | Cries to pain |
| | 2 | Incomprehensible | 2 | Moans to pain |
| | 1 | None | 1 | None |
| **Motor** | 6 | Obeys commands | 6 | Normal spontaneous |
| | 5 | Localizes to pain | 5 | Withdraws to touch |
| | 4 | Withdraws to pain | 4 | Withdraws to pain |
| | 3 | Abnormal flexion | 3 | Abnormal flexion (decorticate) |
| | 2 | Abnormal extension | 2 | Abnormal extension (decerebrate) |
| | 1 | None | 1 | None |

From The Johns Hopkins Children's Center Kids Kard 2005.

# Expert CONSULT

*Online + Print*

## Online access activation instructions

**This Expert Consult** title comes with access to the complete contents online. **Activate your access today** by following these simple instructions:

1. Gently scratch off the surface of the sticker below, using the edge of a coin, to reveal your **activation code.**
2. Visit **www.expertconsultbook.com** and click on the **"Register"** button.
3. **Enter your activation code** along with the other information requested . . . and begin enjoying your access.

**It's that easy!** For technical assistance, email **online.help@elsevier.com** or **call 800-401-9962** (inside the US) or **+1-314-995-3200** (outside the US).

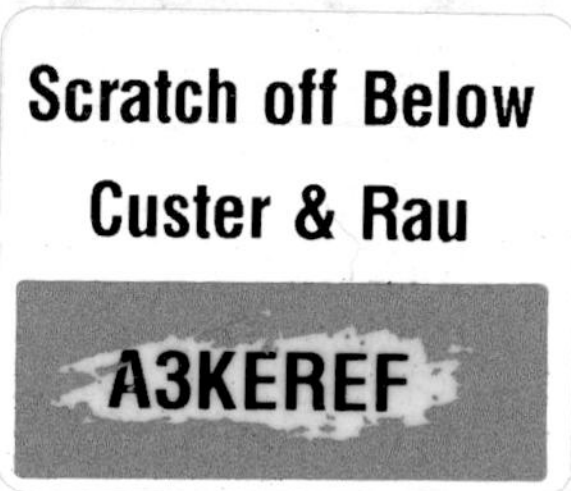

eighteenth
EDITION

# THE HARRIET LANE HANDBOOK

*A Manual for Pediatric House Officers*

The Harriet Lane Service
Children's Medical and Surgical Center of
The Johns Hopkins Hospital

**EDITORS**
**Jason W. Custer, MD**
**Rachel E. Rau, MD**

*with 120 illustrations and over 50 color plates*

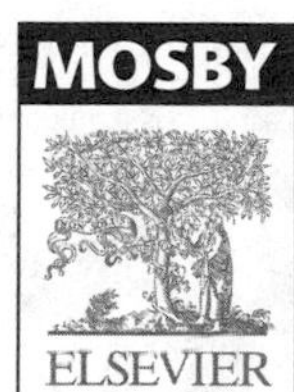

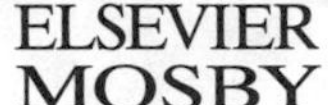

1600 John F. Kennedy Blvd.
Suite 1800
Philadelphia, PA 19103-2899

THE HARRIET LANE HANDBOOK

ISBN: 978-0-323-05303-7
International Edition: 978-0-8089-2415-9



**Notice**

Knowledge and best practice in this field are constantly changing. As new research and experience broaden our knowledge, changes in practice, treatment, and drug therapy may become necessary or appropriate. Readers are advised to check the most current information provided (i) on procedures featured or (ii) by the manufacturer of each product to be administered, to verify the recommended dose or formula, the method and duration of administration, and contraindications. It is the responsibility of the practitioners, relying on their own experience and knowledge of the patients, to make diagnoses, to determine dosages and the best treatment for each individual patient, and to take all appropriate safety precautions. To the fullest extent of the law, neither the Publisher nor the Editors assume any liability for any injury and/or damage to persons or property arising out of or related to any use of the material contained in this book.

The Publisher

**Library of Congress Cataloging-in-Publication Data**

The Harriet Lane handbook : a manual for pediatric house officers / the Harriet Lane Service, Children's Medical and Surgical Center of the Johns Hopkins Hospital ; editors, Jason W. Custer, Rachel E. Rau.—18th ed.
p. ; cm.
Includes bibliographical references and index.
ISBN 978-0-323-05303-7
1. Pediatrics—Handbooks, manuals, etc. I. Custer, Jason W. II. Rau, Rachel E. III. Johns Hopkins Hospital. Children's Medical and Surgical Center.
[DNLM: 1. Pediatrics—Handbooks. WS 29 H297 2009]
RJ48.H35 2009
618.92—dc22

2007042930

*Editor:* James Merritt
*Developmental Editor:* Marybeth Thiel
*Project Manager:* Mary Stermel
*Designer:* Karen O'Keefe Owens
*Illustrations Manager:* Michael Carcel
*Marketing Manager:* Paul Leese

Printed in the United States of America

Last digit is the print number: 9 8 7 6 5 4 3 2 1

**To our loving families:**

*Sharon and Terry Custer,*
*for teaching me the value of hard work and*
*never letting me doubt my dreams;*

*Melissa Custer,*
*my best friend, for her support and encouragement—*
*I love coming home to you;*

*Eddie and Judy Rau,*
*for their selfless love and support, which have made all*
*in my life possible;*

*Peter Wung,*
*my wonderful husband, for ensuring that no matter where*
*life leads, I will be in the best place on earth—by your side.*

*Our daughters,*
*Allison Grace Custer and Abigail Shinyi Wung,*
*who complete our lives.*

**To our patients and their families,**

*who continue to aid us in our development as pediatricians and in the enrichment of our lives.*

**To the consummate pediatrician,**

*Fred Heldrich.*

**To our role model, teacher, and friend**

*Julia McMillan.*

**And to**

*George Dover,*
*Chairman of Pediatrics,*
*The Johns Hopkins Hospital,*
*Devoted advocate for residents, children, and their families.*

# Preface

*The Harriet Lane Handbook* has been in existence since 1953—after Harrison Spencer, chief resident in 1950–1951, suggested that residents develop a pocket-sized "pearl book." As recounted by Henry Seidel, the first editor of *The Harriet Lane Handbook*, "Six of us began without funds and without [the] supervision of our elders, meeting sporadically around a table in the library of the Harriet Lane Home." What they achieved was a concise yet comprehensive handbook that quickly found its way into the pockets of all the residents of the Harriet Lane Home. Residents in subsequent years continued to update and revise the handbook. Ultimately, under the guidance of Robert Cooke (Department Chief from 1956 to 1974), who realized the potential of the handbook, the fifth edition was published for widespread distribution by Year Book. Since its humble beginnings, the handbook has spread not only to pediatricians throughout the country but to a worldwide audience as well. Now translated into many languages, the handbook is still intended as an easy-to-use manual to help pediatricians provide comprehensive and current pediatric care.

Today *The Harriet Lane Handbook* continues to be updated and revised *by* house officers *for* house officers, with each edition improving on the one that came before. Notable changes to this edition include a reorganization of text and figures to improve flow and usability. An important addition is the new "Palliative Care" chapter. Inspired by Dr. Nancy Hutton, who has dedicated her career to improving the quality of care for children with life-limiting conditions and providing essential support for their families, the chapter offers the resources necessary to ensure excellence of care for the patients and their families. In addition, the "Nutrition and Growth" chapter has been reorganized and streamlined to aid the pediatrician in promoting good health through appropriate nutrition. The charts in the "Poisonings" chapter have been revised for easier access to information. The Pediatric Advanced Life Support guidelines have been updated to ensure appropriate management of critically ill children. The "Pulmonology" chapter includes new sections on bronchiolitis and sleep apnea. The "Microbiology and Infectious Disease" and "Immunoprophylaxis" chapters have been updated to include the most current treatment and vaccination recommendations of the Center for Disease Control and the American Association of Pediatrics. To support the growth and development of children's minds as well, a chart for the Reach Out and Read milestones of early literary development has been added to the "Behavior and Development" chapter.

This book, designed for pediatric house staff, would not have been possible without the efforts of this year's senior resident class. We have participated in their growth as pediatricians from their internship and have watched them mature in both clinical skill and character. Each of the residents worked with a faculty advisor, who selflessly dedicated his or her time and expertise to improve the quality and content of this publication.

| Resident | Chapter Title | Faculty Advisor |
|---|---|---|
| Gwyneth Susil, MD | Emergency Management | Allen Walker, MD |
| Amy Valasek, MD | Poisonings | Mitchell Goldstein, MD<br>Suzanne Doyon, MD |
| Jason W. Custer, MD | Procedures | |
| Jennifer L. Jarjosa, MD | Trauma, Burns, and Common Critical Care Emergencies | Allen Walker, MD |
| Nicole Namour, MD, MPH | Adolescent Medicine | Hoover Adger, MD, MPH |
| Hema Dave, MD | Analgesia and Sedation | Jennifer Anders, MD |
| Aisha Frazier, MD, MPH<br>Cozumel Southern Pruette, MD, MS | Cardiology | Jane Crosson, MD<br>William Ravekes, MD<br>W. Reid Thompson, MD |
| Nicole Schumann-Gable MD | Dermatology | Bernard Cohen, MD |
| Martine M. Solages, MD | Behavior and Development | Mary Leppert, MD, MBBCh |
| Sonia Arora Ballal, MD<br>Paul McIntosh, MD | Endocrinology | David Cooke, MD |
| Gregory J. Aune, MD, PhD | Fluids and Electrolytes | Michael Barone, MD |
| Nicole E. Jordan, MD | Gastroenterology | Maria Oliva-Hemker, MD |
| Linda Hayrapetian-Dorsi, MD | Genetics | Ronald Cohn, MD |
| Julia Aquino, MD | Hematology | James Casella, MD |
| Hilary J. Tinkel Vernon, MD, PhD | Immunology and Allergy | Howard Lederman, MD, PhD<br>Robert Wood, MD |
| Nakia Johnson, MD | Immunoprophylaxis | George Siberry, MD, MPH |
| Joelle N. Simpson, MD, MPH | Microbiology and Infectious Disease | George Siberry, MD, MPH |
| Nathaly M. Francisco Sweeney, MD, MPH | Neonatology | Lawrence Nogee, MD |
| Jade M. Tan, MD | Nephrology | Susan Furth, MD |
| Lisa Emrick, MD | Neurology | Thomas Crawford, MD |
| Peter Claybour, MD<br>Jenifer Hampsey, MS, RD, CPS | Nutrition and Growth | Maria Oliva-Hemker, MD |

| Resident | Chapter Title | Faculty Advisor |
|---|---|---|
| Rachel Brennan, MD | Oncology | Kenneth Cohen, MD<br>Patrick Brown, MD |
| Amy Valasek, MD | Palliative Care | Nancy Hutton, MD |
| Fatimah S. Dawood, MD | Pulmonology | Anne Halbower, MD |
| John Holcroft, MD | Radiology | Jane Benson, MD |
| Keith A. Sikora, MD | Rheumatology | Edward Sills, MD |
| Jason W. Custer, MD | Blood Chemistries and Body Fluids | |
| Rachel E. Rau, MD | Biostatistics and Evidence-Based Medicine | |
| Carlton Lee, PharmD, MPH<br>Jason W. Custer MD<br>Rachel E. Rau, MD | Drug Doses | |
| Jason W. Custer, MD | Formulary Adjunct | Carlton Lee, PharmD, MPH |
| Rachel E. Rau, MD | Drugs in Renal Failure | Carlton Lee, PharmD, MPH |

The formulary, which is undoubtedly one of the handbook sections most referred to, is complete, concise, and easy to navigate largely thanks to the efforts of Carlton Lee, PharmD, MPH. With each edition, he carefully updates, revises, and improves the section providing one of the most useful pediatric drug reference texts available.

The Frank Oski Conference Room has been the meeting place for many years of conferences convened to teach and guide residents. The room houses a bookshelf filled with the previous editions of *The Harriet Lane Handbook*. We truly stand on the shoulders of giants as we build on this great work: Drs. Harrison Spencer, Henry Seidel, Herbert Swick, William Friedman, Robert Haslam, Jerry Winkelstein, Dennis Headings, Kenneth Schuberth, Basil Zitelli, Jeffery Biller, Andrew Yeager, Cynthia Cole, Mary Greene, Peter Rowe, Kevin Johnson, Michael Barone, George Siberry, Rob Iannone, Christian Nechyba, Veronica L. Gunn, Jason Robertson, and Nicole Shilkofski. Many of these previous editors continue to contribute to the learning and maturation of the Harriet Lane house staff and have built a tremendous legacy of successful pediatricians. Henry Seidel, Peter Rowe, George Siberry, and Michael Barone are true examples of outstanding clinicians, educators, and mentors.

An undertaking of this magnitude could not have been accomplished without the support and dedication of some very special people. Special thanks go to Megan Brown and Kathy Miller for providing tremendous guidance and support leavened with laughter and friendship. We express our unwavering gratitude to Jeanne Cox for laying the foundation for the "Nutrition and Growth" chapter and for providing support to all of the interns during their journeys through the Neonatal Intensive Care Unit. We are especially grateful to Wayne Reisig for helping us navigate the ever-expanding world of evidence-based medicine. We also offer our deepest gratitude to George Dover, whose tireless work has continued to advance the department greatly and ensure excellence in the care of children and the education of pediatricians. A heartfelt thank-you goes to Dr. Fred Heldrich, whose professionalism and commitment to pediatrics we can only hope to emulate. He will be missed. Our special thanks go to our friend and mentor Janet Serwint, whose leadership continues to enrich our lives. Finally, none of this would have been possible without Julia McMillan, our leader by example, whose passion for the education of the house staff has instilled the love of pediatrics in all of us.

**Residents**
Sarah Aminoff
Kristin Arcara
Eric Balighian
Gia Bradley
J. B. Cantey
Katherine Dahab
Charise Freundlich
Jessica Hebert
Raegan Hunt
Lara Jacobson
Melissa Jerdonek
Candice Jones
Laura Landgraf
Jana Leary
Calvin Lee
Lanier Lopez
Ryan Majcina
Rheanna Platt
Sheila Ravendhran
Ashley Shoemaker
Daniel Sklansky
David Smith
Arvind Srinath
Gwyneth Susil
Megan Tschudy
Michael Walsh
Christine Zimmerman

**Interns**
Hans Bjornsson
Maria Cancio
Jessica Clarke-Pounder
Megan DeCapite
Letitia Dzirasa
Sarah Graham
Stephanie Griese
Rana Hamdy
Jessica Howlett
Khaliah Johnson
Jennifer Johnston
Lisa Kantz
Michael Keller
Amina Khan
Evelyn Kow
Thomas Krupica
Jennifer Leung
Tamorah Lewis
Christina Lindgren
Melanie Nies
Terence Prendiville
Michael Rinke
Amy Sniderman
Katie Sussman
Alison Tribble
Jennifer Webb

**Jason W. Custer**
**Rachel E. Rau**

# Contents

# PART I

# Pediatric Acute Care

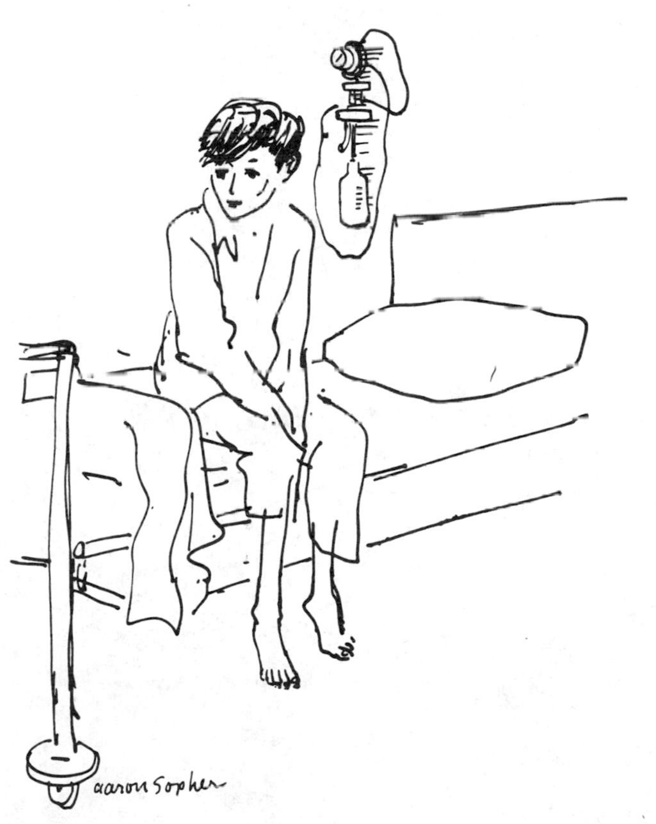

# Emergency Management

*Gwyneth Susil, MD*

When approaching a patient in cardiopulmonary arrest, it is important to remember the basics. Immediately assessing the patient's airway, breathing, and circulation (ABCs) is the most important first step. If at any point the resuscitation is not going as expected, reassess the ABCs, considering the possibility that something has compromised areas that were previously secure.

## I. AIRWAY[1–5]

1

### A. ASSESSMENT

1. **Position the child supine on a flat, hard surface.**
2. **Open airway: Establish an open airway with the head-tilt/chin-lift maneuver. If neck injury is suspected, use jaw thrust with cervical spine (C-spine) immobilization.**
3. **Check for obstruction: Rule out foreign-body, anatomic, or other obstruction.**

### B. MANAGEMENT

1. **Equipment:**

a. Oral airway is used in an unconscious patient.
   (1) Size: With flange at teeth, tip reaches angle of jaw.
   (2) Length: From 4 to 10cm

b. Nasopharyngeal airway is used in a conscious patient.
   (1) Rarely provokes vomiting or laryngospasm.
   (2) Size: Length equals tip of nose to angle of jaw. Check the outer diameter so that the airway does not blanch the alae nasi.
   (3) Diameter: 12 to 36 French (F).
   (4) A shortened endotracheal tube (ETT) may be used.

c. Laryngeal mask airway (LMA) is an option for a secure airway in an unconscious patient that does not require laryngoscopy or tracheal intubation. It allows spontaneous or assisted respiration but **does not prevent aspiration**. It may be useful in patients with abnormal anatomy, difficult airway, or head and neck trauma.

2. **Intubation: Sedation and paralysis are recommended for intubation, except in newborns and in some patients who are unconscious or in cardiorespiratory arrest.**

a. Indications: Obstruction (functional or anatomic), need for prolonged ventilatory assistance or control, respiratory insufficiency, loss of protective airway reflexes, or need for route for approved medications.

b. Equipment (see table on inside front cover): **SOAP** (**S**uction, **O**xygen, **A**irway Supplies, **P**harmacology)

(1) ETT: The following equation should be used to determine the size of the ETT to be used:

(Age [yrs] +16)/4 = internal diameter of ETT tube (mm)

(a) Have one ETT 0.5 mm smaller and one ETT 0.5 mm larger than the estimated size.
(b) An uncuffed ETT should be used in patients ≤8 years old. The depth of insertion (in centimeters; at the teeth or lips) is about three times the ETT size.
(c) Resuscitation tapes based on length may be used to estimate ETT size.

(2) Laryngoscope blade and handle with a functioning light: Generally, a straight blade can be used in all patients. A curved blade may be easier to use in patients >2 years old.
(3) Bag and mask should be attached to 100% oxygen.
(4) ETT stylets should not extend beyond the distal end of the ETT.
(5) Suction: Use a large-bore (Yankauer) suction catheter or 14F to 18F suction catheter.
(6) Nasogastric (or orogastric) tube: Size from nose to angle of jaw to xiphoid process.
(7) Monitoring equipment: Electrocardiography (ECG), pulse oximetry, blood pressure (BP) monitoring, capnometry (end-tidal $CO_2$ monitoring).
(8) Tape to secure the tube.
(9) Consider an LMA for difficult airway.

c. **Procedure:** Attempts should not exceed 30 seconds.

(1) Preoxygenate with 100% $O_2$. Assist ventilation with positive-pressure ventilation only if the patient's effort is inadequate.
(2) Administer intubation medications (Table 1-1 and Fig. 1-1).
(3) Apply cricoid pressure to prevent aspiration (Sellick maneuver) during bag-valve-mask ventilation and intubation.
(4) With patient lying supine on a firm surface, head midline and slightly extended, open mouth with right thumb and index finger using scissoring technique.
(5) Hold laryngoscope blade in left hand. Insert blade into right side of mouth, sweeping tongue to the left out of line of vision.
(6) Advance blade to epiglottis. With straight blade, lift laryngoscope straight up, directly lifting the epiglottis until vocal cords are visible. With curved blade, the tip of the blade rests in the vallecula (between the base of the tongue and epiglottis). Lift straight up to elevate the epiglottis and visualize the vocal cords.
(7) While maintaining direct visualization, pass the ETT from the right corner of the mouth through the cords. The double black marker on the tube should be at the level of the vocal cords.

TABLE 1-1

**RAPID-SEQUENCE INTUBATION MEDICATIONS**

| Drug | Dose (IV) (mg/kg) | Comments |
|---|---|---|
| **ADJUNCTS (FIRST)** | | |
| Atropine (vagolytic) | 0.01–0.02<br>Min: 0.1 mg<br>Max: 1 mg | Vagolytic; prevents bradycardia and reduces oral secretions; may increase HR |
| Lidocaine (optional anesthetic) | 1–2 | Blunts ICP spike, cough reflex, and CV effects of intubation; controls ventricular arrhythmias |
| **SEDATIVE-HYPNOTIC (SECOND)** | | |
| Thiopental | 1–5 | May cause hypotension; myocardial depression (barbiturate); decreases ICP and cerebral blood flow; use low dose in hypovolemia (1–2 mg/kg); may increase oral secretions, cause bronchospasm and laryngospasm; contraindicated in status asthmaticus |
| *or* | | |
| Ketamine | 1–4 | May increase ICP, BP, HR, and oral secretions (general anesthetic); causes bronchodilation, emergence delirium; give with atropine; contraindicated in eye injuries |
| *or* | | |
| Midazolam (benzodiazepine) | 0.05–0.1 | May cause decreased BP and HR and respiratory depression; amnestic properties; reversible with flumazenil (seizure warning applies) |
| *or* | | |
| Fentanyl (opiate) | 1–5 mcg/kg | Fewest hemodynamic effects of all opiates; chest wall rigidity with high-dose or rapid administration; opiates reversible with naloxone (seizure warning applies); don't use with MAO inhibitors |
| *or* | | |
| Etomidate (imidazole/hypnotic) | 0.2–0.3 | Does not cause hypotension or increased ICP; may cause further suppression in patients with adrenal suppression (use cautiously) |
| **PARALYTICS (THIRD)*** | | |
| Rocuronium | 0.6–1.2 | Onset 30–60 sec, duration 30–60 min; administer with sedative; may reverse in 30 min with atropine and neostigmine; minimal effect on HR or BP; precipitates when in contact with other drugs, so flush line before and after use |
| *or* | | |
| Vecuronium | 0.1–0.2 | Onset 70–120 sec, duration 30–90 min; minimal effect on BP or HR; may reverse in 30–45 min with atropine and neostigmine |

*Nondepolarizing neuromuscular blockers, except succinylcholine, which is depolarizing.

BP, Blood pressure; CV, cardiovascular; HR, heart rate; ICP, intracranial pressure; MAO, monoamine oxidase.

*Continued*

TABLE 1-1

RAPID-SEQUENCE INTUBATION MEDICATIONS—cont'd

| Drug | Dose (IV) (mg/kg) | Comments |
|---|---|---|
| PARALYTICS (THIRD)*—cont'd | | |
| *or* | | |
| Succinylcholine | 1–2 | Onset 30–60 sec, duration 3–10 min; increases ICP, irreversible; contraindicated in burns, massive trauma, neuromuscular disease, eye injuries, malignant hyperthermia, and pseudocholinesterase deficiency. *Risk*: Lethal hyperkalemia in undiagnosed muscular dystrophy |

(8) Verify ETT placement: observe chest wall movement, auscultation in both axillae and epigastrium, capnography or colorimetric capnometer, end-tidal $CO_2$ detection (there will be a false-negative response if no effective pulmonary circulation), water vapor in the tube, improvement in oxygen saturation, chest radiograph.

(9) Only when ETT placement is verified should cricoid pressure be removed.

(10) Securely tape ETT in place, noting depth of insertion (cm) at teeth or lips.

### C. RAPID-SEQUENCE INTUBATION MEDICATIONS

**Note** *Titrate drug doses to achieve desired effect (see Fig. 1-1 and Table 1-1).*

## II. BREATHING[1-3]

### A. ASSESSMENT

After the airway is established, evaluate air exchange. Examine for evidence of abnormal chest wall dynamics, such as tension pneumothorax, or central problems such as apnea. Once intubated, deterioration may be caused by **D**isplacement of the ETT, **O**bstruction, **P**neumothorax, or **E**quipment failure (**DOPE**).

### B. MANAGEMENT

Positive-pressure ventilation (application of 100% $O_2$ is never contraindicated in resuscitation situations).

1. **Mouth-to-mouth or mouth-to-nose** breathing is used in situations in which no supplies are available. Provide two slow breaths (1 to 1.5 sec/breath) initially, then 20 breaths/min (30 breaths/min in infants). For newborns, apply 1 breath for every 3 chest compressions. In infants and children, apply 2 breaths after 30 compressions (1 rescuer) or 2 breaths after 15 compressions (2

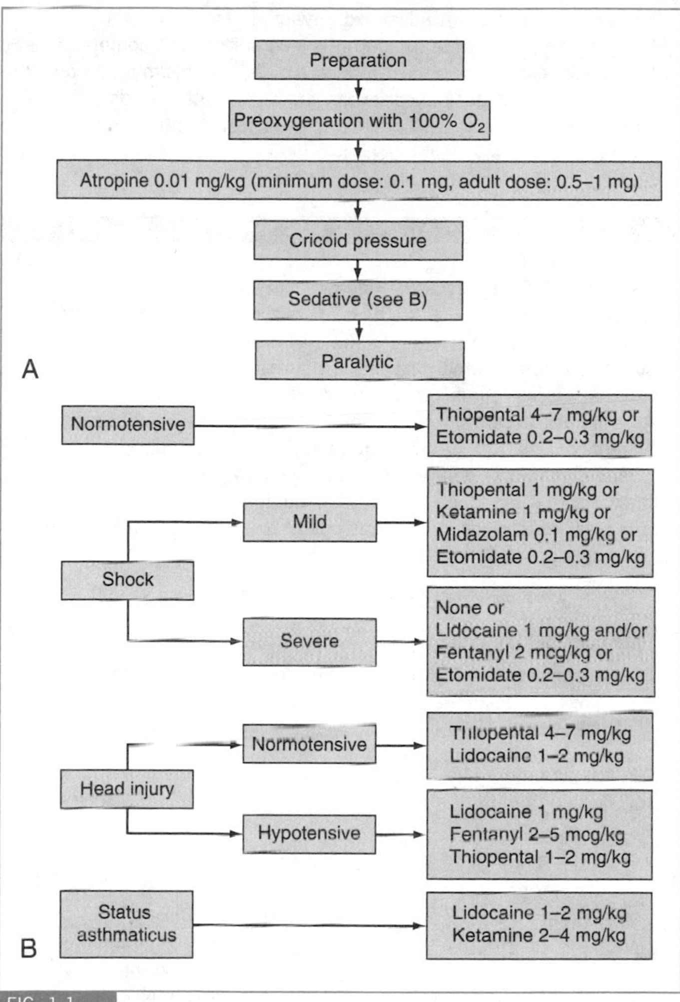


FIG. 1-1

**A,** Treatment algorithm for intubation. **B,** Sedation options. *(Modified from Nichols DG et al [eds]: Golden Hour: The Handbook of Advanced Pediatric Life Support. St. Louis, Mosby, 1996, p 29.)*

rescuers). If there is an advanced airway in place, give 8 to 10 breaths/min. These breaths are not synchronized with compressions.

2. **Bag-mask ventilation** is used at a rate of 20 breaths/min (30 breaths/min in infants). Assess chest expansion and breath sounds. Decompress stomach with orogastric or nasogastric tube with prolonged bag-mask ventilation.
3. **Endotracheal intubation:** See prior section.

## III. CIRCULATION[1,2,4]

### A. ASSESSMENT

1. **Rate:** Assess for bradycardia, tachycardia, or absent heart rate. Generally, bradycardia is <100 beats/min in a newborn and <60 beats/min in an infant or child; tachycardia of >240 beats/min suggests cardiac arrhythmia rather than sinus tachycardia.
2. **Rhythm:** Assess sinus versus abnormal rhythm.
3. **Assess pulses (central and peripheral) and capillary refill (assuming extremity is warm):** <2 sec is normal, 2 to 5 sec is delayed, and >5 sec is markedly delayed, suggesting shock. Decreased or altered mental status may be a sign of inadequate perfusion.
4. **BP:** Measuring blood pressure is one of the least sensitive measures of adequate circulation in children.

$$\text{Hypotension} = \text{systolic BP} < [70 + (2 \times \text{age in years})]$$

### B. MANAGEMENT (Table 1-2)

1. **Chest compressions** (ensure maximum effectiveness of compressions)

a. Press hard and fast (see Table 1-2).
b. Allow for full chest recoil; hands should come fully off the chest between compressions, allowing for venous return.
c. Minimize interruptions to chest compressions.
d. Switch providers often (if available) to limit fatigue.
e. Ensure that backboard is in place.
f. If end tidal $CO_2$ in line: goal is to achieve >10 mm Hg.

TABLE 1-2

MANAGEMENT OF CIRCULATION

| | Location* | Rate (per min) | Compressions: Ventilation |
|---|---|---|---|
| Infants | 1 fingerbreadth below intermammary line | >100 | 15:2 (2 rescuers)<br>30:2 (1 rescuer) |
| Pre-pubertal children | 2 fingerbreadths below intermammary line | 100 | 15:2 (2 rescuers)<br>30:2 (1 rescuer) |
| Adolescents/adults | Lower half of sternum | 100 | 30:2 (1 or 2 rescuers) |

*Depth of compressions should be one third to one half anteroposterior diameter of the chest.

2. **Use of automated external defibrillator (AED):** For children >1 year, use an AED/defibrillator after 5 cycles of cardiopulmonary resuscitation or as soon as available for sudden, witnessed collapse.
3. **Fluid resuscitation with poor perfusion and shock:**
a. If peripheral intravenous (IV) access is not obtained in 90 seconds or after two attempts, *or* if patient is in cardiorespiratory arrest and access is predicted to be difficult, place an intraosseous needle (see Chapter 3). If still unsuccessful, consider central venous access.
b. Initial fluid used should be lactated Ringer's or normal saline (NS) solution. Administer a bolus with 20 mL/kg over 5 to 15 minutes. Reassess. If there is no improvement, consider a repeat bolus with 20 mL/kg of the same fluid. Reassess. If replacement requires more than 40 to 60 mL/kg, or if there is acute blood loss, consider colloids: 5% albumin, plasma, or packed red blood cells at 10 to 15 mL/kg.
c. If cardiogenic etiology is suspected, fluid resuscitation may worsen clinical status. Consider a smaller fluid bolus of 5 to 10 mL/kg.
4. **Pharmacotherapy:** See inside front and back covers for guidelines for drugs to be considered in cardiac arrest and arrhythmia algorithms. Consider early administration of antibiotics or corticosteroids if clinically indicated.

## IV. ALLERGIC EMERGENCIES (ANAPHYLAXIS)[4,6]

### A. DEFINITION

Anaphylaxis is the clinical syndrome of immediate hypersensitivity. It is characterized by cardiovascular collapse, respiratory compromise, and cutaneous and gastrointestinal (GI) symptoms (e.g., urticaria, emesis).

### B. INITIAL MANAGEMENT

1. **ABCs:** Establish airway if necessary. Assess breathing; Supply with 100% $O_2$ with respiratory support as needed. Assess circulation and establish IV access. Place patient on cardiac monitor.
2. **Epinephrine:** Give epinephrine, 0.01 mL/kg (1:1000) intramuscular (IM), maximum dose 0.5 mL. Repeat every 15 min as needed. The site of choice is the lateral aspect of the thigh due to its vascularity.
3. **Albuterol:** Give nebulized albuterol, 0.05 to 0.15 mg/kg in 3 mL NS solution (quick estimate: 2.5 mg for <30 kg, 5 mg for >30 kg) every 15 min as needed.
4. **Histamine-1 receptor antagonist** such as diphenhydramine, 1 to 2 mg/kg through IM, IV, or oral (PO) route (maximum dose, 50 mg). Also, consider a histamine-2 receptor antagonist.
5. **Corticosteroids** help prevent the late phase of the allergic response. Administer methylprednisolone in a 2 mg/kg IV bolus, then 2 mg/kg per day IV or IM divided every 6 hours, or prednisone, 2 mg/kg PO in a bolus once daily. Observe for 6 to 24 hours for late-phase symptoms depending on clinical condition and stability.

6. **Patient should be discharged with an Epi-Pen** (>30 kg), Epi-Pen Junior (<30 kg), or comparable injectable epinephrine product with specific instructions on appropriate use.

### C. HYPOTENSION

1. **Trendelenburg position:** Put patient's head at 30-degree angle below feet.
2. **Fluid:** Administer 20 mL/kg IV NS or lactated Ringer's solution over 5 to 15 min. Repeat bolus as necessary.
3. **Epinephrine:** Give 0.1 mL/kg (1:10,000) IV every 2 to 5 min while an epinephrine or dopamine infusion is being prepared. (See the infusion table on the inside front cover for details of preparation and dosages.)

## V. RESPIRATORY EMERGENCIES[4]

The hallmark of upper airway obstruction is inspiratory stridor, whereas lower airway obstruction is characterized by cough, wheeze, and a prolonged expiratory phase.

### A. ASTHMA

1. **Assessment:** Assess heart rate (HR), respiratory rate, $O_2$ saturation, peak expiratory flow rate, use of accessory muscles, pulsus paradoxus (>20 mm Hg difference in systolic BP for inspiratory versus expiratory phase), dyspnea, alertness, color.
2. **Initial management:**

a. Give $O_2$ to keep saturation >95%.
b. Administer inhaled β-agonists: Nebulized albuterol, 0.05 to 0.15 mg/kg/dose every 20 minutes (or continuously depending on clinical condition) to effect. Albuterol may be given by metered-dose inhaler with aerochamber to a cooperative patient.
c. Additional nebulized bronchodilators include ipratropium bromide, 0.25 to 0.5 mg, nebulized with albuterol (as previously). Benefit has been demonstrated only for moderate to severe exacerbations.
d. If air movement is very poor or the patient is unable to cooperate with a nebulizer, give epinephrine, 0.01 mL/kg SC (1:1000; maximum dose, 0.5 mL) every 15 min up to three doses, or terbutaline, 0.01 mg/kg SC (maximum dose, 0.4 mg) every 15 min up to two doses.
e. Start corticosteroids if there is no response after one nebulized treatment or if patient is steroid dependent or has had a recent emergency department visit or previous admission to an intensive care unit: Prednisone or prednisolone, 2 mg/kg PO every 24 hr or (if severe) methylprednisolone, 2 mg/kg IV/IM bolus, then 2 mg/kg/day divided every 6 hr. Parenteral steroids have not been proven to routinely provide more rapid onset of action or greater clinical effect than oral steroids in children with mild to moderate asthma.

3. **Further management if incomplete or poor response:** Consider obtaining an arterial blood gas value if breath sounds are minimal. Note that a normalizing $Pco_2$ is often a sign of impending respiratory failure.

a. Continue nebulization therapy every 20 to 30 min, and space interval as tolerated.
b. Administer magnesium sulfate, 25 to 75 mg/kg/dose IV or IM (maximum, 2 g) infused over 20 min every 4 to 6 hr up to three to four doses. Many clinicians suggest the higher end of this dosing range (75 mg/kg/dose), although further dosing studies are needed. Do not use in hypotension or renal failure.
c. Administer terbutaline, 2 to 10 mcg/kg IV load, followed by continuous infusion at 0.1 to 0.4 mcg/kg/min titrated to effect (see inside front cover table). Monitor 12-lead ECG, electrolytes, urinalysis, and cardiac enzymes.
d. A helium (≥70%) and oxygen mixture may be of some benefit in the critically ill patient but is more useful in upper airway edema. Avoid use in the severely hypoxic patient.
e. Although aminophylline may be considered, it is no longer considered a preferred mode of therapy for status asthmaticus (see the Formulary for dosage information).

4. **Intubation of those with acute asthma is dangerous and should be reserved for impending respiratory arrest. Indications include deteriorating mental status, severe cyanosis, and respiratory or cardiac arrest. Premedicate with lidocaine, midazolam, and ketamine (see Fig. 1-1 and Table 1-1). Consider using an inhaled anesthetic.**



## B. UPPER AIRWAY OBSTRUCTION

Upper airway obstruction is most commonly caused by foreign-body aspiration or infection.

1. **Epiglottitis is a true emergency. Any manipulation, including aggressive physical examination, attempt to visualize the epiglottis, venipuncture, or IV placement, may precipitate complete obstruction. If epiglottitis is suspected, definitive airway placement should precede all diagnostic procedures. A prototypic "epiglottitis protocol" may include the following:**

a. Unobtrusively give $O_2$ (blow-by). Place patient on NPO status. Pulse oximetry may be used if it does not upset the patient.
b. Have parent accompany child to allay anxiety.
c. Have physician accompany patient at all times.
d. Summon "epiglottitis team" (most senior pediatrician, anesthesiologist, and otolaryngologist in hospital).
e. Management options:
   (1) If patient is unstable (unresponsive, cyanotic, bradycardic), emergently intubate.
   (2) If patient is stable with high suspicion, escort patient with team to operating room for endoscopy and intubation under general anesthesia.
   (3) If patient is stable with moderate or low suspicion, obtain lateral neck radiographs to confirm. An epiglottitis team must accompany the patient at all times.
f. After airway is secured, obtain cultures of blood and epiglottic surface. Begin antibiotics to cover *Haemophilus influenzae* type B,

*Streptococcus pneumoniae*, group A streptococci, *Staphylococcus aureus*. Epiglottitis may be caused by thermal injury.

2. **Croup (laryngotracheobronchitis):**
   a. Mild (no stridor at rest): Treat with cool mist therapy, minimal disturbance, hydration, and antipyretics. Consider steroids (see later).
   b. Moderate to severe:
      (1) Mist or humidified oxygen mask near child's face may be used, although the efficacy of mist therapy is not established. A mist tent may increase a child's anxiety and decrease the physician's ability to observe the patient.
      (2) Administer racemic epinephrine (2.25%), 0.05 mL/kg/dose (maximum dose, 0.5 mL) in 3 mL NS solution *over 15 min*, no more than every 1 to 2 hr, or nebulized epinephrine, 0.5 mL/kg of 1:1000 (1 mg/mL) in 3 mL NS solution (maximum dose, 2.5 mL for ≤4 years old, 5 mL for >4 years old). Observe for a minimum of 2 to 4 hr if discharge is planned after administering nebulized epinephrine. Hospitalize if more than one nebulization is required.
      (3) Administer dexamethasone, 0.3 to 0.6 mg/kg IM or PO once. Prednisolone or prednisone may be adequate but should be administered for several days because of the shorter half-life of these steroid preparations.
      (4) Nebulized budesonide (2 mg) has been shown to be effective in mild to moderate croup and is *equivalent to oral dexamethasone*.
      (5) A helium-oxygen mixture may decrease the work of breathing by decreasing resistance to turbulent gas flow through a narrowed airway. Inspired helium concentration must be ≥70% to be effective.
   c. If a child fails to respond as expected to therapy, consider airway radiography, computed tomography (CT), or evaluation by otolaryngology or anesthesiology. Consider retropharyngeal abscess, bacterial tracheitis, subglottic stenosis, subglottic hemangioma, epiglottitis, or foreign body.
3. **Foreign-body aspiration occurs most often in children <5 years old. It frequently involves hot dogs, candy, peanuts, grapes, or balloons, as well as other small objects. A high index of suspicion, witnessed event, and history of choking are most important for diagnosis.**
   a. If the patient is stable (i.e., forcefully coughing, well oxygenated), removal of the foreign body by bronchoscopy or laryngoscopy should be attempted in a controlled environment.
   b. If the patient is unable to speak, moves air poorly, or is cyanotic, intervene immediately.
      (1) Infant: Place infant over arm or rest on lap. Give five back blows between the scapulae. If unsuccessful, turn infant over and give five chest thrusts, *one per second* (in the same location as external chest compressions). Use tongue-jaw lift to open mouth. Remove

object only if visualized. Attempt to ventilate if unconscious. Repeat sequence as often as necessary.

(2) Child: Perform five abdominal thrusts (Heimlich maneuver) from behind a sitting or standing child or straddled over a child lying supine. Direct thrusts upward in the midline and not to either side of the abdomen.

(3) After back, chest, and/or abdominal thrusts, open mouth and remove foreign body if visualized. Blind finger sweeps are not recommended. Magill forceps may allow removal of foreign bodies in the posterior pharynx.

(4) If the patient is unconscious, remove the foreign body using Magill forceps if needed after direct visualization or laryngoscopy. If there is complete airway obstruction, consider percutaneous (needle) cricothyrotomy (Fig. 1-2)[2] if attempts to ventilate by bag-valve mask or ETT are unsuccessful.



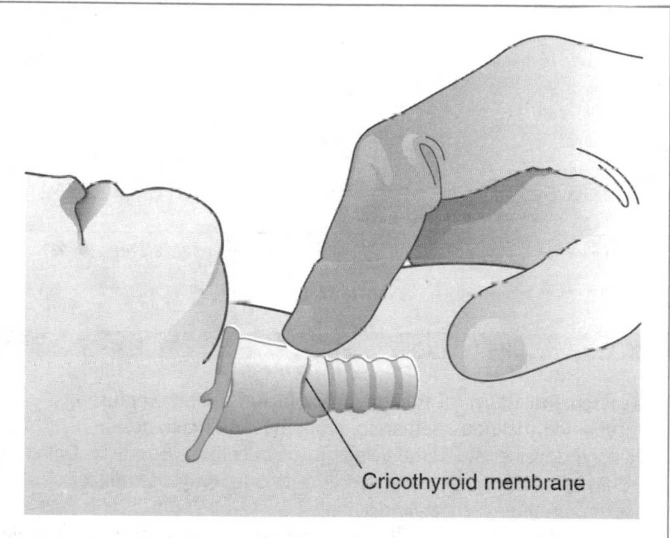


FIG. 1-2

Percutaneous (needle) cricothyrotomy. Extend neck, attach a 3-mL syringe to a 14- to 18-gauge IV catheter, and introduce catheter through the cricothyroid membrane (inferior to the thyroid cartilage, superior to the cricoid cartilage). Aspirate air to confirm position. Remove the syringe and needle, attach the catheter to an adaptor from a 3.0-mm endotracheal tube, which can then be used for positive-pressure oxygenation. *(Modified from Dieckmann RA, Fiser DH, Selbst SM: Illustrated Textbook of Pediatric Emergency and Critical Care Procedures. St. Louis, Mosby, 1997, p 118.)*

BOX 1-1

**DIFFERENTIAL DIAGNOSIS OF ALTERED LEVEL OF CONSCIOUSNESS**

| STRUCTURAL CAUSES |
|---|
| Cerebrovascular accident |
| Cerebral vein thrombosis |
| Hydrocephalus |
| Intracerebral tumor |
| Subdural empyema |
| Trauma (intracranial hemorrhage, diffuse cerebral swelling, shaken baby syndrome) |
| **MEDICAL CAUSES (TOXIC-INFECTIOUS-METABOLIC)** |
| Anoxia |
| Diabetic ketoacidosis |
| Electrolyte abnormality |
| Encephalopathy |
| Hypoglycemia |
| Hypothermia or hyperthermia |
| Hyperammonemia |
| Infection (sepsis) |
| Inborn errors of metabolism |
| Intussusception |
| Meningitis and encephalitis |
| Psychogenic |
| Postictal state |
| Toxins/ingestions |
| Uremia (hemolytic uremic syndrome) |

Modified from Avner, J: Altered states of consciousness. Pediatr Rev 2006;27(9):331–337.

## VI. NEUROLOGIC EMERGENCIES

### A. ALTERED STATES OF CONSCIOUSNESS[7–9]

1. **Assessment: Range of mental status includes alert, confused, disoriented, delirious, lethargic, stuporous, and comatose.**

a. History: Consider structural versus medical causes (Box 1-1). Obtain history of trauma, ingestion, infection, fasting, drug use, diabetes, seizure, or other neurologic disorder.

b. Examination: Assess HR, BP, respiratory pattern, Glasgow Coma Scale, temperature, pupillary response, funduscopy (keep in mind that papilledema is a late finding usually requiring 12 hr to develop; a normal funduscopic examination does not rule out increased intracranial pressure), rash, abnormal posturing, and focal neurologic signs.

2. **Management of coma:**

a. **A**irway (with C-spine immobilization), **B**reathing, **C**irculation, **D**extro stick, **O**xygen, **N**aloxone, **T**hiamine **(ABC DON'T)**.

(1) Naloxone, 0.1 mg/kg IV, IM, SC, or ETT (maximum dose, 2 mg). Repeat as necessary, keeping in mind its short half-life.

(2) Thiamine, 100 mg IV (before starting glucose). Consider in adolescents for deficiencies secondary to alcoholism or eating disorders.
(3) $D_{25}W$, 2 to 4 mL/kg IV bolus if hypoglycemia is present.

b. Laboratory tests: Consider complete blood count, electrolytes, liver function tests, $NH_3$, lactate, toxicology screen (serum and urine), blood gas, serum osmolality, prothrombin time, partial thromboplastin time, and blood and urine culture. If patient is an infant or toddler, consider assessment of plasma amino acids, urine organic acids, and other appropriate metabolic workup.
c. If meningitis or encephalitis is suspected, consider lumbar puncture (LP) and start antibiotics. Consider acyclovir.
d. Request emergent head CT scan after ABCs are stabilized; consider neurosurgical consultation and electroencephalogram (EEG) if indicated.
e. If ingestion is suspected, airway must be protected before GI decontamination (see Chapter 2).
f. Monitor Glasgow Coma Scale and reassess frequently (Table 1-3).

## B. STATUS EPILEPTICUS[10,11]

See Chapter 20 for nonacute evaluation and management of seizures.

1. **Assessment: Common causes of childhood seizures include fever, subtherapeutic anticonvulsant levels, central nervous system (CNS)**

TABLE 1-3

COMA SCALES

| Glasgow Coma Scale | | Modified Coma Scale for Infants | |
|---|---|---|---|
| Activity | Best Response | Activity | Best Response |
| **EYE OPENING** | | | |
| Spontaneous | 4 | Spontaneous | 4 |
| To speech | 3 | To speech | 3 |
| To pain | 2 | To pain | 2 |
| None | 1 | None | 1 |
| **VERBAL** | | | |
| Oriented | 5 | Coos, babbles | 5 |
| Confused | 4 | Irritable | 4 |
| Inappropriate words | 3 | Cries to pain | 3 |
| Nonspecific sounds | 2 | Moans to pain | 2 |
| None | 1 | None | 1 |
| **MOTOR** | | | |
| Follows commands | 6 | Normal spontaneous movements | 6 |
| Localizes pain | 5 | Withdraws to touch | 5 |
| Withdraws to pain | 4 | Withdraws to pain | 4 |
| Abnormal flexion | 3 | Abnormal flexion | 3 |
| Abnormal extension | 2 | Abnormal extension | 2 |
| None | 1 | None | 1 |

Data from Jennet B, Teasdale G: Aspects of coma after severe head injury. Lancet 1977;1:878, and James HE: Neurologic evaluation and support in the child with an acute brain insult. Pediatr Ann 1986;15:16.

infections, trauma, toxic ingestion, and metabolic abnormalities. Less common causes include vascular, neoplastic, and endocrine diseases.

2. **Acute management of seizures (Table 1-4):** If CNS infection is suspected, give antibiotics and/or acyclovir early.

TABLE 1-4

ACUTE MANAGEMENT OF SEIZURES

| Time (min) | Intervention |
|---|---|
| 0–5 | Stabilize the patient<br>Assess airway, breathing, circulation, and vital signs<br>Administer oxygen<br>Obtain intravenous or intraosseous access<br>Correct hypoglycemia if present (dextrose 25% 2–4 mL/kg). In adolescents, give thiamine (100 mg) first<br>Obtain laboratory studies: Consider glucose, electrolytes, calcium, magnesium, BUN, creatinine, and LFTs, CBC, toxicology screen, anticonvulsant levels, blood culture (if infection is suspected)<br>Initial screening history and physical examination |
| 5–15 | Begin pharmacotherapy<br>Lorazepam (Ativan), 0.05–0.1 mg/kg IV, up to 4–6 mg<br>*or*<br>Diazepam (Valium), 0.2–0.5 mg/kg IV (0.5 mg/kg rectally) up to 6–10 mg<br>May repeat lorazepam or diazepam 5–10 min after initial dose |
| 15–35 | If seizure persists, load with:<br>Phenytoin* 15–20 mg/kg IV at rate not to exceed 1 mg/kg/min via central line<br>*or*<br>Fosphenytoin† 15–20 mg PE/kg IV/IM at 3 mg PE/kg/min via peripheral IV live (maximum 150 mg PE/min). If given IM, may require multiple dosing sites<br>*or*<br>Phenobarbital 15–20 mg/kg IV at rate not to exceed 1 mg/kg/min |
| 45 | If seizure persists:<br>Load with phenobarbital if phenytoin was previously used<br>Additional phenytoin or fosphenytoin 5 mg/kg over 12 hr for goal serum level of 10 mg/L<br>Additional phenobarbital 5 mg/kg/dose every 15–30 min (maximum total dose of 30 mg/kg; be prepared to support respirations)<br>Consider IV valproate, especially for partial status epilepticus |
| 60 | If seizure persists,‡ consider pentobarbital, midazolam, or general anesthesia in intensive care unit. Avoid paralytics |

*Phenytoin may be contraindicated for seizures secondary to alcohol withdrawal or most ingestions (see Chapter 2).

†Fosphenytoin dosed as phenytoin equivalent (PE).

‡Pyridoxine 100 mg IV in infant with persistent initial seizure.

BUN, blood urea nitrogen; CBC, complete blood count; CT, computed tomography; EEG, electroencephalogram; LFTs, liver function tests.

Modified from Fischer P: Seizure disorders. Child Adol Psychiatr Clin North Am 1995;4:461.

3. **Diagnostic workup:** When stable, workup may include CT or magnetic resonance imaging, EEG, and LP.

## REFERENCES


1. American Heart Association: Pediatric advanced life support. Pediatrics 2006;117(5):e1005–e1028.
2. Emergency Cardiac Care Committee, American Heart Association: Pediatric advanced life support. JAMA 1992;268:2262–2275.
3. Bledsoe GH, Schexnayder SM: Pediatric rapid sequence intubation. Pediatr Emerg Care 2004;20:339–344.
4. Crain EF, Gersel JC: Clinical Manual of Emergency Pediatrics. New York, McGraw-Hill, 2003.
5. Nichols DG et al (eds): Golden Hour: The Handbook of Advanced Pediatric Life Support. St. Louis, Mosby, 1996.
6. Lieberman P: Use of epinephrine in the treatment of anaphylaxis. Curr Opin Allerg Clin Immunol 2003;3:313–318.
7. Jennet B, Teasdale G: Aspects of coma after severe head injury. Lancet 1977;1:878–881.
8. James HE: Neurologic evaluation and support in the child with an acute brain insult. Pediatr Ann 1986;15:16–22.
9. Avner J: Altered states of consciousness. Pediatr Rev 2006;27(9):331–337.
10. Fischer P: Seizure disorders. Child Adol Psychiatr Clin North Am 1995;4:461–465.
11. Wheless JW: Treatment of status epilepticus in children. Pediatr Ann 2004;33:377–383.

# Poisonings

*Amy Valasek, MD*

2

## I. HISTORY

### A. INTERVIEW

1. Obtain exposure history from family members and/or friends.
2. Important data: Product name, active ingredients, possible contaminants, expiration date, concentration, dose, route, timing and number of exposures (acute, chronic, or repeated ingestion), prior treatments or decontamination efforts.[1,2]
3. Environmental information: Accessible items in the house or garage; open containers; spilled tablets; household members taking medications, herbs, or other complementary medicines.[2]

### B. SUBSTANCE IDENTIFICATION

1. Whenever possible, identify the exact name of the substance ingested and its constituents.[1]
2. Consult local poison control center.
3. If the patient ingested a low-toxicity product, ensure that the patient does not have any signs of toxicity, only one substance was ingested, and appropriate follow-up is arranged.

### C. QUANTITY OF SUBSTANCE INGESTED

Attempt to estimate a missing volume of liquid or the number of missing pills from a container.

## II. LABORATORY FINDINGS

### A. SUBSTANCES WITH DELAYED ONSET OF SYMPTOMS OR DELAYED TOXICITY[1]

Enteric coated formulations, sustained-release preparations, acetaminophen, calcium channel blockers, lithium, theophylline.

### B. TOXIDROMES AND CLINICAL SIGNS (Tables 2-1 and 2-2)

### C. TOXICOLOGY SCREENS

1. Screens include analgesics, amphetamines, antidepressants, barbiturates, cocaine, ethanol, and opiates. If a particular type of ingestion is suspected, verify that the agent is included in the toxicology test.[2]
2. When obtaining a blood or urine toxicology test, consider measuring both aspirin and acetaminophen levels because these are common analgesic ingredients in many medications.[2]
3. Gas chromatography or gas mass spectroscopy can distinguish medications that may cause a false positive toxicology screen for tricyclic antidepressants, such as antihistamines, antipsychotics, and cyclobenzaprine.[3]

*Text continued on p. 25*

TABLE 2-1

TOXIDROMES

| Drug Class | Vital Signs | Neurologic | Skin, Mucous Membranes | GI | GU | Other |
|---|---|---|---|---|---|---|
| **ADRENERGIC/SYMPATHOMIMETIC** | | | | | | |
| Amphetamines, cocaine, sympathomimetics, ephedrine, phenylpropranolamine | ↑ or ↔ RR<br>↑ HR<br>↑ T<br>↑ BP | Alert, agitation, dilated and reactive pupils, hyperreflexia, tremor, delirium, psychosis, seizures | Diaphoresis, wet mucous membranes | Hyperactive bowel sounds, emesis, abdominal pain | Increased urination | |
| **ANTICHOLINERGIC** | | | | | | |
| Antihistamines, atropine, belladonna alkaloids (deadly nightshade), jimsonweed, some mushrooms, phenothiazines, scopolamine, tricyclic antidepressants<br><br>**"Mad as a hatter, red as a beet, blind as a bat, hot as a hare, dry as a bone."** | ↔ RR<br>↑ HR<br>↑ T<br>↔ or ↑ BP | Depressed mental status, confusion, psychosis, paranoid ideation, delirium, ataxia, agitation, seizures, coma, extrapyramidal symptoms, dilated and sluggish pupils, normal DTRs | Dry skin, flushing, dry mucous membranes, decreased sweating | Hypoactive bowel sounds, ileus | Urine retention | Respiratory failure |

| | | | | | | |
|---|---|---|---|---|---|---|
| **ANTICHOLINESTERASE (CHOLINERGIC)** | | | | | | |
| Black widow spider bites, some mushrooms, organophosphate nerve agents, organophosphate and carbamate pesticides, tobacco | ↑ or ↔ RR<br>↓ or ↑ HR<br>↔ T<br>↔ BP | Confusion, depressed mental status, coma, pupillary constriction, normal DTRs or hyporeflexia, seizures, muscle fasciculations, weakness, paralysis | Diaphoresis, wet muccus membranes, salivation, lacrimation | Hyperactive bowel sounds, diarrhea, cramping, emesis | Increased urination | Respiratory failure |
| **SLUDGE:** ***s***alivation, ***l***acrimation, ***u***rination, ***d***efecation, ***g***astric cramping, ***e***mesis | | | | | | |
| **DUMBELS:** ***d***iarrhea, ***u***rination, ***m***iosis, ***b***ronchospasm, ***e***mesis, ***l***acrimation, ***s***alivation | | | | | | |
| **EXTRAPYRAMIDAL** | | | | | | |
| Haloperidol, metoclopramide, phenothiazines | | Tremor rigidity, opisthotonos, torticollis, dysphonia, oculogyric crisis | | | | |
| **HYPERMETABOLIC** | | | | | | |
| Chlorophenoxy herbicides, some phenols, salicylates | ↑ RR<br>↑ HR<br>↑ T | Seizure, restlessness | | | | Metabolic acidosis |

BP, blood pressure; DTR, deep tendon reflex; HR, heart rate; GI, gastrointestinal; GU, genitourinary; RR, respiratory rate; T, temperature.

Data from references 2, 4, 6, 9, and 15.

*Continued*

TABLE 2-1
TOXIDROMES—cont'd

| Drug Class | Vital Signs | Neurologic | Skin, Mucous Membranes | GI | GU | Other |
|---|---|---|---|---|---|---|
| **OPIOID, NARCOTIC** | | | | | | |
| Fentanyl, meperidine, heroin, hydrocodone, oxycodone, propoxyphene, morphine, clonidine | ↓ RR<br>↔ or ↓ HR<br>↔ or ↓ T<br>↔ or ↓ BP | Confusion, lethargy, euphoria, somnolence, seizures, ataxia, coma, pupillary constriction, normal DTRs or hyporeflexia | Normal skin and mucous membranes | Decreased bowel sounds, constipation | Urine retention | Pulmonary edema |
| **SALICYLATES** | | | | | | |
| Aspirin, oil of wintergreen | ↑ RR<br>↑ T | Lethargy, seizures | Emesis | | | Respiratory alkalosis, metabolic acidosis |
| **SEDATIVE-HYPNOTIC** | | | | | | |
| Benzodiazepines, barbiturates | ↓ RR<br>↔ or ↓ HR<br>↔ or ↓ T | Depressed mental status, CNS depression, normal pupils, normal DTRs or hyporeflexia | Normal | Normal | Normal | |
| **THEOPHYLLINE** | | | | | | |
| Aminophylline, caffeine, theophylline | ↑ RR<br>↑ HR<br>↓ BP | Agitation, tremor, seizures | | Emesis | | |
| **WITHDRAWAL** | | | | | | |
| Cessation of alcohol, barbiturates, benzodiazepines, γ-hydroxybutyrate | ↑ HR | Restlessness, hallucinations, anxiety, hyperalgesia, mydriasis | Lacrimation, "goose bumps," sweating | Abdominal cramps, diarrhea | | Yawning, rhinorrhea |

TABLE 2-2

CLINICAL DIAGNOSTIC AIDS

| Clinical Sign | Intoxicant |
|---|---|
| **VITAL SIGNS** | |
| Hypothermia | Alcohols, antidepressants, barbiturates, carbamazepine, carbon monoxide, clonidine, ethanol, hypoglycemics, opioids, phenothiazines, sedative-hypnotics |
| Hyperpyrexia | Amphetamines, anticholinergics, antihistamines, atropinics, β-blockers, cocaine, iron, isoniazid, monoamine oxidase inhibitors (MAOIs), phencyclidine, phenothiazines, quinine, salicylates, sympathomimetics, selective serotonin reuptake inhibitors, theophylline, thyroxine, tricyclic antidepressants (TCAs) |
| Bradypnea | Acetone, alcohol, bartiturates, botulinum toxin, clonidine, ethanol, ibuprofen, narcotics, nicotine, sedative-hypnotics |
| Tachypnea | Amphetamines, barbiturates, carbon monoxide, cyanide, ethylene glycol, isopropanol, methanol, salicylates<br>*Direct pulmonary insult:* hydrocarbons, organophosphates, salicylates |
| Bradycardia | α-Agonists, alcohols, β-blockers, calcium channel blockers, central $\alpha_2$-agonist, clonidine, cyanide, digoxin, narcotics, organophosphates, plants (lily of the valley, foxglove, oleander), sedative-hypnotics |
| Tachycardia | Alcohol, amphetamines, anticholinergics, antihistamines, atropine, cocaine, cyclic antidepressants, cyanide, iron, phencyclidine, salicylates, sympathomimetics, theophylline, TCAs, thyroxine |
| Hypotension | α-Antagonists, ACE inhibitors, barbiturates, carbon monoxide, cyanide, iron, methemoglobinemia, opioids, phenothiazine, sedative-hypnotics, TCAs<br>*Profound hypotension:* β-blockers, calcium channel blockers, clonidine, cyclic antidepressants, digoxin, imidazolines, nitrites, quinidine, propoxyphene, theophylline |
| Hypertension | Amphetamines, anticholinergics, antihistamines, atropinics, clonidine, cocaine, cyclic antidepressants (early after ingestion), diet pills, ephedrine, MAOIs, nicotine, over-the-counter cold remedies, phencyclidine, phenylpropanolamine, pressors, sympathomimetics, TCAs<br>*Delayed hypertension:* thyroxine |
| Hypoxia | Oxidizing agents |
| **NEUROMUSCULAR** | |
| Nervous system instability | *Insidious onset:* acetaminophen, benzocaine, opioids<br>*Abrupt onset:* lidocaine, monocyclic or tricyclic antidepressants, phenothiazines, theophylline<br>*Delayed onset:* atropine, diphenoxylate<br>*Transient instability:* hydrocarbons |

Data from references 1, 2, 4, and 6.

*Continued*

TABLE 2-2

CLINICAL DIAGNOSTIC AIDS—cont'd

| Clinical Sign | Intoxicant |
|---|---|
| **NEUROMUSCULAR—cont'd** | |
| Depression and excitation | Clonidine, imidazolines, phencyclidine |
| Ataxia | Alcohol, anticonvulsants, barbiturates, carbon monoxide, heavy metals, hydrocarbons, solvents, sedative-hypnotics |
| Chvostek/Trousseau signs | Ethylene glycol, hydrofluoric acid-induced hypocalcemia, phosphate-induced hypocalcemia from Fleets enema |
| Coma | Alcohols, anesthetics, anticholinergics (antihistamines, antidepressants, phenothiazines, atropinics, over-the-counter sleep preparations), anticonvulsants, baclofen, barbiturates, benzodiazepines, bromide, carbon monoxide, chloral hydrate, clonidine, cyanide, cyclic antidepressants, γ-hydroxybutyrate (GHB), hydrocarbons, hypoglycemics, inhalants, insulin, lithium, opioids, organophosphate insecticides, phenothiazines, salicylates, sedative-hypnotics, tetrahydrozoline, theophylline |
| Delirium, psychosis | Alcohol, anticholinergics (including cold remedies), cocaine, heavy metals, heroin, LSD, marijuana, mescaline, methaqualone, peyote, phencyclidine, phenothiazines, steroids, sympathomimetics |
| Miosis | Barbiturates, clonidine, ethanol, opioids, organophosphates, phencyclidine, phenothiazines, muscarinic mushrooms |
| Mydriasis | Amphetamines, antidepressants, antihistamines, atropinics, barbiturates (if comatose), botulism, cocaine, glutethimide, LSD, marijuana, methanol, phencyclidine |
| Nystagmus | Barbiturates, carbamazepine, diphenylhydantoin, ethanol, glutethimide, MAOIs, phencyclidine (both vertical and horizontal), sedative-hypnotics |
| Paralysis | Botulism, heavy metals, paralytic shellfish poisoning, plants (poison hemlock). |
| Seizures | Alcohol, ammonium fluoride, amphetamines, anticholinergics, antidepressants, antihistamines, atropine, β-blockers, boric acid, bupropion, caffeine, camphor, carbamates, carbamazepine, carbon monoxide, chlorinated insecticides, cocaine, cyclic antidepressants, diethyltoluamide, ergotamine, ethanol, GHB, *Gyromitra* mushrooms, hydrocarbons, hypoglycemics, ibuprofen, imidazolines, isoniazid, lead, lidocaine, lindane, lithium, LSD, meperidine, nicotine, opioids, organophosphate insecticides, phencyclidine, phenothiazines, phenylpropanolamine, phenytoin physostigmine, plants (water hemlock), propoxyphene, salicylates, strychnine, theophylline |
| **CARDIOVASCULAR** | |
| Hypoperfusion | Calcium channel blockers, iron |
| Wide QRS complex | TCAs |

TABLE 2-2

CLINICAL DIAGNOSTIC AIDS—cont'd

| Clinical Sign | Intoxicant |
|---|---|
| **ELECTROLYTES** | |
| Anion gap metabolic acidosis | Acetaminophen, carbon monoxide, chronic toluene, cyanide, ethanol, ethylene glycol, ibuprofen, iron, isoniazid, lactate, methanol, metformin, paraldehyde, phenformin, salicylates |
| Electrolyte disturbances | Salicylates, theophylline |
| Hypoglycemia | Alcohols, β-blockers, hypoglycemics, salicylates |
| Serum osmolar gap | Acetone, ethanol, ethylene glycol, isopropyl alcohol, methanol, propylene glycol<br>Calculated osmolarity = (2 × serum Na) + BUN/2.8 + glucose/18. Normal osmolarity is 290 mOsm/kg. |
| **GENITOURINARY** | |
| Urine calcium oxalate crystals | Ethyleneglycol |
| **HEMATOLOGIC** | |
| Chocolate brown-colored blood | Methemoglobinemia |
| Methemoglobinemia | Aniline dyes, benzocaine-containing teething products, dapsone, naphthalene, nitrites, pyridium |
| **SKIN** | |
| Asymptomatic cyanosis | Methemoglobinemia |
| Cyanosis unresponsive to oxygen | Aniline dyes, benzocaine, nitrites, nitrobenzene, phenazopyridine, phenacetin |
| Flushing | Alcohols, antihistamines, atropinics, boric acid, carbon monoxide, cyanide, disulfiram |
| Jaundice | Acetaminophen, carbon tetrachloride, heavy metals (iron, phosphorus, arsenic), naphthalene, phenothiazines, plants (mushrooms, fava beans) |
| **ODORS** | |
| Acetone | Acetone, isopropyl alcohol, phenol, salicylates |
| Alcohol | Ethanol |
| Bitter almond | Cyanide |
| Garlic | Heavy metal (arsenic, phosphorus, thallium), organophosphates. |
| Hydrocarbons | Hydrocarbons (gasoline, turpentine, etc.) |
| Oil of wintergreen | Salicylates |
| Pear | Chloral hydrate |
| Violets | Turpentine |
| **RADIOLOGY** | |
| Small opacities on radiograph | Halogenated toxins, heavy metals, iron, lithium, densely packaged products |



4. Recognize drugs not detected by routine toxicology screens.[4]

a. **Coma inducing:** Bromide, carbon monoxide, chloral hydrate, clonidine, cyanide, organophosphates, tetrahydrozoline (in over-the-counter eye drops).

b. **Hypotension inducing:** Colchicines, cyanide, iron.

c. **Hypotension and bradycardia inducing:** β-Blockers, calcium channel blockers, clonidine, digitalis.

## III. ACUTE MANAGEMENT

### A. AIRWAY, BREATHING, CIRCULATION

Establish intravenous (IV) access, contact local poison control center.

### B. SKIN DECONTAMINATION

Indicated if patient was exposed to concentrated lipid-soluble toxins.[1]

### C. EYE FLUSHING[5]

Flush ocular exposures for a minimum of 15 min before re-evaluating. Remove contact lenses.

### D. GASTROINTESTINAL (GI) DECONTAMINATION

1. **Airway protection is extremely important when attempting GI decontamination because of the risk for aspiration. If no gag reflex exists or the patient has altered mental status, intubation is necessary before decontamination efforts.**
2. **Nasogastric/orogastric lavage:**[1,6,7]

a. **Indications:** TCAs, calcium channel blockers, iron, lithium, alcohols, substances that delay gastric emptying.
b. **Risks:** Mechanical trauma to oropharynx or esophagus, aspiration, deoxygenation.
c. **Contraindications:** Ingestion of corrosive substances or hydrocarbons, altered mental status, unprotected airway.
d. Most effective within 60 min of most ingestions.
e. **Procedure/dosage:** Place patient in Trendelenburg or left lateral decubitus position, and pass the largest-bore nasogastric (NG) tube. Confirm tube placement by aspiration of gastric contents. Administer normal saline solution, 50–100 mL in young children or 150–200 mL in adolescents. Withdraw the fluid by aspiration and repeat until lavaged fluid is clear.

3. **Activated charcoal:**[1,4–8]

a. **Indications:** Carbamazepine, barbiturates, dapsone, quinine, and theophylline ingestions. Some evidence for use with digoxin and phenytoin ingestions. Little evidence for use with salicylates.[6]
b. **Risks:** Bowel obstruction, bowel perforation, pulmonary aspiration, hypernatremia, hypermagnesemia.
c. Contraindications: Ileus, mechanical bowel obstruction, altered mental status with unprotected airway, caustic ingestion, hydrocarbon ingestion, ingestion of foreign body.
d. Most effective if the charcoal is given within 1 hr of ingestion.
e. Procedure/dosage: Activated charcoal 1 g/kg PO or via NG tube every 1–6 hr. For adolescents or adults, give 50–100 g. Activated charcoal poorly adsorbs most electrolytes, iron, lithium, mineral acids, mineral bases, alcohols, cyanides, most solvents, and most water-soluble compounds (hydrocarbons).

**4. Whole-bowel irrigation:**[5,6]

a. Consider after consultation with local poison control center or toxicologist.

b. **Indications:** Sustained-release or enteric-coated preparations.

c. **Contraindications:** Altered mental status with unprotected airway, caustic ingestion, hydrocarbon ingestion, ingestion of foreign body, ileus, bowel perforation.

d. **Procedure/dosage**:

(1) Administer 30 mL/kg/hr of osmotically balanced polyethylene glycol electrolyte solution (GoLYTELY, NuLYTELY) to induce liquid stool. Alternatively, can give up to 500 mL/hr.

(2) Continue until rectal effluent is clear. Slow administration and antiemetic medications may be necessary to reduce bloating, nausea, and emesis.

**5. Syrup of ipecac:**[4,5,7,9]

**Not recommended for routine management of poisonings.**

**6. Cathartics:**[4,7,10]

Not recommended for routine management of poisonings.

**7. Simple dilution:**[4]

a. **Indications:** Toxin that causes only local irritation or corrosion.

b. **Contraindications:** Drug ingestions (increased absorption aides a more rapid transit into GI tract).

c. **Diluent:** Water or milk.

## E. ENHANCED ELIMINATION

**1. Urinary alkalinization with forced diuresis**[1,4]

a. **Indications:** Salicylates, isoniazid, dichlorophenoxyacetic acid, phenobarbital, chlorpropamide, chlorophenoxy herbicides.

b. **Procedure/dosage:**

(1) Use this equation to determine dosage:

$$0.6 \times \text{weight (kg)} \times 5\,\text{mEq} = \text{mEq of sodium bicarbonate to be given over 4 hr.}$$

(2) Administer the sodium bicarbonate in intravenous fluid drip containing glucose and KCl.

c. **Alternate dosing:** Sodium bicarbonate, 1–2 mEq/kg IV over 1–2 hr.

d. **Monitor:** Maintain urine pH 7.5–7.8; correct hypokalemia (hypokalemia reduces the ability to alkalinize the urine).

**2. Urinary acidification**

Not recommended secondary to exacerbation of metabolic acidosis and myoglobin deposition.

## F. ACTIVE REMOVAL

**Hemodialysis and hemofiltration:** Consult local poison control center and a pediatric nephrologist.

### G. MEDICATION INGESTIONS (Table 2-3)[11–36]
### H. DRUGS OF ABUSE (Box 2-1)[37–41]
### I. ANTIDOTES (Table 2-4)[42]

## IV. INHALATIONAL INJURIES

### A. PHYSICAL EXAMINATION

Symptoms may be delayed after the inhalational injury occurs. Symptoms that may predict acute inhalational injury include cough, facial burns, inflamed nares, stridor, sputum production, wheezing, and altered mental status.[43]

### B. MANAGEMENT[43]

1. Assess stability of the airway and intubate if there are signs of airway edema.

**Note** *Upper airway obstruction progresses rapidly with thermal or chemical burns to the face, nares, or oropharynx.*

2. Administer supplemental oxygen through a non-rebreather mask. Give aerosolized bronchodilators as needed.
3. Check chest radiograph, arterial blood gases (ABGs) with co-oximetry, and bedside spirometry.

**Note** *Use co-oximetry instead of pulse oximetry to measure oxyhemoglobin. Pulse oximetry cannot distinguish between carboxyhemoglobin or methemoglobin and oxyhemoglobin.*

4. Obtain 12-lead electrocardiogram (ECG) to evaluate for myocardial ischemia or infarction.
5. Observe for at least 24 hr.

*Text continued on p. 64*

TABLE 2-3

MEDICATION INGESTIONS

| Ingestion | Signs and Symptoms | Management |
|---|---|---|
| **Acetaminophen**[11,12] paracetamol, APAP<br><br>a. Rectal administration can lead to toxicity.<br><br>b. High-risk groups for hepatotoxicity: concurrent use of cytochrome P-450 enhancing drugs, current viral illness, diabetes mellitus, or malnourished. | **Phase 1 (first 24 hr):** Anorexia, nausea, malaise, pallor, vomiting, diaphoresis, or normal appearance<br>**Phase 2 (24–72 hr):** Hepatomegaly, RUQ pain, hyperbilirubinemia, elevated liver enzymes, elevated coagulation factors, oliguria<br>**Phase 3 (72–96 hr):** Encephalopathy, cardiomyopathy, hepatic failure and necrosis, coagulopathy, renal failure, emesis, malaise<br>**Phase 4 (4 days–2 weeks):** Recovery or fatal hepatic failure. The end point of liver damage is reached during this phase. | **1. Initial Considerations:**<br>a. No intervention if <200 mg/kg ingested or <10 g in adults<br>b. Hepatotoxicity >200 mg/kg in children or >7.5 g in adolescents<br>c. ALT >1000 IU/L is a marker of severe liver injury, but not prognostic<br>d. *Start treatment immediately if*<br>(1) Single ingestion >150 mg/kg or 7.5 g by history<br>(2) Unknown time of ingestion and acetaminophen level >10 μg/mL<br>(3) Severe clinical symptoms and abnormal liver function<br>(4) Chronic or subacute overdose with risk<br>(5) Acetaminophen level above "possible hepatic toxicity" on nomogram<br>**2. Monitoring:**<br>a. Obtain baseline electrolytes, liver function, coagulation factors, and urinalysis. *Note:* Recheck labs every 12–24 hr.<br>b. Acetaminophen level 4–24 hr after ingestion best predicts hepatotoxicity. *Note:* Levels <4 hr postingestion are unreliable due to drug absorption.<br>c. Recheck levels 8 hr postingestion if extended release ingested.<br>d. Compare measured level with the nomogram (Fig. 2-1). |

*Continued*

TABLE 2-3

MEDICATION INGESTIONS—cont'd

| Ingestion | Signs and Symptoms | Management |
|---|---|---|
| **Acetaminophen—cont'd** | | **3. Supportive Care/Decontamination:**<br>a. *Activated charcoal:* Most useful within 1–2 hr of ingestion and improves outcome if used concurrently with antidote.<br>b. Hemodialysis and hemoperfusion are not recommended.<br>**4. Antidote:** *N*-acetylcysteine (NAC)<br>a. *Drug information:* Increases glutathione stores and conjugates toxic metabolites.<br>b. *PO dosing:* 140 mg/kg PO loading dose, then 70 mg/kg every 4 hr for a total of 17 doses. Repeat the dose if vomiting occurs within 1 hr of administration.<br>*Considerations:* Increase the loading dose by 40% or repeat the loading dose if presentation >6–8 hr postingestion.<br>*Contraindications:* Corrosive ingestion, GI bleed, bowel obstruction<br>c. *IV dosing:*<br>Loading dose: 150 mg/kg diluted in 200 mL $D_5W$ or $D_5$1/2NS administered over 60 min<br>Second dose: 50 mg/kg diluted in 500 mL $D_5W$ administered over 4 hr<br>Third dose: 100 mg/kg diluted in 1000 mL $D_5W$ administered over 16 hr |

| | | |
|---|---|---|
| | | d. *Risks:* Renal tubular damage with both PO and IV forms. Anaphylactoid reactions, bronchospasm, and angioedema with IV form.<br>**5. Adjunct:**<br>a. Use antiemetics (metoclopramide, ondansetron) as necessary.<br>b. Administer NAC via nasogastric or nasoduodenal tube if cannot tolerate oral NAC. |
| **Anticholinergics**[13] (antidepressants, antihistamines, antispasmodics, phenothiazines) | See Table 2-1.<br>Symptoms may develop 12–24 hr after ingestion secondary to decreased GI motility and delayed absorption.<br>Elimination half-life is 8–55 hr. | **1. Supportive Care/Decontamination:**<br>a. If <8 hr of ingestion, give activated charcoal.<br>b. Consider a cathartic, because drug-charcoal complex is excreted in feces.<br>**2. Antidote:** Physostigmine<br>a. See Table 2-4.<br>b. Administer physostigmine only if ECG is normal.<br>c. *Risks:* Seizures, bradycardia, hypotension, bronchospasm. *NOTE:* Risks increase when physostigmine is given rapidly or in large doses.<br>d. *Contraindication:* Ingestion of drug affecting cardiac conduction (TCA)<br>**3. Adjunct:**<br>a. Treat physostigmine seizures with benzodiazepines.<br>b. Treat muscarinic side effects of physostigmine with atropine IV at one half of the dose of physostigmine. |

*Continued*

TABLE 2-3

MEDICATION INGESTIONS—cont'd

| Ingestion | Signs and Symptoms | Management |
|---|---|---|
| **Antidepressants**[14–17]<br>a. *Tricyclic Antidepressants (TCAs):* amitriptyline, clomipramine, desipramine, doxepin, imipramine, nortriptyline, protriptyline, trimipramine<br>b. *Selective Serotonin Reuptake Inhibitors (SSRIs):* amoxapine, citalopram, clomipramine, fluoxetine, fluvoxamine, nefazodone, paroxetine, sertraline, venlafaxine<br>c. *Monoamine Oxidase Inhibitors (MAOIs):* phenelzine, tranylcypromine, isocarboxazid, moclobemide, pargyline, procarbazine, selegiline<br>d. *Serotonin Syndrome:* common with ingestions of two or more drugs: SSRIs, MAOIs, MDMA, amphetamines, meperidine, dextromethrophan | See Table 2-1, *Anticholinergic*<br>*TCAs:* seizures, delirium, arrhythmias (ventricular tachycardia, ventricular fibrillation), hypotension, significantly decreased GI motility<br>*SSRIs*: CNS depression, seizures, coma, agitation, tremor, drowsiness, nystagmus, delirium, arrhythmias, hypertension, emesis, hepatotoxicity<br>*MAOIs:* CNS hyperstimulation, seizures, muscle rigidity, hyperpyrexia, blood pressure instability, rhabdomyolysis<br>*Co-ingestion of MAOIs and food or drugs with biogenic amines (wine, cheese, soy sauce, decongestants):* stroke, seizures, severe hypertension<br>*Serotonin syndrome:* autonomic dysfunction, seizures, muscle rigidity, myoclonus, hyperpyrexia, circulatory collapse, rhabdomyolysis, flushing | **1. Initial Considerations:**<br>a. Ingestions >20–35 mg/kg of TCA are typically fatal.<br>b. TCAs significantly decrease GI motility.<br>c. TCAs have long half-life and slow elimination rates, necessitating prolonged treatment and decontamination.<br>**2. Monitoring:**<br>a. Check 12-lead ECG and continuous cardiac monitoring.<br>b. Monitor potassium levels if administering sodium bicarbonate.<br>**3. Supportive Care/Decontamination:**<br>a. Administer activated charcoal 1 g/kg.<br>b. Consider gastric lavage if <1 hr postingestion.<br>c. If cardiac arrythmias or widened QRS, administer sodium bicarbonate 1–2 mEq/kg bolus with cardiac monitoring. Maintain serum pH 7.45–7.55 with sodium bicarbonate infusion.<br>*NOTE:* Use lidocaine, atenolol, propranolol, or magnesium for arrhythmias. Quinidine and procainamide are contraindicated.<br>**4. Adjunct:**<br>a. If hypotension develops, isotonic saline bolus and sodium bicarbonate are the first-line agents; consider norepinephrine for refractory hypotension.<br>b. Administer benzodiazepines for seizures.<br>*NOTE:* Phenytoin may induce ventricular arrhythmia, and flumazenil precipitates seizures. |

5. **MAOI Overdose: Key Points**
   a. 24-hr observation is recommended due to possible delayed side effects.
   b. Treat hypertension with short-acting antihypertensive (nitroprusside).
   c. Give IV fluids and vasopressors for hypotension.
   d. Treat hyperpyrexia with dantrolene and cooling measures.
   e. Treat severe muscle rigidity and hyperthermia with benzodiazepines and neuromuscular blockade.
   f. Monitor creatine kinase, electrolytes, and urine myoglobin for rhabdomyolysis.
6. **Serotonin Syndrome: Key Points**
   a. Occurs with co-ingestion of MAOIs with sympathomimetic or serotonergic drugs.
   b. Treat seizures with benzodiazepines (diazepam).
   c. Treat hyperthermia with external cooling measures, neuromuscular blockade, and/or mechanical ventilation.
   d. Resolution occurs usually within 72 hr after ingestion.

*Continued*

TABLE 2-3

MEDICATION INGESTIONS—cont'd

| Ingestion | Signs and Symptoms | Management |
|---|---|---|
| **Antihistamines**[18–20]<br>a. *Second/third generation:* Azelastine, brompheniramine, doxylamine, ebastine, fexofenadine, loratidine, mizolastine<br>b. *First generation:* Diphenhydramine, chlorpheniramine, hydroxyzine | See Table 2-1, *Anticholinergic*<br>Paradoxical CNS stimulation, hyperactivity, tremors, dizziness, coma, hypotension, arrhythmias, cardiorespiratory arrest, muscle weakness | **1. Initial Considerations:**<br>a. Antihistamines are in cough syrups, sedatives, antiemetics, drugs to prevent motion sickness, cold preparations, and sleep aids.<br>b. Second-generation antihistamines cause prolonged QT and arrhythmias.<br>c. Observe patient for at least 4 hr postingestion. If ingestion of second generation or slow-release forms, admit and observe regardless of symptoms.<br>**2. Monitoring:**<br>a. 12-lead ECG; continuous cardiac monitoring for second-generation ingestion.<br>b. *NOTE:* May cause false-positive TCA test.<br>**3. Supportive Care/Decontamination:**<br>a. Give activated charcoal if <4 hr postingestion.<br>b. Hemodialysis is not indicated.<br>**4. Antidote:** Physostigmine<br>See Table 2-4<br>**5. Adjunct:**<br>a. First-line treatment for arrhythmia: sodium bicarbonate; then consider magnesium, propranolol.<br>b. Treat seizures with benzodiazepines.<br>c. Treat hyperpyrexia with cooling measures. |

| | | |
|---|---|---|
| **Barbiturates**<br>a. Amobarbital, butalbital, pentobarbital, phenobarbital, secobarbital<br>b. See Box 2-1, *Sedative-Hypnotics*. | Slurred speech, ataxia lethargy, nystagmus, confusion, coma, cutaneous bullae, respiratory depression, flaccid, hyporeflexia; "absent EEG activity" | See Box 2-1, *Sedative-Hypnotics*<br>**1. Initial Considerations:**<br>a. Phenobarbital levels are most useful if measured within 1–2 hr postingestion.<br>b. Ingestion of >6 mg/kg long-acting or >3 mg/kg short-acting barbiturate is usually toxic.<br>**2. Supportive Care/Decontamination:**<br>a. Activated charcoal or multiple doses activated charcoal for phenobarbital.<br>b. Hemodialysis if large doses of phenobarbital ingested.<br>**3. Adjunct:** Sodium bicarbonate to keep urine pH >7.5, which increases phenobarbital elimination. |
| **Benzodiazepines**[21,22]<br>a. Sedatives, anxiolytics, muscle relaxants, hypnotics<br>b. Alprazolam, clorazepate, chlordiazepoxide, clonazepam, diazepam, flurazepam, lorazepam, midazolam, oxazepam, temazepam, triazolam | Coma, dysarthria, ataxia, drowsiness, hallucinations, confusion, agitation, bradycardia, hypotension, respiratory depression | **1. Initial Considerations:** Half-life can be 2 hr to 48 hr.<br>**2. Monitoring:** Levels can be detected in urine and serum toxicology tests.<br>**3. Supportive Care/Decontamination:** Administer activated charcoal if within 1 hr of ingestion and consciousness is not impaired.<br>**4. Antidote:** Flumazenil<br>a. Competitive benzodiazepine antagonist is indicated when the patient cannot protect the airway, is in respiratory distress, or has circulatory compromise.<br>b. See Table 2-4 for side effects and dosing.<br>c. *NOTE:* May cause seizures. |

*Continued*

TABLE 2-3

MEDICATION INGESTIONS—cont'd

| Ingestion | Signs and Symptoms | Management |
|---|---|---|
| **β-Blockers**[23–25]<br>a. $\beta_1$ *selective*: Atenolol, esmolol, metoprolol<br>b. $\beta_1$ and $\beta_2$ *selective:* Labetalol, nadolol, pindolol, timolol | Coma, seizures, altered mental status, hallucinations, cardiac arrhythmia (AV node blockade, accelerated junctional rhythms), bradycardia, CHF, hypotension, respiratory depression, bronchospasm, hypoglycemia | **1. Monitoring:**<br>a. Serial 12-lead ECG for conduction delays every 1–2 hr.<br>b. Observe regular-release preparation for 6 hr postingestion and sustained release for 24 hr.<br>c. Observe ingestions with timolol eye drops for 24 hr.<br>**2. Supportive Care/Decontamination:**<br>a. Activated charcoal recommended if >1 hr postingestion.<br>b. Pretreat bradycardia with atropine before gastric lavage. *NOTE:* Lavage can cause vagal response and worsen bradycardia.<br>c. Whole bowel irrigation for sustained-release preparations.<br>d. Hemodialysis and hemoperfusion not indicated.<br>**3. Antidote**: Glucagon<br>a. See Table 2-4 for side effects and dosing.<br>b. Glucagon infusion should be started at the response dose per hour (e.g., if patient receives 7 mg glucagon before response occurs, then start infusion at 7 mg/hr).<br>c. Glucagon has inotropic and vasopressor effects; administer normal saline during glucagon treatment.<br>**4. Adjunct:**<br>a. Atropine, IV fluids, and vasopressors for hypotension or myocardial depression<br>b. Pacemaker, aortic balloon pump, or cardiopulmonary bypass for unresponsive hypotension. |

<table>
<tr>
<td>Calcium Channel Blockers[24,25]<br>amlodipine, bepridil, diltiazem, isradipine, nicardipine, nifedipine, verapamil</td>
<td>Seizures, coma, dysarthria, lethargy, confusion, decreased myocardial contractility, cardiac arrhythmia, profound hypotension, peripheral vasodilation, apnea, pulmonary edema, bowel infarction, lactic acidosis, hyperglycemia, mild hyperkalemia, flushing, peripheral cyanosis<br>Nifedipine: seizures<br>Bepridil: prolonged QT</td>
<td>1. Initial Considerations: Symptoms may develop hours after ingestion with sustained-release preparation.<br>2. Monitoring:<br>a. Serial 12-lead ECG to evaluate conduction delays.<br>b. Observe regular-release preparation for 6 hr postingestion and sustained-release for 24 hr.<br>3. Supportive Care/Decontamination:<br>a. Gastric lavage if <1 hr postingestion and life-threatening ingestion.<br>b. Activated charcoal recommended.<br>c. Whole-bowel irrigation for sustained-release preparations.<br>d. Hemodialysis and hemoperfusion not indicated.<br>4. Antidote: Calcium Salts<br>a. If unresponsive to atropine, give calcium salts.<br>b. See Table 2-4. Calcium infusion may be necessary.<br>NOTE: Do not exceed serum calcium level of 14 mg/dL or double the normal ionized calcium level.<br>5. Adjunct:<br>a. Atropine, IV fluids, and vasopressors for hypotension or myocardial depression. However, these measures are often ineffective. If severe peripheral vasodilation, norepinephrine, dopamine, epinephrine, or phenylephrine may be necessary.<br>b. Treat nifedipine seizures with lorazepam, diazepam, or calcium.<br>c. Pacemaker, aortic balloon pump, cardiopulmonary bypass.</td>
</tr>
</table>

Continued

TABLE 2-3

MEDICATION INGESTIONS—cont'd

| Ingestion | Signs and Symptoms | Management |
|---|---|---|
| **Carbamazepine**[26] | Coma, seizures, ataxia, motor restlessness, twitching, tremor, athetosis, mydriasis, nystagmus, altered mental status, tachycardia, cardiac conduction abnormalities, hypotension, hypertension, respiratory depression | 1. **Initial Considerations:** Levels increase when coadministered with cytochrome P-450 inhibitors (cimetidine, diltiazem, and erythromycin).<br>2. **Monitoring:**<br>a. Serum carbamazepine level is most useful if obtained 2–4 hr postingestion. However, serum levels do not correlate with clinical toxicity. *NOTE:* Ingestion of multiple anticonvulsants (valproic acid and lamotrigine) with carbamazepine will cause carbamazepine to reach toxic levels sooner.<br>b. Levels >40 mg/L are associated with seizures, coma, and respiratory depression.<br>c. May cause false-positive TCA toxicity test.<br>d. 12-lead ECG to measure QTc.<br>3. **Supportive Care/Decontamination:**<br>a. Activated charcoal recommended. Repeat if serum level is rising.<br>b. Hemodialysis and hemoperfusion indicated in massive overdose. Contact local poison center.<br>4. **Adjunct:** Treat seizures with benzodiazepines. |

| | | |
|---|---|---|
| **Clonidine**[27] | CNS depression, coma, lethargy, hypothermia, miosis, bradycardia, profound hypotension, respiratory depression<br>**Hypertension rarely occurs** | **1. Initial Considerations:**<br>a. Small ingestions cause significant toxicity in children.<br>b. Symptoms occur within 1 hr postingestion and last up to 24 hr.<br>*NOTE:* 10–20 μg/kg = cardiovascular compromise; >20 μg/kg = respiratory depression<br>**2. Monitoring:** 12-lead ECG to evaluate for heart block and continuous cardiac monitoring.<br>**3. Supportive Care/Decontamination:**<br>a. Administer a single dose of activated charcoal.<br>b. Whole-bowel irrigation is effective for clonidine patch ingestions.<br>*NOTE:* Rapid drug absorption makes decontamination effective within 2 hr of ingestion.<br>**4. Antidote:** Naloxone<br>a. Treat for neurologic, cardiovascular, or respiratory symptoms.<br>b. Give 1–2 mg initially. Large amounts (up to 8 mg) may be necessary. If the patient responds to naloxone, continue to give boluses, or start an infusion.<br>c. See Table 2-4.<br>**5. Adjunct:**<br>a. Give atropine if bradycardia does not respond to naloxone.<br>b. Administer IV fluids and vasopressors to treat hypotension. |

*Continued*

TABLE 2-3

MEDICATION INGESTIONS—cont'd

| Ingestion | Signs and Symptoms | Management |
|---|---|---|
| **Digoxin**[28,29] | Seizure, lethargy, headache, disorientation, visual disturbances (blurry, altered color vision, "halos" of color), AV node dissociation and heart block, ventricular or supraventricular escape rhythms, electrolyte imbalances | **1. Initial Considerations:**<br>a. Foxglove, lily of the valley, oleander plant ingestions are similar to digoxin ingestion.<br>b. Chronic ingestions are more likely to be toxic than an acute ingestion.<br>c. Impaired renal function, amiodarone, hypokalemia, hypomagnesemia, and low thyroxine increase digoxin toxicity.<br>**2. Monitoring:**<br>a. Complete absorption takes 2–4 hr postingestion.<br>b. Digoxin levels are most useful if measured 4–6 hr after ingestion.<br>*NOTE:* Complicated pharmacokinetics make serum levels unreliable in predicting clinical toxicity.<br>*Therapeutic serum digoxin concentration*: <2 ng/mL<br>*Toxic serum digoxin concentration:* >4 ng/mL<br>c. 12-lead ECG and continuous cardiac monitoring.<br>d. Monitor electrolytes (calcium, magnesium, potassium) and acid-base status.<br>e. Check urinalysis.<br>**3. Supportive Care/Decontamination:**<br>a. Activated charcoal up to several hours postingestion.<br>b. Hemofiltration, hemodialysis, and hemoperfusion not useful. |

4. **Antidote:** Digoxin Specific Antibody Fragments (Fab)
   a. See Table 2-4.
   b. *Indications:* Progressing clinical toxicity, any arrhythmias, recurring arrhythmias, and progressive bradyarrhythmia, arrhythmias that require electric cardioversion or pacing, or serum potassium 5.5 mEq/L or greater in acute poisoning.

   *NOTE:* Serum digoxin concentration increases after Fab secondary to intravascular diffusion of antibody-bound, inactive digoxin.

   c. *Adverse reactions:* Allergic reaction, rebound hypokalemia, CHF (secondary to the sudden decrease in digoxin's inotropic effect).
5. **Adjunct:**
   a. Electrolyte disturbances (hyperkalemia) typically self-correct after Fab treatment.
   b. *Bradyarrhythmias:* Fab is first-line therapy; consider atropine, dopamine, epinephrine, or isoproterenol for second-line therapy.
   c. *Asystole and pulseless electrical activity (PEA):* Treat according to Pediatric Advanced Life Support (PALS) protocol.
   d. *Life-threatening tachyarrhythmias:* Fab is first-line therapy. If not immediately available, follow standard PALS protocols or overdrive cardiac pacing.

   *NOTE:* Phenytoin has been shown to reverse AV nodal digitalis block. Maximum of 15–20 mg/kg can be infused.



Continued

TABLE 2-3

MEDICATION INGESTIONS—cont'd

| Ingestion | Signs and Symptoms | Management |
| --- | --- | --- |
| **Hypoglycemics**[30]<br>a. *Sulfonylureas:* Glipizide, glyburide, glimepiride, chlorpropamide<br>b. *Biguanides:* Metformin | Status epilepticus, fatigue, dizziness, agitation, confusion, tachycardia, cardiovascular compromise, poor feeding, diaphoresis<br>**Metformin = metabolic acidosis** | **1. Initial Considerations:** Small ingestions can cause significant clinical toxicity.<br>*NOTE:* Hypoglycemia can be delayed 16–24 hr postingestion.<br>**2. Monitoring:** Hourly glucose checks.<br>**3. Supportive Care/Decontamination:**<br>a. Single dose of activated charcoal.<br>b. Hemodialysis and hemoperfusion may be necessary in severe ingestions.<br>**4. Adjunct:**<br>a. Hypertonic glucose ($D_{10}W$, neonates; $D_{25}W$, children; $D_{50}W$, adults) boluses as needed to treat hypoglycemia. Glucose infusion is necessary for several days.<br>b. Octreotide 1–2 μg/kg subcutaneously to treat refractory hypoglycemia. |

| | | |
|---|---|---|
| **Iron**[31,32] | **Phase 1** (0–6 hr postingestion): Encephalopathy, coma, shock, abdominal pain, emesis, GI hemorrhage, diarrhea, hyperglycemia, metabolic acidosis, leukocytosis<br>**Phase 2:** symptoms improve 6–72 hr postingestion.<br>**Phase 3** (6–48 hr postingestion): Following the improvement phase: coma, seizures, shock, cyanosis, abdominal pain, emesis, hepatic dysfunction and necrosis, metabolic acidosis, coagulopathy, hypoglycemia<br>**Phase 4** (4–6 wk after ingestion): GI tract strictures, pyloric stenosis, acute bowel obstruction | **1. Initial Considerations:**<br>a. Ingestions of children's chewable multivitamin with iron, carbonyl iron preparations, and polysaccharide iron preparations are no longer referred to the emergency room.<br>b. If asymptomatic and <30 mg/kg of elemental iron consumed, no treatment necessary beyond observation.<br>c. Refer to emergency room if >40 mg/kg elemental iron consumed or if symptomatic.<br>d. *Toxic reference ranges:*<br>Serum iron 350 μg/dL = minimal toxicity<br>Serum iron 500 μg/dL = moderate toxicity<br>Serum iron 1000 μg/dL = severe life-threatening toxicity<br>**2. Monitoring:**<br>a. Serum iron levels after 6 hr are misleading because liver has cleared free iron.<br>b. Sustained-release preparations need levels at 8 hr postingestion.<br>c. *Serum iron <550 μg/dL:* No further treatment necessary, except GI evacuation as indicated by radiograph.<br>d. *Serum iron, 550–900 μg/dL:* If asymptomatic after 24 hr, no further intervention is necessary.<br>e. *Serum iron >900 μg/dL:* Administer IV desferoxamine.<br>f. Follow abdominal radiograph.<br>g. Monitor electrolytes, anion gap acidosis, CBC. |

*Continued*

TABLE 2-3

MEDICATION INGESTIONS—cont'd

| Ingestion | Signs and Symptoms | Management |
| --- | --- | --- |
| **Iron—cont'd** | | **3. Supportive Care/Decontamination:**<br>a. If asymptomatic, consider gastric decontamination. *NOTE:* Activated charcoal is not indicated.<br>b. Whole-bowel irrigation if iron tablets are visible on radiograph.<br>c. Hemodialysis is indicated in renal impairment.<br>**4. Radiograph Interpretation:**<br>a. If there is radiopaque material on the abdominal x-ray (indicative of significant iron absorption), an anion gap acidosis, and serum iron level greater than 500 μg/dL, start desferoxamine and GI decontamination.<br>b. If the abdominal x-ray is normal, the patient is not acidotic, serum iron level is less than 500 μg/dL, and asymptomatic, then observe the patient.<br>**5. Antidote:** Desferoxamine<br>a. See Table 2-4<br>b. Start immediately if there are signs of organ failure.<br>**6. Adjunct:** Vigorous hydration and maintain adequate urine output. |

| | | |
|---|---|---|
| **NSAIDs**[33]<br>a. *COX-1 and COX-2 Inhibitors:* Salicylates, phenylbutazone, mefenamic acid, meclofenamate, ketorolac, indomethacin, ibuprofen, naproxen<br>b. *COX-2 Inhibitors:* Celecoxib, rofecoxib | Nausea, vomiting, epigastric pain, GI hemorrhage, renal failure, hepatotoxicity | **1. Initial Considerations:**<br>a. Ingestions >400 mg/kg lead to apnea, seizures, acidosis, renal and hepatic toxicity.<br>b. If mefenamic acid or sustained-release NSAID ingested, observe for 12 hr.<br>**2. Monitoring:** Serum electrolytes, lactic acid, BUN, creatinine, and liver function enzymes<br>**3. Supportive Care/Decontamination:**<br>a. Activated charcoal.<br>b. Hemodialysis and hemoperfusion are ineffective.<br>**4. Adjunct:** Treat seizures with diazepam. |
| **Phenothiazines, Butyrophenone**[34]<br>a. Tranquilizers<br>b. Chlorpromazine, fluphenazine, haloperidol, perphenazine, prochlorperazine, promethazine, thioridazine, trifluoperazine | Orthostatic hypotension, akathisia, dystonia, hyperthermia, parkinsonism, tardive dyskinesia, decreased sweating, decreased GI motility, urine retention, miosis, mydriasis | **1. Initial Considerations:**<br>a. Symptoms may occur 6–24 hr after ingestion.<br>b. Risk of neuroleptic malignant syndrome.<br>**2. Monitoring:** 12-lead ECG to evaluate for prolonged QT, ST changes; continuous cardiac monitoring.<br>**3. Supportive Care/Decontamination:**<br>a. Activated charcoal if within 4–6 hr of ingestion.<br>b. Hemodialysis and hemoperfusion not indicated.<br>**4. Antidote:** Benztropine. See Table 2-4.<br>**5. Adjunct:**<br>a. Diphenhydramine for acute dystonic reactions.<br>b. Norepinephrine and phenylephrine for refractory hypotension.<br>c. Nitroprusside to treat hypertension, a rare complication.<br>d. External cooling and sedation for hyperthermia. |

*Continued*

TABLE 2-3

MEDICATION INGESTIONS—cont'd

| Ingestion | Signs and Symptoms | Management |
| --- | --- | --- |
| **Phenytoin, Fosphenytoin**[35] | Nystagmus, ataxia, lethargy, slurred speech, pyramidal or extrapyramidal signs. Seizures are rare.<br>*IV infusion:* Depresses cardiac conduction and may cause hypotension. | **1. Initial Considerations:** If no signs of toxicity and phenytoin levels are not elevated or increasing after 8 hr of observation, can discharge to home.<br>**2. Monitoring:**<br>a. Phenytoin has unpredictable absorption; therefore, serial levels are needed.<br>b. Hypoalbuminemia, hyperbilirubinemia, or uremia disrupt the protein-binding capacity of phenytoin. Therefore, symptoms could develop when serum phenytoin is within the therapeutic range.<br>*NOTE:* Determination of free phenytoin fraction is helpful.<br>**3. Supportive Care/Decontamination:**<br>a. Activated charcoal if levels are increasing or persistently elevated.<br>b. Hemodialysis or hemoperfusion not indicated.<br>**4. Adjunct:** Treat seizures with diazepam, lorazepam, phenobarbital. |

| | | |
|---|---|---|
| **Salicylates**[36] (Fig. 2-2)<br>a. Aspirin, methylsalicylate, nonaspirin salicylate<br>b. Salicylates are also present in cough and cold preparations, topical preparations (oil of wintergreen) and creams, Pepto Bismol, wart and callus treatments | GI upset, vomiting, hyperpyrexia, dizziness, lethargy, dysarthria, seizure, respiratory depression, coma, cerebral edema, hepatic dysfunction, hyperglycemia, hyperkalemia, metabolic acidosis, hyponatremia, coagulopathy<br>Tinnitus, impaired hearing with chronic abuse | **1. Initial Considerations:**<br>a. Ingestions >150 mg/kg are referred to the emergency room.<br>b. Mild symptoms (GI upset, tachypnea, tinnitus) with ingestions of 150–300 mg/kg.<br>c. Moderate toxicity (agitation, fever, diaphoresis) with ingestions of 300–500 mg/kg.<br>d. Severe toxicity (seizure, coma, dysarthria, pulmonary edema, cardiorespiratory arrest) with ingestions >500 mg/kg.<br>e. *Chronic salicylism:* Symptoms of severe toxicity may occur at lower ingestion and serum salicylate levels.<br>**2. Rapid Confirmation of Salicylate Use:**<br>a. *Ferric chloride test ($FeCl_3$):* Several drops of 10% $FeCl_3$ mixed with 1 mL urine turns purple if salicylates are in urine (extremely sensitive test).<br>b. *Trinder Spot Test:* 1 mL Trinder reagent mixed with 1 mL urine will turn violet if salicylates are in urine.<br>**3. Monitoring:**<br>a. Check plasma salicylate level on arrival and every 2 hr until levels decline.<br>b. Monitor levels 6–12 hr postingestion of sustained-released formulation, and every 2 hr until levels begin to decline.<br>*NOTE:* Plasma levels may not correlate with clinical toxicity.<br>c. Monitor electrolytes, ionized calcium, magnesium, phosphorus, liver and renal function, coagulation markers, anion gap, lactic acid. |

*Continued*

TABLE 2-3

MEDICATION INGESTIONS—cont'd

| Ingestion | Signs and Symptoms | Management |
|---|---|---|
| **Salicylates—cont'd** | | d. Monitor urine pH and specific gravity.<br>e. 12-lead ECG and continuous cardiac monitoring.<br>**4. Supportive Care/Decontamination:**<br>a. Gastric lavage indicated up to 4 hr postingestion for large overdoses.<br>b. Activated charcoal for presentations 6–8 hr postingestion.<br>c. Whole-bowel irrigation for enteric-coated ingestions.<br>d. Hemodialysis indicated if patient has unresponsive acidosis, seizures, coma, renal failure, CHF, hepatic compromise with coagulopathy, progressive deterioration, or salicylate level >100 mg/dL after acute ingestion.<br>**5. Adjunct:**<br>a. *Fluid Resuscitation:* Give IV fluids with 5% dextrose, potassium, and 50–100 mEq/L sodium bicarbonate at twice maintenance.<br>*NOTE:* Serum alkalinization increases excretion and decreases CNS entry.<br>b. Alkalinize urine and maintain pH >7.5. Goal urine output is 2 mL/kg/hr.<br>*NOTE:* Monitor for hypokalemia secondary to alkalinization. |

| | | |
|---|---|---|
| **Valproate (VPA)** Divalproex, Depakote | Somnolence, coma, respiratory depression, electrolyte abnormalities, hyperammonemia, acidosis<br>*3–5 days postingestion:* pancytopenia | **1. Initial Considerations:** Absorption of enteric-coated form can be delayed up to 24 hr.<br>**2. Monitoring:**<br>a. VPA serum levels every 6 hr for first 24 hr.<br>*NOTE:* Therapeutic levels: 50–100 mg/L<br>b. Monitor electrolytes and ammonia.<br>**3. Supportive Care/Decontamination:**<br>a. Activated charcoal if levels are rising or massive acute ingestion.<br>b. Whole-bowel irrigation for large ingestions of enteric formulation.<br>c. Hemodialysis and hemoperfusion indicated for rapid deterioration, hepatic dysfunction, and serum levels >1000 mg/L.<br>**4. Adjunct:**<br>a. Carnitine supplementation is recommended for the following children:<br>(1) Children <2 yr receiving >1 anticonvulsant for complex neurologic disorder<br>(2) Failure to thrive<br>(3) Ketogenic diets<br>(4) VPA-induced hepatic dysfunction<br>b. *PO Carnitine Dose:* 100 mg/kg/day divided every 8 hr.<br>c. *IV Carnitine Dose:* 150–500 mg/kg/day divided every 8 hr.<br>d. Carnitine should be continued for 3 days or until clinical improvement. |

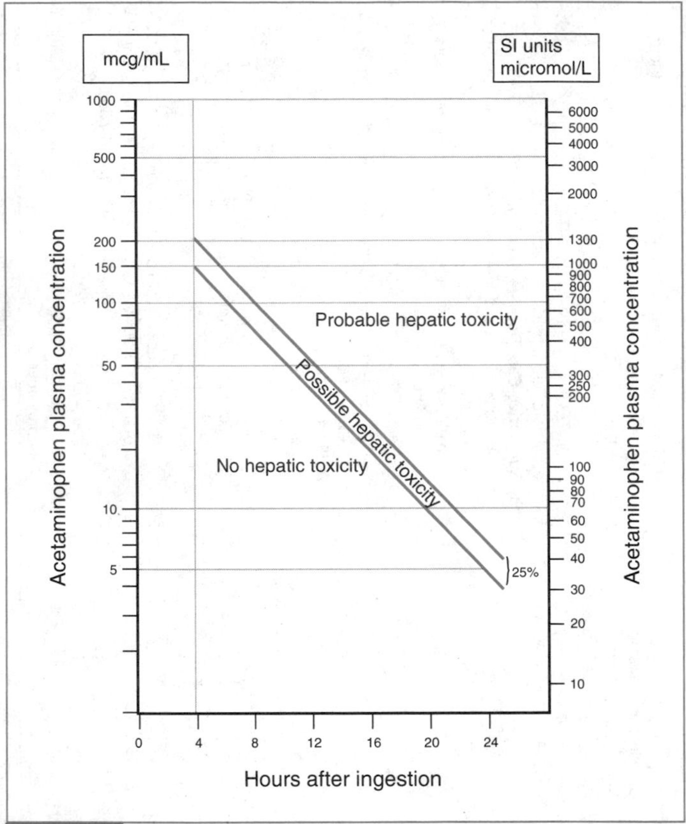


FIG. 2-1

Semilogarithmic plot of plasma acetaminophen levels versus time. *Note:* This nomogram is valid for use after acute ingestions of acetaminophen. The need for treatment cannot be extrapolated based on a level before 4 hours. In chronic overdose, toxicity can be seen with much lower plasma levels. *(From Jones AL: Mechanism of action and value of N-acetylcysteine in the treatment of early and late acetaminophen poisoning: A critical review. J Toxicol Clin Toxicol 1998;36: 277–285.)*

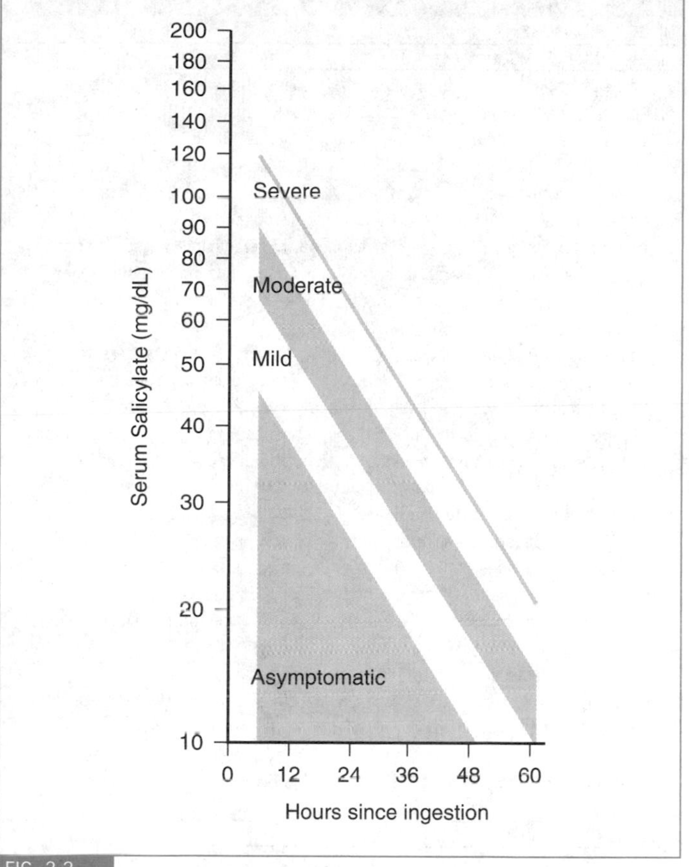


FIG. 2-2

The Done nomogram for estimating severity of salicylate poisoning using serum salicylate levels. *(From Temple AR: Acute and chronic effects of aspirin toxicity and their treatment. Arch Intern Med 1981;141:366.)*

BOX 2-1

## DRUGS OF ABUSE[37–41]

### Amphetamine (Stimulant)

1. **Names:** Amphetamine ("bennies, black beauties, crosses, hearts, speed, uppers"), methamphetamine ("ice, chalk, crank, crystal meth, fire, glass, speed"), dextromethamphetamine, ephedrine ("ma huang, herbal Ecstasy"), methylphenidate ("Ritalin, JIF, MPH, R-ball, Skippy, white dragon, Ciba-19"), phenylpropanolamine ("Propagest, BT 72s, co-pilot"), pseudoephedrine
2. **Routes:** Enteral, intravenous, intranasal, and smoked
3. **Acute Intoxication:** Dilated pupils, euphoria, hyperactivity, pressured speech, hyperthermia/fever, flushing, diaphoresis, hypertension, tachycardia, angina, arrhythmias, tremor, ataxia, dry mouth, diarrhea, bladder sphincter contraction, insomnia, suicidal and homicidal ideations

   **Toxic Ingestion:** Coma, circulatory collapse, hypertensive crisis, cerebral hemorrhage, seizure, psychosis, rhabdomyolysis, violent behaviors

   **Chronic Abuse:** Cardiomyopathy, pulmonary hypertension, vasculitis
4. **Monitoring:** Easily detected in POS (point-of-service) EMIT urine drug screens.

   *NOTE:* Isomers of nasal inhalants/cold preparations cause false positives.

   *NOTE:* Amphetamines are detectable in the urine up to 48 hr after last use.
5. **Supportive Care/Decontamination:**
   a. 12-lead ECG and continuous cardiorespiratory monitoring.
   b. Consider activated charcoal for recent ingestions.
   c. Check abdominal radiograph if body packing or stuffing is suspected.
   d. Hemodialysis indicated for acute renal failure, acidemia, or hyperkalemia.
6. **Adjunct:**
   a. Benzodiazepines are indicated for agitation or seizures.
   b. Treat hypertensive crisis with benzodiazepines, hydralazine, nitroprusside, or phentolamine.
   c. Treat hyperpyrexia with external cooling measures and benzodiazepines.
7. **Withdrawal:** Generalized fatigue, myalgias, poor concentration, confusion, anxiety, depression, insomnia for 1–2 days after use.

### Cocaine (Stimulant)

1. **Names:** Cocaine ("blow, bump, candy, C, Charlie, coke, flake, rock, snow"; "crack and freebase" are smokable forms)
2. **Routes:** Intranasal, intravenous, and smoked
3. **Acute Intoxication:** Dilated pupils, dry mouth, hyperalertness, increased energy, anxiety, insomnia, paranoia, tremors, muscle rigidity, hyperpyrexia/fever, bradycardia (low doses), tachycardia, hypertension, arrhythmia.

   **Acute Intoxication in Infants**: Dystonic posturing, seizure, hyperactivity, altered mental status.

   **Toxic Ingestion:** Psychosis, seizures, hypertensive crisis, cerebrovascular event, myocardial infarction, rhabdomyolysis, pneumothorax, pneumomediastinum.

   **Chronic Abuse:** Nasal septum ulcers, dilated cardiomyopathy, endocarditis, cellulitis, aortic dissection.

BOX 2-1

DRUGS OF ABUSE—cont'd

COCAINE (STIMULANT)—cont'd

4. **Monitoring:**
   a. Urine toxicology: Metabolites are detected in urine 2–3 days after last use.
   b. Serial 12-lead electrocardiogram (ECG) and cardiorespiratory monitoring
   c. Check cardiac enzymes, creatine kinase (CK), electrolytes, blood urea nitrogen (BUN), creatinine.
   d. Consider head computed tomography (CT) to evaluate for acute cerebrovascular accident.
   e. Consider lumbar puncture if subarachnoid hemorrhage suspected and patient has normal head CT.
   f. Abdominal radiograph to locate foreign body ("body packing or stuffing")
5. **Supportive Care/Decontamination:**
   a. Consider multiple doses of activated charcoal or whole-bowel irrigation for body packing or body stuffing.
   b. If body packer or stuffer is symptomatic, immediate surgical removal of foreign bodies is indicated.
   c. Hemodialysis for acute renal failure.
6. **Adjunct:**
   a. Benzodiazepines are indicated for seizures, agitation, hypertension, and tachycardia. Benzodiazepines are associated with decreased mortality from cocaine use.
   b. Treat hypertensive crisis with nitroprusside and benzodiazepines.

   *NOTE:* β-Blockers are not indicated due to risk of unopposed α-induced hypertension.

   c. Treat hyperpyrexia with external cooling and benzodiazepines.
   d. Treat arrhythmias according to Pediatric Advanced Life Support (PALS) protocol.
   e. Treat rhabdomyolysis with aggressive hydration; maintain urine output 2 mL/kg/hr.
7. **Withdrawal:** Drug cravings, depression, dysphoria, irritability, lethargy, and tremors. Symptoms peak 2–3 days after last use.

ECSTASY (STIMULANT)

1. **Names:** 3,4-methylenedioxymethamphetamine (MDMA) ("Adam, clarity, Eve, E, lover's speed, M&M, peace, STP, X, XTC")
2. **Route:** Enteral
3. **Acute Intoxication:** Enhanced empathy, euphoria, increased pyschomotor drive, tachycardia, hypertension, illusions, difficulty concentrating, headaches, palpitations, flushing, hyperthermia, nystagmus, suicidal and homicidal ideations.

   **Toxic Ingestion:** Psychosis, coma, seizures, intracranial hemorrhage, cerebral infarction, asystole, pulmonary edema, multiorgan system failure, renal or hepatic failure, adult respiratory distress syndrome (ARDS), disseminated

*Continued*

BOX 2-1

DRUGS OF ABUSE—cont'd

ECSTASY (STIMULANT)—cont'd

intravascular coagulation (DIC), syndrome of inappropriate antidiuretic hormone secretion (SIADH), death.

**Chronic Abuse:** Paranoid psychosis.

4. **Monitoring:**
   a. Detectable in routine urine toxicology screens.
   b. 12-lead ECG and continuous cardiorespiratory monitoring.
5. **Supportive Care/Decontamination:**
   a. Consider activated charcoal for recent ingestions.
   b. Check abdominal radiograph if body packing or stuffing is suspected.
   c. Hemodialysis is indicated for acute renal failure, acidemia, or hyperkalemia.
6. **Adjunct:**
   a. Treat hyperthermia with external cooling and benzodiazepines.
   b. Treat hypertension with nitroprusside, phentolamine, or benzodiazepines. β-Blockers are not indicated due to risk of unopposed α-induced hypertension.
   c. Treat agitation, seizures, and delirium with abnormal vital signs with benzodiazepines.
   d. Alkalinization or acidification of urine are not indicated.
7. **Withdrawal:** Generalized fatigue, myalgias, poor concentration, confusion, anxiety, depression, insomnia for 1–2 days after use.

ETHANOL (DEPRESSANT)

1. **Route:** Enteral
2. **Legal Intoxication:** 50–80 mg/dL (varies by state).
3. **Mild/Moderate Intoxication:** <100–200 mg/dL; disinhibition, euphoria, impaired coordination, impaired judgment, slurred speech, sedation.
4. **Severe Intoxication:** >300 mg/dL; confusion, stupor, coma, respiratory depression, loss of protective reflexes, death.
5. **Chronic Abuse:** Holiday heart, "wet" beriberi, "dry" beriberi, cirrhosis, pancreatitis, hepatitis, Mallory-Weiss tear.
6. **Initial Considerations:**
   a. 12 oz beer, 4 oz wine, and 1.5 oz liquor increase blood ethanol levels by approximately 0.025 g/dL (varies by weight).
   b. Blood alcohol >500 mg/dL in teens may be fatal.
   c. Blood alcohol >100 mg/dL in infants may cause coma and hypoglycemia.
7. **Monitoring:**
   a. Serum ethanol level and urine toxicology screen.
   b. Monitor electrolytes, dextrostick, bicarbonate, magnesium, and phosphorus.
8. **Supportive Care/Decontamination:**
   a. Gastric lavage is not indicated due to quick absorption.
   b. If coingestion suspected, consider gastric emptying and activated charcoal.
   c. Consider hemodialysis for hemodynamic instability, impaired hepatic function, or severe symptoms.

BOX 2-1

DRUGS OF ABUSE—cont'd

ETHANOL (DEPRESSANT)—cont'd

9. **Adjunct:**
   a. Hypoglycemic seizures can be treated with glucose and anticonvulsants.
   b. IV fluids: $D_5W$ NS + supplements (100 mg thiamine, 2 g folate, magnesium, and possibly potassium if indicated).

γ-HYDROXYBUTYRATE (GHB) (DEPRESSANT), γ-HYDROXYBUTYROLACTONE (GBL)

1. **Names:** GHB ("liquid ecstasy, date rape drug, Georgia home boy, soap, easy lay")
2. **Route:** Enteral
3. **Acute Intoxication:** 10 mg/kg: sleep, 30 mg/kg: memory loss, 50 mg/kg: general anesthesia/coma; nystagmus, myosis, ataxia, hypothermia.
   **Toxic Ingestion:** CNS and respiratory depression, aggressiveness, seizures, bradycardia, agitation, and aggressive versus obtunded.
4. **Initial Considerations:**
   a. Effects typically last 6–8 hr; toxicity prolonged with ethanol ingestion.
   b. Coma lasts 1–2 hr; patients are delirious and vomiting when emerging from the coma.
5. **Monitoring:**
   a. Not detectable in urine screens.
   b. Detectable via gas chromatography or mass spectrometry.
6. **Adjunct:** Treat bradycardia with atropine.
7. **Withdrawal:** Feelings of doom, anxiety, insomnia, disorientation, visual and auditory hallucinations.

HALLUCINOGENS

1. **Names:** Mescaline ("buttons, cactus, mesc, blue cap"), psilocybin ("magic mushrooms, Aztec, purple passion, shrooms"), LSD ("acid, blotter, boomers, cubes, microdot, yellow sunshine"), phencyclidine ("PCP, angel dust, boat, hog, love boat, peace pill"), dimethyltryptamine, diethyltryptamine.
2. **Routes:** Enteral, Inhaled, intravenous
3. **Acute Intoxication:** Psychosis, paranoia, time and visual distortions, depersonalization, hyperreflexia, hyperthermia, dilated pupils, tachycardia, hypertension, facial flushing.
   **LSD Intoxication:** Flashbacks, psychosis, delusions, grandiosity, paresthesias, weakness, drowziness and dizziness, hyperthermia, tachycardia, hypertension.
   **PCP Intoxication:** Possible bradycardia and hypotension, panic, aggression, violence, seizures, cyclic coma, nystagmus, dyskinesia, dystonia, bronchospasm, hypersalivation.
   **Toxic Exposure:** Rhabdomyolysis.
4. **Initial Consideration:** Half-life ranges from 1–3 days.
5. **Monitoring:** PCP is detected by urine screens.
6. **Adjunct:** Treat seizures, anxiety, and agitation with benzodiazepines.

Continued

BOX 2-1

**DRUGS OF ABUSE—cont'd**

**KETAMINE**

1. **Names:** Ketalar ("cat, Valiums, K, K-hole, Special K, vitamin K")
2. **Routes:** Enteral, inhaled
3. **Acute Intoxication:** Nystagmus, analgesia, anxiety, sedation, amnesia, hallucination, hypersalivation, tachycardia, hypertension, emesis.
   **Toxic Exposure:** Rhabdomyolysis, delirium, respiratory depression, respiratory arrest.
4. **Monitoring:** Not detectable in routine toxicology screens; however, detectable by high-performance liquid chromatography.
5. **Adjunct:** Treat emergence reactions or agitation with benzodiazepines.

**MARIJUANA**

1. **Names:** Marijuana ("blunt, dope, ganja, grass, joint, Mary Jane, pot, reefer, Sinsemilla, skunk, weed"), hashish ("boom, chronic, hash, hemp")
2. **Routes:** Enteral, smoked
3. **Acute Intoxication:** Euphoria, relaxation, confusion, increased appetite, impaired motor skills, tachycardia, anxiety, panic attacks, conjunctival injection, depersonalization, mood change, pneumomediastinum, pneumothorax.
   **Toxic Exposure:** Delusion, panic, paranoia, and psychosis.
   **Chronic Abuse:** Cough, frequent respiratory infection, gynecomastia, infertility.
4. **Initial Considerations:**
   a. Co-ingestion with phenytoin increases marijuana's effects.
   b. Smoking is three times more potent than enteral ingestion.
5. **Monitoring:**
   a. Detected in urine toxicology screens for 3 days after single use and up to 10 days after weekly use.
   b. Consider chest radiograph if low oxygen saturation, chest pain, or unequal breath sounds.
6. **Adjunct:**
   a. Treat toxic delirium and psychosis with benzodiazepines.
   b. Treat disabling insomnia with trazodone.
7. **Withdrawal:** Flulike illness, disturbed sleep, tremor, anorexia. Symptoms peak 4–5 days after last use and slowly resolve over 2 weeks.

**OPIOIDS (DEPRESSANT)**

1. **Names:** Buprenorphine, codeine ("Captain Cody, schoolboy, doors and fours, loads, pancakes and syrup"), fentanyl ("Duragesic, china girl, china white, dance fever, goodfella, STP, six pack, TNT, tango and cash"), heroin ("brown sugar, dope, H, horse, junk skag, skunk, smack"), hydrocodone, hydromorphone, meperidine, morphine ("Miss Emma, monkey"), methadone ("orange barrel, dolphin"), opium ("Big O, black stuff, block, gun, dust, yen shee"), oxycodone ("O.C."), pentazocine ("Talwin, Ts"), propoxyphene ("Darvon, lily")
2. **Routes:** Enteral, intranasal, intravenous, intramuscular, subcutaneous, and smoked.

BOX 2-1

DRUGS OF ABUSE—cont'd

OPIOIDS (DEPRESSANT)—cont'd

3. **Acute Intoxication:** Pinpoint pupils, euphoria, sedation, impaired thought, hypothermia, clammy skin, urine retention, constipation, increased anal tone.
   **Toxic Exposure:** Hypotension, arrhythmia, respiratory depression, coma, seizure, death.
   **Chronic IV Abuse:** Cellulitis, septic emboli, endocarditis, abscesses.
4. **Monitoring:**
   a. Not all opioids are detected by urine screens.
   b. Thin-layer chromatography and radioimmunoassay detect opiate metabolites up to 3 days from last use.
   c. 12-lead ECG and cardiorespiratory monitoring.
5. **Antidote:** Naloxone. See Table 2-4.
6. **Adjunct:** Consider methadone or buprenorphine to prevent withdrawal.
7. **Withdrawal:** Drug cravings, depression, irritability, anxiety, tremors, rhinorrhea, muscle aches, diarrhea, insomnia, piloerection.

SEDATIVE-HYPNOTICS (DEPRESSANT)

1. **Names:** Barbiturates (Amytal, Nembutal, Seconal, Phenobarbital: "ace, barbs, reds, red birds, phennies, yellow jackets"), meprobamate ("barns"), methaqualone ("ludes, mandrex, quads, quay, somnafae, soapers, 714"), methyprylon ("roach 19, easter bunny"), flunitrazepam (Rohypnol: "forget me pill, Roche, Rib, roofies, roofinol, rope, rophies, date pill"), benzodiazepines (Ativan, Halcion, Librium, Valium, Xanax: "candy, downers, sleepers")
2. **Routes:** Enteral, intranasal, intravenous.
3. **Acute Intoxication:** Reduced anxiety, lowered inhibitions, shallow breathing, poor concentration, impaired coordination, impaired memory, impaired judgment, sluggish pupillary response.
   **Toxic Exposure:** Hypotension, bradycardia, pulmonary edema, respiratory depression.
4. **Monitoring:** Not all barbiturates or benzodiazepines are detected on urine screens.
5. **Supportive Care/Decontamination:**
   a. Consider multiple doses of activated charcoal
   b. Hemodialysis or hemoperfusion in severe overdoses.
6. **Antidote:** Flumazenil. See Table 2-4.
7. **Adjunct:** Consider methadone to prevent withdrawal.
8. **Withdrawal:** Seizures increased rapid eye movement sleep, tremors, insomnia, apathy, weakness, agitation, anxiety, cravings, and flulike illness. Symptoms peak 5 days after last use.

TABLE 2-4

**ANTIDOTES***

| Indication | Antidote | Preparation | Administration | Adverse Effects |
|---|---|---|---|---|
| Acetaminophen | *N*-acetylcysteine (Mucomyst) | 4-, 10-, 30-, 100-mL vials of 20% solution | *Loading Dose:* 140 mg/kg PO, followed by<br>*Maintenance Doses:* 70 mg/kg PO q4h for 17 doses or discontinue at 36 hr if undetectable serum levels, normal liver function tests (LFTs), and International Normalized Ratio (INR) <2.<br>*Loading Dose:* 150 mg/kg IV over 1 hr.<br>*Maintenance Dose:* 150 mg/kg IV over 4 hr, then 150 mg/kg over 16 hr. | Nausea/vomiting<br>IV form can cause bronchospasm, anaphylaxis/death. |
| Alcohols (ethylene glycol, methanol) | Ethanol | 95% ampule | 1 mL/kg diluted to 10% given over 1 hr, then 0.1 5 mL/kg/hr to target blood ethanol levels 100–150 mg/dL. | Emesis, sedation |
| | Fomepizole (4-methylpyrazole) | 1-g/mL vials | *Loading Dose:* 15 mg/kg.<br>*Maintenance Dose:* 10 mg/kg q12h for 4 doses; then 15 mg/kg q12h until ethylene glycol or methanol levels are <20 mg/dL.<br>*NOTE:* Give q4h if undergoing hemodialysis. | |
| Anticholinesterase (organophosphate) | Atropine | 0.05, 0.2, 0.5, 1.0, 2.0 mg/mL | *Children:* 0.05–0.1 mg/kg IM, IV, endotracheal tube (ETT) every 5–10 min until bronchial or oral secretions terminate.<br>*Adults:* 2–5 mg IM, IV, ETT every 5–10 min until bronchial or oral secretions terminate.<br>*NOTE:* Dilute in 1–2 mL normal saline for ETT administration. | Tachycardia, dry mouth, mydriasis, urine retention |

| | | | | |
|---|---|---|---|---|
| Antihistamines, anticholinergic agents | Physostigmine sulfate | 1 mg/mL | *Children:* 0.5 mg IV over 3–5 min<br>*Adults:* 1–2 mg IV over 5 min<br>*Alternate Dosing:* 0.02 mg/kg IV over 5 min. May repeat every 10–15 min up to a maximum total of 2 mg (children) and 4 mg (adults).<br>*NOTE:* Do not give if co-ingestion of tricyclic antidepressants.<br>*NOTE:* Increased risk of seizures or asystole if given too rapidly.<br>*NOTE:* Atropine reverses side effects. Atropine dose is one half the dose of physostigmine given. | Seizures, headaches, bradycardia, asystole, bronchospasm, emesis, cholinergic crisis |
| Benzodiazepines | Flumazenil (Romazicon) | 0.1 mg/mL | *Children:* 0.01–0.02 mg/kg IV every minute to a maximum of 1 mg cumulative dose.<br>*Adults:* 0.2 mg/kg IV every minute to a maximum of 5 mg cumulative dose.<br>*NOTE:* Consider continuous infusion.<br>*NOTE:* Do not give if co-ingestion of antidepressants or unknown. | Emesis, facial flushing, agitation, headache, seizures |
| β-Blockers | Glucagon | 1-mg, 10-mg vials | *Children Loading Dose:* 0.05–0.15 mg/kg IV<br>*Children Maintenance Infusion:* 0.05 mg/kg/hr<br>*Adult Loading Dose:* 3.5–5 mg IV repeated 2–3 times to a maximum of 10 mg.<br>*Adult Maintenance Infusion:* 1–5 mg/hr | Hyperglycemia, emesis |
| Calcium channel blockers | Calcium chloride | 1 g/10 mL (13.6 mEq) | *Children:* 0.2–0.25 mg/kg/dose every 10 min until a response is seen. | |

*Contact the Poison Control Center for the most current recommendations: 1-800-222-1222.

Data from references 4, 9, 14, 15, and 42.

*Continued*

TABLE 2-4

**ANTIDOTES—cont'd**

<table>
<tr><th>Indication</th><th>Antidote</th><th>Preparation</th><th>Administration</th><th>Adverse Effects</th></tr>
<tr><td>Calcium channel blockers—cont'd</td><td>Glucagon</td><td>See β-blockers</td><td>Adults: 1 g PRN every 10 min until a response is seen.</td><td></td></tr>
<tr><td>Carbon monoxide</td><td>Hyperbaric oxygen</td><td></td><td>100% oxygen via non-rebreather mask or ventilator.</td><td></td></tr>
<tr><td>Cyanide</td><td>Cyanide antidote kit</td><td>Amyl nitrite 0.3-mL pearl<br>Sodium nitrite, 3% 300 mg/10 mL<br>Sodium thiosulfate 25% 12.5 g/50 mL</td><td>Children: Crush pearl and inhale over 30 sec pending administration of IV sodium nitrite.<br>If the hemoglobin (Hb) is known for children, administer:
<table>
<tr><th>Hb</th><th>Sodium nitrite solution 3% (mL/kg)</th><th>Sodium thiosulfate 25% (mg/kg)</th></tr>
<tr><td>7 g</td><td>0.19</td><td>5.8</td></tr>
<tr><td>8 g</td><td>0.22</td><td>6.6</td></tr>
<tr><td>9 g</td><td>0.25</td><td>7.5</td></tr>
<tr><td>10 g</td><td>0.27</td><td>8.3</td></tr>
<tr><td>11 g</td><td>0.30</td><td>9.1</td></tr>
<tr><td>12 g</td><td>0.33</td><td>10</td></tr>
<tr><td>13 g</td><td>0.36</td><td>10.6</td></tr>
<tr><td>14 g</td><td>0.39</td><td>11.6</td></tr>
</table>
If the hemoglobin is not known for children:<br>Give sodium nitrite 3%: 0.33 mL/kg IV</td><td>Tachycardia, hypotension, methemoglobinemia</td></tr>
</table>

| | | | | |
|---|---|---|---|---|
| | | | Give sodium thiosulfate 25%: 1.6 mL (400 mg)/kg IV every 30–60 min to maximum of 50 mL. Administer immediately after sodium nitrite.<br>*Adults:* Crush pearl and inhale over 30 sec pending administration of IV sodium nitrite.<br>Sodium nitrite 3%: 300 mg (10 mL) IV over 10 min<br>Sodium thiosulfate 25%: 12.5 g IV (2.5 mL/min) over 10 min. | |
| Digoxin, digitoxin toxicity | Digoxin-specific antibody fragments | 38-mg vials | ***If dose ingested is known, calculate:***<br>Body Load Digoxin = mg ingested × 0.8<br>Vials to Administer = Body Load/0.5<br>If serum level is known, then calculate:<br>$\text{Vials to Administer} = \frac{\text{dig level (ng/mL)} \times \text{weight (kg)}}{100}$<br>***If digoxin dose or level unknown in children <20 kg:*** 1 vial<br>***If digoxin dose or level unknown in adult acute toxicity:*** 20 vials | Allergic reaction, rebound hypokalemia, CHF |
| Oleander, foxglove, toad venom | Digoxin-specific antibody fragments | 38-mg vials | *Children <20 kg:* 1 vial<br>*Adults—acute toxicity:* 20 vials<br>*Adults—chronic toxicity:* 6 vials | Allergic reaction, rebound hypokalemia, CHF |

*Continued*

TABLE 2-4

**ANTIDOTES—cont'd**

| Indication | Antidote | Preparation | Administration | Adverse Effects |
|---|---|---|---|---|
| Iron | Desferoxamine (Desferal) | 500-mg vial | *Children/adults:* 5–15 mg/kg/hr IV for 6–12 hr (mild-moderate toxicity) or 24 hr (severe toxicity), then reassess.<br>*NOTE:* Maximum dose 360 mg/kg or 6 g/day<br>*NOTE:* Continue chelation until iron level within normal range, resolution of acidosis, or clinical improvement. | Hypotension |
| Methemoglobinemia | Methylene blue | 10 mg/mL (1%) | *Children/adults:* 1–2 mg/kg over 5 min every 30–60 min; repeat to maximum of 7 mg/kg (0.7 mL/kg).<br>*NOTE:* Contraindicated in G6PD deficiency due to possible delayed hemolysis. | Emesis, anxiety, chest pain, tachycardia, hypertension, green-blue urine, headache, factitious cyanosis |
| Opioid | Naloxone | 0.02 mg/mL, 0.4 mg/mL, 1 mg/mL | *Neonates:* 0.01–0.03 mg/kg/dose<br>*Children:* 0.4–2.0 mg/dose<br>*Adults:* 1–2 mg IV or ETT; can be repeated every 2 min to a maximum of 10 mg | Opioid withdrawal, seizures, arrhythmias, hypertension, pulmonary edema |

| | | | | |
|---|---|---|---|---|
| Pesticides (organophosphate, carbamate) | Atropine | 0.05, 0.2, 0.5, 1.0, 2.0 mg/mL | *Children:* 0.05–0.1 mg/kg IM, IV, ETT every 5–10 min until bronchial or oral secretions terminate<br>*Adults:* 2–5 mg IM IV, ETT every 5–10 min until bronchial or oral secretions terminate<br>NOTE: Dilute in 1–2 mL normal saline for ETT administration. | Tachycardia, dry mouth, mydriasis, urine retention |
| | Pralidoxime (2-PAM, Protopam) | 1 g/20 mL | *Children <12 yr:* 25–50 mg/kg over 30 min, then 9–19 mg/kg/hr<br>*Adults:* 1–2 g IV, repeat in 1 hr PRN, then q6–12h PRN for 24–48 hr. Infuse slowly.<br>Alternatively: continuous infusion of 500 mg/hr. | Nausea, headache, bronchospasm, dizziness, tachycardia, muscle rigidity |
| Phenothiazines (acute dystonic reaction) | Diphenhydramine (Benadryl) | 50 mg/mL | *Children:* 1–2 mg/kg/dose IM/IV q6h. Maximum dose 300 mg/day.<br>*Adults:* 25–50 mg IV/IM/PO q–8h. Maximum dose 400 mg/day. | Sedation, ataxia, paradoxical agitation |
| | Benztropine (Cogentin) | | *Children:* 0.02 mg/kg (maximum 1 mg) IV/IM.<br>*NOTE:* Use in patients <3 yr in life-threatening reactions.<br>*Adults:* 1–2 mg IV/IM | Sedation, blurred vision, dry mouth, tachycardia |
| Warfarin (rodenticides) | Vitamin K | 2 mg/mL, 10 mg/mL; 5-mg tablet | *Children:* 2.5–10 mg SQ/PO up to 100 mg/day in divided doses for prolonged time<br>*Adults:* 5–10 mg SQ/PO up to 200 mg/day in divided doses for prolonged time. | |

## V. CARBON MONOXIDE POISONING[44]

### A. CARBON MONOXIDE (CO)

1. A colorless, odorless, nonirritating, tasteless gas.
2. High-affinity hemoglobin binding causes cardiac ischemia and neurologic injury.

### B. ENVIRONMENTAL EXPOSURES

1. Garages, campers, tents, gas furnaces/heaters/ovens/dryers, wood and coal heating, fireplaces, charcoal grills, automobiles, generators, lawn mowers, snow and leaf blowers, paint remover with methylene chloride.
2. Consider exposure to cyanide as well in the setting of a fire.

### C. AFFINITY FOR HEMOGLOBIN

Carbon monoxide has 240-fold greater affinity for hemoglobin than oxygen, leading to decreased oxygen delivery to tissues.

### D. ELIMINATION HALF-LIFE

1. Room air = 320 min.
2. 100% non-rebreather mask = 40–80 min.
3. Hyperbaric chamber = 20 min.

### E. PHYSICAL EXAMINATION

1. **Mild poisoning:** Headache, nausea, vomiting, dizziness, blurred vision.
2. **Moderate poisoning:** Confusion, syncope, chest pain, dyspnea, weakness, tachycardia, tachypnea, rhabdomyolysis.
3. **Severe poisoning:** Palpitations, arrhythmias, respiratory arrest, noncardiogenic pulmonary edema, seizures, coma.
4. **End organ damage:** Cerebral edema, permanent ocular toxicity, cardiac ischemia, muscle necrosis, myoglobinuria, renal failure.

**Note** *Cherry-red mucosal membranes and retinal hemorrhages are late and rare findings.*

### F. MANAGEMENT

1. Secure the airway and avoid hypercapnia.
2. Administer 100% $O_2$ via non-rebreather face mask until carboxyhemoglobin (COHb) is less than 10% and symptoms resolve.
3. If severe respiratory compromise, cardiovascular instability, altered alertness, nervous system dysfunction, or coma is present, intubate and mechanically hyperventilate using 100% $O_2$ and transfer to a facility with a hyperbaric chamber.
4. Measure serum COHb levels, ABG, complete metabolic panel, cardiac enzymes, creatine kinase, and lactate.

**Note** *Guidelines for COHb levels: Symptomatic at >15%, toxicity at >20%, severe neurologic effects at >40%, and irreversible CNS damage at >50%.*

**Note** *Symptoms may not correlate with COHb levels in the blood.*

5. Obtain ECG and chest radiograph to evaluate for myocardial ischemia and noncardiogenic pulmonary edema.
6. Head computed tomography scan may show infarction and bilateral globus pallidus lesions.
7. Consider hyperbaric oxygen therapy in cases of altered mental status, coma, seizures, loss of consciousness, cardiac dysfunction, or pregnancy with >15% COHb, although specific indications are controversial.
8. Perform neuropsychometric testing if clinically indicated or treating with hyperbaric oxygen.



## VI. METHEMOGLOBINEMIA[14]

### A. ETIOLOGIES

1. Congenital hemoglobinopathy: Genetic deficiency of enzymes that reduce methemoglobin.
2. Oxidative hemoglobin injury in ill infants, i.e., diarrheal illness, poisoning, drugs, or environmental exposure.
3. Agents of injury: Aniline dyes, chloroquine, dapsone, fertilizers containing nitrogens, local anesthetics, high doses of methylene blue, metoclopramide, naphthalene, nitrates, nitrites, rifampin, toluidine, contaminated well water.

**Note** *Routine urine toxicology tests generally do not detect the etiology of methemoglobinemia.*

### B. PHYSICAL EXAMINATION

1. Acute-onset methemoglobinemia: CNS depression, cardiac instability, hemolysis, tissue ischemia.
2. Cyanosis unresponsive to oxygen therapy but with normal $PaO_2$ on ABG.
3. Arterial blood has chocolate-brown color and does not turn red on exposure to air.

**Note** *Cyanosis occurs with 1.5 g/dL methemoglobin level or when 10% or more of the hemoglobin is methemoglobin.*

### C. MANAGEMENT

1. Remove the offending agent.
2. Administer 100% $O_2$. Note that pulse oximetry is not accurate.

3. Perform skin decontamination.
4. Give activated charcoal if suspect oxidant ingestion.
5. Perform co-oximetry analysis of the blood to confirm and quantify methemoglobinemia. Estimate the oxygen-carrying capacity based on the percentage of methemoglobin and the total amount of hemoglobin.
6. Serial ECGs to monitor for myocardial ischemia.
7. Obtain electrolytes, creatinine, ABG, complete blood count with differential, blood smear to evaluate for hemolysis, and urinalysis.
8. Methylene blue is indicated for severe tissue hypoxia (beyond cyanotic discoloration), CNS depression, cardiovascular instability, coexisting medical condition that decreases tolerance for low oxygen delivery to tissues, and methemoglobin level greater than 30%. See Table 2-4.

**Note** *Methylene blue is contraindicated in patients with glucose-6-phosphate dehydrogenase deficiency. Consider hyperbaric oxygen therapy or exchange transfusion.*

## REFERENCES

1. Goldfrank LR et al: Toxicologic Emergencies, 8th ed. New York, McGraw-Hill, 2006.
2. Dart RC et al: Poisoning. In Hay WW et al (eds): Current Pediatric Diagnosis and Treatment, 17th ed. New York, McGraw-Hill, 2005, pp 346–410.
3. Hoppe-Roberts JM: Poisoning mortality in United States: Comparison of national mortality statistics and poision control center reports. Ann Emerg Med 2000;35(5):440–448.
4. Bryant S, Singer J: Management of toxic exposure in children. Emerg Med Clin North Am 2003;21(1):101–119.
5. Henry K et al: Deadly ingestions. Pediatr Clin North Am 2006;53(2):293–315.
6. Michael JB et al: Deadly pediatric poisonings: Nine common agents that kill at low doses. 2004;22(4):1019–1050.
7. Osterhoudt KC et al: Activated charcoal administration in pediatric emergency department. Pediatr Emerg Care 2004;20(8):493–498.
8. Mlcak RP et al: Respiratory management of inhalation injury. Burns 2007;33(1):2–13.
9. Kao L, Nanagas K: Carbon monoxide poisoning. Med Clin North Am 2005;89(6):1161–1194.
10. Umbreit J et al: Methemoglobin—it's not just blue. A concise review. Am J Hematol 2007;82(2):134–144.
11. White M et al: Update on antidotes for pediatric poisonings. Pediatr Emerg Care 2006;22(11):740–749.
12. Calello D et al: New and novel antidotes in pediatrics. Pediatr Emerg Care 2006;22(7):523–530.
13. Dart RC: Acetaminophen poisoning: An evidence based concensus guideline for out-of-hospital management. Clin Toxicol (Phila) 2006;44(1):1–18.
14. Kanter MZ: Comparison of oral and IV acetylcysteine in the treatment of acetominophen poisoning. Am J Health-Syst Pharm 2006;63:1821–1827.

15. Spiller H et al: Efficacy of activated charcoal administered more than four hours after acetaminophen overdose. J Emerg Med 2006;30(1):1–5.
16. Patel RJ et al: Prevalence of autonomic signs and symptoms in antimuscarinic drug poisonings. J Emerg Med 2004;26(1):89–94.
17. Scharman EJ et al: Diphenhydramine and dimenhydrinate poisoning: An evidence-based consensus guideline for out-of-hospital management. Clin Toxicol (Phila) 2006;44(3):205–223.
18. Nine JS et al: Fatality from diphenhydramine monointoxication: A case report and review of the infant, pediatric, and adult literature. Am J Forensic Med Phathol 2006;27(1):36–41.
19. Miller J: Managing antidepression overdoses. Emerg Med Serv 2004;33(10): 113–119.
20. Rosenbaum TG et al: Are one or two dangerous? Tricyclic antidepressant exposure in toddlers. J Emerg Med 2005;29(2):169–174.
21. Isbister GK et al: Relative toxicity of selective serotonin reuptake inhibitors (SSRIs) in overdose. J Toxicol 2004;24(3):277–285.
22. Ty EB et al: Neuroleptic malignant syndrome in children and adolescents. J Clin Neurol 2001;16(3):157–163.
23. Centers for Disease Control and Prevention (CDC: Infant deaths associated with cough and cold medications—two states. MMWR 2007;56(1):1–4.
24. Isbister GK et al: Alprazolam is relatively more toxic than other benzodiazepines in overdose. Br J Clin Pharmacol 2004;58(1):88–95.
25. Thomson JS: Use of flumazenil in benzodiazapine overdose. Emerg Med J 2006;23(2):162.
26. Love JN et al: Lack of toxicity from pediatric beta-blocker exposure. Hum Exp Toxicol 2006;25(6):341–346.
27. Shepard G: Treatment of poisoning caused by beta-adrenergic and calcium channel blockers. Am J Health-Syst Pharm 2006;63(19):1828–1835.
28. DeWitt CR et al: Pharmacology, pathophysiology and management of calcium channel blocker and beta-blocker toxicity. Toxicol Rev 2004;23(4):223–238.
29. Bek K et al: Carbamazepine poisoning managed with haemodialysis and haemoperfusion in three adolescents. Nephrology. 2007;12(1):33–35.
30. Horowitz R: Accidental clonidine patch ingestion in a child. Am J Ther 2005;12(3):272–274.
31. Davis JA: Multiple cardiac arrhythmias in a previously healthy child: A case of accidental digitalis intoxication. Pediatr Emerg Care 2006;22(6):430–434.
32. Eyal D: Digoxin toxicity: Pediatric survival after asystolic arrest. Clin Toxicol (Phila) 2005;43(1):51–54.
33. Little GL et al: Are one or two dangerous? Sulfonylurea exposure in toddlers. J Emerg Med 2005;28(3):305–310.
34. Aldridge M et al: Acute iron poisoning: What every pediatric intensive care unit nurse should know. Dimen Crit Care Nurs 2007;26(2):43–48.
35. Manoguerra AS et al: Iron ingestion: An evidence-based consensus guideline for out-of-hospital management. Clin Toxicol (Phila) 2005;43(6):553–570.
36. Marciniak KE et al: Massive ibuprofen overdose requiring extracorporeal membrane oxygenation for cardiovascular support. Pediatr Crit Care Med 2007;8(2):1–3.
37. Love JN et al: Are one or two dangerous? Phenothiazine exposure in toddlers. J Emerg Med 2006;31(1):53–59.
38. Craig S: Phenytoin poisoning. Neurocrit Care 2005;3(2):161–170.

39. Dargan PI et al: An evidence based flowchart to guide the management of acute salicylate (aspirin) overdose. J Emerg Med 2002;19(3):206–209.
40. Hertz JA et al: Prescription drug misuse: A growing national problem. Adolesc Med Clin 2006;17(3):751–769.
41. Williams JF et al: Abuse of proprietary (over-the-counter) drugs. Adolsc Med Clin 2006;17(3):733–750.
42. Kuhen BM: Many teens abusing medications. JAMA 2007;297(6):578–580.
43. Ruha AM et al: Pharmacologic treatment of acute pediatric methamphetamine toxicity. Pediatr Emerg Care 2006;22(12):782–785.
44. Kaul P et al: Substance abuse. In Hay WW et al (ed): Current Pediatric Diagnosis and Treatment, 17th ed. New York, McGraw-Hill, 2005, pp 147–164.

# Procedures

*Jason W. Custer, MD*

3

## I. GENERAL GUIDELINES

### A. CONSENT

It is crucial to obtain informed consent from the parent or guardian before performing any procedure by explaining the procedure, the indications, any risks involved, and any alternatives. Obtaining consent for life-saving emergency procedures is unnecessary.

### B. RISKS

1. All invasive procedures involve pain and risk for infection and bleeding. Specific complications are listed by procedure.
2. Sedation and analgesia should be planned in advance, and the risks of such explained to the parent and/or patient as applicable. In general, 1% lidocaine buffered with sodium bicarbonate is adequate for local analgesia.
3. Universal precautions should be followed for all patient contact that exposes the health care provider to blood, amniotic fluid, pericardial fluid, pleural fluid, synovial fluid, cerebrospinal fluid, semen, or vaginal secretions.
4. Proper sterile technique is crucial to achieve good wound closure, decrease transmittable diseases, and prevent wound contamination.

## II. BLOOD SAMPLING

### A. HEELSTICK AND FINGERSTICK

1. **Indication:** Blood sampling in infants for laboratory studies unaffected by hemolysis.
2. **Complications:** Infection, bleeding, osteomyelitis.
3. **Procedure:**

a. Warm heel or finger.

b. Clean with alcohol.

(1) Puncture heel using a lancet on the lateral part of the heel, avoiding the posterior area.

(2) Puncture finger using a lancet on the palmar lateral surface of the finger near the tip.

c. Wipe away the first drop of blood, and then collect the sample using a capillary tube or container.

d. Alternate between squeezing blood from the leg toward the heel (or from the hand toward the finger) and then releasing the pressure for several seconds.

### B. EXTERNAL JUGULAR PUNCTURE[1]

1. **Indications:** Blood sampling in patients with inadequate peripheral vascular access or during resuscitation.
2. **Complications:** Infection, bleeding, pneumothorax.

3. **Procedure (Fig. 3-1):**

a. Restrain infant securely. Place infant with head turned away from side of blood sampling. Position with towel roll under shoulders or with head over side of bed to extend neck and accentuate the posterior margin of the sternocleidomastoid muscle on the side of the venipuncture.

b. Prepare area in a sterile fashion.

c. The external jugular vein will distend if its most proximal segment is occluded or if the child cries. The vein runs from the angle of the mandible to the posterior border of the lower third of the sternocleidomastoid muscle.

d. With continuous negative suction on the syringe, insert the needle at about a 30-degree angle to the skin. Continue as with any peripheral venipuncture.

e. Apply a sterile dressing, and put pressure on the puncture site for 5 minutes.

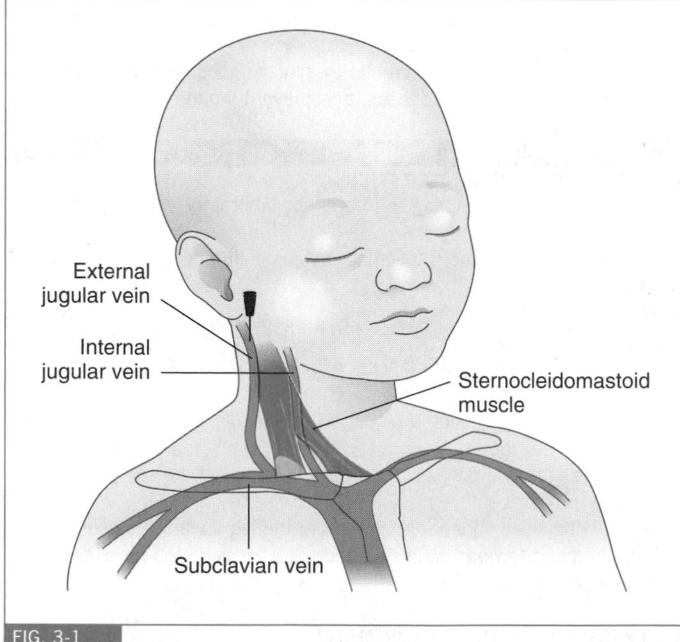


FIG. 3-1

External jugular cannulation. *(From Dieckmann R, Selbst S: Pediatric Emergency and Critical Care Procedures. St. Louis, Mosby, 1997, p 200.)*

## C. FEMORAL ARTERY AND FEMORAL VEIN PUNCTURE[1,2]

1. **Indications:** Venous or arterial blood sampling in patients with inadequate vascular access or during resuscitation.
2. **Contraindications:** Femoral puncture is particularly hazardous in neonates and is not recommended in this age group. There is also a risk in children for trauma to the femoral head and joint capsule. Avoid femoral punctures in children who have thrombocytopenia or coagulation disorders and in those who are scheduled for cardiac catheterization.
3. **Complications:** Infection, bleeding, hematoma of femoral triangle, thrombosis of vessel, osteomyelitis, and septic arthritis of hip.
4. **Procedure (Fig. 3-2):**

a. Hold child securely in frog-leg position with the hips flexed and abducted. It may help to place a roll under the hips.

b. Prepare area in sterile fashion.



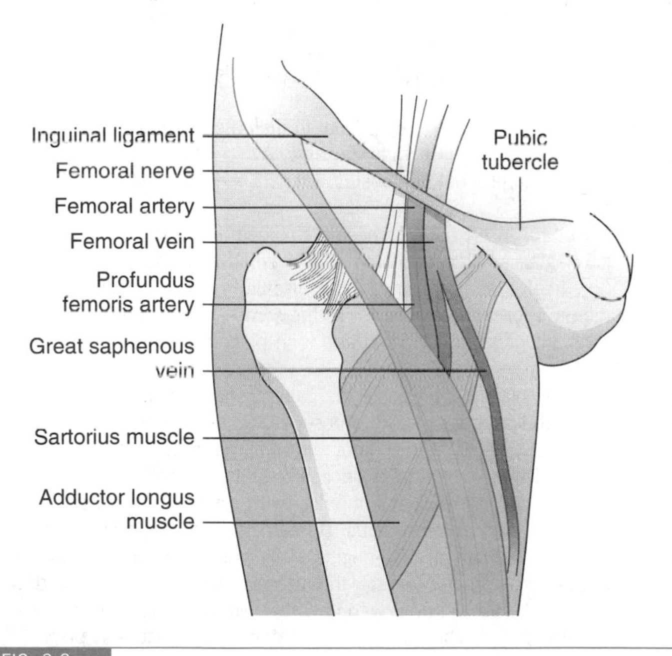


FIG. 3-2

Femoral artery and vein anatomy. *(From Dieckmann R, Selbst S: Pediatric Emergency and Critical Care Procedures. St. Louis, Mosby, 1997, p 199.)*

c. Locate femoral pulse just distal to the inguinal crease (**note that vein is medial to pulse**). Insert needle 2 cm distal to the inguinal ligament and 0.5 to 0.75 cm into the groin. Aspirate while maneuvering the needle until blood is obtained.

**Note** *Right femoral vein is easier to cannulate than the left, owing to a straighter path to the inferior vena cava.*

d. Apply direct pressure for minimum of 5 min.

## D. RADIAL ARTERY PUNCTURE AND CATHETERIZATION[1,2]

1. **Indications: Arterial blood sampling or frequent blood gases and continuous blood pressure monitoring in an intensive care setting.**
2. **Complications: Infection, bleeding, occlusion of artery by hematoma or thrombosis, ischemia if ulnar circulation is inadequate.**
3. **Procedure:**

a. Before procedure, test adequacy of ulnar blood flow with the Allen test. Clench the hand while simultaneously compressing ulnar and radial arteries. The hand will blanch. Release pressure from the ulnar artery, and observe the flushing response. Procedure is safe to perform if entire hand flushes.

b. Locate the radial pulse. It is optional to infiltrate the area over the point of maximal impulse with lidocaine. Avoid infusion into the vessel by aspirating before infusing. Prepare the site in sterile fashion.

   (1) Puncture: Insert butterfly needle attached to a syringe at a 30- to 60-degree angle over the point of maximal impulse; blood should flow freely into the syringe in a pulsatile fashion; suction may be required for plastic tubes. Once the sample is obtained, apply firm, constant pressure for 5 min and then place a pressure dressing on the puncture site.

   (2) Catheter placement: Secure the patient's hand to an arm board. Leave the fingers exposed to observe any color changes. Prepare the wrist with sterile technique and infiltrate over the point of maximal impulse with 1% lidocaine. Make a small skin puncture over the point of maximal impulse with a needle, then discard the needle. Insert an intravenous (IV) catheter with its needle through the puncture site at a 30-degree angle to the horizontal; pass the needle and catheter through the artery to transfix it, then withdraw the needle. Very slowly, withdraw the catheter until free flow of blood is noted. Then advance the catheter and secure in place using sutures or tape. Seldinger technique using a guidewire can also be used. Apply a sterile dressing. Infuse heparinized isotonic fluid (per protocol) at 1 mL/hr. A pressure transducer may be attached to monitor blood pressure.

**Note** *Do not infuse any medications, blood products, or hypotonic or hypertonic solutions through an arterial line.*

### E. POSTERIOR TIBIAL AND DORSALIS PEDIS ARTERY PUNCTURE[2]

1. **Indications:** Arterial blood sampling when radial artery puncture is unsuccessful or inaccessible.
2. **Complications:** Infection, bleeding, ischemia if inadequate circulation.
3. **Procedure (see section II.D for technique):**

a. Posterior tibial artery: Puncture the artery posterior to the medial malleolus while holding the foot in dorsiflexion.
b. Dorsalis pedis artery: Puncture the artery at the dorsal midfoot between the first and second toes while holding the foot in plantar flexion.



## III. VASCULAR ACCESS

### A. PERIPHERAL INTRAVENOUS PLACEMENT

1. **Indications:** To obtain access to peripheral venous circulation to deliver fluid, medications, or blood products.
2. **Complications:** Thrombosis, infection.
3. **Procedure:**

a. Choose IV placement site and prepare with alcohol.
b. Apply tourniquet and then insert IV catheter, bevel up, at angle almost parallel to the skin, advancing until "flash" of blood is seen in the catheter hub. Advance the plastic catheter only, remove the needle, and secure the catheter.
c. After removing tourniquet, attach T connector filled with saline to the catheter; flush with several milliliters of normal saline (NS) to ensure patency of the IV line.

### B. CENTRAL VENOUS CATHETER PLACEMENT[1,3]

1. **Indications:** To obtain emergency access to central venous circulation, to monitor central venous pressure, to deliver high-concentration parenteral nutrition or prolonged IV therapy, or to infuse blood products or large volumes of fluid.
2. **Complications:** Infection, bleeding, arterial or venous perforation, pneumothorax, hemothorax, thrombosis, catheter fragment in circulation, air embolism.
3. **Access sites:**

a. External jugular vein.
b. Subclavian vein: Least common site in children due to increased complications
c. Internal jugular vein: Contraindicated with elevated intracranial pressure (ICP)
d. Femoral vein: Contraindicated with severe abdominal trauma.

4. **Procedure: Seldinger technique**

a. Secure patient, prepare site, and drape in sterile fashion.
b. Insert needle, applying negative pressure to locate vessel.

c. When there is blood return, insert a guidewire through the needle into the vein. Watch cardiac monitor for ectopy.
d. Remove the needle, holding the guidewire firmly.
e. Slip a catheter that has been preflushed with sterile saline over the wire into the vein in a twisting motion. The entry site may be enlarged with a small skin incision or dilator. Pass the entire catheter over the wire until the hub is at the skin surface. Slowly remove the wire, secure the catheter by suture, and attach IV infusion.
f. Apply a sterile dressing over the site.
g. For neck vessels, obtain a chest radiograph to rule out pneumothorax.

5. **Approach:**

a. **External jugular (see Fig. 3-1):** Place patient in 15- to 20-degree Trendelenburg position. Turn the head 45 degrees to the contralateral side. Enter the vein at the point where it crosses the sternocleidomastoid muscle.
b. **Internal jugular:** Place patient in 15- to 20-degree Trendelenburg position. Hyperextend the neck to tense the sternocleidomastoid muscle, and turn head away from the site of line placement. Palpate the sternal and clavicular heads of the muscle and enter at the apex of the triangle formed. An alternative landmark for puncture is halfway between the sternal notch and tip of the mastoid process. Insert the needle at a 30-degree angle to the skin, and aim toward the ipsilateral nipple. When blood flow is obtained, continue with Seldinger technique. Right side is preferable because of straight course to right atrium, absence of thoracic duct, and lower pleural dome on right side.
c. **Subclavian vein (Fig. 3-3):** Position child in Trendelenburg position with a towel roll under the thoracic spine to hyperextend the back. Aim the needle under the distal third of the clavicle toward the sternal notch. When blood flow is obtained, continue with Seldinger technique.
d. **Femoral vein (Fig. 3-4):** Hold child securely with the hip flexed and abducted. Locate the femoral pulse just distal to the inguinal crease. In infants, vein is 5 to 6 mm *medial* to arterial pulse. In adolescents, vein is usually 10 to 15 mm *medial* to the pulse. Place the thumb of the nondominant hand on the femoral artery. Insert the needle medial to the thumb. The needle should enter the skin 2 to 3 cm distal to the inguinal ligament at a 30-degree angle to avoid entering the abdomen. When blood flow is obtained, continue with Seldinger technique.

## C. INTRAOSSEOUS (IO) INFUSION[1,2] (Fig. 3-5)

1. **Indications:** Obtain emergency access in children during life-threatening situations. This is very useful during cardiopulmonary arrest, shock, burns, and life-threatening status epilepticus. IO line can be used to infuse medications, blood products, or fluids. The IO needle should be removed once adequate vascular access has been established.

**2. Complications:**

a. Rare, particularly with correct technique. Frequency of complications increases with prolonged infusions.

b. Extravasation of fluid from incomplete cortex penetration, infection, bleeding, osteomyelitis, compartment syndrome, fat embolism, fracture, epiphyseal injury.

**3. Sites of entry (in order of preference):**

a. Anteromedial surface of the proximal tibia, 2 cm below and 1 to 2 cm medial to the tibial tuberosity on the flat part of the bone (see Fig. 3-5).

b. Distal femur 3 cm above the lateral condyle in the midline.

c. Medial surface of the distal tibia 1 to 2 cm above the medial malleolus (may be a more effective site in older children).

d. Anterosuperior iliac spine at an angle of 90 degrees to the long axis of the body.

**4. Procedure:**

a. Prepare the selected site in sterile fashion if situation allows.

b. If the child is conscious, anesthetize the puncture site down to the periosteum with 1% lidocaine (optional in emergency situations).



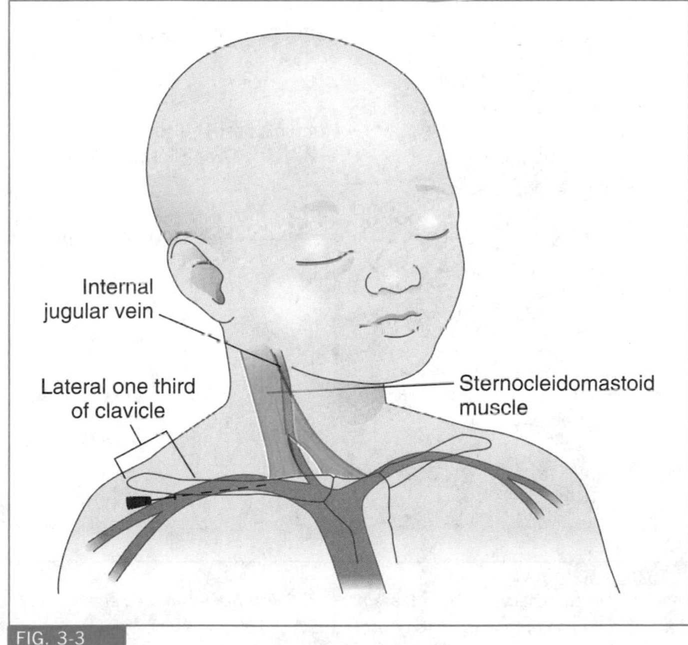


FIG. 3-3

Subclavian vein cannulation. *(From Dieckmann R, Selbst S: Pediatric Emergency and Critical Care Procedures. St. Louis, Mosby, 1997, p 200.)*

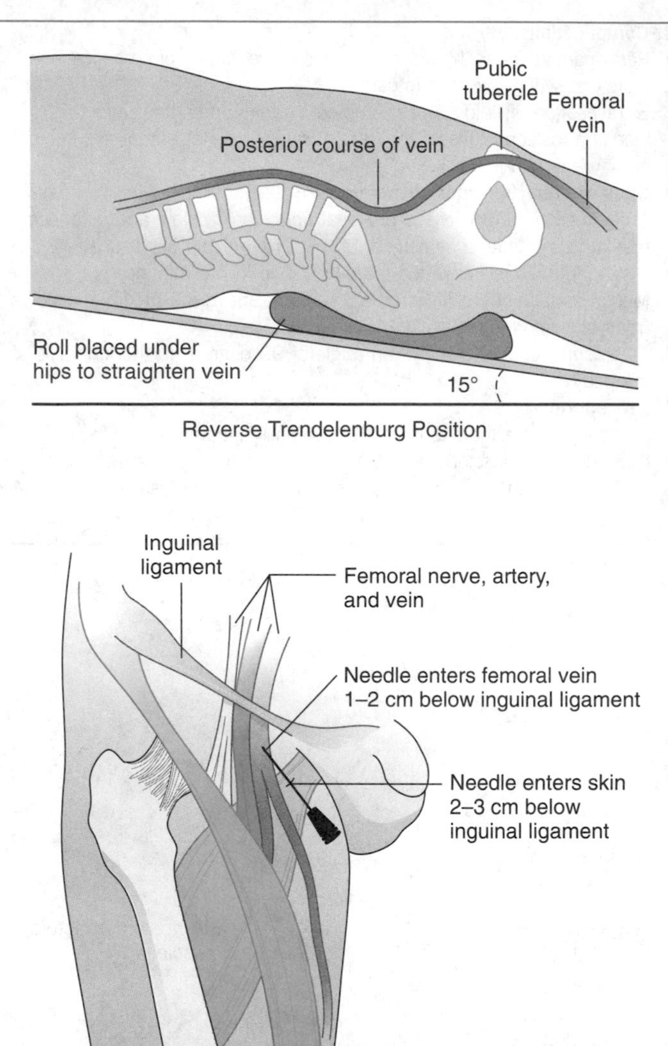


FIG. 3-4

Femoral vein cannulation. *(From Dieckmann R, Selbst S: Pediatric Emergency and Critical Care Procedures. St. Louis, Mosby, 1997, p 199.)*

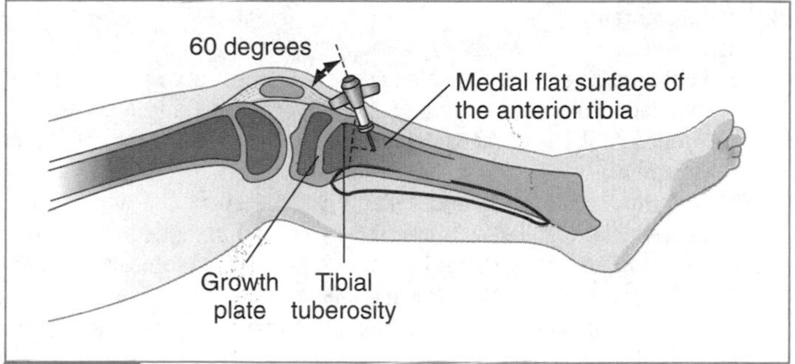


FIG. 3-5

Intraosseous needle placement using standard anterior tibial approach. The insertion point is in the midline on the medial flat surface of the anterior tibia, 1 to 3 cm (2 fingerbreadths) below the tibial tuberosity. *(From Dieckmann R, Selbst S: Pediatric Emergency and Critical Care Procedures. St. Louis, Mosby, 1997, p 222.)*



c. Insert a 15- to 18-gauge IO needle perpendicular to the skin at an angle away from the epiphyseal plate and advance to the periosteum. With a boring rotary motion, penetrate through the cortex until there is a decrease in resistance, indicating that you have reached the marrow. The needle should stand firmly without support. Secure the needle carefully.
d. Remove the stylet, and attempt to aspirate marrow. (Note that it is not necessary to aspirate marrow.) Flush with 10 to 20 mL heparinized NS. Observe for fluid extravasation. Marrow can be sent for determination of glucose levels, chemistries, blood type and cross-match, hemoglobin, blood gas analysis, and cultures.
e. Attach standard IV tubing. Any crystalloid, blood product, or drug that can be infused into a peripheral vein can also be infused into the IO space, but an increased pressure (through pressure bag or push) is needed for infusion. There is a high risk for obstruction if continuous high-pressure fluids are not flushed through the IO needle.

## D. UMBILICAL ARTERY (UA) AND VEIN (UV) CATHETERIZATION[1]

1. **Indications:** Vascular access (via UV), blood pressure (via UA), and blood gas (via UA) monitoring in critically ill neonates.
2. **Complications:** Infection, bleeding, hemorrhage, perforation of vessel; thrombosis with distal embolization; ischemia or infarction of lower extremities, bowel, or kidney; arrhythmia if the catheter is in the heart; air embolus.
3. **Caution:** UA catheterization should never be performed if omphalitis or peritonitis is present. Contraindicated in the presence of possible necrotizing enterocolitis or intestinal hypoperfusion.

**4. Line placement:**

a. Arterial line: Low line versus high line.

(1) **Low line:** The tip of the catheter should lie just above the aortic bifurcation between L3 and L5. This avoids renal and mesenteric arteries near L1, perhaps decreasing the incidence of thrombosis or ischemia.

(2) **High line:** The tip of the catheter should be above the diaphragm between T6 and T9. A high line may be recommended in infants weighing less than 750g, in whom a low line could easily slip out.

b. UV catheters should be placed in the inferior vena cava above the level of the ductus venosus and the hepatic veins and below the level of the right atrium.

c. Catheter length: Determine the length of catheter required using either a standardized graph or the regression formula. Add length for the height of the umbilical stump.

(1) **Standardized graph:** Determine the shoulder-umbilical length by measuring the perpendicular line dropped from the tip of the shoulder to the level of the umbilicus. Use the graph in Figure 3-6 to determine the arterial catheter length, and the graph in Figure 3-7 to determine venous catheter length.

(2) **Birth weight (BW) regression formula:**

$$\text{Low line: UA catheter length (cm)} = \text{BW (kg)} + 7$$

$$\text{High line: UA catheter length (cm)} = [3 \times \text{BW (kg)}] + 9$$

$$\text{UV catheter length (cm)} = [0.5 \times \text{high line UA (cm)}] + 1$$

**Note** *Formula may not be appropriate for small-for-gestational-age or large-for-gestational-age infants.*

5. **Procedure for UA line (Fig. 3-8):**

a. Determine the length of the catheter to be inserted for either high (T6 to T9) or low (L3 to L5) position.

b. Restrain the infant. Prepare and drape the umbilical cord and adjacent skin using sterile technique. Maintaining the infant's temperature is critical.

c. Flush the catheter with a sterile saline solution before insertion.

d. Place sterile umbilical tape around the base of the cord. Cut through the cord horizontally about 1.5 to 2cm from the skin; tighten the umbilical tape to prevent bleeding.

e. Identify the one large, thin-walled umbilical vein and two smaller, thick-walled arteries. Use one tip of open, curved forceps to probe and dilate one artery gently; use both points of closed forceps, and dilate artery by allowing forceps to open gently.

f. Grasp the catheter 1cm from its tip with toothless forceps, and insert the catheter into the lumen of the artery. Aim the tip toward the feet, and gently advance the catheter to the desired distance. Do not force. If resistance is encountered, try loosening umbilical tape; applying steady, gentle pressure; or manipulating the angle of the umbilical cord to skin. Often the catheter cannot be advanced because of creation of a "false luminal tract." There should be good blood return when the catheter enters the iliac artery.

g. Confirm the position of the catheter tip radiographically. Secure the catheter with a suture through the cord, a marker tape, and a tape bridge. The catheter may be pulled back but not advanced once the sterile field is broken.
h. Observe for complications: Blanching or cyanosis of lower extremities, perforation, thrombosis, embolism, or infection. If any complications occur, the catheter should be removed.



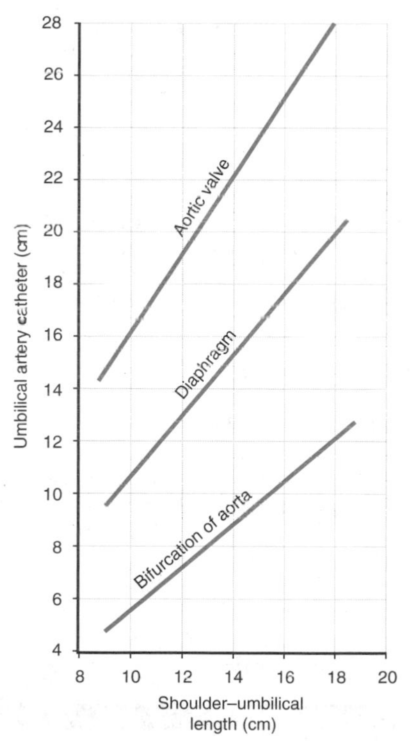


FIG. 3-6
Umbilical artery catheter length.

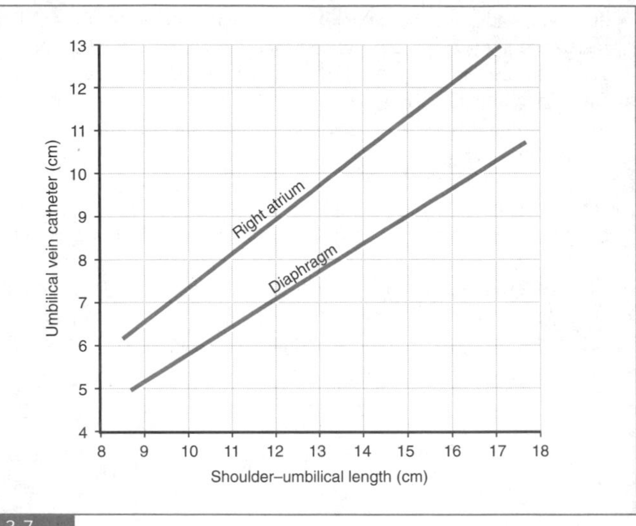


FIG. 3-7

Umbilical vein catheter length.

**Note** *There are no definitive guidelines on feeding with a UA catheter in place. There is concern (up to 24 hours after removal) that the UA catheter or thrombus may interfere with intestinal perfusion. A risk-to-benefit assessment should be individualized. Use isotonic fluids, which contain 0.5 U/mL of heparin. Never use hypo-osmolar fluids in the UA.*

6. **Procedure for UV line (see Fig. 3-8):**

a. Follow steps a–d for UA catheter placement. However, determine catheter length using Figure 3-7.
b. Isolate the thin-walled umbilical vein, clear thrombi with forceps, and insert catheter, aiming the tip toward the right shoulder. Gently advance the catheter to the desired distance. Do not force. If resistance is encountered, try loosening the umbilical tape; applying steady, gentle pressure; or manipulating the angle of the umbilical cord to skin. Resistance is commonly met at the abdominal wall and again at the portal system. Do not infuse anything into the liver.
c. Confirm position of the catheter tip radiographically. Secure catheter as described in step g for UA placement.

## IV. BODY FLUID SAMPLING

### A. LUMBAR PUNCTURE[1,2]

1. **Indications:** **Examination of spinal fluid for suspected infection or malignancy, instillation of intrathecal chemotherapy, or measurement of opening pressure.**

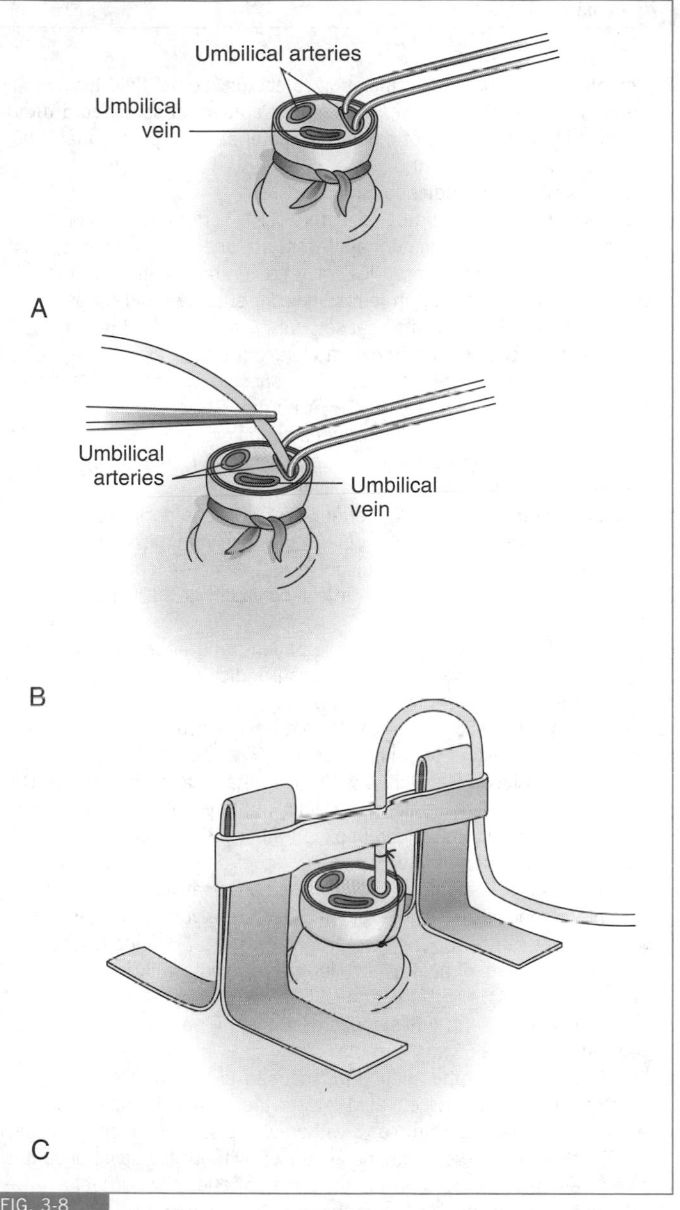


FIG. 3-8

Placement of umbilical arterial catheter. **A,** Dilating the lumen of the umbilical artery. **B,** Inserting the umbilical artery catheter. **C,** Securing the catheter to the abdominal wall using a "bridge" method of taping. *(From Dieckmann R, Selbst S: Pediatric Emergency and Critical Care Procedures. St. Louis, Mosby, 1997, p 504.)*

2. **Complications: Local pain, infection, bleeding, spinal fluid leak, hematoma, spinal headache, or acquired epidermal spinal cord tumor (caused by implantation of epidermal material into spinal canal if no stylet is used on skin entry).**
3. **Cautions and contraindications:**
a. **Increased ICP:** Before lumbar puncture (LP), perform funduscopic examination. The presence of papilledema, retinal hemorrhage, or clinical suspicion of increased ICP may be contraindications to the procedure. A sudden drop in intraspinal pressure by rapid release of cerebrospinal fluid (CSF) may cause fatal herniation. If LP is to be performed, proceed with extreme caution. Computed tomography (CT) may be indicated before LP if there is suspected intracranial bleeding, focal mass lesion, or increased ICP. A normal CT scan does not rule out increased ICP but usually excludes conditions that may put the patient at risk for herniation. Decision to obtain CT should not delay appropriate antibiotic therapy if indicated.
b. **Bleeding diathesis:** A platelet count >50,000/μL is desirable before LP; correction of any clotting factor deficiencies can minimize the risk for bleeding and subsequent cord or nerve root compression.
c. Overlying skin infection may result in inoculation of CSF with organisms.
d. LP should be deferred in an unstable patient, and appropriate therapy should be initiated, including antibiotics if indicated.
4. **Procedure:**
a. Apply local anesthetic cream if sufficient time is available.
b. Position child in either the sitting position (Fig. 3-9) or lateral recumbent position (Fig. 3-10), with hips, knees, and neck flexed. Do not compromise a small infant's cardiorespiratory status by positioning.
c. Locate the desired intervertebral space (either L3–4 or L4–5) by drawing an imaginary line between the top of the iliac crests.
d. Prepare the skin in sterile fashion. Drape conservatively so that it is possible to monitor the infant. Use a 20- to 22-gauge spinal needle with stylet (1.5-inch for children <12 years of age, 3.5 inches for children ≥12 years of age). A smaller-gauge needle will decrease the incidence of spinal headache and CSF leak.
e. The overlying skin and interspinous tissue can be anesthetized with 1% lidocaine using a 25-gauge needle.
f. Puncture the skin in the midline just caudad to the palpated spinous process, angling slightly cephalad toward the umbilicus. Advance several millimeters at a time and withdraw the stylet frequently to check for CSF flow. The needle may be advanced without the stylet once it is completely through the skin. In small infants, one may *not* feel a change in resistance or "pop" as the dura is penetrated.
g. If resistance is met initially (you hit bone), withdraw needle to the skin surface and redirect angle slightly.

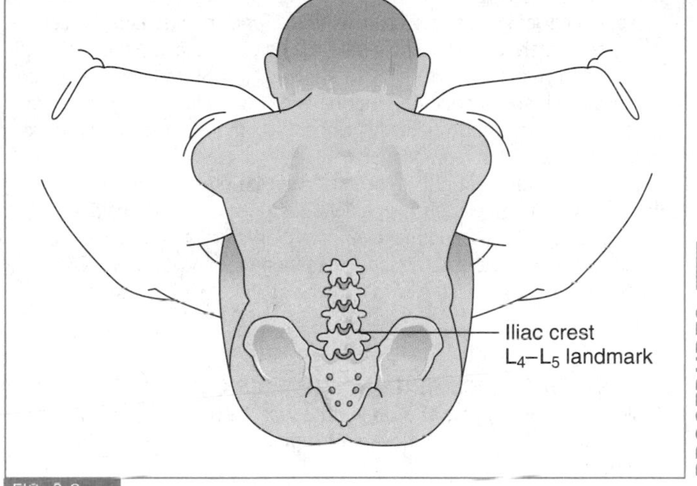


FIG. 3-9
Lumbar puncture site in the sitting position. *(From Dieckmann R, Selbst S: Pediatric Emergency and Critical Care Procedures. St. Louis, Mosby, 1997, p 534.)*

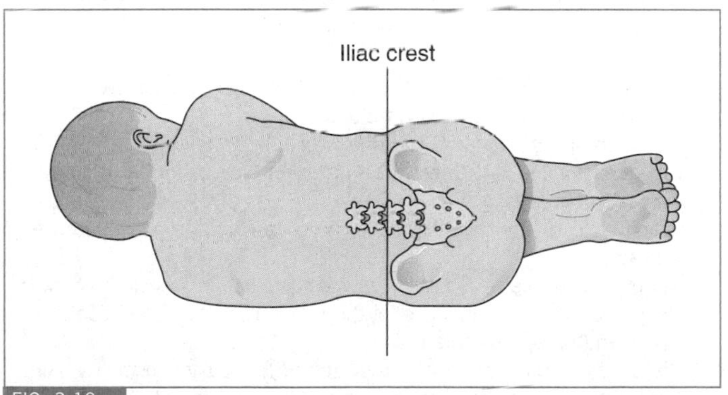


FIG. 3-10
Lumbar puncture site in the lateral (recumbent) position. *(From Dieckmann R, Selbst S: Pediatric Emergency and Critical Care Procedures. St. Louis, Mosby, 1997, p 534.)*

h. Send CSF for appropriate studies (see Chapter 27 for normal values). Send the first tube for culture and Gram stain, the second tube for measurement of glucose and protein levels, and the last tube for cell count and differential. An additional tube can be collected for viral cultures, polymerase chain reaction analysis, or CSF metabolic studies if indicated. If subarachnoid hemorrhage or traumatic tap is suspected, send the first and fourth tubes for cell count, and ask the laboratory to examine the CSF for xanthochromia.
i. Accurate measurement of CSF pressure can be made only with the patient lying quietly on his or her side in an unflexed position. It is not a reliable measurement in the sitting position. Once free flow of spinal fluid is obtained, attach the manometer and measure CSF pressure. Opening pressure is recorded as level at which CSF is steady.

## B. CHEST TUBE PLACEMENT AND THORACENTESIS[1,3]

1. **Indications:** **Evacuation of a pneumothorax, hemothorax, chylothorax, large pleural effusion, or empyema for diagnostic or therapeutic purposes.**
2. **Complications:** **Infection; bleeding; pneumothorax; hemothorax; pulmonary contusion or laceration; puncture of diaphragm, spleen, or liver; bronchopleural fistula.**
3. **Procedure: Needle decompression**

**Note** *For tension pneumothoraces, it is imperative to attempt decompression quickly by inserting a large-bore needle (14- to 22-gauge, based on size) in the anterior second intercostal space in the midclavicular line. Insert needle over superior aspect of rib margin to avoid vascular structures.*

a. When the pleural space is entered, attach catheter to a three-way stopcock and syringe, and aspirate air.
b. Subsequent insertion of a chest tube is still necessary.

4. **Procedure (Fig. 3-11): Chest tube insertion (see inside front cover for chest tube sizes)**

a. Position child supine or with affected side up with arm restrained over the head.
b. Point of entry is the third to fifth intercostal space in the mid to anterior axillary line, usually at the level of the nipple (avoid breast tissue).
c. Prepare and drape in sterile fashion.
d. Patient may require sedation (see Chapter 6). Locally anesthetize skin, subcutaneous tissue, periosteum of rib, chest wall muscles, and pleura with 1% lidocaine.
e. Make a sterile 1- to 3-cm incision one intercostal space below desired insertion point, and bluntly dissect with a hemostat through tissue

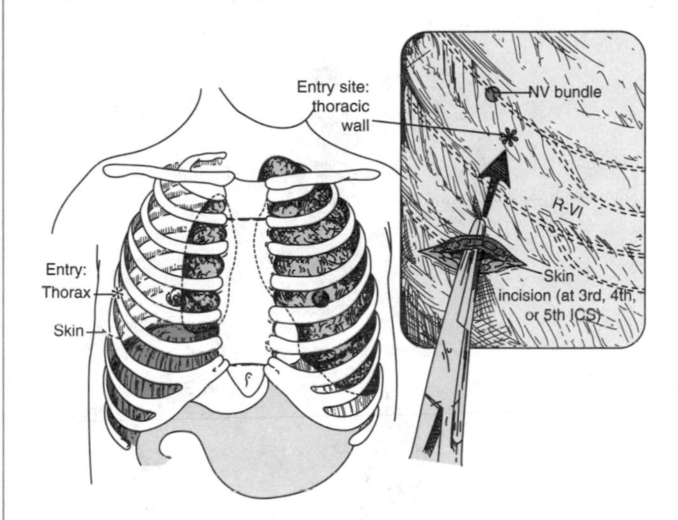


FIG. 3-11

Technique for insertion of chest tube. ICS, intercostal space; NV, neurovascular; R-VI, sixth rib. *(Modified from Fleisher G, Ludwig S: Pediatric Emergency Medicine, 3rd ed. Baltimore, Williams & Wilkins, 2000, p 1905.)*

layers until the superior portion of the rib is reached, avoiding the neurovascular bundle on the inferior portion of the rib.

f. Push the hemostat over the top of the rib, through the pleura, and into the pleural space. Enter the pleural space cautiously and not deeper than 1 cm. Spread hemostat to open, place chest tube in clamp, and guide through entry site to desired distance.
g. For a pneumothorax, insert the tube anteriorly toward the apex. For a pleural effusion, direct the tube inferiorly and posteriorly.
h. Secure the tube with purse-string sutures in which the suture is first tied at the skin, then wrapped around the tube once and tied at the tube.
i. Attach to a drainage system with –20 to –30 cm $H_2O$ pressure.
j. Apply a sterile occlusive dressing.
k. Confirm position and function with chest radiograph.

5. **Procedure: Thoracentesis (Fig. 3-12)**

a. Confirm fluid in pleural space by clinical examination and radiographs or ultrasonography.
b. If possible, place child in sitting position leaning over table; otherwise place supine.

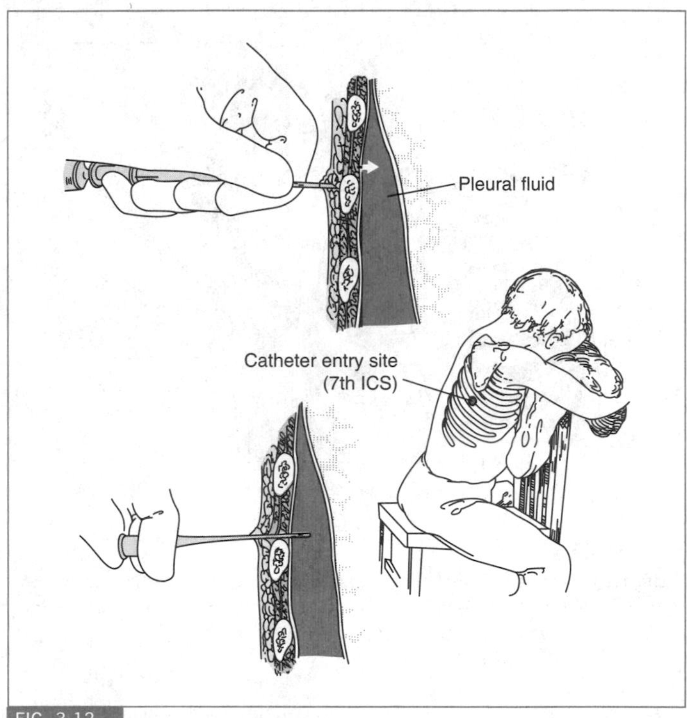


FIG. 3-12

Thoracentesis. ICS, intercostal space. *(Modified from Fleisher G, Ludwig S: Pediatric Emergency Medicine, 3rd ed. Baltimore, Williams & Wilkins, 2000, p 1906.)*

c. Point of entry is usually in the seventh intercostal space and posterior axillary line.
d. Prepare and drape area in sterile fashion.
e. Anesthetize skin, subcutaneous tissue, rib periosteum, chest wall, and pleura with 1% lidocaine.
f. Advance an 18- to 22-gauge IV catheter or large-bore needle attached to a syringe onto the rib, and then "walk" over the superior aspect into the pleural space, while providing steady negative pressure; often a popping sensation is generated. Be careful not to advance too far into the pleural cavity. If an IV or pigtail catheter (with guidewire) is used, the soft catheter may be advanced into the pleural space aiming downward.
g. Attach syringe and stopcock device to remove fluid for diagnostic studies and symptomatic relief (see Chapter 27 for evaluation of pleural fluid.)

h. After removing needle or catheter, place an occlusive dressing over the site and obtain a chest radiograph to rule out pneumothorax.

## C. PERICARDIOCENTESIS[1,3]

1. **Indications: To obtain pericardial fluid in cardiac tamponade emergently or nonemergently for diagnostic or therapeutic purposes.**
2. **Complications: Bleeding, infection, puncture of cardiac chamber, cardiac arrhythmia, hemopericardium or pneumopericardium, pneumothorax, hemothorax, cardiac arrest, death.**
3. **Procedure (Fig. 3-13):**

a. Unless contraindicated, provide sedation and/or analgesia for the patient. Monitor electrocardiogram.
b. Place patient at a 30-degree angle (reverse Trendelenburg). Have patient secured.
c. Prepare and drape puncture site in a sterile fashion. A drape across the upper chest is unnecessary and may obscure important landmarks.
d. Anesthetize the puncture site with 1% lidocaine.
e. Insert an 18- or 20-gauge needle just to the left of the xiphoid process, 1 cm inferior to the bottom rib at about a 45-degree angle to the skin.
f. While gently aspirating, advance needle toward the patient's left shoulder until pericardial fluid is obtained.
g. Upon entering the pericardial space, clamp the needle at the skin edge with hemostat to prevent further penetration. Attach a 30-mL syringe with a stopcock.
h. Gently and slowly remove the fluid. Rapid withdrawal of the pericardial fluid can result in shock or myocardial insufficiency.
i. Send fluid for appropriate laboratory studies (see Chapter 27).
j. In nonemergent conditions, this is best performed under two-dimensional echocardiographic guidance.

## D. PARACENTESIS[2]

1. **Indications: Percutaneous removal of intraperitoneal fluid for diagnostic or therapeutic purposes.**
2. **Complications: Bleeding, infection, puncture of viscera.**
3. **Cautions:**

a. Do not remove a large amount of fluid too rapidly, because hypovolemia and hypotension may result from rapid fluid shifts.
b. Avoid scars from previous surgery; localized bowel adhesions increase the chances of entering a viscus in these areas.
c. The bladder should be empty to avoid perforation.
d. Never perform paracentesis through an area of cellulitis.

4. **Procedure:**

a. Prepare and drape the abdomen as for a surgical procedure. Anesthetize the puncture site.
b. With the patient in semisupine, sitting, or lateral decubitus position, insert a 16- to 22-gauge IV catheter attached to a syringe in midline

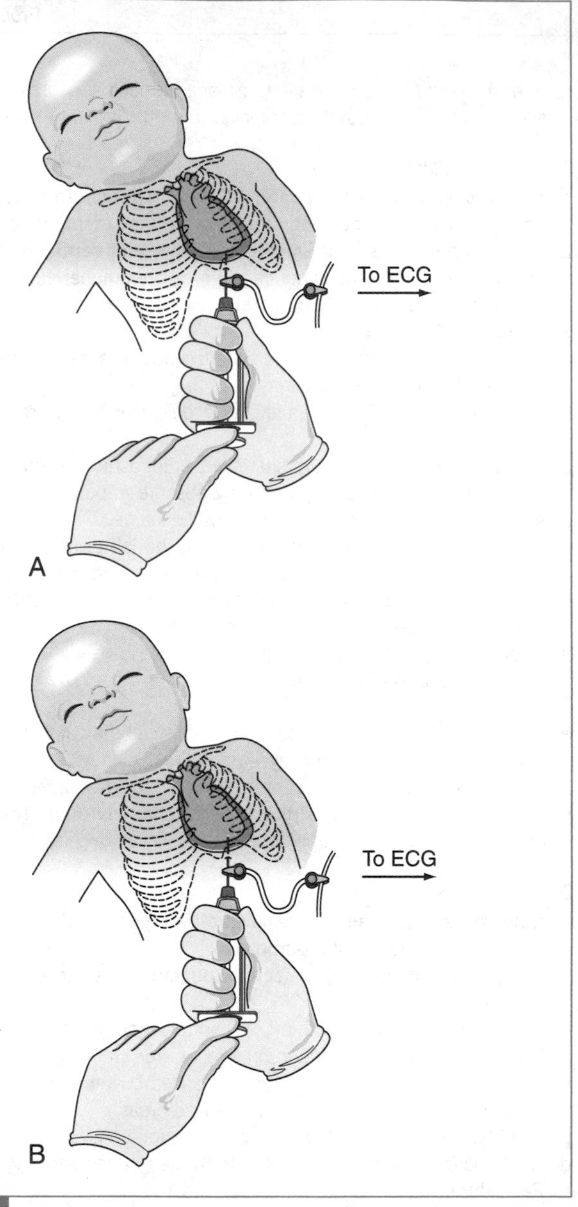


FIG. 3-13

Subxiphoid approach for pericardiocentesis. **A,** Needle in pericardial sac with normal electrocardiogram (ECG). **B,** Needle in heart with current of injury pattern on ECG. *(From Dieckmann R, Selbst S: Pediatric Emergency and Critical Care Procedures. St. Louis, Mosby, 1997, p 594.)*

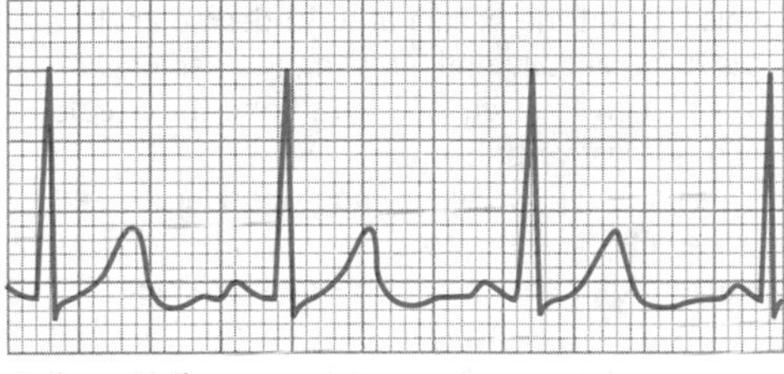
A (cont'd)

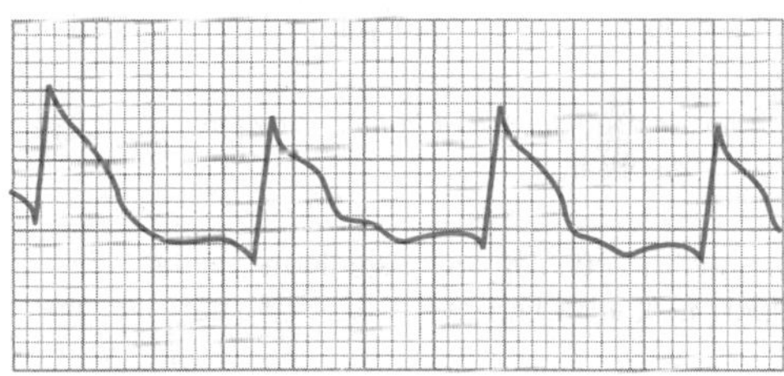
B (cont'd)

FIG. 3-13—cont'd

2 cm below the umbilicus; in neonates, insert just lateral to the rectus muscle in the right or left lower quadrants, a few centimeters above the inguinal ligament.

c. Aiming cephalad, insert the needle at a 45-degree angle while one hand pulls the skin caudally until entering the peritoneal cavity. This creates a Z tract when the skin is released and the needle removed. Apply continuous negative pressure.

d. Once fluid appears in the syringe, remove introducer needle and leave catheter in place. Attach a stopcock and aspirate slowly until an adequate amount of fluid has been obtained for studies or symptomatic relief.

e. If, on entering the peritoneal cavity, air is aspirated, withdraw the needle immediately. Aspirated air indicates entrance into a hollow viscus. (In general, penetration of a hollow viscus during paracentesis does not lead to complications.) Repeat paracentesis with sterile equipment.

f. Send fluid for appropriate laboratory studies (see Chapter 27).

## E. URINARY BLADDER CATHETERIZATION[2]

**1. Indications: To obtain urine for urinalysis and culture sterilely and to accurately monitor hydration status.**

**2. Complications: Hematuria, infection, trauma to urethra or bladder, intravesical knot of catheter (rarely occurs).**

**3. Procedure:**

a. Infant/child should not have voided within 1 hr of procedure.

**Note** *Catheterization is contraindicated in pelvic fractures, known trauma to the urethra, or blood at the meatus.*

b. Prepare the urethral opening using sterile technique.

c. In boys, apply gentle traction to the penis to straighten the urethra.

d. Gently insert a lubricated catheter into the urethra. Slowly advance the catheter until resistance is met at the external sphincter. Continued pressure will overcome this resistance, and the catheter will enter the bladder. In girls, the urethral orifice may be difficult to visualize, but it is usually immediately anterior to the vaginal orifice. Only a few centimeters of advancement is required to reach the bladder in girls. In boys, insert a few centimeters longer than the shaft of the penis.

e. Carefully remove the catheter once the specimen is obtained, and clean iodine from skin.

f. If indwelling Foley catheter is inserted, inflate balloon with sterile water as indicated on bulb, then connect catheter to drainage tubing attached to urine drainage bag. Secure catheter tubing to inner thigh.

## F. SUPRAPUBIC BLADDER ASPIRATION[1]

1. **Indications:** To obtain urine for urinalysis and culture sterilely in children <2 years of age (avoid in children with genitourinary tract anomalies, coagulopathy, or intestinal obstruction). Bypasses distal urethra, thereby minimizing risk for contamination.
2. **Complications:** Infection (cellulitis), hematuria (usually microscopic), intestinal perforation.
3. **Procedure (Fig. 3-14):**

a. Anterior rectal pressure in girls or gentle penile pressure in boys may be used to prevent urination during the procedure. Child should not have voided within 1 hr of procedure.
b. Restrain the infant in the supine, frog-leg position. Prepare suprapubic area in sterile fashion.
c. The site for puncture is 1 to 2 cm above the symphysis pubis in the midline. Use a syringe with a 22-gauge, 1-inch needle, and puncture at a 10- to 20-degree angle to the perpendicular, aiming slightly caudad.
d. Exert suction gently as the needle is advanced until urine enters syringe. The needle should not be advanced more than 1 inch. Aspirate the urine with gentle suction.
e. Clean iodine from skin.

## G. SOFT TISSUE ASPIRATION[4]

1. **Indications:** Cellulitis that is unresponsive to initial standard therapy, recurrent cellulitis or abscesses, immunocompromised patients in whom organism recovery is necessary and may affect antimicrobial therapy.
2. **Complications:** Pain, infection, bleeding.
3. **Procedure:**

a. Select site to aspirate at *point of maximal inflammation* (more likely to increase recovery of causative agent than leading edge of erythema or center).[4]
b. Clean area in sterile fashion.
c. Local anesthesia with 1% lidocaine is optional.
d. Fill tuberculin syringe with 0.1 to 0.2 mL of *nonbacteriostatic* sterile saline and attach to needle.
e. Using 18- or 20-gauge needle (22-gauge for facial cellulitis), advance to appropriate depth and apply negative pressure while withdrawing needle.
f. Send fluid from aspiration for Gram stain and cultures. If no fluid is obtained, you can streak needle on agar plate. Consider acid-fast bacilli and fungal stains in immunocompromised patients.

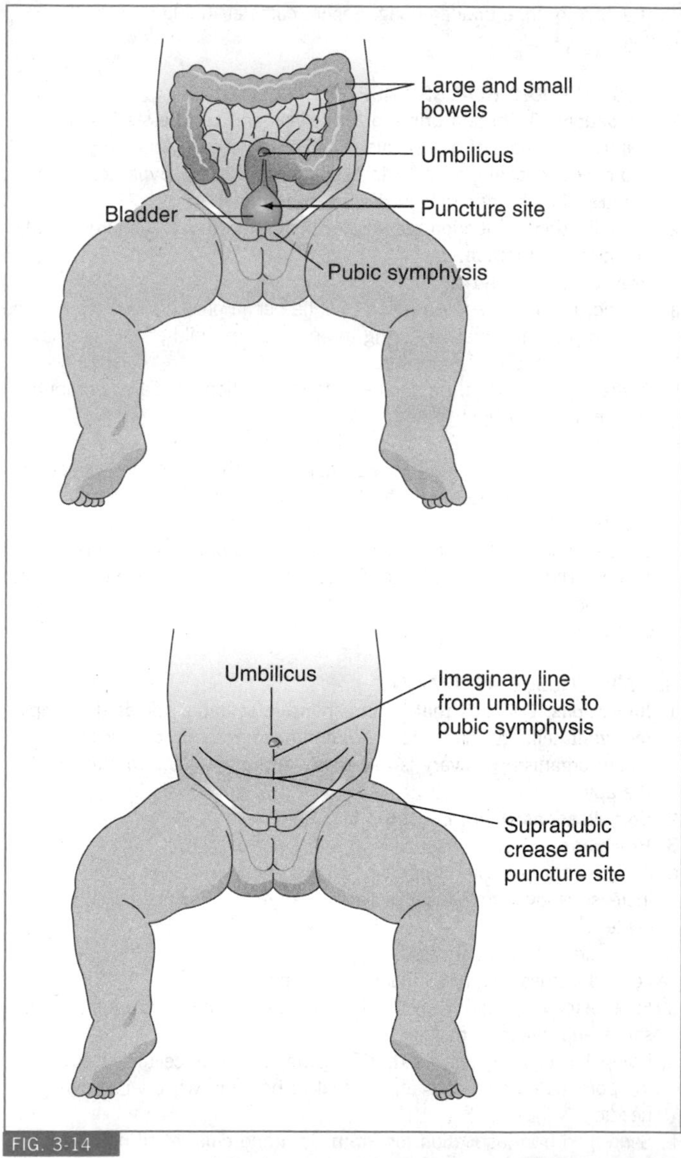


FIG. 3-14

Landmarks for suprapubic bladder aspiration. *(From Dieckmann R, Selbst S: Pediatric Emergency and Critical Care Procedures. St. Louis, Mosby, 1997, p 418.)*

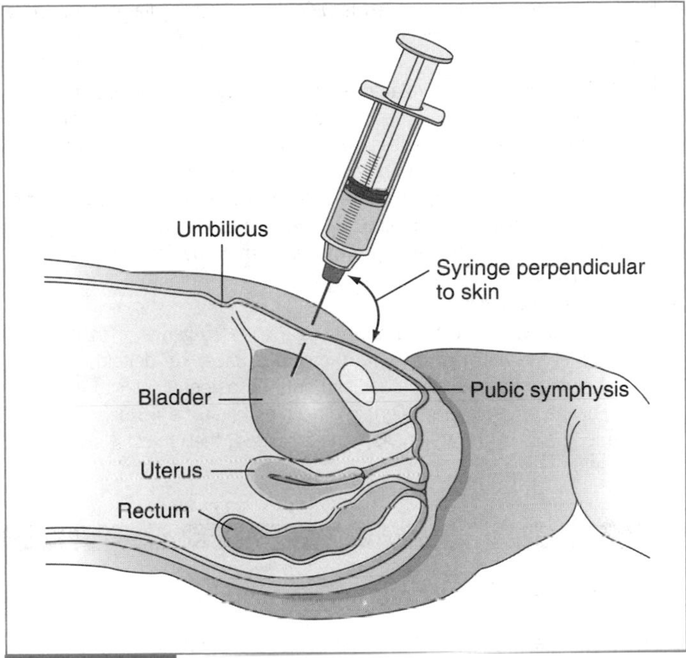


FIG. 3-14—cont'd



## V. IMMUNIZATION AND MEDICATION ADMINISTRATION[2]

### A. SUBCUTANEOUS INJECTIONS

1. **Indications:** Immunizations and other medications.
2. **Complications:** Bleeding, infection, allergic reaction, lipohypertrophy or lipoatrophy after repeated injections.
3. **Procedure:**

a. Locate injection site: Upper outer arm or outer aspect of upper thigh.
b. Clean skin with alcohol.
c. Insert 25- or 27-gauge, 0.5-inch needle into the subcutaneous layer at a 45-degree angle to the skin. Aspirate for blood, then inject medication.

### B. INTRAMUSCULAR INJECTIONS

1. **Indications:** Immunizations and other medications.
2. **Complications:** Bleeding, infection, allergic reaction, nerve injury.
3. **Cautions:**

a. Avoid intramuscular injections in a child with a bleeding disorder or thrombocytopenia.

b. Maximum volume to be injected is 0.5 mL in a small infant, 1 mL in an older infant, 2 mL in a school-aged child, and 3 mL in an adolescent.

4. **Procedure:**

a. Locate injection site: Anterolateral upper thigh (vastus lateralis muscle) in smaller child, or outer aspect of upper arm (deltoid) in older one. The dorsal gluteal region is less commonly used because of risk for nerve or vascular injury. To find the ventral gluteal site, form a triangle by placing your index finger on the anterior iliac spine and your middle finger on the most superior aspect of the iliac crest. The injection should occur in the middle of the triangle formed by the two fingers and the iliac crest.

b. Clean skin with alcohol.

c. Pinch muscle with free hand and insert 23- or 25-gauge, 1-inch needle until the hub is flush with the skin surface. For deltoid and ventral gluteal muscles, the needle should be perpendicular to the skin. For the anterolateral thigh, the needle should be 45 degrees to the long axis of the thigh. Aspirate for blood, then inject medication.

## VI. BASIC LACERATION REPAIR[1]

### A. SUTURING

1. **Techniques (Fig. 3-15):**

a. Simple interrupted.

b. Horizontal mattress: Provides eversion of wound edges.

c. Vertical mattress: For added strength in areas of thick skin or areas of skin movement; provides eversion of wound edges.

d. Running intradermal: For cosmetic closures.

**Note** *Lacerations of the face, lips, hands, genitalia, mouth, or periorbital area may require consultation with a specialist. Ideally, lacerations at increased risk for infection (areas with poor blood supply, contaminated/crush injury) should be sutured within 6 hr of injury. Clean wounds in cosmetically important areas may be closed up to 24 hr after injury in the absence of significant contamination or devitalization. In general, bite wounds should not be sutured except in areas of high cosmetic importance (face). The longer sutures are left in place, the greater the scarring and potential for infection. Sutures in cosmetically sensitive areas should be removed as soon as possible. Sutures in high-tension areas, such as extensor surfaces, should stay in longer (***Table 3-1***).*

2. **Procedure:**

a. Prepare child for procedure with appropriate sedation, analgesia, and restraint.

b. Anesthetize the wound with topical anesthetic or with lidocaine-bicarbonate by injecting the anesthetic into the subcutaneous tissues (see Chapter 6).

c. Forcefully irrigate the wound with copious amounts of sterile NS. Use at least 250 mL for smaller, superficial wounds and more for larger wounds. This is the most important step in preventing infection. Avoid high-pressure irrigation of deep puncture wounds.
d. Prepare and drape the patient for a sterile procedure.

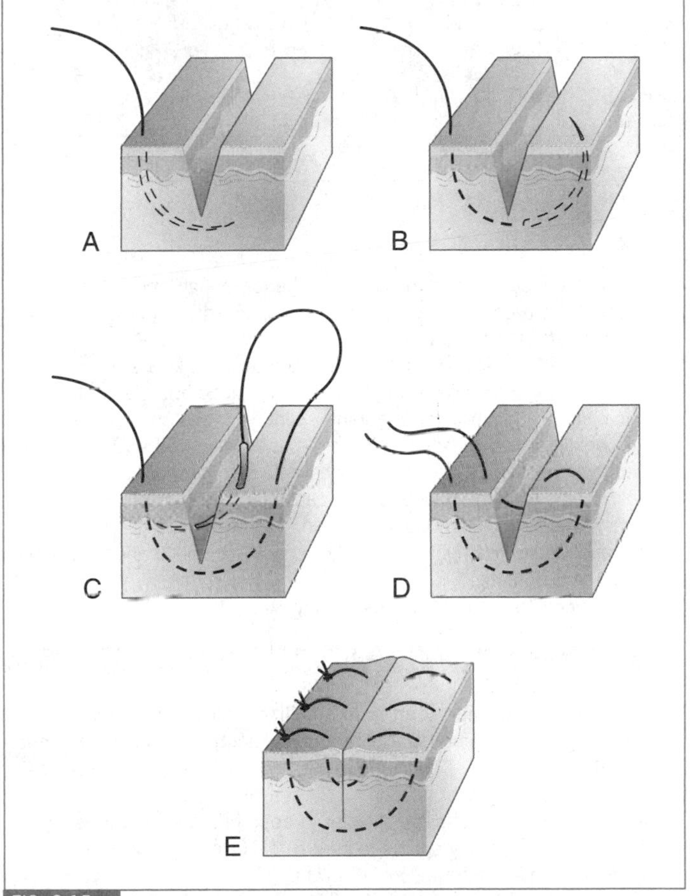


FIG. 3-15

**A-E,** The vertical mattress suture. After initial placement of a simple interrupted stitch with a larger bite, make a backhand pass across the wound, taking small, superficial bites. When the knot is tied, the edges of the laceration should evert slightly. *(From Dieckmann R, Selbst S: Pediatric Emergency and Critical Care Procedures. St. Louis, Mosby, 1997, p 676.)*

TABLE 3-1

**GUIDELINES FOR SUTURE MATERIAL, SIZE, AND REMOVAL**

| Body Region | Monofilament* (for Superficial Lacerations) | Absorbable† (for Deep Lacerations) | Duration (days) |
|---|---|---|---|
| Scalp | 5–0 or 4–0 | 4–0 | 5–7 |
| Face | 6–0 | 5–0 | 3–5 |
| Eyelid | 7–0 or 6–0 | — | 3–5 |
| Eyebrow | 6–0 or 5–0 | 5–0 | 3–5 |
| Trunk | 5–0 or 4–0 | 3–0 | 5–7 |
| Extremities | 5–0 or 4–0 | 4–0 | 7 |
| Joint surface | 4–0 | — | 10–14 |
| Hand | 5–0 | 5–0 | 7 |
| Foot sole | 4–0 or 3–0 | 4–0 | 7–10 |

*Examples of monofilament nonabsorbable sutures: nylon, polypropylene.

†Examples of absorbable sutures: polyglycolic acid and polyglactin 910 (Vicryl).

e. Débride the wound when indicated. Probe for foreign bodies as indicated. Consider obtaining a radiograph if a radiopaque foreign body was involved in the injury.
f. Select suture type for percutaneous closure (see Table 3-1).
g. When suturing is complete, apply topical antibiotic and sterile dressing. If laceration is in proximity of a joint, splinting of the affected area to limit mobility often speeds healing and prevents wound separation.
h. Check wounds at 48 to 72 hr in cases in which wounds are of questionable viability, if wound was packed, or for patients prescribed prophylactic antibiotics. Change dressing at check.
i. For hand lacerations, close skin only; do not use subcutaneous stitches. Elevate and immobilize the hand.
j. Consider child's need for tetanus prophylaxis.

## VII. MUSCULOSKELETAL PROCEDURES

### A. BASIC SPLINTING[1]

1. **Indications: To provide short-term stabilization of limb injuries.**
2. **Complications: Pressure sores, dermatitis, neurovascular impairment.**
3. **Procedure:**

a. Determine style of splint needed.
b. Measure and cut fiberglass or plaster to appropriate length. If using plaster, upper-extremity splints require 8 to 10 layers, and lower-extremity splints require 12 to 14 layers.
c. Pad extremity with cotton Webril, taking care to overlap each turn by 50%. In prepackaged fiberglass splints, additional padding is not generally required. Bony prominences may require additional padding. Place cotton between digits if they are in a splint.
d. Immerse plaster slabs into room-temperature water until bubbling stops. Smooth out wet plaster slab, avoiding any wrinkles.

*Warning:* Plaster becomes hot after drying.

e. Position splint over extremity and wrap externally with gauze. When dry, an elastic wrap can be added.
f. Alternatively, wet one side of fiberglass until saturated. Roll or fold to remove excess water. Mold splint as indicated. *Note*: Using warm water will decrease drying time. This may result in inadequate time to mold splint. Turn edge of the splint back on itself to produce a smooth surface. Take care to cover the sharp edges of fiberglass. When dry, wrap with elastic bandage.
g. Use crutches or slings as indicated.
h. The need for orthopedic referral should be individually assessed.



### B. LONG ARM POSTERIOR SPLINT (Fig. 3-16):

**Indications:** Immobilization of elbow and forearm injuries.

### C. SUGAR TONG FOREARM SPLINT (Fig. 3-17)

Indications: For distal radius and wrist fractures, to immobilize the elbow and minimize pronation and supination.

### D. ULNAR GUTTER SPLINT

1. **Indications:** Nonrotated fourth or fifth (boxer) metacarpal metaphyseal fracture with less than 20 degrees of angulation, uncomplicated fourth and fifth phalangeal fracture.
2. Assess for malrotation, displacement (especially Salter I fractures), angulation, and joint stability before splinting.
3. **Procedure:** Elbow in neutral position, wrist in neutral position, metacarpophalangeal joint at 70 degrees, interphalangeal joint at 20 degrees. Apply splint in U shape from the tip of the fifth digit to 3 cm distal to the volar crease of the elbow. The splint should be wide enough to enclose the fourth and fifth digits.

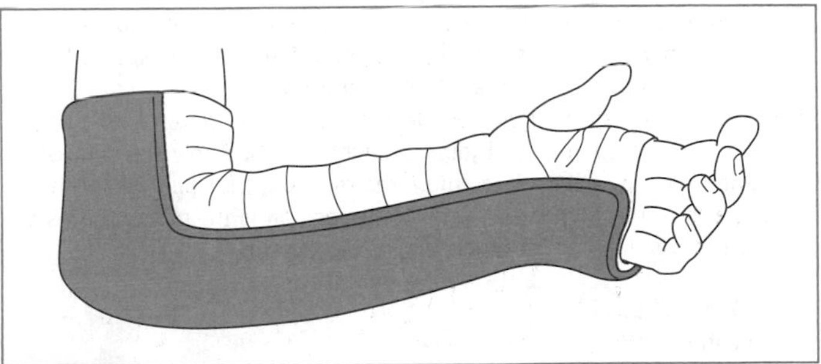

FIG. 3-16

Long arm posterior splint.

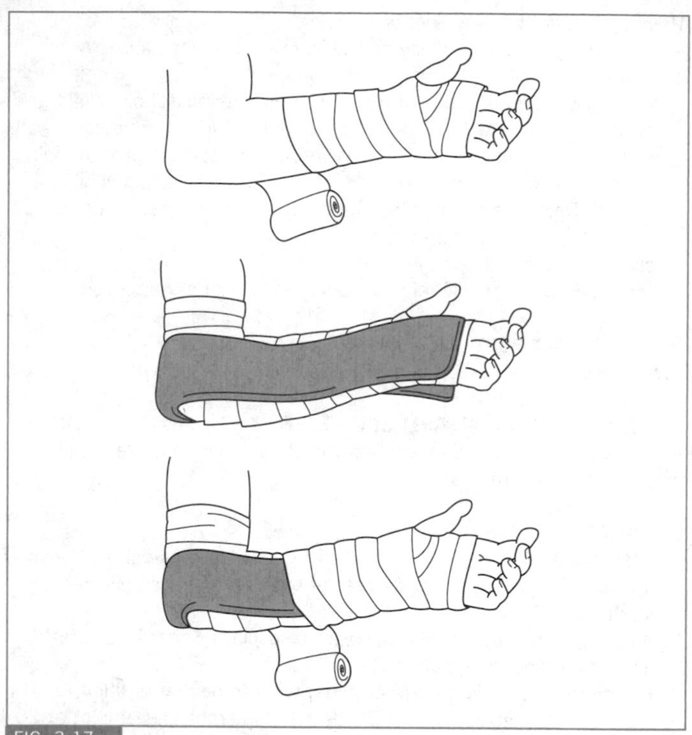

FIG. 3-17
Sugar tong forearm splint.

## E. THUMB SPICA SPLINT

1. **Indications:** Nonrotated, nonangulated, nonarticular fractures of the thumb metacarpal or phalanx, ulnar collateral ligament injury (gamekeeper's or skier's thumb), scaphoid fracture or suspected scaphoid fracture (pain in anatomic snuff box).
2. **Procedure:** Wrist in slight dorsiflexion, thumb in some flexion and abduction, interphalangeal joint in slight flexion. Apply splint in U shape from tip of thumb to mid-forearm. Mold the splint along the long axis of the thumb so that thumb position is maintained. This will result in a spiral configuration along the forearm.

## F. VOLAR SPLINT

1. **Indications:** Wrist immobilization.
2. **Procedure:** Wrist in slight dorsiflexion. Apply splint on palmar surface from the MP joint to 2 to 3 cm distal to the volar crease of the elbow.

It is useful to curve the splint to allow the metacarpophalangeal joint to rest at an 80- to 90-degree angle.

## G. POSTERIOR ANKLE SPLINT

1. **Indications:** Immobilization of ankle sprains and fractures of the foot, ankle, and distal fibula.
2. **Procedure:** Measure leg for appropriate length of plaster. The splint should extend to bases of toes and the upper portion of the calf. A sugar tong (stirrup) splint can be added to increase stability for ankle fractures.

## H. RADIAL HEAD SUBLUXATION (NURSEMAID'S ELBOW) REDUCTION



1. **Presentation:** Commonly occurs in children ages 1 to 4 years with a history of inability to use an arm after it was pulled. The child presents with the affected arm held at the side in pronation with elbow slightly flexed.
2. **Caution:** Rule out a fracture clinically before doing procedure. Consider radiograph if mechanism of injury or history is atypical.
3. **Procedure:**

a. Support the elbow with one hand, and place your thumb laterally over the radial head at the elbow. With your other hand, grasp the child's hand in a handshake position.

b. Quickly and deliberately supinate and externally rotate the forearm, and simultaneously flex the elbow. Alternatively, hyperpronation alone may be used. You may feel a click as reduction occurs.

c. Most children will begin to use the arm within 15 minutes, some immediately after reduction. If reduction occurs after a prolonged period of subluxation, it may take the child longer to recover use of the arm. In this case, the arm should be immobilized with a posterior splint.

d. If procedure is unsuccessful, consider obtaining a radiograph. Maneuver may be repeated if needed.

## REFERENCES


1. Fleisher G, Ludwig S: Pediatric Emergency Medicine, 3rd ed. Baltimore, Williams & Wilkins, 2000.
2. Dieckmann R, Fiser D, Selbst S: Illustrated Textbook of Pediatric Emergency and Critical Care Procedures. St. Louis, Mosby, 1997.
3. Nichols DG et al: Golden Hour: The Handbook of Advanced Pediatric Life Support. St. Louis, Mosby, 1996.
4. Howe PM et al: Etiologic diagnosis of cellulitis: Comparison of aspirates obtained from the leading edge and the point of maximal inflammation. Pediatr Infect Dis J 1987;6(7):685–686.

# Trauma, Burns, and Common Critical Care Emergencies

*Jennifer L. Jarjosa, MD*

4

## I. TRAUMA: OVERVIEW[1]

### A. PRIMARY SURVEY

The primary survey includes assessment of the ABCs: **A**irway, **B**reathing, and **C**irculation. See Chapter 1 for a complete algorithm.

### B. SECONDARY SURVEY

Procedures included in a secondary survey are listed in Table 4-1

### C. "AMPLE" HISTORY

Obtain an AMPLE history: **A**llergies, **M**edications, **P**ast illnesses, **L**ast meal, **E**vents preceding injury.

## II. SPECIFIC TRAUMATIC INJURIES

### A. MINOR CLOSED HEAD TRAUMA (CHT)[2]

1. **Introduction: Head injury can be caused by penetrating trauma, blunt force, rotational acceleration, or acceleration-deceleration injury. CHT can lead to depressed or nondepressed skull fracture, epidural hematoma, subdural hematoma, cerebral contusion, brain edema, increased intracranial pressure (ICP), brain herniation, concussion (mild to moderate diffuse brain injury), and/or coma (diffuse axonal injury [DAI]). See section VI.B for treatment of elevated ICP associated with severe CHT.**
2. **Evaluation:**

a. **Physical examination** (after ABCs and cervical spine [C-spine] immobilization):

(1) Assign Glasgow Coma Scale (GCS) score (see Chapter 1).

(2) Obtain vital signs, with special attention paid to Cushing triad—hypertension, bradycardia, and irregular respiratory pattern.

(3) Perform careful neurologic examination as part of secondary survey (see Table 4-1).

(4) If severe symptoms are present, or if CHT is not minor, follow procedures for emergency management of increased ICP and coma (see section VI.B).

(5) Rule out possible drug or alcohol ingestion/use as etiology of altered mental status.

b. **Associated symptoms:** Altered level or loss of consciousness (LOC), amnesia (before, during, or after the event), mental status change, behavior change, seizure activity, vomiting, headache, gait disturbance, visual change, or lethargy since event.

TABLE 4-1

**SECONDARY SURVEY**

Remove all of patient's clothing, and perform a thorough head-to-toe examination, with special emphasis on the following. Remember to keep the child warm throughout the examination.

| Organ System | Secondary Survey |
|---|---|
| Head | Scalp/skull injury |
| | *Raccoon eyes:* Periorbital ecchymoses; suggest orbital roof fracture |
| | *Battle's sign:* Ecchymoses behind pinna; suggests mastoid fracture |
| | CSF leak from ears/nose or hemotympanum suggests basilar skull fracture |
| | *Pupil size, symmetry, and reactivity:* Unilateral dilation of one pupil suggests compression of cranial nerve III (CNIII) and possible impending herniation; bilateral dilation of pupils is ominous and suggests bilateral CNIII compression or severe anoxia and ischemia |
| | Corneal reflex |
| | Funduscopic examination for papilledema as evidence of increased intracranial pressure |
| | Hyphema |
| Neck | Cervical spine tenderness, deformity, injury |
| | Trachea midline |
| | Subcutaneous emphysema |
| Chest | Clavicle deformity, tenderness |
| | Breath sounds, heart sounds |
| | Chest wall symmetry, paradoxical movement, rib deformity/fracture |
| | Petechiae over chest/head suggest traumatic asphyxia |
| Abdomen | Serial examinations to evaluate tenderness, distention, ecchymosis |
| | Shoulder pain suggests referred subdiaphragmatic process |
| | Orogastric aspirates with blood or bile suggest intra-abdominal injury |
| | Splenic laceration suggested by left upper quadrant rib tenderness, flank pain, and/or flank ecchymoses |
| Pelvis | Tenderness, symmetry, deformity, stability |
| Genitourinary | Laceration, ecchymoses, hematoma, bleeding |
| | Rectal tone, blood, displaced prostate |
| | Blood at urinary meatus suggests urethral injury; do not catheterize |
| Back | Log-roll patient to evaluate spine for step-off along spinal column |
| | Tenderness |
| | Open or penetrating wound |
| Extremities | *Neurovascular status:* Pulse, perfusion, pallor, paresthesias, paralysis, pain |
| | Deformity, crepitus, pain |
| | Motor/sensory examination |
| | *Compartment syndrome:* Pain out of proportion to expected; distal pallor/pulselessness |
| Neurologic | *Quick screen:* **AVPU** (**A**lert, **V**ocal stimulation response, **P**ainful stimulation response, **U**nresponsive) |
| | Glasgow Coma Scale (see Chapter 1) |

TABLE 4-1

SECONDARY SURVEY—cont'd

| Organ System | Secondary Survey |
|---|---|
| Skin | Capillary refill, perfusion<br>Lacerations, abrasions<br>*Contusion:*<br>• Blue-purple: 0–5 days old<br>• Green: 5–7 days old<br>• Yellow: 7–10 days old<br>• Brown: 10–14 days old<br>• Resolution: 2–4 weeks old |

BOX 4-1

**INDICATIONS FOR IMAGING IN MINOR CLOSED HEAD TRAUMA**

**CHILDREN ≤1 YEAR OF AGE**

Normal neurologic examination, no symptoms, no scalp hematoma: no imaging

Normal neurologic examination, no symptoms, scalp hematoma: skull radiographs

If positive for fracture, follow with CT scan

Abnormal neurologic examination, symptoms: CT scan

**CHILDREN >1 YEAR OF AGE**

Normal neurologic examination, no symptoms: no imaging

Normal neurologic examination, symptoms: consider CT scan

Abnormal neurologic examination, with or without seizure: CT scan

Modified from Marx JA: Rosen's Emergency Medicine: Concepts and Clinical Practice, 6th ed. St. Louis, Mosby, 2006, chap. 38.

c. **Mechanism of injury:**
   (1) Linear forces: Less likely to cause LOC; more commonly lead to skull fractures, intracranial hematoma, or cerebral contusion.
   (2) Rotational forces: Commonly cause LOC; occasionally associated with DAI.
   (3) Suspect abuse if mechanism of injury is not consistent with sustained injuries.

3. **Management:**

a. Evaluate C-spine.

b. Obtain computed tomography (CT) scan of head, non-contrast (Box 4-1):
   (1) Always obtain when LOC present.
   (2) In absence of LOC, use clinical judgment based on mechanism of injury, severity of known injuries, and deficits on examination.

c. Observe patient:
   (1) Monitor for 4–6 hr to detect delayed signs or symptoms of intracranial injury, which can occur with epidural bleeds, in which a symptom-free lucid period can precede variable degrees of acute-onset mental status change.

(2) Recommend continued observation at home, or in hospital if clinically unstable or if there are concerns about home environment (care giver reliability, follow-up, etc.). Counsel parents on indications to have patient re-evaluated.

d. Consider patients with the following symptoms for hospitalization:
   (1) Depressed or declining level of consciousness or prolonged unconsciousness (GCS 8–12).
   (2) Neurologic deficit.
   (3) Increasing headache or persistent vomiting.
   (4) Seizures.
   (5) Cerebrospinal fluid otorrhea or rhinorrhea, hemotympanum, Battle's sign, or raccoon eyes.
   (6) Linear skull fracture crossing the groove of the middle meningeal artery, a venous sinus of the dura, or the foramen magnum.
   (7) Compound skull fracture or fracture into the frontal sinus.
   (8) Depressed skull fracture.
   (9) Bleeding disorder or patient receiving anticoagulation therapy.
   (10) Intoxication or illness obscuring neurologic state.
   (11) Suspected child abuse.

e. For sports-related injuries, refer to Centers for Disease Control and Prevention guidelines: "Management of Concussion in Sports" at http://www.cdc.gov/ncipc/pub-res/tbi_toolkit/physicians/concussion_sports.htm.

## B. NECK INJURIES[2]

See Chapter 25 (Radiology) for more in-depth evaluation of cervical trauma.

**1. Immobilize C-spine prior to careful history and physical examination. Due to large occiput in infants, use support under neck/shoulders to maintain neutral position and avoid neck flexion.**

**2. Radiographic studies:**

a. Posteroanterior (PA), lateral views (including C7), and odontoid view.

b. Flexion and extension views of C-spine, if:
   (1) Point tenderness.
   (2) Symptoms on palpation.
   (3) Any suspicion of abnormality on PA or lateral views.
   (4) Unstable C-spine injury not suspected.

c. Magnetic resonance imaging (MRI) indicated to rule out direct spinal cord damage if neurologic symptoms persist and plain films are negative.

d. For details on reading C-spine films, see Chapter 25.

**3. Clinically clear the C-spine:**

a. Patient must be awake, without a distracting injury.

b. Palpate posterior neck for localized tenderness. If there is pain, maintain C-spine collar for immobilization until further evaluation can definitively rule out injury. If there is no pain, assess active and passive range of motion.

## C. BLUNT THORACIC AND ABDOMINAL TRAUMA[3]

1. **Anatomic considerations in children:**
a. Pliable rib cage.
b. Solid organs proportionally larger than those of adults.
c. Underdeveloped abdominal musculature.
2. **Common injuries:**
a. Thoracic: Pneumothorax, hemothorax, pulmonary contusion, fractures; damage to major blood vessels, heart, diaphragm.
b. Abdominal: Hematomas within gastrointestinal (GI) tract; damage to spleen, liver, pancreas, kidneys, genitourinary (GU) system, or major blood vessels.
3. **Evaluation:**
a. Careful history and physical examination.
b. Laboratory studies:
   (1) Type and cross-match.
   (2) Thoracic injury: Complete blood count (CBC), pulse oximetry; consider arterial blood gas (ABG).
   (3) Abdominal injury: CBC (follow serial hemoglobin values), electrolytes, liver function tests, amylase, lipase, urinalysis.
c. Radiologic evaluation:
   (1) Chest radiograph with or without chest CT with IV contrast, if patient is stable.
   (2) Abdominal CT with IV contrast (routine oral contrast is not indicated, secondary to high false-negative rate for hollow viscus injury)
   (3) Consider focused abdominal ultrasound or diagnostic peritoneal lavage when coexisting injuries (e.g., neurologic or significant orthopedic) prevent CT scan. If peritoneal lavage is used, the open method is preferred in small children, with warmed isotonic saline (10–15 mL/kg).
4. **Emergent treatment:**
a. If significant trauma is suspected or diagnosed, consult a pediatric surgeon..
b. Tension pneumothorax:
   (1) Signs: Severe respiratory distress, distended neck veins, contralateral tracheal deviation, diminished breath sounds, compromised systemic perfusion by obstruction of venous return.
   (2) Treatment: Needle decompression followed by chest tube placement directed toward lung apex (see Chapter 3).
c. Open pneumothorax (aka sucking chest wound): Allows free flow of air between atmosphere and hemithorax. Cover defect with an occlusive dressing (i.e., petroleum jelly gauze), give positive-pressure ventilation, and insert chest tube (see Chapter 3).

d. Hemothorax: Provide fluid resuscitation followed by placement of a chest tube directed posteriorly and inferiorly.

## D. ORTHOPEDIC/LONG BONE TRAUMA[4,5]

1. **Fractures:** Some fracture patterns are unique to children (Fig. 4-1); growth-plate injuries are classified by the Salter-Harris classification (Table 4-2). Ligaments are stronger than bones or growth plates in children; thus, dislocations and sprains are relatively uncommon, whereas growth-plate disruption and bone avulsion are more common. For basic splinting techniques, see Chapter 3.
2. **Compartment syndrome:**[1,5] Elevated muscle compartment pressure (enclosed by surrounding fascia) impairs blood flow, resulting in nerve and muscle damage.

a. Can be secondary to crush injury, fractures, burns, infections (necrotizing fasciitis), or hemorrhage. Most commonly seen with tibial fractures.

b. Marked by the 6 Ps: **P**ain (earliest symptom), **P**aresthesias, **P**allor, **P**oikilothermia, **P**aralysis, **P**ulselessness.

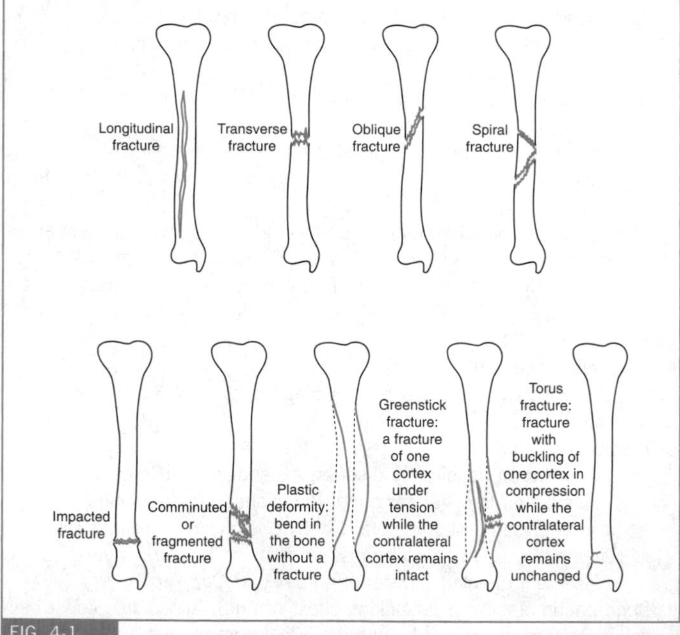


FIG. 4-1

Fracture patterns unique to children. *(Modified from Ogden JA: Skeletal Injury in the Child, 3rd ed. Philadelphia, WB Saunders, 2000.)*

TABLE 4-2

SALTER-HARRIS CLASSIFICATION OF GROWTH-PLATE INJURY

| Class I | Class II | Class III | Class IV | Class V |
|---|---|---|---|---|
| Fracture along growth plate | Fracture along growth plate with metaphyseal extension | Fracture along growth plate with epiphyseal extension | Fracture across growth plate, including metaphysis and epiphysis | Crush injury to growth plate without obvious fracture |
| I | II | III | IV | V |

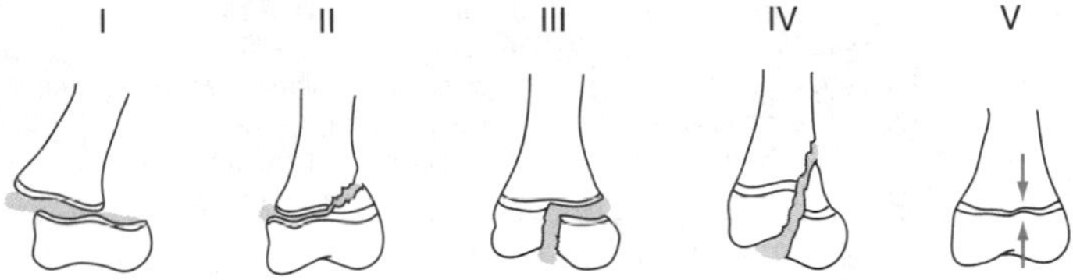

(1) Although traditional signs, the 6 Ps are not reliable, with the exception of pain and paresthesias.
(2) Unremitting pain, even after appropriate analgesia, is the most sensitive sign. Pain with passive muscle stretching is strong clinical indicator.
(3) Palpable pulse does not rule out compartment syndrome.

c. Studies: Measure intracompartmental pressure (normal = 10 mm Hg; 20–30 mm Hg usually produces clinical symptoms).
d. Management: Emergent (within 6 hr of symptom onset) surgical fasciotomy (absolutely indicated if pressure ≥30 mm Hg).
e. Can cause rhabdomyolysis. Follow urinalysis, creatinine kinase, and electrolytes (risk for hyperkalemia). Consider saline resuscitation, urine alkalinization (to keep urine pH > 6.5) and mannitol, 250 to 500 mg/kg, if laboratory studies show evidence of rhabdomyolysis.
f. Outcome: Determined by duration of increased pressure.
(1) <6 hr: Good outcome after fasciotomy in 95% of cases.
(2) >12 hr: Good outcome after fasciotomy in 6% of cases.

## III. ANIMAL BITES[2]

### A. WOUND CONSIDERATIONS

**1. Special considerations:**

a. Deep bites: Possibility of foreign body or fracture—consider radiographs (especially hand or scalp).
b. Periorbital bites: Possibility of corneal abrasion, lacrimal duct involvement, or other ocular damage—consider ophthalmologic evaluation.
c. Hand: Prone to infection—follow for development of osteomyelitis.
d. Nose: Evaluate for cartilage injury.

TABLE 4-3

ANIMAL BITES

| Animal | Common Organism(s) | Special Considerations |
|---|---|---|
| Dog | *Staphylococcus aureus*<br>*Pasteurella multocida* | Crush injury |
| Cat | *P. multocida* | Deep puncture wound<br>Often associated with fulminant infection<br>Slow to respond to treatment |
| Human | *Streptococcus viridans*<br>*S. aureus*<br>Anaerobes<br>Eikenella corrodens | Consider child abuse<br>Assess risk for hepatitis B, herpes sinplex, and human immunodeficiency virus transmission |
| Rodent | *Streptobacillus moniliformis*<br>*Spirillum minus* | Low incidence of secondary infection<br>Rat-bite fever—occurs rarely |

2. **High infection risk:**
a. Puncture wounds.
b. Hand or foot wounds.
c. Cat or human bites.
d. Wounds in asplenic or immunocompromised patients.
e. Wounds with care delayed >12 hr
3. **Animal species (Table 4-3).**

## B. MANAGEMENT

1. **Wound hygiene:**
a. Irrigate with copious amounts of sterile saline using high-pressure syringe irrigation. Do not irrigate puncture wounds.
b. Débride devitalized tissue.
c. Explore for foreign bodies. Consider surgical débridement and exploration for extensive wounds, wounds involving metacarpophalangeal joint, and cranial bites by a large animal.
d. Culture only if evidence of infection is present.
2. **Closure:**
a. Avoid closing wounds of high infection risk (see list at III.A).
b. Wounds that involve tendons, joints, deep fascial layers, or major vasculature should be evaluated by a plastic or hand surgeon and, if indicated, closed in the operating room.
c. Suturing: When indicated, closure should be done with minimal simple, interrupted, nylon sutures. Approximate wound edges loosely. Avoid deep sutures.
   (1) Head and neck: Can usually be safely sutured (with the exceptions noted) after copious irrigation and wound débridement if within 6 to 8 hr of injury and no signs of infection. Facial wounds often require primary closure for cosmetic reasons; infection risk is lower due to good vascular supply.
   (2) Extremities: In large hand wounds, the subcutaneous dead space should be closed with minimal absorbable sutures, with delayed

cutaneous closure in 3 to 5 days if there is no evidence of infection.

3. **Antibiotics: Prophylactic antibiotics are only indicated in cases of high infection risk, as listed at III.A. See Chapter 17 for appropriate antibiotic therapies.**
4. **Rabies and tetanus prophylaxis: See Chapter 16.**
5. **Disposition:**

a. Outpatient care: Obtain careful follow-up of all bite wounds, especially those requiring surgical closure, within 24 to 48 hr. Extremity wounds, especially of the hands, should be immobilized in position of function and kept elevated. Wound should be kept clean and dry.

b. Inpatient care: Consider hospitalization for observation and parenteral antibiotics for significant human bites, immunocompromised or asplenic hosts, established deep or severe infections, bites associated with systemic complaints, bites with significant functional or cosmetic morbidity, and/or unreliable follow-up or care by the parent/guardian.

6. **The infected wound: Wounds that subsequently become infected may require drainage and débridement, possibly under anesthesia. Adjust antibiotic therapy according to Gram stain and culture results.**

## IV. BURNS[1,2,6]

### A. EVALUATION OF PEDIATRIC BURNS (Tables 4-4 and 4-5)

**Note** *The extent and severity of burn injury may change over the first few days after injury; therefore, be cautious in discussing prognosis.*

### B. BURN MAPPING

**Calculate total body surface area (TBSA) burned (Fig 4-2):** Based only on percentage of second- and third-degree burns.

### C. EMERGENT MANAGEMENT OF PEDIATRIC BURNS

1. **Acute stabilization: Special considerations of basic trauma principles.**

a. Airway/breathing:

(1) Intubation: Consider for >20% to 25% BSA burned, or any respiratory distress, which could be indicative of inhalation injury (upper airway edema, parenchymal damage, etc).

**Note** *Avoid late use of succinylcholine, due to increased risk of hyperkalemia (see Chapter 1.)*

(2) Inhalation injury: Assume carbon monoxide poisoning with severe and/or closed-space burns.

(a) Administer humidified 100% $O_2$ until carboxyhemoglobin (COHb) level <10%. Elimination half-life of COHb is dependent on $PaO_2$ (consider hyperbaric $O_2$ if pH < 7.4 and COHb elevated).

TRAUMA, BURNS, AND COMMON CRITICAL CARE EMERGENCIES 4

TABLE 4-4

THERMAL INJURY

| Type of Burn | Description/Comment |
|---|---|
| Flame | Most common type of burn; when clothing burns, the exposure to heat is prolonged, and the severity of the burn is worse. |
| Scald/contact | Mortality is similar to that in flame burns when total body surface area involved is equivalent; see text for description of patterns of scald injury and burns suspicious of intentional injury. |
| Chemical | Tissue damaged by protein coagulation or liquefaction rather than hyperthermic activity. |
| Electrical | Injury is often extensive, involving skeletal muscle and other tissues in addition to the skin damage. Extent of damage may not be initially apparent. The tissues that have the least resistance are the most heat sensitive. Bone has the greatest resistance, nerve tissue the least. Cardiac arrest may occur from passage of the current through the heart. |
| Inhalation | Present in 30% of victims of major flame burns; should be considered when there is evidence of fire in enclosed space: singed nares, facial burns, charred lips, carbonaceous secretions, posterior pharynx edema, hoarseness, cough, or wheezing. Inhalation injury increases mortality. |
| Cold injury/frostbite | Freezing results in direct tissue injury. Toes, fingers, ears, and nose are commonly involved. Initial treatment includes rewarming in tepid (105°–110°F) water for 20–40 min. Excision of tissue should not be done until complete demarcation of nonviable tissue has occurred. |

TABLE 4-5

BURN DEGREE

| Burn Depth/Degree | Description/Comment |
|---|---|
| First degree | Only epidermis involved; tender and erythematous. |
| Second degree (partial-thickness) | Epidermis and dermis involved, but dermal appendages spared.<br>• *Superficial (papillary dermis):* erythematous, tender. Thin-walled blisters.<br>• *Deep (reticular dermis):* can be mixture of red and white; 2-point discrimination diminished, but can feel pressure. |
| Third degree (full-thickness) | Destroys epidermis and all of the dermis; leathery and painless; requires grafting. |
| Fourth degree | Full-thickness destruction of skin and subcutaneous tissue; require extensive débridement and reconstruction. |

(b) Make decisions based on $Pao_2$ rather than pulse oximetry.

b. Circulation: Start IV fluid resuscitation for infants with burns >10% of BSA, children with burns >15% BSA, or children with evidence of smoke inhalation. Consider a bolus of 20 mL/kg lactated Ringer's or

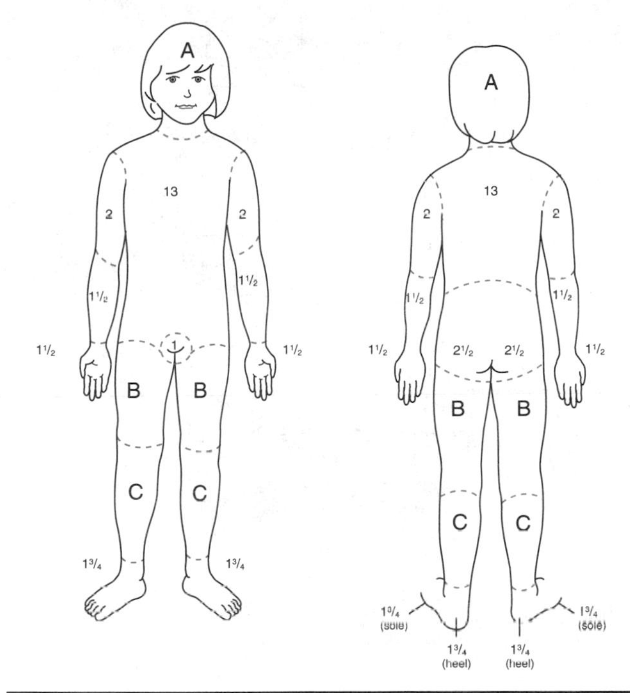


| | < 1 yr | 1 yr | 5 yr | 10 yr | 15 yr | Adult |
|---|---|---|---|---|---|---|
| A half of head | $9\frac{1}{2}$ | $8\frac{1}{2}$ | $6\frac{1}{2}$ | $5\frac{1}{2}$ | $4\frac{1}{2}$ | $3\frac{1}{2}$ |
| B half of thigh | $2\frac{3}{4}$ | $3\frac{1}{4}$ | 4 | $4\frac{1}{4}$ | $4\frac{1}{2}$ | $4\frac{3}{4}$ |
| C half of leg | $2\frac{1}{2}$ | $2\frac{1}{2}$ | $2\frac{3}{4}$ | 3 | $3\frac{1}{4}$ | $3\frac{1}{2}$ |

FIG. 4-2

Burn assessment chart. All numbers are percentages. *(From Barkin RM, Rosen P: Emergency Pediatrics: A Guide to Ambulatory Care, 6th ed. St. Louis, Mosby, 2003.)*

normal saline solutions. Further fluid resuscitation should maintain a urine output >0.5 mL/kg/hr. Use Parkland formula (Fig. 4-3).

c. Secondary survey: Consider associated traumatic injuries. Electrical injury can produce deep tissue damage, intravascular thrombosis, cardiac and respiratory arrest, fractures secondary to muscle

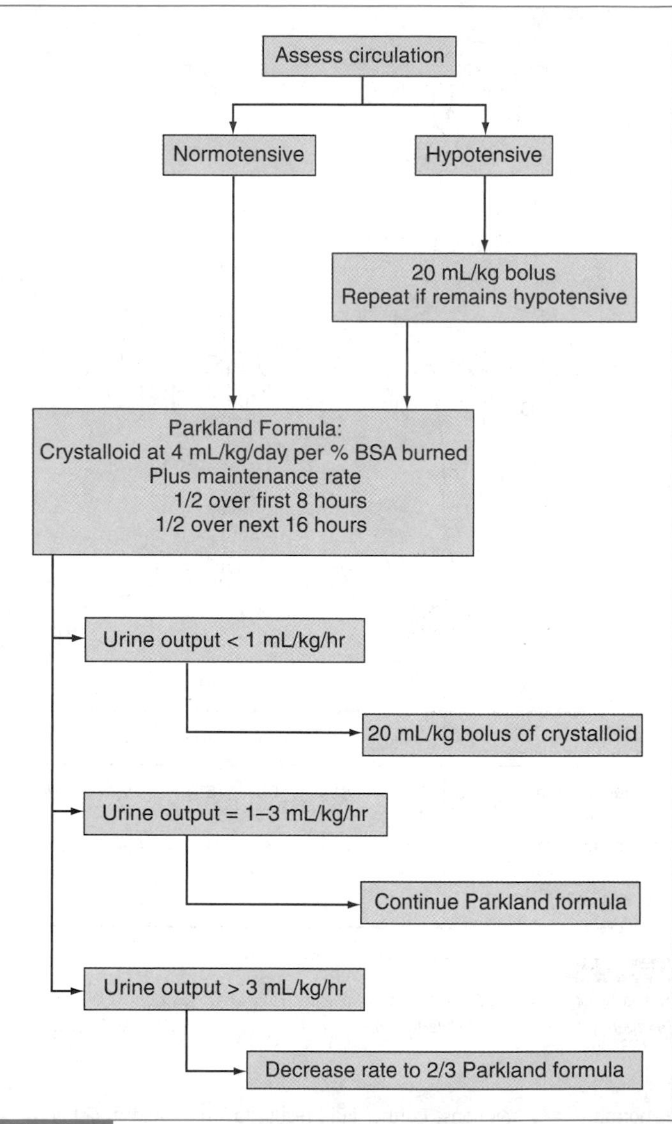


FIG. 4-3

Fluid management of life-threatening burns. *(Modified from Nichols DG et al [eds]: Golden Hour: The Handbook of Pediatric Advanced Life Support. St. Louis, Mosby, 1996, p 460.)*

contraction, and cardiac arrhythmias. Look for exit site for electrical injury.

d. Analgesia: IV narcotic therapy often necessary for pain control.
e. GI: Place nasogastric tube for decompression; begin prophylaxis for Curling's stress ulcers with histamine-2 receptor blockers and/or antacids.
f. GU: Use Foley catheter to monitor urine output, decompress bladder, and prevent possible soiling of wounds.
g. Eye: Ophthalmologic evaluation as necessary. Use topical ophthalmic antibiotics if abrasions are present.
h. Special considerations:
   (1) Tetanus immunoprophylaxis (see Chapter 16).
   (2) Temperature management: Cooling decreases the severity of the burn if administered within 30 min of injury; it also helps to relieve pain. If burns are >10% of BSA, cool for no more than 30 min and apply clean, dry towels to burn to avoid hypothermia.
   (3) Chemical burns: It is important to wash away or neutralize the chemical. Except in rare circumstances, the most efficacious first aid for chemical burns is lavage with copious volumes of water.

## D. FURTHER MANAGEMENT OF PEDIATRIC BURNS

**1. Outpatient management:**

a. Considerations: If burn is <10% of an infant's BSA (or <15% of a child's BSA), is not full-thickness, and does not involve eyes, ears, face, hands/feet, or perineum, treat as outpatient.
b. Management:
   (1) Clean with warm saline or mild soap and water. Débride open wounds and necrotic tissue.
   (2) Apply topical antibacterial agent (Table 4-6). Oral antibiotics not indicated.
   (3) Follow-up within 1 week is recommended.
   (4) Have patient clean burn at home twice daily with mild soap (taking special care to remove previously applied antibacterial agent), followed by application of an antibacterial agent and sterile dressing, as previously.

**2. Inpatient management:**

a. Indications:
   (1) Any partial-thickness burn >10% TBSA or any full-thickness burn >5% TBSA.
   (2) Significant electrical or chemical injury.
   (3) Burns of critical areas, such as face, hands, feet, perineum, or joints.
   (4) Burns leading to suspicions of abuse or unsafe home environment.
   (5) Patient with underlying chronic illness.
   (6) Evidence of significant inhalation injury.
   (7) Circumferential, full-thickness injury.

TABLE 4-6

TOPICAL ANTIBACTERIAL AGENTS

| Agent | Action | Side Effects | Use |
|---|---|---|---|
| Silver sulfadiazine (Silvadene) | Broad antibacterial; painless, fair eschar penetration | Sulfonamide sensitivity, occasional leukopenia; contraindicated in pregnancy | Q12hr; cover with light dressings; leave face and chest open. |
| Bacitracin ointment | Limited antibacterial action, poor eschar penetration; transparent, easy to apply | Rapid development of resistance; conjunctivitis develops if ointment comes into contact with eye | Q12hr; apply to small areas; acceptable with facial burns. |
| Mafenide (Sulfamylon) | Excellent antibacterial for gram-positive and gram-negative bacteria and *Clostridium*; rapid eschar penetration | Painful sulfonamide sensitivity; carbonic anhydrase inhibition may lead to acidosis | Q12hr; cover with light dressings; leave face, chest, abdomen open. |

b. Fluid therapy (see Fig. 4-3):
   (1) Consider central venous access for burns >25% BSA.
   (2) Use the Parkland formula as a guideline to estimate fluid need. Requirements decrease by 25% to 50% after first 24 hr. Determine concentrations and rates by monitoring weight, serum electrolytes, urine output, nasogastric losses.
   (3) Consider adding colloid after 18 to 24 hr (albumin, 1 g/kg/day) to maintain serum albumin >2 g/dL.
   (4) Withhold potassium generally for the first 48 hr because of a large release of potassium from damaged tissues. To manage electrolytes most effectively, monitor urine electrolytes twice weekly and replace urine losses accordingly.

3. **Burn prevention: Install smoke detectors; keep water-heater maximum temperature <52°C (<120°F). It takes 2 min of immersion at 52°C to cause a full-thickness burn, compared with 5 sec of immersion at 60°C.**

## V. CHILD ABUSE

### A. INTRODUCTION

Approach should be multidisciplinary—medical professionals, social worker, and community agencies such as emergency medical service providers, police, social services, and prosecutors.

### B. MANAGEMENT[2,7,8]

The medical professional should suspect, diagnose, treat, report, and document all cases of child abuse, neglect, or maltreatment.

1. **Suspect:** Be suspicious whenever there is inappropriate parental response, delay in seeking medical attention, inadequate history of injury, mechanism of injury inconsistent with physical findings, evidence of neglect or failure to thrive, evidence of disturbed emotions or expressions in a child, prior history of suspicious events, or parental substance abuse.
2. **Diagnose:** Concerning injuries. Attempt to correlate all physical findings with history.

a. Bruises: Shape and color of bruises are important (see Table 4-1). Be suspicious of bruises in protected areas (chest, abdomen, back, buttocks). Looped marks or railroad track marks may indicate injury from cords, belts, and ropes.

b. Bites: Shape, size, and location are important; photodocument, if possible. Intercanine distances of >3 cm are suggestive of human bites, which generally crush more than lacerate.

c. Burns: Absence of splash marks, clearly demarcated edges, stocking glove patterns, symmetrically burned buttocks and/or lower legs, spared inguinal creases, and symmetrical involvement of palms or soles are all suggestive of nonaccidental injury.

d. Bleeding:

(1) Retinal hemorrhages are virtually pathognomonic of abuse (abusive head trauma/shaken-baby syndrome).

(2) Duodenal hematomas are suspicious for nonaccidental trauma; may be secondary to blunt trauma and eventually lead to upper GI obstruction.

e. Skeletal injury: Correlate mechanism of injury with physical finding; rule out any underlying bony pathology.

(1) Long bones: Classic fracture of abuse is the epiphyseal/metaphyseal fracture, seen as the "bucket handle" or "corner" fracture at the end of long bones, secondary to jerking or shaking of a child's limb. Fractures of the femur and humerus may be suspicious of abuse, but spiral fractures can be seen with rotational forces, such as the "toddler's fracture" of the tibia.

(2) Ribs: Nonaccidental trauma may lead to posterior nondisplaced rib fractures, which may not be visible on plain film until callus formation. Fractures are usually secondary to severe squeezing of the rib cage. Closed-chest compressions from cardiopulmonary resuscitation do not appear to cause rib fractures in children.

(3) Skull: Fractures >3 mm wide, complex fractures, bilateral fractures, and nonparietal fractures suggest forces greater than those sustained from minor household trauma.

f. Shaken-baby syndrome: Classically presents with retinal hemorrhages, subdural hematoma, long bone or rib fractures, and central nervous system (CNS) dysfunction, such as seizure, apnea, or lethargy secondary to intracranial injury.

g. Sexual abuse:
   (1) Normal genital examination does not rule out abuse.
   (2) Genital examination should be performed by trained forensic specialist, due to variability in genital anatomy, especially the hymen.
   (3) Document vaginal bleeding in the prepubertal female; injury to external genitalia, especially the posterior region; bruising; or discharge; can be suspicious for abuse.
   (4) Evaluate anus for bruising, laceration, hemorrhoids, scars that extend beyond the anal verge, absence of anal wink, or evidence of infection, such as genital warts. Circumferential hematoma of the anal sphincter is associated with forced penetration.
   (5) When sexual abuse is suspected as having occurred within past 72 hr, defer interview and detailed GU examination until a multidisciplinary forensic team with expertise in the clinical and laboratory evaluation of sexual abuse can be involved. If possible, avoid collection of laboratory specimens without input from this team.

3. **Useful studies:**

a. Skeletal surveys suggested to evaluate suspicious bony trauma in any child; these studies are mandatory for children <2 years of age (see Chapter 25 for components).
b. Bone scan may be indicated to identify early or difficult-to-detect fractures.
c. Noncontrast head CT scan is useful for visualizing intracranial hemorrhage, though unreliable for detection of skull fractures.
d. MRI may identify lesions not detected by CT scan (e.g., posterior fossa injury and DAI).
e. Dilated, indirect ophthalmoscopy by an ophthalmologist is important for accurate detection of retinal hemorrhages in suspected abusive head trauma/shaken-baby syndrome.

4. **Treat:** Medical stabilization is primary goal. Prevention of further injuries is the long-term goal.
5. **Report:** All health care providers are required by law to report suspected child maltreatment to the local police and/or child welfare agency. Suspicion, supported by objective evidence, is criterion for reporting and should first be discussed with not only the rest of the involved medical team but also the family. The professional who makes such reports is immune from any civil or criminal liability.
6. **Document:** Write legibly, carefully documenting the following: reported and suspected history and mechanisms of injury; any history given by the victim in his or her own words (use quotation marks); information provided by other providers or services; and physical examination findings, including drawings of injuries and details of dimensions, color, shape, and texture. Always consider early use of police crime laboratory photography to document injuries.

## VI. COMMON CRITICAL CARE EMERGENCIES

### A. ACUTE HYPERTENSION[9]

1. **Assessment:**

a. Use appropriate cuff size for blood pressure (BP) measurement.

b. Hypertensive *urgency*: More common in children; significant elevation in BP *without* accompanying end-organ damage. Symptoms include headache, blurred vision, and nausea.

c. Hypertensive *emergency*: Elevation of both systolic and diastolic BP *with* acute end-organ damage (e.g., cerebral infarction, pulmonary edema, renal failure, hypertensive encephalopathy, seizures, and cerebral hemorrhage).

d. Possible underlying etiologies: Medication or ingestion, cardiovascular, renovascular, renal parenchymal, endocrine, or CNS.

**Note** *Rule out hypertension secondary to elevated ICP before lowering BP.*

e. Physical examination: Four-extremity BP, funduscopy (papilledema, hemorrhage, exudate), visual acuity, thyroid examination, evidence for congestive heart failure (tachycardia, gallop rhythm, hepatomegaly, edema), abdominal examination (mass, bruit), thorough neurologic examination, evidence of virilization, cushingoid effect.

f. Initial diagnostic evaluation: Urinalysis, blood urea nitrogen, creatinine, electrolytes, chest radiograph, and electrocardiogram.

g. Consider renin level, toxicology screen, thyroid and adrenal testing, urine catecholamines, abdominal ultrasound, renal Doppler ultrasound, head CT

2. **Management:**

a. Hypertensive emergency:

(1) Goal: To lower BP promptly but gradually to preserve cerebral autoregulation. The mean arterial pressure (MAP = 1/3 systolic BP + 2/3 diastolic BP) should be lowered by one third of the planned reduction over 6 hr, an additional one third over the next 24 to 36 hr, and the final one third over the next 48 hr (Table 4-7).

(2) Consult nephrologist and/or cardiologist.

(3) After elevated ICP is ruled out, do not delay treatment because of further diagnostic workup.

b. Hypertensive urgency:

(1) Goal: To lower MAP by 20% over 1 hr and return to baseline levels over 24 to 48 hr (Table 4-8).

(2) An oral route may be adequate. (Note that use of sublingual nifedipine is not recommended because this agent can result in a precipitous, uncontrolled fall in BP.)

### B. INCREASED INTRACRANIAL PRESSURE[10]

See Chapter 20 for evaluation and management of hydrocephalus.

TABLE 4-7

MEDICATIONS FOR HYPERTENSIVE EMERGENCY*

| Drug | Onset (Route) | Duration | Interval to Repeat/ ↑ Dose | Comments |
|---|---|---|---|---|
| Diazoxide (arteriole vasodilator) | 1–5 min (IV) | Variable (2–12 hr) | 15–30 min | May cause edema, hyperglycemia |
| Hydralazine (arteriole vasodilator) | 5–20 min (IV) | 2–6 hr | 4–6 hr | May cause reflex tachycardia, prolonged hypotension, nausea |
| **INFUSIONS** | | | | |
| Nitroprusside (arteriole and venous vasodilator) | <30 sec (IV) | Very short | 30–60 min | Requires ICU setting; follow thiocyanate level |
| Labetalol (α-, β-blocker) | 1–5 min (IV) | Variable (~6 hr) | 10 min | May require ICU setting |
| Nicardipine (calcium channel blocker) | 1 min (IV) | 3 hr | 15 min | May cause edema, headache, nausea, vomiting |

*See Formulary for dosing.
ICU, intensive care unit.

TABLE 4-8

MEDICATIONS FOR HYPERTENSIVE URGENCY*

| Drug | Onset (Route) | Duration | Interval to Repeat | Comments |
|---|---|---|---|---|
| Enalaprilat | 15 min (IV) | 12–24 hr | 8–24 hr | May cause hyperkalemia, hypoglycemia |
| Minoxidil | 30 min (PO) | 2–5 days | 4–8 hr | Contraindicated in pheochromocytoma |

*See Formulary for dosing.
PO, Per os.

1. **Assessment:**
   a. History: Obtain history regarding trauma, vomiting, fever, headache, neck pain, unsteadiness, seizure, vision change, gaze preference, and change in mental status. In infants, look for irritability, vomiting, poor feeding, lethargy, and bulging fontanel.
   b. Physical examination:
      (1) Evaluate vital signs for Cushing's triad (hypertension, bradycardia, irregular respiratory pattern).
      (2) Thorough neurologic examination: Pay special attention to photophobia, neck stiffness, pupillary response, cranial nerve dysfunction (especially paralysis of upward gaze or abduction), papilledema, neurologic deficit, abnormal posturing, altered mental status.

c. Laboratory studies: CBC, electrolytes, glucose, toxicology screen, blood culture.

2. **Management:** **Elevate head of bed 30 degrees. Obtain emergent neurosurgical consult and head CT. Do not lower BP if elevated ICP is suspected. Immobilize C-spine if trauma is suspected.**

a. Stable patient (responsive, stable vital signs, no focal findings): Apply cardiorespiratory monitor.

b. Unstable patient:
   (1) Give normal saline or hyperosmolar solutions for maintenance fluids.
   (2) Give 3% NaCl, 2–5 mL/kg, or mannitol, 0.25 g/kg IV, for temporary reduction of ICP. May increase mannitol gradually to a 1 g/kg/dose if needed, although high-dose mannitol can produce significant hypotension from osmotic diuresis.
   (3) Reserve hyperventilation for acute management; keep $P_{CO_2}$ at 30 to 35 mm Hg. Provide controlled neuroprotective intubation, as outlined in Figure 1-1 and Table 1-1 (avoid ketamine).

c. Lumbar puncture contraindicated due to herniation risk. Do not delay antibiotics if meningitis suspected.

d. In space-occupying lesions (tumors, abscesses), consider dexamethasone to reduce cerebral edema in consultation with neurosurgeon.

e. Consider epinephrine or phenylephrine infusion to maintain and keep systemic pressure above ICP.

$$\text{Cerebral perfusion pressure (CPP)} = \text{MAP} - \text{ICP}$$

f. Prevent hyperthermia: Goal is body temperature <37.5°C.

g. Avoid hypotension, hypoxia, hypercarbia, and hypovolemia.

## C. SHOCK

1. **Definition: Physiologic state characterized by inadequate oxygen and nutrient delivery to meet tissue demands.**

a. Compensated shock: Body maintains perfusion to vital organs; may be hard to detect; tachycardia may be present.

b. Decompensated shock: Poor perfusion, tachycardia, hypotension.

c. See Table 4-9 for categorization.

2. **Causes (Table 4-10):**

a. Hypovolemic shock.

b. Distributive shock, including septic, anaphylactic, and neurogenic shock.

c. Cardiogenic shock.

3. **Management (see Table 4-10).**

## D. RESPIRATORY FAILURE

1. **Definition:** Failure of the lungs to exchange oxygen and/or carbon dioxide

TABLE 4-9

**CATEGORIZATION OF HEMORRHAGE AND SHOCK IN PEDIATRIC TRAUMA PATIENTS**

| System | Mild Hemorrhage, Compensated Shock, Simple Hypovolemia (<30% blood volume loss) | Moderate Hemorrhage, Decompensated Shock, Marked Hypovolemia (30%–45% blood volume loss) | Severe Hemorrhage, Cardiopulmonary Failure, Profound Hypovolemia (>45% blood volume loss) |
|---|---|---|---|
| Cardiovascular | Mild tachycardia | Moderate tachycardia | Severe tachycardia |
| | Weak peripheral pulses | Thready peripheral pulses | Absent peripheral pulses |
| | Strong central pulses | Weak central pulses | Thready central pulses |
| | Low-normal blood pressure | Frank hypotension | Profound hypotension (SBP <50 mm Hg) |
| | (SBP > 70 mm Hg + [2 × age in years]) | (SBP < 70 mm Hg + [2 × age in years]) | Severe acidosis |
| | Mild acidosis | Moderate acidosis | |
| Respiratory | Mild tachypnea | Moderate tachypnea | Severe tachypnea |
| Neurologic | Irritable, confused | Agitated, lethargic | Obtunded, comatose |
| Integumentary | Cool extremities, mottling | Cool extremities, pallor | Cold extremities, cyanosis |
| | Poor capillary refill (>2 sec) | Delayed capillary refill (>3 sec) | Prolonged capillary refill (>5 sec) |
| Excretory | Mild oliguria, increased specific gravity | Marked oliguria, increased blood urea nitrogen | Anuria |

SBP, systolic blood pressure.

Adapted from Advanced Trauma Life Support Course, Chicago, Ill, American College of Surgeons.

TABLE 4-10

**TYPES OF SHOCK, PHYSIOLOGIC RESPONSE, AND BASIC TREATMENT**

| Shock | HR | Preload | Contractility | SVR | Treatment |
|---|---|---|---|---|---|
| Septic (early warm) | ↑ | ↓↓ | +/– | ↓ | Fluid, dopamine, epinephrine |
| Septic (late cold) | ↑ | ↓↓ | ↓ | ↑ | Fluid, dopamine, epinephrine |
| Cardiogenic | ↑ | ↑ | ↓↓ | ↑ | Fluid, dobutamine/milrinone, epinephrine |
| Neurogenic | ↑ | ↓↓ | +/– | ↓↓ | Fluid, norepinephrine |
| Hypovolemic | ↑ | ↓↓ | +/– | ↑ | Fluid, dopamine, epinephrine |
| Anaphylactic | ↑ | ↓↓ | ↓ | ↓ | Fluid, epinephrine |

HR, heart rate; SVR, systemic vascular resistance.

**2. Causes:**

a. Neurologic: Muscle weakness, altered sensorium.

b. Obstruction: Foreign body, inflammation.

c. Parenchymal disease: Pneumonia, pulmonary edema, adult respiratory distress syndrome (ARDS).

d. Mechanical: Abnormal chest wall, trauma.

**3. Management:**

a. Intubation and mechanical ventilation (See Chapter 1 for discussion of intubation).

b. Noninvasive positive-pressure ventilation.

**4. Types of ventilatory support:**

a. Volume limited:

(1) Delivers a preset tidal volume to a patient regardless of pressure required.

(2) Risk for barotrauma reduced by pressure alarms and pressure pop-off valves that limit peak inspiratory pressure (PIP).

b. Pressure limited:

(1) Gas flow is delivered to the patient until a preset pressure is reached and then held for the set inspiratory time (reduces the risk for barotrauma).

(2) Useful for neonatal and infant ventilatory support (<10 kg), in which the volume of gas being delivered is small in relation to the volume of compressible air in the ventilator circuit, which makes reliable delivery of a set tidal volume difficult.

c. High-frequency ventilation:[12]

(1) High-frequency oscillatory ventilation (HFOV):

(a) High-amplitude and high-frequency pressure waveform generated in the ventilator circuit. Tidal volumes are less than dead space. Bias gas flow provides fresh gas at ventilator and maintains airway pressure.

(b) Minimizes barotrauma and oxygen toxicities.

(c) Patient must be euvolemic secondary to risk for decreased venous return.

(2) High-frequency jet ventilation:

(a) Used simultaneously with a conventional ventilator.

(b) A jet injector port delivers short bursts of inspiratory gas.

(c) Adequate gas exchange can be achieved at low airway pressures, providing maintenance of lung volume and minimal risk for barotrauma.

**5. Ventilator parameters:**

a. Peak inspiratory pressure (PIP): Attained during the respiratory cycle.

b. Positive end-expiratory pressure (PEEP): Airway pressure maintained between inspiratory and expiratory phases; prevents alveolar collapse during expiration, decreasing work of reinflation and improving gas exchange.

c. Rate (intermittent mandatory ventilation) or frequency (Hz): Number of mechanical breaths delivered per minute or rate of oscillations in HFOV.
d. Inspired oxygen concentration ($FiO_2$): Fraction of oxygen present in inspired gas.
e. Inspiratory time (Ti): Length of time spent in the inspiratory phase of the respiratory cycle.
f. Tidal volume ($V_T$): Volume of gas delivered during inspiration.
g. Power ($\Delta P$): Amplitude of the pressure waveform in HFOV.
h. Mean airway pressure ($\overline{PAW}$): Average pressure over entire respiratory cycle.

6. **Modes of operation:**

a. Intermittent mandatory ventilation (IMV): A preset number of breaths are delivered each minute. The patient can take breaths on his or her own, but the ventilator may cycle on during a patient breath.
b. Synchronized IMV (SIMV): Similar to IMV, but the ventilator synchronizes delivered breaths with inspiratory effort and allows the patient to finish expiration before cycling on. More comfortable for patient than IMV.
c. Assist control ventilation (AC or AMV): Every inspiratory effort by the patient triggers a ventilator-delivered breath at the set $V_T$. Ventilator-initiated breaths are delivered when the spontaneous rate falls below the backup rate.
d. Pressure support ventilation (PSV): Inspiratory effort opens a valve, allowing airflow at a preset positive pressure. Patient determines rate and inspiratory time. May be used in combination with other modes of operation. Determine effectiveness of ventilation by monitoring tidal volumes.
e. Noninvasive positive-pressure ventilation (NIPPV): Respiratory support provided through face mask.
   (1) Continuous positive airway pressure (CPAP): Delivers airflow (with set $FiO_2$) to maintain a set airway pressure.
   (2) Bilevel positive airway pressure (BiPAP): Delivers airflow to maintain set pressures for inspiration and expiration.

7. **Initial ventilator settings:**

a. Volume limited:
   (1) Rate: Approximately normal range for age (see Table 24-1).
   (2) $V_T$: Approximately 8–10 mL/kg.
   (3) Ti: Generally use inspiration-to-expiration (I/E) ratio of 1:2. More prolonged expiratory phases are required for obstructive diseases to avoid air trapping.
   (4) $FiO_2$: Selected to maintain targeted oxygen saturation and $PaO_2$.
b. Pressure limited:
   (1) Rate: Approximately normal range for age (see Table 24-1).
   (2) PEEP: Start with 3–5 cm $H_2O$ and increase as clinically indicated. (Monitor for decreases in cardiac output with increasing PEEP.)

(3) PIP: Set at pressure required to produce adequate chest wall movement (approximate this using hand-bagging and manometer).
(4) $FiO_2$: Selected to maintain targeted oxygen saturation and $PaO_2$.

c. HFOV:
(1) Frequency: 10 to 15 Hz for neonates, 5 to 8 Hz for children.
(2) Power: Select to achieve adequate chest wall movement.
(3) MAP: 1 to 4 cm $H_2O$ higher than settings on a conventional ventilator.
(4) $FiO_2$: Selected to maintain targeted oxygen saturation and $PaO_2$.

d. High-frequency jet ventilator:
(1) PIP: Increase 2 cm $H_2O$ over conventional ventilator setting.
(2) Ti: Set at 0.02 sec.
(3) Frequency: In neonates, set at 420 cycles/sec.

8. **Further ventilator management:**

a. Follow patient closely with pulse oximetry, end-tidal carbon dioxide measurements, and clinical assessment. Confirm findings with ABGs, and adjust ventilator parameters as indicated (Table 4-11).

b. In cases of ARDS or other condition of poor compliance, or of air leaks, permissive hypercapnia and $V_T$ of 5 mL/kg should be used to avoid barotrauma.

c. Parameters for initiating high-frequency ventilation:
(1) Oxygenation Index (OI) >40 (see section VI.G for calculation of OI).
(2) Inability to provide adequate oxygenation or ventilation with conventional ventilator.

d. Parameters predictive of successful extubation:
(1) $PaCO_2$ appropriate for patient.
(2) PIP generally 14–16 cm $H_2O$.
(3) PEEP 2–3 cm $H_2O$ (infants) or 5 cm $H_2O$ (children).

TABLE 4-11
EFFECTS OF VENTILATOR SETTING CHANGES

| | Typical Effects on Blood Gases | |
|---|---|---|
| Ventilator Setting Changes | $PaCO_2$ | $PaO_2$ |
| ↑ PIP | ↓ | ↑ |
| ↑ PEEP | ↑ | ↑ |
| ↑ Rate (IMV) | ↓ | Minimal ↑ |
| ↑ I:E ratio | No change | ↑ |
| ↑ $FiO_2$ | No change | ↑ |
| ↑ Flow | Minimal ↓ | Minimal ↑ |
| ↑ Power (in HFOV) | ↓ | No change |
| ↑ $\overline{PAW}$ (in HFOV) | Minimal ↓ | ↑ |

$FiO_2$, fraction of inspired oxygen; HFOV, high-frequency oscillatory ventilation; I:E ratio, inspiratory/expiratory ratio; IMV, intermittent mechanical ventilation; $\overline{PAW}$, mean airway pressure; PEEP, positive end-expiratory pressure; PIP, peak inspiratory pressure.

(4) IMV 2 to 4 breaths/min (infants); children may wean to CPAP or pressure support.
(5) $FiO_2$ <40% (maintaining $PaO_2$ >70).
(6) Adequate air leak around endotracheal tube in cases of airway edema or stenosis.
(7) Maximum negative inspiratory pressure (NIF) >20–25 cm $H_2O$.
(8) Minimal secretions.

## E. STATUS EPILEPTICUS (see Chapter 1)

## F. STATUS ASTHMATICUS (see Chapter 1)

## G. CRITICAL CARE REFERENCE DATA

**1. Minute ventilation ($V_E$):**

$$V_E = \text{Respiratory rate} \times \text{tidal volume } (V_T)$$

a. $V_E \times PaCO_2$ = constant (for volume-limited ventilation)
b. Normal $V_T$ = 10–15 mL/kg

**2. Alveolar gas equation:**

$$P_AO_2 = PiO_2 - (P_ACO_2/R)$$

$$PiO_2 = FiO_2 \times (P_B - 47\text{ mm Hg})$$

a. $PiO_2$ = Partial pressure of inspired $O_2$ minus 150 mm Hg at sea level on room air.
b. R = Respiratory exchange quotient ($CO_2$ produced/$O_2$ consumed) = 0.8.
c. $P_ACO_2$ = Partial pressure of alveolar $CO_2$ minus partial pressure of arterial $CO_2$ ($PaCO_2$).
d. $P_B$ = Atmospheric pressure = 760 mm Hg at sea level. Adjust for high-altitude environment.
e. Water vapor pressure = 47 mm Hg.
f. $P_AO_2$ = Partial pressure of $O_2$ in the alveoli.

**3. Alveolar-arterial oxygen gradient (A-a gradient):**

$$\text{A-a gradient} = P_AO_2 - PaO_2$$

a. Obtain ABG, measuring $P_AO_2$ and $P_ACO_2$ with patient on 100% $FiO_2$ for at least 15 min.
b. Calculate the $P_AO_2$ and then the A-a gradient.
c. The larger the gradient, the more serious the respiratory compromise. A normal gradient is 20–65 mm Hg on 100% $O_2$ or 5–20 mm Hg on room air.

**4. Oxygen content ($CaO_2$):**

$$O_2 \text{ content of sample (mL/dL)} = (O_2 \text{ capacity} \times O_2 \text{ saturation [as decimal]}) + \text{dissolved } O_2$$

a. $O_2$ capacity = hemoglobin (g/dL) × 1.34.
b. Dissolved $O_2$ = $PO_2$ (of sample) × 0.003.
c. Hemoglobin carries more than 99% of $O_2$ in blood under standard conditions.

**5. Arteriovenous $O_2$ difference ($AVDo_2$)**

$$AVDo_2 = Cao_2 - Cvo_2 = \text{arterial } O_2 \text{ content} - \text{mixed venous } O_2 \text{ content}$$

a. Usually done after placing patient on 100% $Fio_2$ for 15 min.
b. Obtain ABG and mixed venous blood sample (best obtained from pulmonary artery catheter), and measure $O_2$ saturation in each sample.
c. Calculate arterial and mixed venous oxygen contents and then $AVDo_2$ (normal, 5 mL/100 dL).
d. Used in the calculation of $O_2$ extraction ratio.

**6. $O_2$ extraction ratio:**

$$O_2 \text{ extraction} = (AVDo_2/Cao_2) \times 100$$

Normal range, 28% to 33%.

a. Calculate $AVDo_2$ and $O_2$ contents.
b. Extraction ratios are indicative of the adequacy of $O_2$ delivery to tissues, with increasing extraction ratios suggesting that metabolic needs may be outpacing the oxygen content being delivered.[12]

**7. Oxygenation Index (OI):**

$$OI = \frac{\text{mean airway pressure (cm } H_2O) \times FiO_2 \times 100}{Pao_2}$$

OI > 35 for 5 to 6 hr is one criterion for ECMO (extracorporeal membrane oxygen) support.

**8. Intrapulmonary shunt fraction (Qs/Qt):**

$$\frac{Qs}{Qt} = \frac{(\text{A–a gradient}) \times 0.003}{AVDo_2 + (\text{A–a gradient} \times 0.003)}$$

where Qt is cardiac output and Qs is flow across right-to-left shunt.

a. Formula assumes ABGs obtained on 100% $Fio_2$.
b. Represents the mismatch of ventilation and perfusion and is normally <5%.
c. A rising shunt fraction (usually >15%–20%) is indicative of progressive respiratory failure.

## REFERENCES

1. Marx JA: Rosen's Emergency Medicine: Concepts and Clinical Practice, 6th ed. Philadelphia, Mosby, 2006.
2. Fleisher GR, Ludwig S (eds): Textbook of Pediatric Emergency Medicine, 5th ed. Philadelphia, Lippincott Williams & Wilkins, 2006.
3. Sanchez J, Paidas C: Childhood trauma: Now and in the new millennium. Surg Clin North Am 1999;79(6):1503–1535.
4. Green NE: Skeletal Trauma in Children, 3rd ed. Philadelphia, WB Saunders, 2003.
5. Canale ST: Campbell's Operative Orthopedics, 10th ed. St. Louis, Mosby, 2003.
6. Barkin RM, Rosen P: Emergency Pediatrics: A Guide to Ambulatory Care, 6th ed. St. Louis, Mosby, 2003.

7. Kellogg N: The evaluation of sexual abuse in children. Pediatrics. 2005;116(2):506–512.
8. Section on Radiology: Diagnostic imaging of child abuse. Pediatrics 2000;105(6):1345–1348.
9. Nichols DG et al (eds): Golden Hour: The Handbook of Advanced Pediatric Life Support. St. Louis, Mosby, 1996.
10. Dutton RP, McCunn M: Traumatic brain injury. Curr Opin Crit Care 2003;9(6):503–509.
11. Charney J: Pediatric ventilation outside the operating room. Anesthesiol Clin North Am 2001;19(2):399–404.
12. Rogers M: Textbook of Pediatric Intensive Care, 3rd ed. Baltimore, Williams & Wilkins, 1996.

# PART II

# Diagnostic and Therapeutic Information

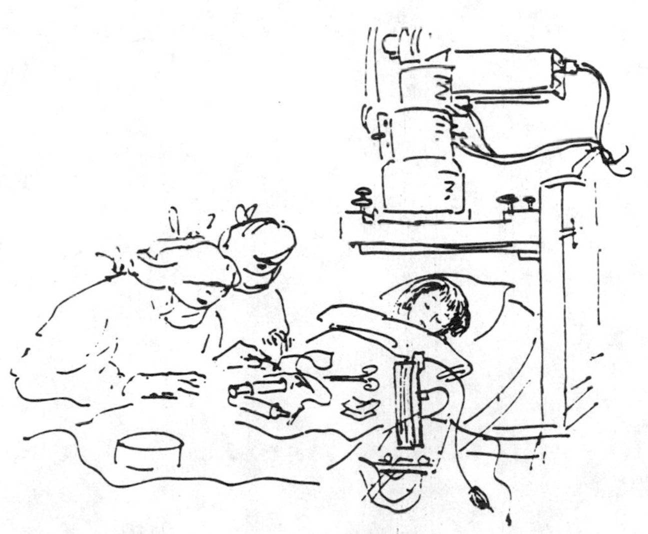

# Adolescent Medicine

Nicole Namour, MD, MPH

5

## I. ADOLESCENT HEALTH MAINTENANCE (Box 5-1)

### A. CHIEF COMPLAINT[1]

Hidden agenda: Adolescents often present with chief complaints that are not the true concern or motivation for the visit. Gentle but persistent questioning ("Is there anything else?") often leads to the actual reason for the visit.

### B. MEDICAL HISTORY[2,3]

Includes information regarding immunizations, chronic illness, trauma or injury (fractures, burns, head injury, fights, sports-related injury), medications (including hormonal contraception, over-the-counter [OTC] drugs, nutritional supplements, and complementary and alternative medicines), recent dental care, hospitalizations, or surgeries.

### C. FAMILY HISTORY[2,3]

Includes any information regarding psychiatric disorders, suicide, alcoholism or substance abuse, and chronic medical conditions or familial risk factors (hypertension, diabetes, cholesterol, heart attack, stroke, cancer, asthma, tuberculosis, human immunodeficiency virus [HIV]).

### D. REVIEW OF SYSTEMS (AREAS OF EMPHASIS WITH AN ADOLESCENT)[2,3]

1. **Nutrition:** Dietary habits, including skipped meals, special diets, purging methods, recent weight gain or loss.
2. **Skin:** Acne, moles, rashes, warts.
3. **Genitourinary:** Dysuria, urgency, frequency, discharge, bleeding.
4. **Menstrual:** Menarche, frequency, duration, pain, menometrorrhagia.

### E. PSYCHOSOCIAL AND MEDICOSOCIAL HISTORY (Table 5-1) (HEADSS)[2–4]

1. **Home:** Household composition; family dynamics and relationships; living and sleeping arrangements; guns in the home; recent changes.
2. **Education:** School attendance, suspensions, grade failure; grades as compared with previous years; attitude toward school; favorite, most difficult, best subjects; special educational needs; goals for the future.
3. **Activities:** Friendships with same or opposite sex, ages of friends, best friend, dating, recreational activities, physical activity, sports participation, hobbies and interests, job, weapon carrying, fighting.
4. **Drugs:** Personal use of tobacco, alcohol, illicit drugs, anabolic steroids; peer substance use; family substance use and attitudes. If personal use, administer **CAGE** questionnaire:

   **C** — Have you ever felt the need to **C**UT down?
   **A** — Have others **A**NNOYED you by commenting on your use?

BOX 5-1

**AAP RECOMMENDATIONS FOR ANNUAL ADOLESCENT PREVENTIVE SERVICES**

Immunizations

Health guidance for teens: Normal development,*,† injury prevention,*,‡ nutrition,* physical activity,* dental health,* breast or testicular self-examination,* skin protection*

Health guidance for parents*

Screening/Counseling:§ Obesity,* contraception,|| tobacco use,* alcohol use,* substance use,* hypertension,* depression/suicide,* eating disorders,* school problems,* abuse,*,†,¶ hearing,* vision*

Tests: Tuberculosis,|| Papanicolaou test,|| human immunodeficiency virus infection,|| sexually transmitted diseases,|| cholesterol,|| urinalysis,|| hematocrit||

*Note:* These are the recommendations of the AAP. Other organizations, including the AAFP, American Academy of Family Physicians; ACIP, Advisory Committee on Immunization Practices; AMA, American Medical Association; BF, Bright Futures; USPSTF, U.S. Preventive Services Task Force, have different recommendations that only suggest some of these services. Refer to Elster AB: Comparison of recommendations for adolescent clinical preventive services developed by national organizations. Arch Pediatr Adolesc Med 1998;152:193 for a comparison list.

*Procedure is recommended for all adolescents/parents.

†This includes providing adolescents with information on normal physical, psychosocial, and sexual development.

‡This includes activities such as promoting the use of safety belts and safety helmets, placement of home smoke detectors, and reducing the risk for injury from firearms and violence. Organizations differ in the activities they include for injury prevention.

§The AAP recommends "development/behavioral assessment."

||Procedure is recommended for selected adolescents who are at high risk for the medical problem.

¶Child abuse is not addressed as a separate screening topic but is included in the general screening for family violence.

**G** — Have you ever felt **G**UILTY about your use or about something you said or did while using?

**E** — Have you ever needed an **E**YE-OPENER (alcohol/drug use first thing in the morning or before noon)?

**Any affirmative answer on CAGE indicates high risk for alcoholism or dependence and requires further assessment.**

**Also helpful in this age group is the CRAFFT questionnaire:**

**C** — Have you ever ridden in a **C**AR driven by someone (or yourself) who was "high" or had been using alcohol or drugs?

**R** — Do you ever use alcohol or drugs to **R**ELAX, feel better about yourself, or fit in?

**A** — Do you ever use alcohol/drugs while you are **A**LONE?

**F** — Do your family or **F**RIENDS ever tell you that you should cut down on your drinking or drug use?

**F** — Do you ever **F**ORGET things you did while using alcohol or drugs?

**T** — Have you gotten into **T**ROUBLE while you were using alcohol or drugs?

TABLE 5-1

PSYCHOSOCIAL DEVELOPMENT OF ADOLESCENTS

| Task | Early Adolescence (10–13 yr) | Middle Adolescence (14–16 yr) | Late Adolescence (>17 yr) |
|---|---|---|---|
| Independence | Less interest in parental activities<br>Wide mood swings | Peak of parental conflicts | Reacceptance of parental advice and values |
| Body image | Preoccupation with self and pubertal changes<br>Uncertainty about appearance | General acceptance of body<br>Concern over making body more attractive | Acceptance of pubertal changes |
| Peers | Intense relationships with same-sex friend | Peak of peer involvement<br>Conformity with peer values<br>Increased sexual activity and experimentation | Peer group less important<br>More time spent in sharing intimate relationships |
| Identity | Increased cognition<br>Increased fantasy world<br>Idealistic vocational goals<br>Increased need for privacy<br>Lack of impulse control | Increased scope of feelings<br>Increased intellectual ability<br>Feeling of omnipotence<br>Risk-taking behavior | Practical, realistic vocational goals<br>Refinement of moral, religious, and sexual values<br>Ability to compromise and to set limits |



Two or more affirmative answers suggest a significant problem.

5. **Sexuality:** Sexual feelings toward opposite or same sex; sexual intercourse or types of sexual practices—age at first intercourse, number of lifetime and current partners, ages of partners, recent change in partners; contraception and sexually transmitted disease (STD) prevention; history of STD, prior pregnancies, abortions; ever fathered a child; history of nonconsensual intimate physical contact or sex; sex for money or drugs.
6. **Suicide/depression:** Feelings about self, both positive and negative; history of depression or other mental health problems; current or prior suicidal thoughts; prior suicide attempts; sleep problems: difficulty getting to sleep, early waking; changes in appetite or weight; anhedonia; irritability; anxiety.

## F. PHYSICAL EXAMINATION (MOST PERTINENT ASPECTS)[2,3,5]

1. **Height, weight (calculate body mass index [BMI]), and blood pressure with percentiles.**

2. **Dentition and gums (smokeless tobacco use, enamel erosion from induced vomiting).**
3. **Skin:** Acne (type and distribution of lesions), scars, piercings, tattoos.
4. **Thyroid.**
5. **Spine:** Scoliosis (see section V).
6. **Breasts:** Tanner stage (Fig. 5-1), masses (females); gynecomastia (males).
7. **External genitalia:**
   a. Visual inspection (human papillomavirus, ulcers, rashes, pubic lice, trauma, discharge).
   b. Pubic hair distribution: Tanner stage (Figs. 5-2 and 5-3).
   c. Testicular examination: Tanner stage (Table 5-2), masses (hydrocele, varicocele, hernia).

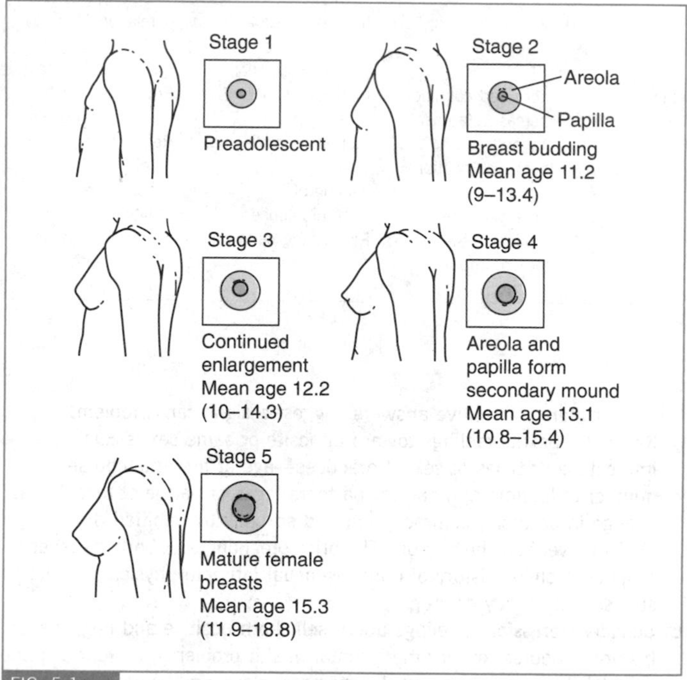


FIG. 5-1

Tanner stages of breast development in females. *(Modified from Johnson TR et al: Children Are Different: Developmental Physiology, 2nd ed. Columbus, Ohio, Ross Laboratories, 1978. Mean age and range [2 standard deviations around mean] from Joffe A: Introduction to adolescent medicine. In McMillan JA et al [eds]: Oski's Pediatrics Principles and Practice, 3rd ed. Philadelphia, Lippincott Williams & Wilkins, 1999, p 531.)*

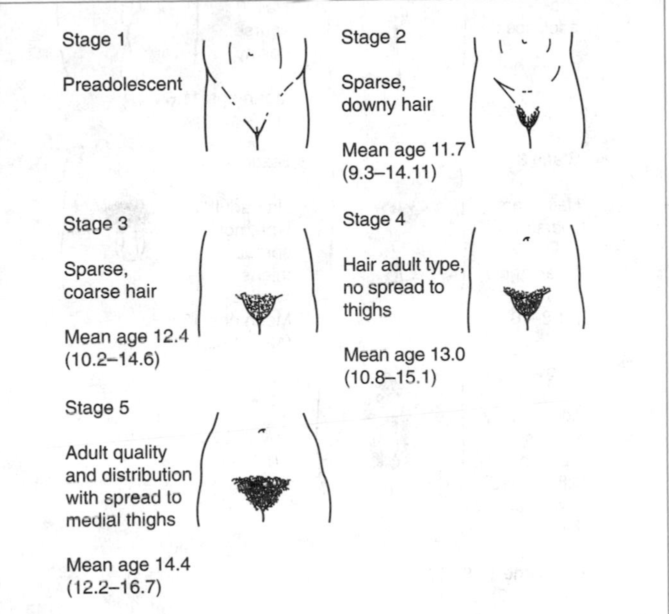


FIG 5-2

Pubic hair development in females. *(Modified from Neinstein LS, Kaufman FR: Normal physical growth and development. In Neinstein LS [ed]: Adolescent Healthcare: A Practical Guide, 4th ed. Philadelphia, Lippincott Williams & Wilkins, 2002, p 28. Age range [2 standard deviations around mean] from Joffe A: Introduction to adolescent medicine. In McMillan JA et al [eds]: Oski's Pediatrics Principles and Practice, 3rd ed. Philadelphia, Lippincott Williams & Wilkins, 1999, p 531.)*

8. **Pelvic examination:** Any age female who is sexually active or has a gynecologic complaint; suggest a screening Papanicolaou (Pap) smear for females who have been sexually active for 3 or more years or any female age ≥21 years. See Table 5-3 for course of action based on results of Pap smear.

## G. LABORATORY TESTS[2,3]

1. **Purified protein derivative (PPD):** If high risk for tuberculosis, see Chapter 17 for screening recommendations.
2. **Hemoglobin and hematocrit:** Once during puberty for males; at least once after menarche for females.

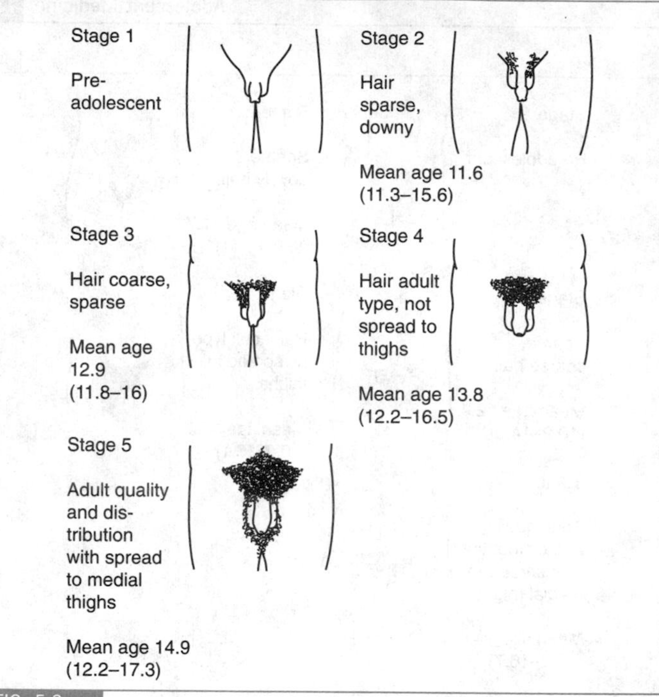


FIG. 5-3

Pubic hair development in males. *(Data from Neinstein LS, Kaufman FR: Normal physical growth and development. In Neinstein LS [ed]: Adolescent Healthcare: A Practical Guide, 4th ed. Philadelphia, Lippincott Williams & Wilkins, 2002, p 30. Age range [2 standard deviations around mean] from Joffe A: Introduction to adolescent medicine. In McMillan JA et al [eds]: Oski's Pediatrics Principles and Practice, 3rd ed. Philadelphia, Lippincott Williams & Wilkins, 1999, p 531.)*

TABLE 5-2

**GENITAL DEVELOPMENT (MALE)**

| Stage | Comment (±2 standard deviation around mean age) |
|---|---|
| 1 | Preadolescent: Testes, scrotum, and penis about same size and proportion as in early childhood |
| 2 | Enlargement of scrotum and testes; skin of scrotum reddens and changes in texture; little or no enlargement of penis; mean age 11.4 yr (9.5–13.8 yr) |
| 3 | Enlargement of penis, first mainly in length; further growth of testes and scrotum; mean age 12.9 yr (10.8–14.9 yr) |
| 4 | Increased size of penis with growth in breadth and development of glans; further enlargement of testes and scrotum and increased darkening of scrotal skin; mean age 13.77 yr (11.7–15.8 yr) |
| 5 | Genitalia adult in size and shape; mean age 14.9 yr (13–17.3 yr) |

Data from Joffe A: Introduction to adolescent medicine. In McMillan JA et al (eds): Oski's Pediatrics Principles and Practice, 3rd ed. Philadelphia, Lippincott Williams & Wilkins, 1999, pp 530–531.

TABLE 5-3

SUMMARY OF TREATMENT RECOMMENDATIONS FOR CYTOLOGIC AND HISTOLOGIC ABNORMALITIES IN ADOLESCENTS

| Diagnosis | ACOG Recommendation for Adolescents |
|---|---|
| ASC-US with positive HPV | Repeat Pap test in 6 and 12 mo or HPV test alone in 12 mo |
| ASC-US with negative HPV | Repeat Pap test in 12 mo |
| ASC-H | Colposcopy |
| LSIL | Repeat Pap test in 6 and 12 mo or HPV test alone in 12 mo |
| HSIL | Colposcopy |
| AGC | Colposcopy, endocervical assessment, possible endometrial evaluation |
| Cancer | Colposcopy with endocervical assessment |
| CIN 1 | Pap test at 6 and 12 mo or HPV test alone at 12 mo, colposcopy for any abnormality |
| CIN 2 | Close follow-up at 4- to 6-mo intervals (cytology or colposcopy) |
| CIN 3 | Ablative or excision therapy |

ACOG, American College of Obstetricians and Gynecologists; AGC, atypical glandular cells; ASC-H, atypical squamous cells, cannot rule out high-grade squamous intraepithelial lesion; ASC-US, atypical squamous cells—undetermined significance; CIN, cervical intraepithelial neoplasia; HPV, human papillomavirus; HSIL, high-grade SIL; LSIL, low-grade squamous intraepithelial lesion.

From ACOG: Evaluation and management of abnormal cervical cytology and histology in the adolescent. Committee Opinion. Obstet Gynecol 2006;107(4):965.

3. **Urinalysis and microscopic evaluation: First encounter or end of puberty; pyuria is an indication for further evaluation for urinary tract infection.**
4. **Sexually active adolescents:**
   a. Serologic tests: Syphilis and HIV annually.
   b. Males: First-part voided urinalysis and leukocyte esterase screen can be used alone with positive results confirmed by detection tests for gonorrhea and *Chlamydia,* including cultures, ligase chain reaction (LCR), and polymerase chain reaction (PCR), or these tests can be sent automatically with the first-voided urine.
   c. Females: Detection tests for gonorrhea and *Chlamydia* (i.e., cultures, LCR, PCR), wet preparation, potassium hydroxide (KOH), cervical Gram stain, Pap smear, mid-vaginal pH.
5. **Cholesterol: Once during puberty or if personal or familial risk factors (refer to Chapter 7 for more information).**

## H. IMMUNIZATIONS[2,3,6]

See Chapter 16 for dosing, route, formulation, and schedules.

1. **Tetanus, diphtheria, and pertussis (Tdap): Booster at age 11 to 12 years and Td vaccine every 10 years thereafter.**
2. **Measles: Two doses of live attenuated vaccine required after first birthday. Use measles, mumps, rubella (MMR) vaccine if not**

previously immunized for mumps or rubella. Assess pregnancy status; do not administer rubella vaccine to any woman anticipating pregnancy within 90 days.

3. **Hepatitis B vaccine (HBV):** Recommended for all adolescents if not previously vaccinated using the three-dose regimen recommended by the Advisory Committee on Immunization Practices (ACIP) and the American Academy of Pediatrics (AAP).
4. **Varicella vaccine:** Recommended if not previously vaccinated and no personal history of disease. Two doses 3 months apart if <13 years; 2 doses 4 to 8 weeks apart if >13 years.
5. **Meningococcal vaccine (MCV4):** Recommended for all adolescents at age 11 to 12 years or at high school entry. If it has not already been received, all adolescents should receive it before entering college or military enlistment, especially if living in dormitories.
6. **Hepatitis A vaccine (HAV):** Recommended for all adolescents who have not received it after age 1 year. Administered as 2 doses 6 months apart.
7. **Human papillomavirus vaccine:** Recommended for adolescent females at age 11 to 12 years, but may be given to any female age 9 to 26 years. Administered as 3 doses within a 6-month period.

### I. ANTICIPATORY GUIDANCE

See Box 5-1.

## II. PUBERTAL EVENTS AND TANNER STAGE DIAGRAMS[2]

### A. PSYCHOSOCIAL DEVELOPMENT (see Table 5-1)

### B. TEMPORAL RELATIONSHIP OF THE BIOLOGIC EVENTS OF ADOLESCENCE (see Figs. 5-1 to 5-3 and Table 5-2) (Age limits for the events and stages are approximations and may differ from those used by other authors)

1. **Precocious puberty:** The onset of secondary sexual characteristics before age 8 years in girls and 9 years in boys.
2. **Delayed puberty:** The lack of secondary sexual development by age 13 years in girls and 14 years in boys.
3. **Mean peak height velocity:**

a. Girls: 12.1 years (±2 standard deviations;10.4 to 13.9 years).
b. Boys: 14.1 years (±2 standard deviations;12.2 to 15.9 years).

## III. CONTRACEPTIVE INFORMATION

### A. METHODS OF CONTRACEPTION (Table 5-4)

### B. COMBINED HORMONAL CONTRACEPTIVES (ESTROGEN AND PROGESTERONE)

1. **Contraindications**[7] (developed for oral contraceptive pill [OCP], but apply to any contraceptive containing estrogen).

a. Refrain from providing (World Health Organization [WHO] category 4): History of thrombophlebitis or thromboembolic disease, stroke, ischemic

TABLE 5-4

METHODS OF CONTRACEPTION

| Method | Failure Rate (%) Typical Use | Failure Rate (%) Perfect Use | Benefits | Risks/Disadvantages |
|---|---|---|---|---|
| **COMBINED HORMONAL** | | | | |
| Oral | 8 | 0.3 | Intercourse-independent; rapid reversibility; daily, weekly, or monthly dosing options; decreased risk for dysmenorrhea, rheumatoid arthritis, iron-deficiency anemia, ovarian and uterine cancers, ovarian cysts, acne, ectopic pregnancy, benign breast disorders | Thromboembolic phenomena, cerebrovascular accident, hypertension, worsening migraines, nausea, weight gain, breast tenderness, breakthrough bleeding, amenorrhea, depression; not a barrier to STD |
| Transdermal | 8 | 0.3 | | |
| Injectable | 0.1 | 0.3 | | |
| Vaginal ring | 8 | | | |
| **PROGESTIN ONLY** | | | | |
| DMPA | 3 | 0.3 | Intercourse-independent; can be used while breast-feeding; no estrogen; decreased risk for ovarian/endometrial cancer; no drug interactions; pill and implant have rapid reversibility | Menstrual irregularity/amenorrhea, weight gain, reversible osteopenia, mood changes, breast tenderness, headaches; not a barrier to STD; DMPA delays return to fertility |
| Progestin pill | 3 | 0.05 | | |
| Implant | 0.05 | 0.05 | | |

*Note:* (1) Emergency contraception decreases the risk of pregnancy by ≥75% if used within 72 hr. (2) The following methods are generally not recommended for adolescents:[13] progesterone-only pill, intrauterine devices, diaphragm, cervical cap, female condom, withdrawal, spermicide, natural family planning.
DMPA, depomedroxyprogesterone acetate; IUD, intrauterine device; PID, pelvic inflammatory disease; STD, sexually transmitted disease; UTI, urinary tract infection.

Data from Neinstein LS, Nelson AL: Contraception. In Neinstein LS (ed): Adolescent Healthcare: A Practical Guide, 4th ed. Philadelphia, Lippincott Williams & Wilkins, 2002, p 836, and Nelson AL, Neinstein LS: Intrauterine devices. In Neinstein LS (ed): Adolescent Healthcare: A Practical Guide, 4th ed. Philadelphia, Lippincott Williams & Wilkins, 2002, pp 884–887.

Continued

TABLE 5-4

METHODS OF CONTRACEPTION—cont'd

| Method | Failure Rate (%) | | Benefits | Risks/Disadvantages |
|---|---|---|---|---|
| | Typical Use | Perfect Use | | |
| **IUD** | | | | |
| CopperT380A | 0.8 | 0.6 | Decreased ectopic pregnancy; intercourse-independent, rapidly reversible, discreet | Practitioner placement/removal required; only appropriate for low risk (parous and monogamous); no STD protection; may increase PID, *Actinomyces* colonization, or infection; increased menstrual bleeding and cramping (CopperT380A only); expulsion, perforation, or embedment |
| Levonorgestrel IUS | 0.1 | 0.1 | | |
| **BARRIER** | | | | |
| Male condom | 15 | 2 | No major risks; low cost, nonprescription; male involved; protects against STD and cervical cancer | Decreased sensation; use with each act of coitus; requires male cooperation |
| Diaphragm with contraceptive cream or jelly | 16 | 6 | Most effective female barrier method; reduced risk for STD; may be placed in anticipation; single insertion for multiple acts of intercourse | Professional fitting and prescription only; requires motivation, preparation, and access; messy; allergies, increased risk for UTI, small risk for toxic shock syndrome |
| Female condom | 21 | 5 | May be inserted up to 8 hr before coitus | Complex and difficult to place; low efficacy; lack of STD reduction evidence; expensive; use with each act of coitus; associated noise |
| **OTHER** | | | | |
| Withdrawal | 27 | | | |
| Spermicide | 29 | | | |
| **NO METHOD** | **85** | | | |

(coronary) heart disease, complicated structural heart disease, breast cancer, estrogen-dependent neoplasia; pregnancy; lactation for <6 weeks; liver disease (including liver cancer, benign hepatic adenoma, active viral hepatitis, severe cirrhosis); diabetes with vascular complications; headaches with focal neurologic symptoms; major surgery with prolonged immobilization; any surgery on the legs; hypertension with pressures higher than 160/100 mm Hg or with vascular disease; thrombogenic mutations, including factor V Leiden, prothrombin mutation; protein C, S, or antithrombin deficiencies.

b. Exercise caution (WHO category 3): Postpartum for <21 days, lactation for 6 weeks to 6 months, use of drugs that affect liver enzymes (e.g., rifampin, griseofulvin, anticonvulsants), gallbladder disease, hypertension with pressures 140–159/90–99 mm Hg, or history of hypertension where pressures could not be evaluated.

c. Advantages generally outweigh disadvantages (WHO category 2): Major surgery without prolonged immobilization, sickle cell disease, undiagnosed abnormal vaginal or uterine bleeding, undiagnosed breast mass, headaches without focal neurologic symptoms, superficial thrombophlebitis, uncomplicated valvular heart disease, smoking and <age 35 years, obese (BMI > 30), cervical cancer or lesions, diabetes without complications, mental retardation, drug or alcohol abuse, severe psychiatric disorders, family history of hyperlipidemia or myocardial infarction before age 50 years.



**2. Serious complications (ACHES):**[8]

a. **A**bdominal pain (pelvic vein or mesenteric vein thrombosis, pancreatitis).

b. **C**hest pain (pulmonary embolism).

c. **H**eadaches (thrombotic or hemorrhagic stroke, retinal vein thrombosis).

d. **E**ye symptoms (thrombotic or hemorrhagic stroke, retinal vein thrombosis).

e. **S**evere leg pain (thrombophlebitis of the lower extremity).

**3. OCP instructions:**[9]

a. Take 1 pill each day, preferably at the same time of day.

b. Take the **first** pill on the first to the seventh day (first day is preferred, Sunday start most common) after the beginning of your menstrual period.

c. Some pill packs have 28 pills; others have 21 pills. When the 28-day pack is empty, immediately start taking pills from a new pack. When the 21-day pack is empty, wait 1 week (7 days) and then begin taking pills from a new pack.

d. If you **vomit** within 30 minutes of taking a pill, take another pill or use a backup method if you have sex during the next 7 days.

e. If you forget to take 1 pill, take it as soon as you remember, even if it means taking 2 pills in 1 day.

f. If you forget to take 2 or more pills, take 2 pills every day until you are back on schedule. Use a backup method (e.g., condoms) or do not have sex for 7 days.
g. If you miss 2 or more menstrual periods, come to the clinic for a pregnancy test.
h. Need backup method for first month.
i. No STD protection; therefore, a barrier method should be used in addition to the pill.

4. **Transdermal (patch) instructions:**[10]
a. Apply within 5 days of the onset of menses anywhere on trunk or upper extremities except breasts.
b. Replace every 7 days for 3 weeks.
c. Allow 7 days without patch for menses, then restart cycle.
d. Rotate location of application to avoid skin irritation.
e. If patch falls off, put on new patch as soon as possible and use backup method of contraception.

5. **Combination monthly injection instructions:**[10,11]
a. First injection during first 5 days of menstrual cycle or 7 days after first- or second-trimester abortion or 21 to 29 days postpartum if not breast-feeding.
b. Reinjection 23 to 33 days after prior injection.
c. Return to clinic for pregnancy test if you have missed two periods.

6. **Vaginal ring instructions:**[10]
a. Ring placed in vagina for 3 weeks.
b. Ring removed for 1 week for withdrawal bleeding.
c. New ring placed in vagina for 3 weeks.
d. If ring is expelled, rinse with water and reinsert; backup contraception is needed if ring is out for >3 hr.

7. **Follow-up recommendations:**[12]
a. Pelvic examination at baseline or during first 3 to 6 months of use, then annually.
b. Two or three follow-up visits per year to monitor patient compliance, blood pressure, and side effects.

### C. LONG-ACTING PROGESTIN METHODS

1. **Contraindications:**[13] Active thrombophlebitic or thromboembolic disorders, undiagnosed abnormal genital bleeding, pregnancy, acute liver disease, carcinoma of the breast, history of intracranial hypertension, hypersensitivity to components, hypertension with pressures greater than 160/100 mm Hg, diabetes with vascular disease, ischemic heart disease, stroke; <6 weeks postpartum.
2. **Not contraindicated:**[13] Breast-feeding, history of thrombosis, hypertriglyceridemia, tobacco abuse, migraine, systemic lupus,

hepatic disease, sickle cell (evidence suggests reduced frequency/severity of painful crises), seizure disorder.

3. **Depomedroxyprogesterone acetate (DMPA) injection instructions:**[13]
a. Initial injection first 5 days after onset of menses.
b. Reinjection every 11 to 13 weeks.
c. Reinjection after 13 weeks or initial injection after first 5 days of cycle (Fig. 5-4).

## D. EMERGENCY CONTRACEPTIVE PILL (ECP) (Table 5-5)

1. **Contraindications:**[14]
a. The contraindications for estrogen-containing emergency contraception regimens are the same as those for OCPs (see section III.B.1), but use over time has shown that such stringent restrictions for single use are not necessary. History of previous thrombosis is not a contraindication for single use, but progesterone-only methods are preferred.
b. Progesterone-only regimen contraindications are pregnancy, undiagnosed abnormal genital bleeding, or hypersensitivity to a component of the product.
c. ECP is contraindicated with pregnancy because of maternal side effects without offsetting benefits; no evidence of teratogenic risk.

2. **Guidelines and instructions for use:**[14,15]
a. Advance prescription should be considered with sexually active teens. New regulations allow OTC use in women ≥age 18 years.
b. May be combined with other ongoing methods of birth control.
  (1) OCP may start 24 hr after second ECP dose.
  (2) DMPA can be given the same day.
c. Recommend diphenhydramine 1 hr before the first dose of ECP to reduce nausea.
d. First ECP dose should be taken as soon as possible. Linear relationship between efficacy and the time from intercourse to treatment. Most effective when used within 72 hr after unprotected sex, but can be used up to 120 hr after intercourse.
e. Second ECP dose should be taken 12 hr after the first dose. With Plan B, both doses can be taken at the same time.
f. Pregnancy test may be administered before taking an ECP, but the dose should not be delayed for this because efficacy diminishes over time to dosing.
g. Take the opportunity to discuss proper use of regular birth control for the future.
h. No absolute limit of ECP frequency during a cycle if there is need, but women using ECP frequently should be advised of other, more effective methods of birth control.
i. Perform pregnancy test if there is no menstrual period within 3 weeks of ECP treatment.

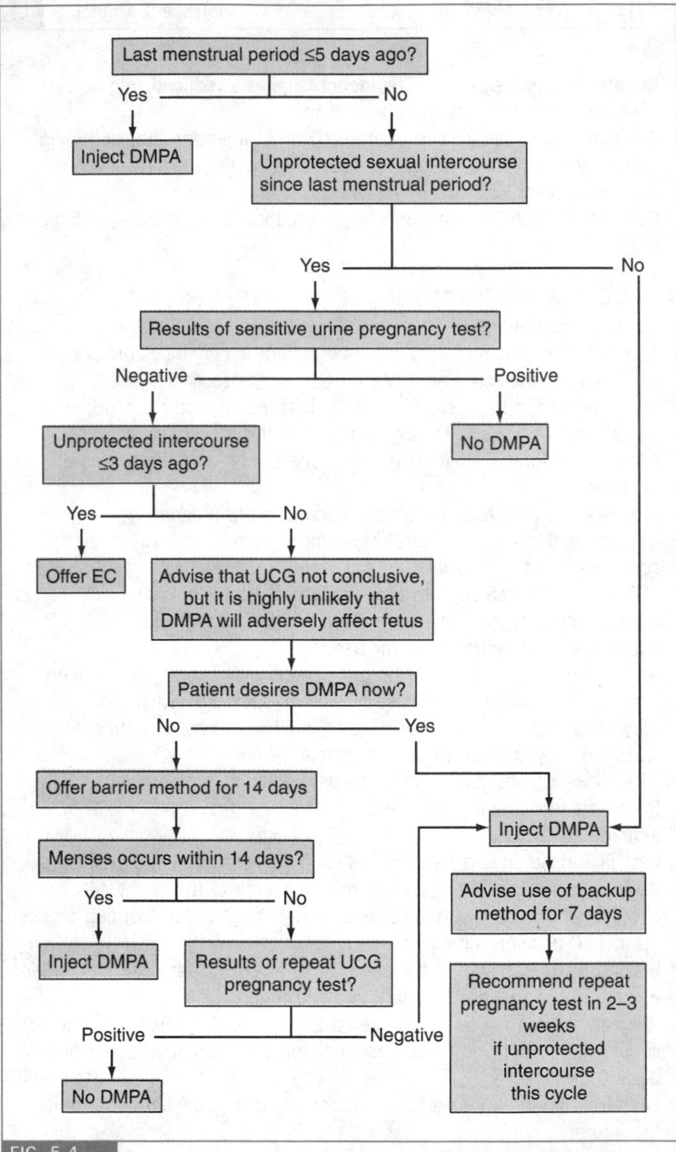


FIG. 5-4

Depomedroxyprogesterone acetate (DMPA) use algorithm for initial or late injection. *(Data from Nelson AL, Neinstein LS: Long acting progestins. In Neinstein LS [ed]: Adolescent Healthcare: A Practical Guide, 4th ed. Philadelphia, Lippincott Williams & Wilkins, 2002, p 931.)*

TABLE 5-5

EMERGENCY CONTRACEPTIVE PILL*

| Trade Name | Ethinyl Estradiol per Dose (mg) | Levonorgestrel per Dose (mg) | Pills per Dose† |
|---|---|---|---|
| Plan B‡ | 0 | 0.75 | 1 white |
| Preven‡ | 0.1 | 0.5 | 2 blue |
| Alesse | 0.1 | 0.5 | 5 pink |
| Aviane | 0.1 | 0.5 | 5 orange |
| Levlen | 0.12 | 0.6 | 4 light-orange |
| Lo-Ovral | 0.12 | 0.6 | 4 white |
| Nordette | 0.12 | 0.6 | 4 light-orange |
| Ovral | 0.1 | 0.5 | 2 white |
| Seasonale | 0.12 | 0.6 | 4 pink |
| Triphasil | 0.12 | 0.5 | 4 yellow |
| Trilevlen | 0.12 | 0.5 | 4 yellow |

*Oral contraceptive pills approved by the FDA for use as emergency contraception.
†All require 2 doses; both doses of Plan B can be given at the same time.
‡Manufactured solely for the purpose of emergency contraception.

Modified from Brill SR, Rosenfeld WD: Med Clin North Am, Adolesc Med 2000;84:12.



## IV. VAGINAL INFECTIONS, GENITAL ULCERS, AND WARTS

See Chapter 17 for discussion of infection with chlamydia, gonorrhea, pelvic inflammatory disease, and HIV and for further discussion of syphilis. See Formulary for additional information and comments regarding specific medications. After diagnosis of an STD, encourage the patient to refrain from intercourse until full therapy is complete, the partner is treated, and all visible lesions are resolved.

### A. DIAGNOSTIC FEATURES AND MANAGEMENT OF VAGINAL INFECTION (Table 5-6)

### B. DIAGNOSTIC FEATURES AND MANAGEMENT OF GENITAL ULCERS AND WARTS (Table 5-7)

## V. SCOLIOSIS[16]

Refer to Figure 5-5 for routine screening for scoliosis. Many curves that are detected on screening are nonprogressive or too slight to be significant.

### A. ASSESSMENT

1. **Radiographic determination of the Cobb angle (Fig. 5-6): If there is clinical suspicion of significant scoliosis on screening, use erect thoracoabdominal spinal view.**
2. **Bone scan with or without magnetic resonance imaging (MRI): If pain is worse at night, progressive, well localized, or otherwise suspicious, obtain bone scan or MRI to look for tumor, infection, or fracture.**

*Text continued on p. 148*

TABLE 5-6

## DIAGNOSTIC FEATURES AND MANAGEMENT OF VAGINAL INFECTIONS

| | Normal Vaginal Examination | Yeast Vaginitis | Trichomoniasis | Bacterial Vaginosis |
|---|---|---|---|---|
| Etiology | Uninfected; *Lactobacillus* predominant | *Candida albicans* and other yeasts | *Trichomonas vaginalis* | Associated with *Gardnerella vaginalis*, various anaerobic bacteria, and mycoplasma |
| Typical symptoms | None | Vulvar itching and/or irritation, increased discharge | Malodorous purulent discharge, vulvar itching | Malodorous, slightly increased discharge |
| Discharge | | | | |
| • Amount | Variable; usually scant | Scant to moderate | Profuse | Moderate |
| • Color* | Clear or white | White | Yellow-green | Usually white or gray |
| • Consistency | Nonhomogeneous, floccular | Clumped; adherent plaques | Homogeneous | Homogeneous, low viscosity; smoothly coating vaginal walls |
| Inflammation of vulvar or vaginal epithelium | No | Yes | Yes | No |
| pH of vaginal fluid[†] | Usually <4.5 | Usually <4.5 | Usually >5.0 | Usually >4.5 |
| Amine ("fishy") odor with 10% KOH | None | None | May be present | Present |

| | | | | |
|---|---|---|---|---|
| Microscopy[‡] | Normal epithelial cells; *Lactobacillus* predominates | Leukocytes, epithelial cells, yeast, mycelia, or pseudomycelia in 40%–80% of cases | Leukocytes; motile trichomonads seen in 50%–70% of symptomatic patients, less often in the absence of symptoms | Clue cells, few leukocytes; *Lactobacillus* outnumbered by profuse mixed flora, nearly always including *G. vaginalis* plus anaerobic species, on Gram stain |
| Usual treatment | None | Single dose of oral fluconazole, or miconazole or clotrimazole vaginal suppository | Metronidazole, single dose or 7-day course | Oral or topical metronidazole or oral clindamycin |
| Usual management of sex partners | None | None; topical treatment if candidal dermatitis of penis is present | Treatment recommended | Examine for sexually transmitted disease; routine treatment not recommended |

*Note:* Gram stain is also excellent for detecting yeasts and pseudomycelia and for distinguishing normal flora from the mixed flora seen in bacterial vaginosis, but it is less sensitive than the saline preparation for detection of *T. vaginalis*. Refer to Formulary for dosing information.

*Color of discharge is determined by examining vaginal discharge against the white background of a swab.

[†]pH determination is not useful if blood is present.

[‡]To detect fungal elements, vaginal fluid is digested with 10% KOH before microscopic examination; to examine for other features, fluid is mixed (1:1) with physiologic saline.

From Holmes KK et al: Sexually Transmitted Diseases. New York: McGraw-Hill; 1990 and Centers for Disease Control and Prevention: Guidelines for treatment of sexually transmitted diseases. MMWR 1998;47(RR-1):1–118.

TABLE 5-7

**DIAGNOSTIC FEATURES AND MANAGEMENT OF GENITAL ULCERS AND WARTS**

| Infection | Clinical Presentation | Presumptive Diagnosis | Definitive Diagnosis | Treatment/Management of Sex Partners |
|---|---|---|---|---|
| Genital herpes | Grouped vesicles, painful shallow ulcers; tender inguinal adenopathy | Tzanck smear looking for multinucleated giant cells | Viral culture | No known cure. Prompt initiation of therapy shortens duration of first episode. For severe recurrent disease, initiate therapy at start of prodrome or within 1 day of onset of lesions. See Formulary for dosing of acyclovir, famciclovir, or valacyclovir. Transmission can occur during asymptomatic periods. |
| Primary syphilis | Indurated, well-defined, usually single painless ulcer or "chancre"; nontender inguinal adenopathy | Nontreponemal serologic test: VDRL, RPR, or STS | Treponemal serologic test: FTA-ABS or MHA-TP; darkfield microscopy or direct fluorescent antibody tests of lesion exudates or tissue | Parenteral penicillin G is preferred treatment; preparation(s), dosage, and length of treatment depend on stage and clinical manifestations (see Chapter 17). All sexual contacts of persons with acquired syphilis should be evaluated. Contacts within the previous 3 months may be falsely seronegative; presumptive treatment recommended. |
| HPV infection (genital warts) | Single or multiple soft, fleshy, papillary or sessile, painless growths around the anus, vulvovaginal area, penis, urethra, or perineum; no inguinal adenopathy | Typical clinical presentation | Papanicolaou smear revealing typical cytologic changes | Treatment does not eradicate infection. *Goal:* Removal of exophytic warts. Exclude cervical dysplasia before treatment. Patient-administered therapies include podofilox and imiquimod cream. Clinician-applied therapies include podophyllin 10%–25% in compound tincture of benzoin, bichloroacetic or trichloroacetic acid, and surgical removal. Podofilox, imiquimod, and podophyllin are contraindicated in pregnancy. Period of communicability is unknown. |

*Note:* Chancroid, lymphogranuloma venereum (LGV), and granuloma inguinale should be considered in the differential diagnosis of genital ulcers if the clinical presentation is atypical and tests for herpes and syphilis are negative.

FTA-ABS, fluorescent treponemal antibody absorbed; HPV, human papilloma virus; MHA-TP, microhemagglutination assay for antibody to *T. pallidum*; RPR, rapid plasma reagin; STS, serologic test for syphilis; VDRL, Venereal Disease Research Laboratory.

Modified from Centers for Disease Control and Prevention: Guidelines for treatment of sexually transmitted diseases. MMWR 1998;47(RR-1):1–118 and Adger H: Sexually transmitted diseases. In Oski FA et al (eds): Principles and Practice of Pediatrics. Philadelphia, Lippincott, Williams & Wilkins, 1999.

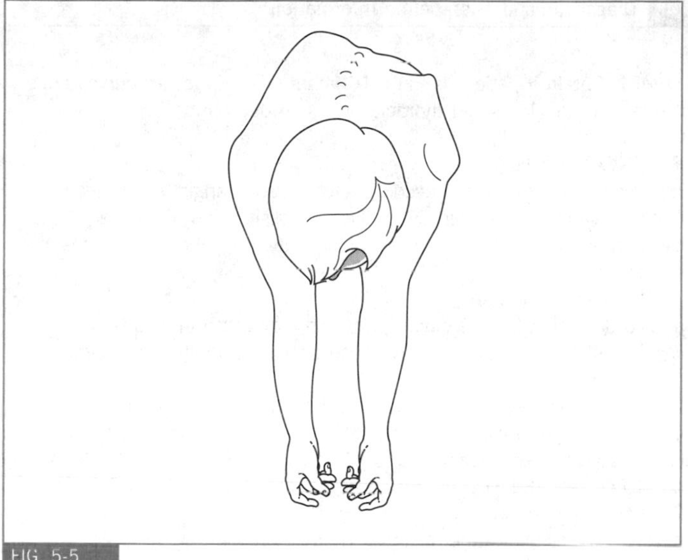

FIG. 5-5

Forward bending test. This emphasizes any asymmetry of the paraspinous muscles and rib cage.

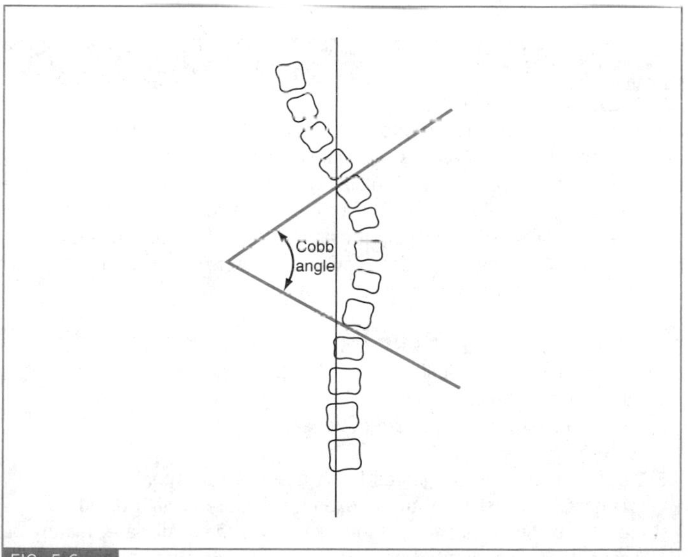


FIG. 5-6

Cobb angle. This is measured using the superior and inferior end plates of the most tilted vertebrae at the end of each curve.

3. **MRI:** Obtain if patient is <age 10 years or if "opposite" curves are present (i.e., left-sided thoracic or right-sided lumbar).

### B. TREATMENT

Treatment plan determined according to the Cobb angle and skeletal maturity, which is assessed by grading the ossification of the iliac crest. It can be estimated in females; skeletal maturity is reached 18 months after menarche.

1. **Skeletally immature:**
   a. <10 degrees: Obtain a single follow-up radiograph in 4 to 6 months to ensure there has been no significant progression of the scoliosis.
   b. 10 to 20 degrees: Obtain follow-up radiographs every 4 to 6 months while still growing.
   c. 20 to 40 degrees: Bracing is required.
   d. >40 degrees: Surgical correction is necessary.
2. **Skeletally mature:**
   a. <40 degrees: No further evaluation or intervention is indicated.
   b. >40 degrees: Surgical correction is required.
3. **Orthopedic referral:** Indicated if the patient is skeletally immature with a curve >20 degrees or skeletally mature with a curve >40 degrees, or in the presence of suspicious pain or neurologic symptoms.

## VI. RECOMMENDED COMPONENTS OF THE PREPARTICIPATION PHYSICAL EVALUATION (PPE)[17,18]

### A. MEDICAL HISTORY

Should include information regarding illnesses/injuries since the last examination; chronic conditions and medications; hospitalizations or surgeries; medications used by athletes (including performance-enhancing agents); use of special equipment or protective devices during sports participation; allergies, particularly those associated with anaphylaxis or respiratory compromise and those provoked by exercise; immunization status (HBV, MMR, tetanus, and varicella).

### B. REVIEW OF SYSTEMS AND PHYSICAL EXAMINATION ITEMS

Examination items are in italics.

1. **Height and weight.**
2. **Vision:** Visual problems, corrective lenses; *visual acuity, pupil equality.*
3. **Cardiac:** History of congenital heart disease; syncope, dizziness, or chest pain during exercise; history of high blood pressure or heart murmurs; family history of heart disease; history of disqualification or limited participation in sports because of a cardiac problem; *blood pressure, heart rate and rhythm, pulses (including*

*radial/femoral lag), auscultation for heart sounds, murmurs—both standing and supine.*

4. **Respiratory:** Asthma, coughing, wheezing, or dyspnea during exercise.
5. **Abdomen:** Organomegaly and single kidney are contraindications for contact sports.
6. **Genitourinary:** Age at menarche, last menstrual period, regularity of menstrual periods, number of periods in the last year, longest interval between periods, dysmenorrhea; *palpation of the abdomen, palpation of the testicles, examination of the inguinal canals.*
7. **Orthopedic:** Previous injuries that have limited sports participation or required medical intervention; screening orthopedic examination (Fig. 5-7).
8. **Neurology:** History of a significant head injury/concussion; numbness or tingling in the extremities; severe headaches; seizure disorder.
9. **Skin:** Rashes; *evidence of contagious infections (e.g., varicella or impetigo).*
10. **Psychosocial:** Weight control and body image; stresses at home or in school; use or abuse of drugs and alcohol; *attention to signs of eating disorders, including oral ulcerations, eroded tooth enamel, edema, lanugo hair, calluses or ulcerations on knuckles.*

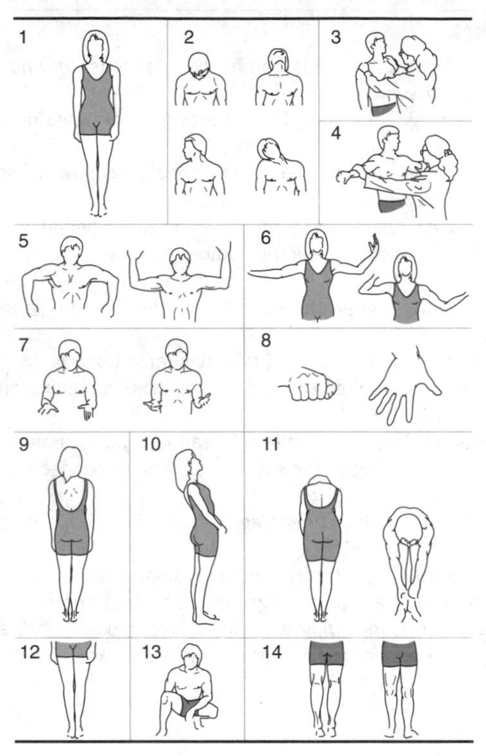


FIG. 5-7

Screening orthopedic examination. The general musculoskeletal screening examination consists of the following: *1,* inspection, athlete standing, facing examiner (symmetry of trunk, upper extremities); *2,* forward flexion, extension, rotation, lateral flexion of neck (range of motion, cervical spine); *3,* resisted shoulder shrug (strength, trapezius); *4,* resisted shoulder abduction (strength, deltoid); *5,* internal and external rotation of shoulder (range of motion, glenohumeral joint); *6,* extension and flexion of elbow (range of motion, elbow); *7,* pronation and supination of elbow (range of motion, elbow and wrist); *8,* clenching of fist, then spreading of fingers (range of motion, hand and fingers); *9,* inspection, athlete facing away from examiner (symmetry of trunk, upper extremities); *10,* back extension, knees straight (spondylolysis and spondylolisthesis); *11,* back flexion with knees straight, facing toward and away from examiner (range of motion, thoracic and lumbosacral spine; spine curvature; hamstring flexibility); *12,* inspection of lower extremities, contraction of quadriceps muscles (alignment symmetry); *13,* "duck walk" four steps (motion of hips, knees, and ankles; strength; balance); *14,* standing on toes, then on heels (symmetry, calf; strength; balance). *(Modified from American Academy of Family Physicians: Preparticipation Physical Examination, 2nd ed. Kansas City, Mo, American Academy of Family Physicians, 1997.)*

## REFERENCES


1. Woods ER, Neinstein LS: Office visit, interview techniques and recommendations to parents. In Neinstein LS (ed): Adolescent Healthcare: A Practical Guide, 4th ed. Philadelphia, Lippincott Williams & Wilkins, 2002, p 64.
2. Joffe A: Introduction to adolescent medicine. In McMillan JA, DeAngelis CD, Feigan RD, Warshaw J (eds): Oski's Pediatrics Principles and Practice, 3rd ed. Philadelphia, Lippincott Williams & Wilkins, 1999, pp 528–535.
3. Rosen DS, Neinstein LS: Preventive healthcare for adolescents. In Neinstein LS (ed): Adolescent Healthcare: A Practical Guide, 4th ed. Philadelphia, Lippincott Williams & Wilkins, 2002, pp 82–117.
4. Fishman M, Bruner A, Adger H: Substance abuse among children and adolescents. Pediatr Rev 1997;18:397–398.
5. ACOG: Evaluation and management of abnormal cervical cytology and histology in the adolescent. Committee Opinion. Obstet Gynecol 2006;107(4):963–968.
6. Centers for Disease Control and Prevention: Immunization of adolescents: Recommendation of the Advisory Committee on Immunization Practices, the American Academy of Pediatrics, the American Academy of Family Physicians, and the American Medical Association. MMWR 1996;45(No. RR-13):5–11.
7. Reproductive Health and Research: Low-dose combined oral contraceptives. In Medical Eligibility Criteria for Contraceptive Use, 3rd ed. Geneva: WHO, 2004, pp 1–10.
8. Hatcher RA et al: Contraceptive Technology, 18th ed. New York, Ardent Media, 2004.
9. Reproline: Combined oral contraceptives (COCs). Available at http://www.reproline.jhu.edu/english/6read/6multi/pg/ci3.htm. Accessed December 10, 2007.
10. Nelson AL, Neinstein LS: Combination hormonal contraceptives. In Neinstein LS (ed): Adolescent Healthcare: A Practical Guide, 4th ed. Philadelphia, Lippincott Williams & Wilkins, 2002, pp 875–878.
11. Reproline: Combined injectable contraceptives (CICs). Available at http://www.reproline.jhu.edu/english/6read/6multi/pg/ci4.htm. Accessed December 10, 2007.
12. Wilson MD: Adolescent pregnancy and contraception. In McMillan JA, DeAngelis CD, Feigan RD, Warshaw J (eds): Oski's Pediatrics Principles and Practice, 3rd ed. Philadelphia, Lippincott Williams & Wilkins, 1999, pp 544–546.
13. Nelson AL, Neinstein LS: Long acting progestins. In Neinstein LS (ed): Adolescent Healthcare: A Practical Guide, 4th ed. Philadelphia, Lippincott Williams & Wilkins, 2002, pp 922–932.
14. Nelson AL, Neinstein LS: Emergency contraception. In Neinstein LS (ed): Adolescent Healthcare: A Practical Guide, 4th ed. Philadelphia, Lippincott Williams & Wilkins, 2002, pp 913–916.
15. Brill SR, Rosenfeld WD: Contraception. Med Clin North Am 2000;84:919–920.
16. Kautz SM, Skaggs DL: Getting an angle on spinal deformities. Contemp Pediatr 1998;15:114–123.
17. Andrews JS: Making the most of the sports physical. Contemp Pediatr 1997;14:188.
18. Hergenroeder AC, Neinstein LS: Guidelines in sports medicine. In Neinstein LS (ed): Adolescent Healthcare: A Practical Guide, 4th ed. Philadelphia, Lippincott Williams & Wilkins, 2002, pp 382–391.

# Analgesia and Sedation

*Hema Dave, MD*

6

## I. PAIN ASSESSMENT (Table 6-1)

### A. INFANT[1]

1. **Physiologic response:** Seen primarily in acute pain; subsides with continuing pain. Is unreliable as an indicator of chronic pain. Increases in blood pressure, heart rate, and respiratory rate; oxygen desaturation; crying; diaphoresis; flushing; pallor.
2. **Behavioral response:**
   a. Observe characteristics and duration of cry, facial expressions, visual tracking, body movements, and response to stimuli.
   b. Neonatal Infant Pain Scale (NIPS): Behavioral assessment tool for the preterm neonate (gestational age <37 weeks) and full-term neonate (gestational age >37 weeks up to 6 weeks after birth).
   c. FLACC scale (Table 6-2): Measures and evaluates pain interventions by quantifying pain behaviors, such as facial expression, leg movement, activity, cry, and consolability, with scores ranging from 0 to 10.[2] Revised FLACC scale reliable for children with cognitive impairment.[3]

### B. PRESCHOOLER

In addition to physiologic and behavioral responses, use the **FACES** pain rating scale to assess pain intensity in children as young as age 3 years.

### C. SCHOOL-AGE AND ADOLESCENT

Evaluate physiologic and behavioral responses; ask about description, location, and character of pain. Children age 7–8 years can use the standard pain rating scale (0 is no pain and 10 is the worst pain ever experienced).

## II. ANALGESICS[1,4]

### A. NONOPIOID ANALGESICS

Weak analgesics with antipyretic activity are commonly used to manage mild to moderate pain of nonvisceral origin. Administer alone or in combination with opiates (Table 6-3).

1. **Acetaminophen:** Weak analgesic with no anti-inflammatory activity; does not affect platelets.
2. **Nonsteroidal anti-inflammatory drugs (NSAIDs):**
   a. Especially useful for sickle cell, bony, rheumatic, and inflammatory pain. Recommend histamine-2-receptor blocker concurrently with prolonged use.
   b. Primary adverse effects are gastrointestinal (epigastric pain, gastritis, and bleeding), interference with platelet aggregation, bronchoconstriction, hypersensitivity reactions, and azotemia. May interfere with bone healing. Should be avoided in patients with several renal disease, dehydration, or heart failure.

TABLE 6-1

DEVELOPMENTAL RESPONSES TO PAIN

| Stage | Age | Response |
|---|---|---|
| INFANT | | |
| | <6 mo | **No expression of anticipatory fear.** Level of anxiety reflects that of the parent. |
| | 6–18 mo | **Anticipatory fear** of painful experiences begins to develop. |
| PRESCHOOLER | | |
| | 18–24 mo | **Verbalization.** Children express pain with words such as "hurt" and "boo-boo." |
| | 3 yr | **Localization and identification of external causes.** Children more reliably assess their pain but continue to depend on visual cues for localization and are unable to understand a reason for pain. |
| SCHOOL-AGE CHILD | | |
| | 5–7 yr | **Cooperation.** Children have improved understanding of pain and ability to localize it and cooperate. |

Data from Hsu DC: Pain Control and Sedation in Children. Uptodate Online 113. Available at www.utdol.com.

TABLE 6-2

FLACC: PAIN ASSESSMENT TOOL

| | Scoring | | |
|---|---|---|---|
| Categories | 0 | 1 | 2 |
| Face | No particular expression or smile | Occasional grimace or frown, withdrawn, disinterested | Frequent to constant frown, quivering chin, clenched jaw |
| Legs | Normal position or relaxed | Uneasy, restless, tense | Kicking or legs drawn up |
| Activity | Lying quietly, normal position, moves easily | Squirming, shifting back and forth, tense | Arched, rigid or jerking |
| Cry | No cry (awake or asleep) | Moans or whimpers, occasional complaint | Crying steadily, screams or sobs, frequent complaints |
| Consolability | Content, relaxed | Reassured by occasional touching, hugging or being talked to; distractible | Difficult to console or comfort |

From Manworren R, Hynan L: Clinical validation of FLACC: Preverbal patient pain scale. Pediatr Nurs 2003;29(2):140–146.

## B. OPIOIDS (Table 6-4)

1. Produce analgesia by binding mu receptors in the brain and spinal cord.
2. Most flexible and widely used analgesics. Side effects include pruritus, nausea, vomiting, constipation, urine retention, and (rarely) respiratory depression and hypotension.
3. Morphine is the gold (unit) standard of this drug class.

TABLE 6-3

NONOPIOID ANALGESICS

| Drug | Route | GI Irritation | Platelet Inhibition | Comments |
|---|---|---|---|---|
| Acetaminophen | PO/PR | No | No | Weak analgesic with excellent antipyretic activity. No anti-inflammatory properties. |
| Aspirin | PO/PR | Yes | Yes | Avoid, owing to Reye, syndrome. |
| Choline magnesium trisalicylate (Trilisate) | PO | Yes | No | Avoid, owing to Reye syndrome. No antiplatelet effect. Useful in patients with leukemia. |
| **NSAIDs** | | | | |
| Ibuprofen | PO | Yes | Yes | Trilisate is similar to ibuprofen with less effect on platelets. |
| Ketorolac | IV/IM, PO | Yes | Yes | Potent analgesic; 1 mg/kg IV is comparable to 0.1 mg/kg morphine. Only parenteral NSAID. |
| Naproxen | PO | Yes | Yes | GI distress |





## C. LOCAL ANESTHETICS[4–7]

Used primarily to anesthetize areas for minor procedures. Administered topically, subcutaneously, into peripheral nerves (e.g., digital nerve, penile nerve block), or centrally (epidural/spinal). They act by blocking nerve conduction at the sodium channel.

1. **For all local anesthetics, 1% solution = 10 mg/mL.**
2. **Topical local anesthetics (Table 6-5):**[8]
   a. EMLA (**E**utectic **M**ixture of **L**ocal **A**nesthetics).
   b. Ela-Max (topical liposomal lidocaine cream).
   c. LET (**L**idocaine, **E**pinephrine, **T**etracaine).
   d. TAC (**T**etracaine, **A**drenaline [epinephrine], **C**ocaine).
   e. Viscous lidocaine.
3. **Injectable local anesthetics (Table 6-6):**
   a. Infiltration of the skin at the site: Used for painful procedures such as wound closure, blood drawing, intravenous (IV) line placement, or lumbar puncture.
   b. To reduce stinging from injection: Use a small needle (27- to 30-gauge). Alkalinize anesthetic: Add 1 mL (1 mEq) sodium bicarbonate to 9 mL lidocaine (or 29 mL bupivacaine), use lowest concentration of anesthetic available, warm solution (between 37° and 42° C), inject anesthetic slowly, and rub skin at injection site first.

*Text continued on p. 160*

TABLE 6-4

**COMMONLY USED OPIATES**

| Drug | Equi-analgesic Doses (mg/kg/dose) | Routes | Onset (min) |
|---|---|---|---|
| Codeine | 1.2 | PO | 30–60 |
| Meperidine (Demerol) | 1.0 | IV | 5–10 |
| | 1.5–2.0 | PO | 30–60 |
| Oxycodone | 0.1 | PO | 30–60 |
| Methadone | 0.1 | IV | 5–10 |
| | 0.1 | PO | 30–60 |
| Morphine | 0.1 | IV | 5–10 |
| | 0.1–0.2 | IM/SC | 10–30 |
| | 0.3–0.5 | PO | 30–60 |
| Hydromorphone | 0.015 | IV/SC | 5–10 |
| | 0.02–0.1 | PO | 30–60 |
| Fentanyl | 0.001 | IV | 1–2 |
| | 0.001 | Transdermal | 12 |
| | 0.01 | Transmucosal | 15 |

Data from Yaster M et al: Pediatric Pain Management and Sedation Handbook. St. Louis, Mosby, 1997, pp 29–50.

| Duration (hr) | Notable Side Effects | Comments |
|---|---|---|
| 3–4 | • Can cause severe nausea and vomiting<br>• Histamine release | Converted in liver to morphine (10%). Newborns and 10% of U.S. population cannot make this conversion. |
| 3–4<br>2–4 | • Catastrophic interaction with **MAO inhibitors**<br>• Tachycardia, histamine release<br>• Metabolite can cause **seizures;** avoid in predisposed patients | Euphoric effects are greater than with morphine. Low doses (0.1–0.25 mg/kg) stop shivering. Not recommended for prolonged use or patient-controlled analgesia. |
| 3–4 | | Available in sustained-release form for chronic pain. Much less nauseating than codeine. |
| 4–24<br>4–24 | | Initial dose may produce analgesia for 3–4 hr; duration of action is increased with repeated dosing. |
| 3–4<br>4–5<br>4–5 | • Seizures in neonates<br>• Can cause significant histamine release | The "gold standard" against which all other opioids are compared. Available in sustained-release form for chronic pain. |
| 3–4 | | Less sedation, nausea, pruritus than morphine. |
| 0.5–1<br>2–3 | • **Pruritus**<br>• Bradycardia<br>• **Chest wall rigidity** with doses >5 μg/kg (but can occur at all doses), treat with naloxone or neuromuscular blockade | Rarely causes cardiovascular instability (relatively safer in hypovolemia, congenital heart disease, or head trauma). Respiratory depressant effect much longer (4 hr) than analgesic effect. Levels of unbound drug are higher in newborns. Most commonly used opioid for short painful procedures. |

TABLE 6-5

COMMONLY USED TOPICAL LOCAL ANESTHETICS[8]

| | Components (1% of any anesthetic = 10 mg/mL) | Intact skin | Nonintact skin | Directions for Use |
|---|---|---|---|---|
| EMLA (eutectic mixture of local anesthetics) | • Lidocaine 2.5%<br>• Prilocaine 2.5% | Yes | No | • Good for venipuncture, circumcision, lumbar puncture, joint aspiration, abscess drainage, and bone marrow aspiration.<br>• Apply to intact skin.<br>• Cover with occlusive dressing at least 90 min. |
| LET | • Lidocaine 4%<br>• Epinephrine 0.1%<br>• Tetracaine 0.5% Mixed with cellulose | Yes | Yes | • Good for scalp and facial wounds <5 cm.<br>• Available in gel or liquid form. Apply 1–3 mL of liquid-saturated cotton ball or gel to wound for 20–30 min.<br>• Do not use in contaminated wounds. |
| TAC | • Tetracaine 0.25%–0.5%<br>• Adrenaline (epinephrine) 0.025%–0.05%<br>• Cocaine 4%–11.8% | Yes | Yes | • Available in gel or liquid form. Apply 1–3 mL of liquid-saturated cotton ball or gel to wound for 15 min. |
| Viscous lidocaine | Lidocaine 2% | Yes | Yes | • Good for superficial mouth and throat ulcerations (e.g., herpetic stomatitis, mucositis).<br>• Do not use for teething. |

| Peak Effect (min) | Approximate Duration (min) | Cautions |
|---|---|---|
| 90 | 60 | **Nonsterile:** Use only on intact skin.<br>**Methemoglobinemia:** Do not use in patients with methemoglobinemia-predisposing conditions (G6PD deficiency, use of methemoglobin-inducing medications such as sulfonamide antibiotics).<br>Infants <3 mo of age have low levels of methemoglobin reductase. Use sparingly; up to 1 g is safe.<br>**Maximum dose:** maximum lidocaine dose, 5 mg/kg. |
| 30 | 45 | **Vasoconstriction:** Contraindicated in areas supplied by end-arteries (e.g., pinna, nose, penis, digits). Avoid contact with mucous membranes.<br>**Maximum dose:** Maximum lidocaine dose, 5 mg/kg. |
| 15 | ? | **Vasoconstriction:** Contraindicated in areas supplied by end-arteries (e.g., pinna, nose, penis, and digits).<br>**Cocaine toxicity:** Avoid contact with mucous membranes and in patients taking monoamine oxidase inhibitors. Reapplication contraindicated. Seizures can occur even with appropriate dosing<br>**Maximum dose:** Maximum cocaine dose, 3 mg/kg. |
| 10 | 30 | **Maximum dose:** Maximum lidocaine dose, 5 mg/kg.<br>*Note:* May combine with Maalox and Benadryl elixir in a 1:1:1 fashion to make formula more palatable.<br>Give 3 mg/kg/dose no more often than q2hr. |

TABLE 6-6

COMMONLY USED INJECTABLE LOCAL ANESTHETICS[1,5]

| Agent | Concentration (%) (1% solution = 10 mg/mL) | Max dose (mg/kg) | Onset (min) | Duration (hr) |
|---|---|---|---|---|
| Lidocaine | 0.5–2 | 5 | 3 | 0.5–2 |
| Lidocaine with epinephrine | 0.5–2 | 7 | 3 | 1–3 |
| Bupivicaine | 0.25–0.75 | 2.5 | 15 | 2–4 |
| Bupivicaine with epinephrine | 0.25–0.75 | 3 | 15 | 4–8 |

***Note:* Max volume = (max mg/kg × weight in kg)/(% solution × 10).**

Data from St. Germaine Brent A: The management of pain in the emergency department. Pediatr Clin North Am 2000;47(3):651–679, and Yaster M et al: Pediatric Pain Management and Sedation Handbook. St Louis, Mosby, 1997, pp 51–72.

c. To enhance efficacy and duration: Add epinephrine to decrease vascular uptake. **Never use local anesthetics with epinephrine in areas supplied by end arteries** (e.g., pinna, digits, nasal tip, and penis).

d. Local anesthetic toxicity: CNS and cardiac toxicity are of greatest concern. CNS symptoms are seen before cardiovascular collapse. Progression of symptoms: Perioral numbness, dizziness, auditory disturbances, muscular twitching, unconsciousness, seizures, coma, respiratory arrest, cardiovascular collapse. It is important to calculate the volume limit of the local anesthetic and always draw up less than the maximum volume.

**Note** *Bupivicaine is associated with more severe cardiac toxicity than lidocaine.*

## D. NONPHARMACOLOGIC MEASURES OF PAIN RELIEF

**1. Sucrose for neonates (Sweet Ease):**

a. Indications: Procedures such as heel sticks, venipuncture, IV line insertion, arterial puncture, insertion of a Foley catheter, and lumbar puncture in neonates and infants <age 6 mo.

b. Procedure: Administer 2 mL of 25% sucrose solution by syringe into the infant's mouth (1 mL in each cheek) or allow infant to suck solution from a nipple (pacifier) no more than 2 min before the start of the painful procedure.

c. May be given for more than one procedure within a relatively short period of time but should not be administered more than twice in 1 hr.

d. Seems to be more effective when given in combination with a pacifier; non-nutritive suck also contributes to calming the infant and decreasing pain-elicited distress.

e. Contraindications—avoid use if patient is under NPO restrictions.

**2. Parental presence.**

**3. Distraction with toys.**

**4. Child life specialists strongly encouraged.**

## III. SEDATION[1,4–7,9]

### A. DEFINITIONS

1. **Mild sedation (anxiolysis):** Intent is anxiolysis with maintenance of consciousness. Practically, obtained when a single drug is given once at a low dose (not chloral hydrate).
2. **Moderate sedation:** Formerly known as *conscious sedation*. A controlled state of depressed consciousness during which airway reflexes and airway patency **are maintained**. Patient responds appropriately to age-appropriate commands ("open your eyes") and light touch. Practically, obtained any time a combination of sedative-hypnotic and analgesic is used.
3. **Deep sedation:** A controlled state of depressed consciousness during which airway reflexes and airway patency **may not be maintained** and the child is unable to respond to physical or verbal stimuli. Practically, required for most painful procedures in children. The following IV drugs always produce deep sedation: Ketamine, propofol, etomidate, thiopental, methohexital.
4. **Mild and moderate sedation can easily progress to deep sedation.**



### B. PREPARATION

1. **Patient must be NPO for solids and clear liquids** (Table 6-7 shows current American Society of Anesthesiologists recommendations).
2. **Obtain written informed consent.**
3. **Obtain a focused patient history:**
   a. Allergies and medications.
   b. Airway (asthma, acute respiratory disease, reactive airway disease), airway obstruction (mediastinal mass, history of noisy breathing, obstructive sleep apnea), craniofacial abnormalities (e.g., Pfeiffer, Crouzon, Apert, Pierre Robin syndromes), recent upper respiratory infection (suggests increased risk of laryngospasm).
   c. Aspiration risk (neuromuscular disease, gastroesophageal reflux disease, altered mental status, obesity, pregnancy).
   d. Prematurity, comorbidities, and adverse reactions to sedatives and anesthesia.

TABLE 6-7
FASTING RECOMMENDATIONS

| Food Type | Minimum Fasting Period (hr) |
|---|---|
| Clear liquids | 2 |
| Breast milk | 4 |
| Nonhuman milk, formula | 6 |
| Solids | 8 |

Data from Practice guidelines for preoperative fasting and the use of pharmacologic agents to reduce the risk of pulmonary aspiration: Application to healthy patients undergoing elective procedures. A report by the American Society of Anesthesiologists Task Force on Preoperative Fasting and Use of Pharmacologic Agents to Reduce the Risk of Pulmonary Aspiration [Online]. Available at http://www.asahq.org/publicationsAndServices/NPO.pdf.

4. **Perform a physical examination** (with specific attention to head, ears, eyes, nose, and throat [HEENT]; lungs; cardiac examination; and neuromuscular function. Assess ability to open mouth and extend neck. If risk for moderate sedation is too high, consider an anesthesia consultation and general anesthesia).
5. **Have an emergency plan ready.** Make sure qualified backup personnel and equipment are close by.
6. **Have personnel available.** At least two individuals must be available: Physician (to administer sedation and perform procedure) and an additional person trained in sedation (e.g., to monitor patient and document vital signs, drug administration).
7. **Ensure IV access.**
8. **Have airway equipment available (SOAP):**

a. **S**uction.

b. **O**xygen.

c. **A**irway equipment: Appropriately sized oral and nasal airways, laryngoscope with blades, endotracheal tubes (ETT) with stylet (ETT size = AGE/4 + 4), bag-valve with mask, and tape (see inside front cover for appropriate equipment sizes)

d. **P**harmacy:

(1) Intubation medications: Atropine, paralytic, induction agent (i.e., sedative-hypnotic).

(2) Emergency medications: Epinephrine, atropine, glucose.

(3) Antagonist ("reversal") agents: Naloxone, flumazenil.

## C. MONITORING

1. **Vital signs:** Obtain baseline vital signs (including pulse oximetry). Continuously monitor heart rate and oxygen saturation; intermittently monitor blood pressure and respiratory rate. Record vital signs at least every 5 min until the patient returns to presedation level of consciousness.

**Note** *Complications most often occur 5 to 10 min after administration of IV medication and immediately after a procedure is completed (when stimuli associated with the procedure are removed).*[7]

2. **Airway:** Assess airway patency and adequacy of ventilation through capnography, auscultation, or direct visualization frequently.

## D. PHARMACOLOGIC AGENTS

1. **Goal of sedation:** To tailor drug combination to provide levels of analgesia, sedation-hypnosis, and anxiolysis deep enough to facilitate the procedure but shallow enough to avoid loss of airway reflexes.
2. **CNS, cardiovascular, and respiratory depression are potentiated by combining sedative drugs and/or opioids and by rapid drug infusion.** Titrate to effect.

3. **Common sedative agents** (Table 6-8):
a. Sedating antihistamines (diphenhydramine, hydroxyzine): Mild sedative-hypnotics used for sedation and treatment of opiate-induced pruritus. See Formulary for dosing.
b. Chloral hydrate: Oral sedative agent often used to produce immobilization for nonpainful procedures. Associated with a high risk for failure and airway obstruction. Not recommended for routine use.
c. Barbiturates (Table 6-9).
d. Benzodiazepines (see Table 6-9).
e. Opiates (see Table 6-4).
f. Ketamine: A phencyclidine derivative that causes potent dissociative anesthesia, analgesia, and amnesia. Causes bronchodilation, maintains ventilatory response to hypoxia, and allows relative maintenance of airway reflexes (Table 6-10).

4. **Reversal agents:**
a. Naloxone: Opioid antagonist. See Box 6-1 for Narcan administration protocol.
b. Flumazenil: Benzodiazepine antagonist. See Formulary for dosing details.

### E. DISCHARGE CRITERIA[10]

1. **Airway patency and stable cardiovascular function.**
2. **Easy arousability with intact protective reflexes (swallows and coughs, gag reflex).**
3. **Ability to talk and sit up unaided (if age appropriate).**
4. **Adequate hydration.**
5. **Recovery after sedation protocols varies but typically ranges from 60 to 120 min.**

### F. EXAMPLES OF SEDATION PROTOCOLS (Tables 6-11 and 6-12)

### G. SEDATIVE-HYPNOTIC AND ANALGESICS QUICK REFERENCE GUIDE (Table 6-13)

## IV. PATIENT-CONTROLLED ANALGESIA (PCA)

### A. DEFINITION

PCA is a device that enables a patient to receive continuous ("basal") opioids and/or self-administer small supplemental doses ("bolus") of analgesics on an as-needed basis. In children < age 6 years, a family member, caregiver, or nurse may administer doses.

### B. INDICATIONS

Moderate to severe pain of acute or chronic nature. Commonly used in sickle cell disease, post-surgery, post-trauma, burns, and cancer. Also for preemptive pain management (e.g., to facilitate dressing changes).

*Text continued on p. 168*

TABLE 6-8

**PROPERTIES OF COMMON SEDATIVE AGENTS**

| Drug/Drug Class | Anxiolysis | Analgesia | Sedation/ Hypnosis |
|---|---|---|---|
| **Sedating antihistamines**<br>Diphenhydramine<br>Hydroxyzine | No | No | Yes |
| **Chloral hydrate*** | No | No | Yes |
| **Barbiturates** | No | No | Yes |
| **Benzodiazepines** | Yes | No | Yes |
| **Opiates** | No | Yes | Yes |
| **Ketamine** | Yes | Yes | Yes |
| **Propofol** | Yes | Yes | Yes |

*High rate of failure of chloral hydrate combined with its adverse effects increase the risk/benefit profile of this agent. We recommend considering alternative sedatives whenever possible. See Formulary for dosing recommendations.
OSA, obstructive sleep apnea.

TABLE 6-9

**COMMONLY USED BENZODIAZEPINES* AND BARBITURATES[1,5,9]**

| Drug Class | Duration of Action | Drug | Route | Onset (min) |
|---|---|---|---|---|
| Benzodiazepines | Short | Midazolam (Versed) | IV | 1–3 |
| | | | IM/IN | 5–10 |
| | | | PO/PR | 10–30 |
| | Intermediate | Diazepam (Valium) | IV (painful) | 1–3 |
| | | | PR | 7–15 |
| | | | PO | 30–60 |
| | Long | Lorazepam (Ativan) | IV | 1–5 |
| | | | IM | 10–20 |
| | | | PO | 30–60 |
| Barbiturates | Short | Methohexital | PR† | 5–10 |
| | | Thiopental | PR† | 5–10 |
| | Intermediate | Pentobarbital | IV | 1–10 |
| | | | IM | 5–15 |
| | | | PO/PR | 15–60 |

*Use IV solution for PO, PR, and intranasal (IN) administration. Rectal diazepam gel (Diastat) is also available.
†IV administration produces general anesthesia; only PR should be used for sedation.

Data from Yaster M et al: Pediatric Pain Management and Sedation Handbook. St. Louis, Mosby, 1997, pp 345–374; St Germaine Brent A: The management of pain in the emergency department. Pediatr Clin North Am 2000;47(3):651–679; and Cote CJ et al: A Practice of Anesthesia for Infants and Children. Philadelphia, WB Saunders, 2001.

| Reversible | Comments |
|---|---|
| No | • Antiemetics and antipruritics often used to treat opioid side effects. |
| No | • May cause severe airway obstruction in children with OSA.<br>• 30%–40% failure rate.<br>• Long and unpredictable onset/duration of action. |
| No | • Contraindicated in patients with porphyria. |
| Yes | |
| Yes | |
| No | • Dissociative agent.<br>• Increases heart rate, blood pressure, intraocular pressure, intracranial pressure.<br>• Administer with benzodiazepine (to counter emergence delirium) and antisialagogue. |
| No | Give 1 mg/kg followed by 0.5 mg/kg IV.<br>Extremely rapid onset and brief recovery (5–15 min) antiemetic and euphoric<br>Caution: Respiratory depression, apnea, hypotension. |

| Duration (hr) | Comments |
|---|---|
| 1–2 | • Has rapid and predictable onset of action, a short recovery time<br>• Causes amnesia<br>• Results in mild depression of hypoxic ventilatory drive |
| 0.25–1<br>2–3<br>2–3 | • Poor choice for procedural sedation<br>• Excellent for muscle relaxation or prolonged sedation<br>• Painful on IV injection<br>• Faster onset than midazolam |
| 3–4<br>3–6<br>3–6 | • Poor choice for procedural sedation<br>• Ideal for prolonged anxiolysis, seizure treatment |
| 1–1.5<br>1–1.5 | • PR form used as sedative for nonpainful procedures<br>• IV form induces general anesthesia; do not use for sedation |
| 1–4<br>2–4<br>2–4 | • Predictable sedation and immobility for nonpainful procedures<br>• Minimal respiratory depression when used alone<br>• Associated with slow wake up and agitation |

TABLE 6-10

**KETAMINE DOSING AND PHARMACOKINETICS[1,5,9]**

| Route | Onset (min) | Duration (min) | Effects | Contraindications | Comments |
|---|---|---|---|---|---|
| IV<br>IM<br>(painful)<br>PO/PR | 0.5–2<br>5–10<br>20–45 | 20–60*<br>30–90<br>60–120+ | • ***CNS effects:*** Increased ICP, emergence delirium with auditory, visual, and tactile hallucinations<br>• ***Cardiovascular effects:*** Inhibits catecholamine reuptake, causing increased HR, BP, SVR, PVR, direct myocardial depression<br>• ***Respiratory effects:*** Bronchodilation, increased secretions (can result in laryngospasm), maintenance of ventilatory response to hypoxia, relative maintenance of airway reflexes<br>• ***Other effects:*** Increased muscle tone, myoclonic jerks, increased IOP, nausea, emesis | • Increased ICP<br>• Increased IOP<br>• Hypertension<br>• Pre-existing psychotic disorders | • Causes bronchodilation (useful in asthmatics)<br>• Nystagmus indicates likely therapeutic effect<br>• Vocalizations/ movement may occur even with adequate sedation<br>• Results in "deep sedation" by any route |

*IV ketamine has a high risk for inducing general anesthesia; this should be used only by providers highly skilled in airway management.

BP, blood pressure; HR, heart rate; ICP, intracranial pressure; IOP, intraocular pressure; PVR, pulmonary vascular resistance; SVR, systemic vascular resistance.

Data from Yaster M et al: Pediatric Pain Management and Sedation Handbook. St. Louis, Mosby, 1997, pp 376–382; St Germaine Brent A: The management of pain in the emergency department. Pediatr Clin North Am 2000;47(3):651–679; and Cote CJ et al: A Practice of Anesthesia for Infants and Children. Philadelphia, WB Saunders, 2001.

BOX 6-1

**NALOXONE (NARCAN) ADMINISTRATION**

**INDICATIONS: PATIENTS REQUIRING NALOXONE (NARCAN) USUALLY MEET ALL OF THE FOLLOWING CRITERIA***

- Unresponsive to physical stimulation
- Shallow respirations or respiratory rate <8 breaths/min†
- Pinpoint pupils

**PROCEDURE**

1. **Stop opioid administration** (as well as other sedative drugs), start the **ABCs** (**A**irway, **B**reathing, **C**irculation), and call for **HELP**.
2. **Dilute naloxone:** Mix 0.4 mg (1 ampule) of naloxone with 9 mL of normal saline (final concentration 0.04 mg/mL = 40 μg/mL). (If child <40 kg, dilute 0.1 mg (one-fourth ampule) in 9 mL of normal saline to make 0.01 mg/mL solution = 10 μg/mL.)
3. **Administer and observe response:** Administer dilute naloxone slowly (1–2 μg/kg/dose IV over 2 min). Observe patient response.
4. **Titrate to effect:** Within 1–2 min, patient should open eyes and respond. If not, continue until a total dose of 10 μg/kg is given. If no response is obtained, evaluate for other cause of sedation/respiratory depression.
5. **Discontinue naloxone administration:** Discontinue naloxone as soon as patient responds (e.g., takes deep breaths when directed).
6. **Caution:** Another dose of naloxone may be required within 30 min of first dose (duration of action of naloxone is shorter than that of most opioids).
7. **Monitor patient:** Assign a staff member to monitor sedation/respiratory status and to remind the patient to take deep breaths as necessary.
8. **Alternative analgesia:** Provide nonopioids for pain relief. Resume opioid administration at half the original dose when the patient is easily aroused and respiratory rate is >9 breaths/min.

*Patients with significant opiate exposure (sickle cell, cancer) should be carefully evaluated for the need for naloxone. The reversal of analgesia could produce hypertension, tachycardia, ventricular arrhythmias, and pulmonary edema. If necessary, give at the lowest dose possible and titrate carefully.

†Respiratory rates that require naloxone vary according to infant's/child's usual rate.

Modified from McCaffery M, Pasero C: Pain: Clinical Manual. St Louis, Mosby, 1999, pp 269–270.

TABLE 6-11

EXAMPLES OF SEDATION PROTOCOLS*

| | Dosage | Comments |
|---|---|---|
| Midazolam + fentanyl | Midazolam 0.1 mg/kg IV × 3 doses PRN<br>Fentanyl 1 mcg/kg IV × 3 doses PRN | • High likelihood of respiratory depression<br>• Infuse fentanyl no faster than 3-min intervals |
| Ketamine + midazolam + atropine ("ketodazzline") | **PO route:** combine<br>Ketamine 5 mg/kg<br>Midazolam 0.5 mg/kg<br>Atropine 0.02 mg/kg<br>**IV route:**<br>Ketamine 0.25 mg/kg × 1 dose†<br>Midazolam 0.1 mg/kg × 3 doses PRN<br>Atropine 0.02 mg/kg × 1 dose<br>**IM route:** combine (use smallest volume possible)<br>Ketamine 1.5–2.0 mg/kg<br>Midazolam 0.15–0.2 mg/kg<br>Atropine 0.02 mg/kg | • Atropine = antisialogogue<br>• Midazolam = counter emergence delirium |

*These examples reflect commonly used current protocols at the Johns Hopkins Children's Center; variations are found at other institutions.

†Ketamine can be given intravenously, but the risk for inducing general anesthesia is very high; this should be used only by providers skilled in airway management.

Data from Yaster M et al: Pediatric Pain Management and Sedation Handbook. St. Louis, Mosby, 1997.

### C. ROUTES OF ADMINISTRATION

IV, subcutaneous, or epidural.

### D. AGENTS (Table 6-14)

### E. COMPLICATIONS

1. Pruritus, nausea, constipation, urine retention, excessive drowsiness, respiratory depression.
2. Consider a low-dose naloxone (Narcan) infusion (0.25 mcg/kg/hr) to reduce pruritus and nausea.[11]

## V. OPIOID TAPERING[4]

### A. INDICATION

Tapering schedule is required if the patient has received frequent opioid analgesics for >5–10 days.

### B. GUIDELINES

1. **Conversion:** Convert all drugs to a single equi-analgesic member of that group (Table 6-15).

TABLE 6-12

SUGGESTED ANALGESIA AND SEDATION PROTOCOLS

| Pain Threshold | Procedure | Suggested Drug Choices |
|---|---|---|
| **Nonpainful** | CT scan/EEG/ECHO | Midazolam* |
| **Mild** | Phlebotomy, LP, IV access | EMLA<br>EMLA + midazolam |
| | BM aspiration | Midazolam |
| | Pelvic exam | TAC/LET |
| | Minor laceration, well vascularized | Lidocaine |
| | Minor laceration, not well vascularized | |
| **Moderate** | Arthrocentesis | Midazolam + fentanyl or ketamine† + fentanyl + atropine or propofol |
| | Dislocation repair | Midazolam + fentanyl |
| | I&D abscess | Midazolam + fentanyl |
| | Fracture reduction | Midazolam + morphine |
| | Major laceration | Ketamine + atropine + midazolam |
| | Burn débridement | Ketamine + atropine + midazolam |
| **Severe** | Consider anesthesia consultation and general anesthesia | Ketamine + midazolam + atropine or propofol |

*Caution for antiepileptics for EEG.

†Ketamine should not be chosen with head injury or open globe eye injury.

BM, bone marrow; CT, computed tomography; ECHO, echocardiogram; EEG, electroencephalogram; I&D, incision and drainage; LP, lumbar puncture; TAC/LET, tetracaine, adrenaline, cocaine/lidocaine, epinephrine, tetracaine.

Data from Yaster M et al: Pediatric Pain Management and Sedation Handbook. St. Louis, Mosby, 1997, 551–552.

2. **PCA wean:** Change drug dosing from continuous/intermittent IV infusion to oral (PO) bolus therapy around the clock. If on PCA, administer first PO dose, then stop basal infusion 30–60 min later. Keep bolus doses, but reduce by 25%–50%. Discontinue PCA if no boluses are required in next 6 hr, increase PO dose, or add adjuvant analgesic (e.g., NSAID).
3. **Slow dose decrease:** During an intermittent IV/PO wean, decrease total daily dose by 10%–20% every 1–2 days (e.g., to taper a morphine dose of 40 mg/day, decrease the daily dose by 4–8 mg every 1–2 days).
4. **Oral regimen:** If not done previously, convert IV dosing to equivalent PO administration 1–2 days before discharge, and continue titration as outlined previously.

## C. EXAMPLES (Box 6-2)

TABLE 6-13

ANALGESICS AND SEDATIVE-HYPNOTIC DRUGS QUICK REFERENCE (ALPHABETICAL)

| Drug | Route | Dose |
|---|---|---|
| SEDATIVE-HYPNOTIC | | |
| **Diazepam** | PO | 0.25–0.3 mg/kg |
| | IV (painful) | 0.1 mg/kg |
| **Diphenhydramine** | PO, IV, IM | 5 mg/kg/day divided q6hr |
| **Hydroxyzine** | PO | 2 mg/kg/day divided q6–8hr |
| | IM | 0.5–1 mg/kg/dose q4–6hr |
| **Lorazapam** | PO, IV, IM | 0.05 mg/kg |
| **Midazolam** | PO | 0.5–0.8 mg/kg |
| | PR | 0.5–1.0 mg/kg |
| | IN | 0.2–0.3 mg/kg |
| | IM | 0.15–0.2 mg/kg |
| | IV sedation | 0.1 mg/kg up to 0.25 mg/kg |
| ANALGESIC | | |
| **Fentanyl** | IV | 1 μg/kg |
| | IV infusion | 1–5 μg/kg/hr |
| | PO oralet | 10–15 μg/kg, max 400 μg |
| **Hydromorphone** | IV | 0.015 mg/kg |
| | IV infusion | 2–4 μg/kg/hr |
| **Ketorolac** | IV, IM | 0.5 mg/kg q6hr |
| **Methadone** | PO, IV, IM, SC | 0.1 mg/kg q8–12hr |
| **Morphine** | IV | 0.05–0.1 mg/kg |
| | IV infusion | 10–40 μg/kg/hr |
| **Oxycodone** | PO | 0.1 mg/kg q4–6hr |
| OTHER | | |
| **Ketamine** | PO | 5 mg/kg |
| | IV | 0.25–0.5 mg/kg |
| | IM | 1.5–2.0 mg/kg |

Data from Fisher QA: Pediatric Anesthesia Pearls. Baltimore, Johns Hopkins Department of Anesthesia and Critical Care Medicine, 2000.

TABLE 6-14

ORDERS FOR PATIENT-CONTROLLED ANALGESIA

| Drug | Basal Rate (μg/kg/hr) | Bolus Dose (μg/kg) | Lockout Period (min) | Boluses (hr) | Max Dose (μg/kg/hr) |
|---|---|---|---|---|---|
| Morphine | 10–30 | 10–30 | 6–10 | 4–6 | 100–150 |
| Hydromorphone | 3–5 | 3–5 | 6–10 | 4–6 | 15–20 |
| Fentanyl | 0.5–1 | 0.5–10 | 6–10 | 2–3 | 2–4 |

Data from Yaster M et al: Pediatric Pain Management and Sedation Handbook. St. Louis, Mosby, 1997, p 100.

TABLE 6-15

**RELATIVE POTENCIES AND EQUIVALENCE OF OPIOIDS**

| Drug | Morphine Equivalence Ratio | IV Dose (mg/kg) | Equivalent PO Dose (mg/kg) |
|---|---|---|---|
| Meperidine | 0.1 | 1 | 1.5–2 |
| Methadone | 0.25–1 | 0.1 | 0.1 |
| Morphine | 1 | 0.1 | 0.3–0.5 |
| Hydromorphone | 5–7 | 0.015 | 0.02–0.1 |
| Fentanyl | 80–100* | 0.001 | NA |

*Note:* Removing a transdermal fentanyl patch does not stop opioid uptake from the skin, and fentanyl will continue to be absorbed for 12–24 hr after patch removal; fentanyl 25-μg patch administers 25 μg/hr of fentanyl.

From Yaster M et al: Pediatric Pain Management and Sedation Handbook. St. Louis, Mosby, 1997, p 40.



BOX 6-2

**EXAMPLES OF OPIOID TAPERING**

**EXAMPLE 1**

Patient on morphine PCA to be converted to PO morphine with home weaning.

For example: morphine PCA basal rate = 2 mg/hr, average bolus rate = 0.5 mg/hr.

Step 1: Calculate daily dose: Basal + bolus = (2 mg/hr × 24 hr) + (0.5 mg/hr × 24 hr) = 60 mg IV morphine.

Step 2: Convert according to drug potency: Morphine IV/morphine oral = approx 3:1 potency. 3 × 60 mg = 180 mg PO morphine.

Step 3: Prescribe 90 mg bid or 60 mg tid; wean 10%–20% of original dose (30 mg) every 1–2 days.

**EXAMPLE 2**

Patient on morphine PCA to be converted to transdermal fentanyl. Morphine PCA basal rate = 2 mg/hr. No boluses.

Step 1: Convert according to drug potency: Fentanyl/morphine = approx 100:1 potency; 2 mg/hr morphine = 2000 μg/hr morphine = 20 μg/hr fentanyl.

Step 2: Prescribe 25 μg fentanyl patch (delivers 25 μg/hr fentanyl).

Step 3: Stop IV morphine 8 hr after patch is applied; prescribe second patch at 72 hr.

Step 4: Prescribe PRN IV morphine with caution.

Data from Yaster M et al: Pediatric Pain Management and Sedation Handbook. St. Louis, Mosby, 1997, pp 29–50.

## REFERENCES

1. Yaster M et al: Pediatric Pain Management and Sedation Handbook. St. Louis, Mosby, 1997.
2. Manworren R, Hynan L: Clinical validation of FLACC: Preverbal patient pain scale. Pediatr Nurs 2003;29(2):140–146.
3. Malviya S, Voepel-Lewis T: The revised FLACC observational pain tool: Improved reliability and validity for pain assessment in children with cognitive impairment. Paediatr Anaesth 2006;16(3):258–265.

4. Yaster M, Maxwell LG: Pediatric regional anesthesia. Anesthesiology 1989;70:324–338.
5. St. Germain Brent A: The management of pain in the emergency department. Pediatr Clin North Am 2000;47(3):651–679.
6. Krauss B, Green S: Procedural sedation and analgesia in children. Lancet 2006;367:766-780.
7. Krauss B, Green SM: Sedation and analgesia for procedures in children. NEJM 2000;342:938.
8. Zempsky W, Cravero J: Relief of pain and anxiety in pediatric patients in emergency medical systems. Pediatrics 2004;114(5):1348–1356.
9. Cote CJ et al: A Practice of Anesthesia for Infants and Children. Philadelphia, WB Saunders, 2001.
10. American Academy of Pediatrics Committee on Drugs: Guidelines for monitoring and management of pediatric patients during and after sedation for diagnostic and therapeutic procedures. Pediatrics 1992;89:1110–1115.
11. Maxwell LG et al: The effects of a small-dose naloxone infusion on opioid-induced side effects and analgesia in children and adolescents treated with intravenous patient-controlled analgesia: A double-blind, prospective, randomized, controlled study. Anesth Analg 2005;100:953–958.

# Cardiology

*Aisha Frazier, MD, MPH, and Cozumel Southern Pruette, MD, MS*

7

## I. WEBSITES

www.americanheart.org (Open the Heart and Stroke Encyclopedia)
www.cincinnatichildrens.org/heartcenter/encyclopedia/
www.pted.org
www.murmurlab.org

## II. THE CARDIAC CYCLE (Fig. 7-1)

## III. PHYSICAL EXAMINATION

### A. BLOOD PRESSURE

1. **Blood pressure:**
   a. Four limb blood pressure measurements can be used to assess for coarctation of the aorta; pressure must be measured in both the right and left arms because of the possibility of an aberrant right subclavian artery.
   b. Pulsus paradoxus: An exaggeration of the normal drop in systolic blood pressure (SBP) seen with inspiration. Determine the SBP at the end of exhalation and then during inhalation; if the difference is >10 mm Hg, consider pericardial effusion, tamponade, pericarditis, severe asthma, or restrictive cardiomyopathies.
   c. **Blood pressure norms:**[1,2] **Figure 7-2, Tables 7-1 and 7-2, and Figure 7-3.**
2. **Pulse pressure = systolic pressure − diastolic pressure.**

See Box 7-1 (pulse pressure differential diagnosis).

3. **Mean arterial pressure (MAP) = diastolic pressure + (pulse pressure/3). In preterm infants and newborns, generally a normal MAP = gestational age in weeks + 5.**

See Figure 7-4.

### B. HEART SOUNDS

1. **$S_1$: Associated with closure of mitral and tricuspid valves; best heard at the apex or left lower sternal border (LLSB).**
2. **$S_2$: Associated with closure of pulmonary and aortic valves, heard best at the left upper sternal border (LUSB) and has normal physiologic splitting that increases with inspiration.**
3. **$S_3$: Heard best at the apex or LLSB.**
4. **$S_4$: Heard at the apex.**

See Box 7-2 for abnormal heart sounds.[3]

### C. SYSTOLIC AND DIASTOLIC SOUNDS

1. **Ejection click: Sounds like splitting of the $S_1$ but is most audible at the apex, in contrast to the normal finding of a split $S_1$, which is**

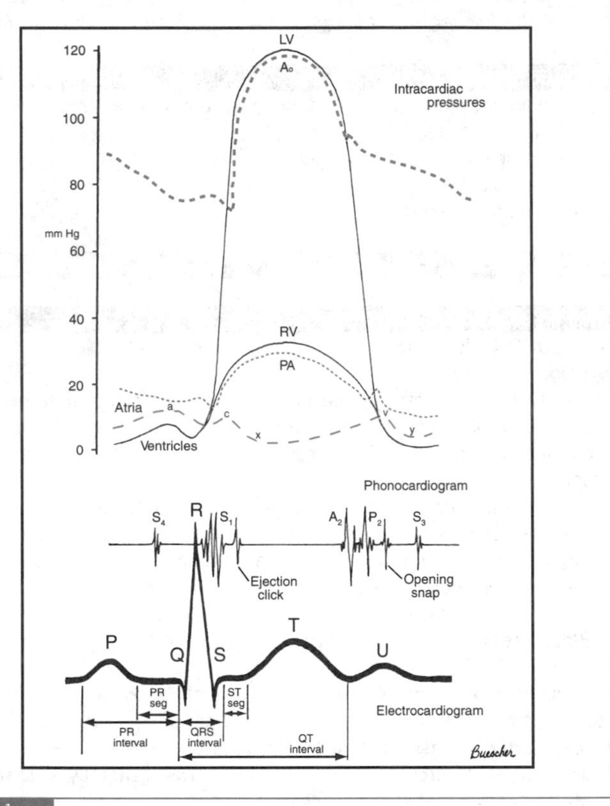


FIG. 7-1

The cardiac cycle.

**best heard at the LLSB. May also be heard at the LUSB with valvular pulmonary stenosis (PS).** Associated with stenosis of the semilunar valves and large great arteries (e.g., systemic hypertension; pulmonary hypertension; idiopathic dilation of the pulmonary artery; tetralogy of Fallot [TOF], in which the aorta is dilated; and persistent truncus arteriosus).

2. **Midsystolic click with or without a late systolic murmur: Heard near the apex in mitral valve prolapse.**
3. **Diastolic opening snap: Audible at the apex or LLSB in mitral stenosis.**

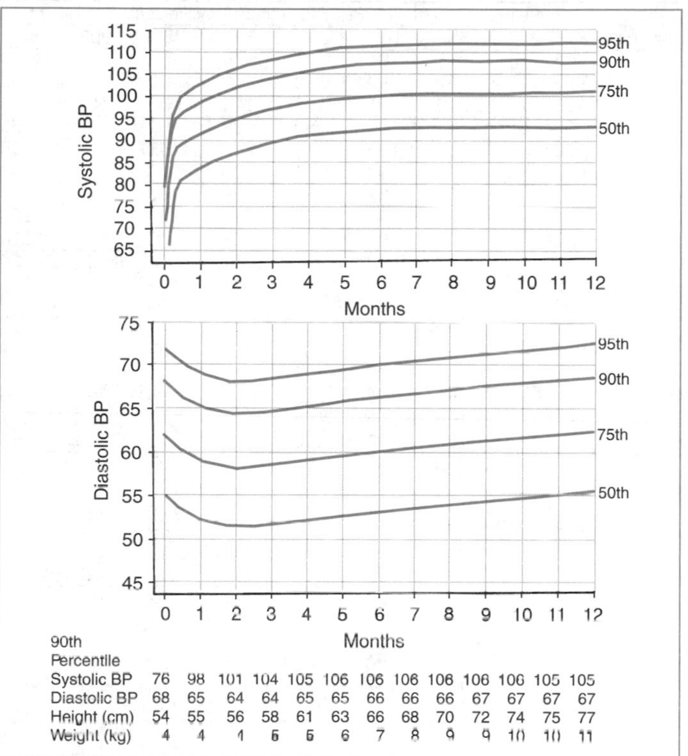


| 90th Percentile | | | | | | | | | | | | | |
|---|---|---|---|---|---|---|---|---|---|---|---|---|---|
| Systolic BP | 76 | 98 | 101 | 104 | 105 | 106 | 106 | 106 | 106 | 106 | 106 | 105 | 105 |
| Diastolic BP | 68 | 65 | 64 | 64 | 65 | 65 | 66 | 66 | 66 | 67 | 67 | 67 | 67 |
| Height (cm) | 54 | 55 | 56 | 58 | 61 | 63 | 66 | 68 | 70 | 72 | 74 | 75 | 77 |
| Weight (kg) | 4 | 4 | 4 | 5 | 5 | 6 | 7 | 8 | 9 | 9 | 10 | 10 | 11 |

FIG. 7-2

Linear regression of mean systolic blood pressure on postconceptional age (gestational age in weeks plus weeks after delivery). *(Data from Zubrow AB et al: Determinants of blood pressure in infants admitted to neonatal intensive care units. A prospective multicenter study. J Perinatol 1995;15:470–479.)*

## D. MURMURS[4] (MURMURLAB.ORG)

1. **Benign heart murmurs:** Caused by a disturbance of the laminar flow of blood, frequently produced as the diameter of the blood's pathway decreases and the velocity increases. More than 80% of children have innocent murmurs sometime during childhood, most commonly beginning at age 3 to 4 years. Innocent murmurs are accentuated in high-output states, especially with fever and anemia, and are associated with normal electrocardiogram (ECG) and radiographic findings. However, note that ECG and chest radiograph are not routinely useful or cost-effective screening tools for distinguishing

*Text continued on p. 181*

TABLE 7-1

**BLOOD PRESSURE LEVELS FOR THE 50TH, 90TH, AND 95TH PERCENTILES OF BLOOD PRESSURE FOR *GIRLS* AGE 1–17 YEARS BY PERCENTILES OF HEIGHT[2]**

| | Height*→ | Systolic BP (SBP) (mm Hg) by Percentile of Height | | | | | | |
|---|---|---|---|---|---|---|---|---|
| Age (yr) | BP[†]↓ | 5% | 10% | 25% | 50% | 75% | 90% | 95% |
| 1 | 50th | 83 | 84 | 85 | 86 | 88 | 89 | 90 |
| | 90th | 97 | 97 | 98 | 100 | 101 | 102 | 103 |
| | 95th | 100 | 101 | 102 | 104 | 105 | 106 | 107 |
| 2 | 50th | 85 | 85 | 87 | 88 | 89 | 91 | 91 |
| | 90th | 98 | 99 | 100 | 101 | 103 | 104 | 105 |
| | 95th | 102 | 103 | 104 | 105 | 107 | 108 | 109 |
| 3 | 50th | 86 | 87 | 88 | 89 | 91 | 92 | 93 |
| | 90th | 100 | 100 | 102 | 103 | 104 | 106 | 106 |
| | 95th | 104 | 104 | 105 | 107 | 108 | 109 | 110 |
| 4 | 50th | 88 | 88 | 90 | 91 | 92 | 94 | 94 |
| | 90th | 101 | 102 | 103 | 104 | 106 | 107 | 108 |
| | 95th | 105 | 106 | 107 | 108 | 110 | 111 | 112 |
| 5 | 50th | 89 | 90 | 91 | 93 | 94 | 95 | 96 |
| | 90th | 103 | 103 | 105 | 106 | 107 | 109 | 109 |
| | 95th | 107 | 107 | 108 | 110 | 111 | 112 | 113 |
| 6 | 50th | 91 | 92 | 93 | 94 | 96 | 97 | 98 |
| | 90th | 104 | 105 | 106 | 108 | 109 | 110 | 111 |
| | 95th | 108 | 109 | 110 | 111 | 113 | 114 | 115 |
| 7 | 50th | 93 | 93 | 95 | 96 | 97 | 99 | 99 |
| | 90th | 106 | 107 | 108 | 109 | 111 | 112 | 113 |
| | 95th | 110 | 111 | 112 | 113 | 115 | 116 | 116 |
| 8 | 50th | 95 | 95 | 96 | 98 | 99 | 100 | 101 |
| | 90th | 108 | 109 | 110 | 111 | 113 | 114 | 114 |
| | 95th | 112 | 112 | 114 | 115 | 116 | 118 | 118 |
| 9 | 50th | 96 | 97 | 98 | 100 | 101 | 102 | 103 |
| | 90th | 110 | 110 | 112 | 113 | 114 | 116 | 116 |
| | 95th | 114 | 114 | 115 | 117 | 118 | 119 | 120 |
| 10 | 50th | 98 | 99 | 100 | 102 | 103 | 104 | 105 |
| | 90th | 112 | 112 | 114 | 115 | 116 | 118 | 118 |
| | 95th | 116 | 116 | 117 | 119 | 120 | 121 | 122 |
| 11 | 50th | 100 | 101 | 102 | 103 | 105 | 106 | 107 |
| | 90th | 114 | 114 | 116 | 117 | 118 | 119 | 120 |
| | 95th | 118 | 118 | 119 | 121 | 122 | 123 | 124 |
| 12 | 50th | 102 | 103 | 104 | 105 | 107 | 108 | 109 |
| | 90th | 116 | 116 | 117 | 119 | 120 | 121 | 122 |
| | 95th | 119 | 120 | 121 | 123 | 124 | 125 | 126 |
| 13 | 50th | 104 | 105 | 106 | 107 | 109 | 110 | 110 |
| | 90th | 117 | 118 | 119 | 121 | 122 | 123 | 124 |
| | 95th | 121 | 122 | 123 | 124 | 126 | 127 | 128 |
| 14 | 50th | 106 | 106 | 107 | 109 | 110 | 111 | 112 |
| | 90th | 119 | 120 | 121 | 122 | 124 | 125 | 125 |
| | 95th | 123 | 123 | 125 | 126 | 127 | 129 | 129 |
| 15 | 50th | 107 | 108 | 109 | 110 | 111 | 113 | 113 |
| | 90th | 120 | 121 | 122 | 123 | 125 | 126 | 127 |
| | 95th | 124 | 125 | 126 | 127 | 129 | 130 | 131 |
| 16 | 50th | 108 | 108 | 110 | 111 | 112 | 114 | 114 |
| | 90th | 121 | 122 | 123 | 124 | 126 | 127 | 128 |
| | 95th | 125 | 126 | 127 | 128 | 130 | 131 | 132 |
| 17 | 50th | 108 | 109 | 110 | 111 | 113 | 114 | 115 |
| | 90th | 122 | 122 | 123 | 125 | 126 | 127 | 128 |
| | 95th | 125 | 126 | 127 | 129 | 130 | 131 | 132 |

*Height percentile determined by standard growth curves.

[†]Blood pressure percentile determined by a single measurement.

| Diastolic BP (DBP) (mm Hg) by Percentile of Height | | | | | | |
|---|---|---|---|---|---|---|
| 5% | 10% | 25% | 50% | 75% | 90% | 95% |
| 38 | 39 | 39 | 40 | 41 | 41 | 42 |
| 52 | 53 | 53 | 54 | 55 | 55 | 56 |
| 56 | 57 | 57 | 58 | 59 | 59 | 60 |
| 43 | 44 | 44 | 45 | 46 | 46 | 47 |
| 57 | 58 | 58 | 59 | 60 | 61 | 61 |
| 61 | 62 | 62 | 63 | 64 | 65 | 65 |
| 47 | 48 | 48 | 49 | 50 | 50 | 51 |
| 61 | 62 | 62 | 63 | 64 | 64 | 65 |
| 65 | 66 | 66 | 67 | 68 | 68 | 69 |
| 50 | 50 | 51 | 52 | 52 | 53 | 54 |
| 64 | 64 | 65 | 66 | 67 | 67 | 68 |
| 68 | 68 | 69 | 70 | 71 | 71 | 72 |
| 52 | 53 | 53 | 54 | 55 | 55 | 56 |
| 66 | 67 | 67 | 68 | 69 | 69 | 70 |
| 70 | 71 | 71 | 72 | 73 | 73 | 74 |
| 54 | 54 | 55 | 56 | 56 | 57 | 58 |
| 68 | 68 | 69 | 70 | 70 | 71 | 72 |
| 72 | 72 | 73 | 74 | 74 | 75 | 76 |
| 55 | 56 | 56 | 57 | 58 | 58 | 59 |
| 69 | 70 | 70 | 71 | 72 | 72 | 73 |
| 73 | 74 | 74 | 75 | 76 | 76 | 77 |
| 57 | 57 | 57 | 58 | 59 | 60 | 60 |
| 71 | 71 | 71 | 72 | 73 | 74 | 74 |
| 75 | 75 | 75 | 76 | 77 | 78 | 78 |
| 58 | 58 | 58 | 59 | 60 | 61 | 61 |
| 72 | 72 | 72 | 73 | 74 | 75 | 75 |
| 76 | 76 | 76 | 77 | 78 | 79 | 79 |
| 59 | 59 | 59 | 60 | 61 | 62 | 62 |
| 73 | 73 | 73 | 74 | 75 | 76 | 76 |
| 77 | 77 | 77 | 78 | 79 | 80 | 80 |
| 60 | 60 | 60 | 61 | 62 | 63 | 63 |
| 74 | 74 | 74 | 75 | 76 | 77 | 77 |
| 78 | 78 | 78 | 79 | 80 | 81 | 81 |
| 61 | 61 | 61 | 62 | 63 | 64 | 64 |
| 75 | 75 | 75 | 76 | 77 | 78 | 78 |
| 79 | 79 | 79 | 80 | 81 | 82 | 82 |
| 62 | 62 | 62 | 63 | 64 | 65 | 65 |
| 76 | 76 | 76 | 77 | 78 | 79 | 79 |
| 80 | 80 | 80 | 81 | 82 | 83 | 83 |
| 63 | 63 | 63 | 64 | 65 | 66 | 66 |
| 77 | 77 | 77 | 78 | 79 | 80 | 80 |
| 81 | 81 | 81 | 82 | 83 | 84 | 84 |
| 64 | 64 | 64 | 65 | 66 | 67 | 67 |
| 78 | 78 | 78 | 79 | 80 | 81 | 81 |
| 82 | 82 | 82 | 83 | 84 | 85 | 85 |
| 64 | 64 | 65 | 66 | 66 | 67 | 68 |
| 78 | 78 | 79 | 80 | 81 | 81 | 82 |
| 82 | 83 | 83 | 84 | 85 | 85 | 86 |
| 64 | 65 | 65 | 66 | 67 | 67 | 68 |
| 78 | 79 | 79 | 80 | 81 | 81 | 82 |
| 82 | 83 | 83 | 84 | 85 | 85 | 86 |

TABLE 7-2

## BLOOD PRESSURE LEVELS FOR THE 50TH, 90TH, AND 95TH PERCENTILES OF BLOOD PRESSURE FOR *BOYS* AGE 1–17 YEARS BY PERCENTILES OF HEIGHT[2]

| | Height* → | Systolic BP (SBP) (mm Hg) by Percentile of Height | | | | | | |
|---|---|---|---|---|---|---|---|---|
| Age (yr) | BP†↓ | 5% | 10% | 25% | 50% | 75% | 90% | 95% |
| 1 | 50th | 80 | 81 | 83 | 85 | 87 | 88 | 89 |
| | 90th | 94 | 95 | 97 | 99 | 100 | 102 | 103 |
| | 95th | 98 | 99 | 101 | 103 | 104 | 106 | 106 |
| 2 | 50th | 84 | 85 | 87 | 88 | 90 | 92 | 92 |
| | 90th | 97 | 99 | 100 | 102 | 104 | 105 | 106 |
| | 95th | 101 | 102 | 104 | 106 | 108 | 109 | 110 |
| 3 | 50th | 86 | 87 | 89 | 91 | 93 | 94 | 95 |
| | 90th | 100 | 101 | 103 | 105 | 107 | 108 | 109 |
| | 95th | 104 | 105 | 107 | 109 | 110 | 112 | 113 |
| 4 | 50th | 88 | 89 | 91 | 93 | 95 | 96 | 97 |
| | 90th | 102 | 103 | 105 | 107 | 109 | 110 | 111 |
| | 95th | 106 | 107 | 109 | 111 | 112 | 114 | 115 |
| 5 | 50th | 90 | 91 | 93 | 95 | 96 | 98 | 98 |
| | 90th | 104 | 105 | 106 | 108 | 110 | 111 | 112 |
| | 95th | 108 | 109 | 110 | 112 | 114 | 115 | 116 |
| 6 | 50th | 91 | 92 | 94 | 96 | 98 | 99 | 100 |
| | 90th | 105 | 106 | 108 | 110 | 111 | 113 | 113 |
| | 95th | 109 | 110 | 112 | 114 | 115 | 117 | 117 |
| 7 | 50th | 92 | 94 | 95 | 97 | 99 | 100 | 101 |
| | 90th | 106 | 107 | 109 | 111 | 113 | 114 | 115 |
| | 95th | 110 | 111 | 113 | 115 | 117 | 118 | 119 |
| 8 | 50th | 94 | 95 | 97 | 99 | 100 | 102 | 102 |
| | 90th | 107 | 109 | 110 | 112 | 114 | 115 | 116 |
| | 95th | 111 | 112 | 114 | 116 | 118 | 119 | 120 |
| 9 | 50th | 95 | 96 | 98 | 100 | 102 | 103 | 104 |
| | 90th | 109 | 110 | 112 | 114 | 115 | 117 | 118 |
| | 95th | 113 | 114 | 116 | 118 | 119 | 121 | 121 |
| 10 | 50th | 97 | 98 | 100 | 102 | 103 | 105 | 106 |
| | 90th | 111 | 112 | 114 | 115 | 117 | 119 | 119 |
| | 95th | 115 | 116 | 117 | 119 | 121 | 122 | 123 |
| 11 | 50th | 99 | 100 | 102 | 104 | 105 | 107 | 107 |
| | 90th | 113 | 114 | 115 | 117 | 119 | 120 | 121 |
| | 95th | 117 | 118 | 119 | 121 | 123 | 124 | 125 |
| 12 | 50th | 101 | 102 | 104 | 106 | 108 | 109 | 110 |
| | 90th | 115 | 116 | 118 | 120 | 121 | 123 | 123 |
| | 95th | 119 | 120 | 122 | 123 | 125 | 127 | 127 |
| 13 | 50th | 104 | 105 | 106 | 108 | 110 | 111 | 111 |
| | 90th | 117 | 118 | 120 | 122 | 124 | 125 | 126 |
| | 95th | 121 | 122 | 124 | 126 | 128 | 129 | 130 |
| 14 | 50th | 106 | 107 | 109 | 111 | 113 | 114 | 115 |
| | 90th | 120 | 121 | 123 | 125 | 126 | 128 | 128 |
| | 95th | 124 | 125 | 127 | 128 | 130 | 132 | 132 |
| 15 | 50th | 109 | 110 | 112 | 113 | 115 | 117 | 117 |
| | 90th | 122 | 124 | 125 | 127 | 129 | 130 | 131 |
| | 95th | 126 | 127 | 129 | 131 | 133 | 134 | 135 |
| 16 | 50th | 111 | 112 | 114 | 116 | 118 | 119 | 120 |
| | 90th | 125 | 126 | 128 | 130 | 131 | 133 | 134 |
| | 95th | 129 | 130 | 132 | 134 | 135 | 137 | 137 |
| 17 | 50th | 114 | 115 | 116 | 118 | 120 | 121 | 122 |
| | 90th | 127 | 128 | 130 | 132 | 134 | 135 | 136 |
| | 95th | 131 | 132 | 134 | 136 | 138 | 139 | 140 |

*Height percentile determined by standard growth curves.

†Blood pressure percentile determined by a single measurement.

| Diastolic BP (DBP) (mm Hg) by Percentile of Height | | | | | | |
|---|---|---|---|---|---|---|
| 5% | 10% | 25% | 50% | 75% | 90% | 95% |
| 34 | 35 | 36 | 37 | 38 | 39 | 39 |
| 49 | 50 | 51 | 52 | 53 | 53 | 54 |
| 54 | 54 | 55 | 56 | 57 | 58 | 58 |
| 39 | 40 | 41 | 42 | 43 | 44 | 44 |
| 54 | 55 | 56 | 57 | 58 | 58 | 59 |
| 59 | 59 | 60 | 61 | 62 | 63 | 63 |
| 44 | 44 | 45 | 46 | 47 | 48 | 48 |
| 59 | 59 | 60 | 61 | 62 | 63 | 63 |
| 63 | 63 | 64 | 65 | 66 | 67 | 67 |
| 47 | 48 | 49 | 50 | 51 | 51 | 52 |
| 62 | 63 | 64 | 65 | 66 | 66 | 67 |
| 66 | 67 | 68 | 69 | 70 | 71 | 71 |
| 50 | 51 | 52 | 53 | 54 | 55 | 55 |
| 65 | 66 | 67 | 68 | 69 | 69 | 70 |
| 69 | 70 | 71 | 72 | 73 | 74 | 74 |
| 53 | 53 | 54 | 55 | 56 | 57 | 57 |
| 68 | 68 | 69 | 70 | 71 | 72 | 72 |
| 72 | 72 | 73 | 74 | 75 | 76 | 76 |
| 55 | 55 | 56 | 57 | 58 | 59 | 59 |
| 70 | 70 | 71 | 72 | 73 | 74 | 74 |
| 74 | 74 | 75 | 76 | 77 | 78 | 78 |
| 56 | 57 | 58 | 59 | 60 | 60 | 61 |
| 71 | 72 | 72 | 73 | 74 | 75 | 76 |
| 75 | 76 | 77 | 78 | 79 | 79 | 80 |
| 57 | 58 | 59 | 60 | 61 | 61 | 62 |
| 72 | 73 | 74 | 75 | 76 | 76 | 77 |
| 76 | 77 | 78 | 79 | 80 | 81 | 81 |
| 58 | 59 | 60 | 61 | 61 | 62 | 63 |
| 73 | 73 | 74 | 75 | 76 | 77 | 78 |
| 77 | 78 | 79 | 80 | 81 | 81 | 82 |
| 59 | 59 | 60 | 61 | 62 | 63 | 63 |
| 74 | 74 | 75 | 76 | 77 | 78 | 78 |
| 78 | 78 | 79 | 80 | 81 | 82 | 82 |
| 59 | 60 | 61 | 62 | 63 | 63 | 64 |
| 74 | 75 | 75 | 76 | 77 | 78 | 79 |
| 78 | 79 | 80 | 81 | 82 | 82 | 83 |
| 60 | 60 | 61 | 62 | 63 | 64 | 64 |
| 75 | 75 | 76 | 77 | 78 | 79 | 79 |
| 79 | 79 | 80 | 81 | 82 | 83 | 83 |
| 60 | 61 | 62 | 63 | 64 | 65 | 65 |
| 75 | 76 | 77 | 78 | 79 | 79 | 80 |
| 80 | 80 | 81 | 82 | 83 | 84 | 84 |
| 61 | 62 | 63 | 64 | 65 | 66 | 66 |
| 76 | 77 | 78 | 79 | 80 | 80 | 81 |
| 81 | 81 | 82 | 83 | 84 | 85 | 85 |
| 63 | 63 | 64 | 65 | 66 | 67 | 67 |
| 78 | 78 | 79 | 80 | 81 | 82 | 82 |
| 82 | 83 | 83 | 84 | 85 | 86 | 87 |
| 65 | 66 | 66 | 67 | 68 | 69 | 70 |
| 80 | 80 | 81 | 82 | 83 | 84 | 84 |
| 84 | 85 | 86 | 87 | 87 | 88 | 89 |

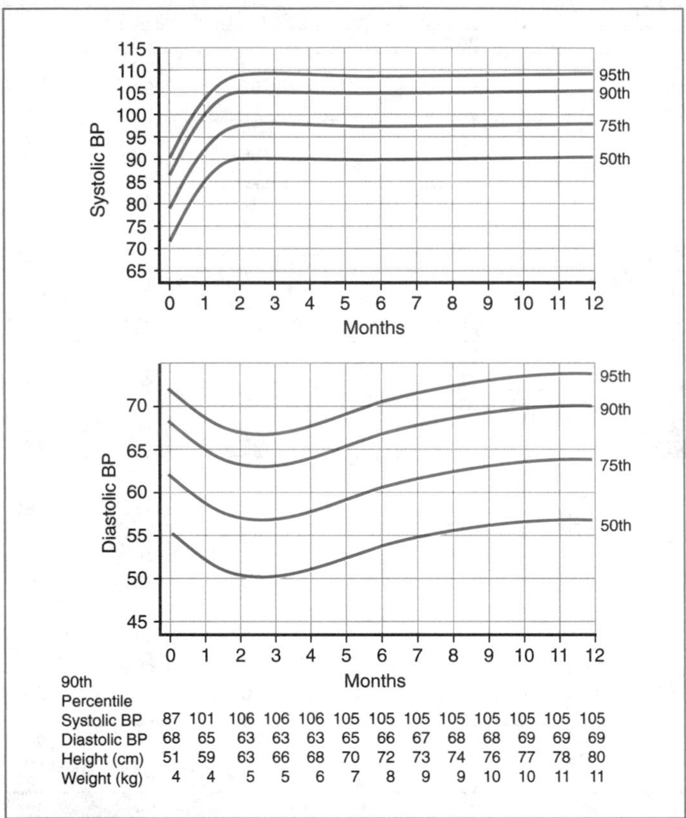


| 90th Percentile | | | | | | | | | | | | | |
|---|---|---|---|---|---|---|---|---|---|---|---|---|---|
| Systolic BP | 87 | 101 | 106 | 106 | 106 | 105 | 105 | 105 | 105 | 105 | 105 | 105 | 105 |
| Diastolic BP | 68 | 65 | 63 | 63 | 63 | 65 | 66 | 67 | 68 | 68 | 69 | 69 | 69 |
| Height (cm) | 51 | 59 | 63 | 66 | 68 | 70 | 72 | 73 | 74 | 76 | 77 | 78 | 80 |
| Weight (kg) | 4 | 4 | 5 | 5 | 6 | 7 | 8 | 9 | 9 | 10 | 10 | 11 | 11 |

FIG. 7-3

Age-specific percentile of blood pressure (BP) measurements in girls from birth to 12 months of age; Korotkoff phase IV (K4) used for diastolic BP. *(From Horan MJ et al: Task Force on Blood Pressure Control in Children: Report of the Second Task Force on Blood Pressure Control in Children. Pediatrics 1987;79[1]:1–25.)*

**BOX 7-1**

**PULSE PRESSURE DIFFERENTIAL DIAGNOSIS**

| Wide Pulse Pressure (>40 mm Hg) | Narrow Pulse Pressure (<25 mm Hg) |
|---|---|
| Aortic insufficiency | Aortic stenosis |
| Arteriovenous fistula | Pericardial effusion |
| Patent ductus arteriosus | Pericardial tamponade |
| Thyrotoxicosis | Pericarditis |
| | Significant tachycardia |



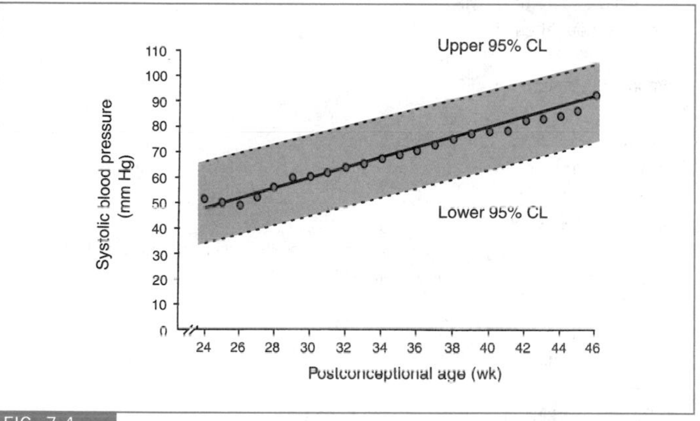


FIG. 7-4

Age-specific percentiles of blood pressure (BP) measurements in boys from birth to 12 months of age; Korotkoff phase IV (K4) used for diastolic BP. *(From Horan MJ et al: Task Force on Blood Pressure Control in Children: Report of the Second Task Force on Blood Pressure Control in Children. Pediatrics 1987;79[1]:1–25.)*

benign from pathologic murmurs. Clinical characteristics of these murmurs are summarized in Table 7-3.[3] When one or more of the following are present, the murmur is likely to be pathologic and require cardiac consultation:

- Symptoms
- Cyanosis
- Systolic murmur that is loud (grade ≥3/6), harsh, and long in duration
- Diastolic murmur
- Abnormal heart sounds
- Presence of a click
- Abnormally strong or weak pulses

2. **Systolic murmurs** (Fig. 7-5).
3. **Diastolic murmurs** (see Fig. 7-5).

BOX 7-2

## SUMMARY OF ABNORMAL HEART SOUNDS

### ABNORMAL SPLITTING

**Widely Split $S_1$**

Ebstein's anomaly

RBBB

**Widely Split and Fixed $S_2$**

Right ventricular volume overload (e.g., ASD, PAPVR)

Abnormal pulmonary valve (e.g., PS)

Electrical delay in RV contraction (e.g., RBBB)

Early aortic closure (e.g., MR)

Occasional normal child

**Narrowly Split $S_2$**

Pulmonary hypertension

AS

Delay in LV contraction (e.g., LBBB)

Occasional normal child

**Single $S_2$**

Pulmonary hypertension

One semilunar valve (e.g., pulmonary atresia, aortic atresia, truncus arteriosus)

P2 not audible (e.g., TGA, TOF, severe PS)

Severe AS

Occasional normal child

**Paradoxically Split $S_2$**

Severe AS

LBBB, Wolff-Parkinson-White syndrome (type B)

**Abnormal Intensity of P2**

Increased P2 (e.g., pulmonary hypertension)

Decreased P2 (e.g., severe PS, TOF, TS)

**$S_3$**

Occasionally heard in healthy children or adults

Dilated ventricles (e.g., large VSD, CHF)

**$S_4$**

Always pathologic

Decreased ventricular compliance

AS, aortic stenosis; ASD, atrial septal defect; LBBB, left bundle-branch block; MR, mitral regurgitation; PAPVR, partial anomalous pulmonary venous return; PS, pulmonary stenosis; RBBB, right bundle-branch block; TGA, transposition of the great arteries; TOF, tetralogy of Fallot; TS, tricuspid stenosis.

Modified from Park MK: Pediatric Cardiology for Practitioners, 4th ed. St. Louis, Mosby, 2002, p 20.

TABLE 7-3

COMMON INNOCENT HEART MURMURS

| Type (Timing) | Description of Murmur | Age Group |
|---|---|---|
| Classic vibratory murmur (Still's murmur; systolic) | Maximal at LMSB or between LLSB and apex<br>Grade 1–2/6 in intensity<br>Low-frequency vibratory, twanging string, groaning, squeaking, or musical | 3–6 yr; occasionally in infancy |
| Pulmonary ejection murmur (systolic) | Maximal at LUSB<br>Early to midsystolic<br>Grade 1–2/6 in intensity<br>Blowing in quality | 8–14 yr |
| Pulmonary flow murmur of newborn (systolic) | Maximal at LUSB<br>Transmits well to left and right chest, axilla, and back<br>Grade 1–2/6 in intensity | Premature and full-term newborns<br>Usually disappears by 3–6 mo |
| Venous hum (continuous) | Maximal at right (or left) supraclavicular and infraclavicular areas<br>Grade 1–2/6 in intensity<br>Inaudible in supine position<br>Intensity changes with rotation of head and disappears with compression of jugular vein | 3–6 yr |
| Carotid bruit (systolic) | Right supraclavicular area over carotids<br>Grade 1–2/6 in intensity<br>Occasional thrill over carotid | Any age |

LLSB, left lower sternal border; LMSB, left middle sternal border; LUSB, left upper sternal border.

From Park MK: Pediatric Cardiology for Practitioners, 4th ed. St. Louis, Mosby, 2002, p 31.

## IV. LIPID MONITORING RECOMMENDATIONS: PREVENTION OF ATHEROSCLEROTIC DISEASE (AMERICAN ACADEMY OF PEDIATRICS RECOMMENDATIONS)

### A. SCREENING OF CHILDREN AND ADOLESCENTS

**Perform targeted screening of fasting lipids in children > 2 years of age with family history of dyslipidemia or premature cardiovascular disease:**

1. **Those whose parents or grandparents, at ≤55 years of age, were found to have coronary atherosclerosis.**
2. **Those whose parents or grandparents, at ≤55 years of age, had a documented myocardial infarction (MI), angina pectoris, peripheral vascular disease, cerebrovascular disease, or sudden cardiac death.**
3. **Those whose parent has an elevated blood cholesterol level (240 mg/dL or higher).**
4. **Those whose parental history is unobtainable, particularly for those with other risk factors, such as smoking, diets high in saturated fats and cholesterol, or obesity.**

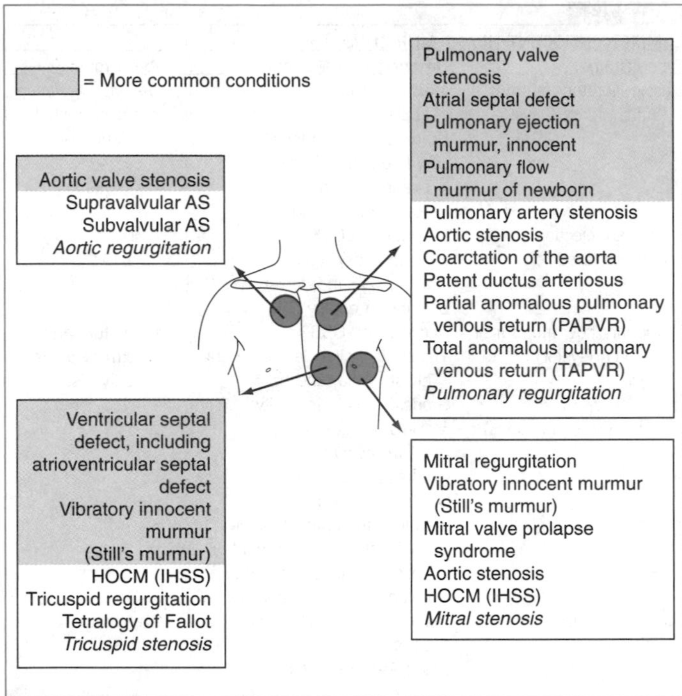


FIG. 7-5

The location at which various murmurs may be heard. Diastolic murmurs are in *italics*. AS, aortic stenosis; HOCM, hypertrophic obstructive cardiomyopathy; IHSS, idiopathic hypertrophic subaortic stenosis. *(From Park MK: Pediatric Cardiology for Practitioners, 4th ed. St. Louis, Mosby, 2002, p 26.)*

## B. GOALS FOR LIPID LEVELS IN CHILDHOOD (Figs. 7-6 and 7-7)

## C. MANAGEMENT OF HYPERLIPIDEMIA

1. **Normal and borderline low-density lipoprotein (LDL) levels:** Education and risk factor intervention, including diet, smoking cessation, and an exercise program. For borderline levels, reevaluate in 1 year.
2. **High LDL levels:** Examine for secondary causes (liver, thyroid, renal disorders) and familial disorders. Then initiate low-fat, low-cholesterol diet, and reevaluate in 3 months.
3. Drug therapy should be considered in children >10 years of age after failure of an adequate trial of diet therapy (6–12 months); LDL >190 mg/dL without other cardiovascular disease risk factors; or >160 mg/dL with risk factors (diabetes, obesity, blood pressure

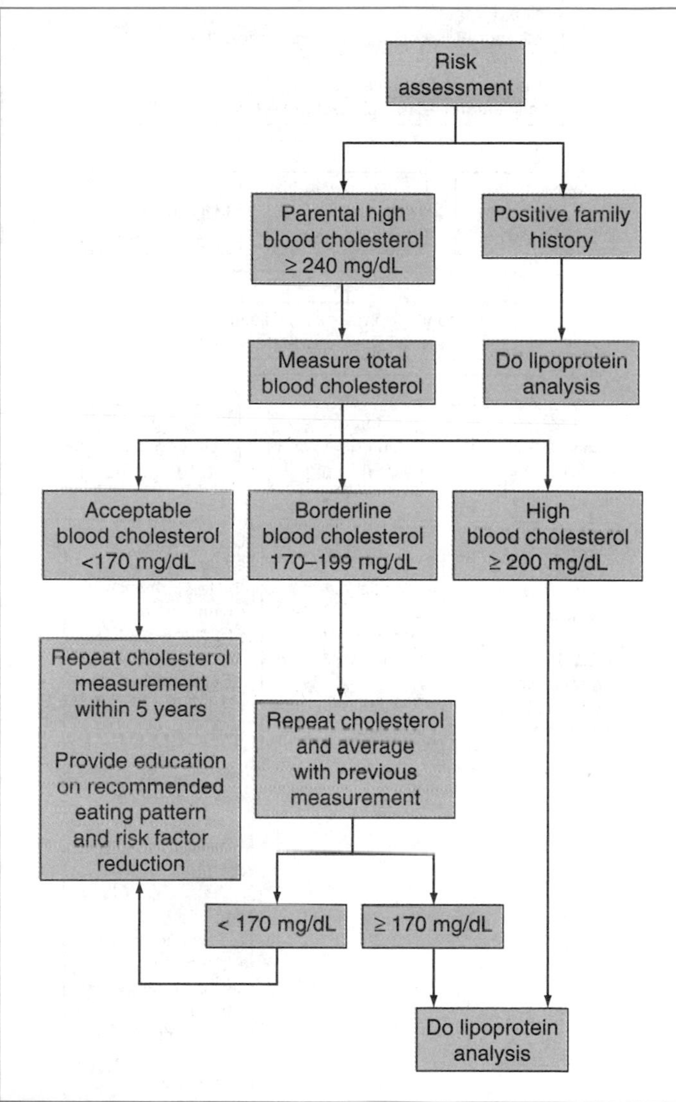


FIG. 7-6
Cholesterol flow chart.

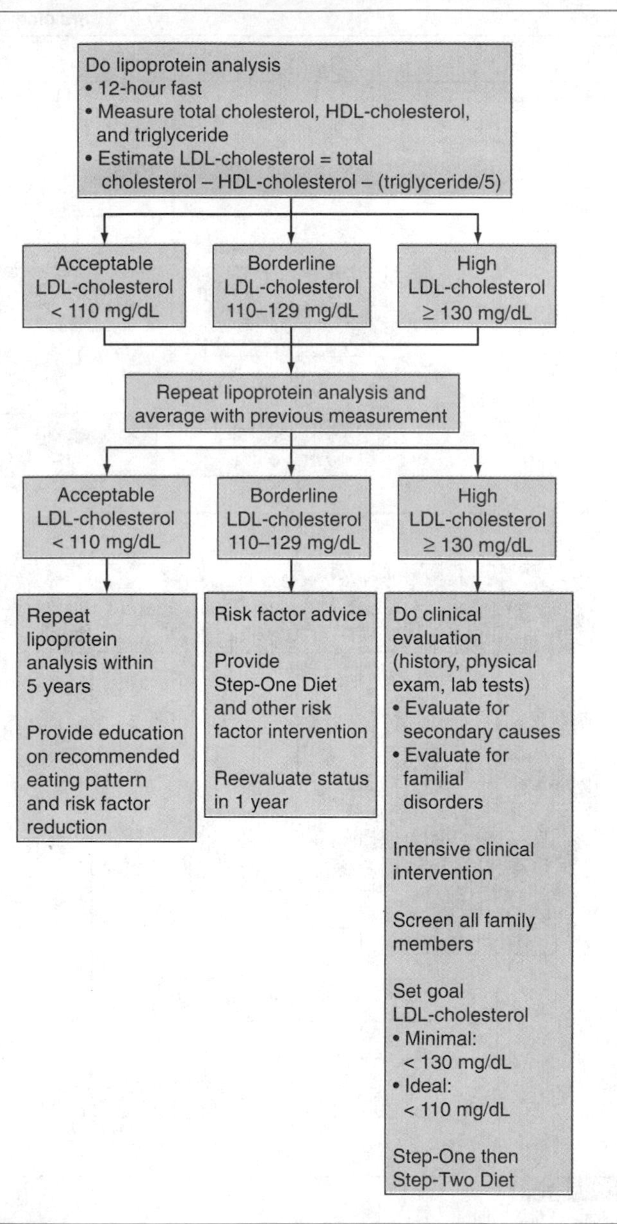


FIG. 7-7

Lipoprotein analysis flow chart.

elevation, strong family history of premature cardiovascular disease). Bile acid sequestrants and statins are the usual first-line drugs for treatment in children.

4. **Persistently high triglycerides (>150 mg/dL) and reduced HDL (<35 mg/dL):** Evaluate for secondary causes (diabetes, alcohol abuse, renal or thyroid disease).

## V. ELECTROCARDIOGRAPHY

### A. BASIC ELECTROCARDIOGRAPHY PRINCIPLES

1. **Lead placement** (Fig. 7-8).
2. **ECG complexes** (see Fig. 7-1).
   a. P wave: Represents atrial depolarization.
   b. QRS complex: Represents ventricular depolarization.
   c. T wave: Represents ventricular repolarization.
   d. U wave: May follow T wave, representing late phases of ventricular repolarization.
3. **Systematic approach for evaluating ECGs (Table 7-4 shows normal ECG parameters):**[3,5]
   a. Rate.
      (1) Standardization: Paper speed is 25 mm/sec. One small square = 1 mm = 0.04 sec. One large square = 5 mm = 0.2 sec. Amplitude standard: 10 mm = 1 mV.
      (2) Calculation: Heart rate (beats per minute) = 60 divided by the average R-R interval in seconds, or 1500 divided by the R-R interval in millimeters.
   b. Rhythm.
      (1) Sinus rhythm: Every QRS complex is preceded by a P wave, normal PR interval (the PR interval may be prolonged, as in



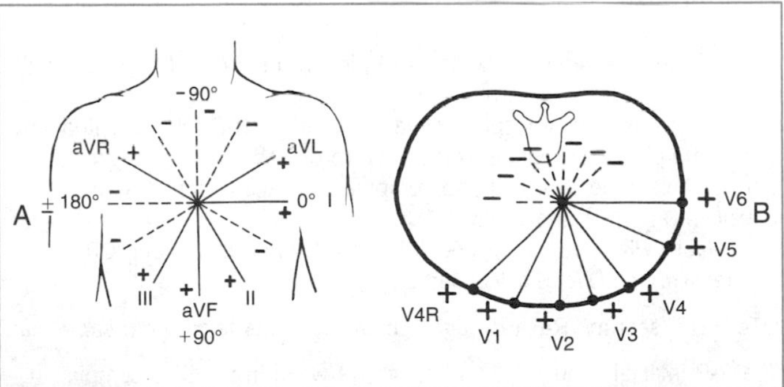


FIG. 7-8

**A,** Hexaxial reference system. **B,** Horizontal reference system. *(Modified from Park MK, Guntheroth WG: How to Read Pediatric ECGs, 4th ed. Philadelphia, Mosby, 2006, p 3.)*

TABLE 7-4
NORMAL PEDIATRIC ECG PARAMETERS

| Age | Heart Rate (bpm) | QRS Axis* | PR Interval (sec)* | QRS Duration (sec)† |
|---|---|---|---|---|
| 0–7 days | 95–160 (125) | +30 to 180 (110) | 0.08–0.12 (0.10) | 0.05 (0.07) |
| 1–3 wk | 105–180 (145) | +30 to 180 (110) | 0.08–0.12 (0.10) | 0.05 (0.07) |
| 1–6 mo | 110–180 (145) | +10 to +125 (+70) | 0.08–0.13 (0.11) | 0.05 (0.07) |
| 6–12 mo | 110–170 (135) | +10 to +125 (+60) | 0.10–0.14 (0.12) | 0.05 (0.07) |
| 1–3 yr | 90–150 (120) | +10 to +125 (+60) | 0.10–0.14 (0.12) | 0.06 (0.07) |
| 4–5 yr | 65–135 (110) | 0 to +110 (+60) | 0.11–0.15 (0.13) | 0.07 (0.08) |
| 6–8 yr | 60–130 (100) | −15 to +110 (+60) | 0.12–0.16 (0.14) | 0.07 (0.08) |
| 9–11 yr | 60–110 (85) | −15 to +110 (+60) | 0.12–0.17 (0.14) | 0.07 (0.09) |
| 12–16 yr | 60–110 (85) | −15 to +110 (+60) | 0.12–0.17 (0.15) | 0.07 (0.10) |
| >16 yr | 60–100 (80) | −15 to +110 (+60) | 0.12–0.20 (0.15) | 0.08 (0.10) |

*Normal range and (mean).
†Mean and (98th percentile).

New data compiled from Park MK: Pediatric Cardiology for Practitioners, 4th ed. St Louis, Mosby, 2002, and Davignon A et al: Normal ECG standards for infants and children. Pediatr Cardiol 1979; 1:123–131.

first-degree atrioventricular [AV] block), and normal P-wave axis (upright P in lead I and aVF).

(2) There is normal respiratory variation of the R-R interval without morphologic changes of the P wave or QRS complex.

c. Axis: Determine quadrant and compare with age-matched normal values (Fig. 7-9; see Table 7-4).

d. Intervals (PR, QRS, QTc): See Table 7-4 for normal PR and QRS intervals. The QTc is calculated as

$$QTc = QT\ (sec)\ m/\sqrt{R\text{-}R}\ \text{(average 3 measurements taken from same lead)}$$

The R-R interval should extend from the R wave in the QRS complex in which you are measuring QT to the preceding R wave. Normal values for QTc are as follows:

(1) 0.44 sec is 97th percentile for infants 3 to 4 days old.[6]

(2) ≤0.45 sec in infants <6 months old.

| Lead $V_1$ | | | Lead $V_6$ | | |
|---|---|---|---|---|---|
| R Wave Amplitude (mm)† | S Wave Amplitude (mm)† | R/S Ratio | R Wave Amplitude (mm)† | S Wave Amplitude (mm)† | R/S Ratio |
| 13.3 (25.5) | 7.7 (18.8) | 2.5 | 4.8 (11.8) | 3.2 (9.6) | 2.2 |
| 10.6 (20.8) | 4.2 (10.8) | 2.9 | 7.6 (16.4) | 3.4 (9.8) | 3.3 |
| 9.7 (19) | 5.4 (15) | 2.3 | 12.4 (22) | 2.8 (8.3) | 5.6 |
| 9.4 (20.3) | 6.4 (18.1) | 1.6 | 12.6 (22.7) | 2.1 (7.2) | 7.6 |
| 8.5 (18) | 9 (21) | 1.2 | 14 (23.3) | 1.7 (6) | 10 |
| 7.6 (16) | 11 (22.5) | 0.8 | 15.6 (25) | 1.4 (4.7) | 11.2 |
| 6 (13) | 12 (24.5) | 0.6 | 16.3 (26) | 1.1 (3.9) | 13 |
| 5.4 (12.1) | 11.9 (25.4) | 0.5 | 16.3 (25.4) | 1.0 (3.9) | 14.3 |
| 4.1 (9.9) | 10.8 (21.2) | 0.5 | 14.3 (23) | 0.8 (3.7) | 14.7 |
| 3 (9) | 10 (20) | 0.3 | 10 (20) | 0.8 (3.7) | 12 |



(3) ≤0.45 sec in males >1 week old and prepubescent females.
(4) ≤0.46 sec for postpubescent females.

e. P-wave size and shape: Normal P wave should be <0.10 sec in children, <0.08 sec in infants, with amplitude < 0.3 mV (3 mm in height, with normal standardization).

f. R-wave progression: There is generally a normal increase in R-wave size and decrease in S-wave size from leads $V_1$ to $V_6$ (with dominant S waves in right precordial leads and dominant R waves in left precordial leads), representing dominance of left ventricular forces. However, newborns and infants have a normal dominance of the right ventricle.

g. Q waves: Normal Q waves are usually <0.04 sec in duration and <25% of the total QRS amplitude. Q waves are <5 mm deep in left precordial leads and aVF and ≤8 mm deep in lead III for children <3 years of age.

h. ST-segment and T-wave evaluation: ST-segment elevation or depression >1 mm in limb leads and >2 mm in precordial leads is consistent with

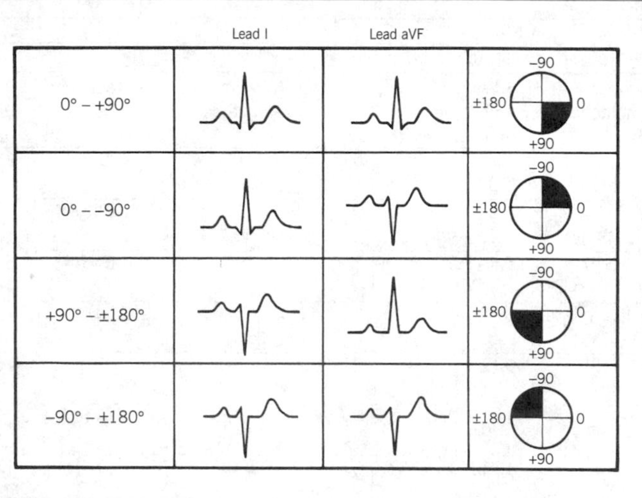


FIG. 7-9

Locating quadrants of mean QRS axis from leads I and aVF. *(From Park MK, Guntheroth WG: How to Read Pediatric ECGs, 4th ed. Philadelphia, Mosby, 2006, p 17.)*

TABLE 7-5

**NORMAL T-WAVE AXIS**

| Age | $V_1$, $V_2$ | AVF | I, $V_5$, $V_6$ |
|---|---|---|---|
| Birth–1 day | ± | + | ± |
| 1–4 days | ± | + | + |
| 4 days to adolescent | – | + | + |
| Adolescent to adult | + | + | + |

+, T wave positive; –, T wave negative; ±, T wave normally either positive or negative.

myocardial ischemia or injury. Tall, peaked T waves may be seen in hyperkalemia. Flat or low T waves may be seen in hypokalemia, hypothyroidism, normal newborn, and myocardial and pericardial ischemia and inflammation (Table 7-5 and Fig. 7-10).

i. Hypertrophy.
   (1) Atrial (Fig. 7-11).
   (2) Ventricular: Diagnosed by QRS axis, voltage, and R/S ratio (Box 7-3; see also Table 7-4).

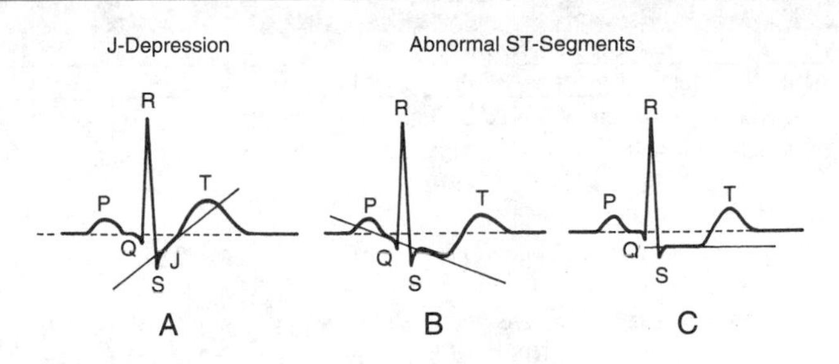


FIG. 7-10

Nonpathologic (nonischemic) and pathologic (ischemic) ST and T changes. **A,** Characteristic nonischemic ST-segment alteration called J depression; note that the ST slope is upward. **B** and **C,** Ischemic or pathologic ST-segment alterations. **B,** Downward slope of the ST segment. **C,** Horizontal segment is sustained. *(From Park MK, Guntheroth WG: How to Read Pediatric ECGs, 4th ed. Philadelphia, Mosby; 2006, p 107.)*

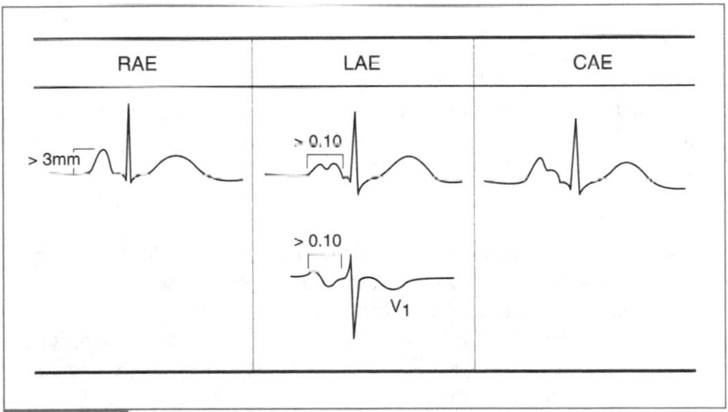

FIG. 7-11

Criteria for atrial enlargement. CAE, combined atrial enlargement; LAE, left atrial enlargement; RAE, right atrial enlargement. *(From Park MK: Pediatric Cardiology for Practitioners, 4th ed. St. Louis, Mosby, 2002, p 44.)*

BOX 7-3

**VENTRICULAR HYPERTROPHY CRITERIA**

**RIGHT VENTRICULAR HYPERTROPHY (RVH) CRITERIA**

**Must Have at Least One of the Following:**

Increased right and anterior QRS voltage (with normal QRS duration):

- R in lead $V_1$, >98th percentile for age
- S in lead $V_6$, >98th percentile for age
- Upright T wave in lead $V_1$ after 3 days of age to adolescence

**Supplemental Criteria**

- Right ventricle strain (associated with inverted T wave in $V_1$ with tall R wave)
- Presence of Q wave in $V_1$ (QR or QRS pattern)
- Right axis deviation (RAD) for patient's age

**LEFT VENTRICULAR HYPERTROPHY (LVH) CRITERIA**

Increased QRS voltage in left leads (with normal QRS duration):

- R in lead $V_6$ (and I, aVL, $V_5$), >98th percentile for age
- S in lead $V_1$, >98th percentile for age
- Left ventricle strain (associated with inverted T wave in leads $V_6$, I, and/or aVF)

**Supplemental Criteria**

- Left axis deviation (LAD) for patient's age
- Volume overload (associated with Q wave >5 mm and tall T waves in $V_5$ or $V_6$)

## B. ECG ABNORMALITIES

1. **Nonventricular arrhythmias** (Table 7-6).[7]
2. **Ventricular arrhythmias** (Table 7-7; Figs. 7-12, 7-13, and 7-14).
3. **Nonventricular conduction disturbances** (Fig. 7-15 and Table 7-8).[8]
4. **Ventricular conduction disturbance** (Table 7-9).

## C. MYOCARDIAL INFARCTION IN CHILDREN

1. **Etiology:** Rare in children but could occur with anomalous origin or aberrant course of a coronary artery, Kawasaki disease, congenital heart disease (presurgical and postsurgical), and dilated cardiomyopathy. It is rarely seen in children with hypertension, lupus, myocarditis, cocaine ingestion, and use of adrenergic drugs (e.g., β-agonists used for asthma).
2. **Frequent ECG findings in children with acute MI:**[9]

a. New-onset wide Q waves (>0.035 sec), seen within first few hours (and persistent over several years).
b. ST-segment elevation (>2 mm), seen within first few hours.
c. Diphasic T waves, seen within first few days (becoming sharply inverted, then normalizing over time).
d. Prolonged QTc interval (>0.44 sec) with accompanying abnormal Q waves.

*Text continued on p. 200*

TABLE 7-6

**NONVENTRICULAR ARRHYTHMIAS**

| Name/Description | Cause | Treatment |
|---|---|---|
| **SINUS** | | |
| **Tachycardia** | | |
| Normal sinus rhythm with HR >95th percentile for age (usually <230 beats/min) | Hypovolemia, shock, anemia, sepsis, fever, anxiety, CHF, PE, myocardial disease, drugs (e.g., β-agonists, albuterol, caffeine, atropine) | Address underlying cause. |
| **Bradycardia** | | |
| Normal sinus rhythm with HR <5th percentile for age | Normal (especially in athletic individuals), increased ICP, hypoxia, hyperkalemia, hypercalcemia, vagal stimulation, hypothyroidism, hypothermia, drugs (e.g., digoxin, β-blockers), long QT syndrome | Address underlying cause; if symptomatic, refer to inside back cover for bradycardia algorithm. |
| **SUPRAVENTRICULAR*** | | |
| **Premature Atrial Contraction** | | |
| Narrow QRS complex; ectopic focus in atria with abnormal P wave morphology | Digitalis toxicity, medications (e.g., caffeine, theophylline, sympathomimetics), normal variant | Treat digitalis toxicity; otherwise no treatment needed. |
| **Atrial Flutter** | | |
| Atrial rate between 250 and 350 beats/min, yielding characteristic sawtooth or flutter pattern with variable ventricular response rate and normal QRS complex | Dilated atria, previous intra-atrial surgery, valvular or ischemic heart disease, idiopathic in newborns | Synchronized cardioversion or overdrive pacing; treat underlying cause. |

*Abnormal rhythm resulting from ectopic focus in atria or AV node, or from accessory conduction pathways. Characterized by different P-wave shape and abnormal P-wave axis. QRS morphology usually normal. See Fig. 7-12.[7]

AV, atrioventricular; CHF, congestive heart failure; HR, heart rate; ICP, intracranial pressure; PE, pulmonary embolism; SA, sinoatrial; SVT, supraventricular tachycardia.

*Continued*

TABLE 7-6

NONVENTRICULAR ARRHYTHMIAS—cont'd

| Name/Description | Cause | Treatment |
|---|---|---|
| **SUPRAVENTRICULAR—cont'd** | | |
| **Atrial Fibrillation** | | |
| Irregular, with atrial rate between 350 and 600 beats/min, yielding characteristic fibrillatory pattern (no discrete P waves) and irregular ventricular response rate of about 110–150 beats/min with normal QRS complex | Wolff-Parkinson-White syndrome and those listed previously (except not idiopathic), alcohol exposure, familial | Synchronized cardioversion; then may need anticoagulation pretreatment. |
| **SVT** | | |
| Sudden run of three or more premature supraventricular beats at >230 beats/min, with narrow QRS complex and abnormal P wave; either sustained (>30 sec) or nonsustained<br>*I. AV Reentrant:* Presence of accessory bypass pathway, in conjunction with AV node, establishes cyclic pattern of reentry independent of SA node; most common cause of nonsinus tachycardia in children (see Wolff-Parkinson-White syndrome, Table 7-9 and Fig. 7-13) | Most commonly idiopathic, but may be seen in congenital heart disease (e.g., Ebstein's anomaly, transposition) | Vagal maneuvers, adenosine; if unstable, need immediate synchronized cardioversion (0.5 j/kg up to 1 j/kg). Consult cardiologist. See "Tachycardia with Poor Perfusion" and "Tachycardia with Adequate Perfusion" algorithms in back of handbook. |
| *II. Junctional:* Automatic focus; simultaneous depolarization of atria and ventricles yields invisible P wave or retrograde P wave | Cardiac surgery, idiopathic | Adjust for clinical situation; consult cardiology. |
| *III. Ectopic atrial tachycardia:* Rapid firing of ectopic focus in atrium | Idiopathic | AV nodal blockade, ablation |
| **Nodal Escape/Junctional Rhythm** | | |
| Abnormal rhythm driven by AV node impulse, giving normal QRS complex and invisible P wave (buried in preceding QRS or T wave) or retrograde P wave (negative in lead II, positive in aVR), seen in sinus bradycardia | | |

TABLE 7-7
VENTRICULAR ARRHYTHMIAS

| Name/Description | Cause | Treatment |
|---|---|---|
| **PVC** | | |
| Ectopic ventricular focus causing early depolarization. Abnormally wide QRS complex appears prematurely, usually with full compensatory pause. May be unifocal or multifocal. **Bigeminy** is alternating normal and abnormal QRS complexes; **trigeminy** is two normal QRS complexes followed by an abnormal one. A **couplet** is two consecutive PVCs. | Myocarditis, myocardial injury, cardiomyopathy, long QT syndrome, congenital and acquired heart disease, drugs (catecholamines, theophylline, caffeine, anesthetics), MVP, anxiety, hypokalemia, hypoxia, hypomagnesemia. **Normal variant.** | None. More worrisome if associated with underlying heart disease or syncope, if worse with activity, or if they are multiform (especially couplets). Address underlying cause, rule out structural heart disease. |
| **VENTRICULAR TACHYCARDIA** | | |
| Series of three or more PVCs at rapid rate (120–250 beats/min), with wide QRS complex and dissociated, retrograde, or no P wave. | See causes of PVCs (70% have underlying cause) | See "Tachycardia with Poor Perfusion" and "Tachycardia with Adequate Perfusion" algorithms in back of handbook. |
| **VENTRICULAR FIBRILLATION** | | |
| Depolarization of ventricles in uncoordinated, asynchronous pattern, yielding abnormal QRS complexes of varying size and morphology with irregular, rapid rate. Rare in children. | Myocarditis, MI, postoperative state, digitalis or quinidine toxicity, catecholamines, severe hypoxia, electrolyte disturbances, long QT syndrome | Requires immediate defibrillation. See algorithm for "Asystole and Pulseless Arrest" inside back cover. |

MI, Myocardial infarction; MVP, mitral valve prolapse; PVC, premature ventricular contraction.

7 CARDIOLOGY

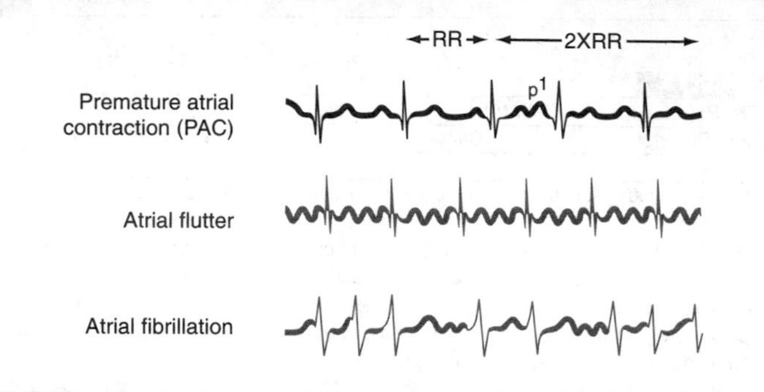


FIG. 7-12

Supraventricular arrhythmias. $p^1$, Premature atrial contraction. *(From Park MK, Guntheroth WG: How to Read Pediatric ECGs, 4th ed. Philadelphia, Mosby, 2006, p 129.)*

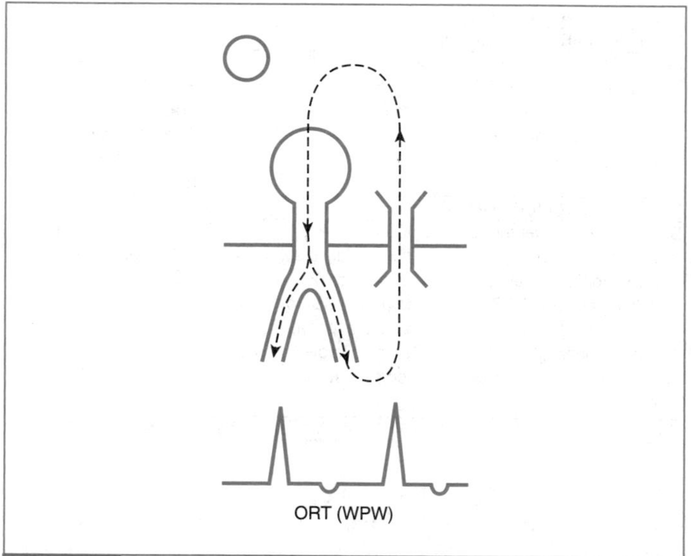


FIG. 7-13

Supraventricular tachycardia pathway: Mechanism for orthodromic reentry (Wolff-Parkinson-White syndrome). Diagram shows the SA node (*upper left circle*), with the AV node (above *the horizontal line*) and bundle branches crossing to the ventricle (below *the horizontal line*). *(Adapted from Walsh EP: Cardiac arrhythmias. In Fyler DC [ed]: Nadas' Pediatric Cardiology. Philadelphia, Hanley & Belfus, 1992, p 384.)*

RR
2XRR
Premature ventricular contraction (PVC)
PVC
Ventricular tachycardia
p
Ventricular fibrillation

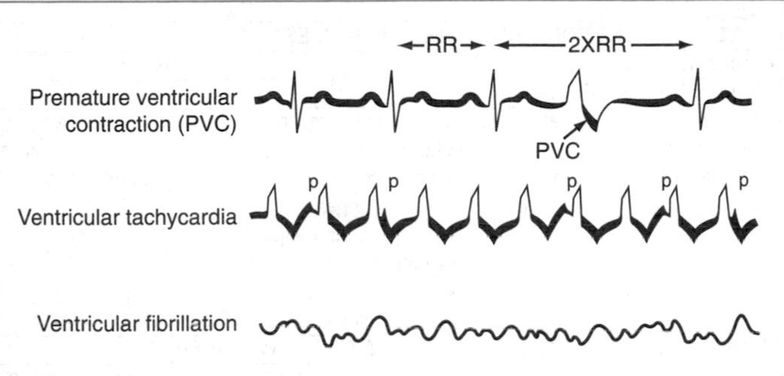

FIG. 7-14
Ventricular arrhythmias. P, P wave. *(From Park MK, Guntheroth WG: How to Read Pediatric ECGs, 4th ed. Philadelphia, Mosby, 2006, p 138.)*



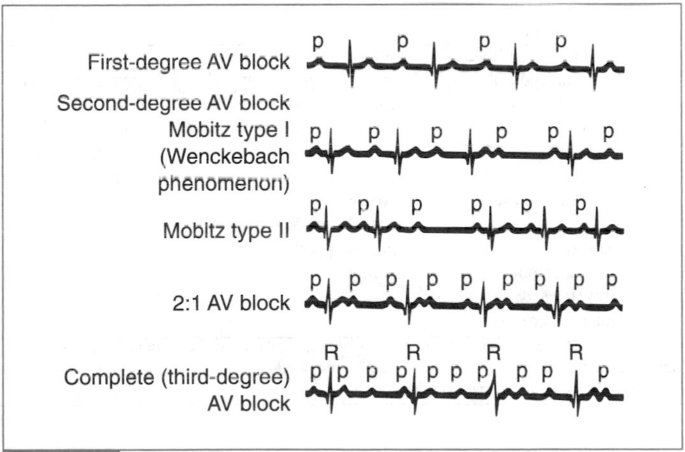

First-degree AV block
Second-degree AV block
Mobitz type I (Wenckebach phenomenon)
Mobitz type II
2:1 AV block
Complete (third-degree) AV block
p
R

FIG. 7-15
Conduction blocks. P, P wave; R, QRS complex. *(From Park MK, Guntheroth WG: How to Read Pediatric ECGs, 4th ed. Philadelphia, Mosby, 2006, p 141.)*

TABLE 7-8

NONVENTRICULAR CONDUCTION DISTURBANCES

| Name/Description* | Cause | Treatment |
|---|---|---|
| **FIRST-DEGREE HEART BLOCK** | | |
| Abnormal but asymptomatic delay in conduction through AV node, yielding prolongation of PR interval | Acute rheumatic fever, tickborne (i.e., Lyme) disease, connective tissue disease, congenital heart disease, cardiomyopathy, digitalis toxicity, postoperative state, normal children | None necessary, except address the underlying cause. |
| **SECOND-DEGREE HEART BLOCK: MOBITZ TYPE I (WENCKEBACH)** | | |
| Progressive lengthening of PR interval until a QRS complex is not conducted. Does not usually progress to complete heart block | Myocarditis, cardiomyopathy, congenital heart disease, postoperative state, MI, toxicity (digitalis, β-blocker), normal children, Lyme disease, lupus | Address underlying cause. |
| **SECOND-DEGREE HEART BLOCK: MOBITZ TYPE II** | | |
| Loss of conduction to ventricle without lengthening of the PR interval. May progress to complete heart block. | Same as for Mobitz Type I | Address underlying cause; may need pacemaker. |
| **THIRD-DEGREE (COMPLETE) HEART BLOCK** | | |
| Complete dissociation of atrial and ventricular conduction. P wave and PR interval regular; RR interval regular and much slower. Width of QRS complex will be narrow and faster with underlying junctional pacemaker, wide and slower with ventricular pacemaker | Congenital due to maternal lupus or other connective tissue disease, structural heart disease; acquired (acute rheumatic fever, myocarditis, Lyme carditis, postoperative, cardiomyopathy, MI, drug overdose) | If bradycardic and symptomatic, consider pacing; see bradycardia algorithm on inside back cover. |

*High-degree AV block: Conduction of atrial impulse at regular intervals, yielding 2:1 block (two atrial impulses for each ventricular response), 3:1 block, etc.
AV, atrioventricular; MI, myocardial infarction.

TABLE 7-9
VENTRICULAR CONDUCTION DISTURBANCES

| Name/Description | Criteria | Causes/Treatment |
|---|---|---|
| **RIGHT BUNDLE-BRANCH BLOCK (RBBB)** | | |
| Delayed right bundle conduction prolongs RV depolarization time, leading to wide QRS | 1. RAD<br>2. Prolonged or wide QRS with terminal slurred R′ (m-shaped RSR′ or RR′) in $V_1$, $V_2$, aVR<br>3. Wide and slurred S wave in leads I and $V_6$ | ASD, surgery with right ventriculostomy, Ebstein's anomaly, coarctation in infants <6 mo, endocardial cushion defect, and partial anomalous pulmonary venous return; occasionally occurs in normal children |
| **LEFT BUNDLE-BRANCH BLOCK (LBBB)** | | |
| Delayed left bundle conduction prolongs septal and LV depolarization time, leading to wide QRS with loss of usual septal signal; there is still a predominance of left ventricle forces. Rare in children. | 1. Wide negative QS complex in lead $V_1$ with loss of septal R wave<br>2. Entirely positive wide R or RR′ complex in lead $V_6$ with loss of septal Q wave | Hypertension, ischemic or valvular heart disease, cardiomyopathy |
| **WOLFF-PARKINSON-WHITE (WPW)** | | |
| Atrial impulse transmitted via anomalous conduction pathway to ventricles, bypassing AV node and normal ventricular conduction system. Leads to premature and prolonged depolarization of ventricles. Bypass pathway is a predisposing condition for SVT. | 1. Shortened PR interval<br>2. Delta wave<br>3. Wide QRS | Acute management of SVT if necessary as previously described; consider ablation of accessory pathway if recurrent SVT. All patients need cardiology referral |

ASD, atrial septal defect; AV, atrioventricular; LV, left ventricle; RAD, right axis deviation; RV, right ventricle; SVT, supraventricular tachycardia.

e. Deep, wide Q waves in leads I, aVL, or $V_6$, without Q waves in II, III, aVF, suggestive of anomalous origin of the left coronary artery.

3. **Other criteria:**

a. Elevated creatinine kinase (CK)/MB fraction, although this is not specific for detection of acute MI in children.

b. Cardiac troponin I is a more sensitive indicator of early myocardial damage in children.[10] It becomes elevated within hours of cardiac injury, persists for 4 to 7 days, and is specific for cardiac injury.

## D. ECG FINDINGS SECONDARY TO ELECTROLYTE DISTURBANCES, MEDICATIONS, AND SYSTEMIC ILLNESSES

1. **Digitalis:**

a. Digitalis effect: Associated with shortened QTc interval, ST depression ("scooped" or "sagging"), mildly prolonged PR interval, and flattened T waves.

b. Digitalis toxicity: Primarily arrhythmias (bradycardia, supraventricular tachycardia, ectopic atrial tachycardia, ventricular tachycardia, AV block).

2. **Other conditions** (Table 7-10).[7,11]

## E. LONG QT SYNDROME

1. **Diagnosis:** QTc >0.44-0.46 sec in absence of other underlying causes (electrolyte disturbances, prematurity). The diagnosis may be supported by associated bradycardia, second-degree AV block, multiform premature ventricular contractions (PVCs), ventricular tachycardia, or abnormal T-wave morphologies. In approximately 10% of cases, patients may have a normal QTc on ECG. Patients may also have a family history of long QT with unexplained syncope, seizure, or cardiac arrest without prolongation of QTc on ECG. Treadmill exercise test may prolong the QTc and will sometimes incite arrhythmias.
2. **Complications:** Associated with the ventricular arrhythmias (torsades de pointes), syncope, and sudden death.
3. **Management:** Patients are most often managed with β-blockers and/or defibrillators; rarely require cardiac sympathetic denervation or demand cardiac pacemakers.

# VI. CONGENITAL HEART DISEASE

Table 7-11 shows common genetic syndromes associated with cardiac lesions.

## A. ACYANOTIC LESIONS (Table 7-12)

## B. CYANOTIC LESIONS (Table 7-13)

An oxygen challenge test is used to evaluate the etiology of cyanosis in neonates. Obtain baseline arterial blood gas (ABG) with saturation at $FiO_2 = 0.21$, then place infant in an oxygen hood at $FiO_2 = 1$ for a minimum of

10 min, and repeat ABG. Pulse oximetry will not be useful for following the change in oxygenation once the saturations reach 100% (approximately $Pao_2$ >90 mm Hg) (Table 7-14).[12–15]

Table 7-15 shows acute management of hypercyanotic spells in TOF.

## C. SURGERIES AND OTHER INTERVENTIONS

1. **Atrial septostomy:** Creates an intra-atrial opening to allow for mixing or shunting between atria (i.e., for transposition of the great arteries [TGA], tricuspid atresia, mitral atresia). Most commonly performed percutaneously with a balloon-tipped catheter (**Rashkind procedure**), in patients with TGA and a small patent foramen ovale, to improve mixing of systemic and pulmonary venous return.
2. **Palliative systemic-to-pulmonary artery shunts,** such as the **Blalock-Taussig shunt:** Use systemic arterial flow to increase pulmonary blood flow in cardiac lesions with impaired pulmonary perfusion (e.g., TOF, hypoplastic right heart, tricuspid atresia, PS) (Fig. 7-16).
3. **Palliative superior vena cava-to-pulmonary artery shunts (Glenn shunt):** Directs a portion of the systemic venous return directly into the pulmonary blood flow (usually performed outside of the neonatal period in infants with lower pulmonary vascular resistance) as an intermediate step to a Fontan procedure (see Fig. 7-16).
4. **Fontan procedure:** Anastomosis of the superior vena cava (SVC) to the right pulmonary artery (RPA) (Glenn shunt), together with anastomosis of the right atria and/or inferior vena cava (IVC) to pulmonary arteries via conduits; separates systemic and pulmonary circulations in patients with functionally single ventricles (tricuspid atresia, hypoplastic left heart syndrome).
5. **Norwood procedure:** Used for hypoplastic left heart syndrome.

a. Stage 1: Anastomosis of the proximal main pulmonary artery (MPA) to the aorta, with aortic arch reconstruction and transection and patch closure of the distal MPA; a modified right Blalock-Taussig shunt (subclavian artery to RPA) to provide pulmonary blood flow; alternatively, a right ventricle to pulmonary artery conduit can be used for pulmonary blood flow (Sano modification). An atrial septal defect is created to allow for adequate left to right flow.

b. Stage 2: Bidirectional Glenn shunt to reduce volume overload of single right ventricle and modified Fontan procedure to correct cyanosis.

6. **Repair of TGA:**

a. Atrial inversion (**Mustard or Senning operation**) (rarely performed today).

b. Arterial switch (of **Jantene**).

7. **Ross procedure:** Pulmonary root autograft for aortic stenosis; autologous pulmonary valve replaces aortic valve, and aortic or pulmonary allograft replaces pulmonary valve.

*Text continued on p. 209*

TABLE 7-10

## SYSTEMIC EFFECTS ON ELECTROCARDIOGRAM

| | Short QT | Long QT-U | Prolonged QRS | ST-T Changes |
|---|---|---|---|---|
| **CHEMISTRY** | | | | |
| Hyperkalemia | | | X | X |
| Hypokalemia | | X | X | X |
| Hypercalcemia | X | | | |
| Hypocalcemia | | X | | |
| Hypermagnesemia | | | | |
| Hypomagnesemia | | X | | |
| **DRUGS** | | | | |
| Digitalis | X | | | X |
| Phenothiazines | | T | | |
| Phenytoin | X | | | |
| Propranolol | X | | | |
| Tricyclics | | T | T | T |
| Verapamil | | | | |
| **MISCELLANEOUS** | | | | |
| CNS injury | | X | | X |
| Friedreich's ataxia | | | | X |
| Duchenne's muscular dystrophy | | | | |
| Myotonic dystrophy | | | X | X |
| Collagen vascular disease | | | | X |
| Hypothyroidism | | | | |
| Hyperthyroidism | | | X | X |
| Other diseases | | Romano-Ward | Lyme disease | |

CNS, central nervous system; T, present only with drug toxicity; X, present.

From Garson A Jr: The Electrocardiogram in Infants and Children: A Systematic Approach. Philadelphia, Lea & Febiger, 1983, p 172, and Walsh EP: Cardiac arrhythmias. In Fyler DC, Nadas A (eds): Pediatric Cardiology. Philadelphia, Hanley & Belfus, 1992, pp 141-143.

| Sinus Tachycardia | Sinus Bradycardia | AV Block | Ventricular Tachycardia | Miscellaneous |
|---|---|---|---|---|
| | | | | |
| | | X | X | Low-voltage Ps; peaked Ts |
| | | | | |
| | X | X | X | |
| X | | X | | |
| | | X | | |
| | | | | |
| | | | | |
| | T | X | T | |
| | | | T | |
| | | | | |
| | X | X | | |
| T | | T | T | |
| | X | X | | |
| | | | | |
| X | X | X | | |
| X | | | | Atrial flutter |
| X | X | | | Atrial flutter |
| X | | X | | |
| | | X | X | |
| | X | | | Low voltage |
| X | | X | | |
| | | Holt-Oram, maternal lupus | | |

TABLE 7-11

**COMMON GENETIC SYNDROMES ASSOCIATED WITH CARDIAC DEFECTS***

| Syndrome | Dominant Cardiac Defect |
|---|---|
| CHARGE | Ventricular, atrioventricular, and ASDs |
| DiGeorge | Aortic arch anomalies, tetralogy of Fallot |
| Down | Atrioventricular septal defects, VSD |
| Marfan | Aortic root dissection, mitral valve prolapse |
| Loeys-Dietz | Aortic root dissection with higher risk of rupture at smaller dimensions |
| Noonan | Supravalvular pulmonic stenosis, ASD |
| Turner | Coarctation of the aorta, bicuspid aortic valve |
| Williams | Supravalvular aortic stenosis |

*See Chapter 13 for details of diagnostic work-up and evaluation of syndromes.

ASD, atrial septal defect; CHARGE, a syndrome of associated defects, including **c**oloboma of the eye, **h**eart anomaly, choanal **a**tresia, **r**etardation, and **g**enital and **e**ar anomalies; VSD, ventricular septal defect.

From Pelech AN: Evaluation of the pediatric patient with a cardiac murmur. Pediatr Clin North Am 1999;46(2):170.

TABLE 7-12

## ACYANOTIC CONGENITAL HEART DISEASE

| Lesion Type | Examination Findings |
|---|---|
| Ventricular septal defect (VSD): 20%–25% of CHD | 2–5/6 holosystolic murmur, loudest at the LLSB<br>A systolic thrill may be felt at the LLSB<br>± Apical diastolic rumble with large shunt<br>$S_2$ may be narrow and P2 may be increased, with large VSD and pulmonary hypertension |
| Atrial septal defect (ASD) | Wide, fixed split $S_2$ with a grade 2–3/6 SEM at the LUSB<br>May have mid-diastolic rumble at LLSB |
| Patent ductus arteriosus (PDA): 5%–10% of CHD in term infants; 40%–60% in preterm infants weighing <1500 g | 1–4/6 continuous "machinery" murmur loudest at the LUSB |
| Atrioventricular septal defects: 30%–60% occur in Down syndrome | Hyperactive precordium with systolic thrill at the LLSB and loud $S_2$. There may be a grade 3–4/6 holosystolic regurgitant murmur along the LLSB<br>May hear systolic murmur of MR at apex<br>May hear mid-diastolic rumble at LLSB or at apex<br>Gallop rhythm may be present |
| Pulmonary stenosis (PS) | Ejection click at LUSB with valvular PS<br>Click intensity will vary with respiration, decreasing with inspiration and increasing with expiration<br>$S_2$ may split widely with P2 diminished in intensity<br>SEM (2–5/6) ± thrill at LUSB with radiation to back and sides |
| Aortic stenosis (AS) | Systolic thrill at RUSB, suprasternal notch, or over carotids<br>Ejection click, which does not vary with respiration, if valvular AS<br>Harsh SEM (2–4/6) at second RICS or third LICS with radiation to the neck and apex<br>May have early diastolic decrescendo murmur as a result of AR<br>Narrow pulse pressure if severe stenosis |
| Coarctation of the aorta: 8%–10% of CHD with male/female ratio of 2:1.<br>May present as (1) infant in CHF (2) child with HTN (3) child with murmur | 2–3/6 SEM at the LUSB with radiation to the left interscapular area<br>Bicuspid valve is often associated and thus may have systolic ejection click at the apex and RUSB<br>BP in lower extremities will be lower than in upper extremities<br>Pulse oximetry discrepancy of >5% between upper and lower extremities is also suggestive of coarctation |

AR, aortic regurgitation; BP, blood pressure; BVH, biventricular hypertrophy; CHD, congenital heart disease; CHF, congestive heart failure; HTN, hypertension; LAE, left atrial enlargement; LICS, left intercostal space; LLSB, left lower sternal border; LUSB, left upper sternal border; LVH, left ventricular hypertrophy; MR, mitral regurgitation; PVM, pulmonary vascular markings; RAD, right axis deviation;

| ECG Findings | Chest Radiograph Findings |
|---|---|
| *Small VSD:* Normal<br>*Medium VSD:* LVH ± LAE<br>*Large VSD:* BVH ± LAE, pure RVH | May show cardiomegaly and increased PVMs dependent on the amount of left to right shunting |
| *Small ASD:* Normal<br>*Hemodynamically significant ASD:* RAD and mild RVH or RBBB with an RSR′ in $V_1$ | May show cardiomegaly with increased PVMs if hemodynamically significant lesion |
| *Small–moderate PDA:* Normal or LVH<br>*Large PDA:* BVH | May have cardiomegaly and increased PVMs, depending on size of shunt (see Chapter 18 for treatment) |
| Superior QRS axis RVH and LVH may be present | Cardiomegaly with increased PVMs |
| *Mild PS:* Normal<br>*Moderate PS:* RAD and RVH<br>*Severe PS:* RAE and RVH with strain | Normal heart size with normal to decreased PVMs |
| *Mild AS:* Normal<br>*Moderate–severe AS:* LVH ± strain | Usually normal |
| *In infancy:* RVH or RBBB<br>*In older children:* LVH | Marked cardiomegaly and pulmonary venous congestion. Rib notching from collateral circulation not seen in infants because collaterals not yet established; usually seen after 5 years of age. |

RAE, right atrial enlargement; RICS, right intercostal space; RBBB, right bundle-branch block; RUSB, right upper sternal border; RVH, right ventricular hypertrophy; SEM, systolic ejection murmur.

TABLE 7-13

CYANOTIC CONGENITAL HEART DISEASE

| Lesion | Examination Findings | ECG Findings | Chest Radiograph Findings |
|---|---|---|---|
| Tetralogy of Fallot:<br>1. Large VSD<br>2. RVOT obstruction<br>3. RVH<br>4. Overriding aorta<br>The degree of RVOT obstruction will determine whether there is clinical cyanosis. If there is only mild PS, there will be a left to right shunt, and the child will be acyanotic. Increased obstruction leads to increased right to left shunting across the VSD and cyanosis. | Loud systolic ejection murmur at left midsternal border and LUSB and a loud, single $S_2$. May also have a thrill at the left midsternal border and LLSB.<br>*Tet spells:* Occur in young infants. As RVOT obstruction increases or systemic resistance decreases, right to left shunting across the VSD occurs. May present with tachypnea, increasing cyanosis, and decreasing murmur. See Table 7-15 for treatment. | RAD and RVH. | Boot-shaped heart with normal heart size ± decreased PVMs |
| Transposition of great arteries | Nonspecific findings. Extreme cyanosis. $S_2$ will be single and loud. May have murmur from associated VSD or PS, but if not present, there may not be a murmur. | Because RV acts as systemic ventricle, patient will have RAD and RVH. Upright T wave in $V_1$ after age 3 days may be only abnormality. | Classic finding: "egg on a string" with cardiomegaly; possible increased PVMs |

ASD, atrial septal defect; CAE, common atrial enlargement; IVC, inferior vena cava; LA, left atrium; LLSB, left lower sternal border; LSB, left upper sternal border; LUSB, left upper sternal border; LVH, left ventricular hypertrophy; PA, pulmonary artery; PDA, patent ductus arteriosus; PFO, patent foramen ovale; PVM, pulmonary vascular markings; PS, pulmonary stenosis; RA, right atrium; RAD, right axis deviation; RAE, right atrial enlargement; RV, right ventricle; RVH, right ventricular hypertrophy; RVOT, right ventricular outflow tract; SEM, systolic ejection murmur; SVC, superior vena cava; VSD, ventriclar septal defect.

*Continued*

TABLE 7-13

CYANOTIC CONGENITAL HEART DISEASE—cont'd

| Lesion | Examination Findings | ECG Findings | Chest Radiograph Findings |
|---|---|---|---|
| Tricuspid atresia: Absent tricuspid valve and hypoplastic RV and PA. Must have ASD, PDA, or VSD for survival. | Single $S_2$. A grade 2–3/6 systolic regurgitation murmur at the LLSB is present if there is a VSD. Occasionally, there is a PDA murmur | Superior QRS axis; RAE or CAE, and LVH | Normal or slightly enlarged heart size; may have boot-shaped heart |
| Total anomalous pulmonary venous return: Pulmonary veins drain into RA or other location besides LA. Must have ASD or PFO for survival. 1. *Supracardiac (most common):* Common pulmonary vein into SVC 2. *Cardiac:* Pulmonary vein into coronary sinus or RA 3. *Subdiaphragmatic:* Common pulmonary vein into IVC, portal vein, ductus venosus, or hepatic vein 4. *Mixed type* | Hyperactive RV impulse, quadruple rhythm, $S_2$ fixed and widely split, 2–3/6 SEM at LUSB, and mid-diastolic rumble at LLSB | RAD, RVH (RSR′ in $V_1$). May see RAE | Cardiomegaly and increased PVMs; classic finding is “snowman in a snowstorm,” but this is rarely seen until after age 4 months |
| **OTHER** | | | |
| Cyanotic CHDs that occur at a frequency of <1% each include pulmonary atresia, Ebstein's anomaly, truncus arteriosus, single ventricle, and double outlet right ventricle. | | | |

TABLE 7-14

**INTERPRETATION OF OXYGEN CHALLENGE TEST**

| Condition | $FiO_2 = 0.21$ $PaO_2$ (% Saturation) | | $FiO_2 = 1.00$ $PaO_2$ (% Saturation) | $PaCO_2$ |
|---|---|---|---|---|
| Normal | 70 (95) | | >200 (100) | 35 |
| Pulmonary disease | 50 (85) | | >150 (100) | 50 |
| Neurologic disease | 50 (85) | | >150 (100) | 50 |
| Methemoglobinemia | 70 (85) | | >200 (85) | 35 |
| Cardiac disease | | | | |
| • Separate circulation* | <40 (<75) | | <50 (<85) | 35 |
| • Restricted PBF† | <40 (<75) | | <50 (<85) | 35 |
| • Complete mixing without restricted PBF‡ | 50 (85) | | <150 (<100) | 35 |
| Persistent pulmonary hypertension | *Preductal* | *Postductal* | | |
| PFO (no R to L shunt) | 70 (95) | <40 (<75) | Variable | 35–50 |
| PFO (with R to L shunt) | <40 (<75) | <40 (<75) | Variable | 35–50 |

*D-Transposition of the great arteries (D-TGA) with intact ventricular septum.

†Tricuspid atresia with pulmonary stenosis or atresia, pulmonary atresia or critical pulmonary stenosis with intact ventricular septum, or tetralogy of Fallot.

‡Truncus, total anomalous pulmonary venous return, single ventricle, hypoplastic left heart, D-TGA with ventricular septal defect, tricuspid atresia without pulmonary stenosis or atresia.

PBF, Pulmonary blood flow; PFO, patent foramen ovale.

From Lees MH: Cyanosis of the newborn infant: Recognition and clinical evaluation. J Pediatr 1970;77:484; Kitterman JA: Cyanosis in the newborn infant. Pediatr Rev 1982;4:13; and Jones RW et al: Arterial oxygen tension and response to oxygen breathing in differential diagnosis of congenital heart disease in infancy. Arch Dis Child 1976;51:667.

TABLE 7-15

TREATMENT OPTIONS FOR "TET SPELLS"

| Treatment | Rationale |
|---|---|
| Oxygen | Reduces hypoxemia, decreases PVR |
| Intravenous fluids | Provides volume resuscitation |
| Calm child | Decreases PVR |
| Encourage knee-chest position | Decreases venous return and increases SVR |
| Phenylephrine (0.02 mg/kg IV) | Increases SVR |
| Propranolol (0.15–0.25 mg/kg slow IV push) | Has negative inotropic effect on infundibular myocardium; may block drop in SVR |
| Morphine (morphine sulfate 0.1–0.2 mg/kg SC or IM) | Decreases venous return, decreases PVR, relaxes infundibulum. Do not try to establish IV access initially. Use the SC route. |
| Methoxamine | Increases SVR |
| Sodium bicarbonate (1 mEq/kg IV) | Reduces metabolic acidosis |
| Correct anemia | Increases delivery of oxygen to tissues |
| Correct pathologic tachyarrhythmias | May abort hypoxic spell |
| Infuse glucose | Avoids hypoglycemia from increased utilization and depletion of glycogen stores |

IM, intramuscular; IV, intravenous; PVR, peripheral venous resistance; SC, subcutaneous; SVR, systemic vascular resistance.



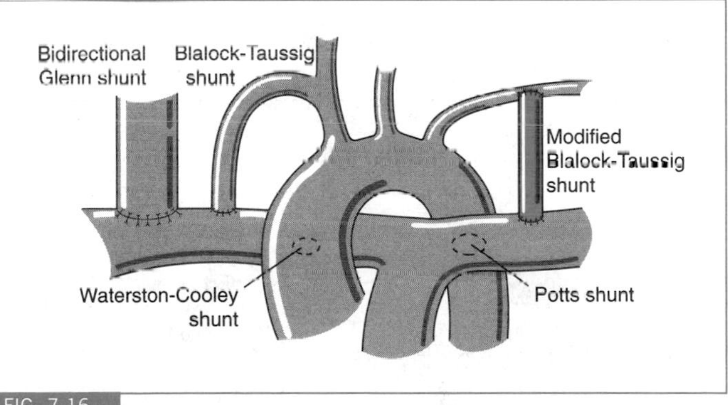


FIG. 7-16

Schematic diagram of cardiac shunts.

## VII. IMAGING

### A. CHEST RADIOGRAPH

**1. Evaluate the heart:**

a. Size: The cardiac shadow should be less than 50% of the thoracic width, which is the maximal width between the inner margins of the ribs, as measured on a posteroanterior radiograph during inspiration.

b. Shape: The shape of the heart can aid in the diagnosis of chamber/vessel enlargement and some congenital heart disease (Fig. 7-17).
c. Situs (levocardia, mesocardia, dextrocardia).

2. **Evaluate the lung fields:**
a. Decreased pulmonary blood flow is seen in pulmonary or tricuspid stenosis/atresia, TOF, pulmonary hypertension ("peripheral pruning").
b. Increased pulmonary blood flow can be seen as increased pulmonary vascular markings (PVMs) with redistribution from bases to apices of lungs and extension to lateral lung fields (see Tables 7-12 and 7-13).
c. Venous congestion, or congestive heart failure (CHF), causes increased PVMs centrally, interstitial and alveolar pulmonary edema (air bronchograms), septal lines, and pleural effusions (see Tables 7-12 and 7-13).

3. **Evaluate the airway: The trachea usually bends slightly to the right above the carina in normal patients with a left-sided aortic arch. A perfectly straight or left-bending trachea suggests a right aortic arch, which may be associated with other defects (TOF, truncus arteriosus, vascular rings, chromosome 22 microdeletion).**

4. **Skeletal anomalies:**
a. Rib notching (e.g., from collateral vessels in patients >5 years of age with coarctation of the aorta).

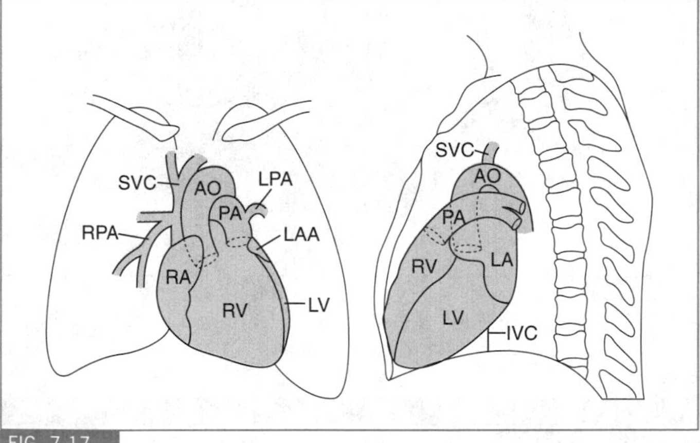


FIG. 7-17

Radiologic contours of the heart. AO, Aorta; IVC, inferior vena cava; LA, left atrium; LAA, left atrial appendage; LPA, left pulmonary artery; LV, left ventricle; PA, pulmonary artery; RA, right atrium; RPA, right pulmonary artery; RV, right ventricle; SVC, superior vena cava.

b. Sternal abnormalities (e.g., Holt-Oram syndrome, pectus excavatum in Marfan Ehlers-Danlos, and Noonan syndromes).
c. Vertebral anomalies (e.g., VATER/VACTERL syndrome: **V**ertebral anomalies, **A**nal atresia, **T**racheoesophageal fistula, **R**adial and **R**enal, **C**ardiac, and **L**imb anomalies).

Please see Chapter 25 for more information on the chest radiograph.

## B. ECHOCARDIOGRAPHY

1. **Approach:**
a. Transthoracic echocardiography (TTE): Does not require general anesthesia, is simpler to perform than transesophageal echocardiography (TEE), but does have limitations in some patients (e.g., uncooperative, obese, or those with suspected endocarditis).
b. TEE: Uses an ultrasound transducer on the end of a modified endoscope to view the heart from the esophagus and stomach, allowing for better imaging of intracardiac structures. It allows for better imaging in obese and intraoperative patients. TEE is also useful for visualizing very small lesions such as some vegetations.
2. **Shortening fraction:** Very reliable index of left ventricular function. Normal values range from approximately 30% to 45%, depending on age.[16]

## C. EXERCISE RECOMMENDATIONS FOR CONGENITAL HEART DISEASE (Table 7-16)

# VIII. ACQUIRED HEART DISEASE

## A. ENDOCARDITIS

1. **Common causative organisms:** About 70% of causes of endocarditis are streptococcal species (*Streptococcus viridans,* enterococci); 20% are staphylococcal species (*Staphylococcus aureus, Staphylococcus epidermidis*); 10% are other organisms (*Haemophilus influenzae,* gram-negative bacteria, fungi).
2. **Clinical findings:** New heart murmur, recurrent fever, splenomegaly, petechiae, fatigue, Osler nodes (tender nodules at fingertips), Janeway lesions (painless hemorrhagic areas on palms or soles), splinter hemorrhages, and Roth spots (retinal hemorrhages).

## B. BACTERIAL ENDOCARDITIS PROPHYLAXIS[15,17]

1. All dental procedures that involve treatment of gingival tissue or periapical region of the teeth or oral mucosal perforation.
2. Invasive procedures that involve incision or biopsy of respiratory mucosa, such as tonsillectomy and adenoidectomy.
3. Not recommended for genitourinary or gastrointestinal tract procedures; solely for bacterial endocarditis prevention.

See Table 7-17 and Box 7-4.

TABLE 7-16

**EXERCISE RECOMMENDATIONS FOR CONGENITAL HEART DISEASE AND SPORTS ALLOWED FOR SOME SPECIFIC CARDIAC LESIONS[18]**

| Diagnosis | Sports Allowed |
|---|---|
| Small ASD or VSD | All |
| Mild aortic stenosis | All |
| MVP (without other risk factors) | All |
| Moderate aortic stenosis | IA, IB, IIA |
| Mild LV dysfunction | IA, IB, IC |
| Moderate LV dysfunction | IA only |
| Hypertrophic cardiomyopathy | None (or IA only) |
| Severe aortic stenosis | None |
| Long QT syndrome | None |

| Sports Classification | Low Dynamic (A) | Moderate Dynamic (B) | High Dynamic (C) |
|---|---|---|---|
| I. Low static | Billiards<br>Bowling<br>Golf<br>Riflery | Baseball<br>Softball<br>Table tennis<br>Volleyball<br>Fencing | Badminton<br>Cross-country skiing<br>Field hockey*<br>Race walking<br>Racquetball<br>Running (long distance)<br>Soccer*<br>Tennis |
| II. Moderate static | Archery<br>Auto racing*,†<br>Diving*,†<br>Equestrian*,†<br>Motorcycling*,† | Fencing<br>Field events (jumping)<br>Figure skating*<br>Football (American)*<br>Surfing<br>Rugby*<br>Running (sprint)<br>Synchronized swimming† | Basketball*<br>Ice hockey*<br>Cross-country skiing (skating technique)<br>Swimming<br>Lacrosse*<br>Running (middle distance)<br>Team handball |
| III. High static | Bobsledding<br>Field events<br>Gymnastics*,†<br>Rock climbing<br>Sailing<br>Windsurfing*,†<br>Waterskiing*,†<br>Weight lifting*,† | Body building*,†<br>Downhill skiing*,†<br>Skateboarding*,† | Boxing*<br>Wrestling*<br>Martial Arts*<br>Speed skating<br>Cycling*,†<br>Rowing |

*Danger of bodily collision.

†Increased risk if syncope occurs.

From Maron BJ et al: 36th Bethesda Conference: Eligibility recommendations for competitive athletes with cardiovascular abnormalities. J Am Coll Cardiol 2005;45(8):1313–1375; and Washington RL et al: Medical conditions affecting sports participation. Pediatrics 2001;107(5):1205–1209.

TABLE 7-17

PROPHYLACTIC REGIMENS FOR DENTAL AND RESPIRATORY TRACT PROCEDURES

| Situation | Agents | Regimen* |
|---|---|---|
| Standard general prophylaxis | Amoxicillin | Adult: 2 g; Children: 50 mg/kg PO 1 hr before procedure |
| Unable to take oral medications | Ampicillin *or* | Adult: 2 g IM or IV; Children: 50 mg/kg IM or IV within 30 min before procedure |
| | Cefazolin or ceftriaxone† | Adult: 1 g IM or IV; Children 50 mg/kg kg IM or IV within 30 min before procedure |
| Allergic to penicillin | Clindamycin *or* | Adult: 600 mg; Children: 20 mg/kg PO 1 hr before procedure |
| | Cephalexin† *or* | Adult: 2 g; Children: 50 mg/kg PO 1 hr before procedure |
| | Azithromycin or clarithromycin | Adult: 500 mg; Children: 15 mg/kg PO 1 hr before procedure |
| Allergic to penicillin and unable to take oral medications | Clindamycin *or* | Adult: 600 mg IM or IV; Children: 20 mg/kg IM or IV within 30 min before procedure |
| | Ceftriaxone or cefazolin† | Adult: 1 g IM or IV; Children: 50 mg/kg IM or IV within 30 min before procedure |

*Total children's dose should not exceed adult dose.

†Cephalosporins should not be used in persons with intermediate-type hypersensitivity reaction to penicillins or ampicillin.

Adapted from Wilson W et al: Prevention of Infective Endocarditis. Guidelines from the American Heart Association: A Guideline from the American Heart Association Rheumatic Fever, Endocarditis, and Kawasaki Disease Committee, Council on Cardiovascular Disease in the Young, and the Council on Clinical Cardiology, Council on Cardiovascular Surgery and Anesthesia, and the Quality of Care and Outcomes Research Interdisciplinary Working Group. Circulation 2007;116:1747.

## C. MYOCARDIAL DISEASE

1. **Dilated cardiomyopathy: End result of myocardial damage, leading to atrial and ventricular dilation with decreased contractile function of the ventricles.**

a. Etiology: Infectious, toxic (alcohol, anthracyclines), metabolic (hypothyroidism, muscular dystrophy), immunologic, collagen vascular disease.

b. Symptoms: Fatigue, weakness, shortness of breath.

c. Examination: Look for signs of CHF, including tachycardia, tachypnea, rales, cold extremities, jugular venous distention, hepatomegaly, peripheral edema, $S_3$ gallop, and displacement of point of maximal impulse to the left and inferiorly.

BOX 7-4

**CARDIAC CONDITIONS FOR WHICH ANTIBIOTIC PROPHYLAXIS IS RECOMMENDED FOR DENTAL, RESPIRATORY TRACT, INFECTED SKIN, SKIN STRUCTURES, OR MUSCULOSKELETAL TISSUE PROCEDURES**

Prosthetic cardiac valve

Previous bacterial endocarditis

Congenital heart disease (CHD)*

- Unrepaired cyanotic defect, including palliative shunts and conduits
- Completely repaired CHD with prosthetic material/device (placed by surgery or catheterization), during first 6 months after procedure†
- Repaired CHD with residual defects at or adjacent to the site of prosthetic patch or device (which inhibit endothelialization)
- Cardiac transplantation patients who develop cardiac valvulopathy

*Antibiotic prophylaxis is not recommended for any other form of CHD except for the conditions just cited that are associated with the highest risk of adverse outcome from endocarditis.
†Endothelialization process of prosthetic material occurs within 6 months after the procedure.

Adapted from Wilson W et al: Prevention of Infective Endocarditis: Guidelines from the American Heart Association: A Guideline from the American Heart Association Rheumatic Fever, Endocarditis, and Kawasaki Disease Committee, Council on Cardiovascular Disease in the Young, and the Council on Clinical Cardiology, Council on Cardiovascular Surgery and Anesthesia, and the Quality of Care and Outcomes Research Interdisciplinary Working Group. Circulation 2007;116:1745.

d. Chest radiograph: Generalized cardiomegaly, pulmonary congestion.
e. ECG: Sinus tachycardia, left ventricular hypertrophy (LVH), possible atrial enlargement, arrhythmias, conduction disturbances, ST-segment and T-wave changes.
f. Echocardiography: Enlarged ventricles (increased end-diastolic and end-systolic dimensions) with little or no wall thickening; decreased shortening fraction.
g. Treatment: Management of CHF (digoxin, diuretics, vasodilation, rest). Consider anticoagulants to decrease risk for thrombus formation.

2. **Hypertrophic cardiomyopathy: Abnormality of myocardial cells leading to significant ventricular hypertrophy, particularly of the left ventricle, with small to normal ventricular dimensions. Contractile function is increased, but filling is impaired secondary to stiff ventricles. The most common type is asymmetrical septal hypertrophy, also called idiopathic hypertrophic subaortic stenosis (IHSS), with varying degrees of obstruction. A 4% to 6% incidence of sudden death in children and adolescents with hypertrophic obstructive cardiomyopathy (HOCM).**

a. Etiology: Genetic (autosomal dominant, 60% of cases) or sporadic (40% of cases).
b. Symptoms: Easy fatigability, anginal pain, shortness of breath, occasional palpitations.
c. Examination: Usually found in adolescents or young adults; signs

include left ventricular heave, sharp upstroke of arterial pulse, murmur of mitral regurgitation, midsystolic ejection murmur along left midsternal border (LMSB) that increases in intensity in the standing position (in patients with midcavity left ventricular obstruction).

d. Chest radiograph: Globular-shaped heart with left ventricular enlargement.
e. ECG: LVH, prominent Q waves (septal hypertrophy), ST-segment and T-wave changes, arrhythmias.
f. Echocardiography: Extent and location of hypertrophy, obstruction, increased contractility.
g. Treatment: Moderate restriction of physical activity, administration of negative inotropes (β-blocker, calcium channel blocker) to help improve filling, and subacute bacterial endocarditis prophylaxis. If at increased risk for sudden death, may consider implantable defibrillator. If symptomatic with subaortic obstruction, may benefit from myectomy.

3. **Restrictive cardiomyopathy: Myocardial or endocardial disease (usually infiltrative or fibrotic) resulting in stiff ventricular walls, with restriction of diastolic filling but normal contractile function. Results in atrial enlargement. Associated with a high mortality rate. Very rare in children.**
4. **Myocarditis: Inflammation of myocardial tissue.**

a. Etiology: Viral (coxsackievirus, echovirus, poliomyelitis, mumps, rubella, cytomegalovirus, human immunodeficiency virus, arbovirus, adenovirus, influenza); bacterial, rickettsial, fungal, or parasitic infection; Immune-mediated disease (Kawasaki disease, acute rheumatic fever); collagen vascular disease; toxin-induced.
b. Symptoms: Nonspecific and inconsistent, depending on severity of disease. Variably anorexia, lethargy, emesis, lightheadedness, cold extremities, shortness of breath.
c. Examination: Look for signs of CHF (tachycardia, tachypnea, jugular venous distention, rales, gallop, hepatomegaly); occasionally, a soft, systolic murmur or arrhythmias may be noted.
d. Chest radiograph: Variable cardiomegaly and pulmonary edema.
e. ECG: Low QRS voltages throughout (<5 mm), ST-segment and T-wave changes (e.g., decreased T-wave amplitude), prolongation of QT interval, arrhythmias (especially premature contractions, first- or second-degree AV block).
f. Laboratory tests: CK, troponin
g. Echocardiography: Enlargement of heart chambers, impaired left ventricular function.
h. Treatment: Bed rest, diuretics, inotropes (dopamine, dobutamine, milrinone), digoxin, gamma globulin (2 g/kg over 24 hr), afterload reducer (e.g., angiotensin-converting enzyme inhibitor), possibly steroids. May require heart transplantation if no improvement (about 20% to 25% of cases).

## D. PERICARDIAL DISEASE

1. **Pericarditis: Inflammation of visceral and parietal layers of pericardium.**

a. Etiology: Viral (especially echovirus, coxsackievirus B), tuberculosis, bacterial, uremic, neoplastic, collagen vascular, post-MI or postpericardiotomy, radiation induced, drug induced (e.g., procainamide, hydralazine), or idiopathic.

b. Symptoms: Chest pain (retrosternal or precordial, radiating to back or shoulder, pleuritic in nature, alleviated by leaning forward, aggravated by supine position), dyspnea.

c. Examination: Pericardial friction rub, distant heart sounds, fever, tachypnea.

d. ECG: Diffuse ST-segment elevation in almost all leads (representing inflammation of adjacent myocardium); PR-segment depression.

e. Treatment: Often self-limited. Treat underlying condition, and provide symptomatic treatment with rest, analgesia, and anti-inflammatory drugs.

2. **Pericardial effusion: Accumulation of excess fluid in pericardial sac.**

a. Etiology: Associated with acute pericarditis (exudative fluid) or serous effusion resulting from increased capillary hydrostatic pressure (e.g., CHF), decreased plasma oncotic pressure (e.g., hypoproteinemia), and increased capillary permeability (transudative fluid).

b. Symptoms: Can present with no symptoms, dull ache in left chest, abdominal pain, or symptoms of cardiac tamponade, discussed subsequently.

c. Examination: Muffled distant heart sounds, dullness to percussion of posterior left chest (secondary to atelectasis from large pericardial sac), hemodynamic signs of cardiac compression (see section VIII. D.3.c).

d. Chest radiograph: Globular, symmetrical cardiomegaly.

e. ECG: Decreased voltage of QRS complexes, electrical alternans (variation of QRS axis with each beat secondary to swinging of heart within pericardial fluid).

f. Echocardiography shows extent and location of hypertrophy, obstruction, increased contractility.

g. Treatment: Address underlying condition. Observe if asymptomatic; use pericardiocentesis if there is sudden increase in volume or hemodynamic compromise. Nonsteroidal anti-inflammatory drugs or steroids may be of benefit, depending on etiology.

3. **Cardiac tamponade: Accumulation of pericardial fluid under high pressure, causing compression of cardiac chambers, limiting filling, and decreasing stroke volume and cardiac output.**

a. Etiology: As for pericardial effusion. Most commonly associated with viral infection, neoplasm, uremia, and acute hemorrhage.

b. Symptoms: Dyspnea, fatigue, cold extremities.

c. Examination: Jugular venous distention, hepatomegaly, peripheral edema, tachypnea, rales (from increased systemic and pulmonary venous pressure), hypotension, tachycardia, pulsus paradoxus (decrease in systolic blood pressure by >10 mm Hg with each inspiration), decreased capillary refill (from decreased stroke volume and cardiac output), quiet precordium, and muffled heart sounds.
d. ECG: Sinus tachycardia, decreased voltage, electrical alternans.
e. Echocardiography: Right ventricle collapse in early diastole, right atrial/left atrial collapse in end-diastole and early systole.
f. Treatment: Pericardiocentesis with temporary catheter left in place if necessary (see Chapter 3), pericardial window or stripping if it is a recurrent condition.



## E. KAWASAKI DISEASE

The leading cause of acquired heart disease in children in developed countries. It is seen almost exclusively in children <8 years of age. Patients present with acute febrile vasculitis, which may lead to long-term cardiac complications from vasculitis of coronary arteries. The number of cases peaks in winter and spring.

1. **Etiology:** Unknown. Thought to be immune-regulated, in response to infectious agents or environmental toxins.
2. **Diagnosis:** Based on clinical criteria. These include high fever lasting 5 days or more, plus at least four of the following five criteria:

a. Bilateral bulbar conjunctival injection without exudate.
b. Erythematous mouth and pharynx, strawberry tongue, or red, cracked lips.
c. Polymorphous exanthem (may be morbilliform, maculopapular, or scarlatiniform).
d. Swelling of the hands and feet, with erythema of the palms and soles.
e. Cervical lymphadenopathy (>1.5 cm in diameter), usually single and unilateral.

**Note** *Atypical Kawasaki disease, more often seen in infants, consists of fever with fewer than four of the criteria just cited but findings of coronary artery abnormalities. Echocardiography should be considered in any infant <6 months with fever of >7 days' duration, laboratory evidence of systemic inflammation, and no other explanation for the febrile illness.*

3. **Other clinical findings:** Often associated with extreme irritability, abdominal pain, diarrhea, vomiting. Also seen are anterior uveitis (80%), arthritis and arthralgias (35%), aseptic meningitis (25%), pericardial effusion or arrhythmias (20%), gallbladder hydrops (<10%), carditis (<5%), and perineal rash with desquamation.
4. **Laboratory findings:** Leukocytosis with left shift, neutrophils with

vacuoles or toxic granules, elevated C-reactive protein (CRP) or erythrocyte sedimentation rate (ESR) (seen acutely), thrombocytosis (after first week, peaking at 2 weeks), normocytic and normochromic anemia, sterile pyuria (70%), increased liver function tests (40%).

5. **Subacute phase (11 to 25 days after onset of illness):** Resolution of fever, rash, and lymphadenopathy. Often, desquamation of the fingertips or toes and thrombocytosis occur.
6. **Cardiovascular complications:** If untreated, 15% to 25% develop coronary artery aneurysms and dilation in this phase (peak prevalence occurs about 2 to 4 weeks after onset of disease; rarely appears after 6 weeks) and are at risk for coronary thrombosis acutely and coronary stenosis chronically. Carditis; aortic, mitral, and tricuspid regurgitation; pericardial effusion; CHF; MI; left ventricular dysfunction; and ECG changes may also occur.
7. **Convalescent phase:** ESR, CRP, and platelet count return to normal.

TABLE 7-18

GUIDELINES FOR TREATMENT AND FOLLOW-UP OF CHILDREN WITH KAWASAKI DISEASE

| Risk Level | Pharmacologic Therapy |
|---|---|
| I (no coronary artery changes at any stage of illness) | None beyond initial 6–8 weeks |
| II (transient coronary artery ectasia that resolves by 8 weeks after disease onset) | None beyond initial 6–8 weeks |
| III (small to medium solitary coronary artery aneurysm) | 3–5 mg/kg/day aspirin, at least until aneurysm resolves |
| IV (one or more large, >6 mm, aneurysms and coronary arteries with multiple small to medium aneurysms, without obstruction) | Long-term aspirin (3–5 mg/kg/day) and warfarin or LMWH for patients with giant aneurysms |
| V (coronary artery obstruction) | Long-term aspirin (3–5 mg/kg/day); warfarin or LMWH if giant aneurysm persists; consider use of β-blockers to reduce myocardial work |

**Those with coronary artery abnormalities are at increased risk for MI, arrhythmias, and sudden death.**

8. **Management** (Table 7-18):[19]
   a. Intravenous immune globulin (IVIG) has been shown to reduce incidence of coronary artery dilation to <3% and decrease duration of fever if given in the first 10 days of illness. Current recommended regimen is a single dose of IVIG, 2 g/kg over 10 to 12 hr.
   b. Aspirin is recommended for both its anti-inflammatory and its antiplatelet effects. AHA recommends initial high-dose aspirin (80 to 100 mg/kg/day divided in four doses) until 48–72 hr after defervescence. Then continue with low-dose aspirin (3 to 5 mg/kg/day as a single daily dose) for 6 to 8 weeks or until platelet count and ESR are normal (if there are no coronary artery abnormalities) or indefinitely if coronary artery abnormalities persist.
   c. Dipyridamole, 4 mg/kg divided in three doses, is sometimes used as

| Physical Activity | Follow-up and Diagnostic Testing | Invasive Testing |
|---|---|---|
| No restrictions beyond initial 6–8 weeks. | Counsel on cardiovascular risk factors every 5 years. | None recommended |
| No restrictions beyond initial 6–8 weeks. | Counsel on cardiovascular risk factors every 3–5 years. | None recommended |
| For patients in first decade of life, no restriction beyond initial 6–8 weeks; during the second decade of life, physical activity guided by stress testing every 2 years; avoid competitive contact and high-impact sports while on antiplatelet therapy. | Annual follow-up with echocardiogram and electrocardiogram. | Angiography, if stress testing or echocardiography suggests stenosis |
| Annual stress testing guides physical activity; avoid competitive contact and high-impact sports while on anticoagulant therapy. | Echocardiogram and electrocardiogram at 6-mo intervals, annual stress testing, atherosclerosis risk factor counseling at each visit. | Cardiac catheterization 6–12 months after acute illness with additional testing if ischemia noted or testing inconclusive |
| Contact sports, isometrics, and weight training should be avoided; other physical activity recommendations guided by outcome of stress testing or myocardial perfusion scan. | Echocardiogram and electrocardiogram at 6-mo intervals, annual Holter and stress testing. | Cardiac catheterization 6–12 months after acute illness to aid in selecting therapeutic options, additional testing if ischemia noted |

BOX 7-5

**GUIDELINES FOR THE DIAGNOSIS OF INITIAL ATTACK OF RHEUMATIC FEVER (JONES CRITERIA)**

| MAJOR MANIFESTATIONS | MINOR MANIFESTATIONS |
|---|---|
| Carditis | *Clinical findings* |
| Polyarthritis | Arthralgia |
| Chorea | Fever |
| Erythema marginatum | *Laboratory findings* |
| Subcutaneous nodule | Elevated acute phase reactants (erythrocyte sedimentation rate, C-reactive protein) |
| | Prolonged PR interval |

***Plus***

**Supporting evidence of antecedent group A streptococcal infection**

Positive throat culture or rapid streptococcal antigen test

Elevated or rising streptococcal antibody titer

*Note:* If supported by evidence of preceding group A streptococcal infection, the presence of two major manifestations or of one major and two minor manifestations indicates a high probability of acute rheumatic fever.

alternative to aspirin, particularly if symptoms of influenza or varicella arise while on aspirin (concern for Reye's syndrome).

d. Follow-up: Serial echocardiography is recommended to assess coronary arteries and left ventricular function (at time of diagnosis, at 2 weeks, at 6 to 8 weeks, and at 12 months [optional]). More frequent intervals and long-term follow-up are recommended if abnormalities are seen on echocardiography (see Table 7-18).

## F. RHEUMATIC HEART DISEASE

1. **Etiology:** Believed to be immunologically mediated delayed sequela of group A streptococcal pharyngitis.
2. **Clinical findings:** History of streptococcal pharyngitis 1 to 5 weeks before onset of symptoms. Often with pallor, malaise, easy fatigability.
3. **Diagnosis:** Jones criteria (Box 7-5).
4. **Management:** Penicillin, bed rest, salicylates, supportive management of CHF (if present) with diuretics, digoxin, morphine.

## G. LYME DISEASE

1. Etiology: Following viral infection with *Borrelia burgdorferi.*
2. Clinical symptoms: Approximately 8% to 10% of patients with Lyme disease will get AV block. Other possible symptoms include myocarditis and pericarditis.

## REFERENCES

1. Zubrow AB et al: Determinants of blood pressure in infants admitted to neonatal intensive care units: A prospective multicenter study. Philadelphia Neonatal Blood Pressure Study Group. J Perinatol 1995;15:470.

2. National High Blood Pressure Education Program Working Group on High Blood Pressure in Children and Adolescents: The fourth report on the diagnosis, evaluation, and treatment of high blood pressure in children and adolescents. Pediatrics 2004;114(2 Suppl):555–576.
3. Park MK: Pediatric Cardiology for Practitioners, 4th ed. St. Louis, Mosby, 2002.
4. Sapin SO: Recognizing normal heart murmurs: A logic-based mnemonic. Pediatrics 1997;99(4):616–619.
5. Davignon A et al: Normal ECG standards for infants and children. Pediatr Cardiol 1979;1:123–131.
6. Schwartz PJ et al: Prolongation of the QT interval and the sudden infant death syndrome. NEJM 1998;338:1709–1714.
7. Garson A Jr: The Electrocardiogram in Infants and Children: A Systematic Approach. Philadelphia, Lea & Febiger, 1983.
8. Park MK, Guntheroth WG: How to Read Pediatric ECGs, 4th ed. Philadelphia, Mosby, 2006.
9. Towbin JA, Bricker JT, Garson A Jr: Electrocardiographic criteria for diagnosis of acute myocardial infarction in childhood. Am J Cardiol 1992;69:1545–1548.
10. Hirsch R et al: Cardiac troponin I in pediatrics: Normal values and potential use in assessment of cardiac injury. J Pediatr 1997;130:872–877.
11. Walsh EP: Cardiac arrhythmias. In Fyler DC, Nadas A (eds): Pediatric Cardiology. Philadelphia, Hanley & Belfus, 1992, p 384.
12. Lees MH: Cyanosis of the newborn infant: Recognition and clinical evaluation. J Pediatr 1970;77:484–498.
13. Kitterman JA: Cyanosis in the newborn infant. Pediatr Rev 1982;4:13–24.
14. Jones RW et al: Arterial oxygen tension and response to oxygen breathing in differential diagnosis of heart disease in infancy. Arch Dis Child 1976;51: 667–673.
15. American Academy of Pediatrics: 2006 Red Book: Report of the Committee on Infectious Diseases, 27th ed. Elk Grove Village, Ill, The Academy, 2006.
16. Colan SD et al: Developmental modulation of myocardial mechanics: Age- and growth-related alterations in afterload and contractility. J Am Coll Cardiol 1992;19:619–629.
17. Wilson W et al: Prevention of Infective Endocarditis: Guidelines from the American Heart Association: A Guideline from the American Heart Association Rheumatic Fever, Endocarditis, and Kawasaki Disease Committee, Council on Cardiovascular Disease in the Young, and the Council on Clinical Cardiology, Council on Cardiovascular Surgery and Anesthesia, and the Quality of Care and Outcomes Research Interdisciplinary Working Group. Circulation 2007;116:1736–1754.
18. Maron BJ et al: 36th Bethesda Conference: Eligibility recommendations for competitive athletes with cardiovascular abnormalities. *J Am Coll Cardiol* 2005;45(8):1313–1375.
19. Newburger JW et al: Diagnosis, treatment, and long term management of Kawasaki disease. Circulation 2004;110:2747–2771.

# Dermatology

*Nicole Schumann-Gable, MD*

8

## I. WEBSITE

www.med.jhu.edu/peds/dermatlas

Please refer to the color plates in this chapter for photographic examples of dermatologic findings.

## II. EVALUATION AND CLINICAL DESCRIPTION OF SKIN FINDINGS

### A. PRIMARY SKIN LESIONS (Fig. 8-1A)

1. Macule/patch: Small flat lesion with altered color (<0.5 cm); large macule (>0.5 cm).
2. Papule/plaque: Elevated, well-circumscribed lesion (<0.5 cm); large papule (>0.5 cm).
3. Nodule/tumor: Mass located in dermis or subcutaneous fat (may be solid or soft); large nodule.
4. Vesicle/bulla: Blister with transparent fluid; large vesicle.
5. Wheal: Erythematous, well-circumscribed, raised, edematous lesion that appears and disappears quickly.

### B. SECONDARY SKIN LESIONS (Fig. 8-1B)

1. Scale: Small, thin plate of horny epithelium.
2. Pustule: Well-circumscribed elevated lesion filled with pus.
3. Crust: Exudative mass consisting of blood, scale, and pus from skin erosions or ruptured vesicles/papules.
4. Ulcer: Erosion of dermis and cutis with clearly defined edges.
5. Scar: Formation of new connective tissue after damage to epidermis and cutis, leaving permanent change in skin.
6. Excoriation: Surface marks often linear secondary to scratching.
7. Fissure: Linear skin crack with inflammation and pain.

## III. SKIN "LUMPS": DIAGNOSIS AND TREATMENT

### A. HEMANGIOMAS

**1. Pathogenesis.**

A phase of rapid proliferation followed by spontaneous involution. During proliferative phase, densely packed endothelial cells form small capillaries; subsequent vessels develop from existing vasculature.

**2. Clinical manifestations:**

a. Appearance:

(1) Newborns may demonstrate pale macules with threadlike telangiectasias.

(2) Most recognizable form is a bright red, slightly elevated, noncompressible plaque. Frequently, both superficial and deep components are present, with deep components appearing bluish in color.

(3) Size: Can range from a few millimeters to several centimeters.

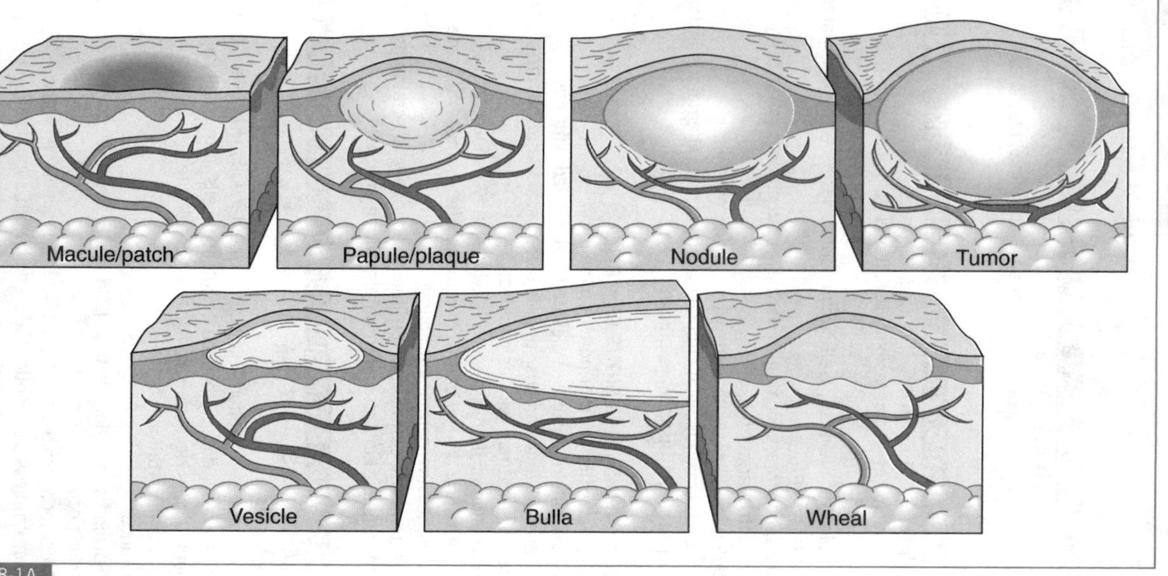


FIG. 8-1A Pattern diagnosis. **A,** Primary skin lesions. (**A** *and* **B,** *From Cohen BA: Pediatric Dermatology, 2nd ed. St. Louis, Mosby, 1999, p 5.*)

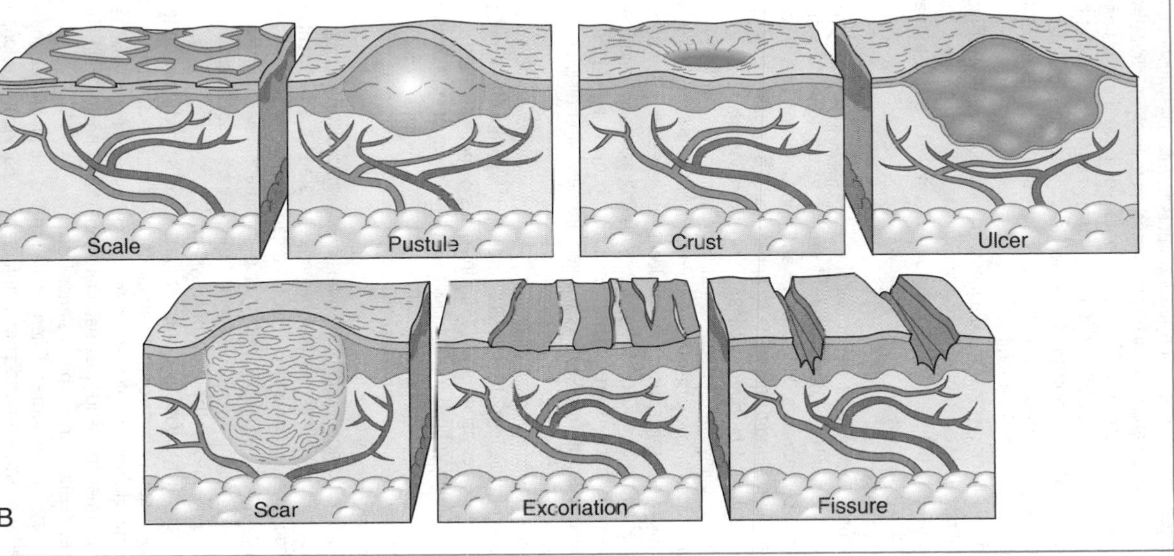


FIG. 8-1B

**B,** Secondary skin lesions.

b. Incidence: Most common soft tissue tumors in infancy, with increased incidence in premature infants; three times more likely in girls than boys. Notably, about 5%–10% of 2-month-olds have these lesions.
c. Natural history: About 5%–10% of hemangiomas are present at birth; remainder develop within the first 4 weeks of life. The most rapid growth phase occurs between ages 2 and 4 months, with regression beginning at age 6–12 months.
d. Diagnosis: Although most are diagnosed clinically, imaging techniques (e.g., ultrasound, computed tomography, magnetic resonance imaging) can be used to differentiate hemangiomas from vascular malformations or neoplastic processes.

3. **Complications:**

a. Ulceration: Most common complication; may result in severe pain, infection, hemorrhage, or scarring; ulceration results from necrosis of superficial components. Hemorrhage and superinfection may also occur. Hemorrhage, although alarming in appearance, is usually minimal and can be controlled by direct pressure. Superinfection may lead to cellulitis, osteomyelitis, or septicemia.
b. Kasabach-Merritt phenomenon: A complication of hemangiopericytoma with rapidly enlarging, usually deep lesions; characterized by anemia, thrombocytopenia, and coagulopathy, requiring aggressive medical management. Lesions are differentiated from benign hemangiomas by their deep red-blue appearance, marked firmness, and histologic appearance.
c. Regionally important lesions:
   (1) Periorbital lesions: May cause amblyopia from obstruction of the visual axis or astigmatism from insidious compression of the globe or extension into the retrobulbar space. Require careful observation and evaluation by an ophthalmologist.
   (2) External auditory canal lesions: May result in otitis or conductive hearing loss.
   (3) Multiple cutaneous hemangiomas and large facial hemangiomas are associated with visceral hemangiomas and may warrant abdominal ultrasound to look for organ involvement (i.e., liver hemangiomas). A high occurrence of hemangiomas in the cervical-tracheal region (PHACES syndrome)[1] may be associated with abnormalities of the urogenital system.[2]
   (4) Visceral hemangiomas: Often characterized by high-flow patterns; may result in high-output cardiac failure and anemia. Large facial hemangiomas are also associated with posterior fossa vascular malformations, and thus patients should have neuroimaging with special attention to the posterior fossa.
   (5) Airway hemangiomas: Often located in the subglottic region; may cause hoarseness and stridor. Infants with cutaneous lesions in a beard distribution (chin, lips, mandibular region, and neck) are at greatest risk for airway involvement.

(6) Lumbosacral hemangiomas that span the midline are associated with spinal malformations, dysraphism, and anomalies of the anorectal and urogenital regions. An ultrasound of the L5 spine in infants <6 months of age is an effective noninvasive screening study.

4. **Management:**

a. Most require no intervention. Decision to treat should be based on location and depth of the lesion, age of patient, and likelihood of complication. Photodocumentation is used to follow the growth and regression process.

b. Systemic corticosteroids are the mainstay of therapy to prevent subsequent complication (i.e., periorbital or subglottic lesions). Usually, 2 to 3 mg/kg/day of prednisone or prednisolone. One third of lesions demonstrate dramatic shrinkage, one third demonstrate stabilization of growth, and one third show no response.

c. Laser ablation: Evidence-based research suggests this is not effective.

d. Interferon: Not often used because of neurologic complications.

e. Embolization: Can be used to treat cutaneous hemangiomas that have not responded to medical therapy.

f. Surgical excision.[3] Used in rare circumstances



## B. WARTS

1. **Pathogenesis.**

Caused by more than 100 types of human papillomavirus (HPV). The virus enters the skin through breaks in the epithelium, causing hyperplasia of the squamous epithelium.

2. **Morphology:**

a. Common warts: Lesions are skin-colored, rough, minimally scaly papules and nodules found on the exposed surfaces of the hands, face, arms, and legs. Lesions can be solitary or multiple, a few millimeters to several centimeters in diameter, and may form large plaques or a confluent, linear pattern secondary to autoinoculation.

b. Flat warts: Occur over the hands, arms, and face; are usually <2 mm wide. Often present in clusters.

c. Plantar warts: Found on the soles of the feet as sometimes painful but often asymptomatic, inward-growing, hyperkeratotic plaques and papules. Trauma on weight-bearing surfaces results in small black dots ("seeds" from thrombosed vessels on the surface of the wart).

d. Anogenital warts: See Chapter 5.

3. **Treatment (Table 8-1):**

a. Spontaneous resolution occurs in >75% of warts in otherwise healthy individuals within 3 years.

b. Keratolytics (i.e., topical salicylates): Work by removing excess scale within and around warts and by triggering an inflammatory reaction. Particularly effective in combination with adhesive tape occlusion; response may take 4 to 6 months.

TABLE 8-1

WART THERAPY

| Treatment | Advantages | Disadvantages |
|---|---|---|
| Keratolytics (lactic acid, salicylic acid, tretinoin) | Available without prescription, home therapy, low cost, low risk, little pain | Slow response, irritation |
| **DESTRUCTIVE AGENTS** | | |
| Cryotherapy | Quick office procedure, relatively low cost | Pain, scarring, recurrence |
| Caustics (topical acids) | Home or office therapy, relatively low cost | Irritation, recurrence, systemic toxicity (podophyllin) |
| Cantharidin (vesicant) | Occasionally effective | High risk for recurrence, prominent pigmentary changes |
| Electrocautery and laser | Usually effective | Pain, scarring, recurrence, requires anesthesia, moderate cost |

From Cohen BA: Warts and children: Can they be separated? Contemp Pediatr 1997;2: 128–149.

c. Destructive techniques depend on destruction of wart and surrounding normal skin and should be used only with the consent of the patient; no evidence that destructive techniques are better than placebo.
   (1) Cryotherapy results in necrosis and blister formation. May produce scarring; warts may recur.
   (2) Caustic agents can be applied after warts have been shaved but require application for several weeks or months.
   (3) Cantharidin is a topical vesicant that causes the formation of intraepidermal blisters. Recurrence risk is high, and blister formation can be difficult to control.
   (4) Electrocautery and $CO_2$ laser ablation require local or general anesthesia. Can be particularly useful for treating large lesions on the trunk and extremities and discrete plantar warts. Both can leave scars, and recurrence is well documented. Open wounds and prolonged healing pose significant problems in weight bearing.
   (5) Intradermal bleomycin has also been used.
   (6) Destructive options for therapy are often not good choices in the treatment of young children.

d. Immunotherapy:
   (1) Involves contact sensitization with a potent allergen initially, followed by application of a low concentration of the allergen in cream form to the wart site. Intralesional injection of antigens has also been recently used.
   (2) Cimetidine (30 to 40 mg/kg/day) divided into two doses for 2 months; however, it may be no better than placebo.[4]

**Note** *As with molluscum contagiosum (discussed subsequently), recalcitrant or widespread lesions should be screened for immunodeficiency (congenital and acquired).*

## C. MOLLUSCUM CONTAGIOSUM

1. **Morphology (Color Plate 1).**

Caused by the pox virus; consists of dome-shaped, often umbilicated, translucent to white papules that range from 1 mm to 1 cm, with a tiny keratotic core at the center. Lesions are often surrounded by scaling and erythema that resemble eczema. They may appear inflamed and secondarily infected when undergoing spontaneous involution. Often occur in children on the trunk, axillary region, face, and diaper regions, often spreading by autoinoculation. In teens, lesions may occur in the genital area as a sexually transmitted disease.

2. **Treatment.**

Lesions are benign and self-limited. Treatment, with the consent of the child, is directed toward symptomatic lesions, because destruction of the individual lesions may lead to scarring and recurrences of new papules are common despite treatment.

a. Use a small curette with gentle pressure to débride the lesion. This treatment is the least likely to cause scarring.
b. Liquid nitrogen may be an option in older children (must only be done with informed consent of the patient).
c. Topical preparations of salicylic-lactic acid combinations, cantharidin, and retinoic acid

## D. PYOGENIC GRANULOMA (Color Plate 2)

1. **Morphology: A benign erythematous, sessile or pedunculated papule, also known as a *lobular capillary hemangioma*. Usually solitary, bright red, soft papules; surface may be weepy, crusty, or completely epithelialized. Papules range in size from 2 mm to 2 cm, and may initially grow rapidly and bleed easily when traumatized. Relatively common in children and young adults; most commonly found on the head and neck, followed by the trunk, upper extremities, and lower extremities, respectively. Biopsy shows proliferating capillaries in a loose edematous fibrous matrix.**
2. **Treatment:**

a. Surgical excision: May recur if not completely removed.
b. Cauterization with silver nitrate.
c. Laser ablation.
d. Shave excision: Electrodessication of the base or pedunculated papule that often has a discernible epithelial collarette.

## E. SCABIES

1. **Pathogenesis: Mites are eight-legged arachnids about the size of a grain of sand. The infecting organism is most commonly *Sarcoptes***

*scabiei.* Spread by skin-to-skin contact and through fomites, as they are able to live for 2 days away from the human body. Activated by warmth, the mite burrows under the skin to the stratum corneum in 2.5 min. Female moves 2–3 mm/day and lays eggs as she tunnels.

2. **Clinical manifestations:** Small papules over female mite bite and/or linear or wavy burrows. Most commonly located in interdigital webs, wrist folds, elbows, axilla, buttocks, and belt line. May cause severe itching, especially at night. May result in secondary phenomena such as uritcaria, excoriation, impetigo, and eczematous plaques.
3. **Treatment:**
   a. Permethrin cream: 5% cream applied from neck down to feet and left on for 8–14 hr. In infants treatment should include scalp, neck, and forehead. Treat all family members with symptoms simultaneously, and advise parents to use topical lubricants generously to treat dryness of the skin produced by scabicide.
   b. Ivermectin: A single oral dose has an efficacy comparable to that of permethrin and may be especially useful in patients with immunodeficiency or crusted scabies. Not yet approved for scabies treatment by the FDA.[5]

### F. REACTIVE ERYTHEMA (Fig. 8-2; Color Plates 3 to 9)

1. **Morphology:** Group of disorders characterized by erythematous patches, plaques, and nodules that vary in size, shape, and distribution.
2. **Etiology:** Represent cutaneous reaction patterns triggered by endogenous and environmental facotrs.

## IV. PAPULOSQUAMOUS LESIONS: DIAGNOSIS AND TREATMENT (Fig. 8-3 and Color Plates 10 to 20)

### A. ATOPIC DERMATITIS (ECZEMA)

1. **Pathogenesis (Color Plates 17 to 20).**

Patients have a genetic predisposition and elevated immunoglobulin E (IgE) levels, which suggests an abnormal response to triggering agents, resulting in the release of histamine, prostaglandins, and cytokines. Inflammation causes itching and subsequent scratching, which produces the clinical lesions of eczema.

2. **Epidemiology:**
   a. Atopic dermatitis affects 15%–25% of children, with the peak prevalence between ages 6 months and 8 to 10 years.
   b. About 95% of children with atopic dermatitis have asthma or allergic rhinitis.
3. **Clinical presentations (Box 8-1).**

Acute changes include erythema, vesicles, crusting, and secondary infection. Chronic changes include lichenification, scaling, and postinflammatory hypopigmentation or hyperpigmentation.

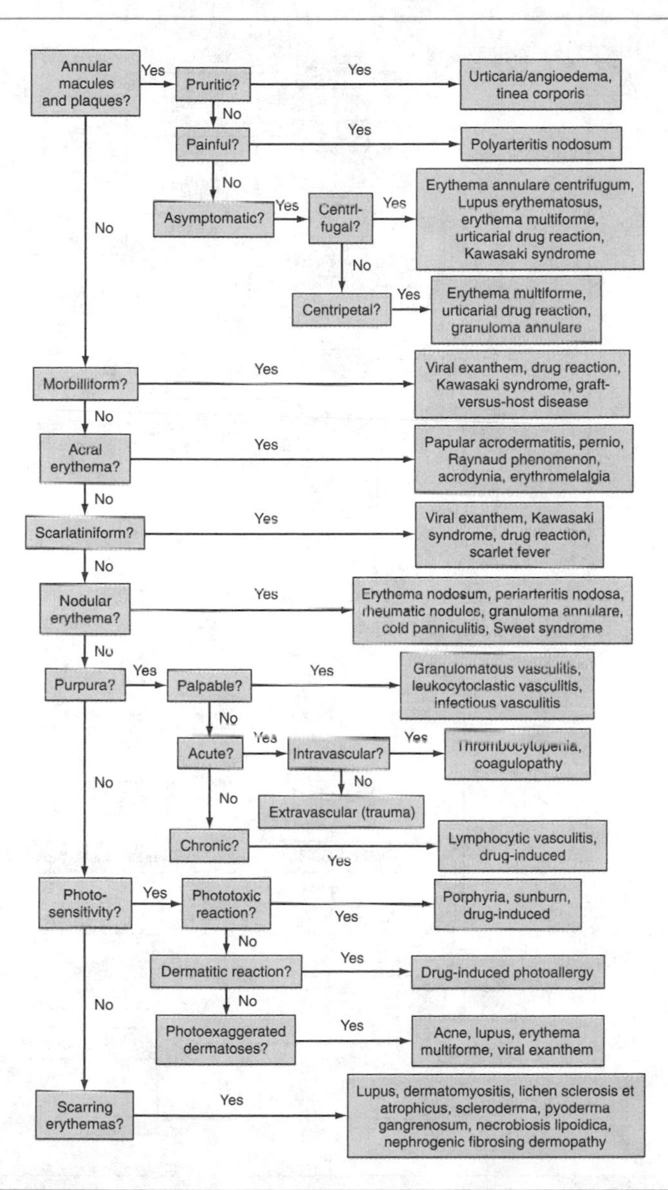


FIG. 8-2

Reactive erythema. *(Modified from Cohen BA: Atlas of Pediatric Dermatology, 3rd ed. St. Louis, Mosby, 2005, p 196.)*

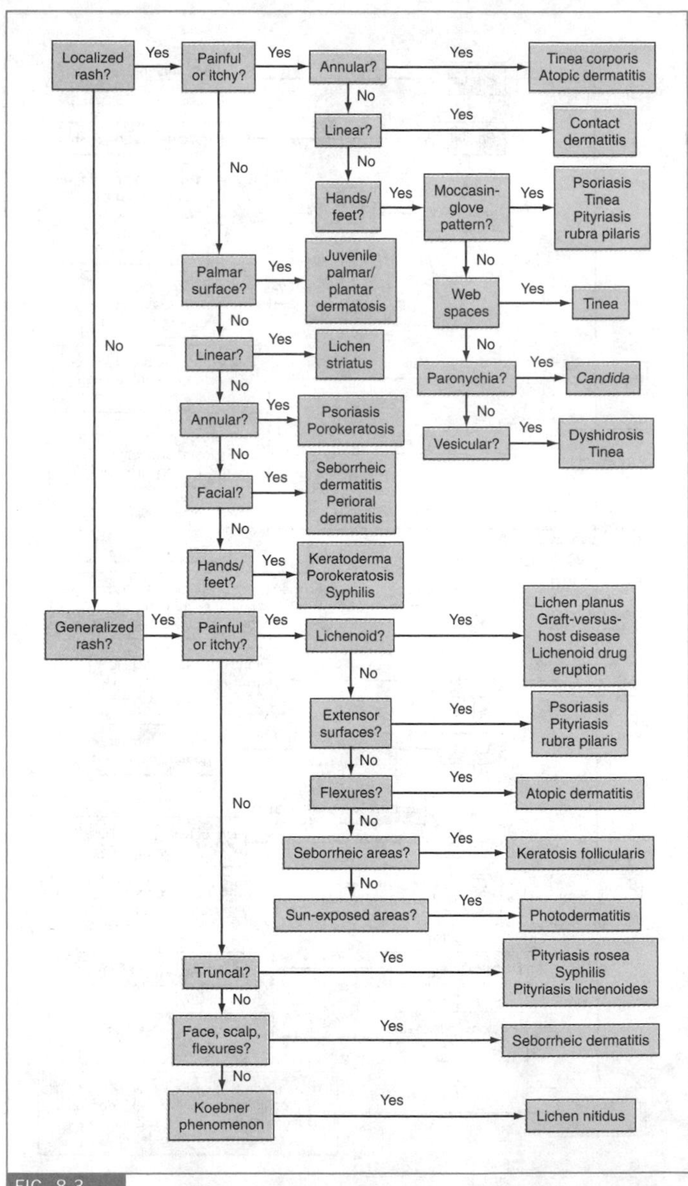


FIG. 8-3

Papulosquamous disorders algorithm. *(Modified from Cohen BA: Atlas of Pediatric Dermatology, 3rd ed. St. Louis, Mosby, 2005, p 97.)*

| BOX 8-1 |
|---|
| **IDENTIFYING CHARACTERISTICS OF ATOPIC DERMATITIS** |
| **MAJOR CRITERIA (SEEN IN ALL PATIENTS)** |
| Pruritus |
| Typical morphology and distribution of lesions |
| Facial and extensor involvement in infants |
| Flexural lichenification in older children and adults |
| Tendency toward chronic or chronically relapsing dermatitis |
| **COMMON FINDINGS (AT LEAST 2)** |
| Personal or family history of atopic disease (asthma, allergic rhinitis, atopic dermatitis) |
| Immediate skin test reactivity |
| White dermatographism and/or delayed blanch to cholinergic agents |
| Anterior subcapsular cataracts |
| **ASSOCIATED FINDINGS (AT LEAST 4)** |
| Xerosis/ichthyosis/hyperlinear palms and soles |
| Pityriasis alba |
| Keratosis pilaris |
| Facial pallor/infraorbital darkening |
| Dennie-Morgan infraorbital fold |
| Elevated serum IgE |
| Tendency toward nonspecific hand dermatitis |
| Tendency toward repeated cutaneous infections |

From Cohen DA: Atopic dermatitis: Breaking the itch-scratch cycle. *Contemp Pediatr* 1992;7:64–81.

a. **Infantile form:** Extensor surfaces are more affected than flexors. Truncal, facial, and scalp involvement is common, with sparing of the diaper area.
b. **Early to middle childhood:** Flexural surfaces are more severely involved.
c. **Late childhood and adolescence:** Lesions tend to be restricted to skin creases and hand dermatitis.

4. **Treatment:**

a. Chronic disease: Bland lubricants, including petroleum jelly, Aquaphor, Eucerin, and vegetable shortening, are mainstays of therapy; may need to be more elegant for older patients. Apply two to three times per day and immediately after bathing or swimming. Bathing time should be short (no more than 5 min); skin should be patted dry, not rubbed, before application of lubricant.
b. Topical steroids:
   (1) Low- and medium-potency steroid creams once or twice per day in the most severely affected areas for eczema flares and for generally no more than 7 days. Severe flares may require a longer duration of therapy followed by a taper to lower-potency steroids. Even with

low-potency steroids, special care is required in areas in which the skin is thin, such as the diaper area, groin, armpits, under the breasts, around the neck, and on the face. High-potency topical steroids should generally be used in consultation with a dermatologist.

(2) Topical steroids can be applied at the same time as lubricants and can be mixed with lubricants when weaning from the topical steroid.

c. Systemic steroids: Should generally be avoided. May be used for short periods of uncontrolled eczema flares or for severe disease requiring hospitalization.

d. Antihistamines: May be used when hives cause scratching, thus exacerbating underlying eczema. Sedating antihistamines (i.e., diphenhydramine, hydroxyzine) more effective for pruritus; no evidence that nonsedating antihistamines are effective in controlling itching. Cetirizine is the most effective of the nonsedating antihistamines.

e. Immunomodulators: Topical tacrolimus (formally known as FK506, currently marketed as Protopic 0.03% and 0.1% ointment) and pimecrolimus (Elidel 1% cream)[6,7] may be used as an alternative to topical steroids. Neither agent causes skin atrophy,[8] allowing for safe alternatives for recalcitrant facial eczema, as well as possibly preventing the need for topical steroids. Can be used safely on patients >2 years of age.[9–11]

f. Protective clothing should be worn.

**Note** *Black box warning placed on Tacrolimus in 2005 due to research showing a potential risk of cancer associated with its use.*

5. **Complications:**

a. Weeping or blistering lesions with no evidence of infection: Cold-water compresses three or four times per day or tepid baths followed by bland lubricant application.

b. Bacterial infection: Usually staphylococcal and sometimes streptococcal; must be recognized quickly. Localized infections can be treated with topical antibiotics; more serious infections require systemic antibiotics.[12]

c. Eczema herpeticum: Must be treated systemically with acyclovir.

## B. PAPULAR URTICARIA (Color Plate 21)

Insect bite-induced hypersensitivity (IBIH)

1. **Morphology: Characterized by chronic or recurrent eruptions of pruritic papules, vesicles, and wheals resulting from a hypersensitivity reaction to biting and stinging insects. Predominance of a T-cell mediated response characterizes its chronic nature. Most commonly grouped in linear clusters and present on exposed areas with sparing of the genital, perianal, and axillary regions. Intense pruritus, resulting**

in excoriation, secondary infection. Scarring and permanent hyperpigmentation and/or hypopigmentation in some patients, particularly in darkly pigmented individuals.

2. **SCRATCH principles:**
   **S: Symmetrical eruption:** Usually in exposed areas; sparing of the diaper region.
   **C: Clustering:** Described as "meal cluster"; linear or triangular groupings of lesions that reflect the biting insect's path along the skin.
   **R: Rover not required:** A history of pets in the home is not a requirement for considering IBIH; exposure may be remote.
   **A: Age:** Rarely seen before age 2 years. Peak age range: 2–10 years, with most children developing tolerance by age 10 years. If patient is <2, rethink diagnosis.
   **T: Target lesions:** Common appearance, especially in darker pigmented patients.
   **Time**: Emphasize chronic nature of eruption and need for watchful waiting.
   **C: Confused pediatrician/parent:** Often diagnosis is met with disbelief by parent and/or referring pediatrician.
   **H: Household:** Because it is a hypersensitivity reaction IBIH often affects only one family member, unlike atopic dermatitis and scabies, in which multiple family members may have a history of symptoms.
3. **Management (The 3 Ps):**

a. **P**revention: Advise patients to wear protective clothing and use insect repellent when outside, launder bedding and mattress pads for bed mites, and maximize flea control for pets.

b. **P**ruritus control: Antihistamines if symptoms are acute and suggest a type 1 nature; not very effective in chronic stages. Topical steroids may also be used for acute lesions; extension into the dermis and fat may make these ineffective. Second-generation antihistamines such as cetirizine (Zyrtec) may be helpful for pruritus.

c. **P**atience: Advise patients of the frustrating, recurrent nature of IBIH reactions; ensure parents of the eventual development of tolerance and resolution of symptoms.

### C. ICHTHYOSIS (see Color Plate 22)

A group of scaling disorders consisting of five major variants: congenital ichthyosiform erythroderma, lamellar ichthyosis, epidermolytic hyperkeratosis, ichthyosis vulgaris, and X-linked ichthyosis. There are also six separate ichthyotic syndromes, of which these lesions are a feature.

### D. TINEA VERSICOLOR (Color Plate 23)

1. **Epidemiology:** Infecting organism is *Pityrosporum (Malassezia)*; commonly colonizes skin by age 4–6 months.

2. **Clinical presentation:** Multiple small oval scaly patches that measure 1–3 cm in diameter in a raindrop pattern on upper chest, back, and proximal portions of the upper extremities of adolescents and young adults. Usually asymptomatic, but some patients may complain of pruritus. Lesions appear light tan, reddish, or white in color; appear hyperpigmented in light-skinned patients and hypopigmented in darker-skinned patients.
3. **Diagnosis:** Based on physical appearance; "spaghetti and meatball" short pseudohyphae on KOH.
4. **Treatment:** Selenium sulfide and propylene glycol; rapidly clear infection; pigmentary changes may take a prolonged time to clear, and recurrence is common.

## V. HAIR LOSS: DIAGNOSIS AND TREATMENT

### A. TINEA CAPITIS (Color Plate 24)

1. **Epidemiology:**

a. *Trichophyton tonsurans* accounts for >90% of tinea capitis in North America. An anthropophilic organism with no known natural reservoir; persists for long periods on fomites, such as hairbrushes, combs, furniture, stuffed toys, and clothing.

b. Most patients are age 1–10 years, but infection may occur at any age.

c. Incidence is highest in African American children and second highest in Hispanic youths. This predisposition is not completely understood, but may be the result of the character of the hair follicle, tight braiding, or the use of pomades.

2. **Clinical presentations:**

a. Classic tinea capitis: Presents as one or more round to oval patches of partial to complete alopecia, with varying degrees of erythema. Scale is present, and the border is slightly raised and more erythematous than the central area.

b. Kerion (Color Plate 25): Inflammatory presentation of tinea capitis. A boggy, tender, edematous plaque or cluster of nodules with erythema; usually solitary and is frequently accompanied by cervical or occipital adenopathy and papular morbilliform eruption, classified as an *id reaction.*

c. Seborrheic dermatitis-like pattern (most common): May produce minimal or no alopecia and show diffuse scaling over the scalp, with pruritus.

d. Follicular pustules with crusting and scaling scattered over the scalp: Pattern seen predominantly in African American children with tight braiding and constant pomade use; often resembles bacterial folliculitis, but bacterial culture is negative.

3. **Diagnosis:** The presumptive clinical diagnosis may be confirmed by either direct microscopic examination or culture of scale (may be collected with a toothbrush on a culture plate or on a moistened culturette swab).

4. **Treatment:**
a. Success requires oral therapy; griseofulvin is the agent of choice. It is best taken with fatty food to promote absorption (see Formulary for dosage information). Standard references suggest 4–6 weeks of therapy, although 8–12 weeks may be required for eradication. Patients should be reevaluated monthly; repeat culture may be obtained 2 weeks *before* therapy is discontinued to document cure. Patients will often develop an eczema-like rash associated with the fungal infection (id reaction); not a drug reaction, and griseofulvin therapy should be continued.
b. Kerions: Treat with prednisone or prednisolone (0.5 mg/kg/day for 10–14 days) if no contraindication exists in addition to standard griseofulvin therapy.
c. The use of sporicidal shampoos in addition to oral therapy promotes rapid elimination of spores, thus decreasing the contagion risk to family members and schoolmates. Selenium sulfide 2.5% shampoo twice weekly is recommended.[13] Ketoconazole 1% and 2% shampoo is also available for this purpose.



## B. ALOPECIA AREATA (Color Plate 26)

1. **Clinical presentation:** Common condition characterized by the sudden onset of asymptomatic, noninflammatory, round, bald patches located on any hair-bearing part of the body, most commonly the scalp. Course is irregular and unpredictable; most patients develop good regrowth of hair within 1 or 2 years.
2. **Diagnosis:** Differentiated by the absence of hair follicles in the bald spot. There is also a lack of scaly erythema, pustules, and crusts.
3. **Treatment:** Topical corticosteroids, topical minoxidil, tar preparations, anthralin, topical sensitizers, and ultraviolet light therapy.[14] Although there is some thought that these treatments may be helpful, there is no research-based evidence that these interventions improve the disease course. Likewise, systemic steroids should generally not be used because they do not alter prognosis. In adolescents and adults, hair loss often resolves over months to years; in younger children, the prognosis is more guarded.

## C. TELOGEN EFFLUVIUM

1. **Pathogenesis:** Growing hair follicles respond to physiologic and pathologic stress (e.g., high fever, severe influenza, infection, surgery, drugs, pregnancy, hypothyroidism) by regressing to the resting, or telogen, state.
2. **Clinical presentation:** A form of alopecia characterized by diffuse hair loss that is usually not clinically obvious to anyone but the patient and parent.
3. **Treatment:** Usually occurs 3–5 months after the stressor and is self-limited.

### D. TRACTION ALOPECIA (Color Plate 27)

1. **Pathogenesis:** Often a result of hairstyles that apply tension for long periods of time.
2. **Clinical presentation:** Noninflammatory linear areas of hair loss at the margins of the hairline, part line, or scattered regions, depending on hair styling procedures used.
3. **Treatment:** Avoidance of styling products or styles resulting in traction.

### E. HAIR PULLING

Hair pulling is a benign, self-limited activity common in young children.

### F. TRICHOTILLOMANIA

1. **Pathogenesis:** Alopecia caused by the compulsion to pull out one's own hair, resulting in irregular areas of incomplete hair loss, mainly on the scalp; eyebrows and eyelashes may also be involved.
2. **Clinical presentation:** Characterized by areas of hair loss within which are short, broken hair shafts of varying lengths.
3. **Treatment:** Most cases spontaneously resolve, but in severe cases a psychiatric evaluation may be warranted.

## VI. ACNE VULGARIS (see Fig. 8-2)

### A. PATHOGENESIS

Results from obstruction of sebaceous follicles, located primarily on the face and trunk, by excessive amounts of sebum and desquamated epithelial cells. The resident anaerobic organism, *Propionibacterium acnes*, proliferates and produces chemotactic and inflammatory mediators that lead to inflammation.

1. **Noninflammatory open comedones, or "blackheads."**
2. **Noninflammatory closed comedones, or "whiteheads."**
3. **Inflammatory papules, pustules, nodules, or cysts.**

### B. TREATMENT (Table 8-2 and Fig. 8-4)

1. **Gentle, nonabrasive cleaning is best.** Vigorous scrubbing, abrasive cleaners, and mechanical devices can promote the development of inflammatory lesions.
2. **Dietary factors play no role in sebum production.**
3. **Comedonal acne:** Treatment goal for noninflammatory acne is first to prevent and second to minimize the formation of new comedones and colonization with *P. acnes.* This type of acne is most common in the preadolescent and early adolescent years.

a. Topical tretinoin or adapalene and benzoyl peroxide (either or both) are treatments of choice. Salicylic acid and topical antibiotics may also be used.

TABLE 8-2

**TOPICAL AND SYSTEMIC ANTIBIOTICS USED TO TREAT ACNE**

| Antibiotic | Characteristics |
|---|---|
| **TOPICAL** | |
| Erythromycin | *P. acnes* very sensitive; least lipophilic |
| Clindamycin | *P. acnes* very sensitive; more lipophilic than erythromycin, but less than benzoyl peroxide |
| Benzoyl peroxide plus erythromycin | *P. acnes* very sensitive; most lipophilic topical agent; less irritating than benzoyl peroxide alone |
| Benzoyl peroxide plus clindamycin | Similar to characteristics for previous benzoyl peroxide plus erythromycin |
| Azelaic acid | *P. acnes* sensitive; minimal lipophilia; can reduce abnormal desquamation |
| Metronidazole | *P. acnes* not sensitive; has anti-inflammatory properties |
| Benzoyl peroxide plus glycolic acid | Glycolic acid may enhance penetration and reduce abnormal desquamation |
| **SYSTEMIC** | |
| Tetracycline | *P. acnes* sensitive; inexpensive; usually needs to be taken two to four times a day; compliance can be a problem because of need to take on an empty stomach |
| Erythromycin | *P. acnes* very sensitive; resistance emerging; gastrointestinal upset common; inexpensive |
| Doxycycline | Lipophilic; *P. acnes* very sensitive; resistance not yet seen; photosensitivity can occur; more expensive than tetracycline and erythromycin |
| Minocycline | Lipophilic; *P. acnes* very sensitive; resistance not yet seen; no photosensitivity; abnormal pigmentation in oral mucosa and skin; vertigo-like symptoms; most expensive |
| Trimethoprim-sulfamethoxazole | Lipophilic; *P. acnes* very sensitive; severe erythema multiforme and toxic epidermal necrolysis limit use |
| Clindamycin | *P. acnes* very sensitive; somewhat lipophilic; pseudomembranous colitis limits use |

From Leyden JJ: Therapy for acne vulgaris. NEJM 1997;16:1156–1162.

b. Apply topical cream or gel sparingly once daily, starting with a low concentration and increasing concentration if local irritation does not occur. Desired clinical results become apparent for several weeks.

c. Continue therapy until it is clear that new lesions are not developing.

**4. Mild inflammatory acne: Scattered small papules or pustules develop, with a minimum of comedones. Proliferation of *P. acnes* occurs at this stage. Often occurs in the early teens and in adult women in their 20s.**

a. Most patients improve after a 2- to 4-week course of topical antibiotics applied twice daily, topical benzoyl peroxide, or a combination.

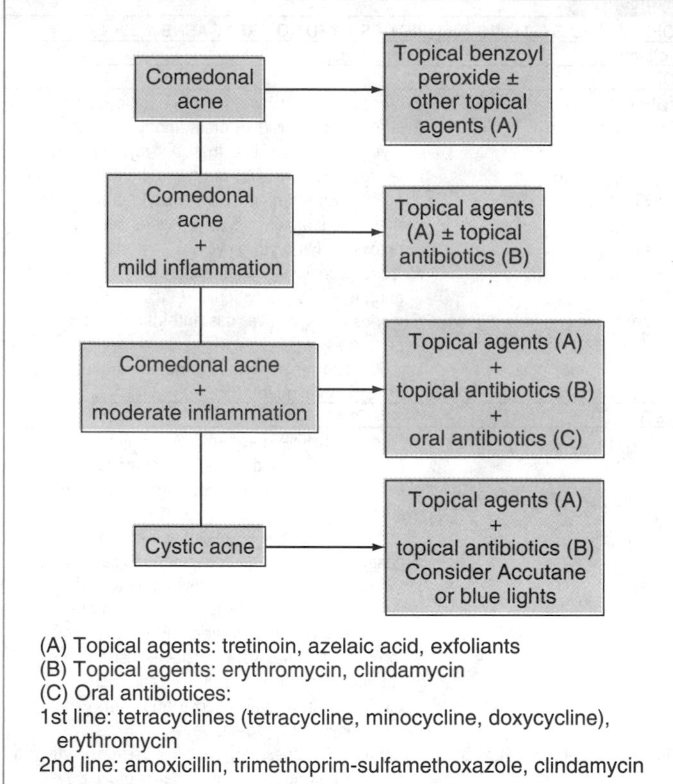


FIG. 8-4

Acne treatment algorithm. *(Courtesy of B. A. Cohen, Johns Hopkins Department of Pediatric Dermatology.)*

b. Treatment should be continued until no new lesions develop and then should be slowly tapered.

5. **Inflammatory acne: Generalized eruption of papules and pustules on the face and trunk. A few patients have a more destructive type of inflammation associated with large, deep inflammatory nodules.**

a. Use a topical retinoid plus a topical and/or systemic antibiotic, depending on the severity of the lesions, for 4–6 weeks.

b. Systemic antibiotics may be used with a topical antibiotic. In general, the dose of the antibiotic should not be reduced for 2–4 months.

c. Patients with nodular, cystic lesions may not respond to systemic antibiotics and may require systemic isotretinoin. Should be used in consultation with a dermatologist such that laboratories may be followed secondary to risk for leukocytosis, to screen for depression, and to ensure that two forms of effective and reliable contraception for women are in place secondary to the medication's teratogenic effects. In addition, use in patients with acute promyelocytic leukemia (APL) is extremely dangerous and can lead to retinoic acid–APL syndrome, characterized by respiratory distress, fever, weight gain, and effusions of the heart and lungs.[15]

d. iPledge Program: Computer-based risk management program; designed to further public health and eliminate fetal exposure to isotretinoin through special restricted distribution program approved by the FDA. Wholesalers, health care professionals, pharmacies, and patients are registered; patients must meet qualifications monthly.

e. Women with persistent acne unresponsive to antibiotics and topical tretinoin may respond to therapy with oral contraceptives after appropriate gynecologic and endocrine evaluation, especially for polycystic ovarian syndrome and other androgen excess conditions.[16]



## VII. COMMON NEONATAL DERMATOLOGIC CONDITIONS (Fig. 8-5 and Color Plates 28 to 36; see also Color Plate 22)

### A. ERYTHEMA TOXICUM NEONATORUM (ET) (see Color Plate 28).

Most common rash (pustular) in infants; is described as a papular rash (2–3 mm in diameter at first), often evolving into vesicles. Rash occurs most often on the second or third days of life (but can emerge as late as 2–3 weeks). Lesions may be clustered and usually resolve in 5–7 days from emergence; recurrences may occur. Vesicular fluid is significant for the presence of eosinophils; treatment is supportive only because rash is self-limited.

### B. TRANSIENT NEONATAL PUSTULAR MELANOSIS (see Color Plates 29 and 30)

Occurs in 4% of infants, especially infants with darker skin tones, and is usually present at birth. This vesicular rash is described as 2–5 mm pustules with a hyperpigmented, nonerythematous base, which over time develops a central crust and leaves a hyperpigmented macule with concurrent scale. Self-limiting, as the name implies.

### C. MILIARIA (see Color Plate 31)

Noted commonly on the nose, these (often erythematous) lesions occur secondary to obstruction of eccrine sweat ducts. May also occur as small papules and pustules secondary to obstruction of these ducts in the mid-epidermis (also known as *prickly heat*). Often occur after the first week of life in areas of high heat production and occlusion by clothes or coverings; course is self-limiting and can be hastened by removal of tight wraps or clothing.

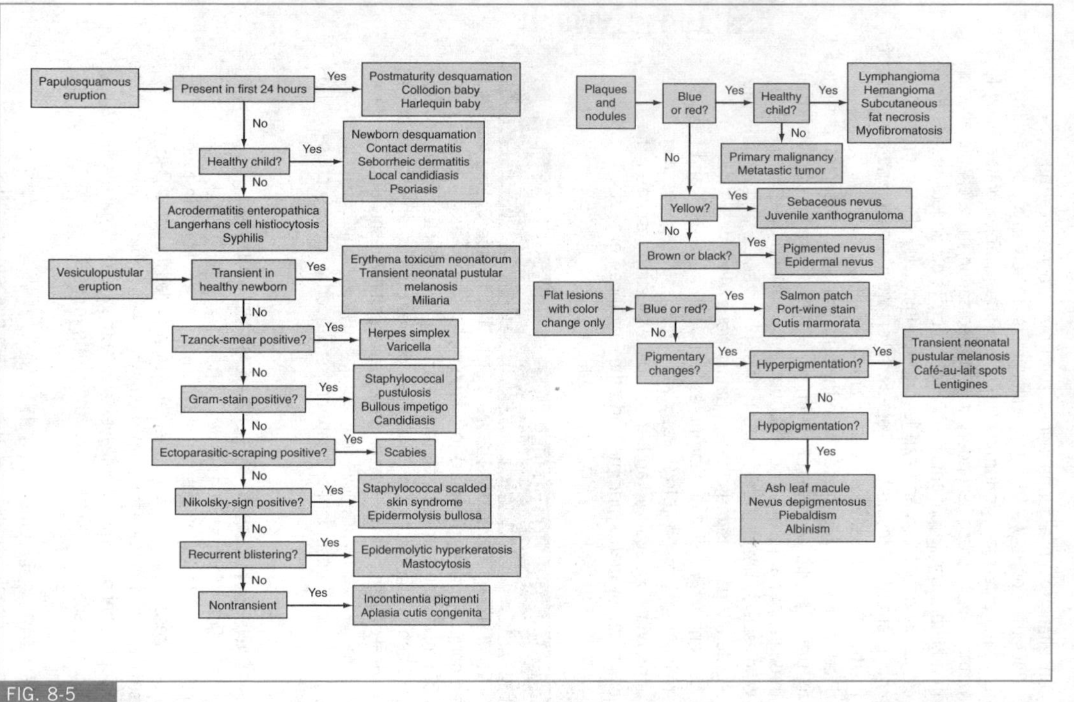


FIG. 8-5 Evaluation of neonatal rashes. *(Modified from Cohen BA: Atlas of Pediatric Dermatology, 3rd ed. St. Louis, Mosby, 2005, p 62.)*

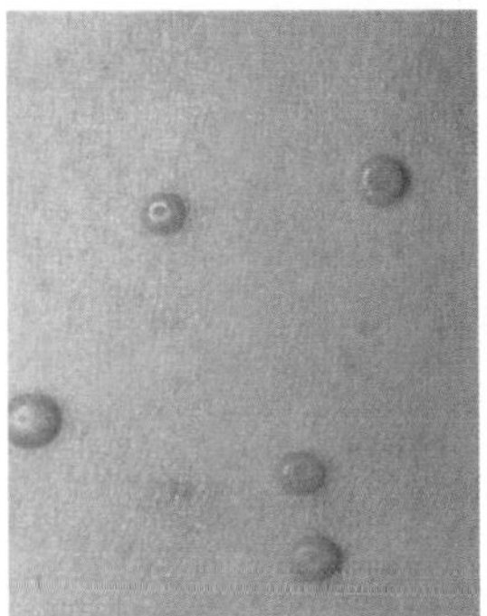

PLATE 1

Molluscum contagiosum. *(From Cohen BA: Pediatric Dermatology. St. Louis, Mosby, 2005, p 126.)*

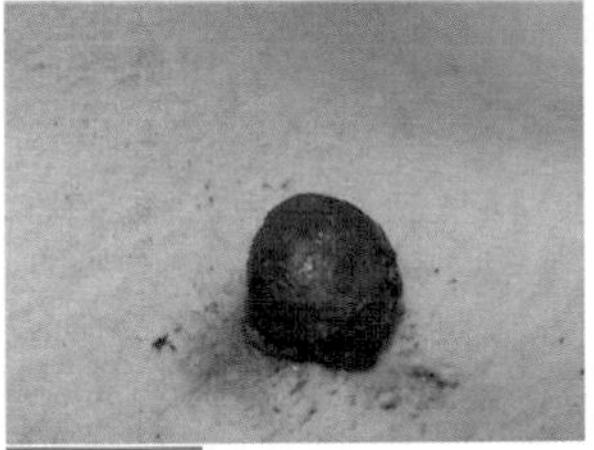

PLATE 2

Pyogenic granuloma. *(From Cohen BA: Dermatology Image Atlas. Available at www.med.jhu.edu/peds/dermatlas, 2001.)*



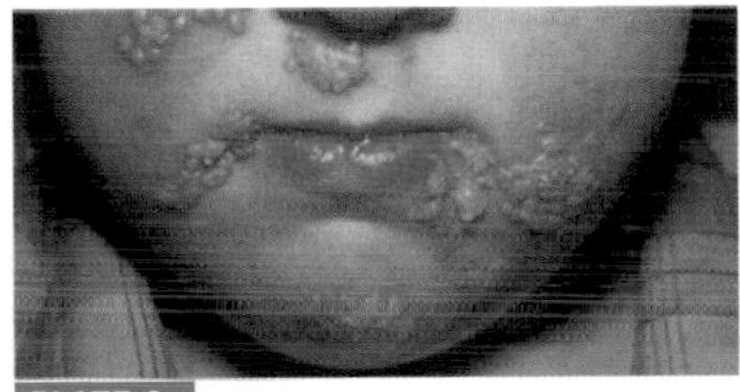

PLATE 3

Herpetic gingivostomatitis. *(From Cohen BA: Pediatric Dermatology. St. Louis, Mosby, 2005, p 103.)*

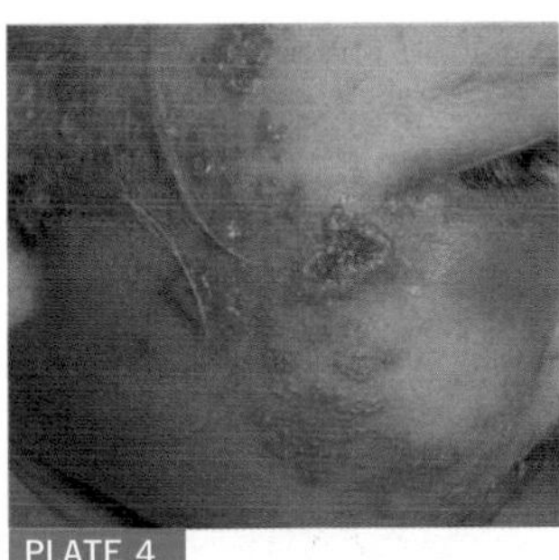

PLATE 4

Herpes zoster. *(From Cohen BA: Pediatric Dermatology. St. Louis, Mosby, 2005, p 106.)*

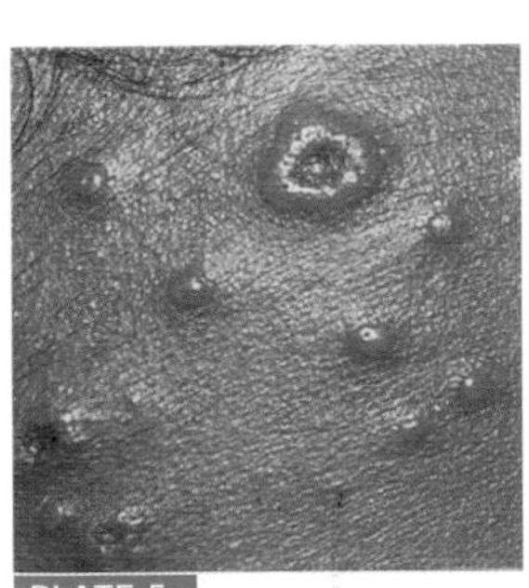

PLATE 5

Varicella. *(From Cohen BA: Pediatric Dermatology. St. Louis, Mosby, 2005, p 104.)*

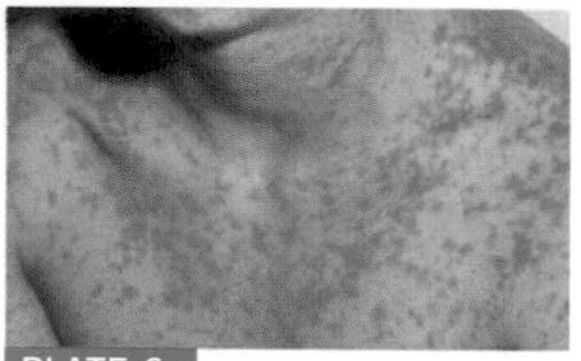

PLATE 6

Measles. *(From Cohen BA: Pediatric Dermatology. St. Louis, Mosby, 2005, p 166.)*

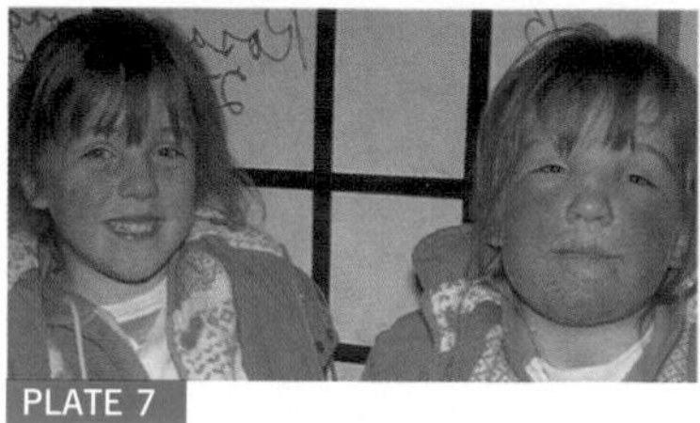

PLATE 7

Fifth disease. *(From Cohen BA: Pediatric Dermatology. St. Louis, Mosby, 2005, p 167.)*

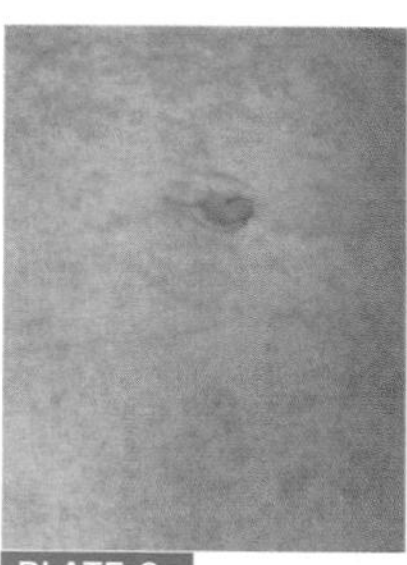

PLATE 8

Roseola. *(From Cohen BA: Pediatric Dermatology. St. Louis, Mosby, 2005, p 168.)*

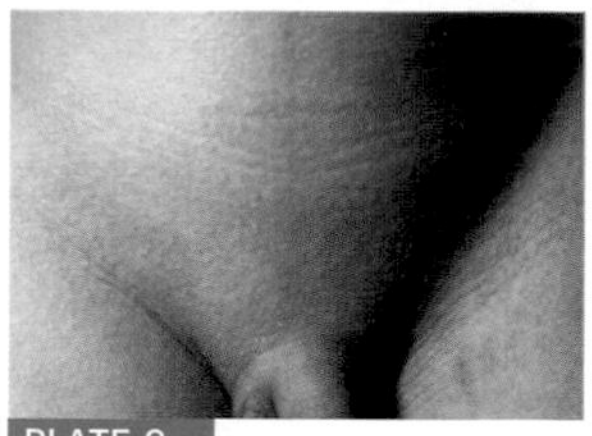

PLATE 9

Scarlet fever. *(From Cohen BA: Dermatology Image Atlas. Available at www.med.jhu.edu/peds/dermatlas, 2001.)*

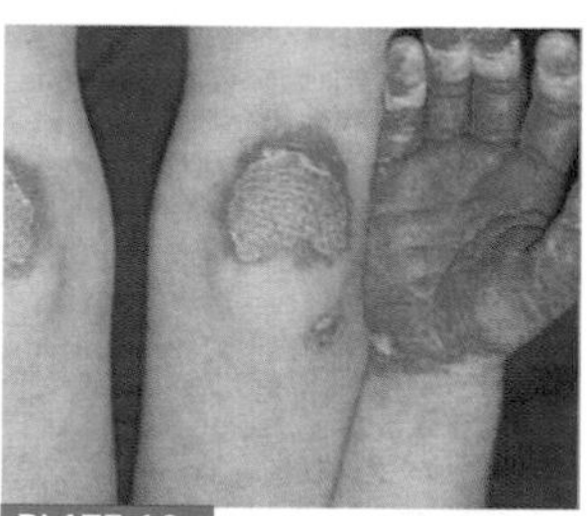

PLATE 10

Psoriasis. *(From Cohen BA: Pediatric Dermatology. St. Louis, Mosby, 2005, p 67.)*

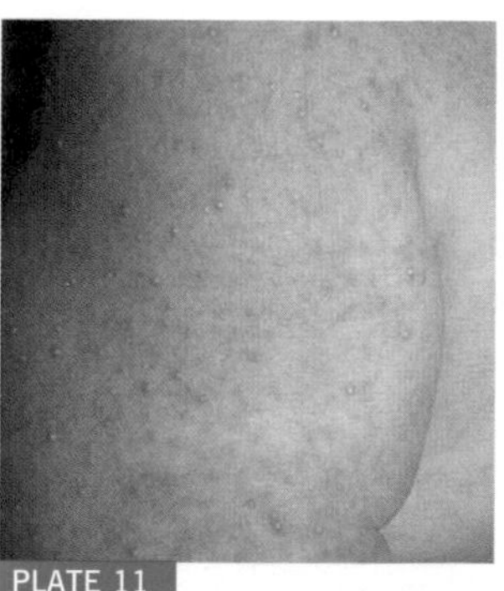

PLATE 11

Keratosis pilaris. *(From Cohen BA: Pediatric Dermatology. St. Louis, Mosby, 2005, p 81.)*

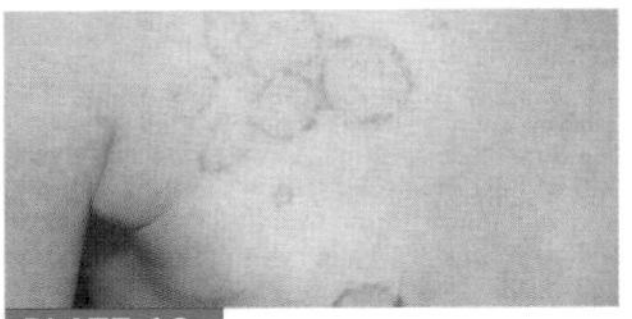

PLATE 12

Tinea corporis. *(From Cohen BA: Pediatric Dermatology. St. Louis, Mosby, 2005, p 94.)*

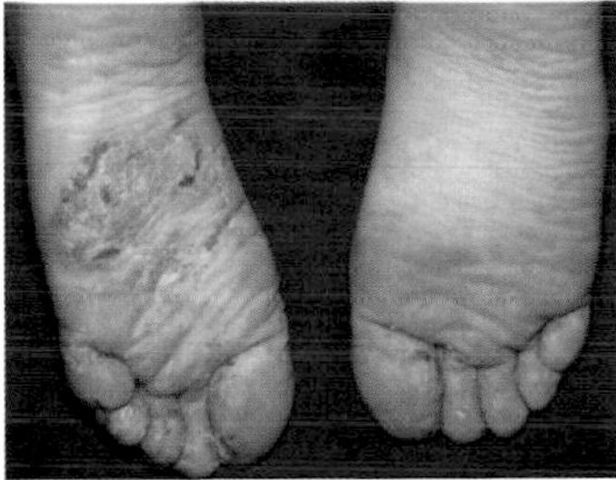

PLATE 13

Tinea pedis. *(From Cohen BA: Dermatology Image Atlas. Available at www.med.jhu.edu/peds/dermatlas, 2001.)*

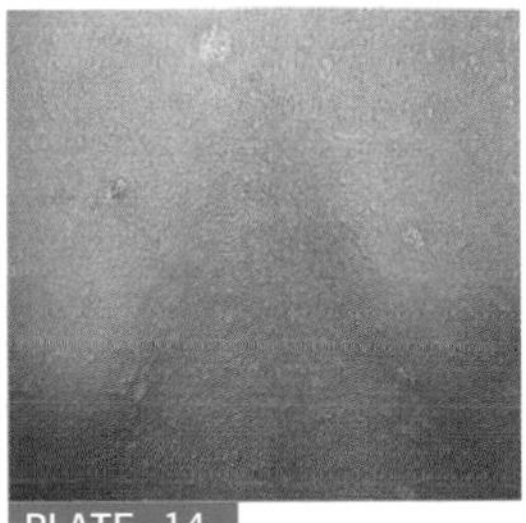

PLATE 14

Pityriasis rosea. *(From Cohen BA: Pediatric Dermatology. St. Louis, Mosby, 2005, p 87.)*



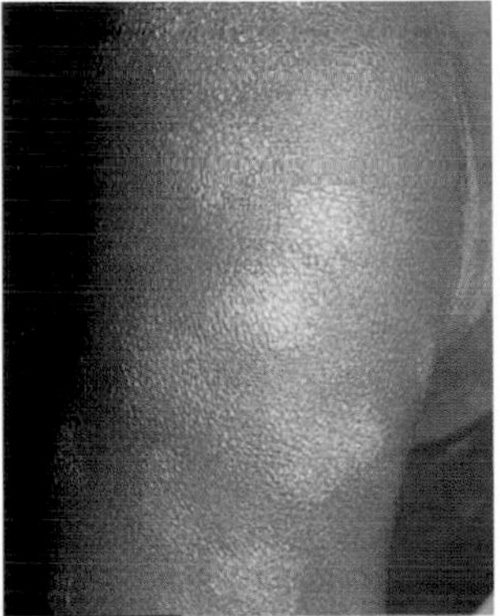

PLATE 15

Pityriasis alba. *(From Cohen BA: Pediatric Dermatology. St. Louis, Mosby, 2005, p 82.)*

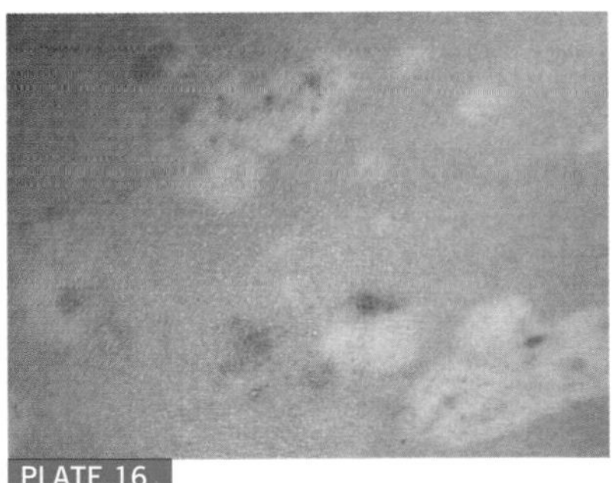

PLATE 16

Postinflammatory hyperpigmentation. *(From Cohen BA: Atlas of Pediatric Dermatology. St. Louis, Mosby, 1993.)*

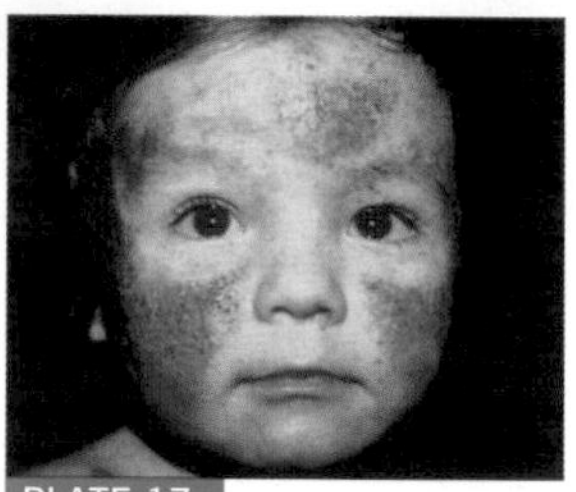
PLATE 17
Infantile eczema. *(From Cohen BA: Pediatric Dermatology. St. Louis, Mosby, 2005, p 79.)*

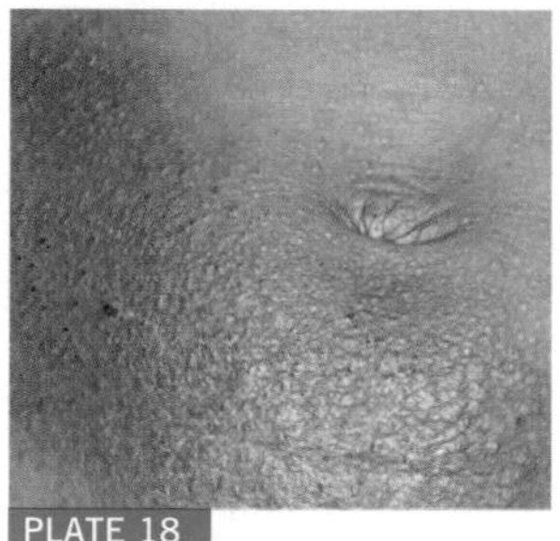
PLATE 18
Childhood eczema. *(From Cohen BA: Dermatology Image Atlas. Available at www.med.jhu.edu/peds/dermatlas, 2001.)*

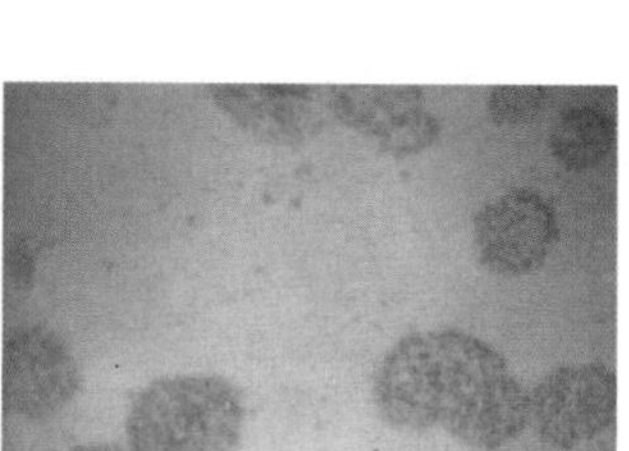
PLATE 19
Nummular eczema. *(From Cohen BA: Pediatric Dermatology. St. Louis, Mosby, 2005, p 80.)*

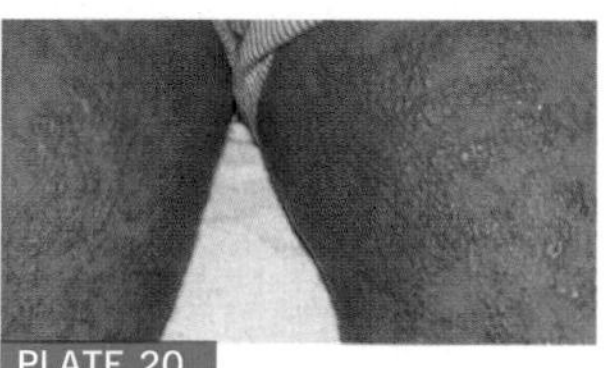
PLATE 20
Follicular eczema. *(From Cohen BA: Pediatric Dermatology. St. Louis, Mosby, 2005, p 80.)*

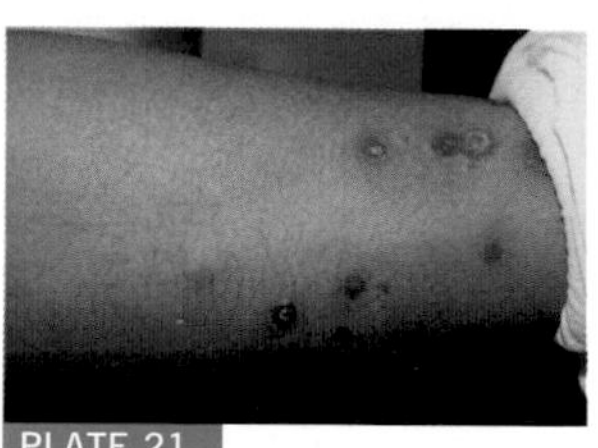
PLATE 21
Papular urticaria. *(From Cohen BA: Dermatology Image Atlas. Available at www.med.jhu.edu/peds/dermatlas, 2001.)*

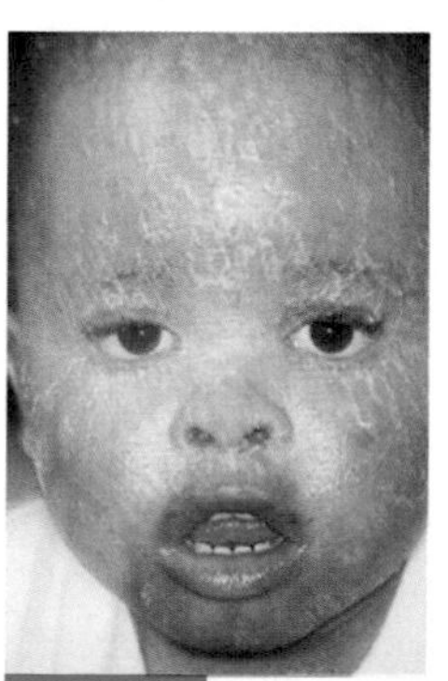
PLATE 22
Congenital ichthyosis erythroderma. *(From Cohen BA: Pediatric Dermatology, St. Louis, Mosby, 2005, p 29.)*

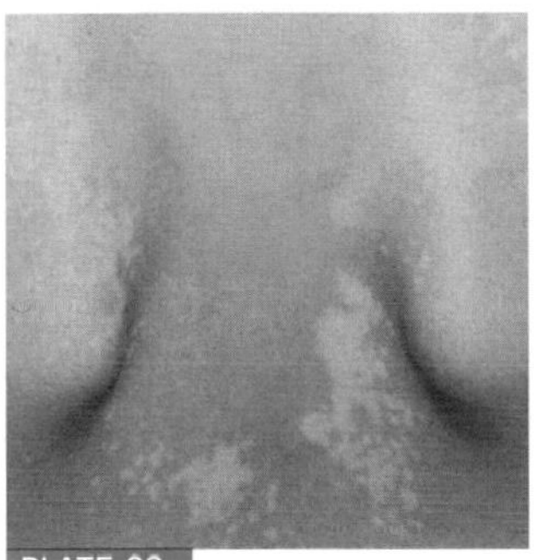

PLATE 23

Tinea versicolor. *(From Cohen BA: Atlas of Pediatric Dermatology. St. Louis, Mosby, 1993.)*

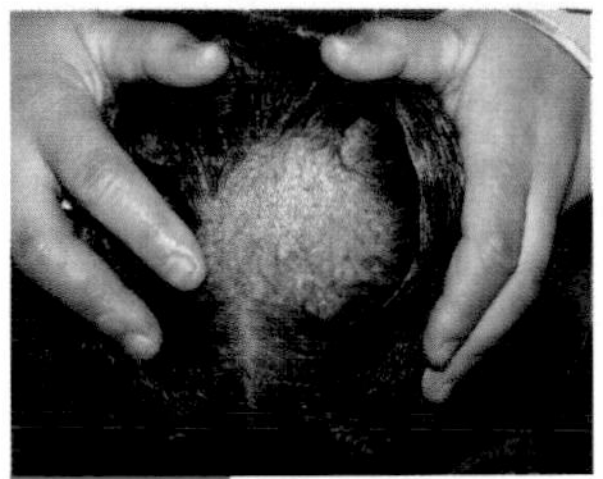

PLATE 24

Tinea capitis. *(From Cohen BA: Atlas of Pediatric Dermatology. St. Louis, Mosby, 1993.)*



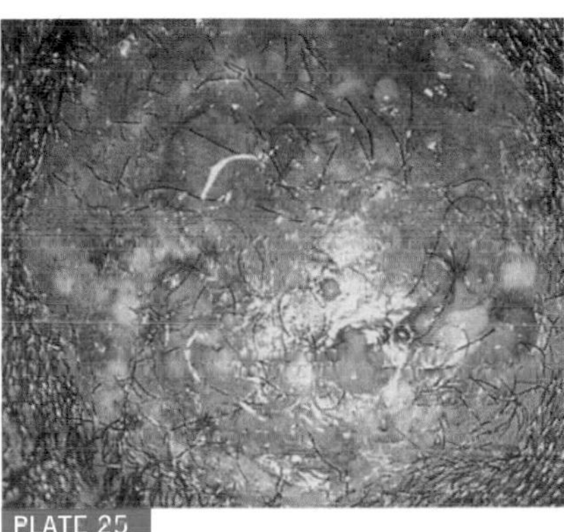

PLATE 25

Kerion. *(From Cohen BA: Pediatric Dermatology. St. Louis, Mosby, 2005, p 207.)*

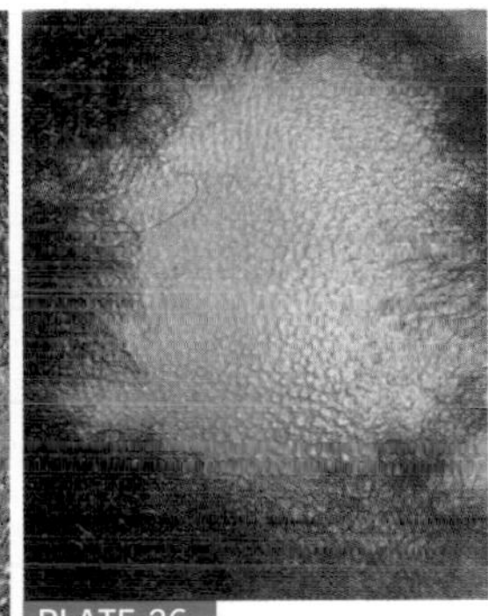

PLATE 26

Alopecia areata. *(From Cohen BA: Pediatric Dermatology. St. Louis, Mosby, 2005, p 208.)*

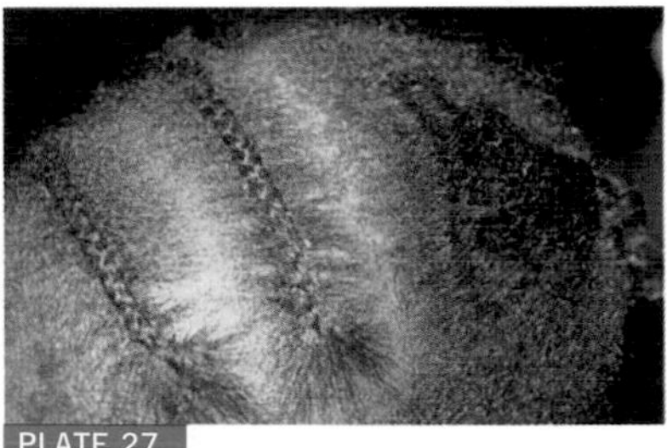

PLATE 27

Traction alopecia. *(From Cohen BA: Pediatric Dermatology. St. Louis, Mosby, 2005, p 209.)*

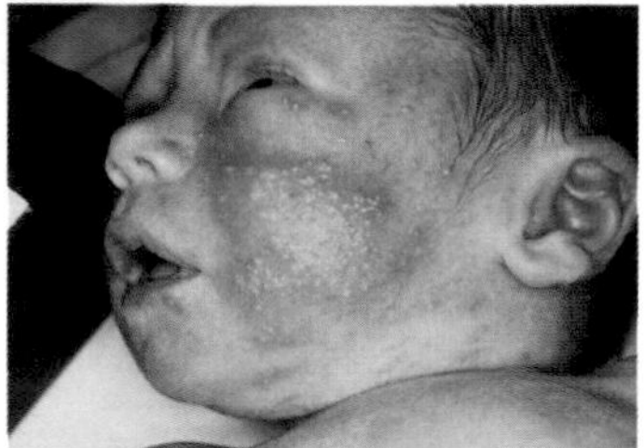

PLATE 28

Erythema toxicum neonatorum. *(From Cohen BA: Pediatric Dermatology. St. Louis, Mosby, 1999, p 18.)*

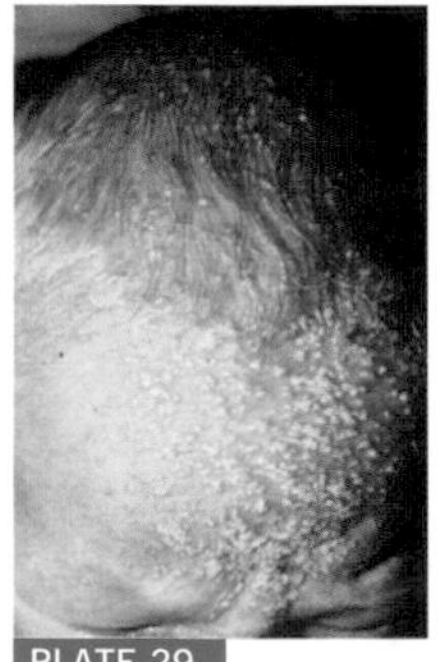

PLATE 29

Transient neonatal pustular melanosis. *(From Cohen BA: Pediatric Dermatology, St. Louis, Mosby, 2005, p 20.)*

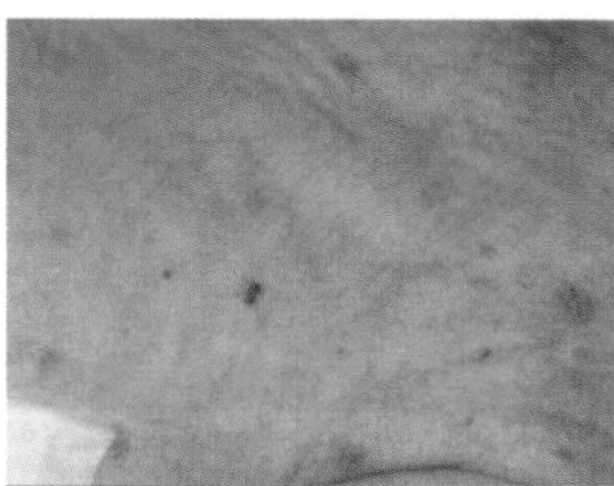

PLATE 30

Hyperpigmentation from resolving transient neonatal pustular melanosis. *(From Cohen BA: Pediatric Dermatology. St. Louis, Mosby, 2005, p 20.)*

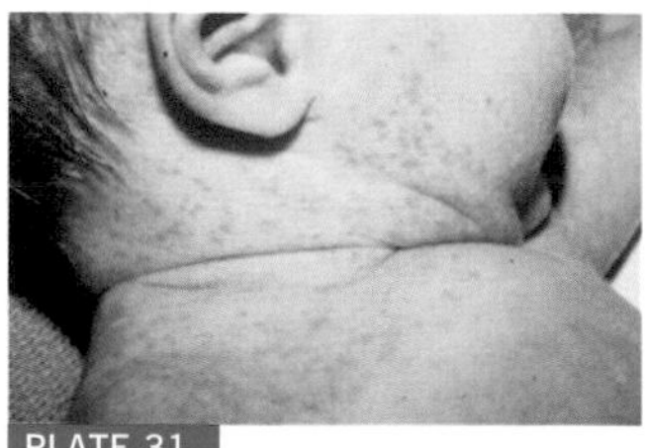

PLATE 31

Miliaria rubra. *(From Cohen BA: Pediatric Dermatology, St. Louis, Mosby, 2005, p 22.)*

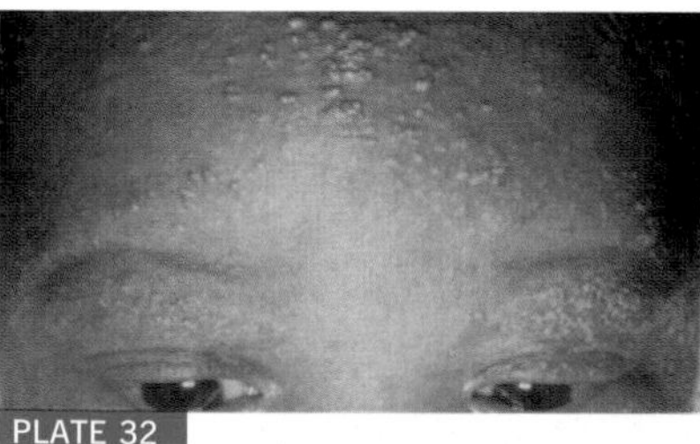

PLATE 32

Milia. *(From Cohen BA: Pediatric Dermatology. St. Louis, Mosby, 2005, p 22.)*

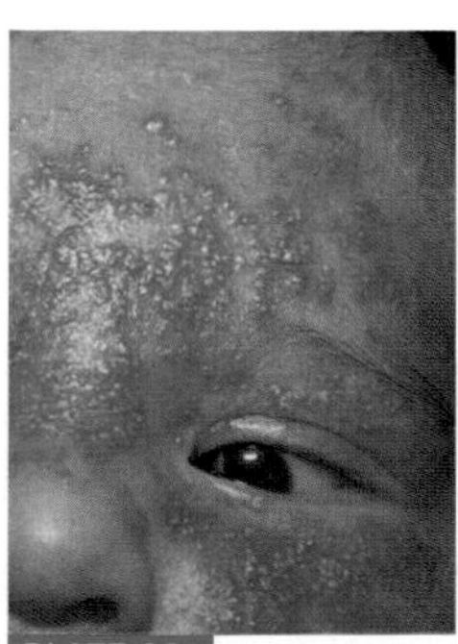

PLATE 33

Neonatal acne. *(From Cohen BA: Pediatric Dermatology. St. Louis, Mosby, 2005, p 23.)*

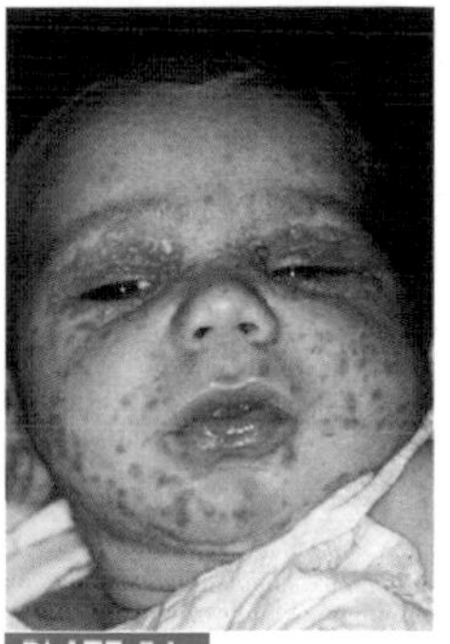

PLATE 34

Seborrheic dermatitis. *(From Cohen BA: Pediatric Dermatology, St. Louis, Mosby, 2005, p 33.)*

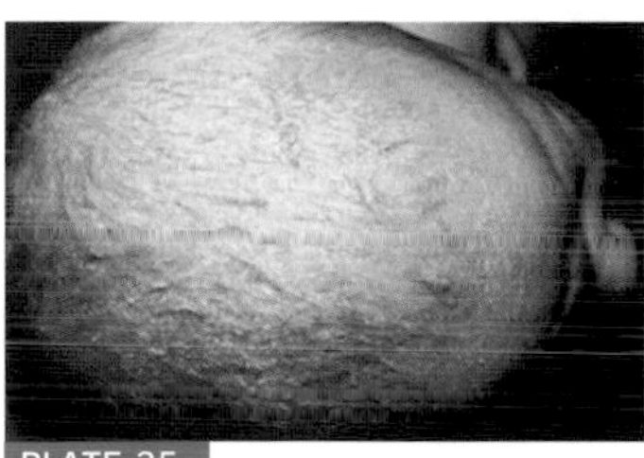

PLATE 35

Seborrheic dermatitis. *(From Cohen BA: Pediatric Dermatology, St. Louis, Mosby, 2005, p 33.)*

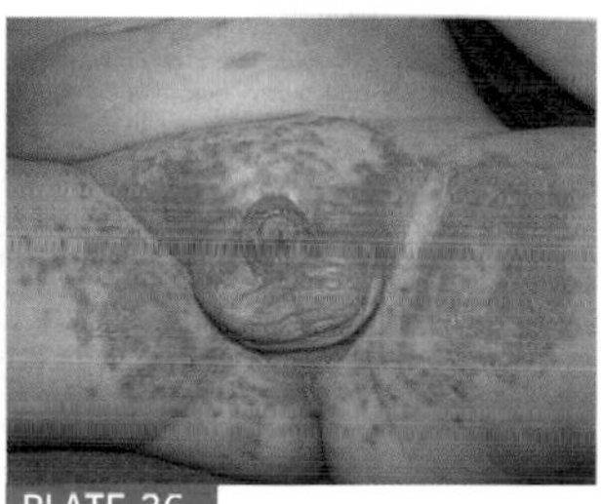

PLATE 36

Diaper candidiasis. *(From Cohen BA: Pediatric Dermatology. St. Louis, Mosby, 2005, p 34.)*

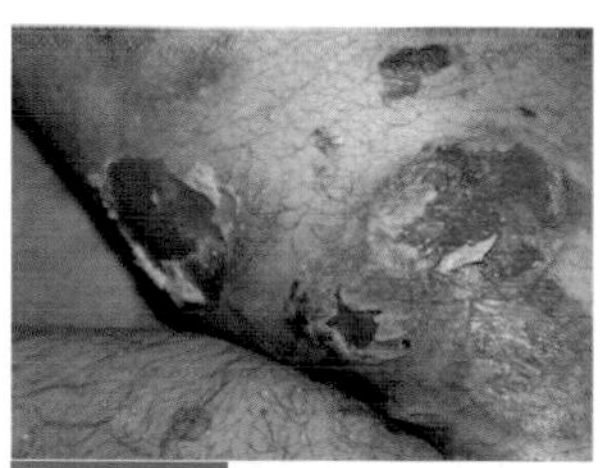

PLATE 37

Pemphigus vulgaris. *(From Cohen BA: Dermatology Image Atlas. Available at www.med.jhu.edu/peds/dermatlas, 2001.)*

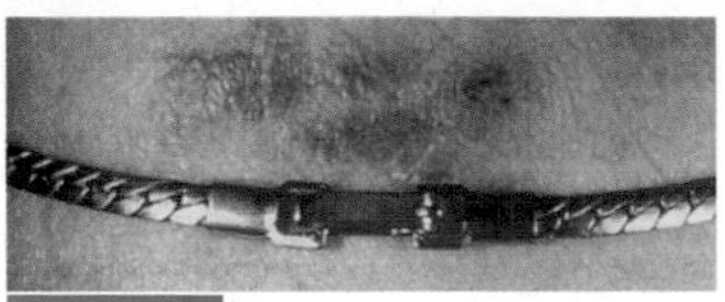

PLATE 38

Allergic contact dermatitis. *(From Cohen BA: Pediatric Dermatology. St. Louis, Mosby, 2005, p 75.)*

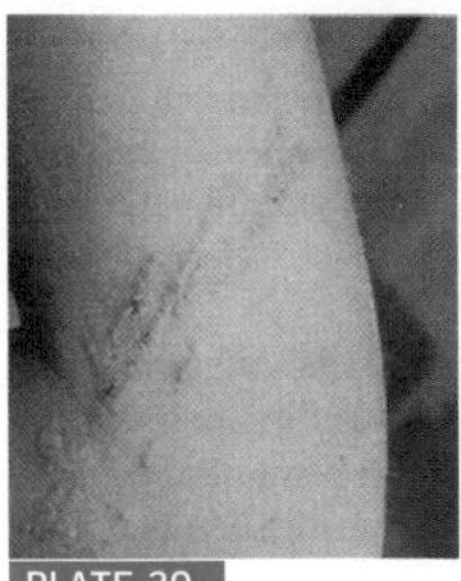

PLATE 39

Poison ivy. *(From Cohen BA: Dermatology Image Atlas. Available at www.med.jhu.edu/peds/dermatlas, 2001.)*

### D. MILIA (see Color Plate 32)

Common lesions (up to 50% occurrence) are 1–3 mm papules (white to yellow in color), occurring mostly on the upper body and face of newborns, usually within the first month of life. Can persist for several months and are epidermal inclusion cysts requiring no treatment.

### E. NEONATAL ACNE (see Color Plate 33)

Often present at birth, these common (occurring in up to 20% of infants), open or closed comedones are thought to be triggered by maternal and endogenous androgens. No treatment is necessary because these lesions are self-limiting.

### F. SEBORRHEIC DERMATITIS (CRADLE CAP) (see Color Plates 34 and 35)

Skin rash characterized by a greasy yellow scale occurring most frequently in the scalp, diaper area, and intertriginous regions; may persist until age 1 year. Affected areas may also have fissuring, weeping, and maceration, although these infants remain otherwise healthy and largely asymptomatic. Specific etiology is unknown. Treatment is unnecessary, although antiseborrheic shampoos (salicylic acid) as well as low-potency corticosteroids may shorten the course.

### G. MONGOLIAN SPOTS

Common skin macules, seen especially in Asian, black, and other dark-skin-toned infants; are seen most often on the buttocks and legs. Resolution is spontaneous, usually within the first year of life.[17]

## VIII. BULLOUS LESIONS: DIAGNOSIS AND TREATMENT

### A. IMPETIGO

1. **Clinical presentation:**

a. Tiny flaccid vesicles or pustules, which enlarge and rupture quickly and are followed by honey-colored crusted plaque, most often overlying insect bite, abrasion, or other skin rashes. Most common bacteria is *Staphylococcus aureus;* at times may be caused by *group A beta-hemolytic streptococci.* May occur anywhere on skin, but more common are sites prone to trauma. Bullae are very infectious and may be inoculated to multiple sites on the patient and other family members. Lesions demonstrate a positive Nikolsky sign. Infection most often from a noncutaneous source such as lungs, bone, meninges, ears.

b. MRSA impetigo: Increasing occurrences within the community and hospital settings. If not improving on standard antibiotics, consider methicillin resistance; may need clindamycin or vancomycin.

2. **Treatment:**
a. Small, localized infections: Topical antibiotics (mupirocin, bacitracin, bacitracin-polymyxin B) along with tepid water compresses.
b. Widespread impetigo: Oral antibiotic with gram-positive coverage (dicloxacillin, cephalexin, clotrimazole, amoxicillin-clavulanate potassium)
c. Parenteral antibiotics, hospitalization and supportive care if any signs of progression to cellulitis or visceral dissemination.

## B. AUTOIMMUNE-BULLOUS LESIONS

1. **Pemphigus vulgaris (Color Plate 37):**
a. Clinical presentation: Bullous disease beginning with intraoral lesions or scalp blisters, which evolve into more widespread disease involving trunk, scalp, face, and extremities. May extend to involve large areas of the body. Blisters heal insidiously without scarring unless they become secondarily infected; 95% have intraoral involvement. Symptoms consist of pruritus, pain, and burning of the skin and mucous membranes; positive Nikolsky sign; downward pressure on existing blisters may cause extension at the periphery (Asbaugh-Hansen sign). May also occur transiently in the newborn period if pemphigus IgG antibody is passed from mother to baby.
b. Pathogenesis: Occurs due to an IgG antibody directed against a transmembrane glycoprotein, desmoglein, on the cell surface of keratinocytes. Desmoglein is a cadherin-type adhesion molecule that comprises desmosomes, which maintain the integrity of the epidermis by acting as adhesive junctions. Disruption of the desmosomes causes blister formation. Positive direct immunofluoresence against IgG detects it.
c. Treatment: Often, admission to the burn unit for management of fluid and electrolyte losses and supportive care. High-dose prednisone to control eruptions. Some patients may require immunosuppressive agents such as cyclophosphamide, azathioprine, mycophenolate. IV immunoglobulin and plasmapheresis have shown promise.

2. **Pemphigus foliaceus:**
a. Clinical presentation: Crops of vesicles, flaccid bullae, and erosions on erythematous base in a seborrheic distribution. Vesicles arise high in the epidermis and quickly crust over. Like pemphigus vulgaris, demonstrates a positive Nikolsky sign but mucous membranes are usually spared. Even with widespread rash patient appears generally well and disease is self-limiting.
b. Pathogenesis: Results from antibodies to desmoglein-1; occurs in the upper half of the epidermis.
c. Treatment: Mild disease may respond to topical steroids. Some cases may require systemic steroids.

3. **Bullous pemphigoid: Large vesiculobullous lesions (>2 cm) located in the subepidermal layer and containing eosinophilic dermal infiltrate.**

These blisters are more likely to be tense. Negative Nikolsky sign. Diagnostic findings are IgG and C3 at the dermal-epidermal junction in the lamina lucida on direct immunofluoresence.

4. **Dermatitis herpetiformis:** Symmetrical, intensely pruritic vesicles approximately 3–4 cm in size clustered on the extensor surfaces. On biopsy, findings of granular IgA deposits in the basement membrane and prominent neurophilic microabcesses at the dermal papillary tips. High incidence of HLA B8 antigens.
5. **Epidermolysis bullosa acquisita:** Blistering results from a disruption of type VII collagen. Resembles bullous pemphigoid clinically with a higher incidence of mucous membrance involvement; may be more resistant to therapy. May occur as isolated autoimmune phenomenon; also associated with systemic lupus erythematosus and inflammatory bowel disease. Often diagnosed by salt-split skin test.



## C. INSECT BITES (see Papular Urticaria, section IV.B)

## D. BURNS (also see Chapter 4)

1. **Chemical:** Produce dry eschar, crust, and form necrotic blisters.
2. **Thermal:** Flame, scald/contact, electrical, cold/frostbite. May produce erythema, moist blistering.
3. **Nonaccidental burns:** Important to evaluate burns for their shape, distribution, inconsistent history, and delay in care, which may point toward a concern for abuse. Symmetrical burns, those from hot water immersion (top of feet and hands may be more involved because skin on palms and soles is thicker), cigarette lesions (punched-out ulcers with dry purple crusts).

**Note** *All burns are susceptible to becoming secondarily infected, which may make it difficult to distinguish the type of burn you are encountering.*

## E. CONTACT DERMATITIS

1. **Irritant dermatitis:** Usually caused by caustic agents such as acid, alkalis, hydrocarbons. Defined on the premise that anyone exposed to these agents for long enough in a high enough concentration would develop a reaction.
2. **Allergic dermatitis (Color Plate 38):**
   a. Pathogenesis: T-cell mediated immune reaction in response to an environmental trigger that comes into contact with the skin. After a sensitization reaction with the initial exposure, an allergic response occurs with subsequent exposures.
   b. Allergens: Most common antigen is poison ivy. Other common allergens include nickel, rubber, glues, dyes in shoes, ethylenediamine in topical lubricants.
   c. Clinical presentation: Most often presents as abrupt erythema, pruritus, and vesiculation; may progress to a chronic stage involving scaling, lichenification, and pigmentary changes. Initial reaction occurs after a

sensitization period of 7–10 days in susceptible individuals. Re-exposure to the antigen will cause a more rapid reactivation reaction.

3. **Poison ivy (Color Plate 39):**

a. Pathogenesis: Often causes a contact dermatitis, which erupts after exposure to a causative plant, most usually of the *Toxicodendron* or *Rhus* genus. Culprit plant is a three-leaved tall shrub or woody rope–like vine that grows within grasses, on trees, on fences, and in vacant areas. Exposure may also occur from contact with item of clothing or pet that has brushed up against the plant.

b. Clinical presentation: Appears often as streaks of erythematous pustules and vesicles; in highly sensitized individuals may appear as large patches. Impressive swelling can ensue. Areas with highest concentration of antigen develop first, and lower doses react in succession. Once on the skin antigen becomes fixed to epithelial cells in 20 min and cannot be spread further. Immediate washing after exposure can reduce eruption; barrier creams may afford some protection.

4. **Diagnosis of contact dermatitis:** *Careful history;* **in some cases, patch testing is helpful.**

5. **Treatment:**

a. Remove causative agent.

b. Topical steroids for local areas of inflammation.

c. If widespread or severe local inflammation involving eyelids, parts of face, genitals, hands, or other areas where swelling can be incapacitating, treat with 2–3 week tapering course of systemic corticosteroids starting at 0.5–1 mg/kg/day.

## REFERENCES


1. Bhattacharya JJ et al: PHACES syndrome: A review of eight previously unreported cases with late arterial occlusions. Neurobiology 2004;46: 227–233.
2. Faranoff AA: Neonatal-Perinatal Medicine: Diseases of the Fetus and Infant, 7th ed. St. Louis, Mosby, 2002.
3. Drolet BA, Esterly NB, Frieden IJ: Hemangiomas and children. Primary Care 1999;3:173–181.
4. Cohen BA: Warts and children: Can they be separated? Contemp Pediatr 1997; 2:128–149.
5. Meinking TL et al: The treatment of scabies with ivermectin. NEJM 1995:333: 26–30.
6. Eichenfield LF et al: Safety and efficacy of pimecrolimus (ASM 981) cream 1% in the treatment of mild and moderate atopic dermatitis in children and adolescents. J Am Acad Dermatol 2002;46:495–504.
7. Wahn U et al: Efficacy and safety of pimecrolimus cream in the long-term management of atopic dermatitis in children. Pediatrics 2002;110:e2, 1–8.
8. Rikkers SM et al: Topical tacrolimus treatment of atopic eyelid disease. Am J Ophthalmol 2003;135:297–302.

9. Boguniewicz M et al, for the Pediatric Tacrolimus Study Group: A randomized, vehicle-controlled trial of tacrolimus ointment for treatment of atopic dermatitis in children. J Allergy Clin Immunol 1998;102:637–644.
10. Reitamo S et al: Efficacy and safety of tacrolimus ointment compared with that of hydrocortisone acetate ointment in children with atopic dermatitis. J Allergy Clin Immunol 2002;109:547–555.
11. Wollenberg A et al: Topical tacrolimus (FK506) leads to profound phenotypic and functional alterations of epidermal antigen-presenting dendritic cells in atopic dermatitis. J Allergy Clin Immunol 2001;107:519–525.
12. Cohen BA: Atopic dermatitis: Breaking the itch-scratch cycle. Contemp Pediatr 1992;7:64–81.
13. Smith ML: Tinea capitis. Pediatr Ann 1996;25:101–105.
14. Cohen BA: Pediatric Dermatology, 3rd ed. London, Mosby, 2005.
15. Mosby's Drug Consult. St. Louis, Mosby, 2004.
16. Leyden JJ: Therapy for acne vulgaris. NEJM 1997;16:1156–1162.
17. Behrman RE: Nelson Textbook of Pediatrics, 17th ed. Philadelphia, Elsevier, 2003.

# Behavior and Development

Martine M. Solages, MD

## I. WEBSITES

www.chadd.org (ADHD)
www.dbpeds.org/handouts
www.disability.gov
www.ninds.nih.gov (cerebral palsy)
www.ldanatl.org (Learning Disabilities Association of America)
www.thearclink.org (ArcLink; mental retardation)
www.brightfutures.org
www.nectac.org (National Early Childhood Technical Assistance Center)
www.reachoutandread.org

9

## II. INTRODUCTION

### A. CHAPTER FOCUS

Developmental disabilities are a group of interrelated, nonprogressive, neurologic disorders occurring in childhood. This chapter focuses on assessment of neurodevelopment to identify possible developmental disability.

### B. DEVELOPMENT

1. Development can be divided into five major streams or skill areas: visual-motor, language (the cognitive streams), motor, social, and adaptive. Each stream has a spectrum of normal and abnormal presentation. Abnormal development in one stream increases the risk for deficit in another and should prompt a careful assessment of all streams. A developmental diagnosis is a functional description and classification that does not specify an etiology or medical diagnosis.
2. Developmental assessment is based on the premise that milestone acquisition occurs at a specific rate and in an orderly and sequential manner. When development is not progressing normally, the pattern of abnormal development usually includes delay, deviancy, or dissociation.

## III. DEFINITIONS[1]

### A. DEVELOPMENTAL QUOTIENT (DQ)

1. A calculation that reflects the rate of development in any given stream. DQ represents the percentage of normal development present at the time of testing. Can be calculated for any given stream as follows:

$$DQ = (\text{developmental age}/\text{chronologic age}) \times 100$$

2. Two separate developmental assessments over time are more predictive than a single assessment.

TABLE 9-1

MENTAL RETARDATION—DSM-IV-TR CLASSIFICATIONS*

| Level | IQ | Academic Potential | Daily Living |
|---|---|---|---|
| Mild | 70–80 | Educable to about the 6th grade level | Fully independent |
| | 50–69 | Reading and writing to 4th–5th grade level or less | Relatively independent with some training |
| Moderate | 35–49 | Limited reading to 1st–2nd grade level | Dress without help, use toilet, prepare food |
| Severe | 20–34 | Very unlikely to read or write | Can be toilet trained, dress with help; may be able to sign name |
| Profound | <20 | None | Occasionally can be toilet trained, dress with help; often nonverbal |

*The American Association on Mental Retardation has moved away from the use of strict categories of mental retardation. It instead advocates an individualized approach that addresses specific limitations in capabilities and functioning.

From American Association on Mental Retardation. Mental Retardation: Definition, Classification and Systems of Supports, 9th ed. Washington, DC, AAMR, 1992, pp 5–34, and American Psychiatric Association: Diagnostic and Statistical Manual of Mental Disorders (DSM-IV-TR), 4th ed., text revision. Washington, DC, American Psychiatric Press, 2000, pp 41–45.

### B. DELAY

Performance significantly below average (DQ < 75) in a given area of skill. May occur in a single stream or several streams.

### C. DEVIANCY

Atypical development within a single stream, such as developmental milestones occurring out of sequence. Deviancy does not necessarily imply abnormality but should alert one to the possibility that problems may exist. Examples: An infant who crawls before sitting, or an infant with early development of hand preference.

### D. DISSOCIATION

A substantial difference in the rate of development between two or more streams. Example: Cognitive-motor difference in some children with mental retardation or cerebral palsy.

## IV. DISORDERS

### A. MENTAL RETARDATION (MR)

Characterized by significantly below-average intellectual functioning (IQ < 70–75) existing concurrently with related limitation in two or more of the following adaptive skill areas: communication, self-care, home living, social skills, community use, self-direction, health and safety, functional academics, leisure, and work (Table 9-1). MR manifests itself before age 18 years. Formal psychometric testing is needed to make the diagnosis. Patients should be referred for diagnosis, review of potential etiology, and guidance if the DQ for any given stream is <70 or if there is significant learning difficulty.

| Work | Expected Mental Age as an Adult (yr) | Intensity of Support |
|---|---|---|
| Employable; may need training to be competitive | — | Intermittent |
| Employable; often need training | 9–11 | Intermittent |
| Likely to need sheltered employment | 5–8 | Limited |
| Sheltered employment | 3–5 | Extensive |
| Very limited | <3 | Pervasive |



## B. COMMUNICATION DISORDERS

Can be subdivided into expressive language disorders, mixed receptive-expressive language disorders, pragmatic language disorders, phonologic disorders, and stuttering. Developmental language disorders can be characterized by deficits of comprehension, interpretation, production, or use of language. Differential diagnosis includes mental retardation, hearing loss, specific language disability, expressive language disorder, mixed expressive-receptive language disorder, selective mutism, and autism (or another pervasive developmental disorder).

## C. LEARNING DISABILITIES (LDs)

A heterogeneous group of disorders that manifest as significant difficulties in one or more of the following seven areas (as defined by the federal government): basic reading skills, reading comprehension, oral expression, listening comprehension, written expression, mathematical calculation, and mathematical reasoning. Specific LDs are diagnosed when the individual's achievement on standardized tests in a given area is substantially below that expected for age, schooling, and level of intelligence.[2]

## D. CEREBRAL PALSY (CP)

A disorder of movement and posture resulting from a permanent, nonprogressive lesion of the immature brain. Manifestations may change with brain growth and development. A child with significant motor impairment can be identified at any age. The diagnosis of CP should be made before age 12 months; however, the mean age of diagnosis is 13 months. CP is classified in terms of physiologic and topographic characteristics as well as severity (Table 9-2). Classification is important because different classifications often have very different etiologies and associated deficits.

## E. ATTENTION DEFICIT/HYPERACTIVITY DISORDER (ADHD)

1. **A neurobehavioral disorder characterized by inattention, distractibility, impulsivity, and hyperactivity, all behaviors that are more frequent and severe than typically observed in children of the same developmental age. Symptoms must persist for at least 6 months, occur before age 7 years, and be evident in two or more settings. See the American Psychiatric Association's *Diagnostic and Statistical Manual of Mental Disorders*, 4th edition, Text Revision (*DSM-IV-TR*) for full diagnostic criteria.[3]**
2. **The differential diagnosis for ADHD is broad. Proper diagnosis, evaluation, and treatment are paramount to ensuring cognitive, academic, behavioral, emotional, and social function. Diagnosis is made using data from history, observation, and behavioral checklists such as the Vanderbilt Assessment Scale. Results of behavioral checklists alone are not sufficient for diagnosis. The Vanderbilt Assessment scale may be downloaded from: http://www.brightfutures.org/mentalhealth/pdf/professionals/bridges/adhd.pdf.**

## F. AUTISM SPECTRUM DISORDERS

Include autism, pervasive developmental disorder NOS, Asperger disorder, childhood disintegrative disorder, and Rett disorder. See the *DSM-IV-TR* for full diagnostic criteria.[3]

TABLE 9-2

**CLINICAL CLASSIFICATION OF CEREBRAL PALSY[4]**

| Type | Pattern of Involvement |
|---|---|
| **I. SPASTIC (Increased tone, clasped knife, clonus, further classified by distribution)** | |
| Hemiplegia | Ipsilateral arm and leg; arm worse than leg |
| Diplegia | Legs primarily affected |
| Quadriplegia | All four extremities impaired; legs worse than arms |
| Double hemiplegia | All four extremities; arms notably worse than legs |
| Monoplegia | One extremity, usually upper; probably reflects a mild hemiplegia |
| Triplegia | One upper extremity and both lower; probably represents a hemiplegia plus a diplegia or incomplete quadriplegia |
| **II. EXTRAPYRAMIDAL (lead pipe or candle wax rigidity, variable tone, +/– clonus)** | |
| Choreathetosis, rigidity, dystonia | Complex movement/tone disorders reflecting basal ganglia pathology |
| Ataxia, tremor | Movement and tone disorders reflecting cerebellar origin |
| Hypotonia | Usually related to diffuse, often severe, cerebral and/or cerebellar cortical damage |

From Capute AJ, Accardo PJ (eds): Cerebral Palsy: Developmental Disabilities in Infancy and Childhood, 2nd ed., vol 2. Baltimore, Paul H. Brookes, 1996, pp 83–86.

1. **Autism:** Essential features are impaired social interaction and communication and a restricted group of activities and interests, with stereotyped behaviors, rituals, or mannerisms. Onset of abnormal functioning occurs before age 3 years. A large proportion of autistic children function in the mentally retarded range. Siblings of children with autism appear to be at greater risk of developing the disorder. Males are disproportionately affected. Assessment scales such as M-CHAT are available for screening (Table 9-3).
2. **Pervasive developmental disorder NOS:** Characterized by impaired social interaction and communication skills and/or repetitive, stereotyped behaviors, but with a symptom profile that does not meet diagnostic criteria for autism or other mental health disorder.
3. **Asperger disorder:** Characterized by impairment in social interactions and restricted, repetitive patterns of behavior with no general delay in language, cognition, or attainment of self-help skills. More common in boys. Those affected have difficulty understanding and responding to social conventions and nonverbal cues and are therefore often unable to develop peer relationships.
4. **Childhood disintegrative disorder:** Characterized by normal development until age 2 years, followed by loss of previously achieved language, social, and motor milestones. Also marked by disordered communication and/or social interaction. Affected individuals may have repetitive movements or stereotypies. Loss of skills occurs before age 10 years.
5. **Rett disorder:** Characterized by normal development in the first 6 months of life; usually described in females. Affected individuals exhibit symptoms of autism, receptive and expressive language delay, psychomotor retardation, decreased head growth, breathing abnormalities, seizures, and poor coordination of gait and trunk movements. Mutations in the *MECP2* gene are strongly associated with Rett disorder.

## V. DEVELOPMENTAL SCREENING AND EVALUATION

### A. DEVELOPMENTAL MILESTONES (Table 9-4)

### B. DEVELOPMENTAL SCREENING GUIDELINES

1. **In assessing for delay, an individual DQ can be calculated for any given developmental stream;** if the quotient is <70%, a diagnosis of delay can be made and warrants further evaluation or referral. For example, a 13-month-old child who does not yet walk alone but is able to walk when led with two hands held (i.e., a 10-month level of motor development) has a DQ of 10/13 = 77% and is not considered delayed.
2. **Developmental surveillance should occur at every well-child visit. Developmental screening using standardized tools should be administered at 9-month, 18-month, and 30-month well-child visits.**[5]

TABLE 9-3

DEVELOPMENTAL SCREENING TESTS BY DIAGNOSIS

| Diagnosis | Screening Tests | Age | Administration Time | Completed by | Weblink |
|---|---|---|---|---|---|
| ADHD | Vanderbilt Scales<br>Connors Scales | 6–12 yr | 10–15 min | Parent and teachers | http://www.brightfutures.org/mentalhealth/pdf/professionals/bridges/adhd.pdf |
| Cognitive/Motor Development | Ages and Stages Questionnaire (ASQ) | 4–60 mo | 10–15 min | Parent | |
| | Parents Evaluation of Developmental Status (PEDS) | 0–8 yr | 2–10 min | Parent | |
| | Child Development Inventory (CDI) | 18 mo–6 yr | 30–50 min | Parent | |
| | Denver II Developmental Screening Test | 0–6 yr | 10–12 min | Clinician | |
| | Capute Scales (CAT/CLAMS) | 3–36 mo | 15–20 min | Clinician | |
| Autism Spectrum Disorders | Modified Checklist for Autism in Toddlers (M-CHAT) | 16–48 mo | 5–10 min | Parent | |
| | Childhood Autism Rating Scale (CARS) | >2 yr | 20–30 min | Parent | |

Adapted from American Academy of Pediatrics. Identifying infants and young children with developmental disorders in the medical home: An algorithm for developmental surveillance and screening. Pediatrics 2006;118:405–420.

### C. COMMONLY USED DEVELOPMENTAL SCREENING AND ASSESSMENT TOOLS

1. Appropriate screening tests vary with age and suspected diagnosis. Significant delays on screening merit referral for formal assessment. Several developmental screening and assessment tools are available (see Table 9-3).
2. **Denver II Developmental Assessment** (see Foldout): A tool for screening the apparently normal child between ages 0 and 6 years. Allows the practitioner to identify those children who may have developmental delay. These children should be further evaluated for the purpose of definitive diagnosis. The test screens the child in four areas: personal-social, fine motor, gross motor, and language. For children born before 38 weeks' gestation, age should be corrected for prematurity, up to age 2 years. A child fails a Denver screen if he or she has two or more delays noted. Indications for referral are a failed test or a classification of untestable on two consecutive screenings.
3. **Capute Scales:** Screening/assessment tools that give quantitative developmental quotients for visual-motor/problem-solving and language abilities. The CLAMS (Clinical Linguistic and Auditory Milestone Scale) was developed for the assessment of language milestones from birth to age 36 months. The CAT (Clinical Adaptive Test) consists of problem-solving items for ages from birth to 36 months, adapted from standardized infant psychological tests.
4. **Goodenough-Harris Draw-a-Person Test:**
   a. Procedure: Give the child a pencil and a sheet of blank paper. Instruct the child to "draw a person; draw the best person you can." Supply encouragement if needed (e.g., "draw a whole person"); however, do not suggest specific supplementation or changes.
   b. Scoring: Ask the child to describe or explain the drawing to you. Give the child one point for each detail present using the guide in Box 9-1 (maximum score: 51) and compare with norms for age.
5. **Gesell figures (**Fig. 9-1**):** When using Gesell figures, the examiner is not supposed to demonstrate the drawing of the figures for the patient.
6. **Gesell block skills:** The structures in Figure 9-2 should be demonstrated for the child. Figure 9-2 includes the developmental age at which each structure can usually be accomplished.

## VI. MEDICAL EVALUATION OF DEVELOPMENTAL DISORDERS

### A. HISTORY

A thorough past medical history should include assessment of risk.

1. **Prenatal and birth:** Toxins, trauma, prematurity, infection.
2. **Past medical problems or trauma:** Infection, medication.

*Text continued on p. 262*

9 BEHAVIOR AND DEVELOPMENT

TABLE 9-4

DEVELOPMENTAL MILESTONES

| Age | Gross Motor | Visual-Motor/Problem Solving |
|---|---|---|
| 1 mo | Raises head from prone position | *Birth*: Visually fixes<br>*1 mo*: Has tight grasp, follows to midline |
| 2 mo | Holds head in midline, lifts chest off table | No longer clenches fists tightly, follows object past midline |
| 3 mo | Supports on forearms in prone position, holds head up steadily | Holds hands open at rest, follows in circular fashion, responds to visual threat |
| 4 mo | Rolls over, supports on wrists, and shifts weight | Reaches with arms in unison, brings hands to midline |
| 6 mo | Sits unsupported, puts feet in mouth in supine position | Unilateral reach, uses raking grasp, transfers objects |
| 9 mo | Pivots when sitting, crawls well, pulls to stand, cruises | Uses immature pincer grasp, probes with forefinger, holds bottle, throws objects |
| 12 mo | Walks alone | Uses mature pincer grasp, can make a crayon mark, releases voluntarily |
| 15 mo | Creeps up stairs, walks backward independently | Scribbles in imitation, builds tower of 2 blocks in imitation |
| 18 mo | Runs, throws objects from standing without falling | Scribbles spontaneously, builds tower of 3 blocks, turns two or three pages at a time |
| 24 mo | Walks up and down steps without help | Imitates stroke with pencil, builds tower of 7 blocks, turns pages one at a time, removes shoes, pants, etc. |
| 3 yr | Can alternate feet when going up steps, pedals tricycle | Copies a circle, undresses completely, dresses partially, dries hands if reminded, unbuttons |
| 4 yr | Hops, skips, alternates feet going down steps | Copies a square, buttons clothing, dresses self completely, catches ball |
| 5 yr | Skips alternating feet, jumps over low obstacles | Copies triangle, ties shoes, spreads with knife |

From Capute AJ, Biehl RF: Functional developmental evaluation: Prerequisite to habilitation. Pediatr Clin North Am 1973;20:3; Capute AJ, Accardo PJ: Linguistic and auditory milestones during the first two years of life: A language inventory for the practitioner. Clin Pediatr 1978;17:847; and Capute AJ et al: The Clinical Linguistic and Auditory Milestone Scale (CLAMS): Identification of cognitive defects in motor delayed children. Am J Dis Child 1986;140:694. Rounded norms from Capute AJ et al: Clinical Linguistic and Auditory Milestone Scale: Prediction of cognition in infancy. Dev Med Child Neurol 1986;28:762.

| Language | Social/Adaptive |
|---|---|
| Alerts to sound | Regards face |
| Smiles socially (after being stroked or talked to) | Recognizes parent |
| Coos (produces long vowel sounds in musical fashion) | Reaches for familiar people or objects, anticipates feeding |
| Laughs, orients to voice | Enjoys looking around |
| Babbles, ah-goo, razz, lateral orientation to bell | Recognizes that someone is a stranger |
| Says "mama, dada" indiscriminately, gestures, waves bye-bye, understands "no" | Starts exploring environment, plays gesture games (e.g., pat-a-cake) |
| Uses two words other than "mama, dada" or proper nouns, jargoning (runs several unintelligible words together with tone or inflection), one-step command with gesture | Imitates actions, comes when called, cooperates with dressing |
| Uses 4–6 words, follows one-step command without gesture | *15–18 mo*: Uses spoon and cup |
| Mature jargoning (includes intelligible words), 7–10 word vocabulary, knows 5 body parts | Copies parent in tasks (sweeping, dusting), plays in company of other children |
| Uses pronouns (I, you, me) inappropriately, follows two-step commands, has a 50-word vocabulary, uses 2-word sentences | Parallel play |
| Uses minimum of 250 words, 3-word sentences, uses plurals, knows all pronouns, repeats two digits | Group play, shares toys, takes turns, plays well with others, knows full name, age, gender |
| Knows colors, says song or poem from memory, asks questions | Tells "tall tales," plays cooperatively with a group of children |
| Prints first name, asks what a word means | Plays competitive games, abides by rules, likes to help in household tasks |

BOX 9-1

## GOODENOUGH-HARRIS SCORING

| | |
|---|---|
| General: | ☐ Head present |
| | ☐ Legs present |
| | ☐ Arms present |
| Trunk: | ☐ Present |
| | ☐ Length greater than breadth |
| | ☐ Shoulders |
| Arms/legs: | ☐ Attached to trunk |
| | ☐ At correct point |
| Neck: | ☐ Present |
| | ☐ Outline of neck continuous with head, trunk, or both |
| Face: | ☐ Eyes |
| | ☐ Nose |
| | ☐ Mouth |
| | ☐ Nose and mouth in two dimensions |
| | ☐ Nostrils |
| Hair: | ☐ Present |
| | ☐ On more than circumference; nontransparent |
| Clothing: | ☐ Present |
| | ☐ Two articles; nontransparent |
| | ☐ Entire drawing (sleeves and trousers) nontransparent |
| | ☐ Four articles |
| | ☐ Costume complete |
| Fingers: | ☐ Present |
| | ☐ Correct number |
| | ☐ Two dimensions; length, breadth |
| | ☐ Thumb opposition |
| | ☐ Hand distinct from fingers and arm |

Normal Values:

| Age (Yr): | 3 | 4 | 5 | 6 | 7 | 8 | 9 | 10 | 11 | 12 | 13 |
|---|---|---|---|---|---|---|---|---|---|---|---|
| Score: | 2 | 6 | 10 | 14 | 18 | 22 | 26 | 30 | 34 | 38 | 42 |

MONTHS 2 4 6 9 12 15 18 24 YEARS 3 4 5 6

# DIRECTIONS FOR ADMINISTRATION

1. Try to get child to smile by smiling, talking or waving. Do not touch him/her.
2. Child must stare at hand several seconds.
3. Parent may help guide toothbrush and put toothpaste on brush.
4. Child does not have to be able to tie shoes or button/zip in the back.
5. Move yarn slowly in an arc from one side to the other, about 8" above child's face.
6. Pass if child grasps rattle when it is touched to the backs or tips of fingers.
7. Pass if child tries to see where yarn went. Yarn should be dropped quickly from sight from tester's hand without arm movement.
8. Child must transfer cube from hand to hand without help of body, mouth, or table.
9. Pass if child picks up raisin with any part of thumb and finger.
10. Line can vary only 30 degrees or less from tester's line. /
11. Make a fist with thumb pointing upward and wiggle only the thumb. Pass if child imitates and does not move any fingers other than the thumb.

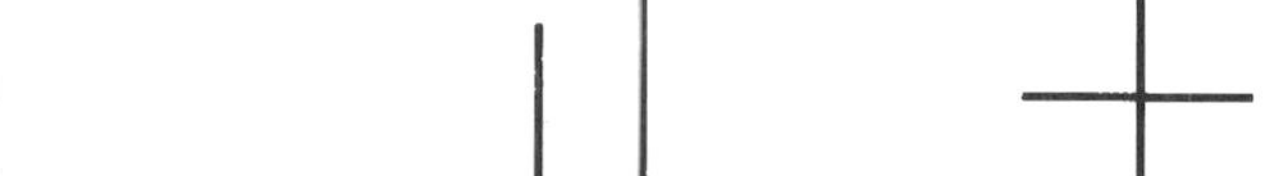

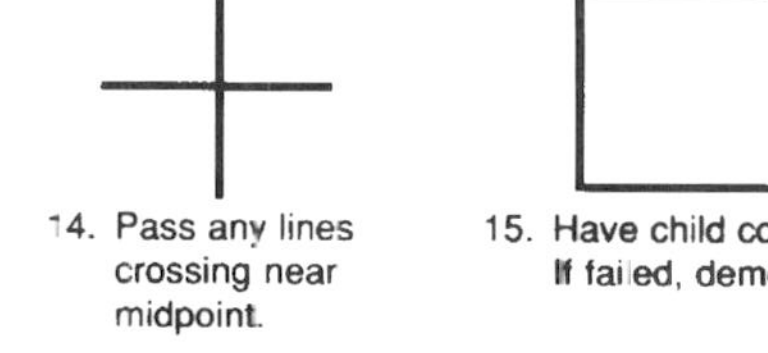

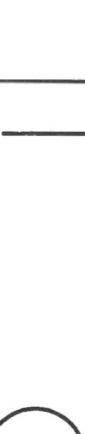

12. Pass any enclosed form. Fail continuous round motions.
13. Which line is longer? (Not bigger.) Turn paper upside down and repeat. (pass 3 of 3 or 5 of 6)
14. Pass any lines crossing near midpoint.
15. Have child copy first. If failed, demonstrate.

When giving items 12, 14, and 15, do not name the forms. Do not demonstrate 12 and 14.

16. When scoring, each pair (2 arms, 2 legs, etc.) counts as one part.
17. Place one cube in cup and shake gently near child's ear, but out of sight. Repeat for other ear.
18. Point to picture and have child name it. (No credit is given for sounds only.) If less than 4 pictures are named correctly, have child point to picture as each is named by tester.

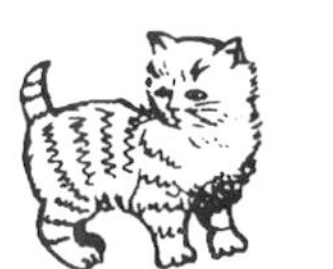
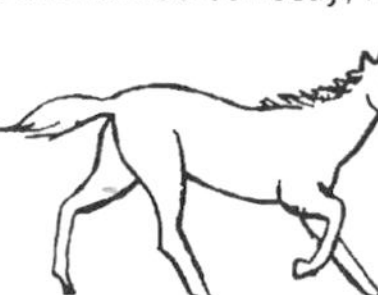
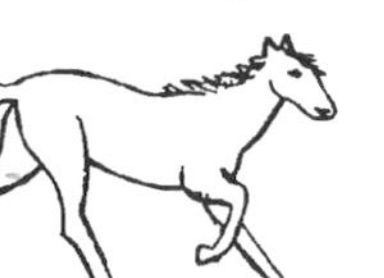
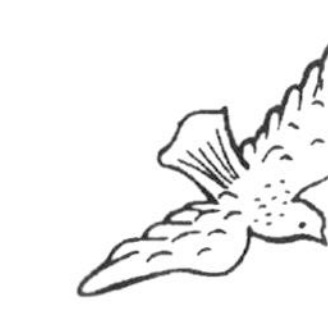
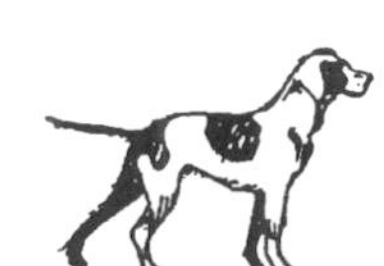
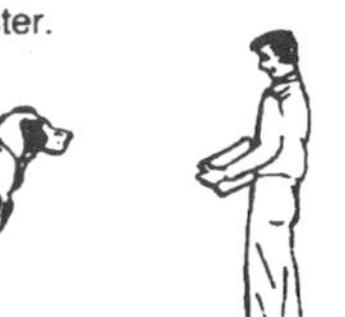

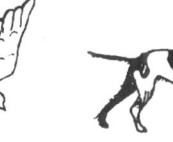

19. Using doll, tell child: Show me the nose, eyes, ears, mouth, hands, feet, tummy, hair. Pass 6 of 8.
20. Using pictures, ask child: Which one flies?... says meow?... talks?... barks?... gallops? Pass 2 of 5, 4 of 5.
21. Ask child: What do you do when you are cold?... tired?... hungry? Pass 2 of 3, 3 of 3.
22. Ask child: What do you do with a cup? What is a chair used for? What is a pencil used for? Action words must be included in answers.
23. Pass if child correctly places <u>and</u> says how many blocks are on paper. (1, 5).
24. Tell child: Put block **on** table; **under** table; **in front of** me, **behind** me. Pass 4 of 4. (Do not help child by pointing, moving head or eyes.)
25. Ask child: What is a ball?... lake?... desk?... house?... banana?... curtain?... fence?... ceiling? Pass if defined in terms of use, shape, what it is made of, or general category (such as banana is fruit, not just yellow). Pass 5 of 8, 7 of 8.
26. Ask child: If a horse is big, a mouse is __? If fire is hot, ice is __? If the sun shines during the day, the moon shines during the __? Pass 2 of 3.
27. Child may use wall or rail only, not person. May not crawl.
28. Child must throw ball overhand 3 feet to within arm's reach of tester.
29. Child must perform standing broad jump over width of test sheet (8 1/2 inches).
30. Tell child to walk forward, ⊂⊃⊂⊃⊂⊃⊂⊃→ heel within 1 inch of toe. Tester may demonstrate. Child must walk 4 consecutive steps.
31. In the second year, half of normal children are non-compliant.

**OBSERVATIONS:**

| | |
|---|---|
| Joints: | ☐ Elbow, shoulder, or both |
| | ☐ Knee, hip, or both |
| Proportion: | ☐ *Head*: 10% to 50% of trunk area |
| | ☐ *Arms*: Approximately same length as trunk |
| | ☐ *Legs:* 1–2 times trunk length; width less than trunk width |
| | ☐ *Feet*: To leg length |
| | ☐ Arms and legs in two dimensions |
| | ☐ Heel |
| Motor coordination: | ☐ Lines firm and well connected |
| | ☐ Firmly drawn with correct joining |
| | ☐ Head outline |
| | ☐ Trunk outline |
| | ☐ Outline of arms and legs |
| | ☐ Features |
| Ears: | ☐ Present |
| | ☐ Correct position and proportion |
| Eye detail: | ☐ Brow or lashes |
| | ☐ Pupil |
| | ☐ Proportion |
| | ☐ Glance directed front in profile drawing |
| Chin: | ☐ Present; forehead |
| | ☐ Projection |
| Profile: | ☐ Not more than one error |
| | ☐ Correct |

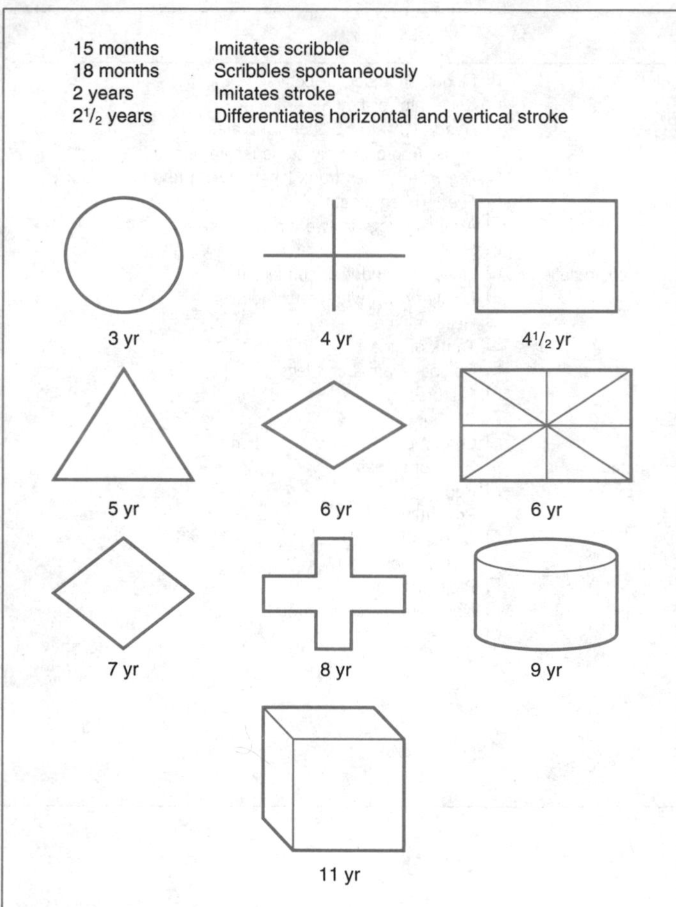


FIG. 9-1

Gesell figures. *(From Illingsworth RS: The Development of the Infant and Young Child, Normal and Abnormal, 5th ed. Baltimore, Williams & Wilkins, 1972, pp 229–232, and Cattel P: The Measurement of Intelligence of Infants and Young Children. New York, Psychological Corporation, 1960, pp 97–261.)*

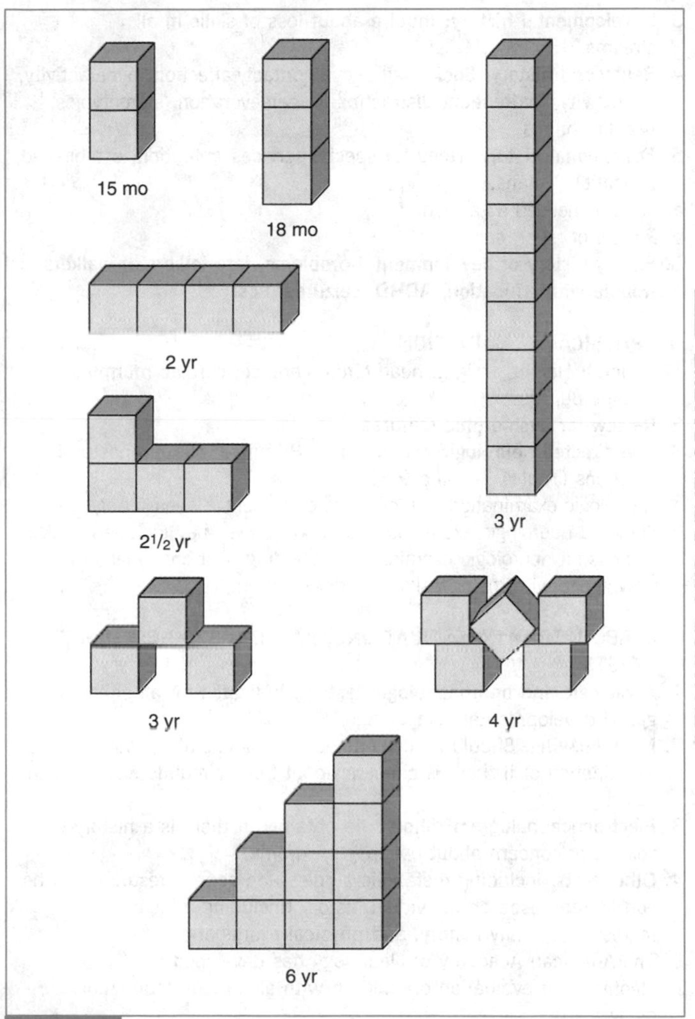


FIG. 9-2

Block skills. *(From Capute AJ, Accardo PJ: The Pediatrician and the Developmentally Disabled Child: A Clinical Textbook on Mental Retardation. Baltimore, University Park Press, 1979, p 122.)*

3. **Developmental history:** Inquire about loss of skills in all streams.
4. **Behavioral history:** Social skills, eye contact, affection, hyperactivity, impulsivity, inattention, distractibility, perseveration, stereotypies, peculiar habits.
5. **Educational history:** Need for special services, retention, established educational plans.
   a. Services needed as a toddler.
   b. Review of report card.
6. **Family history of developmental problems, late talkers or walkers, trouble with education, ADHD, seizures, tics.**

### B. PHYSICAL EXAMINATION

1. **General:** Height, weight, head circumference, cardiac murmurs, midline defects.
2. **Review for dysmorphic features.**
3. **Age-directed neurologic examination:** Primitive reflexes, postural reactions (Tables 9-5 and 9-6).
   a. Neurologic examination in motor age equivalent <1 year of age.
   b. Standard neurologic examination and soft signs (may include nonfocal findings on neurologic examination, including poor coordination and slow speed with motor tasks) in older children.

### C. LABORATORY INVESTIGATIONS, IMAGING STUDIES, OTHER TESTS

1. **Audiologic and ophthalmologic testing:** Indicated for all children with global developmental delay.
2. **Neuroimaging:** Should be considered if child has abnormal neurologic examination or if there is concern about head circumference growth velocity.
3. **Electroencephalogram:** Should be obtained if there is a history of seizure or concern about epilepsy syndrome.
4. **Other tests,** including metabolic studies and genetic testing: May be considered based on individual history (including a history of regression), family history, and physical examination.
5. The American Academy of Neurology has developed an algorithm for evaluation of children with global developmental delay.[6]

## VII. REFERRAL AND INTERVENTION

### A. STATE SUPPORT

1. The Individuals with Disabilities Education Act (IDEA) requires states to provide early intervention services to children.
2. Early intervention services eligibility criteria vary from state to state. The National Early Childhood Technical Assistance Center (www.nectac.org) provides information about criteria in each state.

TABLE 9-5

**POSTURAL REACTIONS**

| Postural Reaction | Age of Appearance | Description | Importance |
|---|---|---|---|
| Head righting | 6 wk–3 mo | Lifts chin from tabletop in prone position | Necessary for adequate head control and sitting |
| Landau response | 2–3 mo | Extension of head, then trunk and legs when held prone | Early measure of developing trunk control |
| Derotational righting | 4–5 mo | Following passive or active head turning, the body rotates to follow the direction of the head | Prerequisite to independent rolling |
| Anterior propping | 4–5 mo | Arm extension anteriorly in supported sitting | Necessary for tripod sitting |
| Parachute | 5–6 mo | Arm extension when falling | Facial protection when falling |
| Lateral propping | 6–7 mo | Arm extension laterally in protective response | Allows independent sitting |
| Posterior propping | 8–10 mo | Arm extension posteriorly | Allows pivoting in sitting |

Modified from Milani-Comparetti A, Gidoni EA: Routine developmental examination in normal and retarded children. Dev Med Child Neurol 1967;9:631; Capute AJ: Early neuromotor reflexes in infancy. Pediatr Ann 1986;15:217; Capute AJ et al: Primitive reflex profile: A quantitation of primitive reflexes in infancy. Dev Med Child Neurol 1984;26:375; and Palmer FB, Capute AJ: Developmental disabilities. In Oski FA (ed): Principles and Practice of Pediatrics. Philadelphia, JB Lippincott, 1994.

### B. RECOMMENDATIONS

1. Facilitate communication between family and school.
2. Advocate for and monitor appropriately.
3. Medical workup when indicated.
4. Provide medication intervention as needed (especially in ADHD and autism).

## VIII. OTHER RESOURCES

### A. AGE-APPROPRIATE BEHAVIORAL ISSUES IN INFANCY AND EARLY CHILDHOOD (Table 9-7)

### B. REACH OUT AND READ MILESTONES OF EARLY LITERACY (Table 9-8)

*Text continued on p. 268*

TABLE 9-6

**PRIMITIVE REFLEXES**

| Primitive Reflexes | Elicitation |
|---|---|
| Moro reflex ("embrace" response) of fingers, wrists, and elbows | *Supine*: Sudden neck extension; allow head to fall back about 3 cm |
| Galant reflex (GR) | *Prone suspension*: Stroking paravertebral area from thoracic to sacral region |
| Asymmetrical tonic neck reflex (ATNR, "fencer" response) | *Supine*: Rotate head laterally about 45–90 degrees |
| Symmetrical tonic neck reflex (STNR, "cat" reflex) | *Sitting*: Head extension/flexion |
| Tonic labyrinthine supine (TLS) | *Supine*: Extension of the neck (alters relation of the labyrinths) |
| Tonic labyrinthine prone (TLP) | *Prone*: Flexion of the neck |
| Positive support reflex (PSR) | Vertical suspension; bouncing hallucal areas on firm surface |
| Stepping reflex (SR, walking reflex) | Vertical suspension; hallucal stimulation |
| Crossed extension reflex (CER) | Prone; hallucal stimulation of an LE in full extension |
| Plantar grasp | Stimulation of hallucal areas |
| Palmar grasp | Stimulation of palm |
| Lower extremity placing (LEP) | Vertical suspension; rubbing tibia or dorsum of foot against edge of tabletop |
| Upper extremity placing (UEP) | Rubbing lateral surface of forearm along edge of tabletop from elbow to wrist to dorsal hand |
| Downward thrust (DT) | Vertical suspension; thrust LEs downward |

LE, lower extremity; UE, Upper extremity.

| Response | Timing |
|---|---|
| Extension, adduction, and then abduction of UEs, with semiflexion | Present at birth, disappears by 3–6 mo |
| Produces truncal incurvature with concavity toward stimulated side | Present at birth, disappears by 2–6 mo |
| Relative extension of limbs on chin side and flexion on occiput side | Present at birth, disappears by 4–9 mo |
| Extension of UEs and flexion of LEs/ flexion of UEs and LE extension | Appear at 5 mo; not present in most normal children; disappears by 8–9 mo |
| Tonic extension of trunk and LEs, shoulder retraction and adduction, usually with elbow flexion | Present at birth, disappears by 6–9 mo |
| Active flexion of trunk with protraction of shoulders | Present at birth, disappears by 6–9 mo |
| *Neonatal*: Momentary LE extension followed by flexion<br>*Mature*: Extension of LEs and support of body weight | Present at birth; disappears by 2–4 mo<br>Appears by 6 mo |
| Stepping gait | Disappears by 2–3 mo |
| Initial flexion, adduction, then extension of contralateral limb | Present at birth; disappears by 9 mo |
| Plantar flexion grasp | Present at birth; disappears by 9 mo |
| Palmar grasp | Present at birth; disappears by 9 mo |
| Initial flexion, then extension, then placing of LE on tabletop | Appears at 1 day |
| Flexion, extension, then placing of hand on tabletop | Appears at 3 mo |
| Full extension of LEs | Appears at 3 mo |

TABLE 9-7

AGE-APPROPRIATE BEHAVIORAL ISSUES IN INFANCY AND EARLY CHILDHOOD

| Age | Behavioral Issue | Symptoms |
|---|---|---|
| 1–3 mo | Colic | Paroxysms of fussiness/crying, 3+ hr per day, 3+ days per wk, may pull knees up to chest, pass flatus |
| 3–4 mo | Trained night feeding | Night awakening |
| 9 mo | Stranger anxiety/ separation anxiety | Distress when separated from parent or approached by a stranger |
| | Developmental night waking | Separation anxiety at night |
| 12 mo | Aggression | Biting, hitting, kicking in frustration |
| | Need for limit setting | Exploration of environment, danger of injury |
| 18 mo | Temper tantrums | Occur with frustration, attention seeking rage, negativity/refusal |
| 24 mo | Toilet training | *Child needs to demonstrate readiness*: shows interest, neurologic maturity (i.e., recognizes urge to urinate or defecate), ability to walk to bathroom and undress self, desire to please/ imitate parents, increasing periods of daytime dryness |
| 24–36 mo | New sibling | Regression, aggressive behavior |
| 36 mo | Nightmare | Awakens crying, may or may not complain of bad dream |
| | Night terrors | Agitation, screaming 1–2 hr after going to bed. Child may have eyes open but not respond to parent. May occur at same time each night. |

From Dixon SD, Stein MT: Encounters with Children: Pediatric Behavior and Development. St. Louis, Mosby, 2000.

| Guidance |
| --- |
| Crying usually peaks at 6 wk and resolves by 3–4 mo. Prevent overstimulation; swaddle infant; use white noise, swing, or car rides to soothe. Avoid medication and formula changes. Encourage breaks for the primary caregiver. |
| Comfort quietly, avoid reinforcing behavior (i.e., avoid night feeds). Do not play at night. Introducing cereal or solid food does not reduce awakening. Develop a consistent bedtime routine. Place baby in bed while drowsy and not fully asleep. |
| Use a transitional object, such as a special toy or blanket; use routine or ritual to separate from parent; may continue until 24 mo but can reduce intensity. |
| Keep lights off. Avoid picking child up or feeding. May reassure verbally at regular intervals or place a transitional object in crib. |
| Say "no" with negative facial cues. Begin time out (1 min/yr of age). No eye contact or interaction, place in a nonstimulating location. May restrain child gently until cooperation is achieved. |
| Avoid punishing exploration or poor judgment. Emphasize child-proofing and distraction. |
| Try to determine cause and react appropriately (i.e., help child who is frustrated, ignore attention-seeking behavior). Make sure child is in a safe location. |
| Age range for toilet training is usually 2–4 yr. Give guidance early; may introduce potty seat but avoid pressure or punishment for accidents. Wait until the child is ready. Expect some periods of regression, especially with stressors. |
| Allow for special time with parent, 10–20 min daily of one-on-one time exclusively devoted to the older sibling(s). Child chooses activity with parent. No interruptions. May not be taken away as punishment. |
| Reassure child, explain that he or she had a bad dream. Leave bedroom door open, use a nightlight, demonstrate there are no monsters under the bed. Discuss dream the following day. Avoid scary movies or television shows. |
| May be familial, not volitional. *Prevention*: For several nights, awaken child 15 min before terrors occur. Avoid overtiredness. *Acute*: Be calm; speak in soft, soothing, repetitive tones; help child return to sleep. Protect child against injury. |

TABLE 9-8

**REACH OUT AND READ MILESTONES OF EARLY LITERACY**

| Age | Motor | Cognitive |
|---|---|---|
| 6–12 mo | Reaches for books, turns pages with help | Looks at pictures, pats pictures |
| 12–18 mo | Carries book, holds book with help, turns several board pages at a time | Points to pictures with a single finger, points to specific items on page, gives book to adult |
| 18–24 mo | Turns one board page at a time | Repeats and retells parts of known stories |
| 24–36 mo | Begins to turn paper pages | Looks at favorite books on his or her own, repeats and retells whole phrases and stories, associates pictures with text of story |
| 3 yr | Turns paper pages easily | Growing attention span, recites favorite stories, begins to identify single letters |
| 4 yr and above | Writes name | Uses past tense and plurals, answers "what will happen next" |

From Reach Out and Read National Center. Available at www.reachoutandread.org.

## REFERENCES

1. Capute AJ et al: Spectrum of developmental disabilities: Continuum of motor dysfunction. Orthop Clin North Am 1981;12:15–21.
2. Shapiro BK, Gallico RP: Learning disabilities. Pediatr Clin North Am 1993;40:491–505.
3. American Psychiatric Association: Diagnostic and Statistical Manual of Mental Disorders, 4th ed, Text Revision. Arlington, Va, American Psychiatric Publishing, 2000.
4. Capute AJ, Accardo PJ (eds): Cerebral Palsy: Developmental Disabilities in Infancy and Childhood, 2nd ed, vol 2. Baltimore, Paul H. Brookes, 1996.
5. American Academy of Pediatrics: Identifying infants and young children with developmental disorders in the medical home: An algorithm for developmental surveillance and screening. Pediatrics 2006;118:405–420.
6. American Academy of Neurology: Practice Parameter: Evaluation of the child with global developmental delay. Neurology 2003;60:367–380.

# Endocrinology

*Sonia Arora Ballal, MD, and Paul McIntosh, MD*

10

## I. DIABETES

### A. DIABETIC KETOACIDOSIS (DKA)

Defined by hyperglycemia, ketonemia, ketonuria, and metabolic acidosis (pH < 7.30, bicarbonate <15 mEq/L).

1. **Assessment:**
a. History: In a *known* diabetic child, determine the usual insulin regimen, last dose, history of infection, or inciting event. In a *suspected* diabetic child, determine whether there is a history of polydipsia, polyuria, polyphagia, weight loss, vomiting, or abdominal pain.
b. Examination: Assess for dehydration, Kussmaul respirations, fruity breath, a change in mental status, and current weight.
c. Laboratory tests: See Figure 10-1 for a management algorithm. In addition, consider assessing the hemoglobin $A_{1c}$ ($HbA_{1c}$) level in a known diabetic as an index of chronic hyperglycemia (normal values are 4.5%–6.1%); in a new-onset diabetic, consider islet cell antibodies, insulin antibodies, thyroid antibodies, and thyroid function tests.
2. **Management: See Figures 10-1 and 10-2. Because the fluid and electrolyte requirements of patients in DKA may vary greatly, the following guidelines should be taken as a starting point; therapy must be individualized based on the dynamics of the patient.**
a. Cerebral edema is the most important complication of DKA; overaggressive hydration and overly rapid correction of hyperglycemia should be avoided because they may play a role in its development.
b. Remember that pH is a good indicator of insulin deficiency; if acidosis is not resolving, the patient may need more insulin. Be cautious: Initial insulin administration will cause a transient worsening of acidosis as potassium is driven into the cells in exchange for hydrogen ions.
c. The degree of hyperglycemia is often a reflection of hydration status.

### B. DIAGNOSTIC CRITERIA

Under the American Diabetes Association guidelines,[1] one of three criteria must be met to make the diagnosis of diabetes mellitus:

Symptoms of diabetes (polyuria, polydipsia, and weight loss) *and*
A random blood glucose ≥200 mg/dL *or*
A fasting blood glucose (no caloric intake for at least 8 hr) ≥126 mg/dL *or*
An oral glucose tolerance test (OGTT) with a 2-hr postload blood glucose of ≥200 mg/dL

(See section VI.A for more information on OGTT.)

### C. DIABETES CLASSIFICIATION (Table 10-1)

Once a diagnosis is made in a child, it is necessary to classify the diabetes as type 1 or type 2.

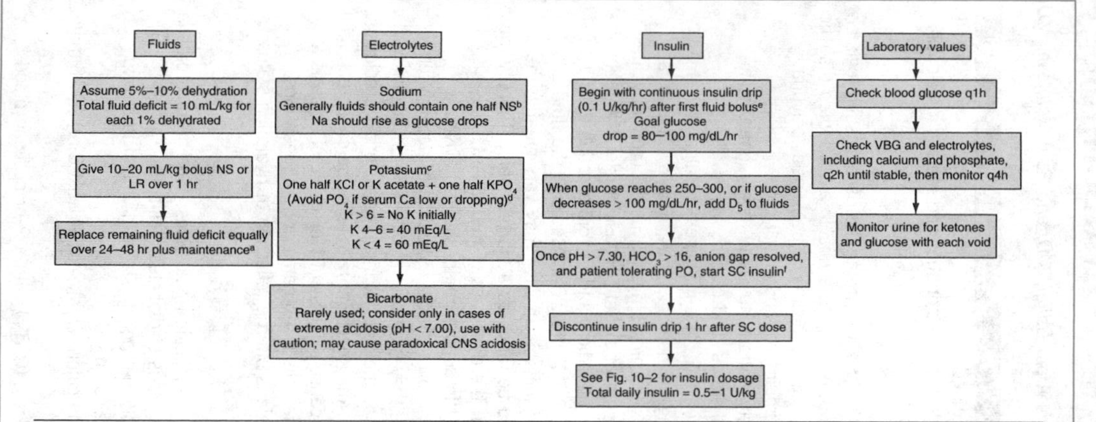

Fluids
Assume 5%–10% dehydration Total fluid deficit = 10 mL/kg for each 1% dehydrated
Give 10–20 mL/kg bolus NS or LR over 1 hr
Replace remaining fluid deficit equally over 24–48 hr plus maintenance[a]
Electrolytes
Sodium Generally fluids should contain one half NS[b] Na should rise as glucose drops
Potassium[c] One half KCl or K acetate + one half KPO4 (Avoid PO4 if serum Ca low or dropping)[d] K > 6 = No K initially K 4–6 = 40 mEq/L K < 4 = 60 mEq/L
Bicarbonate Rarely used; consider only in cases of extreme acidosis (pH < 7.00), use with caution; may cause paradoxical CNS acidosis
Insulin
Begin with continuous insulin drip (0.1 U/kg/hr) after first fluid bolus[e] Goal glucose drop = 80–100 mg/dL/hr
When glucose reaches 250–300, or if glucose decreases > 100 mg/dL/hr, add D5 to fluids
Once pH > 7.30, HCO3 > 16, anion gap resolved, and patient tolerating PO, start SC insulin[f]
Discontinue insulin drip 1 hr after SC dose
See Fig. 10–2 for insulin dosage Total daily insulin = 0.5–1 U/kg
Laboratory values
Check blood glucose q1h
Check VBG and electrolytes, including calcium and phosphate, q2h until stable, then monitor q4h
Monitor urine for ketones and glucose with each void
[a]If urine output is high, include in maintenance until osmotic diuresis slows; therefore maintenance = urine output + insensible losses (one third of standard maintenance calculations).
[b]Some DKA protocols recommend using NS rather than half NS during part of the replacement period in an effort to further decrease risk of cerebral edema.
[c]Patients with DKA are total body K+ depleted and are at risk for severe hypokalemia during DKA therapy. However, serum K+ levels may be normal or elevated as a result of the shift of K+ to the extracellular compartment in the setting of acidosis.
[d]Phosphate is depleted in DKA and will drop further with insulin therapy. Consider replacing half of K as KPO4 for first 8 hr, then all as KCl. Excessive phosphate may induce hypocalcemic tetany.
[e]Lower dose insulin infusions can be considered in very young patients.
[f]Some protocols recommend also waiting for urine ketones to decrease or clear before starting SC insulin.


FIG. 10-1

Management of diabetic ketoacidosis. CNS, central nervous system; LR, lactated Ringer's solution; NS, normal saline; SC, subcutaneous; VBG, venous blood gases. *(Modified from Hafeez W, Vuguin P: Managing diabetic ketoacidosis—a delicate balance. Contemp Pediatr 2000;17[6]:72–83.)*

**Example: A-32 kg patient**

*Total daily SC insulin dose* = 0.5–1.0 units/kg/day
0.75 x 32 = 24 units/day

*Basal insulin dose* = ½ of total daily SC dose:
24 ÷ 2 = 12 units at bedtime as glargine insulin (Lantus) in this example

*Carbohydrate coverage:* 450 ÷ total daily SC insulin dose:
450 ÷ 24 = 18.75;
Insulin: carbohydrate ratio = 1:18.75, or 1:20 in this example

*Correction factor: 1800 rule for insulin lispro (use 1500 for regular insulin)*
1800 ÷ total daily SC insulin dose – 1800 ÷ 24 = 75
1 unit of insulin lispro will decrease blood glucose 75 mg/dL,
or 0.5 units will decrease blood glucose approximately 40 mg/dL,
so that a sliding scale can be made as follows in this example

| For blood glucose | Adjust insulin |
|---|---|
| < 70 mg/dL | subtract 1 unit |
| 71–120 | no adjustment |
| 121–160 | add 0.5 units |
| 161–200 | add 1 unit |
| 201–240 | add 1.5 units |
| each addition increase of 40 mg/dL | add an additional 0.5 units |

FIG. 10-2

Calculations for a starting intermittent subcutaneous (SC) insulin regimen. Calculations are based on empirically determined formulas. Doses are adjusted once responses to starting doses are assessed.

TABLE 10-1

CHARACTERISTICS SUGGESTIVE OF TYPE 1 VERSUS TYPE 2 DIABETES AT PRESENTATION

| Characteristic | Type 1 | Type 2 |
|---|---|---|
| Polydipsia and polyuria | Present for days to weeks | Absent; or present for weeks to months |
| Ethnicity | White | African-American, Hispanic, Asian, Native American |
| Weight | Weight loss | Obese |
| Other physical findings | | Acanthosis nigricans |
| Family history | Negative | Positive |
| Insulin or C-peptide | Low | High |
| Ketoacidosis | More common | Less common |

1. **Patient characteristics:**
a. Typically classified as type 1 if a child has no risk factors for type 2 diabetes and presents in DKA.
b. Type 2 diabetes remains uncommon before the onset of puberty; therefore, prepubertal children are generally diagnosed with type 1 diabetes, although type 2 cannot be excluded.

c. Type 2 diabetes is very unlikely in a nonobese child, but obesity does not protect against type 1 diabetes.

**2. Laboratory characteristics:**

a. Islet cell autoantibodies:
   (1) An absence of these antibodies makes type 1 unlikely.
   (2) As many as 15% of children with type 1 diabetes will not have detectable autoantibodies to a given islet cell autoantigen.
   (3) 5% will not have any detectable islet cell autoantibodies.
   (4) As in adults, a significant fraction of children with type 2 diabetes will have measurable islet cell autoantibodies.

b. Ketoacidosis:
   (1) Presence of DKA does not exclude a diagnosis of type 2 diabetes, because DKA is not uncommon in adolescents with type 2 diabetes and can be just as severe as that which occurs in type 1 diabetes.
   (2) Recurrences of ketosis, especially DKA, should prompt consideration for reclassification in a patient initially designated as type 2.

c. Elevated C-peptide >2 yr after diagnosis is uncommon in type 1 and should prompt reevaluation.

d. Insulin and C-peptide levels are lower in children presenting with type 1 diabetes than in those presenting with type 2 diabetes, but the overlap is large, so that these levels are often not helpful in differentiating early type 1 from type 2 diabetes.

## D. TYPE II DIABETES MELLITUS

1. **There is an increasing prevalence of type 2 diabetes among children, especially among African Americans, Hispanics, and Native Americans; this increase is related to an increased prevalence of childhood obesity.**
2. **Abnormality in glucose levels:** **Caused by insulin resistance and an insulin secretory defect.**
3. **Can present in ketoacidosis** **(chronic high glucose impairs β-cell function and increases peripheral insulin resistance).**
4. **Consider screening by measuring fasting blood glucose levels among children who are overweight (body mass index >85th percentile for age and gender)** ***and*** **have two of the following risk factors:**

a. Family history of type 2 diabetes in a first- or second-degree relative.

b. Race/ethnicity: African American, Native American, Hispanic, or Asian or Pacific Islander.

c. Signs associated with insulin resistance (acanthosis nigricans, hypertension, dyslipidemia, polycystic ovarian disease).

5. **Screening:** **If done, should begin at age 10 years or onset of puberty (whichever occurs first) and repeated every 2 yr.**[2]
6. **Primary treatment: Diet and exercise;** **pharmacologic agents are often necessary for those who fail conservative management or are symptomatic at presentation.**

a. No validated treatment protocols currently exist in children.
b. Metformin has been used for patients with serum glucose levels <350 mg/dL without ketones (see Formulary for additional details).
c. No reported experience in adolescents with acarbose, the newer insulin-sensitizing drugs (i.e., rosiglitazone and pioglitazone), or sulfonylureas. Because of concerns of liver toxicity, the thiazolidinediones are contraindicated in adolescents.

7. **Managing children with diabetes involves close monitoring of daily blood glucose as well as following $HbA_{1c}$ levels.[3] Frequent eye examinations and screening for hypertension, hyperlipidemia, and proteinuria are also important.[4]**



## II. THYROID AND PARATHYROID FUNCTION[5-8]

### A. THYROID TESTS

1. **Interpretation of thyroid function tests (Table 10-2).**
2. **Thyroid scan: Used to assess thyroid clearance and to study structure and function of the thyroid. Localizes ectopic thyroid tissue and hyperfunctioning and nonfunctioning thyroid nodules.**
3. **Technetium uptake: Measures uptake of technetium by thyroid gland; levels are increased in hyperthyroidism and decreased in thyroxine-binding globulin deficiency and in hypothyroidism (except dyshormonogenesis, when it may be increased).**

### B. HYPOTHYROIDISM (Table 10-3)

**Note** *Do not begin treatment of central hypothyroidism until documenting normal ACTH/cortisol function due to risk of inducing an adrenal crisis if there is ACTH deficiency.*

### C. HYPERTHYROIDISM (Table 10-4)

### D. HYPERPARATHYROIDISM AND HYPOPARATHYROIDISM (Table 10-5)

TABLE 10-2

THYROID FUNCTION TESTS: INTERPRETATION

| Disorder | TSH | $T_4$ | Free $T_4$ |
|---|---|---|---|
| Primary hyperthyroidism | L | H | High N to H |
| Primary hypothyroidism | H | L | L |
| Hypothalamic/pituitary hypothyroidism | L, N, H* | L | L |
| TBG deficiency | N | L | N |
| Euthyroid sick syndrome | L, N, H* | L | L to low N |
| TSH adenoma or pituitary resistance | N to H | H | H |
| Compensated hypothyroidism† | H | N | N |

*Can be normal, slightly low, or slightly high.

†Treatment may not be necessary.

H, High; L, low; N, normal; $T_4$, thyroxine; TBG, thyroxine-binding globulin; TSH, thyroid-stimulating hormone.

*Text continued on p. 280*

TABLE 10-3

**HYPOTHYROIDISM**

| Disease and Clinical Symptoms | Onset | Etiology |
|---|---|---|
| **PRIMARY/CONGENITAL** | | |
| Large fontanelles, lethargy, constipation, hoarse cry, hypotonia, hypothermia, jaundice | Symptoms usually develop within first 2 weeks of life and are almost always present by 6 weeks.<br>If the cause is other than absence of the thyroid gland, some infants may be relatively asymptomatic.<br>They are still at risk for developmental delay. | Deficiency of thyrotropin-releasing hormone, thyrotropin (TSH)<br>*or*<br>The most common cause is a defect of fetal thyroid development (athyrosis). Other causes include a mutation in the TSH receptor and thyroid dyshormonogensis. |
| **ACQUIRED** | | |
| Deceleration of growth often the first manifestation; other signs may include coarse, brittle hair; dry, scaly skin; and delayed tooth eruption | Can occur as early as the first 2 years of life | Hashimoto thyroiditis<br>Head/neck radiation |

*Note*: Thyroid hormone levels in premature infants are lower than those seen in full-term infants. Further, the TSH surge seen at approximately 24 hours of age in full-term babies does not appear in preterm infants. In this population, lower levels are associated with increased illness, but the effect of replacement therapy remains controversial.

| Evaluation | Management | Follow-up |
|---|---|---|
| ↓$T_4$<br>↓or ↑ TSH | Replacement with L-thyroxine should begin as soon as diagnosis is confirmed, usually by newborn screens.<br>Goal of therapy is to achieve $T_4$ levels in the upper half of normal range. If hypothyroidism is due to a primary cause, TSH should be kept <5. A minority of infants maintain a persistently high TSH despite correction of $T_4$ level. | Monitor $T_4$ and TSH levels at the end of weeks 1 and 2 of therapy.<br>If levels are adequate, follow every 1–3 months during the first 12 months. |
| ↓$T_4$, ↑TSH<br>The presence of antithyroglobulin and antimicrosomal antibodies suggests Hashimoto thyroiditis | Replacement with L-thyroxine | As for primary/ congenital.<br>After 2 years, monitoring levels every 6 to 12 months should be adequate as dose changes become less frequent. |

TABLE 10-4

**HYPERTHYROIDISM**

| Disease and Clinical Symptoms | Onset | Etiology | Evaluation | Management | Follow-up |
|---|---|---|---|---|---|
| Hyperactivity, irritability, altered mood, insomnia, heat intolerance, increased sweating, pruritus, tachycardia, palpitations, fatigue, weakness, weight loss despite increased appetite, increased stool frequency, oligomenorrhea or amenorrhea, fine tremor, hyperreflexia, hair loss | Prevalence increases with age beginning in adolescence.<br>Has a 4:1 female-to-male predilection. | The most common cause in childhood is Graves disease (see the following table section). Other causes include subacute thyroiditis, factitious hyperthyroidism (intake of exogenous hormone), and rarely a TSH-secreting pituitary tumor.<br>Pituitary resistance to thyroid hormone demonstrates a compensatory rise in $T^4$, but TSH remains within the normal range. | ↓ TSH*<br>↑ $T_4$, $T_3$<br>Further tests include assessment of TSH receptor stimulating antibody, antithyroglobulin and antimicrosomal antibodies, free $T_4$, and free $T_3$. | Treat with propythiouracil (PTU) or methimazole, which inhibit formation of thyroid hormone.<br>Radioactive iodine ($^{131}I$) is an option for refractory cases. | Follow symptoms and level of $T_4$ and TSH. |

*With the rare case of a TSH-secreting tumor, the patient does not have hyperthyroidism if the TSH is not suppressed, regardless of the levels of $T_3$ and $T_4$.

| | | | | |
|---|---|---|---|---|
| **GRAVES DISEASE** | | | | |
| Diffuse goiter, a feeling of grittiness and discomfort in the eye, retrobulbar pressure or pain, eyelid lag or retraction, periorbital edema, chemosis, scleral injection, exophthalmos, extraocular muscle dysfunction, localized dermopathy, and lymphoid hyperplasia | Peak incidence between ages 11 and 15 years.<br>A 5:1 female-to-male ratio.<br>Most children with Graves disease have a family history of some form of autoimmune thyroid disease | Autoimmune | ↑ $T_4$, $T_3$<br>↓ TSH | As for hyperthyroidism |
| **THYROID STORM** | | | | |
| Acute in onset. Manifested by hyperthermia, tachycardia, and restlessness.<br>Untreated, this may progress to delirium, coma, and death. | | | ↑ $T_4$, $T_3$<br>↓ TSH | Propranolol is used to suppress signs and symptoms of thyrotoxicosis.<br>Potassium iodide may also be used for acute hyperthyroid management.<br>Long-term management may include radiation therapy. |

*Continued*

TABLE 10-4

HYPERTHYROIDISM—cont'd

| Disease and Clinical Symptoms | Onset | Etiology | Evaluation | Management | Follow-up |
|---|---|---|---|---|---|
| **NEONATAL THYROTOXICOSIS** | | | | | |
| Microcephaly, frontal bossing, intrauterine growth retardation (IUGR), tachycardia, systolic hypertension leading to widened pulse pressure, irritability, failure to thrive, exophthalmos, goiter, flushing, vomiting, diarrhea, jaundice, thrombocytopenia, and cardiac failure or arrhythmias | Ranges from immediate to delayed for weeks. | Seen exclusively in infants born to mothers with Graves disease. Caused by transplacental passage of maternal thyroid-stimulating immunoglobulin (TSI). Occasionally, mothers are unaware that they have Graves disease. Also, note that if a mother has received definitive treatment (thyroidectomy or radiation therapy), the possible passage of TSI remains. | ↑ $T_4$, $T_3$<br>↓ TSH | As for thyroid storm<br>Digoxin may be indicated for heart failure. | Disease usually resolves by age 6 months |

TABLE 10-5
HYPOPARATHYROIDISM AND HYPERPARATHYROIDISM

| Disease and Clinical Symptoms | Onset | Etiology | Evaluation | Management | Follow-up |
|---|---|---|---|---|---|
| **HYPOPARATHYROIDISM** | | | | | |
| Clinical manifestations range from asymptomatic or mild muscle cramps to hypocalcemic tetany, prolonged QTc, and convulsions. | | Results from a decrease in parathyroid hormone (PTH)<br>Pseudohypoparathyroidism results from PTH resistance; is distinguished by normal or elevated PTH. | ↓ PTH<br>↓ Serum $Ca^2$<br>↑ Serum phos<br>Normal/↓ alkaline phosphatase<br>↓ 1,25-OH-vitamin $D_3$ | Calcium supplementation for documented hypocalcemia<br>Vitamin D supplementation with calcitriol | Carefully monitor serum calcium and phosphorus during therapy. Monitor urine calcium levels to avoid hypercalciuria. |
| **HYPERPARATHYROIDISM** | | | | | |
| Causes hypercalcemia from increased bone and renal resorption and increased intestinal absorption of calcium via increased activated vitamin D.<br>Symptoms of hypercalcemia include vomiting, constipation, abdominal pain, weakness, paresthesias, malaise, and bone pain | Uncommon in childhood | Associated with multiple endocrine neoplasia syndromes (see Box 10-1)<br>Secondary hyperparathyroidism more common; develops in response to hypocalcemic states, such as renal failure or rickets. Distinguishing lab finding in secondary hyperparathyroidism is normal to somewhat decreased calcium levels. | ↑ PTH<br>↑ Serum $Ca^2$<br>↓ Serum phos<br>Normal/↑ alkaline phosphatase | Hydration is mainstay of treatment; enhances calciuria<br>Furosemide may be used with caution if adequate hydration<br>Hydrocortisone, 1 mg/kg q6h, reduces intestinal absorption of calcium<br>Calcitonin transiently opposes bone resorption<br>In severe hypercalcemia, bisphosphates may be considered<br>Surgical removal of parathyroid glands | Beware of hypoparathyroidism following surgical removal of the parathyroid gland. |

### E. MULTIPLE ENDOCRINE NEOPLASIA SYNDROMES (MEN) (Box 10-1)

### F. VITAMIN D DEFICIENCY (Table 10-6)

## III. ADRENAL AND PITUITARY FUNCTION[9-11]

### A. ADRENAL INSUFFICIENCY

Most common causes are congenital adrenal hyperplasia (CAH) and long-term glucocorticoid treatment. Other causes include Addison disease and hypothalamic or pituitary disease secondary to tumors, surgery, radiation therapy, or congenital defects.

1. **Congenital adrenal hyperplasia:**[10,11]

a. Group of autosomal recessive disorders characterized by a defect in one of the enzymes required in the synthesis of cortisol from cholesterol. Cortisol deficiency results in oversecretion of adrenocorticotropic hormone (ACTH) and hyperplasia of the adrenal cortex.
b. The most common cause of ambiguous genitalia in females.
c. 21-Hydroxylase deficiency accounts for 90% of cases.

BOX 10-1

**MULTIPLE ENDOCRINE NEOPLASIA (MEN) SYNDROMES**

**MEN I:** An autosomal dominant condition characterized by hyperplasia of the endocrine pancreas (which usually secretes gastrin, insulin), the anterior pituitary (prolactin, growth hormone, corticotropin or nonhormone-secreting), and the parathyroid glands. Classified as the presence of two of three of the previously cited benign tumors. Hyperparathyroidism is the most common presenting sign. Although asymptomatic cases require no treatment, proton pump inhibitors are the mainstay for gastrinomas, and surgery is the treatment of choice for parathyroid tumors. Any tumors in the head of the pancreas also should be removed.

**MEN IIa:** An autosomal dominant condition characterized by hyperplasia or carcinoma of thyroid C cells in association with pheochromocytoma and primary parathyroid hyperplasia. C-cell hyperplasia or tumors usually appear earlier than pheochromocytoma, and hypercalcemia is a late manifestation indicating hyperparathyroidism.

**MEN IIb:** An autosomal dominant syndrome characterized by the occurrence of multiple neuromas in combination with medullary thyroid carcinoma and pheochromocytoma. The neuromas most often occur on mucosal surfaces. Feeding difficulties, poor sucking, diarrhea, constipation, and failure to thrive may begin in infancy or early childhood, many years before the appearance of neuromas or endocrine symptoms.

*For the MEN II family,* genetic testing is recommended for all family members. For those who test positive, prophylactic thyroidectomy universally is advised owing to the aggressiveness of medullary thyroid tumors. The ideal age for surgery remains unclear. Recommended ages range from infancy up into adolescence, with most experts concurring that thyroid removal in early childhood (age 5 years) is reasonable.

TABLE 10-6

VITAMIN D DEFICIENCY

| Disease, Clinical Symptoms, and Onset | Etiology | Evaluation | Management |
|---|---|---|---|
| **Rickets** (infancy/childhood): Failure of adequate bone mineralization leading to soft bones/skeletal deformities<br>**Osteomalacia** (adults): Bone pain and muscle weakness | Decreased dietary intake<br>Inadequate exposure to sunlight<br>Increased melanin<br>Impaired renal function<br>Fat malabsorption (celiac disease, cystic fibrosis, Crohn's disease) | ↓25–OH vitamin D | Supplementation for:<br>* Breast-fed infants<br>* Those with celiac disease, cystic fibrosis, Crohn's disease, pancreatic deficiency |



d. The enzymatic defect results in impaired synthesis of adrenal steroids beyond the enzymatic block and overproduction of the precursors before the block. Two major classifications:
   (1) Classic (complete enzyme deficiency):
      (a) Occurs with or without salt loss.
      (b) Occurs under basal conditions.
      (c) Adrenal crisis in untreated patients occurs at 1 to 2 weeks of life, with signs and symptoms of adrenal insufficiency rarely occurring before 3 to 4 days of life. (Nonsalt-losing forms have a less severe risk for adrenal crisis owing to preservation of mineralocorticoid synthesis.)
      (d) Diagnosis is based on elevated 17-hydroxyprogesterone (17-OHP) levels.
      (e) Levels of testosterone in girls and androstenedione in boys and girls are also elevated.
   (2) Nonclassic or simple virilizing form (partial enzyme deficiency):
      (a) Adrenal insufficiency tends to occur only under stress; manifests as androgen excess after infancy (precocious pubarche, irregular menses, hirsutism, acne, advanced skeletal maturation).
      (b) Morning 17-OHP levels may be elevated, but diagnosis may require an ACTH stimulation test (see section VI.B). A significant rise in the 17-OHP level 60 min after ACTH injection is diagnostic. Cortisol response will be decreased.
   (3) For infants with ambiguous genitalia, karyotype is an essential feature of the evaluation; for apparent male infants presenting with classic CAH, a karyotype should be evaluated to rule out the possibility of a severely masculinized female infant.

**2. Daily management of adrenal insufficiency:**

a. Glucocorticoid maintenance:

(1) Physiologic glucocorticoid production: Approximately 9–12 $mg/m^2$/day. See Formulary Adjunct for forms of steroids used in physiologic replacement.

(2) For CAH, 12.5 $mg/m^2$/day of hydrocortisone through intravenous (IV) or intramuscular (IM) route or 25 $mg/m^2$/day orally (PO) is recommended for daily maintenance to allow for suppression of the ACTH axis.

(3) For pure adrenal insufficiency, daily oral dosing of 9–12 $mg/m^2$/day of hydrocortisone is often sufficient and helps decrease the toxic effects seen at higher doses.

(4) Doses often are titrated to preserve normal skeletal growth and rate of skeletal maturation. In addition, doses are adjusted to prevent inappropriate adrenergic effects.

b. Mineralocorticoid maintenance:

(1) These patients should have ready access to salt.

(2) For salt-losing forms of adrenal insufficiency, 0.1–0.2 mg/day of oral fludrocortisone acetate once daily is recommended. For patients who cannot take the oral form, IV hydrocortisone at 50 $mg/m^2$/day will supply a maintenance amount of mineralocorticoid activity. (Note that synthetic steroids such as prednisone and dexamethasone do not supply appropriate mineralocorticoid effects.)

(3) Infants also require 1–2 g (17–34 mEq) of sodium supplementation per day.

(4) Always monitor blood pressure and electrolytes when supplementing mineralocorticoids.

c. Stress dose glucocorticoids:

(1) The dose of glucocorticoids should increase in patients with fever or other illness.

(2) Stress dose: 25–50 $mg/m^2$/day of hydrocortisone IV/IM (as a continuous drip or divided q3–6hr) or 75 $mg/m^2$/day PO divided q6–8hr.

(3) For surgery or severe illness, hydrocortisone doses of 50–100 $mg/m^2$/day IV may be indicated.

**3. Acute adrenal crisis:**

a. Often precipitated by acute illness, trauma, surgery, or exposure to excess heat.

b. Characterized by emesis, diarrhea, dehydration, hypotension, metabolic acidosis, and shock.

c. Laboratory values often demonstrate hypoglycemia, hyponatremia, and hyperkalemia. In addition, serum cortisol and aldosterone are decreased, and ACTH and renin are elevated. In infants with CAH, 17-OHP is increased; these studies are useful to perform before steroid administration to confirm the diagnosis, but treatment should not be delayed.

d. Management includes rapid volume expansion to support blood pressure, sufficient dextrose to maintain blood glucose, close monitoring of electrolytes, and corticosteroid administration.
   (1) Give 50 mg/m$^2$ of hydrocortisone by IV bolus (rapid estimate: infants = 25 mg; children = 50–100 mg), followed by 50 mg/m$^2$/24 hr by continuous drip (preferable) or divided q3–4hr.
   (2) *Hydrocortisone and cortisone are the only glucocorticoids that provide the necessary mineralocorticoid effects.*

## B. SYNDROME OF INAPPROPRIATE ANTIDIURETIC HORMONE SECRETION (SIADH)[12] (Table 10-7)

## C. DIABETES INSIPIDUS (DI)[12] (Table 10-8)

**1. Characterized by an impaired ability to concentrate urine. The water-deprivation test (see section VI.C) is diagnostic of DI; the vasopressin**



TABLE 10-7

SYNDROME OF INAPPROPRIATE ANTIDIURETIC HORMONE SECRETION (SIADH)

| Disease and Clinical Symptoms | Etiology | Evaluation | Management |
|---|---|---|---|
| Hallmark is hyponatremia ($Na^+$ < 135 mEq/L) with inappropriately concentrated urine in the setting of euvolemia or mild hypervolemia | Associated with many conditions, including central nervous system (CNS) trauma, CNS infection, pneumonia, and CNS surgery | ↓ Serum $Na^+$ and $Cl^-$ with normal $HCO_3^-$<br>Hypouricemia<br>Inappropriately concentrated urine | Correct hyponatremia slowly with fluid restriction; a reasonable goal is a 10% rise in $Na^+$ per 24 hr.<br>*In the setting of coma or seizures,* more rapid $Na^+$ correction should be undertaken by treating with hypertonic saline. The goal is to acutely raise the serum [$Na^+$] to ~120–125 mEq/L.<br>Definitive therapy is to identify and treat the underlying cause. |

TABLE 10-8

DIABETES INSIPIDUS (DI)[12]

| Disease and Clinical Symptoms | Etiology | Laboratory Findings | Management |
|---|---|---|---|
| **Central DI** | Caused by vasopressin deficiency and is associated with CNS injury, including trauma and tumors | Low urine specific gravity (<1.005)<br>Low urine osmolarity (50–200)<br>Low vasopressin (<0.5 pg/mL) | DDAVP (desmopressin acetate) in nasal spray, IV, PO, or SC preparation. Titrate the DDAVP dosage to urine output, aiming for at least 1-hr period of diuresis per day that is sufficient to stimulate thirst.<br>Monitor electrolytes closely.<br>Infants are often not treated with DDAVP because of difficulties monitoring their input and output. Rather, they are treated with increased free water and salt restriction. |
| **Nephrogenic DI** | Caused by renal tubular resistance to vasopressin; can be genetic or acquired | Low urine specific gravity (<1.005)<br>Low urine osmolarity (50–200) | Cornerstone of therapy in nephrogenic DI: Provision of free water and a low-salt diet |

test (see section VI.D) is used to differentiate between central and nephrogenic DI.

2. Infants with DI may present with failure to thrive, vomiting, constipation, and unexplained fevers; more severe cases show signs of severe dehydration, hypovolemic shock, and convulsions.
3. Following trauma to axons of vasopressin containing neurons, a temporary or permanent DI may result. Due to the initial edema occurring in the area of the hypothalamus and pituitary, a short-lived period (2–5 days) of DI is observed. This is succeeded by a stage of SIADH, as dying neurons release vasopressin. The final stage results in permanent DI, if a significant number of neurons were injured.

## IV. GROWTH AND SEXUAL DEVELOPMENT[13–19]

### A. GROWTH

1. **Target height range: Calculated as midparental stature ± 2 SD (1 SD = 2 inches).**

a. Midparental stature for boys: (paternal height + maternal height + 5 inches)/2.

b. Midparental stature for girls: (paternal height + maternal height + 5 inches)/2.

2. **Short stature (Fig. 10-3):**[13,14]

a. Definition: Height less than the 3rd percentile; decreasing growth velocity; height below the target height.

b. Differential diagnosis: Constitutional growth delay (CGD) and familial short stature (FSS) must be distinguished from pathologic causes of short stature.

(1) FSS: Characterized by slow growth rate during the first 2 to 3 years of life followed by a low-normal growth velocity. Bone age x-rays may be within normal limits for age.

(2) CGD: Typically characterized by similar growth charts as those with FSS; however, a delay in the onset of puberty and skeletal maturation allows for a period of catch-up growth. Family history of delayed puberty is often present. Bone age x-rays may be delayed for age.

(3) Pathologic short stature:

(a) Deceleration of linear growth with no nutritional deficit may suggest growth hormone deficiency, hypothyroidism, or glucocorticoid excess.

(b) Initial weight loss followed by decreased height velocity suggests systemic illness, including malnutrition and other psychosocial influences.

(c) Dysmorphic features may indicate genetic variant, such as trisomy 21 or Turner syndrome.

(d) Disproportionate features or skeletal abnormalities are consistent with skeletal dysplasias or metabolic bone disease.

c. Initial evaluation: In addition to detailed history/physical examination, evaluation of growth curves, and pubertal stage. Initial screening tests include complete blood count, liver function tests, electrolytes, erythrocyte sedimentation rate, and urinalysis (including pH and specific gravity). Also consider thyroid function tests, serum insulin-like growth factor-1 (IGF-1) and IGF binding protein (IGFBP-3), antiendomysial and antigliadin antibodies for celiac disease, bone age (radiograph of left wrist and hand), and karyotype. Consider a skeletal survey in a patient with disproportionate features.

3. **Tall stature: Most common cause is familial tall stature or precocious puberty**

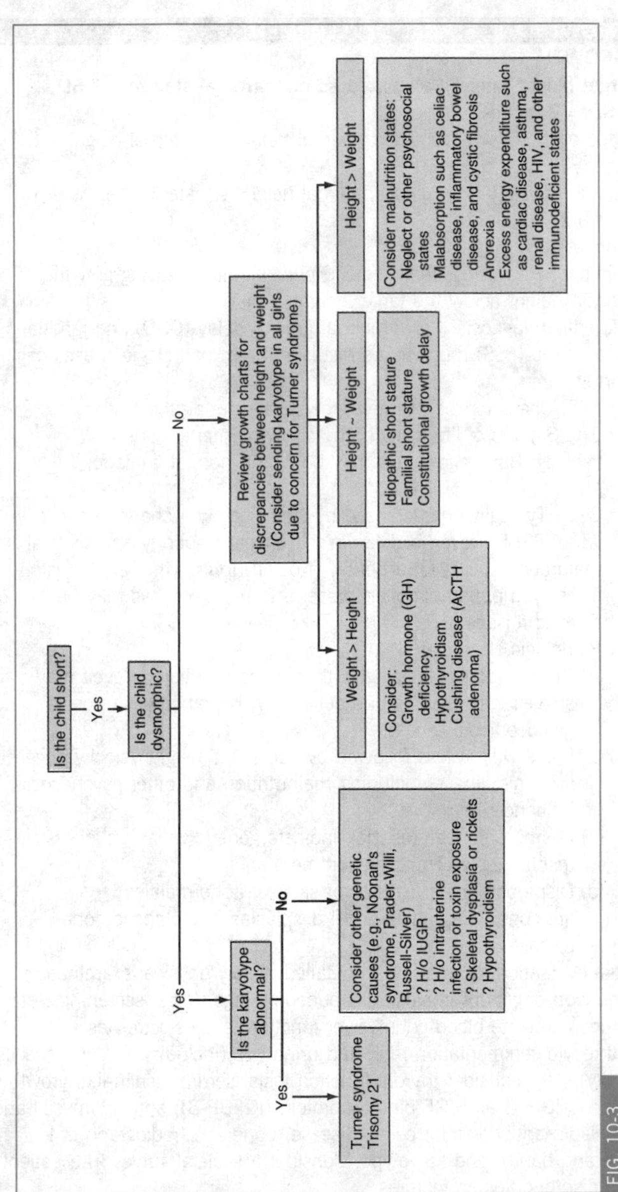


FIG. 10-3

Differential diagnosis of short stature.

4. **Obesity: A growing problem among the pediatric population. Although the majority do not have endocrine etiology, two disease categories may be addressed when approaching the obese patient.**
a. Hypothyroidism: May be evaluated with serum thyroid function tests.
b. Cushing disease: Unlikely without linear growth failure in addition to obesity (see section VI for laboratory testing details).

## B. SEXUAL DEVELOPMENT[15–21]

1. **Delayed puberty: No signs of pubertal development by age 14 years in girls, or >5 yr between thelarche and adrenarche. For boys, delayed puberty implies no testicular enlargement by age 14 years, or >5 yr for genital development. Primary amenorrhea suggests no menarche in the presence of secondary sexual characteristics by age 16 years or no menarche and no secondary sexual characteristics by age 14 years.**
a. Delayed puberty may be divided according to luteinizing hormone (LH) and follicle-stimulating hormone (FSH) levels:
   (1) Hypergonadotropic hypogonadism (high LH and FSH) is secondary to primary gonadal failure, possibly due to Turner syndrome, Klinefelter syndrome, androgen insensitivity, tumor, chemotherapy.
   (2) Hypogonadotropic hypogonadism (low or normal LH/FSH) may be secondary to constitutional delay, or central gonadotropin deficiency. Of the latter cause, etiologies include Kallman's (most common cause of isolated gonadotropin deficiency), central nervous system (CNS) tumors, hypopituitarism.
b. Evaluation of delayed puberty may also be divided into the following categories (Fig. 10-4).
   (1) Constitutional delay.
   (2) Hypopituitarism.
   (3) Chromosomal abnormality.
c. Initial evaluation should include LH and FSH. Bone age and thyroid studies should also be obtained. A gonadotropin-releasing hormone (GnRH) stimulation test can be obtained to rule out hypogonadotropic hypogonadism.
2. **Precocious puberty: Traditionally defined as any sign of secondary sexual maturation before age 8 years in girls and age 9 years in boys. More recent data suggest early puberty may not warrant extensive evaluation or intervention if it occurs after age 6 years in African American girls or after age 7 years in white girls.**
a. Central, true, isosexual, *or* complete precocious puberty (CPP): Involves premature activation of the hypothalamic-pituitary-gonadal axis, leading to increased GnRH and therefore increased LH/FSH; five times more likely to occur in females, and often represents an idiopathic variant of normal puberty. In the majority of males with CPP, a CNS insult or structural anomaly is the cause.

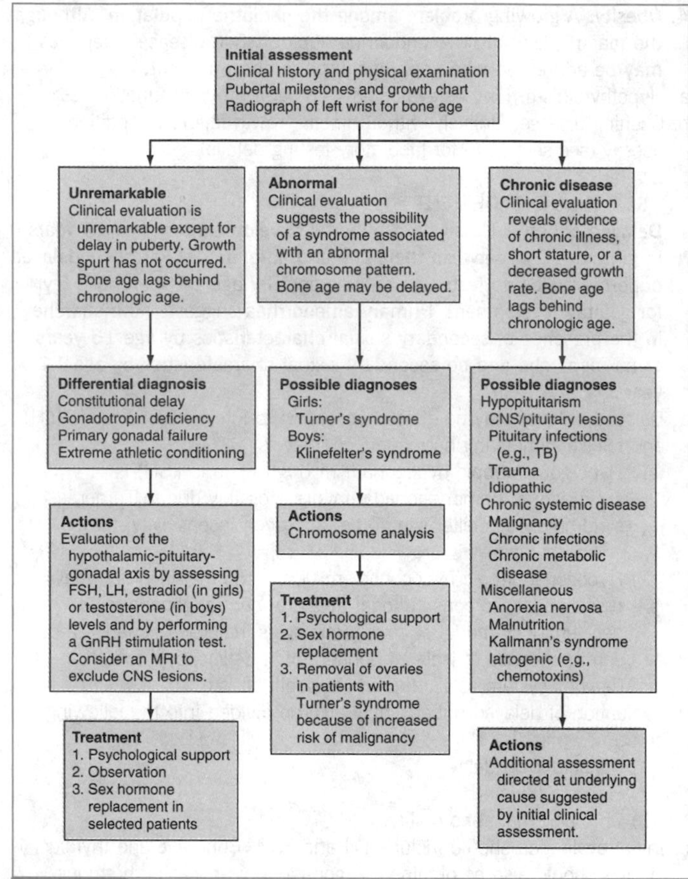


FIG. 10-4

An approach to the child presenting with delayed puberty. CNS, central nervous system; FSH, follicle-stimulating hormone; GnRH, gonadotropin-releasing hormone; LH, luteinizing hormone; MRI, magnetic resonance imaging; TB, tuberculosis.[20] *(From Blondell R et al: Disorders of puberty. Am Family Phys 1999;60(1): 209–218.)*

b. Peripheral *or* pseudoprecocious puberty: GnRH-independent puberty; and involves adrenal, gonadal, ectopic, or exogenous sources of hormone production. Most common causes are CAH, adrenal tumors, McCune-Albright syndrome, gonadal tumors, human chorionic gonadotropin (hCG)-producing tumors, and exogenous sex hormones. Hypothyroidism can also cause GnRH-independent precocity.

Penile length is disproportionately greater than testicular size in pseudo-precocious puberty, whereas testicular volume is disproportionately greater than penile size in normal puberty and in CPP.

c. Initial evaluation: Begin with history (assessing for premature thelarche/adrenarche) physical examination, and growth curves.
   (1) Determine bone age (generally >2 yr in advance of chronologic age in long-standing precocious puberty due to the action of sex hormones).
   (2) Assess degree of estrogenization or virilization; check for pubertal levels of plasma estradiol or plasma testosterone/DHAS, respectively. Check basal and/or GnRH-stimulated LH levels (see section VI.F), estradiol measurement in girls, testosterone levels in boys, 17-OHP levels, dehydroepiandrosterone (DHEA) levels, and urinary 17-ketosteroids (see section VI.G).
   (3) Imaging, such as magnetic resonance imaging of the brain, may help identify a CNS lesion.

3. **Ambiguous genitalia:**

a. Clinical findings in a neonate that indicate possible ambiguous genitalia include anogenital ratio >0.5 (distance between anus and posterior fourchette divided by distance between anus and base of clitoris), phallus length <2.2 cm (mean newborn length – 2 SD), clitoromegaly (length >1 cm), nonpalpable gonads in an apparent male, and hypospadias associated with separation of scrotal sacs or undescended testis.

b. Etiology: Most common cause is CAH (Fig. 10-5). Other causes: testicular regression syndrome, androgen insensitivity, testosterone biosynthesis disorders, and chromosomal abnormalities.

c. Diagnosis: Based on karyotype, measurement of gonadotropins (LH, FSH), adrenal steroids (cortisol, 17-OHP, and ACTH stimulation test), testosterone precursors (DHEA, androstenedione), testosterone, dihydrotestosterone (DHT), and hCG stimulation test (see section VI.H).

d. Cryptorchidism occurs in 3% of term male infants. About 50% of cryptorchid testicles descend by age 3 months, and 80% drop by 12 months. Neoplasm occurs in 48.9% of individuals with untreated cryptorchidism, and 25% of those tumors occur in the contralateral testis. Rule out virilized female with a karyotype. An hCG stimulation test can be used to differentiate cryptorchidism from anorchia (see section VI.H). Treatment is removal of trapped testicle at 1 year of life.

## V. NORMAL VALUES (Tables 10-9 to 10-27)

Normal values may differ among laboratories because of variation in technique and in type of radioimmunoassay used. Unless otherwise noted, the values in these tables are reference ranges from the Johns Hopkins Hospital Laboratories or from SmithKline Beecham clinical laboratories in Baltimore, Maryland.

*Text continued on p. 294*

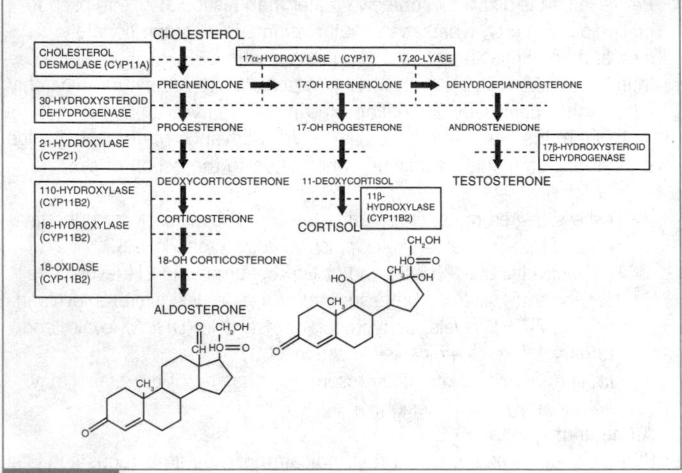


FIG. 10-5

Biosynthetic pathway for steroid hormones.[23] *(From Marshall I et al: Endocrine Hypertension in Childhood. Available at www.endotext.org/pediatrics/pediatrics9/index.html. Accessed December 21, 2007.)*

TABLE 10-9

**GONADOTROPINS**

| Age | FSH (mIU/mL) | LH (mIU/mL) |
|---|---|---|
| Prepubertal children | 0.0–2.8 | 0.0–1.6 |
| Men | 1.4–14.4 | 1.0–10.2 |
| Women, follicular phase | 3.7–12.9 | 0.9–14 |

*Note*: Normal infants have a transient rise in FSH (follicle-stimulating hormone) and LH (luteinizing hormone) to pubertal levels or higher within the first 3 mo, which then declines to prepubertal values by the end of the first year.

TABLE 10-10

**TESTOSTERONE**

| Age | Testosterone, Serum Total (ng/dL) | Testosterone, Unbound (pg/mL) |
|---|---|---|
| Prepubertal children | 10–20 | 0.15–0.6 |
| Men | 275–875 | 52–280 |
| Women | 23–75 | 1.1–6.3 |
| Pregnancy | 35–195 | |

TABLE 10-11

DIHYDROTESTOSTERONE (DHT)

| Age | Males (ng/dL) | Females (ng/dL) |
|---|---|---|
| Cord blood | <2–8 | <2–5 |
| 1–6 mo | 12–85 | <5 |
| Prepubertal | <5 | <5 |
| Tanner stage II–III | 3–33 | 5–19 |
| Tanner stage IV–V | 22–75 | 3–30 |

TABLE 10-12

ESTRADIOL

| Age | Level (pg/mL) |
|---|---|
| Prepubertal children | <25 |
| Men | 6–44 |
| Women | 26–165 |
| Luteal phase | None detected–266 |
| Follicular phase | 118–355 |
| Midcycle | None detected–102 |
| Adult women on OCP | |

*Note:* Normal infants have an elevated estradiol at birth, which decreases to prepubertal values during the first week of life. Estradiol levels increase again between age 1 and 2 months and return to prepubertal values by age 6–12 months.

OCP, oral contraceptive pill.

TABLE 10-13

ANDROSTENEDIONE, SERUM

| Age | Males (ng/dL) | Females (ng/dL) |
|---|---|---|
| Preterm infants | | |
| 26–28 wk to day 4 of life | 92–892 | 92–892 |
| 31–35 wk to day 4 of life | 80–446 | 80–446 |
| Full term infants | | |
| 1–7 day | 20–290 | 20–290 |
| 1–12 mo | 6–68 | 6–68 |
| Prepubertal children | 8–50 | 8–50 |
| Tanner II | 31–65 | 42–100 |
| Tanner III | 50–100 | 80–190 |
| Tanner IV | 48–140 | 77–225 |
| Tanner V | 65–210 | 80–240 |
| Adults | 78–205 | 85–275 |

TABLE 10-14

DEHYDROEPIANDROSTERONE (DHEA)

| Age | DHEA (ng/dL) | DHEA Sulfate (μg/dL) |
|---|---|---|
| Prepubertal children | 25 ± 8 | 2.3–15 |
| Men | 643 ± 112 | 223 ± 93 |
| Women | 516 ± 106 | 138 ± 51 |

Adapted from Bertrand J et al: Pediatric Endocrinology, 2nd ed. Baltimore, Williams & Wilkins, 1993.

TABLE 10-15

**17-HYDROXYPROGESTERONE, SERUM**

| Age | Baseline (ng/dL) | 60 min after ACTH Stimulation (ng/dL) |
|---|---|---|
| Premature infants (31–35 wk) | ≤360 | N/A |
| Term infants, 1st wk of life | ≤63 | N/A |
| 1–5 days | 80–420 | N/A |
| <1 yr | 11–170 | 85–465 |
| 1–5 yr | 4–115 | 50–350 |
| 6–12 yr | 7–69 | 75–220 |
| Male, Tanner stages II–III | 12–130 | 69–310 |
| Female, Tanner stages II–III | 18–220 | 80–420 |
| Male, Tanner stages IV–V | 51–190 | 105–230 |
| Female, Tanner stages IV–V | 36–200 | 80–225 |
| Adult male | 50–250 | 42–250 |
| Adult female, premenopausal | | |
| Follicular phase | 20–100 | 42–250 |
| Midcycle peak | 100–250 | |
| Luteal phase | 100–500 | |

*Note:* 8 AM level is most accurate given diurnal variation. Levels are normally increased in newborns for the first few days of life. Be aware that infant serum contains substances that may cross-react in the assay for 17-hydroxyprogesterone and artificially elevate the level, unless they are separated by chromatography. Before interpreting results on infants, be sure that the laboratory has prepared samples appropriately.

TABLE 10-16

**CORTISOL, SERUM WITH ACTH STIMULATION TEST**

| Condition | Cortisol (μg/dL) |
|---|---|
| Any gender/any age/pre-ACTH, 8 AM | 5.7–16.6 |
| 1 hr post-ACTH | 16–36 |

TABLE 10-17

**17-KETOSTEROIDS, URINE**

| Age | Level (mg/24 hr) |
|---|---|
| <1 mo | <2.0 |
| 1 mo–5 yr | <0.5 |
| 6–8 yr | 1.0–2.0 |
| Men | 9–22 |
| Women | 5–15 |

TABLE 10-18

**17-HYDROXYCORTICOSTEROIDS, URINE**

| Age/Gender | Level |
|---|---|
| Children (body weight variable) | 3 ± 1 $mg/m^2/24$ hr |
| Men | 3–9 mg/24 hr |
| Women | 2–8 mg/24 hr |

TABLE 10-19

**CATECHOLAMINES, URINE**

| Compound | Amount/24-hr Urine Collection |
|---|---|
| Dopamine | 100–440 μg |
| Epinephrine | <15 μg |
| Norepinephrine | 15–86 μg |
| Metanephrines | <0.4 mg |
| Normetanephrines | <0.9 mg |
| Homovanillic acid (HVA) | 0–10 mg |
| Vanillyl mandelic acid (VMA) | 2–10 mg |

*Note:* Catecholamines are elevated in a variety of tumors, including neuroblastoma, ganglioneuroma, ganglioblastoma, and pheochromocytoma.



TABLE 10-20

**CATECHOLAMINES, SERUM**

| Compound | Supine (μg) | Sitting (μg) |
|---|---|---|
| Dopamine | <87 | <87 |
| Epinephrine | <50 | <60 |
| Norepinephrine | 110–410 | 120–680 |

TABLE 10-21

**INSULIN-LIKE GROWTH FACTOR 1 (IGF-1)**

| Age | Males (ng/mL) | Females (ng/mL) |
|---|---|---|
| 2 mo–6 yr | 17–248 | 17–248 |
| 6–9 yr | 88–474 | 88–474 |
| 9–12 yr | 110–565 | 117–771 |
| 12–16 yr | 202–957 | 261–1096 |
| 16–26 yr | 182–780 | 182–780 |
| >26 yr | 123–463 | 123–463 |

*Note:* A clearly normal IGF-1 level argues against growth hormone (GH) deficiency, although in young children, there is considerable overlap between normals and those with GH deficiency.

TABLE 10-22

**INSULIN-LIKE GROWTH FACTOR-BINDING PROTEIN (IGF-BP3)**

| Age (yr) | Males (mg/L) | Females (mg/L) |
|---|---|---|
| 0–2 | 0.94–1.76 | 0.66–2.51 |
| 2–4 | 1.12–2.33 | 0.84–3.77 |
| 4–6 | 1.16–3.13 | 1.32–3.60 |
| 6–8 | 1.32–3.38 | 1.21–4.66 |
| 8–10 | 1.35–3.94 | 1.58–3.99 |
| 10–12 | 1.53–5.02 | 1.93–6.46 |
| 12–14 | 1.73–5.11 | 1.78–6.08 |
| 14–16 | 1.90–6.40 | 2.02–5.44 |
| 16–18 | 1.70–6.04 | 1.88–5.29 |
| 18–20 | 1.52–6.01 | 1.63–6.02 |
| 20–22 | 1.79–5.41 | 1.82–5.35 |
| Adult (continues to vary with age) | 1.15–5.18 | 1.19–5.69 |

*Note:* Levels below the 5th percentile suggest a growth hormone deficiency. This test may have greater discrimination than the IGF-1 test in younger patients.

TABLE 10-23

VITAMIN D

| Compound | Value |
|---|---|
| 25-Hydroxy-vitamin D | (ng/mL) |
| Newborns | 8–21 |
| Children | 17–54 |
| Adults | 10–55 |
| 1,25-Dihydroxy-vitamin D | (pg/mL) |
| Newborns | 8–72 |
| Children | 15–90 |
| Adults | 24–64 |

*Note:* 1,25-dihydroxy-vitamin D is the physiologically active form; however, 25-hydroxy-vitamin D is the value to monitor for vitamin D deficiency, because this approximates body stores of vitamin D.

## VI. TESTS AND PROCEDURES

### A. ORAL GLUCOSE TOLERANCE TEST (OGTT)

1. **Pretest preparation:** A calorically adequate diet is required for 3 days before the test, with 50% of total calories taken as carbohydrate.
2. **Delay test 2 weeks after illness.** *Discontinue all hyperglycemic and hypoglycemic agents (e.g., salicylates, diuretics, oral contraceptives, phenytoin).*
3. **Give 1.75 g/kg (maximum of 75 g) of glucose PO after a 12-hr fast, allowing up to 5 min for ingestion.** Mix glucose with water and lemon juice as a 20% dilution. Quiet activity is permissible during the OGTT. Draw blood samples at 0, 30, 60, 120, 180, and 240 min after ingestion.
4. **Interpretation:** 2-hr blood glucose <140 mg/dL = normal; 140–199 mg/dL = impaired glucose tolerance; ≥200 mg/dL = diabetes mellitus.

### B. ACTH STIMULATION TEST

1. Measures the ability of the adrenal gland to produce cortisol in response to ACTH. It is most useful in diagnosis of adrenal insufficiency.
2. **Method:** For patients >2 years of age, give 250 mcg ACTH. For those <2 years of age, give 125 mcg. Give doses IV over 2 min, and measure cortisol levels at 0, 30, and 60 min.
3. **Interpretation:** With a normal pituitary-adrenal axis, there is a rise in serum cortisol after ACTH administration (see Table 10-1 for values). With ACTH deficiency or prolonged adrenal suppression, there is no rise in cortisol after a single ACTH dose. A blunted cortisol response is indicative of CAH. A lack of response after 3 consecutive days of ACTH stimulation is pathognomonic of Addison disease.

TABLE 10-24

ROUTINE STUDIES (THYROID)

| Test | Age | Normal | Comments |
|---|---|---|---|
| $T_4$ RIA (mcg/dL) | Cord | 6.6–17.5 | Measures total $T_4$ by radioimmunoassay |
| | 1–3 d | 11.0–21.5 | |
| | 1–4 wk | 8.2–16.6 | |
| | 1–12 mo | 7.2–15.6 | |
| | 1–5 yr | 7.3–15.0 | |
| | 6–10 yr | 6.4–13.3 | |
| | 11–15 yr | 5.6–11.7 | |
| | 16–20 yr | 4.2–11.8 | |
| | 21–50 yr | 4.3–12.5 | |
| Free $T_4$ (ng/dL) | 1–10 d | 0.6–2.0 | Metabolically active form; the normal range for free $T_4$ is very assay dependent |
| | >10 d | 0.7–1.7 | |
| $T_3$ RIA (ng/dL) | Cord | 14–86 | Measures $T_3$ by RIA |
| | 1–3 d | 100–380 | |
| | 1–4 wk | 99–310 | |
| | 1–12 mo | 102–264 | |
| | 1–5 yr | 105–269 | |
| | 6–10 yr | 94–241 | |
| | 11–15 yr | 83–213 | |
| | 16–20 yr | 80–210 | |
| | 21–50 yr | 70–204 | |
| TSH (mIU/mL) | Cord | <2.5–17.4 | TSH surge peaks from 80–90 mIU/mL in term newborn by 30 min after birth. Values after 1 wk are within adult normal range. Elevated values suggest primary hypothyroidism, whereas suppressed values are the best indicator of hyperthyroidism. |
| | 1–3 d | <2.5–13.3 | |
| | 1–4 wk | 0.6–10.0 | |
| | 1–12 mo | 0.6–6.3 | |
| | 1–15 yr | 0.6–6.3 | |
| | 16–50 yr | 0.2–7.6 | |
| TBG (mg/dL) | Cord | 0.7–4.7 | |
| | 1–3 d | — | |
| | 1–4 wk | 0.5–4.5 | |
| | 1–12 mo | 1.6–3.6 | |
| | 1–5 yr | 1.3–2.8 | |
| | 6–20 yr | 1.4–2.6 | |
| | 21–50 yr | 1.2–2.4 | |

RIA, radioimmunoassay; RU, resin uptake; $T_3$, triiodothyronine; $T_4$, thyroxine; TBG, thyroxine-binding globulin; TSH, thyroid-stimulating hormone.

From Fisher DA: The thyroid. In Rudolf AM (ed): Pediatrics. Norwalk, Conn, Appleton & Lange, 1991, and LaFranchi SH: Hypothyroidism. Pediatr Clin North Am 1979;26(1):33–51.

## C. WATER DEPRIVATION TEST

1. Determines ability to concentrate urine and is useful in the diagnosis of DI. It requires careful supervision because dehydration and hypernatremia may occur.
2. **Method:** Begin the test after a 24-hr period of adequate hydration

TABLE 10-25

**SERUM $T_4$ IN PRETERM AND TERM INFANTS**

| Age (days) | VLBW (μg/dL) | Birthweight LBW (μg/dL) | Term (μg/dL) |
|---|---|---|---|
| 1–3 | 7.9 ± 3.3 | 11.4 ± 2.5 | 12 ± 1.9 |
| 4–6 | 6.5 ± 2.9 | 9.9 ± 2.5 | 11 ± 2.5 |
| 7–10 | 6.3 ± 3.0 | 9.5 ± 2.3 | |
| 11–14 | 5.7 ± 2.8 | 9.2 ± 2.1 | |
| 15–28 | 7.0 ± 2.5 | 9.1 ± 2.3 | |
| 29–56 | 7.8 ± 2.5 | 9.3 ± 3.3 | |

Low birth weight (LBW): 1500–2499 g; term: 2500–5528 g; very low birth weight (VLBW): 400–1499 g.

From Frank JE et al: Thyroid function in very low birth weight infants: Effects on neonatal hypothyroid screening. J Pediatrics 1996;128(4):548–555.

TABLE 10-26

**MEAN STRETCHED PENILE LENGTH (cm)**

| Age | Mean ± SD | –2.5 SD |
|---|---|---|
| Birth | | |
| 30 wk gestation | 2.5 ± 0.4 | 1.5 |
| 34 wk gestation | 3.0 ± 0.4 | 2.0 |
| Full term | 3.5 ± 0.4 | 2.5 |
| 0–5 mo | 3.9 ± 0.8 | 1.9 |
| 6–12 mo | 4.3 ± 0.8 | 2.3 |
| 1–2 yr | 4.7 ± 0.8 | 2.6 |
| 2–3 yr | 5.1 ± 0.9 | 2.9 |
| 3–4 yr | 5.5 ± 0.9 | 3.3 |
| 4–5 yr | 5.7 ± 0.9 | 3.5 |
| 5–6 yr | 6.0 ± 0.9 | 3.8 |
| 6–7 yr | 6.1 ± 0.9 | 3.9 |
| 7–8 yr | 6.2 ± 1.0 | 3.7 |
| 8–9 yr | 6.3 ± 1.0 | 3.8 |
| 9–10 yr | 6.3 ± 1.0 | 3.8 |
| 10–11 yr | 6.4 ± 1.1 | 3.7 |
| Adult | 13.3 ± 1.6 | 9.3 |

*Note:* Measured from the pubic ramus to the tip of the glans while traction is applied along the length of the phallus to the point of increased resistance.
SD, standard deviation.

From Feldman KW, Smith DW: Fetal phallic growth and penile standards for newborn male infants. J Pediatr 1975;86:395.

TABLE 10-27

**TESTICULAR SIZE**

| Tanner Stage (Genital) | Length (cm) (Mean ± SD) | Volume (mL) |
|---|---|---|
| I | 2.0 ± 0.5 | 2 |
| II | 2.7 ± 0.7 | 5 |
| III | 3.4 ± 0.8 | 10 |
| IV | 4.1 ± 1.0 | 20 |
| V | 5.0 ± 0.5 | 29 |

*Note*: Testicular volume of >4 mL or a long axis >2.5 cm is evidence that pubertal testicular growth has begun.
SD, standard deviation.

and stable weight. Obtain a baseline weight after bladder emptying. Restrict fluids for 7 hours. Measure body weight and urine specific gravity and volume hourly. Check serum $Na^+$ and urine and serum osmolality every 2 hr. Hematocrit and blood urea nitrogen (BUN) levels may also be obtained at these times but are not critical. Monitor carefully to ensure that fluids are not ingested during the test. Terminate the test if weight loss approaches 5%.

3. **Interpretation:**
   a. Normal individuals and those with psychogenic DI who are water deprived will concentrate urine to 500–1400 mOsm/L; plasma osmolality will be 288–291 mOsm/L. Urine specific gravity rises to at least 1.010, urine-to-plasma osmolality ratio is >2, urine volume decreases significantly, and there should be no appreciable weight loss.
   b. In patients with central or nephrogenic DI, specific gravity remains <1.005. Urine osmolality remains <150 mOsm/L, with no significant reduction of urine volume. A weight loss of up to 5% usually occurs. At the end of the test, a serum osmolality >290 mOsm/L, $Na^+$ >150 mEq/L, and a rise of BUN and hematocrit provide evidence that the patient did not receive water.



## D. VASOPRESSIN TEST

1. Used to differentiate between central (antidiuretic hormone [ADH]-deficient) and nephrogenic DI.
2. **Method:** Vasopressin is given subcutaneously, preferably at the end of the water deprivation test. Urine output, urine specific gravity, and water intake are monitored.
3. **Interpretation:** Patients with central DI concentrate their urine (>1.010) and demonstrate a reduction of urine volume and decreased fluid intake in response to exogenous vasopressin. Patients with nephrogenic DI have no significant change in fluid intake or urine volume or specific gravity. Continued fluid intake associated with decreased output and increased specific gravity suggests psychogenic DI.

## E. DEXAMETHASONE SUPPRESSION TEST

1. **Dexamethasone suppresses secretion of ACTH** by the normal pituitary, decreasing endogenous production of cortisol and excretion of 17-hydroxycorticosteroids (17-OHCS) and 17-ketosteroids. Useful in determining the etiology of glucocorticoid or androgen overproduction.
2. **Method:** Give dexamethasone PO for 3 days (low dose, 1.25 $mg/m^2$/day; high dose, 3.75 $mg/m^2$/day divided q6h), and collect 24-hr urine for 17-OHCS.
3. **Interpretation:** In normal patients, low-dose DST causes 17-OHCS to fall to <1 $mg/m^2$/day. In CAH, 17-OHCS levels are suppressed only by

the high-dose DST. 17-OHCS levels are not suppressed even with the high-dose DST in ectopic ACTH production, adrenocortical carcinoma, and some hypothalamic tumors. Incomplete suppression of 17-ketosteroids suggests that the patient has entered puberty. Markedly increased, nonsuppressible 17-ketosteroids suggest the presence of an androgen-producing tumor.

## F. GONADOTROPIN-RELEASING HORMONE (GNRH) STIMULATION TEST

1. **Measures pituitary LH and FSH reserve.** Helpful in the differential diagnosis of precocious or delayed sexual development.
2. **Method:** Give 100 mcg of synthetic GnRH (Factrel) SC, and measure LH and FSH levels at 0 and 40 min.
3. **Interpretation:** Prepubertal children should show no or minimal increase in LH and FSH in response to GnRH. A rise of LH into the adult range occurs in central precocious puberty. See Table 10-9 for normal gonadotropin values.

## G. URINARY 17-KETOSTEROIDS

1. **Measurement of urinary 17-ketosteroid levels** reveals some end products of androgen metabolism; most useful in evaluation of androgen excess.
2. **Method:** Collect and refrigerate 24-hr urine specimen.
3. **Interpretation (see Table 10-17 for normal values):**

a. Increased in CAH (it may take 1–2 weeks for 17-ketosteroids to rise above the normally high newborn levels), virilizing adrenal tumors, androgen-producing gonadal tumors, Cushing syndrome, and stressful illness.
b. Decreased in Addison disease, anorexia nervosa, and panhypopituitarism.

## H. HUMAN CHORIONIC GONADOTROPIN (HCG) STIMULATION TEST

1. **Measures capacity for testosterone biosynthesis;** useful in differentiation of cryptorchidism (undescended testes) from anorchia (absent testes).
2. **Method:** Give 1000 units of hCG IV or IM for 3 days and measure serum testosterone and dihydrotestosterone on day 0 and day 4.
3. **Interpretation:** Testosterone level >100 ng/dL in response to hCG stimulation is evidence for adequate testosterone biosynthesis. In cryptorchidism, testosterone rises to adult levels after hCG administration; in anorchia, there is no rise.

## I. CUSHING EVALUATION

1. **24-hour urine collection** for excess cortisol (normal value range by mass spectrometry is 27–30 ng/mL.

2. **Cortisol level:** Measured at 8 AM; preceded by 1 mg of dexamethasone PO given at 11 PM the night before; level <1.8 mcg/dL (50 nanomol/L) is within normal range of suppression.
3. **Salivary cortisol level:** Measured at 11 PM ("spit in a tube"); levels are akin to free serum cortisol. Normal range is <0.2 mcg/dL.

## J. NEONATAL HYPOGLYCEMIA AND GLUCAGON STIMULATION TEST

1. **Hypoglycemia:** Can be defined as a glucose level that is insufficient to meet metabolic requirements; can vary with perinatal stress, gestational size, and maternal factors. For practical purposes value is defined as <45 mg/dL. A bedside glucometer is inaccurate at levels <40 mg/dL, and a stat serum glucose must be sent.
2. **Symptoms of hypoglycemia:** Abnormal cry, seizures, apnea, hypotonia, bradycardia, hypothermia.
3. Do not delay treatment for serum glucose results.
   a. Asymptomatic infants with plasma glucose level 25–45 mg/dL (1.4–2.5 mM): Begin breast-feeding or nipple/gavage with formula.
   b. Asymptomatic infants with plasma glucose level <25 mg/dL (<1.4 mM), asymptomatic infants who do not tolerate enteral feeding, or symptomatic infants:
      (1) Give IV bolus of glucose 0.25 g/kg (2.5 mL/kg of 10% glucose, or 1.0 mL/kg of 25% glucose) over 1 to 2 min.
      (2) Continue IV glucose at a rate of 6–8 mg/kg/min (3.6–4.8 mL/kg/hr of 10% glucose).
      (3) Increase glucose delivery by 1–2 mg/kg/min if blood glucose is consistently <50 mg/dL during q30–60min interval checks.
4. **If serum glucose is consistently <40 mg/dL,** further endocrine workup is warranted. Obtain serum levels of glucose, insulin, growth hormone, free fatty acids, and β-hydroxybutyrate. Administer glucagon and obtain serum glucose and insulin levels after 15 min. A positive response (i.e., rise in glucose secondary to glucagon) along with elevated insulin levels and a glucose requirement >8 mg/kg/min suggest a diagnosis of hyperinsulinemia. Hypoglycemia with midline defects and micropenis in a male suggest hypopituitarism.

## K. SERUM FREE FRACTIONATED METANEPHRINES

1. This plasma level is a tool for detection of a pheochromocytoma.
2. The upper limits of normal are somewhat assay dependent; however, one study suggests the upper normal limits to be: metanephrine (0.3 nmol/L); normetanephrine (0.6 nmol/L).[22]
3. A pediatric study suggests metanephrines (boys: 0.52; girls: 0.37 nmol/L); normetanephrines (boys: 0.53; girls: 0.42 nmol/L).[23]

## REFERENCES


1. Report of the Expert Committee on the Diagnosis and Classification of Diabetes Mellitus: Diabetes Care 1999;22(Suppl 1):S5–S19.
2. American Diabetes Association: Consensus statement: Type 2 diabetes in children. Diabetes Care 2000;22(12):381.
3. Pinhas-Hamiel O, Zeitler P: Type 2 diabetes: Not just for grownups anymore. Contemp Pediatr 2001;18(1):102–125.
4. American Diabetes Association: Hyperglycemic crises in patients with diabetes mellitus. Diabetes Care 2001;24(1):154–161.
5. Fisher DA: The thyroid. In Rudolf AM (ed): Pediatrics. Norwalk, Conn, Appleton & Lange, 1991.
6. LaFranchi SH: Hyperthyroidism. Pediatr Clin North Am 1979;26(1):33–51.
7. Frank JE et al: Thyroid function in very low birth weight infants: Effects on neonatal hypothyroidism screening. J Pediatr 1996;128(4):548–555.
8. Biswas S: A longitudinal assessment of thyroid hormone concentrations in preterm infants younger than 30 weeks' gestation during the first 2 weeks of life and their relationship to outcome. Pediatrics 2002;109(2):222–227.
9. Orth DN, Kovacs WJ: The adrenal cortex. In Wilson JD (ed): Williams' Textbook of Endocrinology. Philadelphia, WB Saunders, 1998.
10. American Academy of Pediatrics, Section on Endocrinology and Committee on Genetics: Technical report: Congenital adrenal hyperplasia. Pediatrics 2000;106(6):1511–1518.
11. Levine LS: Congenital adrenal hyperplasia. Pediatr Rev 2000;21(5):159–170.
12. Reeves WB et al: Posterior pituitary and water metabolism. In Wilson JD (ed): Williams' Textbook of Endocrinology. Philadelphia, WB Saunders, 1998, pp 311–356.
13. Plotnick L: Growth, growth hormone, and pituitary disorders. In McMillan J (ed): Oski's Pediatrics Principles and Practice. Philadelphia, Lippincott Williams & Wilkins, 1999, pp 1776–1783.
14. MacGillivray MH: The basics for the diagnosis and management of short stature: A pediatric endocrinologist's approach. Pediatr Ann 2000;29(9):570–575.
15. Styne DM: New aspects in the diagnosis and treatment of pubertal disorders. Pediatr Endocrinol 1997;44(2):505–529.
16. Root AW: Precocious puberty. Pediatr Rev 2000;21(1):10–19.
17. Rosen DS, Foster C: Delayed puberty. Pediatr Rev 2001;22(9):309–314.
18. American Academy of Pediatrics, Committee on Genetics, Sections on Endocrinology and Urology: Evaluation of newborn with developmental anomalies of the external genitalia. Pediatrics 2000;106(1):138–142.
19. Ross JL et al: Psychological adaptation in children with idiopathic short stature treated with growth hormone or placebo. J Clin Endocrinol Metab 2004;89(10):4873–4878.
20. Blondell R et al: Disorders of puberty. Am Family Phys1999;60(1):209–218.
21. Master-Hunter T et al: Amenorrhea: Evaluation and treatment. Am Family Phys 2006;73(8):1374–1382.
22. Lenders JW et al: Biomedical diagnosis of pheochromocytoma: Which test is best? JAMA 2002;287:1427–1434.
23. Weise M et al: Utility of plasma free metanephrines for detecting childhood pheochromocytoma. JCEM 2002;87:1955–1960.
24. Cooke DW: Metabolism and endocrinology. In Seidel HM, Rosenstein BJ, Pathak A (eds): Primary Care of the Newborn, 4th ed. Philadelphia, Mosby, 2006.

# Fluids and Electrolytes

*Gregory J. Aune, MD, PhD*

## I. OVERALL GOALS OF FLUID AND ELECTROLYTE MANAGEMENT

### A. ESTIMATE FLUID AND ELECTROLYTE DEFICITS, MAINTENANCE REQUIREMENTS, AND ONGOING LOSSES.

### B. SELECT AND ADMINISTER APPROPRIATE FLUIDS

Select fluids for the following:

1. **Initial replacement: Always with isotonic fluid (i.e., normal saline or lactated Ringer's solution).**
2. **Maintenance requirements and ongoing losses.**

11

## II. MAINTENANCE REQUIREMENTS

Stem from basal metabolism. Metabolism creates two by-products, heat and solute, that need to be eliminated to maintain homeostasis. Heat dissipation through insensible losses and solute excretion in urine each can be considered as representing 50% of maintenance needs; i.e., in the management of children who have anuric renal failure, maintenance fluid needs decrease by 50% because the only fluids that need to be replaced are insensible losses.[1]

### A. CALORIC EXPENDITURE METHOD

Based on the understanding that water and electrolyte requirements more accurately parallel caloric expenditure than body weight or body surface area (BSA). This method is effective for all ages, types of body habitus, and clinical states.

1. **Determine the child's estimated energy requirements (see Table 21-1 in Chapter 21).**
2. **Adjust caloric expenditure needs by various factors (e.g., fever, activity) as described in Chapter 21.**
3. **For each 100 calories metabolized in 24 hr, the average patient will need 100–120 mL $H_2O$, 2–4 mEq $Na^+$, and 2–3 mEq $K^+$, as seen in Table 11-1.**

### B. HOLLIDAY-SEGAR METHOD (Table 11-2 and Box 11-1)

Estimates caloric expenditure in fixed weight categories; it assumes that for each 100 calories metabolized, 100 mL of $H_2O$ will be required. Specifically, for each 100 kcal expended, about 50 mL of fluid is required to provide for skin, respiratory tract, and basal stool losses, and 55–65 mL of fluid is required for the kidneys to excrete an ultrafiltrate of plasma at 300 mOsm/L without having to concentrate the urine.

**Note** *The Holliday-Segar method is not suitable for neonates <14 days old; generally, it overestimates fluid needs in neonates compared with the caloric expenditure method.*

TABLE 11-1

AVERAGE WATER AND ELECTROLYTE REQUIREMENTS PER 100 CALORIES PER 24 HOURS

| Clinical State | $H_2O$ (mL) | $Na^+$ (mEq) | $K^+$ (mEq) |
|---|---|---|---|
| Average patient receiving parenteral fluids* | 100–120 | 2–4 | 2–3 |
| Anuria | 45 | 0 | 0 |
| Acute CNS infections and inflammation | 80–90 | 2–4 | 2–3 |
| Diabetes insipidus | Up to 400 | Var | Var |
| Hyperventilation | 120–210 | 2–4 | 2–3 |
| Heat stress | 120–240 | Var | Var |
| High-humidity environment | 80–100 | 2–4 | 2–3 |

*Adequate maintenance solution: dextrose 5%–10% (as needed) in 0.2% NaCl + 20 mEq/L KCl or K acetate.

CNS, central nervous system; Var, variable requirement.

TABLE 11-2

HOLLIDAY-SEGAR METHOD

| | Water | | Electrolytes |
|---|---|---|---|
| Body Weight | mL/kg/day | mL/kg/hr | (mEq/100 mL $H_2O$) |
| First 10 kg | 100 | ~4 | $Na^+$ 3 |
| Second 10 kg | 50 | ~2 | $Cl^-$ 2 |
| Each additional kg | 20 | ~1 | $K^+$ 2 |

BOX 11-1

HOLLIDAY-SEGAR METHOD

Example: Based on the Holliday-Segar method, determine the correct fluid rate for an 8-year-old child weighing 25 kg:

| | |
|---|---|
| 4 mL/kg/hr × 10 kg = 40 mL/hr (for first 10 kg) | 100 mL/kg/day × 10 kg = 1000 mL/day (for first 10 kg) |
| 2 mL/kg/hr × 10 kg = 20 mL/hr (for second 10 kg) | 50 mL/kg/day × 10 kg = 500 mL/day (for second 10 kg) |
| 1 ml/kg/hr × 5 kg = 5 mL/hr (per additional kg) | 20 mL/kg/day × 5 kg = 100 mL/day (per additional kg) |
| 25 kg 65 mL/hr | 25 kg 1600 mL/day |
| Answer: 65 mL/hr | Answer: 1600 mL/day |

### C. BODY SURFACE AREA METHOD

Based on the assumption that caloric expenditure is related to BSA (Table 11-3). It should not be used for children <10 kg. See BSA nomogram in Formulary Adjunct.

## III. DEFICIT THERAPY

### A. CALCULATED ASSESSMENT

The most precise method of assessing fluid deficit is based on pre-illness weight. If this is not available, clinical observation may be used, as described subsequently.

TABLE 11-3

**STANDARD VALUES FOR USE IN BODY SURFACE AREA METHOD**

| | |
|---|---|
| $H_2O$ | 1500 mL/m²/24 hr |
| $Na^+$ | 30–50 mEq/m²/24 hr |
| $K^+$ | 20–40 mEq/m²/24 hr |

Data from Finberg L et al: Water and Electrolytes in Pediatrics. Philadelphia, WB Saunders, 1982, and Hellerstein S: Fluids and electrolytes: Clinical aspects. Pediatr Rev 1993;14(3): 103–115.

TABLE 11-4

**CLINICAL OBSERVATIONS IN DEHYDRATION***

| | Older Child | | |
|---|---|---|---|
| | 3% (30 mL/kg) | 6% (60 mL/kg) | 9% (90 mL/kg) |
| | Infant | | |
| **Examination** | **5% (50 mL/kg)** | **10% (100 mL/kg)** | **15% (150 mL/kg)** |
| Dehydration | Mild | Moderate | Severe |
| Skin turgor | Normal | Tenting | None |
| Skin (touch) | Normal | Dry | Clammy |
| Buccal mucosa/lips | Moist | Dry | Parched/cracked |
| Eyes | Normal | Deep set | Sunken |
| Tears | Present | Reduced | None |
| Fontanelle | Flat | Soft | Sunken |
| CNS | Consolable | Irritable | Lethargic/obtunded |
| Pulse rate | Normal | Slightly increased | Increased |
| Pulse quality | Normal | Weak | Feeble/impalpable |
| Capillary refill | Normal | ~2 sec | >3 sec |
| Urine output | Normal | Decreased | Anuric |

*For the same degree of dehydration, clinical symptoms are generally worse for hyponatremic dehydration than for hypernatremic dehydration.

CNS, central nervous system.

Data from Behrman RE et al: Nelson Textbook of Pediatrics, 17th ed. Philadelphia, WB Saunders, 2003, and Oski FA: Principles and Practice of Pediatrics, 4th ed. Philadelphia, JB Lippincott, 2006.

$$\text{Fluid deficit (L)} = \text{pre-illness weight (kg)} - \text{illness weight (kg)}$$

$$\text{\% Dehydration} = (\text{pre-illness weight} - \text{illness weight})/\text{pre-illness weight} \times 100\%$$

### B. CLINICAL ASSESSMENT (Table 11-4)

## IV. GUIDELINES FOR DEHYDRATION CALCULATION

The extracellular fluid space is about 20% of the body's weight (40% in the newborn) and is divided 3:1 between interstitial (15% of body weight) and intravascular (5% of body weight) space.[2]

### A. INTRACELLULAR FLUID (ICF) AND EXTRACELLULAR FLUID (ECF) COMPARTMENTS

1. **Normal ICF and ECF composition (Table 11-5).**

TABLE 11-5

**INTRACELLULAR AND EXTRACELLULAR FLUID COMPOSITION**

| | Intracellular (mEq/L) | Extracellular (mEq/L) |
|---|---|---|
| $Na^+$ | 20 | 133–145 |
| $K^+$ | 150 | 3–5 |
| $Cl^-$ | — | 98–110 |
| $HCO_3^-$ | 10 | 20–25 |
| $PO_4^{3-}$ | 110–115 | 5 |
| Protein | 75 | 10 |

**2. In dehydration, there are variable losses from the extracellular and intracellular compartments. The percentage deficit from these compartments is based on the total duration of illness.**

a. Illness < 3 days: 80% ECF deficit, 20% ICF deficit.

b. Illness ≥ 3 days: 60% ECF deficit, 40% ICF deficit.

**3. Electrolyte deficit (from ECF and ICF losses):**

a. $Na^+$ deficit is the amount of $Na^+$ that was lost from the $Na^+$-containing ECF compartment during the dehydration period (see Table 11-5). Intracellular $Na^+$ is negligible as a proportion of total; therefore, it can be disregarded.

$$\textbf{Na}^+ \textbf{ deficit (mEq)} = \textbf{fluid deficit (L)} \times \textbf{proportion from ECF} \times \textbf{Na}^+ \textbf{ concentration (mEq/L) in ECF}$$

b. $K^+$ deficit is the amount of $K^+$ that was lost from the $K^+$-containing ICF compartment during the dehydration period (see Table 11-5). Extracellular $K^+$ is negligible as a proportion of total; therefore it can be disregarded.

$$\textbf{K}^+ \textbf{ deficit (mEq)} = \textbf{fluid deficit (L)} \times \textbf{proportion from ICF} \times \textbf{K}^+ \textbf{ concentration (mEq/L) in ICF}$$

## B. ELECTROLYTE DEFICITS (IN EXCESS OF ECF/ICF ELECTROLYTE LOSSES)

$$\textbf{mEq required} = \textbf{(CD} - \textbf{CP)} \times \textbf{fD} \times \textbf{wt (kg pre-illness)}$$

CD = concentration desired (mEq/L)

CP = concentration present (mEq/L)

fD = distribution factor as fraction of body weight (L/kg): $HCO_3^-$ (0.4–0.5); $Cl^-$ (0.2–0.3); $Na^+$ (0.6–0.7)

## C. PROBABLE DEFICITS OF WATER AND ELECTROLYTES IN SEVERE DEHYDRATION (Table 11-6)

## D. ONGOING LOSSES IN DEHYDRATION (Table 11-7)

## E. DEFICIT CALCULATIONS (Table 11-8; Fig. 11-1; Tables 11-9 and 11-10)

TABLE 11-6

DEFICITS OF WATER AND ELECTROLYTES IN SEVERE DEHYDRATION

| Condition | $H_2O$ (mL/kg) | $Na^+$ (mEq/kg) | $K^+$ (mEq/kg) | $Cl^-$ (mEq/kg) |
|---|---|---|---|---|
| **DIARRHEAL DEHYDRATION** | | | | |
| *Hyponatremic* [$Na^+$]* <130 mEq/L | 100–120 | 10–15 | 8–15 | 10–12 |
| *Isotonic* [$Na^+$]* 130–150 mEq/L | 100–120 | 8–10 | 8–10 | 8–10 |
| *Hypernatremic* [$Na^+$]* >150 mEq/L | 100–120 | 2–4 | 0–6 | 0–3 |
| **PYLORIC STENOSIS** | 100–120 | 8–10 | 10–12 | 10–12 |
| **DIABETIC KETOACIDOSIS** | 100 | 8 | 6–10 | 6 |

*[Na], serum or plasma sodium concentration.

Data from Hellerstein S: Fluid and electrolytes: Clinical aspects. Pediatr Rev 1993;14(3):103–115.

TABLE 11-7

ELECTROLYTE COMPOSITION OF VARIOUS BODY FLUIDS*

| Fluid | $Na^+$ (mEq/L) | $K^+$ (mEq/L) | $Cl^-$ (mEq/L) |
|---|---|---|---|
| Gastric | 20–80 | 5–20 | 100–150 |
| Pancreatic | 120–140 | 5–15 | 90–120 |
| Small bowel | 100–140 | 5–15 | 90–130 |
| Bile | 120–140 | 5–15 | 80–120 |
| Ileostomy | 45–135 | 3–15 | 20–115 |
| Diarrhea | 10–90 | 10–80 | 10–110 |
| Burns† | 140 | 5 | 110 |
| Sweat | | | |
| Normal | 10–30 | 3–10 | 10–35 |
| Cystic fibrosis | 50–130 | 5–25 | 50–110 |

*This table is useful in determining ongoing electrolyte losses in dehydration.
†3–5 g/dL of protein may be lost in fluid from burn wounds.

Data from Behrman RE et al: Nelson Textbook of Pediatrics, 17th ed. Philadelphia, WB Saunders, 2003.

## F. SELECTION OF APPROPRIATE MAINTENANCE FLUIDS

1. Hypotonic fluids offer adequate amounts of water and electrolytes to match maintenance requirements. Many hospitalized patients have water and electrolyte deficits and can retain free water due to various disease processes. Therefore, hypotonic fluids (i.e., 0.225% normal saline [NS]) should be used for matching maintenance needs only.
2. Due to >50 reported deaths or severe neurologic injury from iatrogenic hyponatremia since the mid-1990s, some experts have suggested using NS in all patients receiving maintenance IV fluids.[3]
3. NS may be used to provide water and electrolytes for certain patients (i.e., postoperative neurosurgical and traumatic brain injury patients), but the safety of routinely using NS as maintenance fluid has not been adequately studied in randomized, controlled trials.

*Text continued on p. 311*

TABLE 11-8

## EXAMPLE OF ISONATREMIC DEHYDRATION

Determine an adequate fluid schedule for a 7-kg (pre-illness weight) infant who has been ill for ≥3 days and clinically appears 10% dehydrated. Current weight is 6.3 kg. Serum $Na^+$ = 137. An IV line has just been placed, and no IVF has been administered.

| Deficit Replacement | | $H_2O$ (mL) | $Na^+$ (mEq) | $K^+$ (mEq) |
|---|---|---|---|---|
| **Fluid deficit** | | | | |
| % Dehydration × wt (kg) = 10% × 7 kg × (1000 mL/kg) | | 700 | | |
| *$Na^+$ deficit* | | | | |
| 0.7 × 0.6 × 145 = | | | 61 | |
| *$K^+$ deficit* | | | | |
| 0.7 × 0.4 × 150 = | | | | 21 |
| **Maintenance** | | | | |
| $H_2O$ | | | | |
| 7 kg × 100 mL/kg/day = | | 700 | | |
| *$Na^+$* | | | | |
| 700 mL/day × 3 mEq/100 mL = | | | 21 | |
| *$K^+$* | | | | |
| 700 mL/day × 2 mEq/100 mL = | | | | 14 |
| **24-hr total** | | 1400 | 82 | 56 |
| **Fluid Schedule** | | | | |
| First 8 hr | $^1/_3$ maintenance | 233 | 7 | 5 |
| | $^1/_2$ deficit | 350 | 31 | 21 |
| First 8-hr total | | 583 | 38 | 26 |
| Next 16 hr | $^2/_3$ maintenance | 467 | 14 | 9 |
| | $^1/_2$ deficit | 350 | 30 | 21 |
| Next 16-hr total | | 817 | 44 | 30 |

**Answer**

| | |
|---|---|
| Therefore, first 8 hr: | Next 16 hr: |
| Rate: 583 mL/8 hr = 73 mL/hr | Rate: 817 mL/16 hr = 51 mL/hr |
| $Na^+$: 38 mEq/0.583 L = 65 mEq/L | $Na^+$: 44 mEq/0.817L = 54 mEq/L |
| $K^+$: 26 mEq/0.583 L = 45 mEq/L | $K^+$: 30 mEq/0.817 L = 37 mEq/L |
| $D_5$ $^1/_2$ NS + 40 mEq/L of KCl or K acetate @ ~75 mL/hr × 8 hr | $D_5$ $^1/_2$ NS + 40 mEq/L of KCl or K acetate @ ~50 mL/hr × 16 hr |

In the absence of hypokalemia, 20–30 mEq/L of potassium is commonly used and is usually adequate; monitor carefully for hyperkalemia and adequate urine output if high concentrations of potassium are used. Potassium infusion rates should not exceed 1 mEq/kg/hr. If rate exceeds 0.5 mEq/kg/hr, the patient should be placed on a cardiorespiratory monitor.

**Note:** Remember to account for ongoing losses. They should be replaced concurrently ("piggybacked") with a solution that matches the fluid being lost (see Table 11-7)

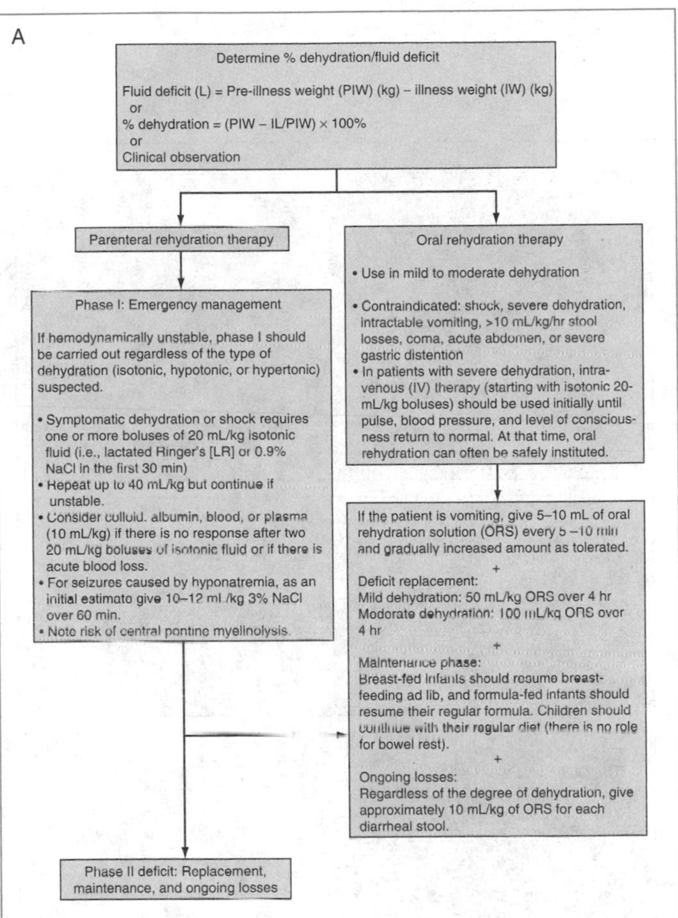

A
Determine % dehydration/fluid deficit
Fluid deficit (L) = Pre-illness weight (PIW) (kg) – illness weight (IW) (kg)
or
% dehydration = (PIW – IL/PIW) × 100%
or
Clinical observation
Parenteral rehydration therapy
Oral rehydration therapy
• Use in mild to moderate dehydration
• Contraindicated: shock, severe dehydration, intractable vomiting, >10 mL/kg/hr stool losses, coma, acute abdomen, or severe gastric distention
• In patients with severe dehydration, intravenous (IV) therapy (starting with isotonic 20-mL/kg boluses) should be used initially until pulse, blood pressure, and level of consciousness return to normal. At that time, oral rehydration can often be safely instituted.
Phase I: Emergency management
If hemodynamically unstable, phase I should be carried out regardless of the type of dehydration (isotonic, hypotonic, or hypertonic) suspected.
• Symptomatic dehydration or shock requires one or more boluses of 20 mL/kg isotonic fluid (i.e., lactated Ringer's [LR] or 0.9% NaCl in the first 30 min)
• Repeat up to 40 mL/kg but continue if unstable.
• Consider colloid: albumin, blood, or plasma (10 mL/kg) if there is no response after two 20 mL/kg boluses of isotonic fluid or if there is acute blood loss.
• For seizures caused by hyponatremia, as an initial estimate give 10–12 mL/kg 3% NaCl over 60 min.
• Note risk of central pontine myelinolysis.
If the patient is vomiting, give 5–10 mL of oral rehydration solution (ORS) every 5–10 min and gradually increased amount as tolerated.
+
Deficit replacement:
Mild dehydration: 50 mL/kg ORS over 4 hr
Moderate dehydration: 100 mL/kg ORS over 4 hr
+
Maintenance phase:
Breast-fed infants should resume breast-feeding ad lib, and formula-fed infants should resume their regular formula. Children should continue with their regular diet (there is no role for bowel rest).
+
Ongoing losses:
Regardless of the degree of dehydration, give approximately 10 mL/kg of ORS for each diarrheal stool.
Phase II deficit: Replacement, maintenance, and ongoing losses


FIG. 11-1A

**A** and **B,** Algorithm for dehydration correction.

*Continued*

B

Phase II deficit: Replacement, maintenance, and ongoing losses*

**Hyponatremic dehydration:**
Implies excess $Na^+$ loss ($Na^+ < 130$ mEq/L)

Replacement:
Fluid deficit (L) = % dehydration × Wt (kg)

$Na^+$ deficit (mEq) = [Fluid deficit (L )] × [Proportion $Na^+$ from ECF] × [$Na^+$ concentration (mEq/L) in ECF]

Excess $Na^+$ deficit = (CD – CP) × fD × Wt (pre-illness weight in kg):
CD = concentration $Na^+$ desired (mEq/L)
CP = concentration $Na^+$ present (mEq/L)
fD = distribution factor as fraction of body weight (L/kg). Example: $Na^+$: 0.6–0.7

+

$K^+$ deficit = [Fluid deficit (L) × [Proportion $K^+$ from ICF] × [$K^+$ concentration (mEq/L) in ICF]

+

Maintenance: Calculate maintenance fluids and electrolytes using Holliday-Segar method

Ongoing losses: Use Table 11-7 to estimate ongoing electrolyte losses for various body fluids. Significant losses should be measured and may require replacement every 6–8 hr.

* Phase cross-reference Table 11-5 for calculations.

**Isonatremic dehydration:**
implies proportional losses of $Na^+$ and free water (FW). ($Na^+$ 130–149 mEq/L)

Replacement:
Fluid deficit (L) = % dehydration × Wt (kg)

$Na^+$ deficit (mEq) = [Fluid deficit (L)] × [Proportion $Na^+$ from ECF] × [$Na^+$ concentration (mEq/L) in ECF]

$K^+$ deficit = [Fluid deficit (L)] × [Proportion $K^+$ from ICF] × [$K^+$ concentration (mEq/L) in ICF]

+

Maintenance: Calculate maintenance fluids and electrolytes using Holliday-Segar method

+

Ongoing losses: Use Table 11-7 to estimate ongoing electrolyte losses for various body fluids. Significant losses should be measured and may require replacement every 6–8 hr.

**Hypernatremic dehydration:**
Implies excess FW loss. Note: The skin may appear thick and doughy, with normal turgor, and children may be excessively irritable on examination. ($Na^+ \geq 150$ mEq/L)

Replacement:
FW deficit (FWD) estimated (L) : 4 mL/kg needed to decrease serum $Na^+$ by 1 mEq/L OR 3 mL/kg if $Na^+ > 170$ because less FW is required to decrease serum $Na^+$ at higher concentrations.
Therefore: FWD = [4 mL/kg (or 3 mL/kg)] × weight × [concentration $Na^+$ present – concentration $Na^+$ desired]

Solute fluid deficit (SFD) (L) = Total fluid deficit (L) – FWD(L)

Solute $Na^+$ deficit = SFD × [Proportion $Na^+$ from ECF] × [$Na^+$ concentration (mEq/L) in ECF]

Solute $K^+$ deficit = SFD × [Proportion $K^+$ from ICF] × [$K^+$ concentration (mEq/L) in ICF]

+

Maintenance: Calculate maintenance fluids and electrolytes using Holliday-Segar method

+

Ongoing losses: Use Table 11-7 to estimate ongoing electrolyte losses for various body fluids. Significant losses should be measured and may require replacement every 6–8 hr.

Give half of the replacement therapy in addition to the maintenance needs over the first 8 hr and the second half over the next 16 hr.

Rapid correction of hyponatremia may be associated with central pontine myelinolysis. Rapid increases in serum $Na^+$ level should therefore be reserved for symptomatic patients only. In asymptomatic patients, the target rate of rise should not exceed 2–4 mEq/L q4h, or about 10–20 mEq/L in 24 hr.

Note: To calculate volume of 3% NaCl needed to raise the serum $Na^+$ by 'X' mEq/L:
Amount of 3% NaCl (mL) = ['X' mEq/L × body weight (kg)] × 0.6 L/kg
Where 'X' = (125 mEq/L – actual serum [Na] to initially raise the serum $Na^+$ rapidly to 125 mEq/L

Give half of the replacement therapy in addition to the maintenance needs over the next 16 hr.

Half of the FW deficit and all of the solute deficit can be replaced over 24 hr. Replace the remainder of the FWD + maintenance during the next 24 hr.

Note: Avoid dropping the serum $Na^+$ > 15 mEq/L per 24 hr to minimize the risk of cerebral edema. Thus for total $Na^+$ corrections of > 30 (i.e., serum $Na^+$ > 175), FW deficit replacement should be spread over > 48 hr. Follow serum $Na^+$ levels at least every 4 hr initially.

FIG. 11-1B

TABLE 11-9

**EXAMPLE OF HYPONATREMIC DEHYDRATION**

Determine an adequate fluid schedule for a 7-kg (pre-illness weight) infant who has been ill for ≥3 days and clinically appears 10% dehydrated. Current weight is 6.3 kg. Serum $Na^+$ = 115. An IV line has just been placed, and no IVF has been administered.

| Deficit Replacement | $H_2O$ (mL) | $Na^+$ (mEq) | $K^+$ (mEq) |
|---|---|---|---|
| *Fluid deficit* | | | |
| % Dehydration × wt (kg) = 10% × 7kg × (1000 mL/kg) | 700 | | |
| *$Na^+$ deficit* | | | |
| 0.7 × 0.6 × 145 = | | 61 | |
| Excess $Na^+$ deficit: | | | |
| (135–115) × 0.6 × 7 = | | 84 | |
| *$K^+$ deficit* | | | |
| 0.7 × 0.4 × 150 = | | | 42 |
| **Maintenance** | | | |
| (See Table 11-8 for exact calculations) | 700 | 21 | 14 |
| **24-hr total** | 1400 | 166 | 56 |
| **Fluid Schedule** | | | |
| First 8 hr — $^1/_3$ maintenance | 233 | 7 | 5 |
| $^1/_2$ deficit | 350 | 73 | 21 |
| First 8-hr total | 583 | 80 | 26 |
| Next 16 hr — $^2/_3$ maintenance | 467 | 14 | 9 |
| $^1/_2$ deficit | 350 | 72 | 21 |
| Next 16-hr total | 817 | 86 | 30 |

**Answer**

Therefore, first 8 hr:
Rate: 583 mL/8 hr = 73 mL/hr
$Na^+$: 80 mEq/0.583 L = 137 mEq/L
$K^+$: 26 mEq/0.58 3L = 45 mEq/L
$D_5$ NS + 40 mEq/L of KCl or
K acetate @ ~75 mL/hr × 8 hr

Next 16 hr:
Rate: 817 mL/16hr = 51 mL/hr
$Na^+$: 86 mEq/0.817 L = 105 mEq/L
$K^+$: 30 mEq/0.817 L = 37 mEq/L
$D_5$ $^1/_2$ NS + 40 mEq/L of KCl or
K acetate @ ~50 mL/hr × 16 hr

In the absence of hypokalemia, 20–30 mEq/L of potassium is commonly used and is usually adequate; monitor carefully for hyperkalemia and adequate urine output if high concentrations of potassium are used. Potassium infusion rates should not exceed 1 mEq/kg/hr. If rate exceeds 0.5 mEq/kg/hr, the patient should be placed on a cardiorespiratory monitor.

**Note:** Remember to account for ongoing losses. They should be replaced concurrently ("piggybacked") with a solution that matches the fluid being lost (see Table 11-7).

TABLE 11-10

**EXAMPLE OF HYPERNATREMIC DEHYDRATION**

Determine an adequate fluid schedule for a 7-kg (pre-illness weight) infant who has been ill for ≥3 days and clinically appears between 10% and 15% dehydrated. Current weight is 6.1 kg. Serum $Na^+$ = 160.

| Replacement | $H_2O$ (mL) | $Na^+$ (mEq) | $K^+$ (mEq) |
|---|---|---|---|
| *Free-water deficit (FWD)* | | | |
| 4 mL/kg × 7kg × [160–145] – | 420 | | |
| *Solute fluid deficit (SFD)* | | | |
| [Total fluid deficit (900)] – [FWD] | 480 | | |
| *Solute $Na^+$ deficit* | | | |
| 0.48 × 0.6 × 145 = | | 42 | |
| *Solute $K^+$ deficit* | | | |
| 0.48 × 0.4 × 150 = | | | 29 |
| **Maintenance** | | | |
| (See Table 11-8 for exact calculations) | 700 | 21 | 14 |
| **Fluid Schedule** | | | |
| First 24 hr | | | |
| 24-hr maintenance | 700 | 21 | 14 |
| $^1/_2$ FWD | 210 | | |
| Solute fluid and electrolyte deficit | 480 | 42 | 29 |
| First 24-hr total | 1390 | 63 | 43 |
| Second 24hr 24-hr maintenance | 700 | 21 | 14 |
| $^1/_2$ FWD | 210 | | |
| Second 24-hr total | 910 | 21 | 14 |

**Answer**

| Therefore, first 24hr: | Second 24 hr: |
|---|---|
| Rate: 1390 mL/24hr = 58 mL/hr | Rate: 910 mL/24 hr = 38 mL/hr |
| $Na^+$: 63 mEq/1.39 L = 45 mEq/L | $Na^+$: 21 mEq/0.91 L = 23 mEq/L |
| $K^+$: 43 mEq/1.39 L = 31 mEq/L | $K^+$: 14 mEq/0.91 L = 15 mEq/L |
| $D_5$ $^1/_4$ NS + 30 mEq/L KCl or | D5 $^1/_4$ NS + 10 mEq/L KCl or |
| K acetate @ 58 mL/hr × 24 hr | K acetate @ 38 mL/hr × 24 hr |

Follow serum $Na^+$ and adjust fluid composition and rate based on clinical response. The second half of the FWD may be replaced subsequently over the next 24 hr, or more rapidly depending on the rate of decline of serum $Na^+$ (avoid decline of >15 mEq/L in 24 hr).

**Note:** In severe hypernatremic dehydration initial lactated Ringer's/normal saline solution resuscitation boluses should be accounted for in order to minimize dropping serum sodium >15 mEq/L per 24 hr to minimize risk of cerebral edema.

### G. PARENTERAL FLUID COMPOSITION (Table 11-11)

### H. ORAL FLUID COMPOSITION (Tables 11-12 and 11-13)

## V. SERUM ELECTROLYTE DISTURBANCES

### A. POTASSIUM

**1. Hypokalemia:**

a. Etiologies and laboratory data (Table 11-14).

b. Clinical manifestations: Skeletal muscle weakness or paralysis, ileus, and cardiac arrhythmias.[4,5] Electrocardiogram (ECG) changes include

TABLE 11-11

**COMPOSITION OF FREQUENTLY USED PARENTERAL FLUIDS**

| Liquid | CHO (g/100 mL) | Protein* (g/100 mL) | Cal/L | $Na^+$ (mEq/L) | $K^+$ (mEq/L) | $Cl^-$ (mEq/L) | $HCO_3^{-}$† (mEq/L) | $Ca^{2+}$ (mEq/L) | mOsm/L |
|---|---|---|---|---|---|---|---|---|---|
| $D_5W$ | 5 | — | 170 | — | — | — | — | — | 252 |
| $D_{10}W$ | 10 | — | 340 | — | — | — | — | — | 505 |
| NS (0.9% NaCl) | — | — | — | 154 | — | 154 | — | — | 308 |
| 1/2 NS (0.45% NaCl) | — | — | — | 77 | — | 77 | — | — | 154 |
| $D_5$ 1/4 NS (0.225% NaCl) | 5 | — | 170 | 34 | — | 34 | — | — | 329 |
| 3% NaCl | — | — | — | 513 | — | 513 | — | — | 1027 |
| 8.4% sodium bicarbonate (1 mEq/mL) | — | — | — | 1000 | — | — | 1000 | — | 2000 |
| Ringer's solution | 0–10 | — | 0–340 | 147 | 4 | 155.5 | — | ≈4 | — |
| Lactated Ringer's | 0–10 | — | 0–340 | 130 | 4 | 109 | 28 | 3 | 273 |
| Amino acid 8.5% (Travasol) | — | 8.5 | 340 | 3 | — | 34 | 52 | — | 880 |
| Plasmanate | — | 5 | 200 | 110 | 2 | 50 | 29 | — | — |
| Albumin 25% (salt poor) | — | 25 | 1000 | 100–160 | — | <120 | — | — | 300 |
| Intralipid‡ | 2.25 | — | 1100 | 2.5 | 0.5 | 4.0 | — | — | 258–284 |

*Protein or amino acid equivalent.

†Bicarbonate or equivalent (citrate, acetate, lactate).

‡Values are approximate; may vary from lot to lot. Also contains <1.2% egg-phosphatides.

CHO, carbohydrate; $HCO_3^-$, bicarbonate; NS, normal saline.

TABLE 11-12

## ORAL REHYDRATION SOLUTIONS

| | CHO (g/dL) | $Na^+$ (mEq/L) | $K^+$ (mEq/L) | $Cl^-$ (mEq/L) | Base (mEq/L) | mOsm/kg $H_2O$ |
|---|---|---|---|---|---|---|
| Ceralyte | 4 | 70 | 20 | 60 | 30 | 220 |
| Infalyte | 3 | 50 | 25 | 45 | 30 | 200 |
| Naturalyte | 2.5 | 45 | 20 | 35 | 48 | 265 |
| Pedialyte | 2.5 | 45 | 20 | 35 | 30 | 250 |
| Rehydralyte | 2.5 | 75 | 20 | 65 | 30 | 310 |
| WHO Solution UNICEFORS* | 2 | 90 | 20 | 80 | 30 | 310 |

*Available from Jianas Bros. Packaging Co., 2533 SW Boulevard, Kansas City, MO 64108.
CHO, carbohydrate.

Data from Snyder J: A clinical pathway for pediatric gastroenteritis. Semin Pediatr Infect Dis 1994;5:231.



TABLE 11-13

## APPROXIMATE ELECTROLYTE COMPOSITION OF COMMONLY CONSUMED FLUIDS (NOT RECOMMENDED FOR ORAL REHYDRATION THERAPY)*

| | CHO (g/dL) | $Na^+$ (mEq/L) | $K^+$ (mEq/L) | $Cl^-$ (mEq/L) | $HCO_3^-$ (mEq/L) | mOsm/kg $H_2O$ |
|---|---|---|---|---|---|---|
| Apple juice | 11.9 | 0.4 | 26 | — | — | 700 |
| Coca-Cola | 10.9 | 4.3 | 0.1 | — | 13.4 | 656 |
| Gatorade | 5.9 | 21 | 2.5 | 17 | — | 377 |
| Ginger ale | 9 | 3.5 | 0.1 | — | 3.6 | 565 |
| Milk | 4.9 | 22 | 36 | 28 | 30 | 260 |
| Orange juice | 10.4 | 0.2 | 49 | — | 50 | 654 |

*Values vary slightly depending on source.

TABLE 11-14

## CAUSES OF HYPOKALEMIA

| | Decreased Stores | | |
|---|---|---|---|
| | Normal Blood Pressure | | |
| Hypertension | Renal | Extrarenal | Normal Stores |
| Renovascular disease | RTA | Skin losses | Metabolic alkalosis |
| Excess renin | Fanconi syndrome | GI losses | Increased insulin |
| Excess mineralocorticoid | Bartter syndrome | High CHO diet | Leukemia |
| Cushing syndrome | DKA | Enema abuse | $\beta_2$ Catecholamines |
| | Antibiotics | Laxative abuse | Familial hypokalemic periodic paralysis |
| | Diuretics | Anorexia nervosa | |
| | Amphotericin B | Malnutrition | |
| **LABORATORY DATA** | | | |
| ↑ Urine $K^+$ | ↑ Urine $K^+$ | ↓ Urine $K^+$ | ↑ Urine $K^+$ |

CHO, carbohydrate; DKA, diabetic ketoacidosis; GI, gastrointestinal; RTA, renal tubular acidosis.

delayed depolarization, with flat or absent T waves and, in extreme cases, U waves.

c. Diagnostic studies:
   (1) Blood: Electrolytes, with blood urea nitrogen/creatinine (BUN/Cr), creatine kinase (CK), glucose, renin, arterial blood gases (ABGs), cortisol
   (2) Urine: Urinalysis, $K^+$, $Na^+$, $Cl^-$, osmolality, 17-ketosteroids.
   (3) Other: ECG.

d. Management: Rapidity of treatment should be proportional to severity of symptoms.
   (1) Acute: Calculate electrolyte deficiency and replace with potassium acetate or potassium chloride. See Formulary for dosage information. Enteral replacement is safer when feasible, with less risk for iatrogenic hyperkalemia. Follow serum $K^+$ closely.
   (2) Chronic: Calculate daily requirements and replace with potassium chloride or potassium gluconate. See Formulary for dosage information.

2. **Hyperkalemia:**

a. See Table 11-15 for etiologies of hyperkalemia and Table 11-16 for clinical manifestations.

b. Management: Immediately stop all IV infusions containing potassium; see algorithm in Figure 11-2.
   (1) **Abnormal ECG** calls for rapid temporizing therapy: Antagonize the effect of $K^+$ on membrane potentials, and redistribute $K^+$ internally into cells.
   (2) **Normal ECG** calls for slow, long-term therapy: Remove $K^+$ from the body.

TABLE 11-15

CAUSES OF HYPERKALEMIA

| Increased Stores | | |
|---|---|---|
| Increased Urine $K^+$ | Decreased Urine $K^+$ | Normal Stores |
| Transfusion with aged blood | Renal failure | Tumor lysis syndrome |
| | Hypoaldosteronism | Leukocytosis (>100 K/μL) |
| Exogenous $K^+$ (e.g., salt substitutes) | Aldosterone insensitivity | Thrombocytosis (>750 K/μL) |
| | ↓ Insulin | Metabolic acidosis* |
| Spitzer syndrome | $K^+$-sparing diuretics | Blood drawing (hemolyzed sample) |
| | Congenital adrenal hyperplasia | Type IV RTA |
| | | Rhabdomyolysis/crush injury |
| | | Malignant hyperthermia |
| | | Theophylline intoxication |

*For every 0.1-unit reduction in arterial pH, there is an approximately 0.2–0.4 mEq/L increase in plasma $K^+$.

RTA, renal tubular acidosis.

TABLE 11-16

CLINICAL MANIFESTATIONS OF $K^+$ DISTURBANCES

| Serum $K^+$ (mEq/L) | ECG Changes | Other Symptoms |
|---|---|---|
| ~2.5 | AV conduction defect, prominent U wave, ventricular arrhythmia, ST-segment depression | Apathy, weakness, paresthesias |
| ~7.5 | Peaked T waves | Weakness, paresthesias |
| ~8.0 | Loss of P wave, widening of QRS | — |
| ~9.0 | ST-segment depression, further widening of QRS | Tetany |
| ~10 | Bradycardia, sine wave QRS-T, first-degree AV block, ventricular arrhythmias, cardiac arrest | — |

AV, atrioventricular; ECG, electrocardiogram.

Data from Feld LG et al: Pediatric fluid and electrolyte therapy. Adv Pediatr 1988;35:497–535.





## B. SODIUM

1. **Hyponatremia:**

a. Etiologies, diagnostic studies, and management (Table 11-17).

b. Factitious etiologies.

(1) Hyperlipidemia: $Na^+$ decreased by 0.002 × lipid (mg/dL).

(2) Hyperproteinemia: $Na^+$ decreased by 0.25 × [protein (g/dL) – 8].

(3) Hyperglycemia: $Na^+$ decreased 1.6 mEq/L for each 100-mg/dL rise in glucose.

2. **Hypernatremia: Etiologies, diagnostic studies, and management (Table 11-18).**

## C. CALCIUM

1. **Hypocalcemia:**

a. Etiologies (Box 11-2).

b. Clinical manifestations: Tetany, neuromuscular irritability with weakness, paresthesias, fatigue, cramping, altered mental status, seizures, laryngospasm, cardiac arrhythmias.[4,5]

(1) ECG changes (prolonged QT interval).

(2) Trousseau's sign (carpopedal spasm after aterial occlusion of an extremity for 3 min).

(3) Chvostek sign (muscle twitching with percussion of facial nerve).

c. Diagnostic studies:

(1) Blood: Total and ionized $Ca^{2+}$, alkaline phosphatase, $Mg^{2+}$, total protein, BUN, creatinine, 25-OH vitamin D.

(a) Albumin: $\Delta$ of 1 g/dL changes total serum $Ca^{2+}$ in the same direction by 0.8 mg/dL.

(b) pH: Acidosis increases ionized calcium.

(2) Urine: $Ca^{2+}$, phosphate, creatinine.

(3) Other: Chest x-ray (visualize thymus), ankle and wrist films (assess for rickets), ECG (calculate QT interval).

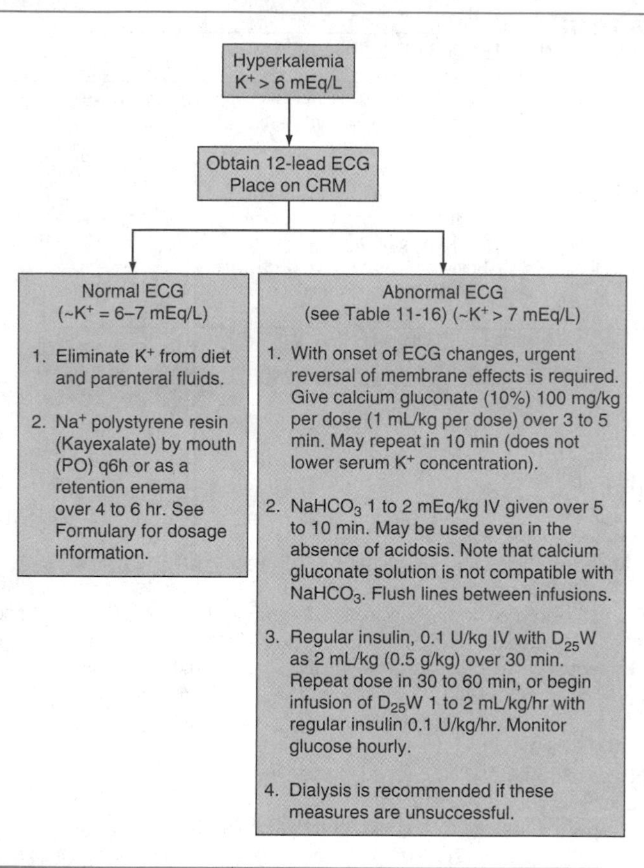


FIG. 11.2
Algorithm for hyperkalemia.

TABLE 11-17

HYPONATREMIA*

| Decreased Weight | | |
|---|---|---|
| **Renal Losses** | **Extrarenal Losses** | **Increased or Normal Weight** |
| $Na^+$-losing nephropathy | GI losses | Nephrotic syndrome |
| Diuretics | Skin losses | Congestive heart failure |
| Adrenal insufficiency | Third spacing | SIADH (see Table 10-7) |
| Cerebral salt-wasting syndrome | Cystic fibrosis | Acute/chronic renal failure |
| | | Water intoxications |
| | | Cirrhosis |
| | | Excess salt-free infusions |
| **LABORATORY DATA** | | |
| ↑ Urine $Na^+$ | ↓ Urine $Na^+$ | ↓ Urine $Na^{+\dagger}$ |
| ↑ Urine volume | ↓ Urine volume | ↓ Urine volume |
| ↓ Specific gravity | ↑ Specific gravity | ↑ Specific gravity |
| ↓ Urine osmolality | ↑ Urine osmolality | ↑ Urine osmolality |
| **MANAGEMENT** | | |
| Replace losses | Replace losses | Restrict fluids |
| Treat cause | Treat cause | Treat cause |

*Hyperglycemia and hyperlipidemia cause spurious hyponatremia.

†Urine $Na^+$ may be appropriate for level of $Na^+$ intake in patients with SIADH and water intoxication.

GI, gastrointestinal; SIADH, syndrome of inappropriate antidiuretic hormone secretion.

TABLE 11-18

HYPERNATREMIA

| Decreased Weight | | |
|---|---|---|
| **Renal Losses** | **Extrarenal Losses** | **Increased Weight** |
| Nephropathy | GI losses | Exogenous $Na^+$ |
| Diuretic use | Skin losses | Mineralocorticoid excess |
| Diabetes insipidus | Respiratory* | Hyperaldosteronism |
| Postobstructive diuresis | | |
| Diuretic phase of ATN | | |
| **LABORATORY DATA** | | |
| ↑ Urine $Na^+$ | ↓ Urine $Na^+$ | Relative ↓ urine $Na^{+\dagger}$ |
| ↑ Urine volume | ↓ Urine volume | Relative ↓ urine volume |
| ↓ Specific gravity | ↑ Specific gravity | Relative ↑ specific gravity |

**CLINICAL MANIFESTATIONS**

Predominantly neurologic symptoms: Lethargy, weakness, altered mental status, irritability, and seizures.[4,5] Additional symptoms may include muscle cramps, depressed deep tendon reflexes, and respiratory failure.

**MANAGEMENT**

Replace free water losses based on calculations in text and treat cause. Consider a natriuretic agent if there is increased weight.

*This cause of hypernatremia is usually secondary to free water loss, so that the fractional excretion of sodium may be decreased or normal.

†Exogenous $Na^+$ administration will cause an increase in the fractional excretion of sodium.

ATN, acute tubular necrosis; GI, gastrointestinal.

BOX 11-2

**ETIOLOGIES OF HYPOCALCEMIA AND HYPERCALCEMIA**

| HYPOCALCEMIA | HYPERCALCEMIA |
|---|---|
| Hypoparathyroidism | Hyperparathyroidism |
| Vitamin D deficiency | Vitamin D intoxication |
| Hyperphosphatemia | Excessive exogenous calcium administration |
| Pancreatitis | Malignancy |
| Malabsorption states (malnutrition) | Prolonged immobilization |
| Drugs (anticonvulsants, cimetidine, aminoglycosides, calcium channel blockers) | Thiazide diuretics |
| | Subcutaneous fat necrosis |
| | Williams syndrome |
| Hypomagnesemia/hypermagnesemia | Granulomatous disease (i.e., sarcoidosis) |
| Maternal hyperparathyroidism if patient is a neonate | Hyperthyroidism |
| | Milk-alkali syndrome |
| Calcitriol (activated vitamin D) insufficiency | |
| Tumor lysis syndrome | |
| Ethylene glycol ingestion | |

d. Management:
   (1) Acute: Consider IV replacement (calcium gluconate, calcium gluceptate, or calcium chloride [cardiac arrest dose]). See Formulary for dosage information.
   (2) Chronic: Consider use of oral supplements of calcium carbonate, calcium gluconate, calcium glubionate, or calcium lactate. See Formulary for dosage information.

e. Special considerations:
   (1) Symptoms of hypocalcemia that are refractory to $Ca^{2+}$ supplementation may be caused by hypomagnesemia.
   (2) Significant hyperphosphatemia should be corrected before correction of hypocalcemia because soft tissue calcification may occur if total $[Ca^{2+}] \times [PO_4^{3-}] \leq 80$.

**2. Hypercalcemia:**

a. Etiologies (see Box 11-2).

b. Clinical manifestations: Weakness, irritability, lethargy, seizures, coma, abdominal cramping, anorexia, nausea, vomiting, polyuria, polydipsia, renal calculi, pancreatitis, ECG changes (shortened QT interval).

c. Diagnostic studies:
   (1) Blood: Total and ionized $Ca^{2+}$, phosphate, alkaline phosphatase, total protein, albumin, BUN, creatinine, parathyroid hormone (PTH), vitamin D.
   (2) Urine: $Ca^{2+}$, phosphate, creatinine.
   (3) Other: ECG (calculate QT interval), KUB radiograph or renal ultrasound (assess for renal calculi).[6]

d. Management:
  (1) Treat the underlying disease.
  (2) Hydrate to increase urine output and $Ca^{2+}$ excretion. If glomerular filtration rate and blood pressure are stable, give NS with maintenance $K^+$ at two to three times maintenance rate until $Ca^{2+}$ is normalized.
  (3) Diuresis with furosemide.
  (4) Consider hemodialysis for severe or refractory cases.
  (5) Steroids may be indicated in malignancy, granulomatous disease, and vitamin D toxicity to decrease vitamin D and $Ca^{2+}$ absorption. Consult appropriate specialists before administering steroids for these conditions.
  (6) For severe or persistently elevated $Ca^{2+}$, give calcitonin or bisphosphonate in consultation with an endocrinologist.



## D. MAGNESIUM

### 1. Hypomagnesemia:

a. Etiologies (Box 11-3).
b. Clinical manifestations: Anorexia, nausea, weakness, malaise, depression, nonspecific psychiatric symptoms, hyperreflexia, carpopedal spasm, clonus, tetany, ECG changes (atrial and ventricular ectopy; torsades de pointes).

BOX 11-3

**ETIOLOGIES OF HYPOMAGNESEMIA AND HYPERMAGNESEMIA**

| Hypomagnesemia | Hypermagnesemia |
|---|---|
| **Increased urinary losses** | **Renal failure** |
| Diuretic use, renal tubular acidosis, hypercalcemia, chronic adrenergic stimulants, chemotherapy | **Excessive administration** |
| **Increased gastrointestinal losses** | Status asthmaticus, eclampsia/pre-eclampsia, cathartics, enemas, phosphate binders |
| Malabsorption syndromes, severe malnutrition, diarrhea, vomiting, short bowel syndromes, enteric fistulas | |
| **Endocrine etiologies** | |
| Diabetes mellitus, parathyroid hormone disorders, hyperaldosterone states | |
| **Decreased intake** | |
| Prolonged parenteral fluid therapy with $Mg^{2+}$-free solutions | |

c. Diagnostic studies:
   (1) Blood: $Mg^{2+}$, total and ionized $Ca^{2+}$.
   (2) Other: Consider evaluation for renal/gastrointestinal losses or endocrine etiologies.

d. Management:
   (1) Acute: Give magnesium sulfate. (See Formulary for dosing and side effects.)
   (2) Chronic: Magnesium oxide or magnesium sulfate. (See Formulary for dosing.)

**2. Hypermagnesemia:**

a. Etiologies (see Box 11-3).

b. Clinical manifestations: Depressed deep tendon reflexes, lethargy, confusion, respiratory failure (in extreme cases).

**Note** *Neonates born prematurely after tocolysis with magnesium sulfate are at high risk for respiratory sequelae, but serum magnesium levels tend to normalize within 72 hr.*

c. Diagnostic studies: $Mg^{2+}$, total and ionized $Ca^{2+}$, BUN, creatinine.

d. Management:
   (1) Stop supplemental $Mg^{2+}$.
   (2) Diuresis.
   (3) Give $Ca^{2+}$ supplements such as calcium chloride (use cardiac arrest doses), calcium gluceptate, or calcium gluconate. (See Formulary for dosing.)
   (4) Dialysis if life-threatening levels are present.

## E. PHOSPHATE

**1. Hypophosphatemia:**

a. Etiologies (Box 11-4).

b. Clinical manifestations: Symptomatic only at very low levels (<1 mg/dL) with irritability, paresthesias, confusion, seizures, myocardial depression, apnea in very low birth weight infants, and coma.

c. Diagnostic studies
   (1) Blood: Phosphate, total and ionized $Ca^{2+}$, BUN, creatinine, Na, K, $Mg^{2+}$. Consider PTH and vitamin D.
   (2) Urine: $Ca^{2+}$, phosphate, creatinine, pH.

**d. Management:**
   (1) Insidious onset of symptoms: Give oral potassium phosphate or sodium phosphate. (See Formulary for dosing.)
   (2) Acute onset of symptoms: Give IV potassium phosphate or sodium phosphate. (See Formulary for dosing.)

**2. Hyperphosphatemia**

a. Etiologies (see Box 11-4).

BOX 11-4

**ETIOLOGIES OF HYPOPHOSPHATEMIA AND HYPERPHOSPHATEMIA**

| Hypophosphatemia | Hyperphosphatemia |
|---|---|
| Starvation | Hypoparathyroidism (rarely in the absence of renal insufficiency) |
| Protein-energy malnutrition | Excessive administration of phosphate (PO, IV, or enemas) |
| Malabsorption syndromes | Tumor lysis syndrome |
| Intracellular shifts associated with respiratory or metabolic alkalosis | Reduction of glomerular filtration rate to <25% (may occur at smaller reductions in neonates) |
| Treatment of diabetic ketoacidosis | |
| Corticosteroid administration | |
| Increased renal losses (i.e., renal tubular defects, diuretic use) | |
| Vitamin D-deficient and vitamin D-resistant rickets | |
| Very-low-birth weight infants when intake does not meet demand | |



b. Clinical manifestations: Symptoms of the resulting hypocalcemia **(see page 315).**

c. Diagnostic studies:
   (1) Blood: Phosphate, total and ionized $Ca^{2+}$, BUN, creatinine, Na, K, $Mg^{2+}$. Consider PTH, vitamin D, complete blood count, ABGs.
   (2) Urine: $Ca^{2+}$, phosphate, creatinine, urinalysis.

d. Management:
   (1) Restrict dietary phosphate.
   (2) Give phosphate binders (calcium carbonate, aluminum hydroxide; use with caution in renal failure). (See Formulary for dosing.)
   (3) For cell lysis (with normal renal function), give an NS bolus and IV mannitol. See Chapter 22 for management of tumor lysis syndrome.
   (4) If patient has poor renal function, consider dialysis.

## VI. ACID-BASE/OSMOLAR GAP DISTURBANCES

### A. DEFINITIONS

1. **Serum osmolality: Number of particles per liter. Can be calculated as follows:**

$$2[Na^+] + \text{glucose (mg/dL)}/18 + \text{BUN (mg/dL)}/2.8$$

a. Normal range: 275 to 295 mOsm/L.

b. Serum osmolar gap = calculated serum osmolality – laboratory measured osmolality.

May be elevated in some anion gap acidosis, but a markedly elevated osmolar gap in the setting of an anion gap acidosis is highly suggestive of acute methanol or ethylene glycol intoxication.

2. **Anion gap (AG):** **Represents anions other than bicarbonate and chloride required to balance the positive charge of $Na^+$. $K^+$ is considered negligible in AG calculations. Clinically, it is calculated as follows:**

$$AG = Na^+ - (Cl^- + HCO_3^-)$$

$$(\text{Normal: } 12\ \text{mEq/L} \pm 2\ \text{mEq/L})$$

3. **Acidosis: pH <7.35:**

a. Respiratory acidosis: Occurs when $Pco_2$ is higher than normal (>45 mm Hg).

b. Metabolic acidosis: Occurs when arterial bicarbonate level is less than normal (<22 mmol/L).

4. **Alkalosis: pH >7.45:**

a. Respiratory alkalosis: Occurs when $Pco_2$ is lower than normal (<35 mm Hg).

b. Metabolic alkalosis: Occurs when arterial bicarbonate level is greater than normal (>26 mmol/L).

## B. RULES FOR DETERMINING PRIMARY ACID-BASE DISORDERS[7]

1. **Determine the pH:** **The body does not fully compensate for primary acid-base disorders; therefore, the primary disturbance will shift the pH away from 7.40. Examine the $Pco_2$ and $HCO_3^-$ to determine whether the primary disturbance is a metabolic acidosis/alkalosis or respiratory acidosis/alkalosis.**
2. **Calculate the anion gap:** **If the anion gap is ≤20 mmol/L, there is a primary metabolic acidosis regardless of pH or serum bicarbonate concentration. (The body does not generate a large anion gap to compensate for a primary disorder.)**
3. **Calculate the excess anion Gap (i.e., "ΔGap" or "Gap–Gap"):**

$$\Delta Gap = [\text{calculated anion gap} - \text{normal anion gap (i.e., 12) mmol/L}] + \text{measured } HCO_3^-$$

a. If the ΔGap is greater than a normal serum bicarbonate concentration (>30 mmol/L), there is an underlying metabolic alkalosis.

b. If the ΔGap is less than a normal bicarbonate concentration (<23 mmol/L), there is an underlying nonanion gap metabolic acidosis *(1 mmol of unmeasured acid titrates 1 mmol of bicarbonate) (+ anion gap* $-\Delta[HCO_3^-]$*).*

## C. ETIOLOGY OF ACID–BASE DISTURBANCES (Fig. 11-3)

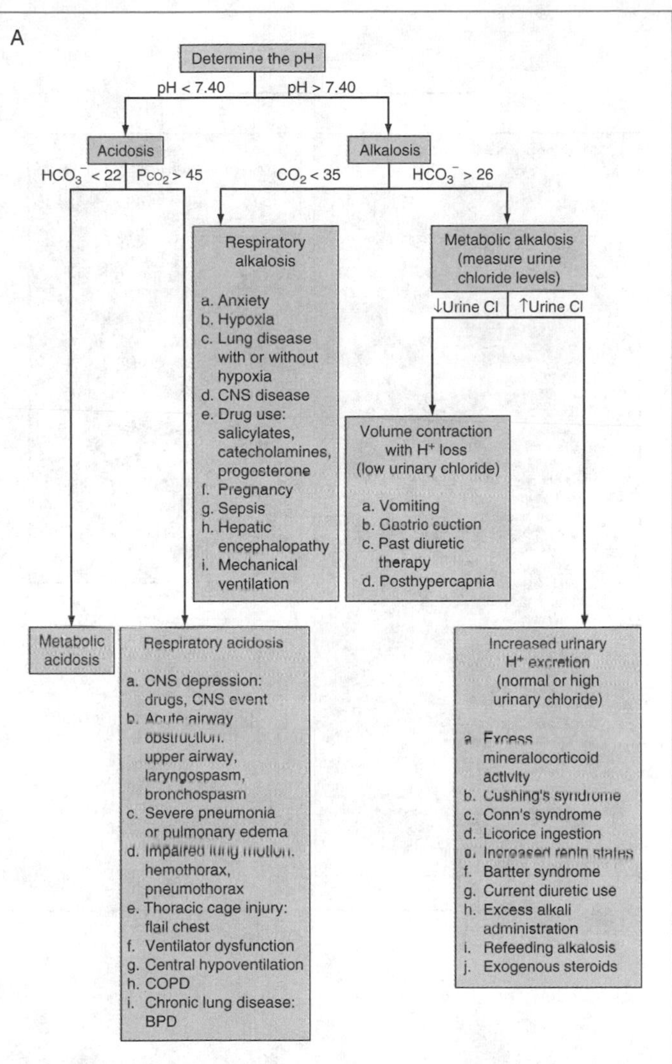


FIG. 11-3A

**A** and **B,** Etiology of acid-base disturbances.

*Continued*

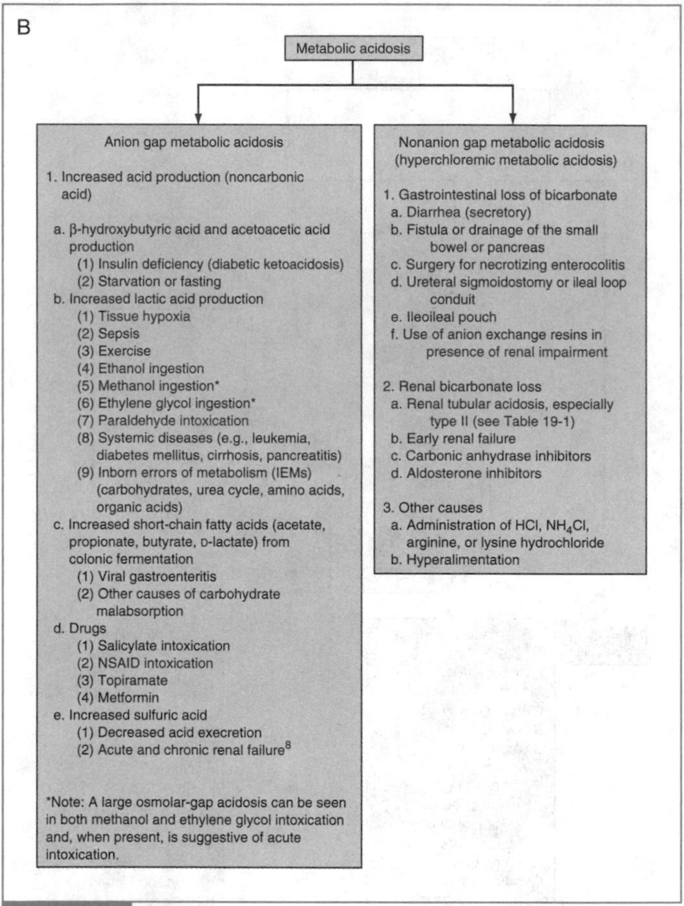

B

Metabolic acidosis

**Anion gap metabolic acidosis**

1. Increased acid production (noncarbonic acid)
   a. β-hydroxybutyric acid and acetoacetic acid production
      (1) Insulin deficiency (diabetic ketoacidosis)
      (2) Starvation or fasting
   b. Increased lactic acid production
      (1) Tissue hypoxia
      (2) Sepsis
      (3) Exercise
      (4) Ethanol ingestion
      (5) Methanol ingestion*
      (6) Ethylene glycol ingestion*
      (7) Paraldehyde intoxication
      (8) Systemic diseases (e.g., leukemia, diabetes mellitus, cirrhosis, pancreatitis)
      (9) Inborn errors of metabolism (IEMs) (carbohydrates, urea cycle, amino acids, organic acids)
   c. Increased short-chain fatty acids (acetate, propionate, butyrate, D-lactate) from colonic fermentation
      (1) Viral gastroenteritis
      (2) Other causes of carbohydrate malabsorption
   d. Drugs
      (1) Salicylate intoxication
      (2) NSAID intoxication
      (3) Topiramate
      (4) Metformin
   e. Increased sulfuric acid
      (1) Decreased acid execretion
      (2) Acute and chronic renal failure[8]

*Note: A large osmolar-gap acidosis can be seen in both methanol and ethylene glycol intoxication and, when present, is suggestive of acute intoxication.

**Nonanion gap metabolic acidosis (hyperchloremic metabolic acidosis)**

1. Gastrointestinal loss of bicarbonate
   a. Diarrhea (secretory)
   b. Fistula or drainage of the small bowel or pancreas
   c. Surgery for necrotizing enterocolitis
   d. Ureteral sigmoidostomy or ileal loop conduit
   e. Ileoileal pouch
   f. Use of anion exchange resins in presence of renal impairment

2. Renal bicarbonate loss
   a. Renal tubular acidosis, especially type II (see Table 19-1)
   b. Early renal failure
   c. Carbonic anhydrase inhibitors
   d. Aldosterone inhibitors

3. Other causes
   a. Administration of HCl, $NH_4Cl$, arginine, or lysine hydrochloride
   b. Hyperalimentation

FIG. 11-3B

## REFERENCES

1. Roberts KB: Fluids and electrolytes: Parenteral fluid therapy. Pediatr Rev 2001;22:380–387.
2. Nichols DG et al: Golden Hour: The Handbook of Advanced Pediatric Life Support. Philadelphia, Elsevier, 1996.
3. Moritz ML, Ayus JC: Prevention of hospital-acquired hyponatremia: A case for using isotonic saline. Pediatrics 2003;111:227–230.
4. Barkin R: Pediatric Emergency Medicine, 2nd ed. St. Louis, Mosby, 1997.
5. Feld LG et al: The approach to fluid and electrolyte therapy in pediatrics. Adv Pediatr 1988;35:497–535.
6. Fleisher G, Ludwig S, Henretig F: Textbook of Pediatric Emergency Medicine. Baltimore, Williams & Wilkins, 2005.
7. Haber RJ: A practical approach to acid-base disorders. West J Med 1991;155:146–151.
8. Segar WE: Parenteral fluid therapy. Curr Probl Pediatr 1972;3:23–40.
9. American Academy of Pediatrics: Practice parameter: The management of acute gastroenteritis in young children. Pediatrics 1996;97:424–431.
10. Saavedra J: Probiotics and infectious diarrhea. Am J Gastroenterol 2000;95:S16–S18.
11. Hanna J et al: The kidney in acid-base balance. Pediatr Clin North Am 1995;42(61):1365–1395.

# Gastroenterology

*Nicole E. Jordan, MD*

12

## I. WEBSITES

www.aap.org (American Academy of Pediatrics)
www.naspghan.org (North American Society for Pediatric Gastroenterology, Hepatology, and Nutrition)
www.acg.gi.org (American College of Gastroenterology)

## II. GASTROINTESTINAL EMERGENCIES

### A. GASTROINTESTINAL BLEEDING

Blood loss from the gastrointestinal (GI) tract occurs in four ways: Hematemesis, hematochezia, melena, and occult bleeding.

1. **Initial evaluation (Fig. 12-1):**
   a. Assess airway, breathing, and circulation and hemodynamic stability.
   b. Perform physical examination, looking for evidence of bleeding.
   c. Verify bleeding with rectal examination and/or testing of stool or emesis for occult blood. Obtain baseline laboratory tests. Consider the following laboratory studies: Complete blood count (CBC), prothrombin time/ partial thromboplastin time (PT/PTT), blood type and cross-match, reticulocyte count, blood smear, blood urea nitrogen/creatinine, electrolytes, and a panel to assess for disseminated intravascular coagulation.
   d. Consider gastric lavage to differentiate upper from lower GI bleeding and to assess for ongoing bleeding.
   e. Provide specific therapy based on assessment and site of bleeding.
   f. Begin initial fluid resuscitation with normal saline or lactated Ringer's solution. Consider transfusion if there is continued bleeding, symptomatic anemia, and/or a hematocrit level <20%. Initiate intravenous acid suppression therapy, preferably with a proton pump inhibitor (PPI).
2. **Differential diagnosis of GI bleeding:** Table 12-1.

### B. ACUTE ABDOMEN[1]

1. **Differential diagnosis:**
   a. GI source: Appendicitis, pancreatitis, intussusception, malrotation with volvulus, inflammatory bowel disease, gastritis, bowel obstruction, mesenteric lymphadenitis, irritable bowel syndrome, abscess, hepatitis, perforated ulcer, Meckel diverticulitis, cholecystitis, choledocholithiasis, constipation, gastroenteritis.
   b. Renal source: Urinary tract infection, pyelonephritis, nephrolithiasis.
   c. Gynecologic source: Ectopic pregnancy, ovarian cyst/torsion, pelvic inflammatory disease.
   d. Oncologic source: Wilms tumor, neuroblastoma, rhabdomyosarcoma, lymphoma.

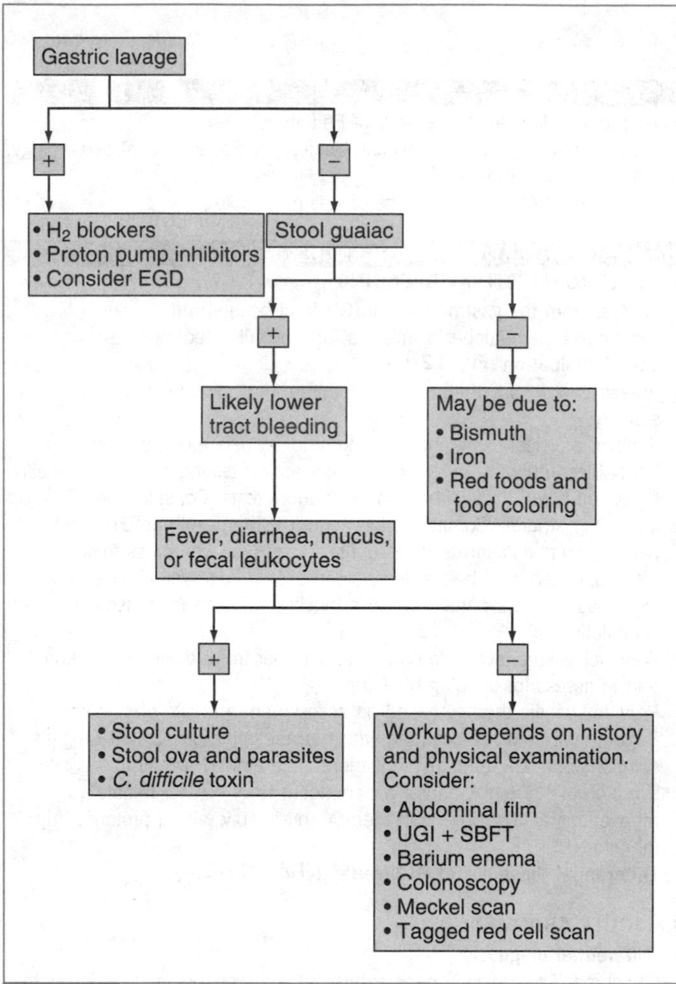


FIG. 12-1

Evaluation of GI bleeding. May use gastrostomy tube (G tube) if present; use nasogastric tube with caution if esophageal varices suspected. EGD, esophagogastroduodenoscopy; SBFT, small-bowel follow-through; UGI, upper gastrointestinal.

TABLE 12-1

DIFFERENTIAL DIAGNOSIS OF GI BLEEDING

| Age | Upper GI Tract | Lower GI Tract |
|---|---|---|
| Newborns (0–30 days) | Swallowed maternal blood<br>Gastritis | Necrotizing enterocolitis<br>Malrotation with midgut volvulus<br>Anal fissure<br>Hirschsprung disease |
| Infant (30 days–1 year) | Gastritis<br>Esophagitis<br>Peptic ulcer disease | Anal fissure<br>Allergic proctocolitis<br>Intussusception<br>Meckel's diverticulum<br>Lymphonodular hyperplasia<br>Intestinal duplication<br>Infectious colitis |
| Preschool (1–5 years) | Gastritis<br>Esophagitis<br>Peptic ulcer disease<br>Esophageal varices<br>Epistaxis | Juvenile polyps<br>Lymphonodular hyperplasia<br>Meckel's diverticulum<br>Hemolytic-uremic syndrome<br>Henoch-Schönlein purpura<br>Infectious colitis<br>Anal fissure |
| School age and adolescent | Esophageal varices<br>Peptic ulcer disease<br>Epistaxis<br>Gastritis | Inflammatory bowel disease<br>Infectious colitis<br>Juvenile polyps<br>Anal fissure<br>Hemorrhoids |

Modified from Pearl R: The approach to common abdominal diagnoses in infants and children. Part II. Pediatr Clin North Am 1998;45:1287–1326.

e. Other sources: Henoch-Schönlein purpura, pneumonia, sickle cell anemia, diabetic ketoacidosis, juvenile rheumatoid arthritis.

2. **Diagnosis:**

a. History: Course and characterization of pain, diarrhea, melena, hematochezia, fever, last oral intake, menstrual history, vaginal discharge/bleeding, urinary symptoms, and respiratory symptoms. Assess past GI history, travel history, and diet.

b. Physical examination:
   (1) General: Vital signs, toxicity, rashes, arthritis, jaundice.
   (2) Abdominal: Moderate to severe abdominal tenderness on palpation, rebound/guarding, rigidity, masses, change in bowel sounds.
   (3) Rectal: Include testing stool for occult blood.
   (4) Pelvic: Discharge, masses, adnexal/cervical motion tenderness.

3. **Studies:**

a. Radiology: First obtain plain abdominal radiographs to assess for obstruction, constipation, free air, gallstones, and kidney stones, and chest radiographs to check for pneumonia. Then consider abdominal/pelvic ultrasonography, abdominal spiral computed tomography with contrast (include rectal contrast for appendicitis evaluation), other contrast studies, and endoscopy.

b. Laboratory: Electrolytes, chemistry panel, CBC, liver and kidney function tests, coagulation studies, blood type and screen/cross-match, urinalysis, amylase, lipase, gonorrhea/chlamydia cultures (or polymerase chain reaction probes), beta-human chorionic gonadotropin (β-hCG), erythrocyte sedimentation rate (ESR), C-reactive protein.

4. **Management:**

a. Immediate: Patient should be placed on nothing by mouth (NPO) status. Begin rehydration. Consider nasogastric decompression, serial abdominal examinations, surgical/gynecologic/GI evaluation as indicated, pain control, and antibiotics as indicated.

b. Definitive: Surgical or endoscopic exploration as warranted.

## III. VOMITING

See Table 12-2 for evaluation of vomiting.

## IV. GASTROESOPHAGEAL REFLUX DISEASE[2]

Gastroesophageal reflux (GER) is passage of gastric contents into the esophagus, and gastroesophageal reflux disease (GERD) is defined as symptoms or complications of GER.

### A. DIAGNOSIS

1. **History and physical examination: Usually sufficient to reliably diagnose GER, identify complications, and initiate management.**
2. **Esophageal pH monitoring: Valid and reliable method of measuring acid reflux.**

TABLE 12-2

**EVALUATION OF VOMITING**

| Type | Etiology | Evaluation |
|---|---|---|
| Typically bilious | Obstruction<br>Intussusception<br>Malrotation ± volvulus<br>Pancreatitis<br>Intestinal dysmotility<br>Peritoneal adhesions<br>Incarcerated inguinal hernia<br>Intestinal atresia, stenosis<br>Superior mesenteric artery syndrome<br>Incarcerated inguinal hernia | Review feeding and medication history.<br>NG/OG tube for decompression if GI obstruction is suspected.<br>If bilious and/or hematemesis, consider surgical consultation.<br>BMP, CBC, ±UA, β-hCG, pancreatic enzymes.<br>Plain abdominal film with upright or cross-table lateral views to rule out obstruction, free air.<br>Abdominal ultrasound if pyloric stenosis is suspected.<br>Upper GI series to rule out pyloric stenosis, obstruction, anomalies snd evaluate GI motility.<br>Neurologic evaluation and imaging. |
| Typically nonbilious | Overfeeding<br>GERD<br>Milk-protein sensitivity<br>Infection (GU, respiratory, gastrointestinal)<br>Peptic disease<br>Drugs<br>Electrolyte imbalance<br>Eating disorders<br>Necrotizing enterocolitis<br>Metabolic abnormality<br>Pyloric stenosis<br>CNS lesion<br>Esophageal/gastric atresia, stenosis<br>Hirschsprung disease<br>Annular pancreas<br>Web<br>Pregnancy | Consider feeding modifications ± medications if GERD is suspected.<br>Avoid antiemetics unless specific, benign etiology is identified. |
| Either bilious or nonbilious | Ileus<br>Appendicitis | |

BMP, basic metabolic panel; CBC, complete blood count; CNS, central nervous system; GERD, gastroesophageal reflux disease hCG- human chorionic gonadotropin; NG/OG, nasogastric/orogastric; UA, urinalysis.

Modified from Saavedra J: Gastroenterology. In Seidel H et al (ed): Primary Care of the Newborn, 4th ed. St. Louis, Mosby, 2006, and Sondheimer JM: Vomiting. In Walker WA et al (eds): Pediatric Gastrointestinal Disease, 3rd ed. New York, BC Decker, 2000.

3. Esophageal impedance monitoring:[3] Combined with esophageal pH monitoring; by nature of its ability to detect both acid as well as nonacid reflux, impedance pH monitoring has greater sensitivity than pH monitoring alone in the detection of GER.
4. Upper GI series: Neither sensitive nor specific for GER but may be useful for the evaluation of anatomic abnormalities.

### B. TREATMENT OPTIONS

1. Diet: Milk-thickening agents (e.g., cereal) may decrease frequency of vomiting. Trial of hypoallergenic formula (e.g., protein hydrolysate) in formula-fed infants.
2. Lifestyle: Children and adolescents with GERD should avoid caffeine, chocolate, and spicy foods that provoke symptoms. Obesity, exposure to tobacco smoke, and alcohol are also associated with GER.
3. Acid-suppressant therapy: PPIs and histamine-2 receptor antagonists ($H_2$RAs) are effective in relieving symptoms and promoting mucosal healing when acid reflux is present. PPIs are superior to $H_2$RAs for this purpose.
4. Prokinetic therapy:[4,5] Literature supports use of erythromycin; if use of a prokinetic agent is warranted, erythromycin in combination with acid suppression should be considered. Current literature insufficient to either support or oppose use of metoclopramide for GERD in infants, and given lack of prospective controlled studies demonstrating metoclopramide's efficacy and safety in the treatment of GER in children, it should not be considered a treatment option.

## V. CELIAC DISEASE[6]

An immune-mediated enteropathy caused by a permanent sensitivity to gluten of the GI tract in genetically susceptible individuals.

### A. ASSOCIATED CONDITIONS

Increased occurrence in children with type 1 diabetes mellitus, autoimmune thyroiditis, Down syndrome, Turner syndrome, Williams syndrome, selective IgA deficiency, and in first-degree relatives of those with celiac disease.

### B. SYMPTOMS

Variable GI presentations, including diarrhea, vomiting, abdominal pain, constipation, abdominal distension, and failure to thrive. Non-GI symptoms include dermatitis herpetiformis, dental enamel hypoplasia of permanent teeth, osteoporosis, short stature, delayed puberty, and iron-deficient anemia resistant to oral iron.

### C. DIAGNOSIS

Measurement of IgA antibody to human recombinant tissue transglutaminase (TTG) recommended for initial testing. Measurement of

IgA antibody to endomysium (EMA) is observer dependent and therefore more subject to interpretation error and added cost. Because of inferior accuracy of antigliadin antibody tests (AGA), use of AGA IgA and AGA IgG test is no longer recommended. Those with IgA deficiency will not have abnormally elevated levels of TTG IgA or EMA IgA; therefore, measurement of quantitative serum IgA can facilitate interpretation when TTG IgA is low. If known selective IgA deficiency and symptoms are suggestive of celiac disease, testing with TTG IgG recommended. Confirmation requires an intestinal biopsy in all cases with findings of villous atrophy as a characteristic histopathologic feature.

### D. MANAGEMENT

Gluten-free diet for life remains the only scientifically proven treatment available.



## VI. EVALUATION OF LIVER TESTS

### A. STUDY RESULTS SUGGESTIVE OF LIVER CELL INJURY

Elevation of aspartate aminotransferase, alanine aminotransferase, lactate dehydrogenase.

### B. STUDY RESULTS SUGGESTIVE OF CHOLESTASIS

Increased bilirubin, urobilinogen, γ-glutamyltransferase, alkaline phosphatase, 5′-nucleotidase, serum bile acids.

### C. TESTS OF SYNTHETIC FUNCTION

Albumin, prealbumin, PT, activated PTT, cholesterol. Elevated $NH_3$ is evidence of decreased ability to detoxify ammonia. See Table 12-3 for evaluation and interpretation of liver tests.

## VII. HYPERBILIRUBINEMIA[7,8]

Bilirubin is the product of hemoglobin metabolism. There are two forms: direct (conjugated) and indirect (unconjugated). Hyperbilirubinemia is usually the result of increased hemoglobin load, reduced hepatic uptake, reduced hepatic conjugation, or decreased excretion. Direct hyperbilirubinemia is defined as direct bilirubin >20% of total or direct bilirubin >2 mg/dL. See Box 12-1 for differential diagnosis of hyperbilirubinemia. Refer to Chapter 18 for evaluation and treatment of newborn hyperbilirubinemia.

## VIII. DIARRHEA[9]

### A. DEFINITION

Usual stool output is 10 g/kg/day in children and 200 g/day in adults. Diarrhea is characterized by passage of loose or watery stools. The volume of fluid lost through stools can vary from 10 mL/kg/day (approximately normal) to >200 mL/kg/day. Acute diarrhea is >3 loose or watery stools per day. Chronic diarrhea is diarrhea lasting more than 14 days.

TABLE 12-3

**EVALUATION OF LIVER FUNCTION TESTS**

| Enzyme | Source | Increased | Decreased | Comments |
|---|---|---|---|---|
| AST/ALT | Liver<br>Heart<br>Skeletal muscle<br>Pancreas<br>RBCs<br>Kidney | Hepatocellular injury<br>Rhabdomyolysis<br>Muscular dystrophy<br>Hemolysis<br>Liver cancer | Vitamin $B_6$ deficiency<br>Uremia | ALT more specific than AST for liver<br>AST > ALT in hemolysis<br>AST/ALT >2 in 90% of alcohol disorders in adults |
| Alkaline phosphatase | Liver<br>Osteoblasts<br>Small intestine<br>Kidney<br>Placenta | Hepatocellular injury<br>Bone growth, disease, trauma<br>Pregnancy<br>Familial | Low phosphate<br>Wilson disease<br>Zinc deficiency<br>Hypothyroidism<br>Pernicious anemia | Highest in cholestatic conditions<br>Must be differentiated from bone source |
| GGT | Bile ducts<br>Renal tubules<br>Pancreas<br>Small intestine<br>Brain | Cholestasis<br>Newborn period<br>Induced by drugs | Estrogen therapy<br>Artificially low in hyperbilirubinemia | Not found in bone<br>Increased in 90% primary liver disease<br>Biliary obstruction<br>Intrahepatic cholestasis<br>Induced by alcohol<br>Specific for hepatobiliary disease in nonpregnant patient |
| 5′-NT | Liver cell membrane<br>Intestine<br>Brain<br>Heart<br>Pancreas | Cholestasis | | Specific for hepatobiliary disease in nonpregnant patient |
| $NH_3$ | Bowel<br>Bacteria<br>Protein metabolism | Hepatic disease secondary to urea cycle dysfunction<br>Hemodialysis<br>Valproic acid therapy<br>Urea cycle enzyme deficiency<br>Organic acidemia and carnitine deficiency | | Converted to urea in liver |

AST/ALT, aspartate aminotransferase/alanine aminotransterase; 5′-NT, 5′-nucleotidase; GGT, γ-glutamyl transpeptidase; RBCs, red blood cells.

BOX 12-1

**DIFFERENTIAL DIAGNOSIS OF HYPERBILIRUBINEMIA**

INDIRECT HYPERBILIRUBINEMIA

**Transient Neonatal Jaundice**
Breast milk jaundice
Physiologic jaundice
Polycythemia
Reabsorption of extravascular blood

**Hemolytic Disorders**
Autoimmune disease
Blood group incompatibility
Hemoglobinopathies
Microangiopathies
Red cell enzyme deficiencies
Red cell membrane disorders

**Enterohepatic Recirculation**
Cystic fibrosis
Hirschsprung disease
Ileal atresia
Pyloric stenosis

**Disorders of Bilirubin Metabolism**
Acidosis
Crigler-Najjar syndrome
Gilbert syndrome
Hypothyroidism
Hypoxia

**Miscellaneous**
Dehydration
Drugs
Hypoalbuminemia
Sepsis

DIRECT HYPERBILIRUBINEMIA

**Biliary Obstruction**
Biliary atresia
Choledochal cyst
Fibrosing pancreatitis
Gallstones or biliary sludge
Inspissated bile syndrome
Neoplasm
Primary sclerosing cholangitis

**Infection**
Cholangitis
Cytomegalovirus
Epstein-Barr virus
Herpes simplex virus

*Continued*

BOX 12-1

**DIFFERENTIAL DIAGNOSIS OF HYPERBILIRUBINEMIA—cont'd**

DIRECT HYPERBILIRUBINEMIA—cont'd

Histoplasmosis
Human immunodeficiency virus
Leptospirosis
Liver abscess
Sepsis
Syphilis
Toxocariasis
Toxoplasmosis
Tuberculosis
Urinary tract infection
Varicella-zoster virus
Viral hepatitis

**Genetic/Metabolic Disorders**

$\alpha_1$-Antitrypsin deficiency
Alagille syndrome
Caroli disease
Cystic fibrosis
Dubin-Johnson syndrome
Galactokinase deficiency
Galactosemia
Glycogen storage disease
Hereditary fructose intolerance
Hypothyroidism
Niemann-Pick disease
Rotor syndrome
Tyrosinemia
Wilson disease

**Chromosomal Abnormalities**

Trisomy 18
Trisomy 21
Turner syndrome

**Drugs**

Acetaminophen
Aspirin
Erythromycin
Ethanol
Iron
Isoniazid
Methotrexate
Oxacillin
Rifampin

| BOX 12-1 |
|---|
| **DIFFERENTIAL DIAGNOSIS OF HYPERBILIRUBINEMIA—cont'd** |
| DIRECT HYPERBILIRUBINEMIA—cont'd |
| **Drugs—cont'd** |
| Steroids |
| Sulfonamides |
| Tetracycline |
| Vitamin A |
| **Miscellaneous** |
| Neonatal hepatitis syndrome |
| Parenteral alimentation |
| Reye syndrome |



## B. ETIOLOGY

1. Diarrhea may be infectious or malabsorptive, and the mechanism is either osmotic or secretory. Underlying etiology should be determined to further assist in management.
2. Osmotic diarrhea: Stool volume depends on diet and decreases with fasting (fecal ion gap ≥100 mOsm/kg).
3. Secretory diarrhea: Stool volume is increased and does not vary with diet (fecal ion gap <100 mOsm/kg).

## C. MANAGEMENT

1. Oral rehydration therapy (ORT): Mainstay of initial management regardless of etiology. Parenteral hydration is indicated in severe dehydration, hemodynamic instability, or failure of ORT. See Chapter 11 for oral rehydration solutions and for calculation of deficit and maintenance fluid requirements.
2. Diet: Breast-feeding should continue, and regular diet should be restarted as soon as the patient is rehydrated, unless found to be the source of the diarrhea (e.g., gluten in CD, lactose in lactose intolerance).
3. Other: Nonspecific antidiarrheal agents (e.g., adsorbents such as kaolin-pectin), antimotility agents (e.g., loperamide), antisecretory drugs, and toxin binders (e.g., cholestyramine) have limited data regarding efficacy. If infectious, antimicrobial therapy may be indicated. If malabsorptive disorder (e.g., celiac disease, inflammatory bowel disease), therapy should be tailored to that disease process (e.g., gluten-free diet, steroids). Probiotics (defined as live microorganisms in fermented foods that promote optimal health by establishing an improved balance in intestinal microflora) are not regulated by the federal government and limited data are available on their use.

## IX. CONSTIPATION AND ENCOPRESIS[10]

### A. DEFINITIONS

1. Constipation: A delay or difficulty in defecation, present for 2 or more weeks. The most common cause is functional, without objective evidence of a pathologic condition. See Box 12-2 for differential diagnosis of constipation.
2. Encopresis: Leakage of stool around impaction. This occurs with chronic constipation, in which there is a loss of sensation in the distended rectal vault.
3. Goal of treatment of functional constipation: Weaning of medication once normal colorectal sensation and stooling patterns have been established. The general approach includes the following steps:

### B. DISIMPACTION (2–5 DAYS)

1. Fecal impaction: A hard mass in lower abdomen identified during physical examination, a dilated rectum filled with large amount of stool found during rectal examination, or excessive stool in the colon identified by abdominal radiography.
2. Oral/nasogastric approach: Shown to be effective when magnesium citrate, oral phosphate soda, and polyethylene glycol (PEG) electrolyte solutions are used.
3. Rectal approach: May be performed with phosphate soda enemas, saline enemas, or mineral oil enemas. Use of soap suds, tap water, and magnesium enemas is not recommended because of their potential toxicity. Rectal disimpaction has also been performed with glycerin suppositories in infants and bisacodyl suppositories in older children although they may be less effective than enemas.

### C. MAINTENANCE THERAPY (USUALLY 3–12 MONTHS)

1. Focuses on the prevention of recurrence; consists of dietary interventions, behavioral modifications, and medications to ensure that bowel movements occur at normal intervals with good evacuation. Only when regular bowel movements have been achieved should gradual discontinuation of maintenance therapy be considered.
2. Dietary changes: Include increased intake of fluids and absorbable and nonabsorbable carbohydrate as a method to soften stools. A balanced diet that includes whole grains, fruits, and vegetables is recommended. Data to support a definitive recommendation for fiber supplementation in the treatment of constipation are too weak.
3. Behavioral modifications: Include regular toilet habits, positive reinforcement, and proper positioning on toilet with stable seating, feet firmly planted, and knees and hips at 90-degree angles. Referral to a mental health care provider may be helpful in situations in which

BOX 12-2

**DIFFERENTIAL DIAGNOSIS OF CONSTIPATION**

FUNCTIONAL

**Developmental**
Attention deficit disorders
Cognitive handicaps

**Situational**
Excessive parental interventions
School bathroom avoidance
Sexual abuse
Toilet phobia

**Depression**

**Constitutional**
Colonic inertia
Genetic predisposition

**Reduced Stool Volume and Dryness**
Dehydration
Low fiber in diet
Underfeeding or malnutrition

NONFUNCTIONAL

**Anatomic Malformations**
Anal stenosis
Anterior displaced anus
Imperforate anus
Pelvic mass (e.g., sacral teratoma)

**Metabolic and Gastrointestinal**
Cystic fibrosis
Diabetes mellitus
Gluten enteropathy
Hypercalcemia
Hypokalemia
Hypothyroidism
Multiple endocrine neoplasia type 2B

**Neuropathic Conditions**
Neurofibromatosis
Spinal cord abnormalities
Spinal cord trauma
Static encephalopathy
Tethered cord

**Intestinal Nerve or Muscle Disorders**
Hirschsprung disease
Intestinal neuronal dysplasia
Visceral myopathies
Visceral neuropathies

*Continued*

BOX 12-2

**DIFFERENTIAL DIAGNOSIS OF CONSTIPATION—cont'd**

**NONFUNCTIONAL—cont'd**

**Abnormal Abdominal Musculature**

Down syndrome

Gastroschisis

Prune belly

**Connective Tissue Disorders**

Ehlers-Danlos syndrome

Scleroderma

Systemic lupus erythematosus

**Drugs**

Antacids

Anticholinergics

Antidepressants

Antihypertensives

Opiates

Phenobarbital

Sucralfate

Sympathomimetics

**Other**

Botulism

Cow's milk protein intolerance

Heavy-metal ingestion (lead)

Vitamin D intoxication

Modified from Constipation Guideline Committee of the North American Society for Pediatric Gastroenterology, Hepatology and Nutrition: Evaluation and treatment of constipation in infants and children. J Pediatr Gastroenterol Nutr 2006;43:e1–e13.

**motivational or behavioral problems are interfering with successful treatment.**

4. **Medications: PEG (osmotic laxatives), lactulose, magnesium hydroxide, or sorbitol is recommended. Prolonged use of stimulant laxatives not recommended.**

## D. SPECIAL CONSIDERATIONS IN INFANTS <1 YEAR OF AGE

Increased intake of fluids, particularly of juices containing sorbitol, such as prune, pear, and apple juices, is recommended within the context of a healthy diet. Barley malt extract, corn syrup, lactulose, or sorbitol can be used as stool softeners. Mineral oil, stimulant laxatives, and phosphate enemas are not recommended. Glycerin suppositories can be useful, and enemas are to be avoided.

## X. PANCREATITIS[11]

Inflammatory disease of the pancreas; falls into two major categories, acute and chronic.

### A. ACUTE PANCREATITIS

1. Defined clinically as sudden onset of abdominal pain associated with rise of pancreatic digestive enzymes in serum or urine with or without radiographic changes in the pancreas. It is a reversible process. Although it is not common in children, when it does occur, most common causes are trauma, multisystem disease, and idiopathic. See Box 12-3 for conditions associated with acute pancreatitis.
2. Diagnosis depends on typical clinical manifestations (e.g., abdominal pain, anorexia, nausea, vomiting, ascites, localized epigastric tenderness, Gray-Turner sign, Cullen's sign), increased serum concentrations of pancreatic enzymes (3 to 4 times above the upper limits of normal), and sonographic or radiologic evidence of pancreatic inflammation.



### B. CHRONIC PANCREATITIS

Defined clinically as a condition characterized by recurring or persisting abdominal pain, with development of pancreatic exocrine or endocrine insufficiency in some patients. It produces irreversible changes in the architecture and function of the pancreas and is a progressive process. Two major morphologic forms: calcific and obstructive. See Box 12-4 for proposed etiologies of chronic pancreatitis in childhood. Common complications include chronic pain, malnutrition, malabsorption, and diabetes mellitus.

### C. MANAGEMENT

The treatment of acute exacerbations of both acute and chronic pancreatitis includes pancreatic rest and entails nasogastric decompression, analgesia, IV fluid hydration, and oral intake restriction. Antibiotics are only indicated in the most severe cases.

## XI. MISCELLANEOUS TESTS

### A. OCCULT BLOOD

1. **Purpose:** To screen for the presence of blood through detection of heme in stool.
2. **Method:** Smear a small amount of stool on the test areas of an occult blood test card and allow to air dry. Apply developer as directed.
3. **Interpretation:** A blue color resembling that of the control indicates the presence of heme. Brisk transit of ingested red meat and inorganic iron may yield a false-positive result. Fruits and vegetables associated with false-positive results include cantaloupes, radishes, bean sprouts, cauliflower, broccoli, and grapes. Screening for the

BOX 12-3

**CONDITIONS ASSOCIATED WITH ACUTE PANCREATITIS**

**SYSTEMIC DISEASES**

**Infections**
Coxsackie
Epstein-Barr
Hepatitis
Influenza A or B
Leptospirosis
Mycoplasma
Rubella
Typhoid fever
Varicella

**Inflammatory and Vasculitic Disorders**
Collagen vascular diseases
Hemolytic uremic syndrome
Henoch-Schönlein purpura
Inflammatory bowel disease
Kawasaki disease

**Sepsis/Peritonitis/Shock**

**Transplantation**

**MECHANICAL/STRUCTURAL**

**Trauma**
Blunt trauma
Child abuse
ERCP

**Perforation**

**Anomalies**
Choledochal cyst
Pancreatic divisum
Stenosis
Other

**Obstruction**
Parasites
Stones
Tumors

**METABOLIC AND TOXIC FACTORS**

**Cystic Fibrosis**

**Diabetes Mellitus**

**Drugs/Toxins**
Chlorothiazides
Furosemide
Tetracyclines
Sulfonamides
Valproic acid
6-Mercaptopurine

BOX 12-3

**CONDITIONS ASSOCIATED WITH ACUTE PANCREATITIS—cont'd**

| METABOLIC AND TOXIC FACTORS—CONT'D |
|---|
| Hypercalcemia |
| Hyperlipidemia |
| Hypothermia |
| Malnutrition |
| Organic Acidemia |
| Renal Disease |

ERCP, endoscopic retrograde cholangiopancreatography

Modified from Robertson MA: Pancreatitis. In Walker WA et al (eds): Pediatric Gastrointestinal Disease, 3rd ed. New York, BC Decker, 2000, pp 1321–1344.



BOX 12-4

**PROPOSED ETIOLOGIES OF CHRONIC PANCREATITIS IN CHILDHOOD**

| CALCIFIC |
|---|
| Cystic fibrosis |
| Hereditary pancreatitis |
| Hypercalcemia |
| Hyperlipidemia |
| Idiopathic |
| Juvenile tropical pancreatitis |
| **OBSTRUCTIVE (NONCALCIFIC)** |
| Congenital anomalies |
| Idiopathic fibrosing pancreatitis |
| Renal disease |
| Sclerosing cholangitis |
| Sphincter of Oddi dysfunction |
| Trauma |

Modified from Robertson MA: Pancreatitis. In Walker WA et al (eds): Pediatric Gastrointestinal Disease, 3rd ed. New York, BC Decker, 2000, pp 1321–1344.

**presence of blood in gastric aspirates or vomitus should be performed using Gastroccult, not stool Hemoccult, cards.**

## B. QUANTITATIVE FECAL FAT

1. **Purpose:** **To screen for fat malabsorption by quantitating fecal fat excretion.**
2. **Method:** **Patient should be on a normal diet (35% fat) with the amount of calories and fat ingested recorded for 2 days before the test and during the test itself. Collect and freeze all stools passed within 72 hours, and send to the laboratory for determination of total fecal fatty acid content.**
3. **Interpretation**

a. Total fecal fatty acid excretion of >5 g fat per 24 hours may suggest malabsorption. Results will vary with amount of fat ingested, and normal values have not been established for children <2 years old.

b. The coefficient of absorption (CA) is a more accurate indicator of fat malabsorption and does not vary with fat intake:

$$CA = (\text{grams of fat ingested} - \text{grams of fat excreted})/(\text{grams of fat ingested}) \times 100$$

Infants <6 months of age should absorb >85% of fat intake. By age 1 year, the fat absorption should be at an adult level of >95%. Quantitative fecal fat is recommended over qualitative methods (e.g., staining with Sudan III), which depend on spot checks and are thus unreliable for diagnosing fat malabsorption.

## REFERENCES

1. Moir CR: Abdominal pain in infants and children. Mayo Clin Proc 1996;71(10):984–989.
2. Rudolph CD et al: Guidelines for evaluation and treatment of gastroesophageal reflux in infants and children: Recommendations of the North American Society for Pediatric Gastroenterology and Nutrition. J Pediatr Gastroenterol Nutr 2001;32:S1–S31.
3. Hirano I et al: ACG practice guidelines: Esophageal reflux testing. Am J Gastroenterol 2007;102:668–685.
4. Chicella MF et al: Prokinetic drug therapy in children: A review of current options. Ann Pharmacother 2005;39:706–711.
5. Hibbs AM et al: Metoclopramide for the treatment of gastroesophageal reflux disease in infants: A systematic review. Pediatrics 2006;118:746–752.
6. Hill ID et al: Guideline for the diagnosis and treatment of celiac disease in children: Recommendations of the North American Society for Pediatric Gastroenterology, Hepatology and Nutrition. J Pediatr Gastroenterol Nutr 2005;40:1–19.
7. Harb R et al: Conjugated hyperbilirubinemia: Screening and treatment in older infants and children. Pediatr Rev 2007;28:83–91.
8. Moyer V et al: Guideline for the evaluation of cholestatic jaundice in infants: Recommendations of the North American Society for Pediatric Gastroenterology, Hepatology and Nutrition. J Pediatr Gastroenterol Nutr 2004;39:115–128.

9. King CK et al: Managing acute gastroenteritis among children: Oral rehydration, maintenance, and nutritional therapy. MMWR Recomm Rep 2003;52:1–16.
10. Constipation Guideline Committee of the North American Society for Pediatric Gastroenterology, Hepatology and Nutrition: Evaluation and treatment of constipation in infants and children: Recommendations of the North American Society for Pediatric Gastroenterology, Hepatology and Nutrtion. J Pediatr Gastroenterol Nutr 2006;43:e1–e13.
11. Lowe ME: Pancreatitis in childhood. Curr Gastroenterol Rep 2004;6:240–246.

# Genetics

*Linda Hayrapetian-Dorsi, MD*

When evaluating a child for a genetic disorder, the three-generation pedigree is a valuable tool. Specifically ask about family history of neonatal or childhood deaths, mental retardation, developmental delay, birth defects, seizure disorders, known genetic disorders, ethnicity, consanguinity, infertility, miscarriages, and stillbirths.



## I. WEBSITES

http://genes-r-us.uthscsa.edu/resources.htm (National Newborn Screening and Genetics Resource Center)

www.ncbi.nlm.nih.gov/omim (Online Mendelian Inheritance in Man [OMIM] website). Includes a search engine for identifying genetic diseases based on clinical phenotype, gene, and OMIM number.

www.genetests.org. Includes information on genetic diagnostic tests, genetic clinics in the United States and laboratories that perform genetic testing.

www.acmg.net/resources/policies/ACT/condition-analyte-links.htm. Includes ACT sheets and algorithm to help guide physicians after a positive newborn metabolic screen.

www.rarediseases.org (National Organization for Rare Disorders)

## II. NEWBORN METABOLIC SCREEN[1-3]

All states screen for phenylketonuria, hypothyroidism, galactosemia, and hemoglobinopathies. (For a list of screening tests and number of states that use each test, see website: http://genes-r-us.uthscsa.edu/resources.htm.)

### A. TIMING

Screen all infants before hospital discharge.

1. **Normal term infants: Screen as close as possible to hospital discharge, and preferably after at least 24 hours of normal protein and lactose feeding. Formula-fed infants may not have a diagnostic abnormality before 36 hours of age. Breast-fed infants may not have a diagnostic abnormality before 48 to 72 hours of age.**
2. **Premature or ill infants: Perform initial screen at or near 7 days of age regardless of feeding status and repeat screen at 28 days of age or at hospital discharge, whichever comes first.**
3. **All infants should be screened by 7 days of age. If first screen is before 24 hours of age, send repeat by 14 days of age. Most geneticists recommend rescreening all infants 2–4 weeks of age.**

### B. RESULTS

1. **Positive results: Immediate follow-up and confirmatory testing, including more specific testing for the particular disease. If a genetic**

disease is suspected, a consult with a geneticist is recommended. See ACT sheets for more information (www.acmg.net/resources/policies/ACT/condition-analyte-links.htm).

2. Negative results: **A normal newborn screen does not imply that there are no genetic abnormalities.**

## III. MANAGEMENT OF GENETIC DISEASES WITH ACUTE PRESENTATION: INBORN ERRORS OF METABOLISM[1,2,4,5]

Inborn errors of metabolism (IEMs) may present any time from the neonatal period to adulthood. Although often thought of as rare, when considered collectively, these disorders represent significant treatable causes of morbidity and mortality.

### A. PRESENTATIONS

1. Neonatal onset: Often presents with anorexia, lethargy, vomiting, seizures, and/or shock. Symptoms often develop at 24–72 hours of age. One in five sick full-term neonates with no risk factors for infection will have metabolic disease.
2. Late onset (>28 days old): Some IEMs characteristically present late, whereas other IEMs may present late if the defect is partial.
   a. Typical findings: Failure to thrive, developmental delay, vomiting, respiratory distress, psychomotor abnormalities, and changes in mental status, including confusion, lethargy, irritability, aggressive behavior, hallucinations, seizures, and coma.
   b. Symptoms are usually brought on by intercurrent illness, prolonged fast, dietary indiscretion, or any process causing increased catabolism.

### B. EVALUATION OF SUSPECTED METABOLIC DISEASE

1. For laboratory tests recommended to detect IEMs, see Box 13-1. For sample collection requirements, see Table 13-1.
2. If the initial evaluation is suspicious for metabolic disease, obtain further testing as listed in Box 13-1 and consult a geneticist. Early diagnosis and appropriate therapy are essential for preventing irreversible brain damage and death.

### C. DIFFERENTIAL DIAGNOSIS

1. Differential diagnosis of hyperammonemia (Fig. 13-1).
2. Differential diagnosis of hypoglycemia (see section III.E).
3. Positive urine reducing substances (Box 13-2).

### D. GENERAL ACUTE MANAGEMENT OF INBORN ERRORS OF METABOLISM

1. Stop dietary sources of protein.
2. Start intravenous (IV) fluids: 10% dextrose (D10) at 1.5 to 2 times maintenance dose delivers 10 to 15 mg/kg/min of glucose to stop catabolism. Add $Na^+/K^+$ based on the degree of dehydration and

electrolyte levels. In severe dehydration, give a normal saline bolus in addition to $D_{10}$ at 1.5 to 2 times the maintenance dose.

3. Provide $HCO_3^-$ replacement for severe acidosis (pH <7.1) only.
4. In cases of hyperammonemia, the following drugs may be used only in consultation with a geneticist (overdoses may be lethal): Sodium benzoate 250 mg/kg (5.5 g/m$^2$) IV; sodium phenylacetate 250 mg/kg (5.5 g/m$^2$) IV; and arginine HCl (10% solution) 6 mL/kg (12 g/m$^2$) IV. Give these doses as a bolus over 90 min. Repeat the same doses over 24 hours as a maintenance dose. Ondansetron may be used to decrease nausea and vomiting associated with these drugs. (Benzoate and phenylacetate are substrates for alternate pathways of nitrogen excretion; arginine supplementation allows continued operation of the urea cycle in defects in which the block is proximal to arginine.)
5. If the patient's condition is unresponsive to this management, hemodialysis should be initiated. Hemodialysis is often required in neonates because of their inherently catabolic state. Exchange transfusion should not be used.



## E. HYPOGLYCEMIA

1. **Definitions: Glucose concentration <40 mg/dL typically is considered hypoglycemia.** Potential causes include endocrine disorders or IEMs, including defects in gluconeogenesis, glycogen breakdown (glycogen

BOX 13-1

LABORATORY TESTS FOR INBORN ERRORS OF METABOLISM

| Initial Tests |
|---|
| Complete blood count with differential |
| Serum electrolytes (calculate anion gap) |
| Blood glucose |
| Aspartate aminotransferase (AST) |
| Alanine aminotransferase (ALT) |
| Total and direct bilirubin |
| Blood gas |
| Plasma ammonium |
| Plasma lactate |
| Urine dipstick: pH, ketones, glucose, protein, bilirubin |
| Urine-reducing substances (Clinitest tablet [Ames Co.], identifies all reducing substances in urine; see Box 13-2) |
| Acylcarnitine profile |
| **Further Testing If Workup Is Suspicious** |
| Plasma amino acids |
| Quantitative plasma carnitine |
| Urine organic acids |
| Carbohydrate deficient transferrin test |
| If lactate level is elevated, serum pyruvate and repeat lactate level. |

TABLE 13-1

SAMPLE COLLECTION

| Specimen | Volume (mL) | Tube* | Handling |
|---|---|---|---|
| Plasma ammonium | 1–3 | Green or purple top (check with your laboratory) | On ice; immediate transport to laboratory; levels rise rapidly on standing. |
| Plasma amino acids[†] | 1–3 | Green top | On ice; if must store, spin down, separate plasma, and freeze. |
| Plasma carnitine | 1–3 | Green top | On ice |
| Acylcarnitine profile | Saturate newborn screen filter paper with blood | | Dry and mail to reference laboratory |
| Lactate | 3 | Gray top | On ice |
| Karyotype | 3 | Green top | Room temperature |
| Very-long-chain fatty acids | 3 | Purple top | Room temperature |
| White blood cells for enzymes/DNA | 3 | Purple top | Room temperature |
| Urine organic acids | 5–10 | — | Deliver immediately or freeze. |
| Urine amino acids | 5–10 | — | Deliver immediately or freeze. |
| Carbohydrate-deficient transferrin test | 1–3 | Red top | Frozen and sent on dry ice. |
| Skin biopsy | | Tissue culture medium or patient's plasma | Refrigerate; do not freeze. |

*Additives in tubes: purple, K3EDTA; green, lithium heparin; gray, potassium oxalate and sodium fluoride.

[†]Obtain after a 3-hour fast.

storage diseases), and fatty acid oxidation, or toxic impairment of gluconeogenesis (organic acidemias).

2. **History questions:** What is the patient's age? What is the relationship between the hypoglycemia and caloric intake? (Does it occur postprandially or after prolonged fasting, or is it constant?) Is the patient septic? Does the patient have hepatomegaly?
3. **Laboratory evaluation** (ideally, collect samples before glucose administration): Complete metabolic panel, including liver function tests (LFTs), insulin, cortisol, growth hormone, acylcarnitine profile, and urinary ketones. Hypoglycemia with inappropriately low urinary ketones is the hallmark of fatty acid oxidation disorders. Consult a geneticist to help interpret laboratory results and guide the workup.

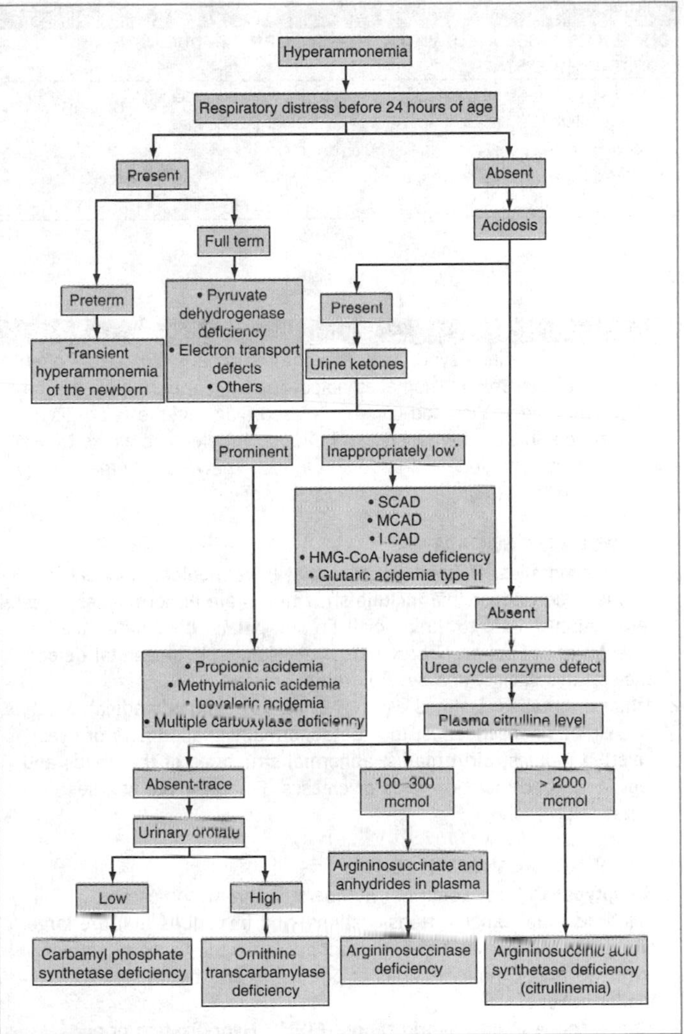


FIG. 13-1

Differential diagnosis of hyperammonemia. *Indicates inappropriately low urinary ketones in settling of symptomatic hypoglycemia. HMG-CoA, hydroxymethylglutaryl-CoA; LCAD, long-chain acyl-CoA dehydrogenase; MCAD, medium-chain acyl-CoA dehydrogenase; SCAD, short-chain acyl-CoA dehydrogenase.

BOX 13-2

**DISORDERS ASSOCIATED WITH A POSITIVE URINE-REDUCING SUBSTANCES TEST**

*Galactose:* Galactosemia, galactokinase deficiency, severe liver disease
*Fructose:* Hereditary fructose intolerance, essential fructosuria
*Glucose:* Diabetes mellitus, renal tubular defects
*p-Hydroxyphenylpyruvic acid:* Tyrosinemia
*Xylose:* Pentosuria

## IV. DYSMORPHOLOGY

The suspicion for many syndromes and chromosomal anomalies is often raised by major or minor anomalies noted on physical examination. The most common anomalies and commonly used diagnostic tests are listed here. More complete information can be found in reference works by Hall and colleagues[6] and Jones.[7] In addition to well-known syndromes, many rare genetic disorders are listed in reference works.[7,8]

### A. PHYSICAL EXAMINATION

1. **Major anomalies:** Defined as those that have medical, surgical, or cosmetic consequences; include structural brain abnormalities, mental retardation, failure to thrive, cleft lip and palate, congenital heart defects, abnormal secondary sexual development, urogenital defects, skeletal dysplasias, and severe limb anomalies.
2. **Minor anomalies:** Defined as not having any serious medical, surgical, or cosmetic consequence; include abnormally shaped ears or eyes, inverted nipples, birth marks, abnormal structures of the hands and feet, and abnormal skin folds or creases. For complete list, see Jones.[7]

### B. GENETIC DIAGNOSTIC TESTS

1. **Karyotype:** Detects abnormal numbers of chromosomes and deletions, duplications, translocations, and inversions that are large enough to be seen by light microscopy. Indicated in every patient with two major malformations or one major and two minor malformations.
2. **Fluorescence in situ hybridization (FISH):** Hybridization of a fluorescently tagged DNA probe to chromosomes allows detection of submicroscopic deletions and duplications. FISH assays are commonly available for the following syndromes: Williams (7q11), Prader-Willi and Angelman (15q11), Miller-Dieker (17p13.3), Smith-Magenis (17p11.2), velocardiofacial and DiGeorge (22q11). For a complete, updated online list of genetic diagnostic tests, see www.genetests.org.

3. **Deoxyribonucleic acid (DNA) analysis:** Many monogenic disorders now have DNA tests available. Contact your laboratory or www.genetests.org for a list of those available.
4. **BAC-CGH arrays:** In addition to conventional chromosomal analysis, the suggestion has been made to send the patient's DNA for BAC-CGH arrays. The novel technology has been developed to detect chromosomal copy number changes on a genome wide and/or high resolution scale, allowing the detection of very small chromosomal abnormalities.

### C. STRUCTURAL DIAGNOSTIC TESTS

1. Brain magnetic resonance imaging (MRI).
2. Ophthalmologic examination: Optic atrophy, coloboma, cataracts, retinal abnormalities, lens subluxation, corneal abnormalities.
3. Echocardiogram.
4. Abdominal ultrasound: Polysplenia or asplenia, absent or horseshoe kidney, ureteral or bladder defects, abdominal situs.
5. Skeletal survey: Abnormalities of bone length or structure.



## V. COMMON SYNDROMES

For more information on common syndromes and other chromosomal abnormalities and syndromes, see Jones, 2006.[7]

### A. TRISOMY 21[7,9]

1. **Features:** Presence of 6 of the following 10 cardinal features in the neonate is highly suggestive of the diagnosis: Hypotonia, poor Moro reflex, hyperflexibility, excess skin on back of the neck, flat facies, slanted palpebral fissures, anomalous auricles, pelvic dysplasia, dysplasia of the mid-phalanx of the fifth finger, and a single transverse palmar (simian) crease.
2. **Associated findings:** Mental retardation (100%), hearing loss (66%), eye disease (60%), serous otitis media (60%–80%), cardiac defects (40%), thyroid disease, gastrointestinal atresias (12%), atlantoaxial instability (12%–20%), and leukemia (1%).
3. **Testing:** Karyotype for diagnosis, echocardiogram, yearly thyroid function tests, LFTs, complete blood count, ophthalmologic and audiologic evaluation; radiographs of the atlanto-occipital junction by age 3 to 5 years.
4. **Health care:** Information about ongoing health care can be found at www.ndss.org.

### B. TURNER SYNDROME—45,X[7,10]

1. **Features:** Short female with broad chest, wide-spaced nipples, webbed neck, congenital lymphedema.
2. **Associated findings:** Gonadal dysgenesis (90%), renal anomalies (60%), cardiac defects (10%–30%), hearing loss (50%).

3. **Testing:** Karyotype for diagnosis. Baseline echocardiogram, renal ultrasound; blood pressure, hearing, growth parameters, and scoliosis screen with each examination; thyroid function tests and echocardiogram every 1 to 2 years.

### C. FRAGILE X SYNDROME[7,11]

1. **Features:** Boys: Mild to profound mental retardation, cluttered speech, autism (60%), macrocephaly, large ears, prognathism, postpubertal macro-orchidism, tall stature. Phenotype most prominent in boys; girls may have only learning disabilities.
2. **Testing:** X-linked inheritance; caused by an expansion of a CGG nucleotide repeat in the *FMR1* gene. The size of the repeat correlates with disease severity. Diagnosis is established by DNA analysis.

### D. MARFAN SYNDROME[7,12,13]

1. **Features:** Major and minor diagnostic criteria involving the skeletal, ocular, cardiovascular, and pulmonary systems, and skin or integument. Features include but are not limited to tall stature, low upper-to-lower segment ratio, arachnodactyly, joint laxity, scoliosis, pectus excavatum or carinatum, lens subluxation, glaucoma, retinal detachment, dilation with or without dissecting aneurysm of ascending aorta, mitral valve prolapse, lumbosacral dural ectasia by computed tomography or MRI scans, and inguinal and/or femoral hernias. For a complete list of criteria for diagnosis in both an index case and a family member, see Scriver and associates[5] and De Paepe and colleagues.[12]
2. **Testing:** Genetic evaluation; routine ophthalmologic evaluation, including slit-lamp examination; and echocardiogram.

### E. 22Q11 SYNDROME[7]

1. **Synonyms:** DiGeorge syndrome, velocardiofacial syndrome (VCFS), Shprintzen syndrome, conotruncal anomaly face syndrome (CTAF).
2. **Features:** Congenital heart defects (85%), palatal abnormalities, immune deficiency (defective T-cell function), hypocalcemia (parathyroid involvement), characteristic facial features.
3. **Testing:** FISH analysis for 22q11.2 deletion and routine cytogenetics to evaluate for chromosomal rearrangement (<1% cases). Measure serum calcium, absolute lymphocyte count, B- and T-cell subsets if lymphopenic, renal ultrasound for structural abnormalities, chest x-ray for thoracic vertebral anomalies, baseline cardiac evaluation, including echocardiogram. Parents should also be tested to determine whether they are carriers of the deletion.

### F. PRADER-WILLI SYNDROME[7,14]

1. **Features:** Hypotonia, poor feeding, and failure to thrive during infancy; short stature, mental retardation, obesity (onset 6 months to

6 years), bizarre and binge-type eating habits, small hands and feet, small genital structures, characteristic facial features.

2. **Testing:** High-resolution karyotype followed by methylation studies specific for Prader-Willi syndrome. Follow growth parameters, routine ophthalmologic evaluation, dietary supervision, physical activity plans.

### G. TRISOMY 18

1. **Features:** Clenched hand (index finger overlapping third and fifth fingers overlapping fourth), intrauterine growth retardation, decreased fetal activity, low-arch dermal ridge pattern, inguinal or umbilical hernia, cardiac defects, prominent occiput, low-set ears, micrognathia, rocker-bottom feet.
2. **Testing:** Karyotype with FISH analysis.
3. **Natural history:** Apnea, severe failure to thrive; 50% die by 1 week, 90% by 1 year.

### H. TRISOMY 13

1. **Features:** Holoprosencephaly, polydactyly, scalp skin defects, seizures, deafness, microcephaly, sloping forehead, cleft lip, cleft palate, retinal anomalies, microphthalmia, abnormal ears, single umbilical artery, inguinal hernia, omphalocele, cardiac defects, urinary tract malformations.
2. **Testing:** Karyotype with FISH analysis.
3. **Natural history:** 44% die within 1 month; 70% die by 1 year.

## VI. DEGENERATIVE DISORDERS

**Note** *Many are progressive neurodegenerative disorders; an exhaustive list is beyond the scope of this chapter.*

### A. LYSOSOMAL DISORDERS (E.G., THE MUCOPOLYSACCHARIDOSES)

Include neurodegeneration with systemic storage resulting from lysosomal enzyme defects (e.g., Hurler, Hunter, Scheie, Sanfilippo, and Sly syndromes).

1. **Presentation:** Hepatosplenomegaly, corneal clouding (except Hunter syndrome), dysostosis multiplex, coarse features, neurologic deterioration.
2. **Laboratory findings:** Inclusion bodies on peripheral blood smear, positive urine mucopolysaccharide spot; characteristic findings on eye examination and skeletal survey.
3. **Definitive diagnosis:** Assay of skin fibroblasts for specific lysosomal hydrolases.
4. **Therapy:** Experimental therapy with exogenous enzyme; bone marrow transplantation may provide some enzyme activity but cannot reverse brain damage.

### B. PEROXISOMAL DISORDERS

Include Refsum syndrome, X-linked adrenoleukodystrophy, Zellweger syndrome, and others.

1. **Presentation:** Seizures, loss of milestones, loss of white matter on MRI scans. Progressive neurodegeneration and eventually death.
2. **Laboratory findings:** Elevated very-long-chain fatty acids, pipecolic acid, phytanic acid, and plasmalogens.
3. **Definitive diagnosis:** Enzyme assays in cultured skin fibroblasts and microscopy of peroxisomes.
4. **Therapy:** Treat adrenal insufficiency if present; provide vitamin K. Research protocols include dietary lipid therapy, bone marrow transplantation, and immunosuppression.

## VII. GENETIC CONSULTATION

### A. INDICATIONS FOR REFERRAL

1. Known or suspected hereditary disorder.
2. Major physical anomalies, unusual body proportions, short stature, dysmorphic features.
3. Major organ malformation.
4. Developmental delay or mental retardation; learning disabilities in females who have brothers with mental retardation.
5. Complete or partial blindness or hearing loss.
6. Deterioration of motor or speech abilities in a previously thriving child.
7. Maternal exposure to drugs, alcohol, or radiation during pregnancy.
8. Strong family history of cancer.
9. Failure to thrive if routine evaluation is unrevealing.

### B. INDICATIONS FOR PRENATAL COUNSELING[1]

1. Genetic disorder or birth defect in one partner.
2. Known carrier of a genetic disorder.
3. Parent with balanced translocation.
4. Previous child with known or suspected genetic disorder.
5. Maternal age >35 years.
6. Abnormal results on triple screening.
7. Family history of known or suspected chromosomal anomaly.
8. Multiple early miscarriages, stillbirths, or neonatal deaths.
9. Member of an ethnic group known to have a high incidence of a specific genetic disorder.
10. Exposures to teratogen or infections.

### C. INDICATIONS FOR KARYOTYPE

1. Two major *or* one major and two minor malformations (include small for gestational age and mental retardation as major).
2. Features of a specific chromosomal syndrome.

3. At risk for familial chromosomal aberration.
4. Ambiguous genitalia.
5. More than two spontaneous abortions or infertility (karyotype both partners).
6. Girls with short stature.

## REFERENCES


1. McMillan JA et al: Oski's Pediatrics: Principles and Practice, 4th ed. Philadelphia, Lippincott Williams & Wilkins, 2006.
2. Seidel HM et al: Primary Care of the Newborn, 3rd ed. St. Louis, Mosby, 2001.
3. Kaye CI and Committee on Genetics: Introduction to the Newborn Screening Fact Sheets. Pediatrics 2006;118:1304–1312.
4. Fernandes J et al: Inborn Metabolic Diseases, 3rd ed. Berlin, Springer-Verlag, 2000.
5. Scriver CR et al: The Molecular and Metabolic Bases of Inherited Disease, 8th ed. New York, McGraw-Hill, 2001.
6. Hall JG et al: Handbook of Normal Physical Measurements. Oxford, UK, Oxford Medical Publications, 1989.
7. Jones KL: Smith's Recognizable Patterns of Human Malformation, 6th ed. Philadelphia, Elsevier, 2006.
8. Gorlin R et al: Syndromes of the Head and Neck, 4th ed. New York, Oxford University Press, 2001.
9. American Academy of Pediatrics, Committee on Genetics: Health supervision for children with Down syndrome. Pediatrics 2001;107:442–449.
10. American Academy of Pediatrics, Committee on Genetics: Health supervision for children with Turner syndrome. Pediatrics 2003;111:692–702.
11. American Academy of Pediatrics, Committee on Genetics: Health supervision for children with Fragile X syndrome. Pediatrics 1996;98:297–300.
12. De Paepe A et al: Revised diagnostic criteria for the Marfan syndrome. Am J Med Genet 1996;62:417–426.
13. American Academy of Pediatrics, Committee on Genetics: Health supervision of children with Marfan syndrome. Pediatrics 1996;98:978–982.
14. Wattendorf DJ, Muenke M: Prader-Willi syndrome. Am Fam Phys 2005;72:827–830.

# Hematology

*Julia Aquino, MD*

14

## I. ANEMIA

### A. GENERAL EVALUATION

Anemia is defined by age-specific norms (Table 14-1 and Fig. 14-1). Evaluation includes the following:

1. **Complete history: Includes blood loss, fatigue, pica, medication exposure, growth and development, nutritional history, menstrual history, ethnic background, history of hyperbilirubinemia and family history of anemia, splenectomy, or cholecystectomy.**
2. **Physical examination: Includes pallor, jaundice, glossitis, tachypnea, tachycardia, cardiac murmur, hepatosplenomegaly, and signs of systemic illness.**
3. **Initial laboratory tests: May include a complete blood count with red blood cell (RBC) indices, reticulocyte count, blood smear, stool for occult blood, urinalysis, and serum bilirubin.**

### B. DIAGNOSIS

Anemias may be categorized as macrocytic, microcytic, or normocytic. Table 14-2 gives an approach to diagnosis based on RBC production and cell size. Note that normal ranges for hemoglobin (Hb) and mean corpuscular volume (MCV) are age dependent.

### C. EVALUATION OF SPECIFIC CAUSES OF ANEMIA

1. **Iron-deficiency anemia: Hypochromic/microcytic anemia with a low reticulocyte count and an elevated red cell distribution width (RDW).**
   a. Serum ferritin reflects total body iron stores after age 6 months and is the first value to fall in iron deficiency; may be falsely elevated with inflammation or infection.
   b. Other indicators: Low serum iron and/or transferrin levels and an elevated total iron-binding capacity (TIBC).
   c. Iron therapy should result in an increased reticulocyte count in 2–3 days and an increase in hematocrit (HCT) after 1–4 weeks of therapy. Iron stores are generally replete with 3 months of therapy.
   d. **Mentzer index (MCV/RBC):** Index >13.5 suggests iron deficiency; Mentzer index <11.5 suggests thalassemia minor. Increased RDW also helps distinguish iron-deficiency anemia from thalassemia.
2. **Hemolytic anemia: Rapid RBC turnover. Etiologies: Congenital membranopathies, hemoglobinopathies, enzymopathies, metabolic defects, and immune-mediated destruction. Useful studies include the following:**
   a. **Reticulocyte count:** Usually elevated; indicates increased production of RBCs to compensate for increased destruction. Corrected reticulocyte count (CRC) accounts for differences in HCT and is an indicator of

TABLE 14–1

AGE-SPECIFIC BLOOD CELL INDICES

| Age | Hb (g/dL)* | HCT (%)* | MCV (fL)* |
|---|---|---|---|
| 26–30 wk gestation[‡] | 13.4 (11) | 41.5 (34.9) | 118.2 (106.7) |
| 28 wk | 14.5 | 45 | 120 |
| 32 wk | 15.0 | 47 | 118 |
| Term[§] (cord) | 16.5 (13.5) | 51 (42) | 108 (98) |
| 1–3 day | 18.5 (14.5) | 56 (45) | 108 (95) |
| 2 wk | 16.6 (13.4) | 53 (41) | 105 (88) |
| 1 mo | 13.9 (10.7) | 44 (33) | 101 (91) |
| 2 mo | 11.2 (9.4) | 35 (28) | 95 (84) |
| 6 mo | 12.6 (11.1) | 36 (31) | 76 (68) |
| 6 mo–2 yr | 12.0 (10.5) | 36 (33) | 78 (70) |
| 2–6 yr | 12.5 (11.5) | 37 (34) | 81 (75) |
| 6–12 yr | 13.5 (11.5) | 40 (35) | 86 (77) |
| 12–18 yr | | | |
| Male | 14.5 (13) | 43 (36) | 88 (78) |
| Female | 14.0 (12) | 41 (37) | 90 (78) |
| Adult | | | |
| Male | 15.5 (13.5) | 47 (41) | 90 (80) |
| Female | 14.0 (12) | 41 (36) | 90 (80) |

*Data are mean (–2 SD).

[†]Data are mean (±2 SD).

[‡]Values are from fetal samplings.

[§]1 mo, capillary hemoglobin exceeds venous: 1 hr: 3.6 g difference; 5 dy: 2.2 g difference; 3 wk: 1.1 g difference.

[||]Mean (95% confidence limits).

Hb, hemoglobin; HCT, hematocrit; MCHC, mean cell hemoglobin concentration; MCV, mean corpuscular volume; RBC, red blood cell; WBC, white blood cell.

erythropoietic activity. A CRC >1.5 suggests increased RBC production as a result of hemolysis or blood loss.

CRC = % reticulocytes × patient HCT/normal HCT

b. **Plasma aspartate aminotransferase and lactate dehydrogenase:** Increased from release of intracellular enzymes.
c. **Haptoglobin:** Binds free Hb; decreased with intravascular and extravascular hemolysis. Also decreased in neonates and with liver dysfunction due to decreased synthesis.
d. **Direct Coombs test:** Tests for the presence of antibody or complement on patient RBCs. Can be falsely negative if affected cells have already been destroyed or antibody titer is low.
e. **Indirect Coombs test:** Tests for free autoantibody in the patient's serum after RBC antibody binding sites are saturated.
f. **Osmotic fragility test:** Useful in diagnosis of hereditary spherocytosis. Can also be positive in ABO incompatibility.
g. **Glucose-6-phosphate dehydrogenase (G6PD) assay:** Quantitative test used to diagnose G6PD deficiency, an X-linked disorder affecting 10%–14% of African American males. May be normal immediately after a

| MCHC (g/dL RBC)* | Reticulocytes | WBCs ($\times10^3/\mu L$)† | Platelets ($10^3/\mu L$)† |
|---|---|---|---|
| 37.9 (30.6) | — | 4.4 (2.7) | 254 (180–327) |
| 31.0 | (5–10) | — | 275 |
| 32.0 | (3–10) | — | 290 |
| 33.0 (30.0) | (3–7) | 18.1 (9–30)‖ | 290 |
| 33.0 (29.0) | (1.8–4.6) | 18.9 (9.4–34) | 192 |
| 31.4 (28.1) | — | 11.4 (5–20) | 252 |
| 31.8 (28.1) | (0.1–1.7) | 10.8 (4–19.5) | — |
| 31.8 (28.3) | — | — | — |
| 35.0 (32.7) | (0.7–2.3) | 11.9 (6–17.5) | — |
| 33.0 (30.0) | — | 10.6 (6–17) | (150–350) |
| 34.0 (31.0) | (0.5–1.0) | 8.5 (5–15.5) | (150–350) |
| 34.0 (31.0) | (0.5–1.0) | 8.1 (4.5–13.5) | (150–350) |
| 34.0 (31.0) | (0.5–1.0) | 7.8 (4.5–13.5) | (150–350) |
| 34.0 (31.0) | (0.5–1.0) | 7.8 (4.5–13.5) | (150–350) |
| 34.0 (31.0) | (0.8–2.5) | 7.4 (4.5–11) | (150–350) |
| 34.0 (31.0) | (0.8–4.1) | 7.4 (4.5–11) | (150–350) |

Data from Forestier F et al: Hematologic values of 163 normal fetuses between 18 and 30 weeks of gestation. Pediatr Res 1986;20:342; Oski FA, Naiman JL: Hematological Problems in the Newborn Infant. Philadelphia, WB Saunders, 1982; Nathan D, Oski FA: Hematology of Infancy and Childhood. Philadelphia; WB Saunders, 1998; Matoth Y et al: Postnatal changes in some red cell parameters. Acta Paediatr Scand 1971;60:317; and Wintrobe MM: Clinical Hematology. Baltimore, Williams & Wilkins, 1999.

hemolytic episode because older, more enzyme-deficient cells have been lysed. See Chapter 30 for a list of oxidizing drugs.

h. **Heinz body preparation:** Detects precipitated Hb within RBCs; present in unstable hemoglobinopathies and enzymopathies during oxidative stress (e.g., G6PD deficiency).

3. **Red cell aplasia: Variable cell size, low reticulocyte count, variable platelet and white blood cell (WBC) counts. Bone marrow aspiration evaluates RBC precursors in the marrow to look for marrow dysfunction, neoplasm, or specific signs of infection.**

a. **Acquired aplasias:**
   (1) **Infectious causes:** Include parvovirus in children with rapid RBC turnover (infects RBC precursors), Epstein-Barr virus, cytomegalovirus (CMV), human herpesvirus type 6, or human immunodeficiency virus (HIV).
   (2) **Transient erythroblastopenia of childhood (TEC):** Occurs from age 6 months to 4 years, with >80% of cases presenting after age 1 year with a normal or slightly low MCV and low reticulocyte count. Spontaneous recovery usually within 4–8 weeks.
   (3) **Exposures:** Include radiation and various drugs and chemicals.

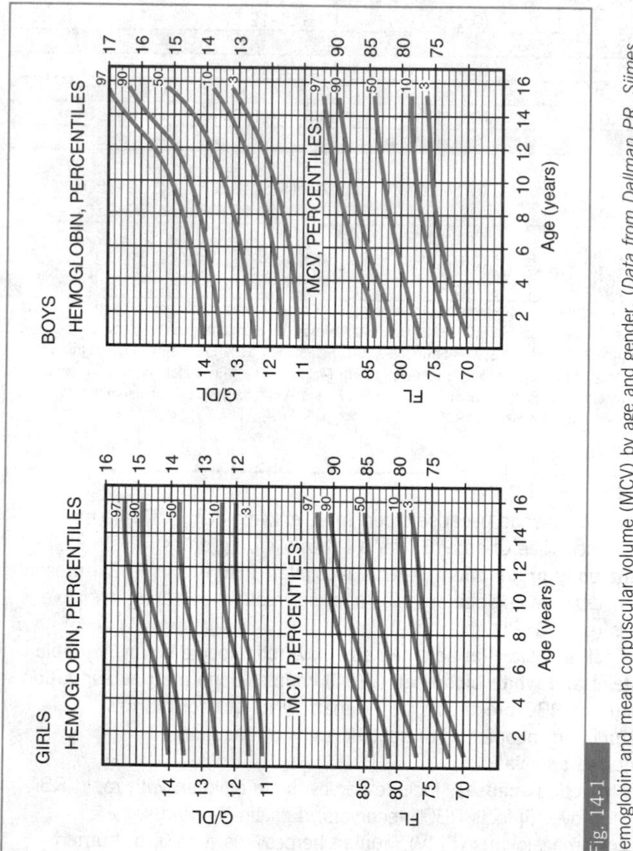


Fig. 14-1 Hemoglobin and mean corpuscular volume (MCV) by age and gender. (*Data from Dallman PR, Siimes MA: Percentile curves for hemoglobin and red cell volume in infancy and childhood. J Pediatr 1979;94:26.*)

TABLE 14-2

CLASSIFICATION OF ANEMIA

| Reticulocyte Count | Microcytic Anemia | Normocytic Anemia | Macrocytic Anemia |
|---|---|---|---|
| Low | Iron deficiency<br>Lead poisoning<br>Chronic disease<br>Aluminum toxicity<br>Copper deficiency<br>Protein malnutrition | Chronic disease<br>RBC aplasia (TEC, infection, drug induced)<br>Malignancy<br>Juvenile rheumatoid arthritis<br>Endocrinopathies<br>Renal failure | Folate deficiency<br>Vitamin $B_{12}$ deficiency<br>Aplastic anemia<br>Congenital bone marrow dysfunction (Diamond-Blackfan or Fanconi syndromes)<br>Drug induced<br>Trisomy 21<br>Hypothyroidism |
| Normal | Thalassemia trait<br>Sideroblastic anemia | Acute bleeding<br>Hypersplenism<br>Dyserythropoietic anemia II | — |
| High | Thalassemia syndromes<br>Hemoglobin C disorders | Antibody-mediated hemolysis<br>Hypersplenism<br>Microangiopathy (HUS, TTP, DIC, Kasabach-Merritt)<br>Membranopathies (spherocytosis, elliptocytosis)<br>Enzyme disorders (G6PD, pyruvate kinase)<br>Hemoglobinopathies | Dyserythropoietic anemia I, III<br>Active hemolysis |

DIC, disseminated intravascular coagulation; G6PD, glucose-6-phosphate dehydrogenase; HUS, hemolytic-uremic syndrome; TEC, transient erythroblastopenia of childhood; TTP, thrombotic thrombocytopenic purpura.

Data from Nathan D, Oski FA: Hematology of Infancy and Childhood, 6th ed. Philadelphia, WB Saunders, 2003.

b. **Congenital aplasias:** Typically macrocytic anemias.

(1) **Fanconi anemia:** Autosomal recessive disorder, usually presents before age 10 years; may present with pancytopenia. Patients may have thumb abnormalities, renal anomalies, microcephaly, or short stature. Chromosomal fragility studies may be diagnostic.

(2) **Diamond-Blackfan-Oski syndrome:** Autosomal recessive pure RBC aplasia; presents in the first year of life. Associated with congenital anomalies in one third of cases including triphalangeal thumb, short stature, and cleft lip.

c. **Aplastic anemia:** Idiopathic bone marrow failure, usually macrocytic.

4. **Physiologic anemia of infancy (physiologic nadir): Decrease in Hb until oxygen needs are greater than oxygen delivery, usually at Hb of 9–11 mg/dL. Normally occurs between age 8–12 weeks for full-term infants and age 3–6 weeks for preterm infants.**
5. **Anemia of chronic inflammation: Usually normocytic with normal to low reticulocyte count. Iron studies reveal low iron, TIBC, and transferrin, and elevated ferritin.**

## II. HEMOGLOBINOPATHIES

### A. HEMOGLOBIN ELECTROPHORESIS

Involves separation of Hb variants based on molecular charge and size. All positive sickle preparations and solubility tests for sickle Hb (e.g., Sickledex) should be confirmed with electrophoresis or isoelectric focusing (a component of the mandatory newborn screen in many states). See Table 14-3 for interpretation of neonatal Hb electrophoresis patterns.

TABLE 14-3

NEONATAL HEMOGLOBIN (Hb) ELECTROPHORESIS PATTERNS*

| Pattern | Interpretation |
|---|---|
| FA | Fetal Hb and adult normal Hb; the normal newborn pattern. |
| FAV | Indicates the presence of both HbF and HbA. However, an anomalous band (V) is present, which does not appear to be any of the common Hb variants. |
| FAS | Indicates fetal Hb, adult normal HbA and HbS, consistent with benign sickle cell trait. |
| FS | Fetal and sickle HbS without detectable adult normal HbA. Consistent with clinically significant homozygous sickle Hb genotype (S/S) or sickle β-thalassemia, with manifestations of sickle cell anemia during childhood. |
| FC† | Designates the presence of HbC without adult normal HbA. Consistent with clinically significant homozygous HbC genotype (C/C), resulting in a mild hematologic disorder presenting during childhood. |
| FSC | HbS and HbC present. This heterozygous condition could lead to the manifestations of sickle cell disease during childhood. |
| FAC | HbC and adult normal HbA present, consistent with benign HbC trait. |
| $FSAA_2$ | Heterozygous HbS/β-thalassemia, a clinically significant sickling disorder. |
| $FAA_2$ | Heterozygous HbA/β-thalassemia, a clinically benign hematologic condition. |
| F† | Fetal HbF is present without adult normal HbA. Although this may indicate a delayed appearance of HbA, it is also consistent with homozygous β-thalassemia major, or homozygous hereditary persistence of fetal HbF. |
| FV† | Fetal HbF and an anomalous Hb variant (V) are present. |
| AF | May indicate prior blood transfusion. Submit another filter paper blood specimen when the infant is 4 mo of age, at which time the transfused blood cells should have been cleared. |

*Note:* HbA: $\alpha_2\beta_2$; HbF: $\alpha_2\gamma_2$; $HbA_2$: $\alpha_2\delta_2$

*Hemoglobin variants are reported in order of decreasing abundance; for example, FA indicates more fetal than adult hemoglobin.

†Repeat blood specimen should be submitted to confirm the original interpretation.

## B. SICKLE CELL ANEMIA

Caused by a genetic defect in β-globin. 8% of African Americans are carriers; 1 in 500 African Americans have sickle cell anemia.

1. **Diagnosis: Often made on newborn screen with Hb electrophoresis. The sickle preparation and Sickledex: Rapid tests that are positive in all sickle hemoglobinopathies. False-negative test results may be seen in neonates and other patients with a high percentage of fetal Hb.**
2. **Complications (Table 14-4): A hematologist should generally be consulted.**
3. **Health maintenance:[2] Ongoing consultation and clinical involvement with a pediatric hematologist and/or with a sickle cell program are essential.**

a. Pneumococcal vaccine: Provide heptavalent protein-conjugate vaccine according to routine childhood schedule; provide a 23-valent polysaccharide vaccine after age 2 years of age, with a booster 3–5 years after the previous dose (see Chapter 16)
b. Influenza vaccine: Yearly for those ≥age 6 months.
c. Meningococcal vaccine: Also recommended.
d. Begin prophylaxis with penicillin as soon as diagnosis is made; prophylaxis may be discontinued by age 5 years if patient has had no prior severe pneumococcal infections or splenectomy and has documented pneumococcal vaccinations, including second 23-valent vaccination. Practice patterns vary. Some continue penicillin indefinitely.
e. Consider supplementation with folic acid.
f. Consider hydroxyurea for severe disease. Increases levels of fetal Hb and decreases HbS content in cells. Has been shown to significantly decrease episodes of vaso-occlusive crises, hemolytic crises, acute chest syndrome, number of transfusions, and days spent in the hospital.[3] May decrease mortality in adults.
g. Ophthalmologic examination: Perform annually after age 10 years.
h. Transcranial Doppler examination: Perform annually between ages 2 and 16 years in patients with SS disease to screen for increased risk for cerebrovascular accident (CVA).
i. Closely follow growth, development, and school performance.

## C. THALASSEMIAS

Defects in α- or β-globin production. Imbalance in production of globin chains leads to precipitation of excess chains, causing ineffective erythropoiesis and shortened survival of mature RBCs.

1. **α-Thalassemias:**

a. **Hb Barts hydrops fetalis (–/–):** Hb Barts ($\gamma_4$) cannot deliver oxygen; usually fatal.
b. **HbH disease ($\beta_4$) (α-/–):** Causes moderately severe anemia.

TABLE 14-4

SICKLE CELL DISEASE COMPLICATIONS

| Complication | Evaluation | Treatment |
|---|---|---|
| **Fever (T ≥38.5°C)** | History and physical<br>CBC with differential<br>Reticulocyte count<br>Blood cultures<br>Chest x-ray, other cultures as indicated | IV antibiotics (third-generation cephalosporin, other antibiotics as indicated)<br>Admit if ill appearing, <3 yr of age, concerning lab results, or complications<br>Some centers use antibiotics with a long half-life and re-evaluate in 24 hr as an outpatient. |
| **Vaso-occlusive crisis**<br>Children <2 yr, dactylitis<br>Children >2 yr, unifocal or multifocal pain | History and physical<br>CBC with differential<br>Reticulocyte count<br>Type and screen | Oral analgesics as an outpatient, as tolerated<br>IV analgesics and IV fluids if outpatient therapy fails (parenteral narcotics in form of PCA and parenteral NSAIDs usually used in combination)<br>Aggressive early treatment of pain is essential. |
| **Acute chest syndrome**<br>New pulmonary infiltrate with fever, cough, chest pain, tachypnea, dyspnea, or hypoxia | History and physical<br>CBC with differential<br>Reticulocyte count<br>Blood cultures<br>Chest x-ray<br>Type and screen | Admit<br>$O_2$, incentive spirometry, bronchodilators<br>IV antibiotics (third-generation cephalosporin and macrolide)<br>Analgesia, IV fluids<br>Simple transfusion for moderately severe illness, exchange transfusion for severe or rapidly progressing illness<br>High-dose dexamethasone controversial[1] |
| **Splenic sequestration**<br>Acutely enlarged spleen and Hb level ≥2 g/dL below patient's baseline | History and physical<br>CBC<br>Reticulocyte count<br>Type and hold | Serial abdominal exams<br>IV fluids and fluid resuscitation as necessary<br>RBC transfusion or, in severe cases, exchange transfusion for cardiovascular compromise and Hb <4.5 g/dL. (Autotransfusion may occur with recovery, leading to increased Hb and CHF. Transfuse cautiously.) |

*Note:* CVA requires emergency transfusion guided by a hematologist and a neurologist experienced with sickle cell disease.

CHF, congestive heart failure; CVA, cerebrovascular accident; Hb, hemoglobin; NSAIDs, nonsteroidal anti-inflammatory drugs; PCA, patient-controlled analgesia; PRBCs, packed red blood cells; RBC, red blood cells; TIA, transient ischemic attack.

*Continued*

TABLE 14-4

SICKLE CELL DISEASE COMPLICATIONS—cont'd

| Complication | Evaluation | Treatment |
|---|---|---|
| **Aplastic crisis**<br>Acute illness with Hb below patient's baseline and low reticulocyte count. May follow viral illnesses, especially parvovirus B19 | History and physical<br>CBC with differential<br>Reticulocyte count<br>Type and screen<br>Parvovirus serology and polymerase chain reaction | Admit<br>IV fluids<br>PRBCs for symptomatic anemia<br>Isolation to protect susceptible individuals and women of childbearing age until parvovirus excluded |
| **Other complications**<br>Priapism, CVA, TIA, gallbladder disease, avascular necrosis | | |



c. **α-Thalassemia trait (α-/α-) or (αα/–):** Occurs in 1.5% of African Americans; causes mild microcytic anemia.

d. **Silent carriers (α-/αα):** Not anemic.

2. **β-Thalassemia: Found throughout the Mediterranean, Middle East, India, and Southeast Asia. Ineffective erythropoiesis is more severe in β-thalassemia than α thalassemia because excess α chains are more unstable than β chains.**

a. **Thalassemia major/Cooley's anemia (β0/β0):** Presence of anemia within the first 6 months of life with hepatosplenomegaly and progressive bone marrow expansion, which may lead to frontal bossing and other skeletal deformities. Regular transfusions required to avoid anemia.

b. **Thalassemia intermedia (β+/β+):** Presents at about age 2 years with moderate, compensated anemia, which may become symptomatic, leading to heart failure, pulmonary hypertension, splenomegaly, and bony expansion, usually in the second or third decade of life.

c. **Thalassemia trait/thalassemia minor (β/β+) or (β/β0):** Usually asymptomatic with microcytosis out of proportion to anemia, sometimes with erythrocytosis.

## III. NEUTROPENIA

An absolute neutrophil count (ANC) <1500/μL, although neutrophil counts vary with age (Table 14-5). Severe neutropenia is defined as an ANC <500/μL. Children with significant neutropenia are at risk for bacterial and fungal infections. Granulocyte colony-stimulating factor may be indicated. Transient neutropenia secondary to viral illness rarely causes significant morbidity. For management of fever and neutropenia in oncology patients, see Chapter 22. See Box 14-1 for causes.

TABLE 14-5

## AGE-SPECIFIC LEUKOCYTE DIFFERENTIAL

| Age | Total Leukocytes* Mean (range) | Neutrophils† Mean (range) | % |
|---|---|---|---|
| Birth | 18.1 (9–30) | 11 (6–26) | 61 |
| 12 hr | 22.8 (13–38) | 15.5 (6–28) | 68 |
| 24 hr | 18.9 (9.4–34) | 11.5 (5–21) | 61 |
| 1 wk | 12.2 (5–21) | 5.5 (1.5–10) | 45 |
| 2 wk | 11.4 (5–20) | 4.5 (1–9.5) | 40 |
| 1 mo | 10.8 (5–19.5) | 3.8 (1–8.5) | 35 |
| 6 mo | 11.9 (6–17.5) | 3.8 (1–8.5) | 32 |
| 1 yr | 11.4 (6–17.5) | 3.5 (1.5–8.5) | 31 |
| 2 yr | 10.6 (6–17) | 3.5 (1.5–8.5) | 33 |
| 4 yr | 9.1 (5.5–15.5) | 3.8 (1.5–8.5) | 42 |
| 6 yr | 8.5 (5–14.5) | 4.3 (1.5–8) | 51 |
| 8 yr | 8.3 (4.5–13.5) | 4.4 (1.5–8) | 53 |
| 10 yr | 8.1 (4.5–13.5) | 4.4 (1.5–8.5) | 54 |
| 16 yr | 7.8 (4.5–13.0) | 4.4 (1.8–8) | 57 |
| 21 yr | 7.4 (4.5–11.0) | 4.4 (1.8–7.7) | 59 |

*Numbers of leukocytes are × $10^3/\mu L$; ranges are estimates of 95% confidence limits; percents refer to differential counts.

†Neutrophils include band cells at all ages and a small number of metamyelocytes and myelocytes in the first few days of life.

BOX 14-1

## DIFFERENTIAL DIAGNOSIS OF CHILDHOOD NEUTROPENIA

| ACQUIRED | CONGENITAL |
|---|---|
| Infection | Cyclic neutropenia |
| Immune mediated | Severe congenital neutropenia (Kostmann syndrome) |
| Hypersplenism | Chronic benign neutropenia of childhood |
| Vitamin $B_{12}$, folate, copper deficiency | Schwachman syndrome |
| Drugs or toxic substances | Fanconi syndrome |
| Aplastic anemia | Metabolic disorders (amino acidopathies, glycogenolysis) |
| Malignancies or preleukemic disorders Ionizing radiation | Osteopetrosis |

| Lymphocytes | | Monocytes | | Eosinophils | |
|---|---|---|---|---|---|
| Mean (range) | % | Mean | % | Mean | % |
| 5.5 (2–11) | 31 | 1.1 | 6 | 0.4 | 2 |
| 5.5 (2–11) | 24 | 1.2 | 5 | 0.5 | 2 |
| 5.8 (2–11.5) | 31 | 1.1 | 6 | 0.5 | 2 |
| 5.0 (2–17) | 41 | 1.1 | 9 | 0.5 | 4 |
| 5.5 (2–17) | 48 | 1.0 | 9 | 0.4 | 3 |
| 6.0 (2.5–16.5) | 56 | 0.7 | 7 | 0.3 | 3 |
| 7.3 (4–13.5) | 61 | 0.6 | 5 | 0.3 | 3 |
| 7.0 (4–10.5) | 61 | 0.6 | 5 | 0.3 | 3 |
| 6.3 (3–9.5) | 59 | 0.5 | 5 | 0.3 | 3 |
| 4.5 (2–8) | 50 | 0.5 | 5 | 0.3 | 3 |
| 3.5 (1.5–7) | 42 | 0.4 | 5 | 0.2 | 3 |
| 3.3 (1.5–6.8) | 39 | 0.4 | 4 | 0.2 | 2 |
| 3.1 (1.5–6.5) | 38 | 0.4 | 4 | 0.2 | 2 |
| 2.8 (1.2–5.2) | 35 | 0.4 | 5 | 0.2 | 3 |
| 2.5 (1–4.8) | 34 | 0.3 | 4 | 0.2 | 3 |

Adapted from Cairo MS, Brauho F: Blood and blood-forming tissues. In Randolph AM (ed): Pediatrics, 21st ed. New York, McGraw-Hill, 2003.



## IV. THROMBOCYTOPENIA

### A. DEFINITION

A platelet count <150,000/µL. Clinically significant bleeding is unlikely with platelet counts >20,000/mm$^3$ in the absence of other complicating factors.

### B. CAUSES OF THROMBOCYTOPENIA

1. **Idiopathic thrombocytopenic purpura (ITP):** A diagnosis of exclusion; can be acute or chronic. WBC count and Hb levels are normal. Indications for treatment of patients without significant bleeding are not well established, many require no therapy. Treatment options include Rh (D) immune globulin (WinRho; useful only in Rh-positive, nonsplenectomized patients), intravenous immune globulin (see Formulary for IVIG dosing), or corticosteroids (i.e., prednisone 2 mg/kg/day or up to 30 mg/kg methylprednisolone for up to 3 days). Splenectomy or chemotherapy may be considered in chronic cases. Platelet transfusions not generally helpful but are necessary in life-threatening bleeding.
2. **Neonatal thrombocytopenia:** May be caused by the following:

a. **Decreased production:** Results from aplastic disorders, congenital malignancy such as leukemia, and viral infections.

b. **Increased consumption:** Usually result of disseminated intravascular coagulation (DIC) from infection or asphyxia.
c. **Immune mediated:** IgG or complement attach to platelets and cause destruction. Specific causes include pre-eclampsia, sepsis, maternal ITP, and platelet alloimmunization.

3. **Neonatal alloimmune thrombocytopenia (NAIT):** Transplacental maternal antibodies (usually against PLA-1 antigen/HPA-1a) cause fetal platelet destruction. If severe, a transfusion of maternal platelets will be more effective in raising the platelet count than random donor platelets. Diagnosis may be confirmed as follows:
a. A mixing study of maternal or neonatal plasma and paternal platelets.
b. Absence of maternal PLA-1 antigen/HPA-1a.
c. A mixing study with patient plasma and a panel of known minor platelet antigens.

4. **Other causes** of thrombocytopenia include microangiopathic hemolytic anemias, such as DIC and hemolytic-uremic syndrome (HUS), infection causing marrow suppression, malignancy, HIV, drug-induced thrombocytopenia, marrow infiltration, cavernous hemangiomas (Kasabach-Merritt syndrome), thrombocytopenia with absent radii syndrome (TAR), thrombosis, hypersplenism, and other rare inherited disorders (e.g., Wiskott-Aldrich syndrome, Noonan syndrome, chromosomal abnormalities).

## V. COAGULATION (Fig. 14-2)

### A. TESTS OF COAGULATION

An incorrect anticoagulant-to-blood ratio will give inaccurate results. See Table 14-6 for normal hematologic values.

1. **Activated partial thromboplastin time (aPTT):** Measures intrinsic system; requires factors V, VIII, IX, X, XI, XII, fibrinogen, and prothrombin. May be prolonged in heparin administration, in hemophilia, in von Willebrand disease (vWD), in DIC, and in the presence of circulating inhibitors (e.g., lupus anticoagulants or other antiphospholipid antibodies).
2. **Prothrombin time (PT):** Measures extrinsic pathway; requires factors V, VII, X, fibrinogen, and prothrombin. May be prolonged in warfarin administration, in deficiencies of vitamin K–associated factors, in malabsorption, in liver disease, in DIC, and in the presence of circulating inhibitors.
3. **Bleeding time (BT):** Evaluates clot formation, including platelet number and function, and von Willebrand factor (vWF). Performed at patient's bedside. Always assess the platelet number and history of ingestion of platelet inhibitors, such as nonsteroidal anti-inflammatory drugs, before a BT test. The Platelet Function Analyzer-100 (PFA-100) system is another in vitro method for measuring platelet and vWF function.

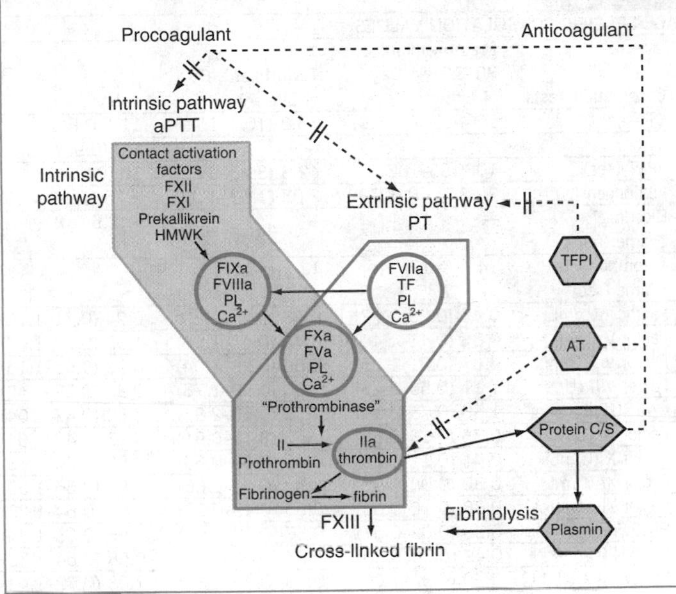


Fig. 14-2

Coagulation cascade. AT, antithrombin; F, factor; HMWK, high molecular weight kininogen; PL, phospholipid; TF, tissue factor; TFPI, tissue factor pathway inhibitor. (*Adaptation courtesy of James Casella and Clifford Takemoto.*)



## B. HYPERCOAGULABLE STATES

Present clinically as venous or arterial thrombosis (Box 14-2).

**1. Laboratory evaluation:**[4]

a. Initial laboratory screening includes PT, high-sensitivity aPTT, circulating anticoagulants, and, if the PT or aPTT are prolonged, a mixing study.

b. Extended workup for hypercoagulable states (Box 14-3): A hematologist should be consulted.

c. The identification of one risk factor, such as an indwelling vascular catheter, does not preclude the search for others, especially when accompanied by a family or personal history of thrombosis.

**2. Treatment of thromboses:**

a. **Heparin:** Used for deep venous thrombus or pulmonary embolus.

(1) See Table 14-7 for heparin bolus and drip adjustment guidelines.

(2) Heparin may be reversed with protamine.

TABLE 14-6

## AGE-SPECIFIC COAGULATION VALUES

| Coagulation Tests | Preterm Infant 30–36 wk, Day of Life #1 | Term Infant, Day of Life #1 | 1–5 yr |
|---|---|---|---|
| PT (sec) | 15.4 (14.6–16.9) | 13.0 (10.1–15.9) | 11 (10.6–11.4) |
| INR | — | — | 1.0 (0.96–1.04) |
| aPTT (sec) | 108 (80–168) | 42.9 (31.3–54.3) | 30 (24–36) |
| Fibrinogen (g/L) | 2.43 (1.50–3.73) | 2.83 (1.67–3.09) | 2.76 (1.70–4.05) |
| Bleeding time (min) | — | — | 6 (2.5–10) |
| Thrombin time (sec) | 14 (11–17) | 12 (10–16) | — |
| Factor II (U/mL) | 0.45 (0.20–0.77) | 0.48 (0.26–0.70) | 0.94 (0.71–1.16) |
| Factor V (U/mL) | 0.88 (0.41–1.44) | 0.72 (0.43–1.08) | 1.03 (0.79–1.27) |
| Factor VII (U/mL) | 0.67 (0.21–1.13) | 0.66 (0.28–1.04) | 0.82 (0.55–1.16) |
| Factor VIII (U/mL) | 1.11 (0.50–2.13) | 1.00 (0.50–1.78) | 0.90 (0.59–1.42) |
| vWF (U/mL) | 1.36 (0.78–2.10) | 1.53 (0.50–2.87) | 0.82 (0.47–1.04) |
| Factor IX (U/mL) | 0.35 (0.19–0.65) | 0.53 (0.15–0.91) | 0.73 (0.47–1.04) |
| Factor X (U/mL) | 0.41 (0.11–0.71) | 0.40 (0.12–0.68) | 0.88 (0.58–1.16) |
| Factor XI (U/mL) | 0.30 (0.08–0.52) | 0.38 (0.10–0.66) | 0.97 (0.56–1.50) |
| Factor XII (U/mL) | 0.38 (0.10–0.66) | 0.53 (0.13–0.93) | 0.93 (0.64–1.29) |
| PK (U/mL) | 0.33 (0.09–0.57) | 0.37 (0.18–0.69) | 0.95 (0.65–1.30) |
| HMWK (U/mL) | 0.49 (0.09–0.89) | 0.54 (0.06–1.02) | 0.98 (0.64–1.32) |
| Factor XIIIa (U/mL) | 0.70 (0.32–1.08) | 0.79 (0.27–1.31) | 1.08 (0.72–1.43) |
| Factor XIIIs (U/mL) | 0.81 (0.35–1.27) | 0.76 (0.30–1.22) | 1.13 (0.69–1.56) |
| D-Dimer | — | — | — |
| FDPs | — | — | — |
| **COAGULATION INHIBITORS** | | | |
| ATIII (U/mL) | 0.38 (0.14–0.62) | 0.63 (0.39–0.97) | 1.11 (0.82–1.39) |
| $\alpha_2$–M (U/mL) | 1.10 (0.56–1.82) | 1.39 (0.95–1.83) | 1.69 (1.14–2.23) |
| C1–Inh (U/mL) | 0.65 (0.31–0.99) | 0.72 (0.36–1.08) | 1.35 (0.85–1.83) |
| $\alpha_2$–AT (U/mL) | 0.90 (0.36–1.44) | 0.93 (0.49–1.37) | 0.93 (0.39–1.47) |
| Protein C (U/mL) | 0.28 (0.12–0.44) | 0.35 (0.17–0.53) | 0.66 (0.40–0.92) |
| Protein S (U/mL) | 0.26 (0.14–0.38) | 0.36 (0.12–0.60) | 0.86 (0.54–1.18) |
| **FIBRINOLYTIC SYSTEM** | | | |
| Plasminogen (U/mL) | 1.70 (1.12–2.48) | 1.95 (1.60–2.30) | 0.98 (0.78–1.18) |
| TPA (ng/mL) | — | — | 2.15 (1.0–4.5) |
| $\alpha_2$–AP (U/mL) | 0.78 (0.4–1.16) | 0.85 (0.70–1.0) | 1.05 (0.93–1.17) |
| PAI (U/mL) | — | — | 5.42 (1.0–10.0) |

$\alpha_2$–AP, $\alpha_2$–antiplasmin; $\alpha_2$–AT, $\alpha_2$–antitrypsin; $\alpha_2$–M, $\alpha_2$–macroglobulin; aPTT, activated partial thromboplastin time; ATIII, antithrombin III; FDPs, fibrin degradation products; HMWK, high-molecular-weight kininogen; INR, International Normalized Ratio; PAI, plasminogen activator inhibitor; PK, prekallikrein; PT, prothrombin time; TPA, tissue plasminogen activator; VIII, factor VIII procoagulant; vWF, von Willebrand factor.

| 6–10 yr | 11–16 yr | Adult |
|---|---|---|
| 11.1 (10.1–12.1) | 11.2 (10.2–12.0) | 12 (11.0–14.0) |
| 1.0 (0.91–1.11) | 1.02 (0.93–1.10) | 1.10 (1.0–1.3) |
| 31 (26–36) | 32 (26–37) | 33 (27–40) |
| 2.79 (1.57–4.0) | 3.0 (1.54–4.48) | 2.78 (1.56–4.0) |
| 7 (2.5–13) | 5 (3–8) | 4 (1–7) |
| — | — | 10 |
| 0.88 (0.67–1.07) | 0.83 (0.61–1.04) | 1.08 (0.70–1.46) |
| 0.90 (0.63–1.16) | 0.77 (0.55–0.99) | 1.06 (0.62–1.50) |
| 0.85 (0.52–1.20) | 0.83 (0.58–1.15) | 1.05 (0.67–1.43) |
| 0.95 (0.58–1.32) | 0.92 (0.53–1.31) | 0.99 (0.50–1.49) |
| 0.95 (0.44–1.44) | 1.00 (0.46–1.53) | 0.92 (0.50–1.58) |
| 0.75 (0.63–0.89) | 0.87 (0.59–1.22) | 1.09 (0.55–1.63) |
| 0.75 (0.55–1.01) | 0.79 (0.50–1.17) | 1.06 (0.70–1.52) |
| 0.86 (0.52–1.20) | 0.74 (0.50–0.97) | 0.97 (0.67–1.27) |
| 0.92 (0.60–1.40) | 0.81 (0.34–1.37) | 1.08 (0.52–1.64) |
| 0.99 (0.66–1.31) | 0.99 (0.53–1.45) | 1.12 (0.62–1.62) |
| 0.93 (0.60–1.30) | 0.91 (0.63–1.19) | 0.92 (0.50–1.36) |
| 1.09 (0.65–1.51) | 0.99 (0.57–1.40) | 1.05 (0.55–1.55) |
| 1.16 (0.77–1.54) | 1.02 (0.60–1.43) | 0.97 (0.57–1.37) |
| — | — | Positive titer ≥ 1:8 |
| — | — | Borderline titer = 1:25–1:50<br>Positive titer < 1:50 |
| 1.11 (0.90–1.31) | 1.05 (0.77–1.32) | 1.0 (0.74–1.26) |
| 1.69 (1.28–2.09) | 1.56 (0.98–2.12) | 0.86 (0.52–1.20) |
| 1.14 (0.88–1.54) | 1.03 (0.68–1.50) | 1.0 (0.71–1.31) |
| 1.00 (0.69–1.30) | 1.01 (0.65–1.37) | 0.93 (0.55–1.30) |
| 0.69 (0.45–0.93) | 0.83 (0.55–1.11) | 0.96 (0.64–1.28) |
| 0.78 (0.41–1.14) | 0.72 (0.52–0.92) | 0.81 (0.60–1.13) |
| 0.92 (0.75–1.08) | 0.86 (0.68–1.03) | 0.99 (0.7–1.22) |
| 2.42 (1.0–5.0) | 2.16 (1.0–4.0) | 4.90 (1.40–8.40) |
| 0.99 (0.89–1.10) | 0.98 (0.78–1.18) | 1.02 (0.68–1.36) |
| 6.79 (2.0–12.0) | 6.07 (2.0–10.0) | 3.60 (0–11.0) |

Data from Andrew M et al: Development of the human anticoagulant system in the healthy premature infant. Blood 1987;70:165–172; Andrew M et al: Development of the human anticoagulant system in the healthy premature infant. Blood 1988;72:1651–1657; and Andrew M et al: Maturation of the hemostatic system during childhood. Blood 1992;8:1998–2005.

BOX 14-2

**HYPERCOAGULABLE CONDITIONS**

| CONGENITAL | ACQUIRED |
|---|---|
| **Protein C and S deficiency:** Hereditary, autosomal dominant disorder. Heterozygotes have threefold to sixfold increased risk for venous thrombosis. | **Endothelial damage:** Causes include vascular catheters, smoking, diabetes, hypertension, surgery, hyperlipidemia |
| **Antithrombin III deficiency:** Hereditary, autosomal dominant disorder. Homozygotes die in infancy. | **Hyperviscosity:** Macroglobulinemia, polycythemia, sickle cell disase |
| **Factor V Leiden (activated protein C resistance):** 2%–5% of whites are heterozygotes with fivefold to tenfold increased risk for venous thrombosis; 1 in 1000 are homozygotes, with 80-fold to 100-fold increased risk for venous thrombosis. | **Antiphospholipid syndromes:** Common in patients with systemic lupus erythematosus; can occur idiopathically. Associated with venous and arterial thromboses and spontaneous abortions. |
| **Homocystinemia:** Increased levels of homocystine associated with arterial and venous thromboses, often due to MTHFR abnormalities. | **Platelet activation:** Caused by essential thrombocytosis, oral contraceptives |
| **Others:** Prothrombin mutation *(G20210A),* plasminogen abnormalities, fibrinogen abnormalities | **Others:** Drugs, malignancy, liver disease, inflammatory disease such as inflammatory bowel disease, paroxysmal nocturnal hemoglobinuria, lipoprotein A, heparin-induced thrombocytopenia |

MTHFR, methyltetrahydrofolate reductase.

BOX 14-3

**EXTENDED WORKUP FOR HYPERCOAGULABLE STATES***

Factors VIII, IX, XI
Activated protein C resistance assay (screening test for factor V Leiden)
Factor V Leiden (DNA-based assay for factor V Leiden)
Factor II 20210A (prothrombin mutation)
Homocystine
Methlytetrahydrofolate reductase (MTHFR) genetic testing if homocystine elevated
Dilute Russel viper venom test (antiphospholipid antibody syndrome)
Platelet neutralization procedure (lupus anticoagulant)
Anticardiolipin screening ELISA assay (anticardiolipin antibodies)
Protein C activity and antigen (protein C deficiency and dysfunction)
Protein S activity and antigen (protein S deficiency and dysfunction)
Antithrombin III activity and antigen (antithrombin III deficiency and dysfunction)
Plasminogen activity
Tissue plasminogen activator (TPA) antigen
Plasminogen activator inhibitor activity (measures activity of this TPA inhibitor)
$\alpha_2$–Antiplasmin activity (measures activity of this plasmin inhibitor)

*Where necessary, abnormality tested for is listed in parenthesis.
ELISA, enzyme-linked immunosorbent assay.

TABLE 14-7

**ADJUSTMENT AND MONITORING OF HEPARIN THERAPY**

**Initial bolus: 75 units/kg (max 7500 units)**
**Initial infusion rate: <1 year of age: 28 unit/kg/h (max 1600 units/h)**
**Initial infusion rate: >1 year of age: 20 unit/kg/h (max 1600 units/h)**

| aPTT Control Ratio | Rebolus/Dose Interruption | Heparin Infusion Adjustment |
|---|---|---|
| <1.2 × | Repeat original bolus | Increase by 4 U/kg/hr |
| 1.2–1.4 × | Repeat half original bolus | Increase by 2 U/kg/hr |
| 1.5-2.5 × | None | No change |
| 2.6–3.2 × | None | Decrease by 2 U/kg/hr |
| 3.3–4.0 ×* | Stop infusion, recheck aPTT in 1 hr<br>Restart infusion when aPTT is in or is projected to be in therapeutic range | Decrease by 4 U/kg/hr |
| 4.1–5.0 ×* | Stop infusion, recheck aPTT in 2 hr<br>Restart infusion when aPTT is in or is projected to be in therapeutic range | Decrease by 6 U/kg/hr |
| >5.0 ×* | Stop infusion; call hematologist immediately | |

*Note:* Check aPTT q6hr until in theraputic range on two consecutive lab values; then check aPTT q12hr ×2, then daily. Check aPTT 4–6 hr after every dose adjustment. Check Heme 8 daily until heparin is discontinued.

*Make sure sample not drawn from heparinized line.

From Streiff MB, Kickler TS: The Johns Hopkins Hospital Hemostatic Testing and Antithrombotic Therapy Manual. Baltimore, 2007.

(3) Heparin therapy should continue for at least 5–7 days while initiating warfarin for treatment of venous thrombosis.

b. **Low-molecular-weight heparin (LMWH):**[5] LMWH (enoxaparin) is routinely used in children, although less studied and more costly than heparin. LMWH has more specific anti-Xa activity, a longer half-life, a more predictable dose-to-efficacy ratio, and requires less monitoring.
  (1) Dose depends on preparation. See Formulary for enoxaparin dosage information.
  (2) Monitor LMWH therapy by following anti-Xa activity. Therapeutic range is 0.5–1.0 U/mL for full anticoagulation and 0.2–0.4 U/mL for prophylactic dosing. Anti-Xa activity should be drawn 4 hours after dose.
  (3) LMWH-induced bleeding can be treated with protamine.

c. **Warfarin:** Used for long-term anticoagulation, although it carries significant risk for morbidity and mortality. Patient must receive heparin while initiating warfarin therapy secondary to hypercoagulability from decreased protein C and S levels.

(1) Usually administered orally at a loading dose for 2–3 days, followed by a daily dose sufficient to maintain the PT/INR in the desired range. Infants often require higher daily doses. In all patients, levels should be measured every 1–2 weeks. See Table 14-8 for dose adjustment guidelines and Table 14-9 for management of excessive anticoagulation.

(2) Efficacy is greatly affected by dietary intake of vitamin K. Patients should receive appropriate dietary education.

(3) See Box 14-4 for a list of medicines that influence warfarin therapy.

d. Anticoagulant therapy alters many coagulation tests.

(1) Heparin alters aPTT, thrombin time, heparin level (anti-Xa), mixing studies, and fibrinogen.

(2) Warfarin alters PT, aPTT, dilute Russell Viper Venom test (dRVVT), and vitamin K-dependent factors (II, VII, IX, X, protein C and S).

e. Consult a hematologist for thrombolytic therapy.

**Note** *Children receiving anticoagulation therapy should be protected from trauma. Intramuscular injections are contraindicated. The use of antiplatelet agents and arterial punctures should be avoided.*

TABLE 14-8

**ADJUSTMENT AND MONITORING OF WARFARIN TO MAINTAIN AN INR BETWEEN 2 AND 3***

| I. Day 1 | |
|---|---|
| If the baseline INR is 1.0–1.3: | |
| Dose = 0.2 mg/kg orally | |
| **II. Loading Days 2 to 4: If the INR is** | |
| **INR** | **Action** |
| 1.1–1.3 | Repeat initial loading dose |
| 1.4–1.9 | 50% of initial loading dose |
| 2.0–3.0 | 50% of initial loading dose |
| 3.1–3.5 | 25% of initial loading dose |
| >3.5 | Hold until INR <3.5, then restart at 50% less than previous dose |
| **III. Maintenance Oral Anticoagulation Dose Guidelines** | |
| **INR** | **Action** |
| 1.1–1.4 | Increase by 20% of dose |
| 1.5–1.9 | Increase by 10% of dose |
| 2.0–3.0 | No change |
| 3.1–3.5 | Decrease by 10% of dose |
| >3.5 | Hold until INR <3.5, then restart at 20% less than the previous dose |

*Onset of action of warfarin is 36–72 hr, peak effects in 5–7 days. Because of this long half-life, avoid making dose adjustments with excessive frequency. Slow onset and offset of action allow for flexible dosing schedule.

From Streiff MB, Kickler TS: The Johns Hopkins Hospital Hemostatic Testing and Antithrombotic Therapy Manual, 3rd ed. Baltimore, 2007.

TABLE 14-9

**MANAGEMENT OF EXCESSIVE WARFARIN ANTICOAGULATION**

| | |
|---|---|
| INR <5 without significant bleeding | Hold warfarin<br>Recheck INR in 12–24 hr<br>When INR approaches therapeutic range, resume warfarin at 15%–20% lower dose and follow INR daily |
| INR ≥5 but <9 without significant bleeding | Hold warfarin<br>Recheck INR q12h<br>If high risk for bleeding, consider low dose of vitamin K orally (1–2.5 mg PO in adults)<br>When INR approaches therapeutic range, resume warfarin at 20% lower dose and follow INR daily |
| INR ≥9 without significant bleeding | Hold warfarin<br>Recheck INR q12h<br>Give vitamin K orally (5 mg in adults)<br>May use additional doses of vitamin K as needed (1–2 mg PO in adults)<br>When INR approaches therapeutic range, resume warfarin at dose at least 20% lower and follow INR daily |
| Serious bleeding at any INR elevation | Hold warfarin<br>Give vitamin K IV over 1 hr (10 mg IV in adults)<br>Vitamin K may be repeated in 12 hr as needed<br>Monitor INR q6h<br>Consider use of FFP, or NovoSeven (20 μg/kg IV), or FEIBA (50 units/kg IV) |

***Note:* Always evaluate for bleeding risks and potential drug interactions.**

FEIBA, Factor eight inhibitor bypassing activity

From Streiff MB, Kickler TS: The Johns Hopkins Hospital Hemostatic Testing and Antithrombotic Therapy Manual, 3rd ed. Baltimore, 2007.

14

HEMATOLOGY

BOX 14-4

MEDICATIONS THAT INFLUENCE WARFARIN THERAPY

| Significant Increase in the INR | Significant Decrease in the INR |
|---|---|
| Amiodarone | Amobarbital |
| Anabolic steroids | Aprepitant |
| Bactrim (TMP/SMZ) | Butabarbital |
| Chloramphenicol | Carbamazepine |
| Disulfiram | Dicloxacillin |
| Fluconazole | Griseofulvin |
| Isoniazid | Methimazole |
| Metronidazole | Phenobarbital |
| Miconazole | Phenytoin |
| Phenylbutazone | Primidone |
| Quinidine | Propylthiouracil |
| Sulfinpyrazone | Rifabutin |
| Sulfisoxazole | Rifampin |
| Tamoxifen | Secobarbital |
| **Moderate Increase in the INR** | **Moderate Decrease in the INR** |
| Cimetidine | Atazanavir |
| Ciprofloxacin | Efavirenz |
| Clarithromycin | Nafcillin |
| Delavirdine | Ritonavir |
| Efavirenz | |
| Itraconazole | |
| Lovastatin | |
| Omeprazole | |
| Propafenone | |
| Ritonavir | |

## C. BLEEDING DISORDERS (Fig. 14-3 and Box 14-5)

1. **Factor VIII deficiency (hemophilia A):** X-linked disorder characterized by prolonged aPTT and reduced factor VIII activity. PT and BT are normal. Treat with factor VIII concentrate. Recombinant factor VIII is preferred to reduce risk for infection. The factor level usually recovers by 2% per 1 unit of factor VIII per kilogram of body weight (Table 14-10 shows desired level). Factor may need to be redosed based on the clinical scenario. The first dose has a shorter half-life; a second dose, if needed, is given after 4–8 hr. Thereafter, the half-life is approximately 8–12 hr, and subsequent doses are usually given every 12 hr. Continuous infusion often required for surgical patients, usually with a 50 U/kg loading dose, followed by 3–4 U/kg/hr. For suspected intracranial bleeding, replace to 100% before diagnostic procedures, such as CT scan.

Units of factor VIII = weight (kg) × desired % replacement × 0.5

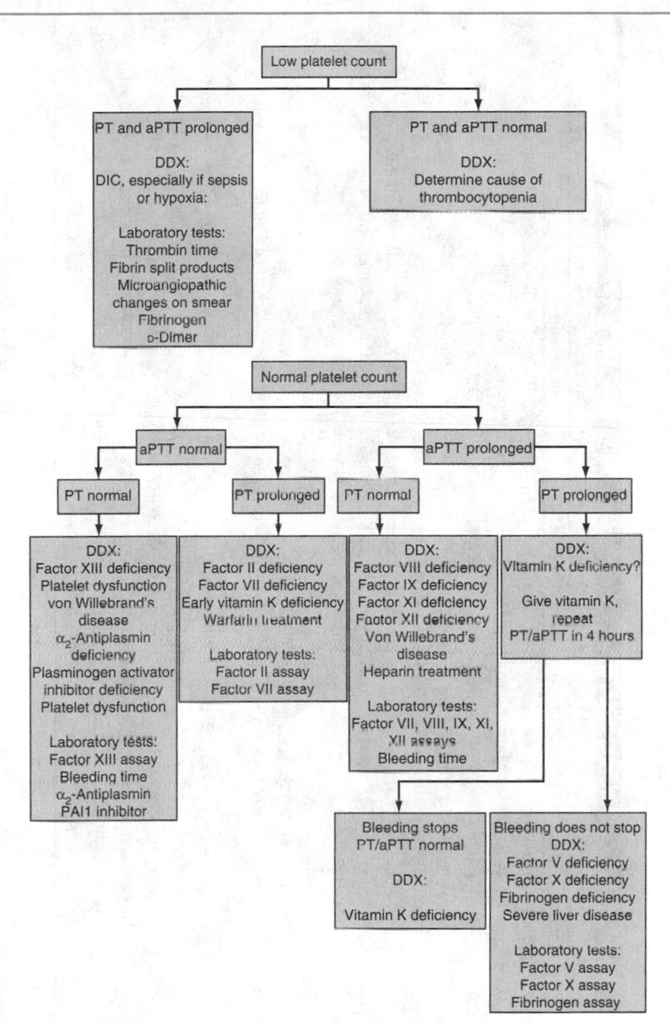


Fig. 14-3
Differential diagnosis of bleeding disorders.

BOX 14-5

**BLEEDING DISORDERS**

| CONGENITAL | ACQUIRED |
|---|---|
| Disorder of platelet number or function | **Disseminated intravascular coagulation:** Characterized by prolonged PT and aPTT, decreased fibrinogen and platelets, increased fibrin degradation products, and elevated D-dimers. Treatment includes identifying and treating underlying disorder. Replacement of depleted coagulation factors with FFP may be necessary in severe cases, especially when bleeding is present; 10–15 mL/kg will raise clotting factors 20%. Fibrinogen, if depleted, can be given as cryoprecipitate. Platelet transfusions may also be necessary. |
| **Thrombocytopenia:** Secondary to bone marrow disease or defective megakaryocyte maturation | **Liver disease:** The liver is the major site of synthesis of factors V, VII, IX, X, XI, XII, XIII, prothrombin, plasminogen, fibrinogen, protein C and S, and ATIII. Treatment with FFP and platelets may be needed, but this will increase hepatic protein load. Vitamin K should be given to patients with liver disease and clotting abnormalities. |
| **Disorders of platelet function:** Bernard-Soulier syndrome, Glanzmann thrombasthenia, storage pool diseases | **Vitamin K deficiency:** Factors II, VII, IX, X, protein C, and protein S are vitamin K dependent. Early vitamin K deficiency may present with isolated prolonged PT because factor VII has the shortest half-life. Fibrinogen should be normal. |
| **Factor VIII deficiency:** See text | **Hemolytic-uremic syndrome/thrombotic thrombocytopenic purpura (HUS/TTP):** Characterized by the triad of microangiopathic hemolytic anemia, uremia, and thrombocytopenia. HUS/TTP is often triggered by bacterial enteritis, especially caused by *Escherichia coli* O157:H7, although there are a variety of causes. HUS does not typically include coagulation abnormalities, such as those seen in DIC. Avoid blood products in patients with HUS thought to be secondary to pneumococcal infection. TTP includes the triad of HUS in addition to fever and CNS changes and is more common in older adolescents and adults. |
| **Factor IX deficiency:** See text | |
| **Von Willebrand disease:** See text | |

TABLE 14-10

DESIRED FACTOR REPLACEMENT IN HEMOPHILIA

| Bleeding Site | Desired Level (%) |
|---|---|
| Joint or simple hematoma | 20–40 |
| Simple dental extraction | 50 |
| Major soft tissue bleed | 80–100 |
| Serious oral bleeding | 80–100 |
| Head injury | 100+ |
| Major surgery (dental, orthopedic, other) | 100+ |

*Note:* A hematologist should be consulted for all major bleeding and before surgery.



2. **Factor IX deficiency (hemophilia B or Christmas disease):** X-linked disorder characterized by prolonged aPTT and low factor IX activity. Treat with factor IX concentrate. The factor level usually recovers by 1% for each unit of factor IX concentrate per kilogram of body weight; it has a half-life of 18–24 hr. As with factor VIII, a second dose, if needed, should be given at a shorter interval. Recombinant factor IX has a shorter half-life; consider evaluation of in vivo factor survival in each patient. Replace to 100% before diagnostic procedures if intracranial bleed suspected.

$$\text{Units of factor IX} = \text{weight (kg)} \times \text{desired \% replacement}$$

**Note** *All patients with hemophilia should be vaccinated with hepatitis A and hepatitis B vaccines.*

3. **Von Willebrand disease:** vWF binds platelets to subendothelial surfaces and carries and stabilizes factor VIII.

a. **Type 1:** Characterized by decreased quantity of vWF typically without identifiable gene mutation, decreased ristocetin cofactor activity proportional to vWF, and mild to moderate bleeding. Typically prolonged BT, normal platelet count, and mild to moderate prolongation of aPTT.

b. **Type 2:** Characterized by four subtypes all with various functional abnormalities of vWF molecule, a more marked decrease in ristocetin cofactor activity compared to decrease in vWF, and moderate to severe bleeding.

c. **Type 3:** Characterized by more severe decrease in vWF secondary to genetic mutations and severe bleeding.

d. Factor VIII and vWF levels are decreased in type 1 and 3 disease but may be normal in variants with dysfunctional vWF.

e. In patients with a proven response to desmopressin acetate (DDAVP), bleeding or minor surgical procedures may be treated with DDAVP intravenously over 20–30 min or intranasally (see Formulary for dosage information).

**Note** *DDAVP may be contraindicated in vWD type 2b because it may exacerbate thrombocytopenia.*

f. For more severe disease or patients with dysfunctional vWF (type 2), treatment of choice is Humate P (heat-inactivated vWF-enriched concentrate: 40 IU/kg), a similar product containing active vWF, or cryoprecipitate. Concentrates are preferred because they are virally inactivated.
g. Aminocaproic acid 100 mg/kg IV or PO every 4–6 hr (up to 24 g/day) may be useful for treatment of oral bleeding and as prophylaxis for dental extractions.

## VI. BLOOD COMPONENT REPLACEMENT

### A. BLOOD VOLUME

Requirements are age specific (Table 14-11).

### B. BLOOD PRODUCT COMPONENTS

1. **RBCs: The decision to transfuse RBCs should be made with consideration of clinical symptoms and signs, the degree of cardiorespiratory or CNS disease, the cause and course of anemia, and options for alternative therapy, noting the risks for transfusion-associated infections and reactions.**

a. **Packed RBC (PRBC) transfusion:** Concentrated RBCs, with HCT of 55%–70%. A typed and cross-matched blood product is preferred when possible; O-negative (or O-positive) blood may be used if transfusion cannot be delayed. O-negative is preferred for females of child-bearing age to reduce risk for Rh sensitization.
   (1) Unless rapid replacement is required for acute blood loss or shock, infuse no faster than 2–3 mL/kg/hr (generally 10 mL/kg aliquots over 4 hr) to avoid congestive heart failure.

TABLE 14-11

ESTIMATED BLOOD VOLUME (EBV)

| Age | Total Blood Volume (mL/kg) |
|---|---|
| Preterm infants | 90–105 |
| Term newborns | 78–86 |
| 1–12 mo | 73–78 |
| 1–3 yr | 74–82 |
| 4–6 yr | 80–86 |
| 7–18 yr | 83–90 |
| Adults | 68–88 |

Data from Nathan D, Oski FA: Hematology of Infancy and Childhood. Philadelphia, WB Saunders, 1998.

(2) A rule of thumb in severe compensated anemia is to give an $X$ mL/kg aliquot, where $X$ = patient Hb (g/dL); for example, if Hb = 5 g/dL, transfuse 5 mL/kg over 4 hr.

(3) To calculate the volume of PRBC to achieve a desired HCT, use the following equation:

$$\text{Volume of PRBCs (mL)} = \frac{\text{EBV (mL)} \times (\text{desired HCT} - \text{actual HCT})}{\text{HCT of PRBCs}}$$

where EBV is the estimated blood volume (see Table 14-11 for age-specific EBV) and HCT of PRBCs is usually 55%–70%.

b. **Leukocyte-poor PRBCs:**

(1) **Filtered RBCs:** 99.9% of WBCs removed from product; used for CMV-negative patients to reduce risk for CMV transmission. Also reduces likelihood of a nonhemolytic febrile transfusion reaction.

(2) **Washed RBCs:** 92%–95% of WBCs removed from product. Similar advantages to leukocyte-poor filtered RBCs. Although filtered leukocyte-poor blood is now more commonly used, washing may be helpful if a patient has pre-existing antibodies to blood products (e.g., patients who have complete IgA deficiency or a history of urticarial transfusion reactions).

c. **Irradiated blood products:**

(1) Many blood products (PRBCs, platelet preparations, leukocytes, fresh frozen plasma [FFP], and others) contain viable lymphocytes capable of proliferation and engraftment in the recipient, causing graft-versus-host disease (GVHD). Irradiation with 1500 cGy before transfusion may prevent GVHD but does not prevent antibody formation against donor white cells. Engraftment most likely in young infants, immunocompromised patients, and patients receiving blood from first-degree relatives.

(2) Indications: Intensive chemotherapy, leukemia, lymphoma, bone marrow transplantation, solid organ transplantation, known or suspected immune deficiencies, intrauterine transfusions, and transfusions in neonates.

d. **CMV-negative blood:** Obtained from donors who test negative for CMV. May be given to neonates or other immunocompromised patients, including those awaiting organ or marrow transplant who are CMV negative.

2. **Platelets: Indicated to treat severe or symptomatic thrombocytopenia. Should not be refrigerated because this promotes premature platelet activation and clumping.**

a. **Single-donor product:** Preferred over pooled concentrate for patients with antiplatelet antibodies.

b. **Leukocyte-poor:** Use if there is a history of significant acute, febrile platelet transfusion reactions.

c. Usually give 4 U/m$^2$, or approximately 10 mL/kg of normally concentrated platelet product. The platelet count is raised by 10,000 to

15,000/μL by giving 1 U/m$^2$. For infants and children, 10 mL/kg will increase the platelet count by approximately 50,000/μL.

d. Hemorrhagic complications are rare with platelet counts >20,000/μL. A transfusion "trigger" of 10,000/μL is recommended by many in the absence of serious bleeding complications. A platelet count >50,000/μL is advisable for minor procedures; >100,000/μL is advisable for major surgery or intracranial operation.

3. **FFP:** Contains all clotting factors except platelets. Used in severe clotting factor deficiencies with active bleeding or to reverse effects of warfarin. Also replaces anticoagulant factors (antithrombin III, protein C, protein S). Used in treatment of DIC, vitamin K deficiency with active bleeding, or thrombotic thrombocytopenic purpura (TTP). 1 mL of FFP expected to provide 1 unit of activity of all factors except labile factor V and VIII, but individual units may vary. The usual amount is 10 to 15 mL/kg; repeat doses as needed. In acquired TTP, plasma exchange is the treatment of choice.
4. **Cryoprecipitate:** Enriched for factor VIII (5–10 U/mL), vWF, and fibrinogen. Historically useful for children with factor VIII or vWF deficiency in the context of active bleeding, but concentrates or recombinant products now preferred because of lower risk for viral transmission.
5. **Monoclonal factor VIII:** Highly purified factor, derived from pooled human blood.
6. **Recombinant factor VIII or IX:** Highly purified, with less theoretical infectious risk than pooled human products risk for inhibitor formation, as with other products.

## C. PRBC EXCHANGE TRANSFUSION

1. Partial PRBC exchange transfusion may be indicated for sickle cell patients with acute chest syndrome, stroke, intractable pain crisis, or refractory priapism. Replace with Sickledex-negative cells. Goal is to reduce percentage of HbS to <40%. Follow HCT carefully during transfusion to avoid hyperviscosity, maintaining HCT <35%.
2. Indications for double-volume PRBC exchange transfusion include severe acute chest and CVA. Goal is to reduce percentage of HbS to <30%. Expected reduction in percentage of circulating sickle cells is 60%–80%.
3. To calculate the volume of PRBC needed for a double-volume exchange, use the following equation:

$$\frac{\text{EBV (mL)} \times \text{Patient HCT} \times 2}{\text{HCT of PRBC}}$$

where EBV is the age-dependent estimated blood volume (see Table 14-11) and HCT of PRBC is 55%–70%

### D. COMPLICATIONS OF TRANSFUSIONS

1. **Acute transfusion reactions:**

a. **Acute hemolytic reaction:** Most often the result of blood group incompatibility. Signs and symptoms include fever, chills, tachycardia, hypotension, and shock. Treatment includes immediate cessation of blood transfusion and institution of supportive measures. Laboratory findings include DIC, hemoglobinuria, and positive Coombs test.

b. **Febrile nonhemolytic reaction:** Usually the result of host antibody response to donor leukocyte antigens, common in previously transfused patients. Symptoms include fever, chills, and diaphoresis. Stop transfusion and evaluate. Prevention includes premedication with antipyretics, antihistamines, corticosteroids, and, if necessary, use of leukocyte-poor PRBCs.

c. **Urticarial reaction:** Reaction to donor plasma proteins. Stop transfusion immediately; treat with antihistamines, and epinephrine and steroids if there is respiratory compromise (see also treatment of anaphylaxis, Chapter 1). Use washed or filtered RBCs with the next transfusion.

d. **Evaluation of acute transfusion reaction:**

(1) Patient's urine: Test for hemoglobin.

(2) Patient's blood: Confirm blood type, screen for antibodies, and repeat DCT on pretransfusion and post-transfusion sera.

(3) Donor blood: Culture for bacteria.

2. **Delayed transfusion reaction:** Usually due to minor blood group antigen incompatibility with low or absent titer of antibodies at time of transfusion. Occurs 3–10 days after transfusion. Symptoms include fatigue, jaundice, and dark urine. Laboratory findings include anemia, a positive Coombs test, new RBC antibodies, and hemoglobinuria. The need for acute intervention is much less likely than with acute reactions.

3. **Transmission of infectious diseases:**[6] Blood supply is tested for HIV types 1 and 2, HTLV types I and II, hepatitis B, hepatitis C, syphilis, and West Nile virus. Data from 2006 estimate the risk for transmitting infection as follows: HIV (1 in 2 million); HTLV (1 in 641,000); hepatitis B (1 in 63,000–500,000); hepatitis C (1 in 250,000–500,000); parvovirus (1 in 10,000). CMV, hepatitis A, parasitic, tickborne, and prion diseases may also be transmitted by blood products.

4. **Sepsis:** Sepsis occurs with products that are contaminated with bacteria, particularly platelets, because they are stored at room temperature.

## VII. INTERPRETING BLOOD SMEARS

See Color Plates 1 to 12 in this chapter for examples of blood smears. Examine the blood smear in an area where the RBCs are nearly touching but do not overlap.

### A. RBC

Examine size, shape, and color.

### B. WBC

A rough estimate of the WBC count can be made by looking at the smear under high power (100× magnification). Each one cell per high power field correlates with approximately 500 WBC/cubic mm.

### C. PLATELETS

A rough estimate of platelet count is one platelet per high power field corresponds to 10,000–15,000/μL. Platelet clumps usually indicate >100,000 platelets/μL.

## REFERENCES


1. Bernini JC et al: Beneficial effect of intravenous dexamethasone in children with mild to moderately severe acute chest syndrome complicating sickle cell disease. Blood 1998;92(9):3082–3089.
2. American Academy of Pediatrics, Section on Hematology/Oncology Committee on Genetics: Health supervision in children with sickle cell disease. Pediatrics 2002;109:526–535.
3. Koren A et al: Effect of hydroxyurea in sickle cell anemia: A clinical trial in children and teenagers with severe sickle cell anemia and sickle beta-thalassemia. Pediatr Hematol Oncol 1999;16(3):221–232.
4. Streiff MB, Kickler TS: The Johns Hopkins Hospital Hemostatic Testing and Antithrombotic Therapy Manual, 3rd ed. Baltimore, 2007.
5. Monagle P et al: Antithrombotic therapy in children: Seventh ACCP Consensus Conference on antithrombotic and thrombolytic therapy. Chest 2004;126:645S–687S.
6. American Academy of Pediatrics: Red book: 2006 Report of the committee on infectious diseases, 27th ed. Elk Grove Village, Ill, AAP, 2006.

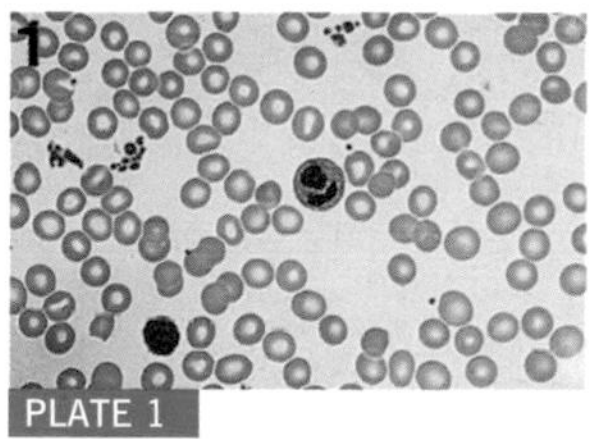

PLATE 1

Normal smear. Round RBCs with central pallor about one third of the cell's diameter, scattered platelets, occasional white blood cells.

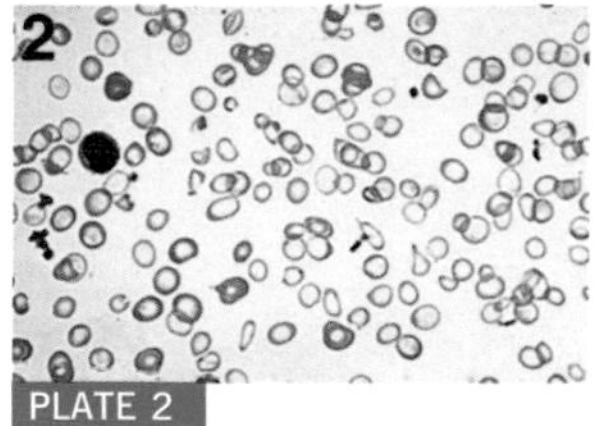

PLATE 2

Iron deficiency. Hypochromic/microcytic RBCs, poikilocytosis, plentiful platelets, occasional ovalocytes and target cells.



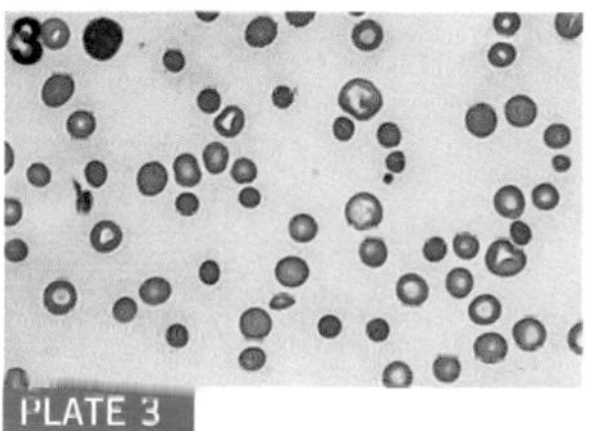

PLATE 3

Spherocytosis. Microspherocytes a hallmark (densely stained RBCs with no central pallor).

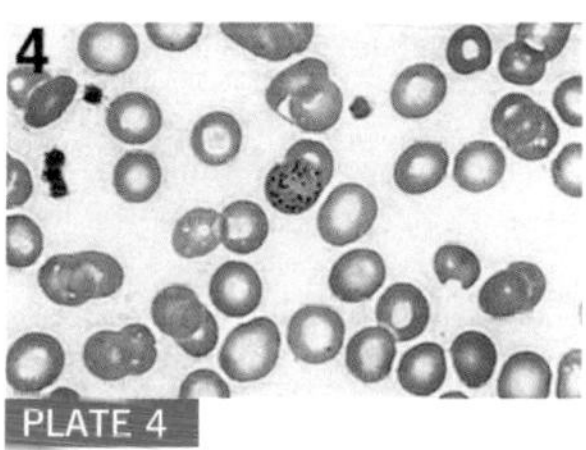

PLATE 4

Basophilic stippling as a result of precipitated RNA throughout the cell; seen with heavy metal intoxication, thalassemia, iron deficiency, and other states of ineffective erythropoesis.

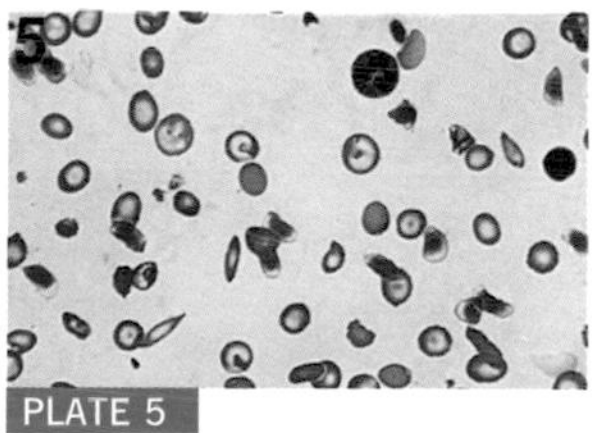

PLATE 5

Hemoglobin SS disease. Sickled cells, target cells, hypochromia, poikilocytosis, Howell-Jolly bodies; nucleated RBCs common (not shown).

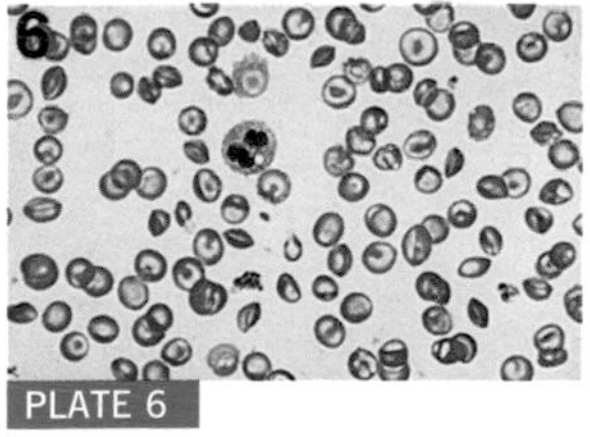

PLATE 6

Hemoglobin SC disease. Target cells, "oat cells," poikilocytosis; sickle forms rarely seen.

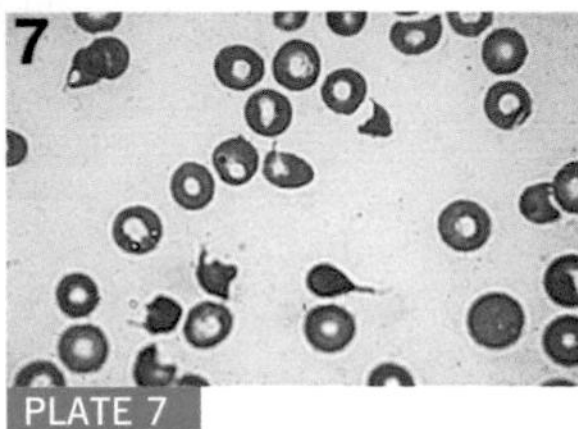


PLATE 7

Microangiopathic hemolytic anemia. RBC fragments, anisocytosis, polychromasia, decreased platelets.

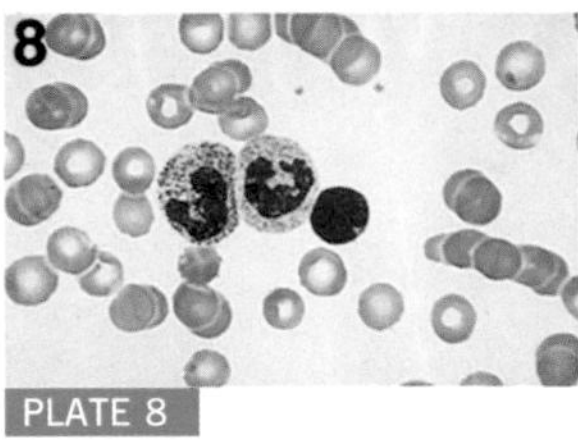


PLATE 8

Toxic granulations. Prominent dark blue primary granules; commonly seen with infection and other toxic states, such as Kawasaki disease.

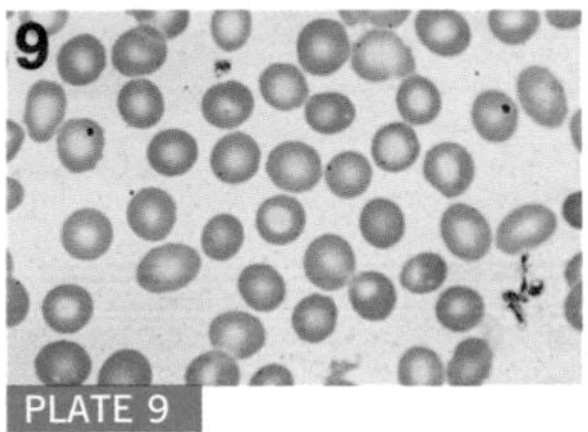


PLATE 9

Howell-Jolly body. Small, dense nuclear remnant in an RBC; suggests splenic dysfunction or asplenia.

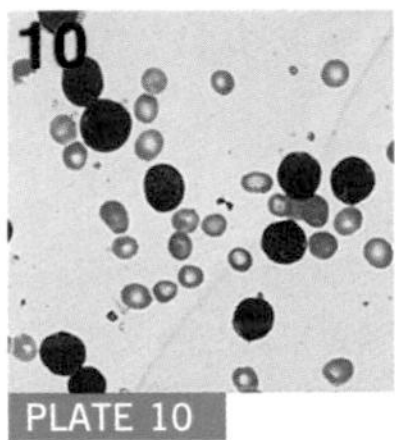


PLATE 10

Leukemic blasts showing large nucleus-to-cytoplasm ratio.

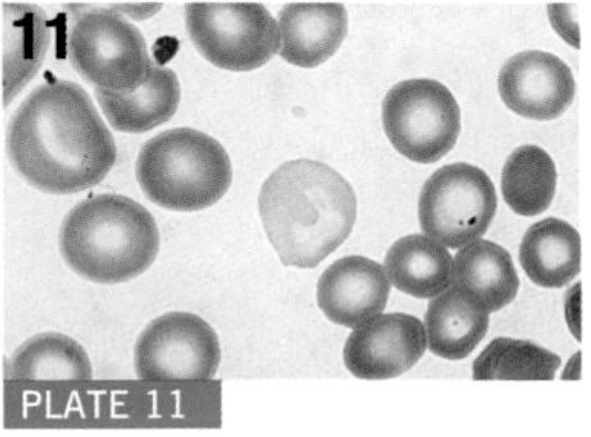


PLATE 11

Polychromatophilia. Diffusely basophilic because of RNA staining; seen with early release of reticulocytes from the marrow.

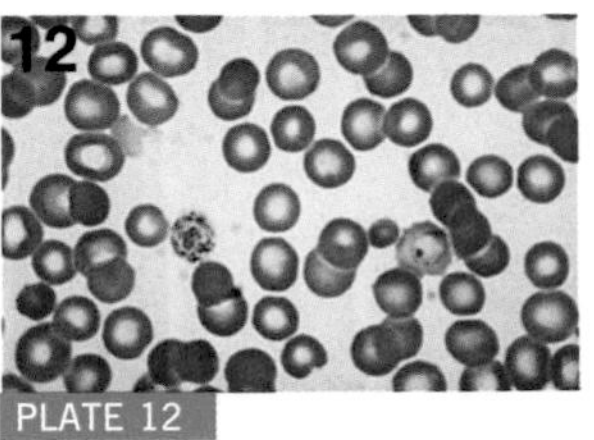


PLATE 12

Malaria. Intraerythrocytic parasites.

# Immunology and Allergy

*Hilary J. Tinkel Vernon, MD, PhD*

15

## I. ALLERGIC RHINITIS

### A. EPIDEMIOLOGY

1. **Most common chronic condition.**
2. **Significant impact on quality of life including school performance, sleep patterns, demonstrated in multiple studies.**
3. **Increases risk for recurrent otitis media, and acute and chronic sinusitis.**

### B. DIAGNOSIS

1. **History:**

a. Symptoms:
   (1) Nasal: Congestion, rhinorrhea, pruritus.
   (2) Ocular: Pruritus, tearing.
   (3) Postnasal drip: Sore throat, cough, pruritus.

b. Patterns:
   (1) Seasonal: Depends on local allergens.
   (2) Perennial.

c. Coexisting atopic diseases common (eczema, asthma, food allergy).

2. **Physical examination:**

a. "Allergic facies" with shiners, mouth breathing, transverse nasal crease.
b. Nasal mucosa may be normal to pink to pale gray
c. Injected sclera with or without clear discharge.

3. **Laboratory studies:**

a. Nasal smear for eosinophils: Quick, easy screen with good positive predictive value.
b. Total immunoglobulin E (IgE): Nonspecific due to wide overlap between atopic and nonatopic subjects.
c. Peripheral blood eosinophil count.
d. Skin testing: Gold standard.
e. Radio allergosorbent testing (RAST): Identifies presence of serum IgE to selected antigens.
f. Imaging studies: Not useful.
g. Nasal provocative test: Research test only.

### C. DIFFERENTIAL DIAGNOSIS

1. **Vasomotor rhinitis:** Symptoms made worse by scents, alcohol, or changes in temperature or humidity.
2. **Adenoid hypertrophy.**
3. **Rhinitis medicamentosa:** Rebound rhinitis from prolonged use of nasal vasoconstrictors.
4. **Sinusitis:** Acute or chronic.
5. **Nonallergic rhinitis with eosinophilia syndrome (NARES).**
6. **Nasal polyps.**

### D. TREATMENT

1. **Allergen avoidance:**
   a. Relies on identification of triggers.
   b. Difficult to avoid ubiquitous airborne allergens.
   c. Thorough house cleaning and allergy-proof bed coverings can be useful.
2. **Topical corticosteroids (fluticasone, mometasone, budesonide):**
   a. Most effective maintenance therapy for nasal congestion.
   b. Minimal benefit for ocular symptoms.
   c. No proven adverse effect on long-term growth.
   d. Adverse effects: Nasal irritation, sneezing, bleeding.
3. **Oral antihistamines (diphenhydramine, cetirizine):**
   a. Second-generation preparations preferable (cetirizine, loratidine, desloratidine, fexofenadine).
   b. Adverse effects: Sedation, anticholinergic side effects, risk for development of tolerance.
4. **Leukotriene inhibitors (montelukast).**
5. **Mast cell stabilizers (cromolyn):**
   a. Inexpensive and easily available.
   b. Most effective as prophylaxis.
   c. Few adverse effects.
6. **Intranasal antihistamines (azelastine):**
   a. Effective for acute symptoms.
   b. Not studied in children under age 5 years.
   c. Adverse effects: Bitter taste, systemic absorption with sedation.
7. **Decongestants (pseudoephedrine):**
   a. May be effective in the short term.
   b. Adverse effects: Anxiety, insomnia, rebound symptoms, tachycardia.
8. **Anticholinergics (ipratropium):**
   a. Useful for rhinorrhea only.
   b. Adverse effects: Drying of nasal mucosa.
9. **Immunotherapy:**
   a. Success rate is high when patients are chosen carefully and when performed by an allergy specialist.
   b. Consider when drug side effects are limiting or triggering allergens are difficult to avoid.
   c. Not recommended in poorly compliant patients or those with asthma.
   d. Not well studied in children under age 5 years.
10. **Nasal rinsing:**
   a. Hypertonic saline.
   b. Tolerable and inexpensive.

## II. FOOD ALLERGY

### A. EPIDEMIOLOGY

1. **5%–8% in pediatric population.**
2. **Most common allergens in children:** Milk, eggs, peanuts, tree nuts, soy, wheat.

## B. MANIFESTATIONS OF FOOD ALLERGY

Often a combination of several syndromes.

1. **Anaphylaxis:**
a. Uniphasic, biphasic, or protracted patterns.
b. Risk factors for fatal outcome:
   (1) History of asthma.
   (2) Peanut or tree nut allergy.
   (3) Delayed administration of epinephrine.

2. **Skin syndromes:**
a. Urticaria/angioedema:
   (1) Chronic urticaria rarely related to food allergy.
   (2) Acute urticaria predicts risk for future anaphylaxis.
b. Atopic dermatitis/eczema:
   (1) Food allergy more common in patients with atopic dermatitis.
   (2) Acute and chronic skin changes often coexist.

3. **Gastrointestinal syndromes:**
a. Oral allergy syndrome:
   (1) Edema of oral mucosa after ingestion of certain fresh fruits and vegetables in patients with pollen allergies.
   (2) Inciting antigens destroyed by cooking.
   (3) Caused by cross-reactivity of antibodies to pollens.
   (4) Rarely progresses beyond the mouth.
b. Allergic eosinophilic gastroenteritis, esophagitis:
   (1) Reflux, abdominal pain, diarrhea, early satiety.
   (2) Characterized by eosinophilic infiltration of digestive tract.
c. Food-induced enterocolitis:
   (1) Presents in infancy.
   (2) Vomiting and diarrhea (may contain blood); when severe, may lead to lethargy, dehydration, hypotension, acidosis.
   (3) Most commonly associated with milk, soy.
d. Infantile proctocolitis:
   (1) Confined to distal colon and presents with only diarrhea.
   (2) Symptoms of short duration; rarely leads to anemia.

4. **Respiratory syndromes:**
a. Rhinitis.
b. Asthma.
c. Heiner syndrome:
   (1) Precipitating IgG antibody to cow's milk.
   (2) Results in pulmonary infiltrates, hemosiderosis, anemia, recurrent pneumonia, and failure to thrive.

## C. DIAGNOSIS OF FOOD ALLERGY (Fig. 15-1)

1. **History:**
a. Identify specific foods.
b. Establish timing and nature of reactions; patient should keep a food diary.

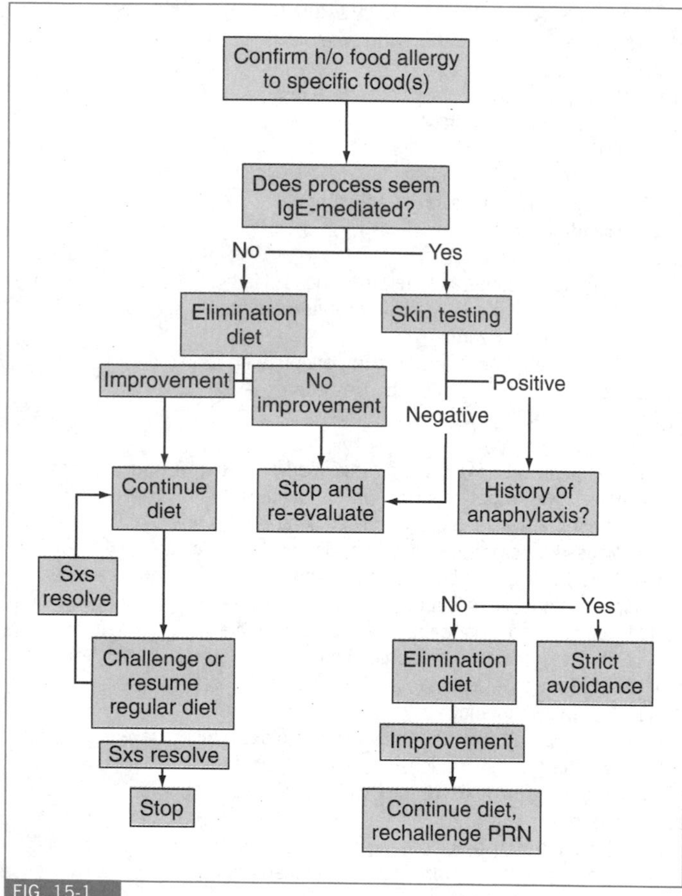


FIG. 15-1

Evaluation and management of food allergy. *(Data from Wood RA: The natural history of childhood food allergy. Pediatrics 2003;111[6]:1631–1637, and Wood RA: Up to Date 2007. Available at www.uptodate.com.)*

2. **Physical examination.**
3. **Skin testing:**
a. Skin prick test has poor positive predictive value, but very good negative predictive value.
b. Patient must not be taking antihistamines.
c. Intradermal tests have high false-positive rates.
4. **RAST (specific IgE levels):**
a. Like skin tests, RAST has poor positive predictive value, excellent negative predictive value.
b. Levels above a certain range have increasing positive predictive value.
c. IgG testing not useful.
5. **Oral food challenges:**
a. Must be done under medical supervision with intravenous (IV) access for giving emergency medications if needed.
b. Patient must not be taking antihistamines.
c. Most effective when double-blinded using graded doses of disguised food.

## D. DIFFERENTIAL DIAGNOSIS

1. **Food intolerance:**
a. Nonimmunologic.
b. Based on toxins or other properties of foods.
2. **Malabsorption syndromes:**
a. Cystic fibrosis, celiac disease, lactase deficiency.
b. GI malformations

## E. TREATMENT

1. **Allergen avoidance:**
a. Most important intervention.
b. Patients must pay close attention to food ingredients.
c. Infants with milk, soy allergies may be placed on elemental formula.
2. **Anaphylaxis:**
a. Immediate intervention required.
b. Epinephrine first; then consider antihistamines, fluids, bronchodilators, corticosteroids.
c. Vasopressors if necessary for hypotension.
3. **Angioedema, urticaria:**
a. Antihistamines, corticosteroids.
b. Broad differential.
4. **Atopic dermatitis: Symptomatic control.**
5. **Natural history:**
a. About one third of allergies are lost in a 1- to 2-year period (peanut, tree nut, and shellfish allergies are rarely outgrown).
b. Most likely to be outgrown with complete avoidance.
c. Skin tests and RAST may remain positive even though symptoms resolve.

## III. PENICILLIN ALLERGY (Fig. 15-2)

## IV. IMMUNOGLOBULIN THERAPY

### A. INTRAVENOUS IMMUNE GLOBULIN (IVIG)

**1. Indications:**

a. Replacement therapy for antibody-deficient disorders:
   (1) 400–500 mg/kg IV every month to start.
   (2) Adjust dosing to maintain trough IgG level of at least 500 mg/dL.

b. Immune thrombocytopenic purpura:
   (1) 400–1000 mg/kg IV as a single dose, then repeat dose as needed.
   (2) May also use Rh (D) immunoglobulin (WinRho) in Rh-positive patients.

c. Kawasaki disease:
   (1) 2 g/kg × 1 dose over 8–12 hr.
   (2) If signs and symptoms persist, consider second dose of 2 g/kg.
   (3) Should be started within first 10 days of symptoms.

d. Pediatric human immunodeficiency virus (HIV) infection: 400 mg/kg every 28 days for hypogammaglobulinemia (IgG concentration <250 mg/dL), recurrent serious bacterial infections, failure to form antibodies to common antigens, or measles prophylaxis.

e. Bone marrow transplantation:
   (1) 400–500 mg/kg/dose to start, adjust dosing to maintain trough IgG level of at least 500 mg/dL.
   (2) May decrease incidence of infection and death but not acute graft-versus-host disease.

f. Other potential uses:
   (1) Guillain-Barré syndrome.
   (2) Refractory dermatomyositis and polymyositis.
   (3) Chronic inflammatory demyelinating polyneuropathy.

**2. Precautions and adverse reactions:**

a. Severe systemic symptoms (hemodynamic changes, respiratory difficulty, anaphylaxis).

b. Less severe systemic reactions (headache, myalgia, fever, chills, nausea, vomiting) may be alleviated by decreasing infusion rate or premedication with IV corticosteroids, antihistamines, and/or antipyretics.

c. Aseptic meningitis syndrome.

d. Acute renal failure (increased risk with preexisting renal insufficiency and with sucrose-containing IVIG).

e. Acute venous thrombosis (increased risk with sucrose-containing IVIG).

f. Use with caution in patients with undetectable IgA level due to trace amounts of IgA in IVIG, although routine screening for IgA deficiency is not recommended in potential recipients.

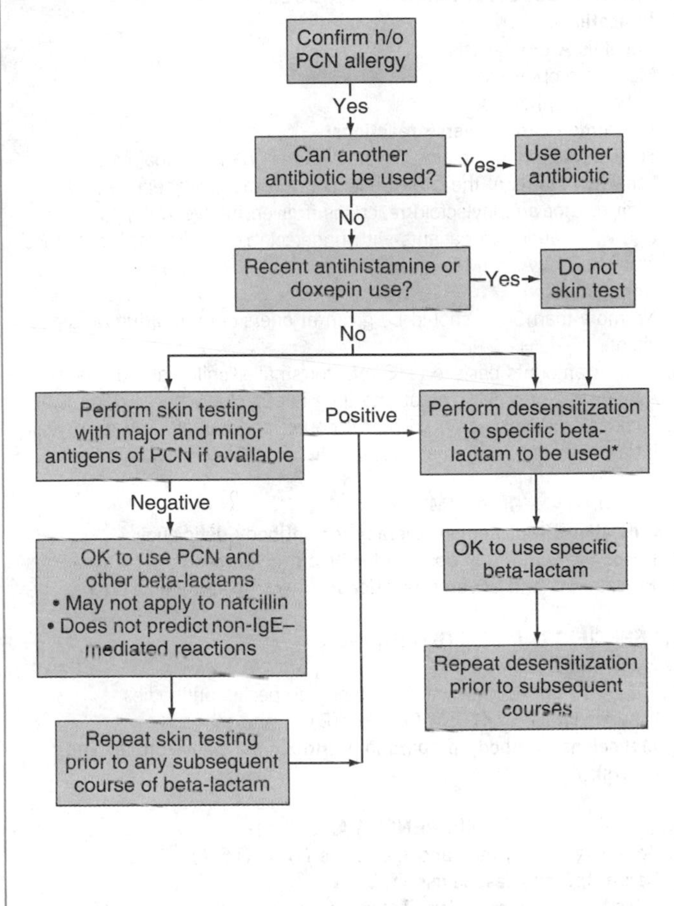


FIG. 15-2

Evaluation and management of penicillin allergy. *(Adapted from O'Dowd LC: Penicillin and related antibiotic allergy; skin testing; and desensitization. Up to Date 2007. Available at www.uptodate.com.)*

### B. INTRAMUSCULAR IMMUNE GLOBULIN (IMIG)

1. **Indications:**
   a. Hepatitis A prophylaxis.
   b. Measles prophylaxis.
   c. Rubella prophylaxis.
2. **Precautions and adverse reactions:**
   a. Severe systemic symptoms (hemodynamic changes, anaphylaxis).
   b. Local symptoms at the site of injection increase with repeated use.
   c. High risk for anaphylactoid reactions if given intravenously.
   d. Use with caution in patients with undetectable IgA levels due to trace amounts of IgA in IMIG.
3. **Administration:**
   a. No more than 5 mL should be given at one site in an adult or large child.
   b. Smaller amounts per site (1–3 mL) for smaller children and infants.
   c. Administration of >15 mL at one time is essentially never warranted.
   d. Peak serum levels achieved by 48 hours, and half-life is 3 to 4 weeks
   e. Intravenous or intradermal use of IMIG is absolutely contraindicated.

### C. SUBCUTANEOUS IMMUNE GLOBULIN

1. **Indication:** Replacement therapy for antibody deficiency.
2. **Dose:** Same monthly dose as for IV but given every 3–7 days.
3. **Precautions and adverse reactions:** Similar to IMIG and IVIG.

### D. SPECIFIC IMMUNE GLOBULINS

1. **Hyperimmune globulins:**
   a. Prepared from donors with high titers of specific antibodies.
   b. Includes HBIG, VZIG, CMV-IG, Rho(D)IG, and others.
2. **Monoclonal antibody preparations (rituximab, palivizumab, and others).**

### E. IMMUNOLOGIC REFERENCE VALUES

1. **Serum IgG, IgM, IgA, and IgE levels (Table 15-1).**
2. **Serum IgG subclass levels (Table 15-2).**
3. **Lymphocyte enumeration (Table 15-3).**
4. **Serum complement levels (Table 15-4).**

## V. EVALUATION OF A SUSPECTED IMMUNODEFICIENCY (Table 15-5)

*Text continued on p. 400*

TABLE 15-1

SERUM IMMUNOGLOBULIN LEVELS*

| Age | IgG (mg/dL) | IgM (mg/dL) | IgA (mg/dL) | IgE (IU/ml) |
|---|---|---|---|---|
| Cord blood (term) | 1121 (636–1606) | 13 (6.3–25) | 2.3 (1.4–3.6) | 0.22 (0.04–1.28) |
| 1 mo[‖] | 503 (251–906) | 45 (20–87) | 13 (1.3–53) | |
| 6 wk | | | | 0.69 (0.08–6.12) |
| 2 mo | 365 (206–601) | 46 (17–105) | 15 (2.8–47) | |
| 3 mo | 334 (176–581) | 49 (24–89) | 17 (4.6–46) | 0.82 (0.18–3.76) |
| 4 mo | 343 (196–558) | 55 (27–101) | 23 (4.4–73) | |
| 5 mo | 403 (172–814) | 62 (33–108) | 31 (8.1–84) | |
| 6 mo | 407 (215–704) | 62 (35–102) | 25 (8.1–68) | 2.68 (0.44–16.3) |
| 7–9 mo | 475 (217–904) | 80 (34–126) | 36 (11–90) | 2.36 (0.76–7.31) |
| 10–12 mo | 594 (294–1069) | 82 (41–149) | 40 (16–84) | |
| 1 yr | 679 (345–1213) | 93 (43–173) | 44 (14–106) | 3.49 (0.80–15.2) |
| 2 yr | 685 (424–1051) | 95 (48–168) | 47 (14–123) | 3.03 (0.31–29.5) |
| 3 yr | 728 (441–1135) | 104 (47–200) | 66 (22–159) | 1.80 (0.19–16.9) |
| 4–5 yr | 780 (463–1236) | 99 (43–196) | 68 (25–154) | 8.58 (1.07–68.9)[†] |
| 6–8 yr | 915 (633–1280) | 107 (48–207) | 90 (33–202) | 12.89 (1.03–161.3)[‡] |
| 9–10 yr | 1007 (608–1572) | 121 (52–242) | 113 (45–236) | 23.6 (0.98–570.6)[§] |
| 14 yr | | | | 20.07 (2.06–195.2) |
| Adult | 994 (639–1349) | 156 (56–352) | 171 (70–312) | 13.2 (1.53–114) |

*Numbers in parentheses are the 95% confidence intervals (CIs).

[†]IgE data for 4 yr.

[‡]IgE data for 7 yr.

[§]IgE data for 10 yr.

[‖]For data on LBW preterm infants, see Ballow M et al: Development of the immune system in very low birth weight (less than 1500 g) premature infants: Concentrations of plasma immunoglobulins and patterns of infections. Pediatr Res 1986;9:899–904.

From Kjellman NM et al: Serum IgE levels in healthy children quantified by a sandwich technique (PRIST). Clin Allergy 1976;6:51–59; Jolliff CR et al: Reference intervals for serum IgG, IgA, IgM, C3, and C4 as determined by rate nephelometry. Clin Chem 1982;28:126–128; and Zetterström O, Johansson SG: IgE concentrations measured by PRIST in serum of healthy adults and in patients with respiratory allergy: A diagnostic approach. Allergy 1981;36(3)537–547.

TABLE 15-2

**SERUM IgG SUBCLASS LEVELS***

| Age (yr) | IgG1 (mg/dL) | IgG2 (mg/dL) | IgG3 (mg/dL) | IgG4 (mg/dL) |
|---|---|---|---|---|
| 0.5–1 | 290 (140–620) | 58 (41–130) | 41 (11–85) | 0.2 (0–0.8) |
| 1–1.5 | 350 (170–650) | 62 (40–140) | 42 (12–87) | 3 (0–26) |
| 1.5–2 | 400 (220–720) | 80 (50–180) | 44 (14–91) | 7 (0–41) |
| 2–3 | 450 (240–780) | 95 (55–200) | 46 (15–93) | 14 (0–69) |
| 3–4 | 480 (270–810) | 115 (65–220) | 48 (16–96) | 20 (1–94) |
| 4–6 | 500 (300–840) | 130 (70–250) | 50 (17–97) | 26 (2–116) |
| 6–9 | 570 (350–910) | 170 (85–330) | 54 (20–100) | 37 (3–158) |
| 9–12 | 600 (370–930) | 210 (10–400) | 58 (22–109) | 47 (4–190) |
| 12–18 | 580 (370–910) | 260 (110–480) | 63 (24–116) | 49 (5–196) |
| Adult | 500 (280–800) | 300 (115–570) | 64 (24–120) | 35 (5–125) |

*Numbers in parentheses are the 95% confidence intervals (CIs).

From Schauer U et al: IgG subclass concentrations in certified reference material 470 and reference values for children and adults determined with the binding site reagents. Clin Chem 2003;49(11):1924–1929.

TABLE 15-3

**T AND B LYMPHOCYTES IN PERIPHERAL BLOOD**

| Age | CD3 (Total T cell) Count*,† (%)† | CD4 count*,† (%)† | CD8 Count*,† (%)† | CD19 (B cell) Count*,† (%)† |
|---|---|---|---|---|
| 0–3 mo | 2.50–5.50 (53–84) | 1.60–4.00 (35–64) | 0.56–1.70 (12–28) | 0.12–2.10 (14–76) |
| 3–6 mo | 2.50–5.60 (51–77) | 1.80–4.00 (35–56) | 0.59–1.60 (12–23) | 0.00–2.80 (00–84) |
| 6–12 mo | 1.90–5.90 (49–76) | 1.40–4.30 (31–56) | 0.50–1.70 (12–24) | 0.02–2.30 (01–80) |
| 1–2 yr | 2.10–6.20 (53–75) | 1.30–3.40 (32–51) | 0.62–2.00 (14–30) | 0.00–2.30 (00–80) |
| 2–6 yr | 1.40–3.70 (56–75) | 0.70–2.20 (28–47) | 0.49–1.30 (16–30) | 0.02–1.40 (02–76) |
| 6–12 yr | 1.20–2.60 (60–76) | 0.65–1.50 (31–47) | 0.37–1.10 (18–35) | 0.00–0.74 (00–67) |
| 12–18 yr | 1.00–2.20 (56–84) | 0.53–1.30 (31–52) | 0.33–0.92 (18–35) | 0.00–0.39 (00–60) |
| Adult‡ | 0.70–2.10 (55–83) | 0.30–1.40 (28–57) | 0.20–0.90 (10–39) | 0.10–0.50 (6–19) |

*Absolute counts (number of cells per microliter × $10^{-3}$).

†Normal values (10th to 90th percentile).

‡From Comans-Bitter WM et al: Immunophenotyping of blood lymphocytes in childhood. Reference values for lymphocyte subpopulations. J Pediatr 1997;130(3):388–393.

From Shearer WT et al: Lymphocyte subsets in healthy children from birth through 18 years of age: The Pediatric AIDS Clinical Trials Group P1009 study. J Allergy Clin Immunol 2003;112: 973–980.

TABLE 15-4

SERUM COMPLEMENT LEVELS*

| Age | C3 (mg/dL) | C4 (mg/dL) |
|---|---|---|
| Cord blood (term) | 83 (57–116) | 13 (6.6–23) |
| 1 mo | 83 (53–124) | 14 (7.0–25) |
| 2 mo | 96 (59–149) | 15 (7.4–28) |
| 3 mo | 94 (64–131) | 16 (8.7–27) |
| 4 mo | 107 (62–175) | 19 (8.3–38) |
| 5 mo | 107 (64–167) | 18 (7.1–36) |
| 6 mo | 115 (74–171) | 21 (8.6–42) |
| 7–9 mo | 113 (75–166) | 20 (9.5–37) |
| 10–12 mo | 126 (73–180) | 22 (12–39) |
| 1 yr | 129 (84–174) | 23 (12–40) |
| 2 yr | 120 (81–170) | 19 (9.2–34) |
| 3 yr | 117 (77–171) | 20 (9.7–36) |
| 4–5 yr | 121 (86–166) | 21 (13–32) |
| 6–8 yr | 118 (88–155) | 20 (12–32) |
| 9–10 yr | 134 (89–195) | 22 (10–40) |
| Adult | 125 (83–177) | 28 (15–45) |

*Numbers in parentheses are the 95% confidence intervals (CIs).

Modified from Jolliff CR et al: Reference values for serum IgG, IgA, IgM, C3, and C4 as determined by rate nephelometry. Clin Chem 1982;28:126–128.

TABLE 15-5

EVALUATION OF A SUSPECTED IMMUNODEFICIENCY

| Suspected Functional Abnormality | Clinical Findings | Initial Tests | More Advanced Tests |
|---|---|---|---|
| Antibody (e.g., common variable immunodeficiency, X-linked agammaglobulinemia, IgA deficiency) | Sinopulmonary and systemic infections (pyogenic bacteria)<br>Enteric infections (enterovirus, other viruses, *Giardia* sp.)<br>Autoimmune disease (immune thrombocytopenia, hemolytic anemia, inflammatory bowel disease) | Immunoglobulin levels (IgG, IgM, IgA)<br>Antibody titers to T-cell dependent protein antigens<br>Antibody titers to T-cell independent polysaccharide antigens in a child ≥2 yr (e.g., Pneumovax) | B-cell enumeration<br>Immunofixation electrophoresis<br>IgG subclass levels |
| Cell-mediated immunity (e.g., severe combined immunodeficiency, DiGeorge syndrome) | Pneumonia (pyogenic bacteria, fungi, *Pneumocystis jerovicii*, viruses) | Total lymphocyte counts<br>HIV ELISA/Western blot/PCR<br>Delayed type hypersensitivity skin tests (*Candida* sp., tetanus toxoid, mumps, *Cryptosporidium* sp.) | T-cell enumeration (CD3, CD4, CD8)<br>In vitro T-cell proliferation to mitogens, antigens or allogenic cells<br>FISH 22q11 for DiGeorge deletion |
| Phagocytosis (chronic granulomatous disease, leukocyte adhesion deficiency, Chediak-Higashi syndrome) | Cutaneous infections, abscesses, lymphadenitis (staphylococci, enteric bacteria, fungi, mycobacteria), poor wound healing | WBC/neutrophil count and morphology | Nitroblue tetrazolium (NBT) test or dihydro-rhodamine (DHR) reduction test<br>Chemotactic assay<br>Phagocytic assay |
| Spleen | Bacteremia/hematogenous infection (pneumococcus, other streptococci, *Neisseria* sp.) | Peripheral blood smear for Howell-Jolly bodies<br>Hemoglobin electrophoresis (HbSS) | Technetium-99 spleen scan or sonogram |
| Complement | Bacterial sepsis and other blood-borne infections (encapsulated bacteria, especially *Neisseria* sp.)<br>Lupus, glomerulonephritis<br>Angioedema | CH50 (total hemolytic complement) | Alternative pathway assays (AH 50)<br>Mannose-binding lectin level<br>Individual complement component assays |

ELISA, enzyme-linked immunosorbent assay; FISH, fluorescent in situ hybridization; HIV, human immunodeficiency virus; PCR, polymerase chain reaction; WBC, white blood cell.

From Rosen FS et al: The primary immunodeficiencies: Recent advances in the genetics of primary immunodeficiency syndromes. N Engl J Med 1995;333(7):431–440, and Shyur SD, Hill HR: Recent advances in the genetics of primary immunodeficiency syndromes. J Pediatr 1996;129(1):8–24.

## REFERENCES


1. Barrett DJ: Approach to the child with recurrent infections. Up to Date 2006. Available at www.uptodate.com.
2. Blaiss MS: Antihistamines: Treatment selection criteria for pediatric seasonal allergic rhinitis. Allergy Asthma Proc 2005;26(2):95–102.
3. Bonilla FB, Geha RS: Primary immunodeficiency diseases. J Allergy Clin Immunol 2003;111(2 Suppl):S571–S581.
4. Fireman P: Therapeutic approaches to allergic rhinitis: Treating the child. J Allergy Clin Immunol 2000;105:S616–S621.
5. Garavello DW et al: Nasal rinsing with hypertonic solution: An adjunctive treatment for pediatric seasonal allergic rhinoconjunctivitis. Int Arch Allergy Immunol 2005;137(4):310–314.
6. Gelfand EW: Pediatric allergic rhinitis: Factors affecting treatment choice. Ear Nose Throat J 2005;84(3):163–168.
7. Lifschitz CH: Dietary protein-induced proctitis/colitis, enteropathy, and enterocolitis of infancy. Up to Date 2006. Available at www.uptodate.com.
8. O'Dowd LC, Atkins P: Penicillin and other antibiotic allergy, skin testing, and desensitization. Up to Date 2006. Available at www.uptodate.com.
9. Orange J et al: Use of intravenous immunoglobin in human disease: A review of evidence by members of the Primary Immunodeficiency Committee of the American Academy of Allergy, Asthma, and Immunology. J Allergy Clin Immunol 2006;117(4):S525–S553.
10. Passali D et al: Consensus conference of allergic rhinitis in childhood. Allergy 1999;54:4–34.
11. Pickering LK (ed): Red Book: 2003 Report of the Committee on Infectious Diseases, 26th ed. Elk Grove Village, Ill, American Academy of Pediatrics, 2003.
12. Ressel GW: AHRQ releases review of treatments for allergic and nonallergic rhinitis. Am Family Phys 2002;66(11):2164– 2167.
13. Sampson HA et al: American Gastroenterology Association technical review on the evaluation of food allergy in gastrointestinal disorders. Gastroenterology 2001;120(4):1023–1025.
14. Sicherer SH: Manifestations of food allergy: Evaluation and management. Am Family Phys1999;59(2):415–424.
15. Stone KD: Atopic diseases of childhood. Curr Opin Pediatr 2002;14:634–646.
16. Wood RA: The natural history of food allergy. Pediatrics 2003;111(6):1631–1637.

# Immunoprophylaxis

*Nakia Johnson, MD*

## I. SOURCES OF INFORMATION

### A. PRINTED SOURCES

American Academy of Pediatrics. *Red Book: 2006 Report of the Committee on Infectious Diseases,* 26th ed. Elk Grove Village, Ill, AAP, 2006.

Updated Recommended Childhood Vaccination Schedule is published each January in *Pediatrics* and *Morbidity and Mortality Weekly Report*.

Current issues of *Morbidity and Mortality Weekly Report*.

Vaccine package inserts.

16

### B. ELECTRONIC AND TELEPHONE SOURCES

State health departments.

The Centers for Disease Control and Prevention (CDC): Can provide telephone consultation and send printed material on vaccines. Call 1-800-232-SHOT.

American Academy of Pediatrics (AAP) website: www.aap.org.

Vaccine Adverse Event Reporting System (VAERS) website: www.vaers.org. To submit a report about an adverse event or for questions, call 1 800-822-7967.

National Network for Immunization Information website: www.immunizationinfo.org.

Immunization Action Coalition website: www.immunize.org.

## II. IMMUNIZATION SCHEDULES

### A. RECOMMENDED CHILDHOOD IMMUNIZATION SCHEDULE (Fig. 16-1)

### B. CATCH-UP IMMUNIZATION SCHEDULES

1. Lapsed immunizations: **Resume immunization schedule as if the usual interval had elapsed. Repeating doses is not indicated.**
2. **Catch-up immunization schedules (Tables 16-1 and 16-2).**

a. *Haemophilus influenzae* type b (Hib): See section V.C.

b. Pneumococcal conjugate vaccine (PCV7): See Table 16-3.

### C. MINIMUM AGE FOR INITIAL VACCINATION AND MINIMUM INTERVALS BETWEEN DOSES OF VARIOUS VACCINES (Table 16-4)

### D. GUIDELINES FOR SPACING LIVE AND INACTIVATED ANTIGENS (Table 16-5)

## III. IMMUNIZATION GUIDELINES

### A. VACCINE INFORMED CONSENT

Vaccine information statements (VISes) can be obtained from local health departments, the CDC, the AAP, and vaccine manufacturers. For vaccines

FIG. 16-1A

A

## Recommended Immunization Schedule for Persons Aged 0–6 Years—UNITED STATES•2007

| Vaccine ▼ Age ▶ | Birth | 1 mos | 2 mos | 4 mos | 6 mos | 12 mos | 15 mos | 18 mos | 19–23 mos | 2–3 yrs | 4–6 yrs |
|---|---|---|---|---|---|---|---|---|---|---|---|
| Hepatitis B[1] | HepB | HepB | | *see footnote 1* | | HepB | | | | HepB Series | |
| Rotavirus[2] | | | Rota | Rota | Rota | | | | | | |
| Diphtheria,Tetanus,Pertussis[3] | | | DTaP | DTaP | DTaP | | DTaP | | | | DTaP |
| *Haemophilus influenzae* type b[4] | | | Hib | Hib | *Hib[4]* | Hib | | | Hib | | |
| Pneumococcal[5] | | | PCV | PCV | PCV | PCV | | | | PCV PPV | |
| Inactivated Poliovirus | | | IPV | IPV | | IPV | | | | | IPV |
| Influenza[6] | | | | | | | Influenza (Yearly) | | | | |
| Measles, Mumps, Rubella[7] | | | | | | MMR | | | | | MMR |
| Varicella[8] | | | | | | Varicella | | | | | Varicella |
| Hepatitis A[9] | | | | | | | HepA (2 doses) | | | HepA Series | |
| Meningococcal[10] | | | | | | | | | | MPSV4 | |

Range of recommended ages

Catch-up immunization

Certain high-risk groups

This schedule indicates the recommended ages for routine administration of currently licensed childhood vaccines, as of December 1, 2006, for children aged 0–6 yrs. Additional information is available at http://www.cdc.gov/nip/recs/child-schedule.htm. Any dose not administered at the recommended age should be administered at any subsequent visit, when indicated and feasible. Additional vaccines may be licensed and recommended during the yr. Licensed combination vaccines may be used whenever any components of the combination are indicated and other components of the vaccine are not contraindicated and if approved by the Food and Drug Administration for that dose of the series. Providers should consult the respective Advisory Committee on Immunization Practices statement for detailed recommendations. Clinically significant adverse events that follow immunization should be reported to the Vaccine Adverse Event Reporting System (VAERS). Guidance about how to obtain and complete a VAERS form is available at http://www.vaers.hhs.gov or by telephone, 800-822-7967.

**1. Hepatitis B vaccine (HepB).** *(Minimum age: birth)*

**At birth:**

- Administer monovalent HepB to all newborns before hospital discharge.
- If mother is hepatitis surface antigen (HBsAg)-positive, administer HepB and 0.5 mL of hepatitis B immune globulin (HBIG) within 12 hours of birth.
- If mother's HBsAg status is unknown, administer HepB within 12 hours of birth.Determine the HBsAg status as soon as possible and if HBsAg-positive, administer HBIG (no later than age 1 wk).
- If mother is HBsAg-negative, the birth dose can only be delayed with physician's order and mother's negative HBsAg laboratory report documented in the infant's medical record.

**After the birth dose:**

- The HepB series should be completed with either monovalent HepB or a combination vaccine containing HepB. The second dose should be administered at age 1–2 mos. The final dose should be administered at age ≥24 wks. Infants born to HBsAg-positive mothers should be tested for HBsAg and antibody to HBsAg after completion of ≥3 doses of a licensed HepB series, at age 9–18 mos (generally at the next well-child visit).

**4-mo dose:**

- It is permissible to administer 4 doses of HepB when combination vaccines are administered after the birth dose. If monovalent HepB is used for doses after the birth dose, a dose at age 4 mos is not needed.

**2. Rotavirus vaccine (Rota).** *(Minimum age: 6 wks)*

- Administer the first dose at age 6–12 wks. Do not start the series later than age 12 wks.
- Administer the final dose in the series by age 32 wks. Do not administer a dose later than age 32 wks.
- Data on safety and efficacy outside of these age ranges are insufficient.

**3. Diphtheria and tetanus toxoids and acellular pertussis vaccine (DTaP).** *(Minimum age: 6 wks)*

- The fourth dose of DTaP may be administered as early as age 12 mos, provided 6 mos have elapsed since the third dose.Administer the final dose in the series at age 4–6 yrs.

**4. *Haemophilus influenzae* type b conjugate vaccine (Hib).** *(Minimum age: 6 wks)*

- If PRP-OMP (PedvaxHIB® or ComVax® [Merck]) is administered at ages 2 and 4 mos, a dose at age 6 mos is not required. TriHiBit®(DTaP/Hib) combination products should not be used for primary immunization but can be used as boosters following any Hib vaccine in children aged ≥ 12 mos.

**5. Pneumococcal vaccine.** *(Minimum age: 6 wks for pneumococcal conjugate vaccine [PCV]; 2 yrs for pneumococcal polysaccharide vaccine [PPV])*

- Administer PCV at ages 24–59 mos in certain high-risk groups. Administer PPV to children aged ≥2 yrs in certain high-risk groups. See *MMWR* 2000; 49(No. RR-9):1–35.

**6. Influenza vaccine.** *(Minimum age: 6 mos for trivalent inactivated influenza vaccine [TIV]; 5 yrs for live, attenuated influenza vaccine [LAIV])*

- All children aged 6–59 mos and close contacts of all children aged 0–59 mos are recommended to receive influenza vaccine.
- Influenza vaccine is recommended annually for children aged ≥59 mos with certain risk factors, health-care workers, and other persons (including household members) in close contact with persons in groups at high risk. See *MMWR* 2006; 55(No. RR-10):1–41.
- For healthy persons aged 5–49 yrs, LAIV may be used as an alternative to TIV.
- Children receiving TIV should receive 0.25 mL if aged 6–35 mos or 0.5 mL if aged ≥3 yrs.
- Children aged <9 yrs who are receiving influenza vaccine for the first time should receive 2 doses (separated by ≥4 wks for TIV and ≥6 wks for LAIV).

**7. Measles, mumps, and rubella vaccine (MMR).** *(Minimum age: 12 mos)*

- Administer the second dose of MMR at age 4–6 yrs. MMR may be administered before age 4–6 yrs, provided ≥4 wks have elapsed since the first dose and both doses are administered at age ≥12 mos.

**8. Varicella vaccine.** *(Minimum age: 12 mos)*

- Administer the second dose of varicella vaccine at age 4–6 yrs. Varicella vaccine may be administered before age 4–6 yrs, provided that ≥3 mos have elapsed since the first dose and both doses are administered at age ≥12 mos. If second dose was administered ≥28 days following the first dose, the second dose does not need to be repeated.

**9. Hepatitis A vaccine (HepA).** *(Minimum age: 12 mos)*

- HepA is recommended for all children aged 1 yr (i.e., aged 12–23 mos). The 2 doses in the series should be administered at least 6 mos apart.
- Children not fully vaccinated by age 2 yrs can be vaccinated at subsequent visits.
- HepA is recommended for certain other groups of children, including in areas where vaccination programs target older children. See *MMWR* 2006; 55(No. RR-7):1–23.

**10. Meningococcal polysaccharide vaccine (MPSV4).** *(Minimum age: 2 yrs)*

- Administer MPSV4 to children aged 2–10 yrs with terminal complement deficiencies or anatomic or functional asplenia and certain other high-risk groups. See *MMWR* 2005; 54(No. RR-7):1–21.

**A** and **B,** Recommended childhood immunization schedule, United States, 2006. *Dark bars* indicate vaccines to be given if previous recommended doses were missed or given earlier than the recommended minimum age. Combination vaccines may be used when vaccine components are indicated, as long as other components are not contraindicated. Note that DTaP/IPV/HepB (Pediarix) given according to the vaccination schedule will result in the administration of an extra dose of HepB, which is acceptable according to the American Academy of Pediatrics (AAP). Most recent recommendations can be found on the Centers for Disease Control and Prevention (CDC) or AAP websites. *(Modified from the CDC Advisory Committee on Immunization Practices [Online]. Available at www.cdc.gov/nip/acip.)*

B

## Recommended Immunization Schedule for Persons Aged 7–18 Yrs—UNITED STATES•2007

| Vaccine ▼ / Age ▶ | 7–10 yrs | 11–12 yrs | 13–14 yrs | 15 yrs | 16–18 yrs |
|---|---|---|---|---|---|
| Tetanus, Diphtheria, Pertussis[1] | see footnote 1 | Tdap | | Tdap | |
| Human Papillomavirus[2] | see footnote 2 | HPV (3 doses) | | HPV Series | |
| Meningococcal[3] | MPSV4 | MCV4 | | MCV4[3] MCV4 | |
| Pneumococcal[4] | | PPV | | | |
| Influenza[5] | | Influenza (Yearly) | | | |
| Hepatitis A[6] | | HepA Series | | | |
| Hepatitis B[7] | | HepB Series | | | |
| Inactivated Poliovirus[8] | | IPV Series | | | |
| Measles, Mumps, Rubella[9] | | MMR Series | | | |
| Varicella[10] | | Varicella Series | | | |

Range of recommended ages

Catch-up immunization

Certain high-risk groups

This schedule indicates the recommended ages for routine administration of currently licensed childhood vaccines, as of December 1, 2006, for children aged 7–18 yrs. Additional information is available at http://www.cdc.gov/nip/recs/child-schedule.htm. Any dose not administered at the recommended age should be administered at any subsequent visit, when indicated and feasible. Additional vaccines may be licensed and recommended during the year. Licensed combination vaccines may be used whenever any components of the combination are indicated and other components of the vaccine are not contraindicated and if approved by the Food and Drug Administration for that dose of the series. Providers should consult the respective Advisory Committee on Immunization Practices statement for detailed recommendations. Clinically significant adverse events that follow immunization should be reported to the Vaccine Adverse Event Reporting System (VAERS). Guidance about how to obtain and complete a VAERS form is available at http://www.vaers.hhs.gov or by telephone, 800-822-7967.

**1. Tetanus and diphtheria toxoids and acellular pertussis vaccine (Tdap).** *(Minimum age: 10 yrs for BOOSTRIX® and 11 yrs for ADACEL™)*
- Administer at age 11–12 yrs for those who have completed the recommended childhood DTP/DTaP vaccination series and have not received a tetanus and diphtheria toxoids vaccine (Td) booster dose.
- Adolescents aged 13–18 yrs who missed the 11–12 yr Td/Tdap booster dose should also receive a single dose of Tdap if they have completed the recommended childhood DTP/DTaP vaccination series.

**2. Human papillomavirus vaccine (HPV).** *(Minimum age: 9 yrs)*
- Administer the first dose of the HPV vaccine series to females at age 11–12 yrs.
- Administer the second dose 2 mos after the first dose and the third dose 6 mos after the first dose.
- Administer the HPV vaccine series to females at age 13–18 yrs if not previously vaccinated.

**3. Meningococcal vaccine.** *(Minimum age: 11 yrs for meningococcal conjugate vaccine [MCV4]; 2 yrs for meningococcal polysaccharide vaccine [MPSV4])*
- Administer MCV4 at age 11–12 yrs and to previously unvaccinated adolescents at high school entry (at approximately age 15 yrs).
- Administer MCV4 to previously unvaccinated college freshmen living in dormitories; MPSV4 is an acceptable alternative.
- Vaccination against invasive meningococcal disease is recommended for children and adolescents aged ≥2 yrs with terminal complement deficiencies or anatomic or functional asplenia and certain other high-risk groups. See *MMWR* 2005; 54(No. RR-7):1–21. Use MPSV4 for children aged 2–10 yrs and MCV4 or MPSV4 for older children.

**4. Pneumococcal polysaccharide vaccine (PPV).** *(Minimum age: 2 yrs)*
- Administer for certain high-risk groups. See *MMWR* 1997; 46 (No. RR-8):1–24, and *MMWR* 2000; 49(No. RR-9):1–35.

**5. Influenza vaccine.** *(Minimum age: 6 mos for trivalent inactivated influenza vaccine [TIV]; 5 yrs for live, attenuated influenza vaccine [LAIV])*
- Influenza vaccine is recommended annually for persons with certain risk factors, health-care workers, and other persons (including household members) in close contact with persons in groups at high risk. See *MMWR* 2006; 55(No.RR-10):1–41.
- For healthy persons aged 5–49 yrs, LAIV may be used as an alternative to TIV.
- Children aged <9 yrs who are receiving influenza vaccine for the first time should receive 2 doses (separated by ≥4 wks for TIV and ≥6 wks for LAIV).

**6. Hepatitis A vaccine (HepA).** *(Minimum age: 12 mos)*
- The 2 doses in the series should be administered at least 6 mos apart.
- HepA is recommended for certain other groups of children, including in areas where vaccination programs target older children. See *MMWR* 2006; 55(No.RR-7):1–23.

**7. Hepatitis B vaccine (HepB).** *(Minimum age: birth)*
- Administer the 3-dose series to those who were not previously vaccinated.
- A 2-dose series of Recombivax HB® is licensed for children aged 11–15 yrs.

**8. Inactivated poliovirus vaccine (IPV).** *(Minimum age: 6 wks)*
- For children who received an all-IPV or all oral poliovirus (OPV) series, a fourth dose is not necessary if the third dose was administered at age ≥4 yrs.
- If both OPV and IPV were administered as part of a series, a total of 4 doses should be administered, regardless of the child's current age.

**9. Measles, mumps, and rubella vaccine (MMR).** *(Minimum age: 12 mos)*
- If not previously vaccinated, administer 2 doses of MMR during any visit, with ≥4 wks between the doses.

**10. Varicella vaccine.** *(Minimum age: 12 mos)*
- Administer 2 doses of varicella vaccine to persons without evidence of immunity.
- Administer 2 doses of varicella vaccine to persons aged <13 yrs at least 3 mos apart. Do not repeat the second dose, if administered ≥28 days after the first dose.
- Administer 2 doses of varicella vaccine to persons aged ≥13 yrs at least 4 wks apart.

**The Recommended Immunization Schedules for Persons Aged 0–18 Yrs are approved by the Advisory Committee on Immunization Practices (http://www.cdc.gov/nip/acip), the American Academy of Pediatrics (http://www.aap.org), and the American Academy of Family Physicians (http://www.aafp.org).**

**SAFER • HEALTHIER • PEOPLE™**

FIG. 16-1B

TABLE 16-1

**RECOMMENDED IMMUNIZATION SCHEDULES FOR CHILDREN (AGE 4 MO–6 YR) WHO ARE LATE OR ARE >1 MO BEHIND**

| | Dose 1–2 | Dose 2–3 | Dose 3–4 |
|---|---|---|---|
| DTaP* | 4 wk | 4 wk | 6 mo |
| IPV | 4 wk | 4 wk | 4 wk |
| HepB | 4 wk | 3 wk (at 8 wk after dose 1) | |
| MMR | 4 wk | | |
| Hib | 4 wk (if dose 1 given at <1 yr) | 4 wk (if current age ≤1 yr) | 8 wk (final dose; give only in children 1–5 yr who got 3 doses before age 1 yr) |
| | 8 wk (final dose; if dose 1 given at 12–14 mo of age) | If current age ≥1 yr and dose 1 given at <15 mo | |
| | No further doses if dose 1 given at ≥15 mo | No further doses if previous dose given at ≥15 mo | |
| PCV7 | 4 wk (if dose 1 at <1 yr and current age <2 yr | 4 wk (if current age <1 yr) | 8 wk (final dose; give only in children 1–5 yr who got 3 doses before age 1 yr) |
| | 8 wk (final dose, if dose 1 given at ≥12 mo or currently 24–59 mo) | 8 wk (final dose if current age ≥12 mo) | |
| | No further doses in healthy children if dose 1 given at ≥24 mo | No further doses in healthy children if dose 1 given at ≥24 mo | |

*Allow 6 mo between doses 4 and 5. Dose 5 is not needed if dose 4 is given after 4 yr of age.
DTaP, diphtheria and tetanus toxoids and acellular pertussis; HepB, hepatitis B virus; Hib, *H. influenzae* type B; IPV, inactivated poliovirus vaccine; MMR, measles/mumps/rubella; PCV7, pneumococcal conjugate vaccine.

Data from American Academy of Pediatrics: Red Book: 2006 Report of the Committee on Infectious Diseases, 27th ed. Elk Grove Village, Ill, AAP, 2006.

that do not currently have VISes, the CDC produces “important information” statements. The most recent VIS must be provided to the patient (nonminor) or parent/guardian with documentation of version date and date vaccine administered.

## B. VACCINE ADMINISTRATION

**1. Preferred sites of administration of intramuscular (IM) and subcutaneous (SC) vaccines:**

a. <18 months old: Anterolateral thigh.

b. Toddlers: Anterolateral thigh or deltoid (deltoid preferred if large enough).

c. Adolescents and young adults: Deltoid.

TABLE 16-2

**RECOMMENDED IMMUNIZATION SCHEDULES FOR ADOLESCENTS (AGE 7–18 YR) WHO ARE LATE OR ARE >1 MO BEHIND**

| Vaccine | Dose 1–2 | Dose 2–3 | Dose 3–Booster |
|---|---|---|---|
| Td | 4 wk | 6 mo | 6 mo: if dose 1 given <12 mo and current age <11 yr<br>5 yr: if dose 1 given at >12 mo and dose 3 given at <7 yr and current age 11 yr (give Tdap)<br>10 yr: if dose 3 given at ≥7 yr (give Tdap) |
| IPV | 4 wk | 4 wk | |
| HepB | 4 wk | 8 wk (and 16 wk after dose 1) | |
| MMR | 4 wk | | |
| Varicella | 4 wk | | |

HepB, hepatitis B virus; IPV, inactivated poliovirus vaccine; MMR, measles/mumps/rubella; Td, tetanus and diphtheria toxoids; Tdap, tetanus and diphtheria toxoids and acellular pertussis vaccine.

Data from American Academy of Pediatrics: Red Book: 2006 Report of the Committee on Infectious Diseases, 27th ed. Elk Grove Village, Ill, AAP, 2006.

TABLE 16-3

**CATCH-UP IMMUNIZATION SCHEDULE FOR PCV7 IN PREVIOUSLY UNVACCINATED CHILDREN**

| Age at First Dose | Primary Series | Booster Dose |
|---|---|---|
| 2–6 mo | 3 doses, 6–8 wk apart | 1 dose at 12–15 mo of age |
| 7–11 mo | 2 doses, 6–8 wk apart | 1 dose at 12–15 mo of age |
| 12–23 mo | 2 doses, 6–8 wk apart | |
| ≥24 mo | 1 dose | |

*Booster doses to be given at least 6–8 weeks after the final dose of the primary series.

Data from American Academy of Pediatrics: Red Book: 2006 Report of the Committee on Infectious Diseases, 27th ed. Elk Grove Village, Ill, AAP, 2006.

2. Route:
   a. IM: Deep into muscle to avoid tissue damage from adjuvants, usually with a 22- to 25-gauge (22G to 25G) needle, 7/8 inch to 1 inch long in infants and toddlers and 1 inch to 2 inches long in adolescents and young adults.
   b. SC: Into pinched skinfold with a 23G to 25G needle 5/8 inch to 3/4 inch long.
3. **Simultaneous administration:** **Routine childhood vaccines, including live-virus vaccines, are safe and effective when administered simultaneously at different sites, generally 1 inch to 2 inches apart. If given at separate times, the interval between administration of live-virus vaccines should be >1 month.**

TABLE 16-4

MINIMUM AGE FOR INITIAL VACCINATION AND MINIMUM INTERVAL BETWEEN VACCINE DOSES, BY TYPE OF VACCINE

| Vaccine | Minimum Age for First Dose* | Minimum Interval from Dose to Dose | | |
|---|---|---|---|---|
| | | 1 to 2* | 2 to 3* | 3 to 4 |
| DTaP[†,‡] | 6 wk | 1 mo | 1 mo | 6 mo |
| Hib (PRP-OMP)[‡] | 6 wk | 1 mo | 2 mo[§] | — |
| PCV7 | 6 wk | 1 mo[‖] | 1 mo[‖] | 2 mo[‖] |
| IPV | 6 wk | 1 mo | 1 mo | 1 mo[¶] |
| MMR | 12 mo[#] | 1 mo | — | — |
| HBV[‡] | Birth | 1 mo | 2 mo** | — |
| Varicella | 12 mo | 1 mo[††] | — | — |
| HAV | 12 mo | 6 mo | — | — |
| Influenza[‡‡] | 6 mo | 1 mo | — | — |
| Rotavirus | 6 wk | 4 mo | 4 mo | — |

*These minimum acceptable ages and intervals may not correspond with the optimal recommended ages and intervals for vaccination. See Fig. 16-1.

†The total number of doses of diphtheria and tetanus toxoids should not exceed six each before the seventh birthday. If the fourth dose is given after the fourth birthday, the fifth (booster) dose is not needed.

‡The combination vaccines Pediarix (DTaP/IPV/HepB) and Comvax (HepB-Hib) should not be given to infants <6 weeks of age.

§The booster dose of Hib vaccine recommended after the primary vaccination series should be administered no earlier than age 12 mo.

‖See Table 16-3 for recommendations of number of doses at different ages.

¶If the third dose is given after the fourth birthday, the fourth (booster) dose is not needed.

#Although the age for measles vaccination may be as young as 6 mo in outbreak areas where cases are occurring in children 1 yr of age, children initially vaccinated before the first birthday should be revaccinated at 12–15 mo of age, and an additional dose of vaccine should be administered at the time of school entry or according to local policy. Doses of MMR or other measles-containing vaccine should be separated by at least 1 mo.

**This final dose is recommended at least 4 mo after the first dose, at least 2 mo after the second dose, and no earlier than 6 mo of age.

††A second dose of varicella is indicated for all children who received only one dose of the vaccine.

‡‡Two doses of influenza are recommended for children 6 mo–9 yr of age who have never received the vaccine. Only one dose is required for children 9 yr or older, as well as children 6 mo–9 yr who have received the vaccine in the past.

DTaP, diphtheria and tetanus toxoids and acellular pertussis; HAV, hepatitis A virus; HBV, hepatitis B virus; Hib, *H. influenzae* type B; IPV, inactivated poliovirus vaccine; MMR, measles/mumps/rubella; PCV7, pneumococcal conjugate vaccine.

Data from American Academy of Pediatrics: Red Book: 2006 Report of the Committee on Infectious Diseases, 27th ed. Elk Grove Village, Ill, AAP, 2006.

TABLE 16-5

GUIDELINES FOR SPACING LIVE AND INACTIVATED VACCINES

| Antigen Combination | Minimum Interval Between Doses |
|---|---|
| ≥2 inactivated or inactivated and live | None, can give simultaneously |
| ≥2 live parenteral | 28-day minimum interval, if not given at same time |

Data from American Academy of Pediatrics: Red Book: 2006 Report of the Committee on Infectious Diseases, 27th ed. Elk Grove Village, Ill, AAP, 2006, table 1.6, p 24.

### C. MISCONCEPTIONS REGARDING VACCINE ADMINISTRATION

Vaccines may be given despite the presence of the following:

1. Mild acute illness, regardless of fever.
2. Convalescent phase of illness.
3. Recent exposure to infectious disease.
4. Mild to moderate local reaction to previous dose of vaccine (soreness, redness, swelling).
5. Current antimicrobial therapy.
6. Prematurity (see also section IV.D).
7. Malnutrition.
8. Allergy to penicillin or other antibiotics, except anaphylactic reaction to neomycin or streptomycin.
9. Pregnancy of mother or another household contact (except varicella vaccine may be deferred if there is a pregnant, varicella-susceptible household contact).
10. Breast-feeding.
11. Unimmunized household contact.
12. Family history of adverse event to immunization.



### D. EGG ALLERGIES

1. Skin testing is *not* needed in children with egg allergies before the administration of the measles/mumps/rubella (MMR) vaccine (refer to section V.H for details).
2. Skin testing with yellow fever vaccine is recommended before administration in children with a history of immediate hypersensitivity reaction (e.g., anaphylaxis or generalized urticaria) to eggs.
3. Immediate hypersensitivity reaction to eggs is a contraindication to both the parenteral and intranasal influenza vaccines.

Less severe or local manifestations of allergy to egg are not contraindications to influenza vaccine.

## IV. IMMUNOPROPHYLAXIS GUIDELINES FOR SPECIAL HOSTS

### A. IMMUNOCOMPROMISED HOSTS

1. **Congenital immunodeficiency disorders:**
   a. Live bacterial and live-virus vaccines are generally contraindicated. See the *AAP Red Book*[1] for details regarding individual immunodeficiencies.
   b. Inactivated vaccines should be given according to the routine schedule. Immune response may vary and may be inadequate.
   c. Immunoglobulin (Ig) therapy may be indicated.
   d. Household contacts: Immunize according to the routine childhood immunization schedule; yearly influenza vaccine is recommended.
2. **Known or suspected human immunodeficiency virus (HIV) disease:**
   a. Inactivated vaccines should be given according to the routine immunization schedule (see Fig. 16-1).

b. See Table 16-6 (see also table 3.17 in *AAP Red Book*).[1]

c. MMR vaccine should be given to asymptomatic or mildly symptomatic patients with CD4+ T-lymphocyte counts ≥15%. Immunize at age 12 months; second dose should be administered 1 month after first dose to ensure optimal seroconversion.

d. Varicella vaccine should be considered in asymptomatic or mildly symptomatic patients with CD4+ T-lymphocyte counts ≥25%. Give two doses 3 months apart.

e. A booster dose of the 23-valent pneumococcal polysaccharide vaccine (23PS) is recommended at age 2 and 5 years, in addition to routine PCV7.

f. Immunize all patients at the start of the influenza season as early as age 6 months and yearly thereafter.

g. Passive immunoprophylaxis or chemoprophylaxis should be considered in all HIV-infected children after exposure to any vaccine-preventable disease.

3. **Oncology patients** (Table 16-7).

4. **Functional or anatomic asplenia (including sickle cell disease):**

a. Penicillin prophylaxis: See Chapter 14.

b. Pneumococcal vaccine:

(1) Children ≤5 years at diagnosis (Table 16-8).

(2) Children >5 years at diagnosis: Immunization with a single dose of either PCV7 or 23PS is acceptable. If both vaccines are given, their administration should be separated by 6–8 weeks. A second dose of 23PS may be given in 5 years. Data are insufficient for the most effective combination of the pneumococcal vaccines in older children.

c. Meningococcal vaccine: At age 2 years or at diagnosis if ≥2 years old.

TABLE 16-6

**RECOMMENDATIONS FOR ROUTINE IMMUNIZATION OF HIV-INFECTED CHILDREN**

| HIV Status | Administer | Consider | Do Not Administer |
|---|---|---|---|
| Known asymptomatic HIV infection | HepB, DtaP, IPV, MMR, Hib, PCV, influenza | Varicella* | BCG |
| Symptomatic HIV infection | HepB, DtaP, IPV, MMR, Hib, PCV, influenza | Varicella* | BCG |

*Consider giving in patients with no symptoms or mild symptoms of HIV with a CD4+ lymphocyte percentage >25% for >6 months. If applicable, give 2 doses 3 months apart.

BCG, bacille Calmetté-Guerin; DtaP, diphtheria and tetanus toxoids and acellular pertussis; HepB, hepatitis B virus vaccine; Hib, *H. influenzae* type B; IPV, inactivated poliovirus vaccine; MMR, measles/mumps/rubella; PCV, pneumococcal conjugate vaccine.

Data from American Academy of Pediatrics: Red Book: 2006 Report of the Committee on Infectious Diseases, 27th ed. Elk Grove Village, Ill, AAP, 2006.

TABLE 16-7

IMMUNIZATION FOR ONCOLOGY PATIENTS

| Vaccine | Indications and Comments |
|---|---|
| DtaP | Indicated for incompletely immunized children <7 yr, even during active chemotherapy |
| Td | Indicated 1 yr after completion of therapy in children 7 yr |
| Hib | Indicated for incompletely immunized children if <7 yr |
| HBV | Indicated for incompletely immunized children |
| 23PS | Indicated for asplenic patients |
| PCV7 | Indicated for incompletely immunized children <5 yr |
| Meningococcus | Consider in asplenic patients |
| IPV | Indicated for incompletely immunized children; also recommended for all household contacts requiring immunization to reduce the risk for vaccine-associated polio |
| MMR | Contraindicated until child is in remission and finished with all chemotherapy for 3–6 mo; may need to reimmunize after chemotherapy if titers have fallen below protective levels |
| Influenza | Defer in active chemotherapy; may give as early as 3–4 wk after remission and off chemotherapy if during influenza season; peripheral granulocyte and lymphocyte counts should be >1000/μL; should also be given to household contacts of children with cancer |
| Varicella | Consider immunizing children who have remained in remission and have finished chemotherapy for >1 yr; with absolute lymphocyte count of >700/μL and platelet count of >100,000/μL within 24 hr of immunization; check titers of previously immunized children to verify protective levels of antibodies |

*Note:* Immune reconstitution is slower for oncology patients who have received bone marrow transplants. See Centers for Disease Control and Prevention: MMWR 2000;49(No. RR-10):1–147 for vaccine schedule.

DtaP, diphtheria and tetanus toxoids and acellular pertussis; HBV, hepatitis B virus; Hib, H. influenzae type B; IPV, inactivated poliovirus vaccine; MMR, measles/mumps/rubella; 23PS, 23-valent pneumococcal polysaccharide vaccine; PCV7, pneumococcal conjugate vaccine; Td, tetanus and diphtheria toxoids.

d. Ensure that Hib series is completed; children ≥5 years of age who never received Hib immunization should receive one dose.
e. Children ≥2 years of age undergoing elective splenectomy should receive one or both of the pneumococcal vaccines and the meningococcal vaccine at least 2 weeks before surgery to ensure optimal immune response. Children <2 years of age should receive PCV7 before surgery.

## B. CORTICOSTEROID ADMINISTRATION

Only live viral and live bacterial vaccines are potentially contraindicated (see Table 16-9 for details).

TABLE 16-8

**RECOMMENDATIONS FOR PNEUMOCOCCAL IMMUNIZATION WITH PCV7 OR 23PS VACCINE FOR CHILDREN AT HIGH RISK OF PNEUMOCOCCAL DISEASE**

| Age | Previous Doses | Recommendations |
|---|---|---|
| ≤23 mo | None | PCV7 as in Table 16-3 |
| 24–59 mo | 1–3 doses of PCV7 | 1 dose of PCV7 |
| | | First dose of 23PS vaccine at 24 mo, at least 8 wk after last dose of PCV7 |
| | | Second dose of 23PS vaccine 3–5 yr after first dose of 23PS vaccine |
| 24–59 mo | 4 doses of PCV7 | First dose of 23PS vaccine at 24mo, at least 8 wk after last dose of PCV7 |
| | | Second dose of 23PS vaccine 3–5 yr after first dose of 23PS vaccine |
| 24–59 mo | None | Two doses of PCV 8 wk apart |
| | | First dose of 23PS vaccine 6–8 wk after last dose of PCV7 |
| | | Second dose of 23PS vaccine 3–5 yr after first dose of 23PS vaccine |
| 24–59 mo | 1 dose of 23PS | Two doses of PCV 7, 8 wk apart, beginning at last dose of 23PS vaccine |
| | | One dose of 23PS vaccine 3–5 yr after first dose of 23PS vaccine |

Data from American Academy of Pediatrics: Red Book: 2006 Report of the Committee on Infectious Diseases, 27th ed. Elk Grove Village, Ill, AAP, 2006.

TABLE 16-9

**LIVE-VIRUS IMMUNIZATION FOR PATIENTS RECEIVING CORTICOSTEROID THERAPY**

| Steroid Dose | Recommended Guidelines |
|---|---|
| Topical or inhaled therapy or local injection of steroids | Live-virus vaccines may be given unless there is clinical evidence of immunosuppression; if suppressed, wait 1 mo after cessation of therapy to give live-virus vaccines. |
| Physiologic maintenance doses of steroids | Live-virus vaccines may be given. |
| Low-dose steroids (<2 mg/kg/day prednisone or equivalent, or <20 mg/day if >10 kg) | Live-virus vaccines may be given. |
| High-dose steroids (≥2 mg/kg/day prednisone or equivalent, or 20 mg/day if >10 kg) | |
| Duration of therapy <14 days | May give live-virus vaccines immediately after cessation of therapy. (Consider 2-wk delay in administration.) |
| Duration of therapy ≥14 days | Do not give live-virus vaccines until therapy has been discontinued for 1 mo. |
| Children with immunosuppressive disorders receiving steroid therapy | Live-virus vaccines are contraindicated, except in special circumstances. |

From American Academy of Pediatrics: Red Book: 2006 Report of the Committee on Infectious Diseases, 27th ed. Elk Grove Village, Ill, AAP, 2006, p 77.

## C. PATIENTS TREATED WITH IMMUNOGLOBULIN OR OTHER BLOOD PRODUCTS

See the *AAP Red Book*[1] for suggested intervals between immunoglobulin or blood product administration and MMR or varicella immunization.

## D. PRETERM AND LOW BIRTH WEIGHT INFANTS (<2500 g)

Immunize according to chronologic age using regular vaccine dosage.

1. **Hepatitis B virus (HBV):** Initiation of HBV vaccine may be delayed for infants of hepatitis B surface antigen (HBsAg)-negative mothers until the child is >2 kg or age 2 months, whichever is earlier. See Figure 16-2 for management of preterm infant born to mother with hepatitis B.
2. **Influenza:** Give 2 doses 1 month apart each fall to all preterm infants >6 months of age. Household contacts should also receive influenza vaccine.

## E. PREGNANCY

Live viral vaccines are generally contraindicated during pregnancy.

1. **Influenza:** Inactivated influenza vaccine should be given to all women who will be pregnant during the influenza season; considered safe at any stage of pregnancy. Intranasal form contraindicated during pregnancy.
2. **Tetanus/diphtheria/pertussis:** Any pregnant woman who has not received a tetanus booster within 10 years prior to pregnancy should receive Tdap.
3. **Polio:** Pregnant women not immunized or incompletely immunized against polio should receive the inactivated poliomyelitis vaccine (IPV).
4. **Hepatitis A and B viruses:** When indicated, hepatitis A virus (HAV) and HBV vaccines may be given to pregnant women.
5. **Pneumococcal and meningococcal disease:** Vaccines should be given during pregnancy if a high risk of serious complications due these diseases exists.

## F. ADOLESCENT AND COLLEGE POPULATION

1. **Meningococcal conjugate vaccine (MCV4):** Vaccination recommended for all children ages 11–12 years. Previously unvaccinated adolescents should receive the vaccine prior to high school entry. All college freshmen living in dormitories with no history of meningococcal immunization should be immunized.
2. **Tdap:** Tetanus and diphtheria toxoids and acellular pertussis vaccine should be given to children age 11–12 years. Older adolescents who missed vaccination at age 11–12 years should receive a single dose of Tdap.
3. **Varicella:** Adolescents without a history of varicella disease, immunization, or immunity should receive two doses of the varicella vaccine.

4. **HPV:** See section V.H.
5. **See Chapter 5 for more details.**

## V. IMMUNOPROPHYLAXIS GUIDELINES FOR SPECIFIC DISEASES

### A. GUIDE TO CONTRAINDICATIONS AND PRECAUTIONS TO IMMUNIZATIONS (Table 16-10)

### B. DIPHTHERIA/TETANUS/PERTUSSIS VACCINES AND TETANUS IMMUNOPROPHYLAXIS

1. **Description:**
a. DTaP: Diphtheria and tetanus toxoids combined with acellular pertussis vaccine; preferred formulation for children <7 years of age.
b. DT: Diphtheria and tetanus toxoids without pertussis vaccine; use in children <7 years of age in whom pertussis vaccine is contraindicated.
c. Td: Tetanus toxoid with one third to one sixth the dose of diphtheria toxoid of other preparations; use in individuals ≥7 years of age.
d. TdaP (Boostrix and Adacel): Tetanus and diphtheria toxoids combined with acellular pertussis vaccine; for children age 11–18 years.
2. **Indications:**
a. Routine (see Fig. 16-1).
b. Tetanus prophylaxis in wound management (Table 16-11).
3. **Precautions/contraindications (see Table 16-10).**
4. **Children with neurologic disorders:**
a. Seizures:
(1) Poorly controlled or new-onset seizures: Defer pertussis immunization until seizure disorder is well controlled and progressive neurologic disorder is excluded; then use DTaP and antipyretics for 24 hours after immunization.
(2) Personal or family history of febrile seizures: Use DTaP and antipyretics for 24 hours after immunization.
b. Known or suspected progressive neurologic disorder: Defer pertussis immunization until diagnosis and treatment are established and neurologic condition is stable. Progressive disorders may merit permanent deferral of pertussis immunization. Reconsider pertussis immunization at each visit. Use DT if pertussis vaccine is permanently deferred.

**Note** *Children <1 year with neurologic disorders necessitating temporary deferment of pertussis vaccine should not receive DT because the risk for diphtheria and tetanus is low in the first year of life. After the first birthday, initiate either DT or DTaP immunization as clinically indicated previously.*

5. **Side effects:**
a. Minor side effects within 3 days: Erythema (26%–39%), drowsiness (40%–47%), swelling (15%–30%), anorexia (19%–25%), fussiness

*Text continued on p. 417*

TABLE 16-10

**GUIDE TO CONTRAINDICATIONS AND PRECAUTIONS TO IMMUNIZATIONS, 2006**

| Vaccine | Contraindications | Precautions* | Not Contraindications (Vaccines May Be Given) |
|---|---|---|---|
| General for all vaccines (DTaP, IPV, MMR, Hib, pneumococcal, hepatitis B, varicella, hepatitis A, influenza) | Anaphylactic reaction to a vaccine contraindicates further doses of that vaccine.<br>Anaphylactic reaction to a vaccine constituent contraindicates the use of vaccines containing that substance. | Moderate or severe illnesses with or without a fever<br>Latex allergy† | Mild to moderate local reaction (soreness, redness, swelling) after a dose of an injectable antigen<br>Low-grade or moderate fever after a previous vaccine dose<br>Mild acute illness with or without low-grade fever<br>Current antimicrobial therapy<br>Convalescent phase of illnesses<br>Prematurity (same dosage and indications as for healthy, full-term infants)<br>Recent exposure to an infectious disease |

*Note:* This information is based on the recommendations of the Advisory Committee on Immunization Practices (ACIP) and the Committee on Infectious Diseases of the AAP. Sometimes, these recommendations vary from those in the manufacturers' package inserts. For more detailed information, health care professionals should consult the published recommendations of the ACIP, AAP, and the manufacturers' package inserts. These guidelines, originally issued in 1993, have been updated to give current recommendations as of 2003 (based on information available as of February 2003).

*The events or conditions listed as precautions, although not contraindications, should be reviewed carefully. The benefits and risks of administering a specific vaccine to a person under the circumstances should be considered. If the risks are believed to outweigh the benefits, the immunization should be withheld; if the benefits are believed to outweigh the risks (e.g., during an outbreak or foreign travel), the immunization should be given. Whether and when to administer DTaP to children with proven or suspected underlying neurologic disorders should be decided on an individual basis.

†If a person reports a severe (anaphylactic) allergy to latex, vaccines supplied in vials or syringes that contain natural rubber should not be administered unless the benefits of immunization outweigh the risks of an allergic reaction to the vaccine. For latex allergies other than anaphylactic allergies (e.g., a history of contact allergy to latex gloves), vaccines supplied in vials or syringes that contain dry natural rubber or latex can be administered.

From American Academy of Pediatrics: Red Book: 2006 Report of the Committee on Infectious Diseases, 27th ed. Elk Grove Village, Ill, AAP, 2006, appendix 3, p 847.

*Continued*

TABLE 16-10

**GUIDE TO CONTRAINDICATIONS AND PRECAUTIONS TO IMMUNIZATIONS, 2006—cont'd**

| Vaccine | Contraindications | Precautions* | Not Contraindications (Vaccines May Be Given) |
|---|---|---|---|
| | | | History of penicillin or other nonspecific allergies or fact that relatives have such allergies<br>Pregnancy of mother or household contact<br>Unimmunized household contact<br>Immunodeficient household contact<br>Breast-feeding (nursing infant OR lactating mother) |
| DTaP | Encephalopathy within 7 days of administration of previous dose of DTaP/DTP | Temperature of 40.5°C (104.8°F) within 48 hr after immunization with a previous dose of DTaP/DTP<br>Collapse or shocklike state (hypotonic-hyporesponsive episode) within 48 hr of receiving a previous dose of DTaP/DTP<br>Seizures within 3 days of receiving a previous dose of DTaP/DTP[‡]<br>Persistent inconsolable crying lasting 3 hr, within 48 hr of receiving a previous dose of DTaP/DTP<br>GBS within 6 wk after a dose[§] | Family history of seizures[‡]<br>Family history of sudden infant death syndrome<br>Family history of an adverse event after DTaP/DTP administration |
| IPV | Anaphylactic reactions to neomycin, streptomycin, or polymyxin B | Pregnancy | |

| | | | |
|---|---|---|---|
| MMR[||,¶] | Pregnancy<br>Anaphylactic reaction to neomycin or gelatin<br>Known altered immune function (hematologic and solid tumors, congenital immunodeficiency, severe HIV infection, long-term immunosuppressive therapy) | Recent (within 3–11 mo, depending on product and dose) immune globulin administration[7]<br>Thrombocytopenia or history of thrombocytopenic purpura[#]<br>Tuberculosis or positive PPD** | Simultaneous tuberculin skin testing[††]<br>Breast-feeding<br>Pregnancy of mother of recipient<br>Immunodeficiency in a family member or household contact<br>HIV infection<br>Nonanaphylactic reactions to gelatin or neomycin |
| Hib | None | — | — |
| Hepatitis B | Anaphylactic reaction to baker's yeast | Prematurity[‡‡] | Pregnancy |
| Pneumococcal | None | — | — |

[‡]Acetaminophen given before administering DTaP and thereafter q4hr for 24 hr should be considered for children with a personal or family (i.e., siblings or parents) history of seizures.

[§]The decision to give additional doses of DTaP should be made on the basis of consideration of benefit of further immunization versus risk of recurrence of GBS. For example, completion of the primary series in children is justified.

[||]A theoretical risk exists that the administration of multiple live-virus vaccines within 30 days (4 weeks) of one another if not given on the same day will result in suboptimal immune response. No data substantiate this risk, however.

[¶]An anaphylactic reaction to egg ingestion previously was considered a contraindication unless skin testing and, if indicated, desensitization had been performed. However, skin testing is no longer recommended as of 1997.

[#]The decision to immunize should be made on the basis of consideration of the benefits of immunity to measles, mumps, and rubella versus the risk of recurrence or exacerbation of thrombocytopenia after immunization or from natural infections of measles or rubella. In most instances, the benefits of immunization will be much greater than the potential risks and justify giving MMR, particularly in view of the even greater risk of thrombocytopenia after measles or rubella disease. However, if previous episode of thrombocytopenia occurred in temporal proximity to immunization, not giving a subsequent dose may be prudent.

**A theoretical basis exists for concern that measles vaccine might exacerbate tuberculosis. Consequently, before administering MMR to people with untreated active tuberculosis, initiating antituberculosis therapy is advisable.

[††]Measles immunization may suppress tuberculin reactivity temporarily. MMR vaccine may be given after, or on the same day as, tuberculin testing. If MMR has been given recently, postpone the tuberculin skin test until 4–6 weeks after administration of MMR.

[‡‡]For preterm infants weighing <2 kg at birth and born to hepatitis B surface antigen (HBsAg)-negative mothers, initiation of immunization should be delayed until just before hospital discharge if the infant weighs 2 kg or more, or until approximately 2 months of age, when other routine immunizations are given, to improve response. All preterm infants born to HBsAg-positive mothers should receive immunoprophylaxis (hepatitis B immune globulin and vaccine) beginning as soon as possible after birth, followed by appropriate postimmunization testing.

*Continued*

TABLE 16-10

**GUIDE TO CONTRAINDICATIONS AND PRECAUTIONS TO IMMUNIZATIONS, 2006—cont'd**

| Vaccine | Contraindications | Precautions* | Not Contraindications (Vaccines May Be Given) |
|---|---|---|---|
| Varicella[5] | Pregnancy<br>Anaphylactic reaction to neomycin or gelatin<br>Infection with HIV[§§]<br>Known altered immune function (hematologic and solid tumors, congenital immunodeficiency, long-term immunosuppressive therapy)[\|\|\|\|] | Recent immune globulin administration<br>Family history of immunodeficiency[¶¶] | Pregnancy of mother of recipient<br>Immunodeficiency in a household contact<br>Household contact with HIV infection |
| Hepatitis A | Anaphylactic reaction to 2-phenoxyethanol or alum | Pregnancy | — |
| Influenza | Anaphylactic reaction to eggs | GBS within 6 wk after a previous influenza immunization | Pregnancy |

[§§]Varicella vaccine should be considered for asymptomatic or mildly symptomatic HIV-infected children, specifically children in Centers for Disease Control and Prevention class N1 or A1, with age-specific T-cell percentages of 25% or higher.

[||||]Varicella vaccine should not be administered to people who have cellular immunodeficiencies, but people with impaired humoral immunity may be immunized.

[¶¶]Varicella vaccine should not be administered to a person who has a family history of congenital or hereditary immunodeficiency in parents or siblings unless that person's immune competence has been substantiated clinically or verified by a laboratory.

DtaP, diphtheria and tetanus toxoids and acellular pertussis; DTP, diphtheria and tetanus toxoids and pertussis; GBS, Guillain-Barré syndrome; Hib, *Haemophilus influenzae* type b; HIV, human immunodeficiency virus; IPV, inactivated poliovirus; MMR, measles/mumps/rubella; PPD, purified protein derivative (tuberculin).

TABLE 16-11

INDICATIONS FOR TETANUS PROPHYLAXIS

| Prior Tetanus | Clean, Minor Wounds | | All Other Wounds | |
|---|---|---|---|---|
| Toxoid Doses | Tetanus Vaccine* | TIG | Tetanus Vaccine* | TIG |
| Unknown or <3 | Yes | No | Yes | Yes |
| ≥3, last <5 yr ago | No | No | No | No† |
| ≥3, last 5–10 yr ago | No | No | Yes | No† |
| ≥3, last >10 yr ago | Yes | No | Yes | No† |

*Vaccine choice for child <7 yr of age is DTaP (DT if pertussis is contraindicated). For child >7 yr and <11 yr of age, Td is the vaccine of choice. Consider Tdap in children ≥11 yr of age if pertussis is not contraindicated.

†Any child with HIV infection or who is within the first year after bone marrow transplantation should receive TIG for any tetanus-prone wound regardless of vaccination status.

TIG, tetanus immune globulin: 250 U IM.

Data from American Academy of Pediatrics: Red Book: 2006 Report of the Committee on Infectious Diseases, 27th ed. Elk Grove Village, Ill, AAP, 2006.

(14%–19%), vomiting (7%–13%), pain (4%–11%), body temperature >38.3°C (3%–5%).

b. Moderate to severe side effects: Persistent crying >3 hours (1/100), seizures (1/1750), hypotonic-hyporesponsive episode (1/1750), anaphylaxis (1/50,000), body temperature >40.5°C (rare).

6. **Administration: DTaP, DT, Td, and TdaP are all given in a dose of 0.5 mL IM.**

7. **Special considerations:**

a. Pertussis exposure: Immunize all unimmunized or partially immunized close contacts <7 years.
   (1) Give fourth dose of DTaP if third dose was given >6 months prior.
   (2) Give booster dose of DTaP if last dose was given >3 years prior and child is <7 years old.

b. Chemoprophylaxis for all household and other close contacts: Treat with erythromycin for 14 days to limit secondary transmission regardless of immunization status because pertussis immunity may wane. Estolate preparation may be better tolerated (see Formulary). Azithromycin, clarithromycin, and trimethoprim-sulfamethoxazole are possible alternatives.

**Note** *The total number of DT and DTaP immunizations should not exceed six by the 7th birthday.*

## C. *HAEMOPHILUS INFLUENZAE* TYPE B IMMUNOPROPHYLAXIS

1. **Description:** **The three licensed vaccines consist of a capsular polysaccharide antigen (PRP) conjugated to a carrier protein. It is not necessary to use the same formulation for the entire series. Vaccines do not confer protection against the disease associated with the carrier (e.g., PRP-T does not protect against tetanus).**

a. PRP-OMP: Conjugated to outer membrane protein of *Neisseria meningitidis;* requires only two doses in primary series (2 and 4 months) plus booster at 12–15 months. If PRP-OMP is used only for part of the immunization series, the recommended number of doses to complete the series is based on the other Hib conjugate vaccine used. Children without prior DTaP vaccine may respond better to PRP-OMP than to other formulations.
b. HbOC: Conjugated to mutant diphtheria toxin.
c. PRP-T: Conjugated to tetanus toxoid.
d. PRP-OMP/HepB (Comvax): See section V.P.

2. **Indications:**

a. Routine (see Fig. 16-1).
b. Children not immunized against Hib before age 7 months: Give all doses 2 months apart (minimum of 1 month apart). If initiating Hib immunization at age 7–11 months, give three doses; at age 12–14 months, give two doses; and at age 15–59 months, give one dose. Immunization is not necessary for immunocompetent children ≥60 months of age.
c. Unimmunized children >15 months of age with underlying conditions predisposing to invasive Hib disease (e.g., IgG2 deficiency, HIV) require two doses of vaccine given 2 months apart.
d. Children undergoing splenectomy: May benefit from an additional dose 7–10 days before procedure, even if series was previously completed.
e. Children with invasive Hib disease at age <24 months: Begin Hib immunization 1 month after acute illness, and continue as if previously unimmunized. Vaccination is not required if invasive disease develops after age 24 months.

**Note** *Consider immunologic workup for children who contract invasive Hib disease after completing the immunization series.*

3. **Precautions/contraindications** (see Table 16-10).
4. **Side effects:** Local pain, redness, and swelling in 25% of recipients (mild, lasting <24 hours).
5. **Administration:** Dose is 0.5 mL IM.
6. **Special considerations:** Consider prophylactic rifampin to selected household and child care contacts of children with invasive Hib disease; see the *AAP Red Book*[1] for details because this issue is controversial.

## D. HEPATITIS A VIRUS IMMUNOPROPHYLAXIS

1. **Description:** HAV vaccine is an inactivated adsorbed vaccine; two brands are available, Havrix and Vaqta (preservative-free). Licensed only for children ≥12 months of age.

2. **Indications:**
a. All children ≥12 months of age (see Fig. 16-1 for schedule). Programs established to vaccinate children age 2–18 years should continue giving catch-up vaccinations during routine visits.
b. Travelers to or residents of endemic areas.
c. After exposure to HAV if future exposure is likely.
d. Military personnel.
e. Homosexual or bisexual men.
f. Users of illicit injection drugs.
g. Patients with clotting factor disorders.
h. Patients with chronic liver disease, including HBV or hepatitis C (HCV).
i. Persons at risk for occupational exposure.
j. Immunocompromised individuals; may be immunized, although efficacy is not established in immunocompromised children.
k. Consider use in staff of institutions with ongoing or recurrent outbreaks.
3. **Precautions/contraindications (see Table 16-10).**
4. **Side effects: Local reactions are typically mild; include induration, redness, swelling (18%); headache (12%); fever (6%); fatigue, malaise, anorexia, nausea (1%–10%). No serious adverse events have been reported.**
5. **Administration:** See Table 16-12 **for dose and schedule; give IM.**
6. **Special considerations:**
a. Pre-exposure immunoprophylaxis for travelers
(1) HAV vaccine is preferred for travelers ≥12 months old; a single dose usually provides adequate immunity if time does not allow further doses before travel.
(2) Ig, given IM, is protective for up to 5 months; see the *AAP Red Book*[1] for dosing. Ig can be given without vaccine to children <12 months of age before travel.
b. Postexposure immunoprophylaxis: Ig 0.02 mL/kg IM is 80%–90% effective in preventing symptomatic infection if given within 2 weeks of exposure. Maximum dose per site is 3 mL for infants and small children and 5 mL for large children and adults.

## E. HEPATITIS B VIRUS IMMUNOPROPHYLAXIS
1. **Description:**
a. Hepatitis B immune globulin (HBIG): Prepared from plasma containing high-titer anti-HBsAg antibodies and negative for antibodies to HIV and HCV. Dose: Infants, 0.5 mL IM; older children, 0.06 mL/kg IM.
b. HBV vaccine: Adsorbed HBsAg produced recombinantly. Different recombinant vaccines may be used interchangeably.
c. See section V.P for information on combination vaccines containing hepatitis B (Pediarix, Twinrix, Comvax).
2. **Indications:**
a. Routine (see Fig. 16-1).

TABLE 16-12

RECOMMENDED DOSAGES AND SCHEDULES FOR HAV VACCINES

| Age (yr) | Vaccine | Antigen | Volume (mL) | No. of Doses | Schedule |
|---|---|---|---|---|---|
| 1–18 | Havrix (SB) | 720 ELU | 0.5 | 2 | Initial and 6–12 mo later |
| | Vaqta (Merck) | 25 U | 0.5 | 2 | Initial and 6–18 mo later |
| ≥19 | Havrix (SB) | 1440 ELU | 1.0 | 2 | Initial and 6–12 mo later |
| | Vaqta (Merck) | 50 U | 1.0 | 2 | Initial and 6–12 mo later |
| >18 | Twinrix* (SB) | 720 ELU | 1.0 | 3 | Initial and 1 and 6 mo later |

*Twinrix is a combination of hepatitis B (Energix-B, 20 μg) and hepatitis A (Havrix, 720 ELU) vaccines.

ELU, enzyme-linked immunoassay units; SB, SmithKline Beecham; U, antigen units.

Data from American Academy of Pediatrics: Red Book: 2006 Report of the Committee on Infectious Diseases, 27th ed. Elk Grove Village, Ill, AAP, 2006, p 330.

b. Infants of mothers who are HBsAg positive or indeterminate (Fig. 16-2).

3. **Precautions/contraindications (see Table 16-11).**
4. **Side effects: Pain at injection site (3%–29%) or fever >37.7°C (1%–6%); immediate hypersensitivity reaction is very rare.**
5. **Administration:**

a. See Table 16-13 for dose; give IM in the anterolateral thigh or deltoid; administration in the buttocks or intradermally is not recommended due to decreased immunogenicity.

b. HBV vaccines are interchangeable between different manufacturers, but interchangeability of Pediarix may be limited by the DTaP component. See section V.P.

6. **Special considerations: See Table 16-14 for HBV prophylaxis after percutaneous exposure to blood.**

## F. HUMAN PAPILLOMA VIRUS IMMUNOPROPHYLAXIS

1. **Description: Human papilloma virus (HPV) vaccine is a quadrivalent, inactivated vaccine to prevent genital warts, cervical adenocarcinoma, cervical squamous cell carcinoma, vaginal intraepithelial neoplasia, vulvar intraepithelial neoplasia, cervical intraepithelial neoplasia, and low- to high-grade cervical dysplasia caused by HPV types 6, 11, 16, and 18. It is a 3-dose series.**
2. **Indications:**

a. Routine (see Figure 16-2).

b. Females age 11 to 36 years (can be given to girls as young as age 9 years).

3. **Precautions/contraindications:**

a. Contraindications include history of immediate hypersensitivity to yeast or vaccine component.

b. Precautions include deferring vaccine in the case of moderate to severe acute illnesses.

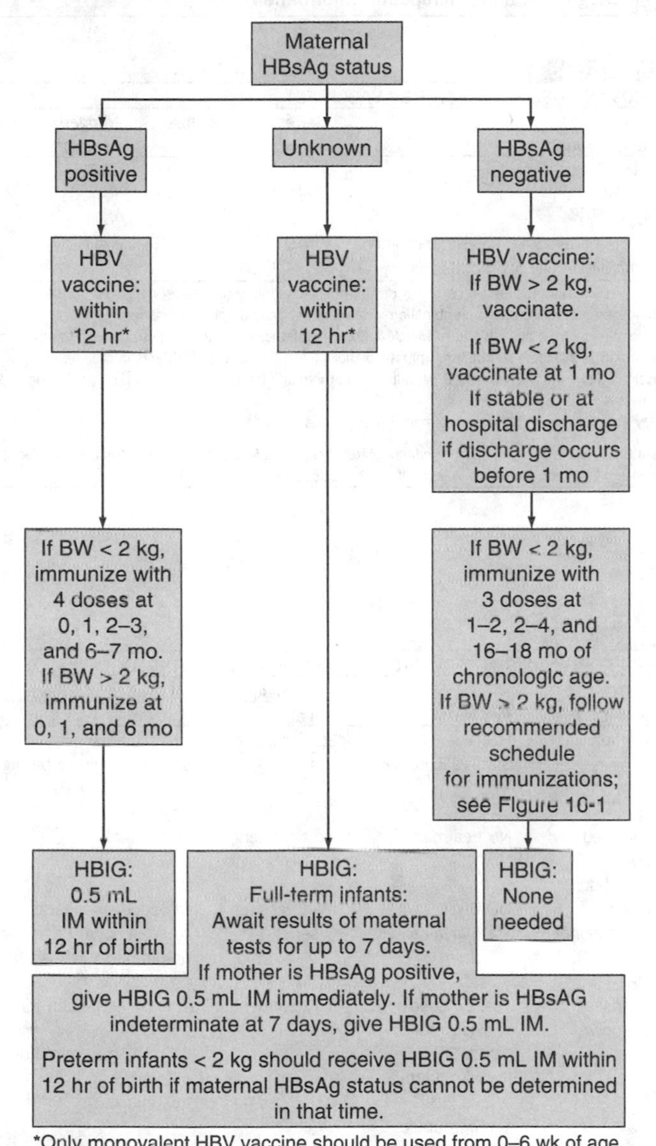


FIG. 16-2

Management of neonates born to mothers with unknown or positive HbsAg status. BW, birth weight. *(Data from American Academy of Pediatrics: Red Book: 2006 Report of the Committee on Infectious Diseases, 26th ed. Elk Grove Village, Ill, AAP, 2006, p 347.)*

TABLE 16-13

RECOMMENDED DOSE FOR HBV VACCINES*

| Patient Group | Recombivax Dose (mcg)† | Engerix-B Dose (mcg)‡ |
|---|---|---|
| Up to 19 yr | 5 | 10 |
| 11–15 yr§ | 10‡ | — |
| ≥20 yr | 10 | 20 |
| Patients undergoing dialysis and other immunosuppressed adults | 40 | 40 |

*Vaccines are administered on a three- or four-dose schedule. Four doses are given if HBV is administered at birth, and a combination vaccine is used to complete the series.

†Recombivax HB is available from Merck & Co. in pediatric, adult, and dialysis patient formulations.

‡Engerix-B is available from GlaxoSmithKline Biologicals; it is also available as combination vaccines: (1) Twinrix (hepatitis B/hepatitis A); (2) Pediarix (DTap/IPV/hepatitis B). See section IV.P for details.

§May use alternative two-dose regimen 6 months apart.

Data from American Academy of Pediatrics: Red Book: 2006 Report of the Committee on Infectious Diseases, 27th ed. Elk Grove Village, Ill, AAP, 2006, p 342.

TABLE 16-14

HBV PROPHYLAXIS AFTER PERCUTANEOUS EXPOSURE TO BLOOD

| | HBsAg Status of Source of Blood | | |
|---|---|---|---|
| Exposed Person | Positive | Negative | Unknown |
| Unimmunized | HBIG<br>Start vaccine series | Start vaccine series | Start vaccine series; if source known to be high risk, treat as HBsAg positive |
| Immunized<br>Known responder | No treatment | No treatment | No treatment |
| Known nonresponder* | HBIG<br>Start vaccine series | Start vaccine series | Start vaccine series; if source known to be high risk, treat as HBsAg positive |
| Response unknown | Test exposed person for anti-HBs:<br>If <10 mIU/mL, give HBIG, reimmunize<br>If ≥10 mIU/mL, no treatment | No treatment | Test exposed person for anti-HBs:<br>If <10 mIU/mL, reimmunize<br>If ≥10 mIU/mL, no treatment |

*If patient has previously failed to respond to second vaccine series, two doses of HBIG (0.06 mL/kg) given 1 mo apart recommended.

Data from American Academy of Pediatrics: Red Book: 2003 Report of the Committee on Infectious Diseases, 26th ed. Elk Grove Village, Ill, AAP, 2003.

**4. Side effects:**

a. Pain, swelling, and erythema at injection site (83%, 25%, and 25%, respectively).

b. Fever (10% of recipients).

c. Nausea (6%).

d. Dizziness (4%).

**5. Administration: Dose is 0.5 mL IM.**

a. First dose can be given at age 9 years but recommended to give the first dose at age 11–12 years.

b. Second dose should be given 2 months after the first dose.

c. Third dose should be given 6 months after the initial dose.

**6. Special considerations:**

a. The series can be given to females with an equivocal or abnormal Pap smear or genital warts; no clinical trials indicate that the vaccine will lend therapeutic benefit in these situations.

b. Can be given to immunocompromised patients.

c. Not recommended for pregnant women; effect of vaccine on fetus is unknown.

## G. INFLUENZA VACCINE AND CHEMOPROPHYLAXIS

**1. Description:**

a. Activated and inactivated influenza vaccines are produced in embryonated eggs.

b. Vaccines contain three viral strains (usually two type A and one type B), based on expected prevalent influenza strains for the upcoming winter.

c. Preparations:

(1) Split-virus vaccines: Subvirion or purified surface antigen vaccines available; licensed for children ≥6 months of age.

(2) Live, attenuated intranasal vaccine (LAIV): Introduced in 2003; not approved for children <60 months of age. Licensed for use in healthy persons age 5–49 years, with no preference given to the inactivated or the intranasal vaccine.[2]

**2. Indications:**

a. High-risk children:

(1) Asthma and other chronic pulmonary diseases.

(2) Hemodynamically significant cardiac disease.

(3) Immunosuppressive disorders and therapy.

(4) HIV infection.

(5) Sickle cell anemia and other hemoglobinopathies.

(6) Diseases requiring long-term aspirin therapy.

(7) Chronic renal disease.

(8) Chronic metabolic disease, including diabetes mellitus.

(9) Conditions that compromise respiratory function or handling of secretions (e.g., spinal cord injury, neuromuscular disorders, cognitive dysfunction, or seizure disorder).

b. Close contacts of high-risk children, children younger than age 24 months, and adults, including household contacts, health care workers, and daycare providers. Consider chemoprophylaxis of these individuals.
c. Consider immunization for other high-risk persons.
   (1) Women who are pregnant during influenza season (only the IM inactivated vaccine is approved for administration to pregnant women).
   (2) International travel to areas with influenza outbreaks.
   (3) Institutional settings, including colleges and other residential facilities.
d. Annual immunization should be encouraged in healthy children age 6 to 59 months of age and their close contacts.

3. **Precautions/contraindications (see Table 16-10).**
4. **Side effects:**

a. Fever 6–24 hours after immunization in children <2 years of age; rare in children >2 years of age.
b. Local reactions uncommon in children <13 years of age; 10% in children ≥13 years of age.
c. Side effects and immunogenicity are similar for whole and split-virus vaccines in children >12 years of age.
d. Guillain-Barré syndrome (GBS): Influenza immunization has been associated with GBS in approximately 1 per 1 million persons ≥45 years of age; GBS has not been associated with influenza immunization in children.
e. LAIV: Nasal congestion (20%–75%), headache (2%–46%), fever (0%–26%), and abdominal pain (2%).

5. **Administration:**

a. Administer annually during the fall in preparation for winter influenza season.
b. Dosage and schedule (Table 16-15); give inactivated vaccine IM.

6. **Special considerations:**

a. Children receiving chemotherapy have poor seroconversion rates until chemotherapy is discontinued for 3–4 weeks and absolute neutrophil and lymphocyte counts are >1000/μL.

TABLE 16-15

INFLUENZA VACCINE DOSAGE AND SCHEDULE

| Age | Volume (mL) | Number of Doses |
|---|---|---|
| 6–35 mo | 0.25 | 1 or 2* |
| 3–8 yr | 0.5 | 1 or 2* |
| ≥9 yr | 0.5 | 1 |

*Two doses, at least 1 mo apart, recommended for children <9 yr receiving influenza vaccine for the first time. Try to give the second dose before December.

Data from American Academy of Pediatrics: Red Book: 2006 Report of the Committee on Infectious Diseases, 27th ed. Elk Grove Village, Ill, AAP, 2006, table 3.29, p 406.

b. Immunization may be delayed in patients on prolonged high-dose steroids (equivalent to 2 mg/kg/day or >20 mg/day of prednisone) until dose is decreased, only if time allows before the influenza season.
c. Infants <6 months of age with high-risk conditions should not be immunized and should not receive chemoprophylaxis. However, close contacts of these infants should receive both vaccine and chemoprophylaxis.
d. LAIV should not be administered until >48 hours after completing antiviral therapy for influenza.[2]

**7. Chemoprophylaxis for influenza A and B:**

a. Oseltamivir and zanamivir: Approved for use in the United States for chemoprophylaxis against influenza A and B in children.
   (1) Oseltamivir: Approved for children ≥1 year of age.
   (2) Zanamivir: Can be given to children ≥5 years of age.
b. Indications:
   (1) High-risk children immunized after influenza is present in the community or if likely to be exposed to individuals infected with influenza: In children <9 years of age, give for 6 weeks after first dose of vaccine or 2 weeks after second dose, depending on whether child is scheduled for 1 or 2 doses of vaccine.
   (2) Unimmunized individuals in close contact with or providing care to high-risk individuals.
   (3) Immunodeficient individuals unlikely to have protective response to vaccine.
   (4) Individuals at high risk for influenza infection with contraindication to vaccine.
   (5) Immunized high-risk individuals if vaccine strain different from circulating strain.
   (6) Healthy children with severe illness from influenza.
c. Chemoprophylaxis is not a substitute for immunization and does not interfere with the immune response to the inactivated virus vaccine.
d. Do not administer chemoprophylaxis until at least 2 weeks after administration of LAIV.

## H. MEASLES/MUMPS/RUBELLA IMMUNOPROPHYLAXIS

**1. Description:**

a. MMR: Combination vaccine composed of live, attenuated viruses. Measles and mumps vaccines are grown in chick embryo cell culture; rubella vaccine is prepared in human diploid cell culture.
b. Monovalent measles, rubella, and measles/rubella (MR) formulations available.
c. Ig: Intramuscular and intravenous immunoglobulin (IVIG) preparations contain similar concentration of measles antibody.

**2. Indications:**

a. Routine (see Fig. 16-1).

b. Screen all women of childbearing age for susceptibility to rubella. People are considered susceptible to rubella unless they have documentation of one dose of rubella-containing vaccine or serologic evidence of immunity. If susceptible, immunize with one dose of MMR unless pregnant.

c. Screen all adolescents and young adults for susceptibility to measles. People are considered susceptible to measles unless they have had two measles-containing vaccines given 1 month apart after age 12 months, physician-diagnosed disease, or laboratory evidence of immunity.

d. Immunize people traveling to foreign countries with MMR. Young children may need to be immunized at a younger age than recommended for routine immunization. See the *AAP Red Book*[1] for details.

**3. Precautions/contraindications (see Table 16-10).**

**4. Misconceptions: The following are *not* contraindications to MMR administration:**

a. Anaphylactic reaction to eggs: Consider observing patient for 90 min after vaccine administration. Skin testing is not predictive of hypersensitivity reaction and therefore is not recommended.

b. Allergy to penicillin.

c. Exposure to measles.

d. History of seizures: There is a slightly increased risk for seizure after immunization. Temperature should be followed and treated with antipyretics.

**5. Side effects:**

a. Minor side effects 7–12 days after immunization: Body temperature to 39.4°C develops 6–12 days after MMR vaccine and lasts 1–5 days (5%–15%); transient rash (5%).

b. Moderate to severe side effects: Febrile seizures (rare); transient thrombocytopenia (1 in 25,000 to 1 in 2 million) 2–3 weeks after immunization; encephalitis and encephalopathy (<1 in 1 million).

**6. Administration:**

a. Dose is 0.5 mL SC.

b. See *AAP Red Book*[1] for suggested intervals between Ig administration and MMR vaccination.

c. Purified protein derivative (PPD) testing may be done on the day of immunization; otherwise, postpone PPD 4–6 weeks because of suppression of response.

**7. Special considerations:**

a. Measles postexposure immunoprophylaxis:

(1) Vaccine prevents or modifies disease if given within 72 hours of exposure.

(2) Ig prevents or modifies disease if given within 6 days of exposure; Indicated in susceptible household contacts, pregnant women,

children <1 year of age, and immunocompromised individuals. Dosage is as follows:
(a) Standard-dose Ig for children and pregnant women: 0.25 mL/kg (maximum dose, 15 mL) IM.
(b) High-dose Ig for immunocompromised children (including those with HIV infection): 0.5 mL/kg (maximum dose, 15 mL) IM. Not required if IVIG received within 3 weeks before exposure.

b. Rubella postexposure immunoprophylaxis: Ig may modify rubella disease but does not prevent congenital rubella syndrome; not recommended for exposed pregnant women.

## I. MENINGOCOCCUS IMMUNOPROPHYLAXIS



1. **Description: Two meningococcal vaccines are now available.**
a. A quadrivalent serogroup-specific vaccine made from purified capsular polysaccharide antigen from groups A, C, Y, and W-135 (MPSV4); intended for use in patients age 2–10 years.
b. A tetravalent conjugate vaccine with antigen from groups A, C, Y, and W-135 (MCV4); intended for use in patients >11 years of age.
c. Immunogenicity of serogroup antigens varies with age of child. No vaccine is available for group B because of poor immunogenicity.
2. **Indications:**
a. Routine immunization of adolescents at age 11–12 years or at high school entry with MCV4 (for more detail, see section IV.F)
b. High-risk groups ≥2 years of age include the following:
(1) Functional or anatomic asplenia.
(2) Terminal complement or properdin deficiencies.
c. Possible adjunct to postexposure chemoprophylaxis in an outbreak setting.
d. College freshmen, particularly those living in dormitories or residence halls, should receive MCV4.
e. Travelers to endemic or hyperendemic areas.
f. U.S. military recruits.
3. **Precautions/contraindications** (see Table 16-10).
4. **Side effects:** Mild; localized erythema lasting 1–2 days occurs infrequently.
5. **Administration:** Dose is 0.5 mL SC for MPSV4 and 0.5 mL IM for MCV4.
6. **Postexposure chemoprophylaxis:** Antibiotics should be given to exposed household, child care, and nursery school contacts within 24 hours of primary case diagnosis. Individuals with potential contact with oral secretions of infected patient should also receive chemoprophylaxis.
a. Rifampin is the drug of choice (see Formulary for dosage information).
b. Ciprofloxacin (500 mg single dose) may be given to persons ≥18 years.
c. Ceftriaxone (125 mg single dose in children <15 years, 250 mg single dose in children ≥15 years).

## J. PNEUMOCOCCAL IMMUNOPROPHYLAXIS

**1. Description:**

a. PCV7: Pneumococcal conjugate vaccine includes seven purified capsular polysaccharides of *Streptococcus pneumoniae,* each coupled to a variant of diphtheria toxin. Serotypes are 4, 9V, 14, 19F, 23F, 18C, and 6B, which account for 88% of cases of bacteremia, 82% of cases of meningitis, and >70% of acute otitis media (AOM) among children <6 years of age.

b. 23PS: Purified capsular polysaccharide includes antigen from 23 serotypes of *S. pneumoniae;* not approved for use in children <2 years of age.

**2. Indications:**

a. Routine (see Fig. 16-1).

b. See Table 16-8 for catch-up schedule for previously unvaccinated children ages 7–24 months.

c. See Table 16-6 for an immunization schedule of high-risk children ages 23–59 months, including those with the following conditions:

(1) Sickle cell disease, functional or anatomic asplenia.

(2) HIV infection.

(3) Congenital immune deficiency.

(4) Chronic renal insufficiency, including nephrotic syndrome.

(5) Immunosuppression, including malignant neoplasms, leukemias, lymphomas, and Hodgkin disease, and solid organ transplantation.

(6) Chronic cardiac disease.

(7) Chronic pulmonary disease (including asthma treated with high-dose oral corticosteroid therapy).

(8) Cerebrospinal fluid leaks.

(9) Diabetes mellitus.

d. Consider immunization in the following children, who are considered to be at moderate risk for invasive pneumococcal infection:

(1) All children ages 24–35 months.

(2) Children ages 36–59 months attending out-of-home care.

(3) Children ages 36–59 months who are of American Indian, Alaska Native, or African American descent.

**3. Precautions/contraindications** (see Table 16-10).

**4. Side effects: Pain and erythema at injection site (common); fever within 1–2 days after administration (less common); severe systemic reactions such as anaphylaxis (rare).**

**5. Administration:**

a. Dose for both PCV7 and 23PS is 0.5 mL given IM.

b. Concurrent administration of PCV7 and 23PS vaccines is not recommended. Either vaccine may be given concurrently with other vaccines in a separate syringe at a separate injection site.

c. Give vaccine 2 weeks or more before elective splenectomy, chemotherapy, radiotherapy, or immunosuppressive therapy; or give 3 months after chemotherapy or radiotherapy.

6. **Special considerations:**
a. Passive immunoprophylaxis with IVIG is recommended for some children with congenital or acquired immune deficiencies.
b. See discussion of functional or anatomic asplenia in section IV.A.
c. PCV7 may provide a modest decrease in recurrent AOM; may therefore be beneficial in children age 24–59 months with either recurrent AOM or with AOM requiring tympanostomy tube placement.

## K. POLIOMYELITIS IMMUNOPROPHYLAXIS

1. **Description:**
a. IPV: Trivalent enhanced-potency vaccine of formalin-inactivated poliovirus types 1, 2, and 3 grown in human diploid or Vero cells.
b. OPV: No longer available in the United States. Children who have received the appropriate number of doses of OPV in other countries should be considered adequately immunized.
c. Combination vaccine (DTaP, HepB, Pediarix, IPV): See section V.P.
2. **Indications:**
a. Routine (see Fig. 16-1).
b. Unimmunized or partially immunized individuals who are at imminent risk for exposure to poliovirus (dose interval may be 4 weeks).
3. **Precautions/contraindications (see Table 16-10).**
4. **Side effects: No serious side effects have been associated with use of IPV.**
5. **Administration:** Dose is 0.5 mL SC.

## L. RABIES IMMUNOPROPHYLAXIS (Table 16-16)

1. **Description:**
a. Three rabies vaccines are available for prophylaxis:
 (1) Human diploid cell vaccine (HDCV).
 (2) Rabies vaccine adsorbed (RVA).
 (3) Purified chicken embryo cell (PCEC).
b. Human rabies immune globulin (RIG): Anti-rabies Ig prepared from plasma of donors hyperimmunized with rabies vaccine.
2. **Indications:**
a. Pre-exposure prophylaxis: Indicated for high-risk groups, including veterinarians, animal handlers, laboratory workers, children living in high-risk environments, those traveling to high-risk areas, and spelunkers.
 (1) Three injections of HDCV or PCEC vaccine on days 0, 7, and 21 or 28.
 (2) Rabies serum antibody titers should be followed at 6-month intervals for those at continuous risk and at 2-year intervals for those with risk for frequent exposure; give booster doses only if titers are nonprotective.
b. Postexposure prophylaxis (see Table 16-16).

TABLE 16-16
RABIES POSTEXPOSURE PROPHYLAXIS

| Animal Type | Evaluation and Disposition of Animal | Postexposure Prophylaxis Recommendations |
|---|---|---|
| Dogs, cats, ferrets | Healthy and available for 10 days' observation | Do not begin prophylaxis unless animal develops symptoms of rabies. |
| | Rabid or suspected rabid; euthanize animal and test brain | Provide immediate immunization and RIG. |
| | Unknown (escaped) | Consult public health officials. |
| Skunk, raccoon, bat,* fox, most other carnivores | Regard as rabid unless animal is euthanized and brain is negative for rabies by fluorescein antibody test | Provide immediate immunization and RIG.[†] |
| Livestock, rodents, rabbit, other mammals | Consider individually | Consult public health officials; these bites rarely require treatment. |

*In the case of direct contact between a human and a bat, consider prophylaxis even if a bite, scratch, or mucous membrane exposure is not apparent.
[†]Treatment may be discontinued if animal fluorescent antibody is negative.

Data from American Academy of Pediatrics: Red Book: 2006 Report of the Committee on Infectious Diseases, 27th ed. Elk Grove Village, Ill, AAP, 2006.

3. **Precautions/contraindications** (see Table 16-10).
4. **Side effects:** Uncommon in children. Local reactions in 25%; mild systemic reactions, such as headache, abdominal pain, and dizziness in 20%; neurologic illness similar to GBS or focal central nervous system (CNS) disorder (reported with HDCV, but not believed to be causally related); immune complex-like reaction (urticaria, arthralgia, angioedema, vomiting, fever, and malaise) 2–21 days after immunization with HDCV, rare in primary series, 6% after booster dose.
5. **Administration:** Dose is 1 mL IM for HDCV, RVA, and PCEC.
6. **Postexposure prophylaxis:**

a. General wound management:
   (1) Clean immediately with soap and water.
   (2) Avoid suturing wound unless indicated for functional reasons.
   (3) Consider tetanus prophylaxis and antibiotics if indicated.

b. Indications: Infectious exposures include bites, scratches, or contamination of open wound or mucous membrane with infectious material of a rabid animal or human.

**Note** *Report all patients suspected of rabies infection to public health authorities.*

c. Administration:
   (1) Vaccine and RIG should be given jointly except in previously immunized patients (no RIG required). If vaccine is not immediately available, give RIG alone and vaccinate later. If RIG is not available, give the vaccine alone. RIG may be given later, if it can be administered within 7 days after initiating immunization.
   (2) Vaccine for postexposure prophylaxis:
      (a) Do not administer in same part of body or in same syringe as RIG.
      (b) Deltoid muscle, except in infants, in whom anterolateral thigh is appropriate.
      (c) Routine serologic testing not indicated.
      (d) Unimmunized: 1 mL IM on days 0, 3, 7, 14, and 28.
      (e) Previously immunized: 1 mL IM on days 0 and 3. Do not give RIG.
   (3) RIG: Recommended dose of 20 IU/kg should not be exceeded. Infiltrate around the wound and give remainder IM.

## M. RESPIRATORY SYNCYTIAL VIRUS (RSV) IMMUNOPROPHYLAXIS

1. **Description:**

a. No vaccine available.

b. Palivizumab (monoclonal RSV-Ig): Humanized mouse monoclonal IgG to RSV, recombinantly produced for IM administration.

c. Polyclonal RSV-IVIG: Ig pooled from donors with high serum titers of RSV-neutralizing antibody, for IV administration. Provides some protection against other respiratory viruses.

2. **Indications:**

a. Infants and children <2 years of age with chronic lung disease (CLD) who have required medical therapy (oxygen, bronchodilators, diuretics, or corticosteroids) within the 6 months before the RSV season: Palivizumab is preferred. Data are limited, but these patients may also benefit from prophylaxis during a second RSV season.

b. Infants ≤32 weeks' estimated gestational age (EGA) at birth who do not have CLD: May benefit from prophylaxis with palivizumab.
   (1) EGA ≤28 weeks: Consider until age 12 months.
   (2) EGA 29–32 weeks: Consider until age 6 months.

c. Prophylaxis should be considered in infants born between 32 and 35 weeks' gestation with two or more of the following risk factors:
   (1) Child care attendance.
   (2) School-aged siblings.
   (3) Exposure to environmental air pollutants, such as tobacco smoke.
   (4) Congenital abnormalities of airways.
   (5) Severe neuromuscular disease.

**Note** *These risk factors are considered additive.*

d. Children ≤24 months of age with significant cyanotic and acyanotic heart disease should be considered for prophylaxis with palivizumab.
e. Children <24 months of age with congenital heart disease should be considered for prophylaxis with palivizumab, especially if they:
   (1) Are receiving medication for the treatment of congestive heart failure.
   (2) Have moderate to severe pulmonary hypertension.
   (3) Have a cyanotic heart lesion.
f. Children with severe immunodeficiency may benefit from RSV-IVIG, although its use has not been evaluated in randomized trials.

3. **Precautions/contraindications** (see Table 16-10).
4. **Side effects:**

a. Palivizumab: Side effects are comparable to placebo.
b. RSV-IVIG: See Formulary.
   (1) Fever in 6% (2% in placebo group).
   (2) 8% of children with CLD require extra diuretics around the time of administration.

5. **Administration: Give RSV-IVIG or palivizumab at onset of RSV season, typically in November, and then monthly during season, which usually ends in March. In general, five total doses are given. Consult local health department for optimal schedule.**

a. Palivizumab: Dose is 15 mg/kg IM monthly.
b. Polyclonal RSV-IVIG: Dose is 15 mL/kg (750 mg/kg) IV monthly. Must defer live-virus vaccines (e.g., MMR and varicella) for 9 months after the last dose.

## N. ROTAVIRUS IMMUNOPROPHYLAXIS

1. **Description: Pentavalent, live viral vaccine containing five reassortant human and bovine rotavirus strains in the form of an oral solution (RotaTeq).**
2. **Indications** (see Fig. 16-1).
3. **Precautions/contraindications:**

a. Contraindications: Hypersensitivity to any vaccine component.
b. Precautions:
   (1) Infants on immunosuppressive therapy, including high-dose steroids and infants with suspected or diagnosed immunodeficiencies (congenital and acquired). For infants who received antibody-containing products, the first dose of rotavirus vaccine can be given at >42 days after product was given.
   (2) Acute moderate to severe gastroenteritis.

4. **Side effects: Diarrhea (24%), vomiting (15%), otitis media (14.5%), nasopharyngitis (7%), and bronchospasm (1%).**
5. **Administration:**

a. Dose is 2 mL PO. Vaccine is packaged in single-dose tubes to be administered directly to the patient without dilution. Should not be

given with other liquids. Do not readminister if infant spits out or vomits dose.
b. Should be administered with 2-month, 4-month, and 6-month vaccines.
c. Infants can receive the first dose of the series between age 6 and 12 weeks.
d. Second dose should be given 4–10 weeks from first dose.
e. Third dose should be given 4–10 weeks from second dose to complete the entire series by age 32 weeks.
6. **Special considerations: Premature infants can begin the series at 6 weeks of chronologic age if clinically stable.**





## O. VARICELLA IMMUNOPROPHYLAXIS

1. **Description:**
a. Vaccine: Cell-free live attenuated varicella virus vaccine.
b. Varicella-zoster immune globulin (VZIG): Prepared from plasma containing high-titer anti-varicella antibodies.
2. **Indications:**
a. Routine (see Fig. 16-1).
b. Aim to immunize before the 13th birthday because two doses are needed after that time.
c. Give second dose to children, adolescents, and adults who only received one dose of the vaccine.
3. **Precautions/contraindications** (see Table 16-10).
4. **Side effects:**
a. Local reaction, 20% to 35%; mild varicelliform rash within 5 to 26 days of vaccine administration, 3% to 5%.
b. Vaccine rash often very mild, but patient may be infectious, reversion to wild-type virus has not been reported. Most varicelliform rashes that occur within 2 weeks of vaccination are due to wild-type VZV infection.
5. **Administration:**
a. Dose is 0.5 mL SC.
b. May give simultaneously with MMR; otherwise, allow at least 1 month between MMR and varicella vaccines.
c. Do not give for 5 months after VZIG; do not give concurrently with VZIG.
d. Avoid salicylates for 6 weeks after vaccine administration if possible.
6. **Special considerations: Vaccine may be given in the following circumstances:**
a. Certain children with acute lymphoblastic leukemia in remission >1 year may be immunized under a research protocol. Approval must be obtained by the appropriate institutional review board.
b. Household contacts of immunocompromised hosts: If a rash develops in the immunized child, avoid direct contact if possible.
c. Household contacts of pregnant women.
7. **Postexposure prophylaxis:**

a. Indications: VZIG should be administered within 96 hours of exposure to individuals who are at high risk for severe varicella and who have had a significant exposure (see later). Repeat VZIG every 3 weeks if exposure is ongoing or repeated.
   (1) Individuals at high risk for severe varicella include the following:
      (a) Immunocompromised individuals without a history of varicella.
      (b) Susceptible pregnant women.
      (c) Newborn infant with onset of varicella in mother from 5 days before to 2 days after delivery (even if mother received VZIG during pregnancy).
      (d) Hospitalized preterm infant who was born before 28 weeks' gestation or who weighs <1000g, regardless of maternal history.
      (e) Hospitalized preterm infant who was born at ≥28 weeks' gestation to a susceptible mother.
   (2) Significant exposures include the following:
      (a) Household contact.
      (b) Face-to-face indoor play.
      (c) Onset of varicella in the mother of a newborn from 5 days before to 2 days after delivery.
      (d) Hospital exposures: Roommate, face-to-face contact with infectious individual, visit by contagious individual, or intimate contact with person with active zoster lesions.

**Note** *For VZIG recipients, incubation period may be up to 28 days instead of 21 days.*

b. VZIG dose is 12.5U/kg IM (maximum dose, 625U; minimum dose, 125U). Do not give intravenously. Local discomfort is common.
c. Varicella vaccine should be administered to susceptible immunocompetent children within 72 hours after varicella exposure. If the child was exposed at the same time as the index case, the vaccine may not protect against the disease. Susceptible immunocompromised children should receive VZIG as soon as possible.

## P. COMBINATION VACCINES

### 1. DTaP/HepB/IPV (Pediarix):

a. Description: DTap, IPV, and hepatitis B (Energix-B, 20μg).
b. Indications:
   (1) Routine: Use when vaccine components are indicated, so long as other components are not contraindicated. Administered in a three-dose schedule, preferably at age 2, 4, and 6 months. See Figure 16-1.
   (2) Should not be administered to infants <6 weeks of age or to children >7 years of age.

c. If used as the third dose to complete the hepatitis B series, should be administered at age 6 months or older.
d. Pediarix should not be used as a booster dose following the three-dose primary DTaP series; insufficient data on safety and efficacy of use as a booster dose.
e. Side effects: Higher rates of fever are reported with combination vaccine than with three vaccines administered separately.
f. Precautions/contraindications (see Table 16-10).

**2. Hep A/Hep B (Twinrix):**

a. Description: Energix-B (20 μg) and Havrix (720 ELU).
b. Indications (see Fig. 16-1).
c. Licensed for use in patients ≥18 years of age.
d. Administered in a three-dose schedule given at 0, 1 month, and at least 6 months later.

**3. Measles/mumps/rubella/varicella (Proquad):**

a. Description: Measles, mumps, rubella, and varicella live viral vaccine.
b. Indications: Use when vaccine components are indicated, so long as other component is not contraindicated See Fig. 16-1.
c. Licensed for patients age 12 months to 12 years.

**Note** *Doses of varicella should be given at least 3 months apart.*

**4. PRP-OMP/HepB (Comvax):**

a. Description: PRP-OMP and Recombivax (5 μg).
b. Indications (see Fig. 16-1).
c. Licensed for use at 2, 4, and 12–15 months of age.



## REFERENCES

1. American Academy of Pediatrics: Red Book: 2006 Report of the Committee on Infectious Diseases, 27th ed. Elk Grove Village, Ill, AAP, 2006.
2. Centers for Disease Control and Prevention: Prevention and control and influenza: Recommendations of the Advisory Committee on Immunization Practices (ACIP). MMWR 2006;55(RR-10):1–32.
3. Centers for Disease Control and Prevention: Guidelines for preventing opportunistic infections among hematopoietic stem cell transplant recipients: Recommendations of CDC, the Infectious Disease Society of America, and the American Society of Blood and Marrow Transplantation. MMWR 2000;49(RR-10):1–147.
4. Centers for Disease Control and Prevention. Available at www.cdc.org.
5. Centers for Disease Control and Prevention: Preventing tetanus, diphtheria, and pertussis among adolescents: Use of tetanus toxoid, reduced diphtheria toxoid and acellular pertussis vaccines: recommendations of the Advisory Committee on Immunization Practices (ACIP). MMWR 2006;55(RR-3):1–30.
6. Centers for Disease Control and Prevention: Prevention of hepatitis A through active or passive immunization: recommendations of the Advisory Committee on Immunization Practices (ACIP). MMWR 2006;55(RR-7):1–23.

7. Centers for Disease Control and Prevention: Prevention of rotavirus gastroenteritis among infants and children: Recommendations of the Advisory Committee on Immunization Practices (ACIP). MMWR 2006;55(RR-12):1–13.
8. Merck package insert for Gardasil (HPV vaccine).
9. Merck package insert for RotaTeq (rotavirus vaccine).
10. Merck package insert for ProQuad (measles, mumps, rubella, and varicella live virus vaccine).

# Microbiology and Infectious Disease

*Joelle N. Simpson, MD, MPH*

17

## I. MICROBIOLOGY

### A. COLLECTION OF SPECIMENS FOR BLOOD CULTURE

1. **Preparation:** Proper specimen collection essential to minimize contamination. Clean venipuncture site with 70% isopropyl ethyl alcohol. Apply tincture of iodine or 10% povidone-iodine and allow to dry for at least 1 min, or scrub site with 2% chlorhexidine. Clean blood culture bottle injection site with alcohol only.
2. **Collection:** Obtain 1–2 mL for a neonate, 2–3 mL for an infant, 3–5 mL for a child, and 10–20 mL for an adolescent. There is a higher culture yield with higher volume blood cultures.

### B. RAPID MICROBIOLOGIC IDENTIFICATION OF COMMON AEROBIC BACTERIA (Fig. 17-1)

### C. CHOOSING APPROPRIATE ANTIBIOTIC BASED ON SENSITIVITIES

1. **Definitions:**[1,2]
   a. **Minimum inhibitory concentration (MIC):** Lowest concentration of an antimicrobial agent that prevents visible growth after an 18- to 24-hr incubation period.
   b. **Minimum bactericidal concentration (MBC):** Lowest concentration of an antimicrobial agent that kills the organism, as measured by subculturing to antibiotic free media after 18- to 24-hr incubation.
2. **Common pitfalls (Table 17-1):** Clinically significant, common discrepancies between in vitro (laboratory reported) and in vivo antibiotic sensitivity profiles.

## II. INFECTIOUS DISEASE

### A. FEVER EVALUATION AND MANAGEMENT GUIDELINES (Figs. 17-2 and 17-3)

### B. COMMON PEDIATRIC INFECTIONS: GUIDELINES FOR INITIAL MANAGEMENT (Table 17-2)

### C. CONGENITAL INFECTIONS

1. **Intrauterine infections:** TORCH infections (toxoplasmosis; syphilis, varicella-zoster [VZV]; rubella; cytomegalovirus; and herpes simplex virus [HSV]) often present in the neonate with overlapping findings: intrauterine growth restriction, hematologic involvement (anemia, neutropenia, thrombocytopenia, petechiae, purpura), ocular signs (chorioretinitis, keratoconjunctivitis, glaucoma, microphthalmos), CNS signs (microcephaly, hydrocephaly, intracranial calcifications), other organ system involvement (pneumonia, myocarditis, nephritis, hepatosplenomegaly, jaundice), and nonimmune hydrops.[6]

*Text continued on p. 451*

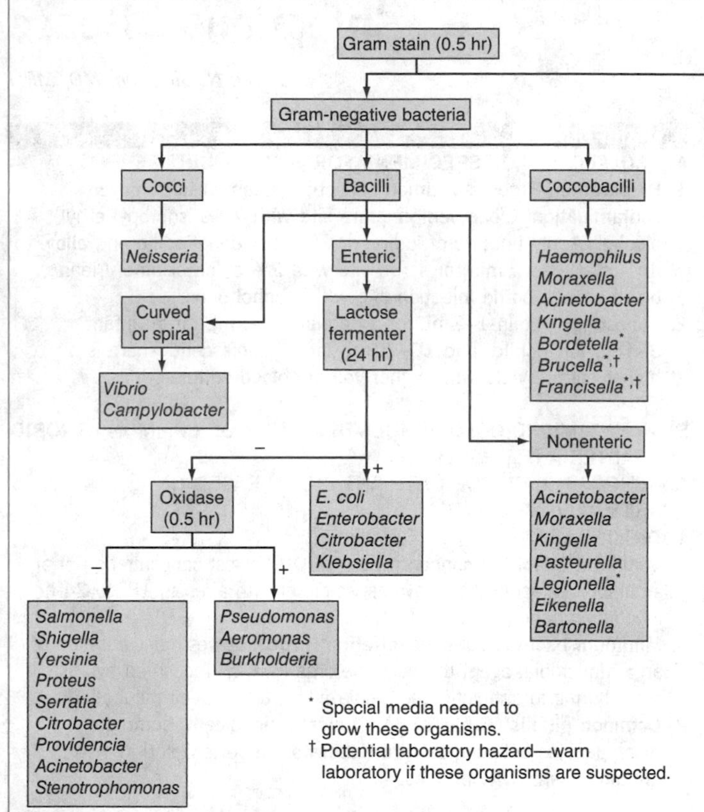


FIG. 17-1

Algorithm demonstrating identification of aerobic bacteria. *Numbers in parentheses* indicate the time required for the tests.

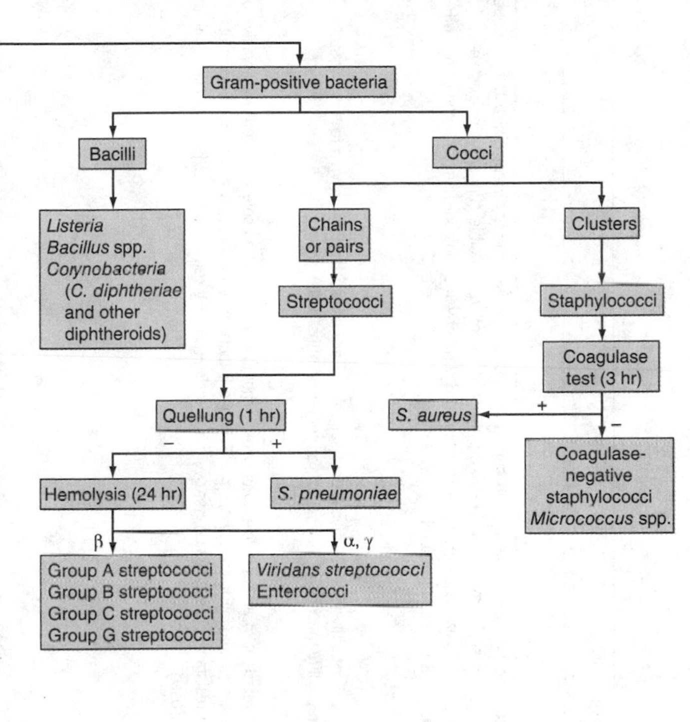
Gram-positive bacteria
Bacilli
Cocci
Listeria
Bacillus spp.
Corynobacteria
(C. diphtheriae
and other
diphtheroids)
Chains
or pairs
Clusters
Streptococci
Staphylococci
Coagulase
test (3 hr)
Quellung (1 hr)
S. aureus
+
−
−
+
Coagulase-
negative
staphylococci
Micrococcus spp.
Hemolysis (24 hr)
S. pneumoniae
β
α, γ
Group A streptococci
Group B streptococci
Group C streptococci
Group G streptococci
Viridans streptococci
Enterococci

TABLE 17-1

**COMMON PITFALLS BETWEEN IN VITRO AND IN VIVO ANTIBIOTIC SENSITIVITY PROFILES**

| Bacteria | In Vivo Resistance | Recommendations |
| --- | --- | --- |
| Staphylococci | Methicillin-resistant *Staphylococcus aureus* (MRSA) | If MRSA is reported to be susceptible to clindamycin in vitro, but resistant to erythromycin, a D test (double disk diffusion assay) is recommended to look for in vitro macrolide-inducible clindamycin resistance. If D test is positive, MRSA may have inducible resistance to clindamycin; consider using vancomycin, TMP-SMX, or linezolid for serious infections. |
| Salmonella | Aminoglycosides | Despite in vitro susceptibility to aminoglycosides, salmonella are not susceptible in vivo to this class of antibiotics. Ampicillin/amoxicillin, TMP-SMX, or cephalosporins preferred. |
| *Enterobacter* spp.<br>*Citrobacter* spp.<br>*Pseudomonas aeruginosa*<br>*Serratia* spp.<br>*Providencia* spp.<br>*Morganella spp.* | Cephalosporins | All are inducibly resistant to all cephalosporins, which should not be used as sole treatment for invasive or serious infections caused by these organisms. Because β-lactamase inhibitors are potent inducers of cephalosporin resistance, and they do not overcome resistance in these organisms, β-lactamase inhibitors should not be used.[3] |

| | | |
|---|---|---|
| *Burkholderia cepacia* *Stenotrophomonas maltophilia* | Aminoglycosides | *Stenotrophomonas* species are often only susceptible to TMP-SMX, the drug of choice in most cases for these organisms. *Burkholderia* often requires a carbapenem plus additional agents. |
| *P. aeruginosa* *Acinetobacter* spp. | TMP-SMX | *P. aeruginosa* and *Acinetobacter* species are usually susceptible to aminoglycosides, but are resistant to TMP-SMX (despite reported in vitro susceptibility). |
| Enterococci | Most single-agent antibiotic classes | Usually requires double-agent therapy for synergy and bacterial killing for invasive infections. Recommended therapy is ampicillin (vancomycin if ampicillin resistant). Add an aminoglycoside (preferably gentamicin or streptomycin) for serious invasive infections. Other antibiotics with activity against enterococci include amoxicillin, penicillin, piperacillin, and imipenem. |
| | Vancomycin-resistant enterococcus (VRE) | VRE is usually *Enterococcus faecium*, although rarely *E. faecalis*. Linezolid is active against most enterococcal isolates, including VRE. Quinupristin/dalfopristin (Synercid) is active against most *E. faecium*, including VRE, but not against *E. faecalis*. The following antibiotics are *not* clinically active against enterococci: all cephalosporins, antistaphylococcal penicillins (e.g., oxacillin), macrolides, clindamycin, and quinolones. |

TMP-SMX, trimethoprim-sulfamethoxazole.

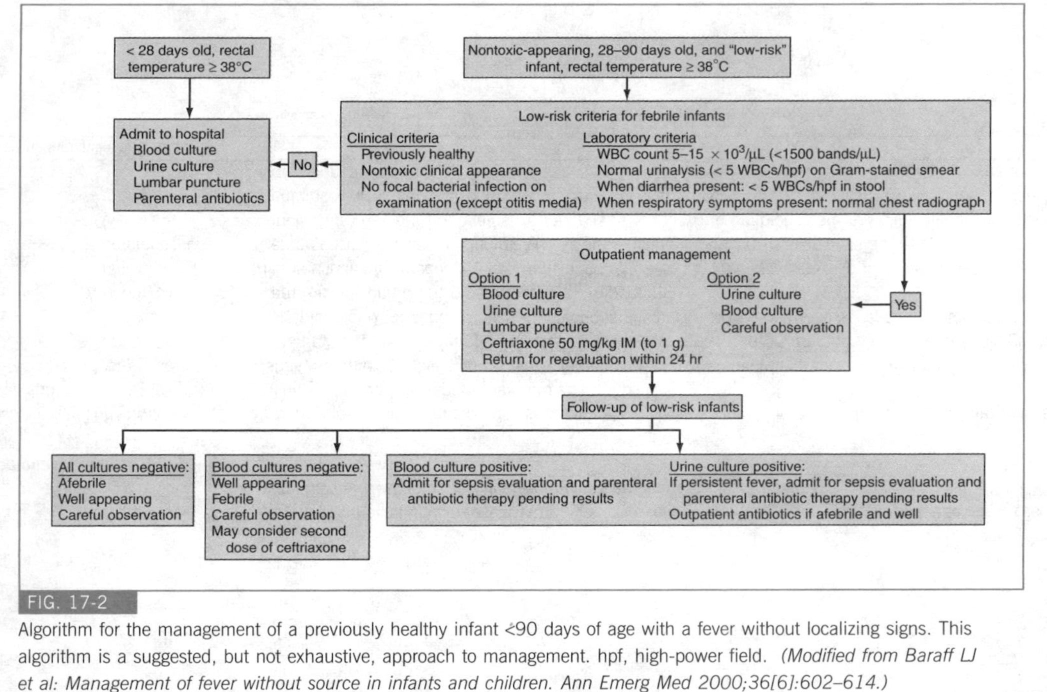


FIG. 17-2

Algorithm for the management of a previously healthy infant <90 days of age with a fever without localizing signs. This algorithm is a suggested, but not exhaustive, approach to management. hpf, high-power field. *(Modified from Baraff LJ et al: Management of fever without source in infants and children. Ann Emerg Med 2000;36[6]:602–614.)*

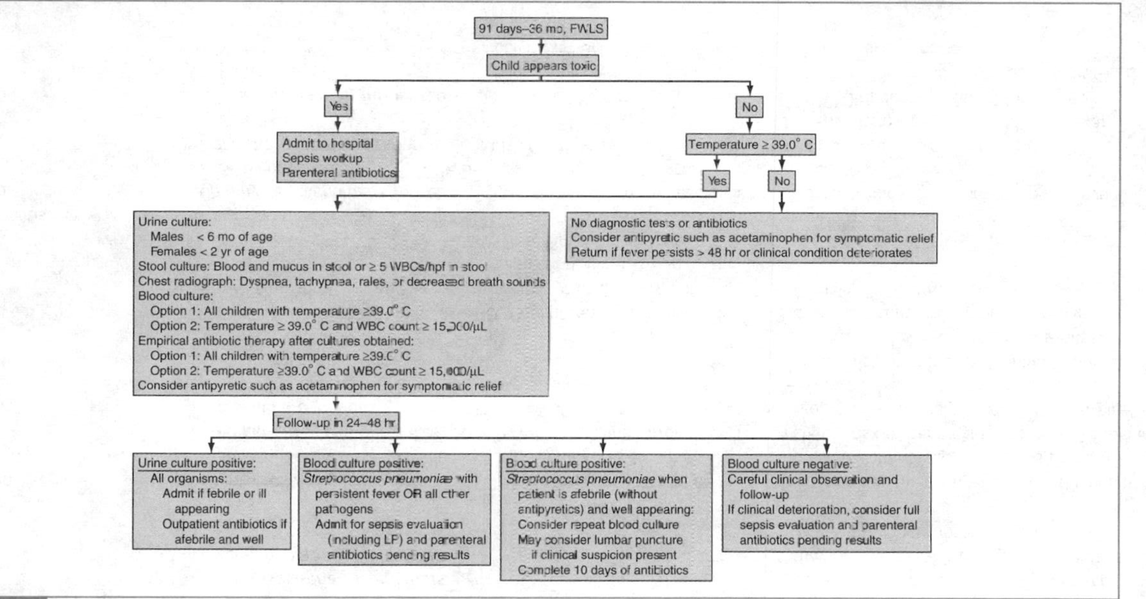
91 days–36 mo, FWLS
Child appears toxic
Yes
No
Admit to hospital
Sepsis workup
Parenteral antibiotics
Temperature ≥ 39.0° C
Yes
No
Urine culture:
Males < 6 mo of age
Females < 2 yr of age
Stool culture: Blood and mucus in stool or ≥ 5 WBCs/hpf in stool
Chest radiograph: Dyspnea, tachypnea, rales, or decreased breath sounds
Blood culture:
Option 1: All children with temperature ≥39.0° C
Option 2: Temperature ≥ 39.0° C and WBC count ≥ 15,000/μL
Empirical antibiotic therapy after cultures obtained:
Option 1: All children with temperature ≥39.0° C
Option 2: Temperature ≥39.0° C and WBC count ≥ 15,000/μL
Consider antipyretic such as acetaminophen for symptomatic relief
No diagnostic tests or antibiotics
Consider antipyretic such as acetaminophen for symptomatic relief
Return if fever persists > 48 hr or clinical condition deteriorates
Follow-up in 24–48 hr
Urine culture positive:
All organisms:
Admit if febrile or ill appearing
Outpatient antibiotics if afebrile and well
Blood culture positive:
Streptococcus pneumoniae with persistent fever OR all other pathogens
Admit for sepsis evaluation (including LP) and parenteral antibiotics pending results
Blood culture positive:
Streptococcus pneumoniae when patient is afebrile (without antipyretics) and well appearing:
Consider repeat blood culture
May consider lumbar puncture if clinical suspicion present
Complete 10 days of antibiotics
Blood culture negative:
Careful clinical observation and follow-up
If clinical deterioration, consider full sepsis evaluation and parenteral antibiotics pending results

FIG. 17-3

Algorithm for the management of a previously healthy child age 91 days to 36 months with a fever without localizing signs. This algorithm is a suggested, but not exhaustive, approach to management. *(Modified from Baraff LJ et al: Management of infants and children 3 to 36 months of age with fever without a source. Pediatr Ann 1993;22[8]:497–498, 501–504.)*

TABLE 17-2

COMMON PEDIATRIC INFECTIONS: GUIDELINES FOR INITIAL MANAGEMENT

| Infectious Syndrome | Usual Etiology | Suggested Empirical Therapy | Suggested Length of Therapy/Comments |
|---|---|---|---|
| **Bacteremia** (outpatient) | *Streptococcus pneumoniae,* GAS, *Neisseria meningitidis, Escherichia coli, Salmonella* | Ceftriaxone or cefotaxime | 7–10 days (longer for some pathogens). Occult bacteremia with susceptible *S. pneumoniae* may be treated with amoxicillin if afebrile, well, and without focal complications. |
| **Bites** | | | |
| Human | Streptococci, *Staphylococcus aureus, Staphylococcus epidermidis*, oral anaerobes, *Eikenella corrodens* | PO: Amoxicillin/clavulanate or cefotaxime + clindamycin; Alt: TMP/SMX + clindamycin<br>IV: Ampicillin/sulbactam | 5–7 days. Cleaning, irrigation, and débridement most important. Assess tetanus immunization status, risk of hepatitis B and HIV. Antibiotic prophylaxis routinely used for human bites. |
| Dog/cat | Human bite pathogens plus *Pasteurella multocida* | Same | 7–10 days. Assess tetanus immunization status, risk of rabies. Antibiotic prophylaxis for all cat bites and selected dog bites. |
| **Cellulitis** | GAS, *S. aureus* (MSSA or MRSA) | PO: Cephalexin. If penicillin-allergic or MRSA common in population, clindamycin<br>IV: Oxacillin; Alt: Clindamycin | 3 days after acute inflammation resolves (usually 7–10 days). |
| **Conjunctivitis** | | | |
| Neonatal | *Chlamydia trachomatis* (onset 3–10 days) | PO: Erythromycin, other macrolides | 14 days. Topical form ineffective in preventing pneumonia. |
| | *Neisseria gonorrhoeae* (onset 2–4 days) | IM/IV: Ceftriaxone, cefotaxime | Localized to eye: Single dose.<br>Disseminated: 7 days of parenteral therapy. |
| Suppurative | *S. pneumoniae, H. influenzae* (nontypeable) | Ophthalmic: Erythromycin, bacitracin/polymyxin B, or polymyxin B/TMP | 5 days. Ointments preferred for infants or young children and eyedrops for older children and adolescents. |

| | | | |
|---|---|---|---|
| Dacrocystitis | *S. pneumoniae*, *H. influenzae*, *S. aureus*, *S. pyogenes*, *P. aeruginosa* | PO: Dicloxacillin or cephalexin | Consider ophthalmologic evaluation to relieve obstruction. |
| **Dental abscesses** | Oral flora, including anaerobes | Clindamycin or amoxicillin/clavulanic acid | Consider dental evaluation for surgical drainage. |
| **Gastroenteritis** | | | |
| Community acquired | Viruses, *E. coli* | Antibiotic therapy strongly discouraged because of possible increased risk for hemolytic-uremic syndrome occurring in patients with *E. coli* 0157:H7 treated with antibiotics[4] | Primary treatment: Fluid and electrolyte replacement. |
| | *Salmonella* | Cefotaxime or ceftriaxone; Alt: Azithromycin | 10–14 days for infants <6 mo, bacteremia, toxicity, or immunocompromised status. Antibiotics generally not indicated otherwise. |
| | *Shigella* | TMP/SMX; Alt: Ceftriaxone or oral cefixime, azithromycin | 5 days. Fluroquinolone if resistant to other antibiotics. |
| | *Yersinia* | TMP/SMX, aminoglycosides, cefotaxime, tetracycline (>8 yr) | Usually no antibiotic therapy is recommended except with bacteremia, extraintestinal infections, or immunocompromised hosts. |
| | *Campylobacter* | Azithromycin or erythromycin | 5–7 days. Shortens duration and fecal excretion. |
| Nosocomial | *Clostridium difficile* | Metronidazole | 7 days. Community organisms unlikely after 72 hr of hospitalization. |

Alt, alternative; flu, influenza; GAS, group A streptococci; GBS, group B streptococci; Hib, *Haemophilus influenzae* type b; TMP/SMX, trimethoprim-sulfamethoxazole.

*Continued*

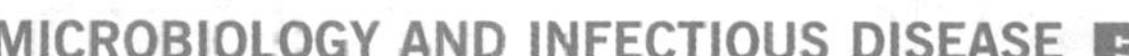

TABLE 17-2

COMMON PEDIATRIC INFECTIONS: GUIDELINES FOR INITIAL MANAGEMENT—cont'd

| Infectious Syndrome | Usual Etiology | Suggested Empirical Therapy | Suggested Length of Therapy/Comments |
|---|---|---|---|
| **Genital warts** | See Chapter 5 | | |
| **Lymphadenitis** | Viruses, GAS, *Mycobacterium tuberculosis, S. aureus,* anaerobes, atypical mycobacteria, *Actinomyces, Bartonella henselae* (cat-scratch disease) | PO: Amoxicillin/clavulanic acid or cloxacillin; Alt: Cephalexin<br>IV: Oxacillin or nafcillin; Alt: Cefazolin | Surgical incision with *M. tuberculosis*. Needle aspiration with *B. henselae.* Clindamycin if penicillin-allergic or MRSA prevalent. |
| **Mastoiditis** (acute) | *S. pneumoniae, Streptococcus pyogenes, S. aureus, H. influenzae (nontypeable)* | Oxacillin + cefotaxime or ceftriaxone; Alt: Amoxicillin/ clavulanic acid | 10 days. Vancomycin or clindamycin if MRSA prevalent. |
| **Meningitis** | | | |
| Neonate <1 mo | GBS, Enterobacteriaceae, (esp. *E. coli*), *Listeria monocytogenes* | Ampicillin and cefotaxime; Alt: Ampicillin and gentamicin | 14–21 days for GBS and *Listeria*. 21 days for Enterobacteriaceae (cefotaxime, aminoglycoside). |
| Neonate 1–3 mo | GBS, *S. pneumoniae, H. influenzae, N. meningitidis*, Enterobacteriaceae | Ampicillin and cefotaxime | 10–14 days for *S. pneumoniae*, 7 days for *N. meningitidis*, 7–10 days for *H. influenzae*. |

| | | | |
|---|---|---|---|
| Infants >3 mo and children | *S. pneumoniae, N. meningitidis, H. influenzae,* neonatal pathogens | Cefotaxime or ceftriaxone. Vancomycin should also be added empirically for possible penicillin-resistant *S. pneumoniae*, until susceptibility is known. | Dexamethasone use except for *H. influenzae* uncertain. Recommended with evidence of increased ICP to be given before or with first antibiotic dose.<br>See *Red Book 2006*[5] for chemoprophylaxis recommendations for contacts of meningococcal and Hib disease. |
| **Orbital cellulitis** | *S. pneumoniae, H. influenzae* (nontypeable), *Moraxella catarrhalis, S aureus,* GAS | Cefotaxime or ceftriaxone + clindamycin or oxacillin | 10 days. Monitor for cavernous thrombosis. |
| **Osteomyelitis** | *S. aureus,* GAS | Semisynthetic penicillin (oxacillin, nafcillin); Alt: Clindamycin or vancomycin | 4–6 wk. |
| Foot puncture | Add *Pseudomonas* | Add ceftazidime. | |
| Sickle cell disease | Add *Salmonella* | Add cefotaxime. | |
| **Otitis media** (acute) | *S. pneumoniae, H. influenzae* (nontypeable), *M. catarrhalis*, viruses | First-line: High-dose amoxicillin (80–100 mg/kg/day).<br>Alt for penicillin allergy: Cefuroxime, cefdinir, cefprozil, azithromycin<br>Persistent otitis media (after 3 days): Amoxicillin/clavulanic acid, cefuroxime, or ceftriaxone (IM/IV) | 5–10 days. For persistent otitis media (at 2–3 days follow-up) despite antibiotic therapy, consider tympanocentesis.<br>Short course 5–7 days for >2 yr old without language or hearing deficit. |
| **Otitis externa** (uncomplicated) | *Pseudomonas* Enterobacteriaceae, *Proteus* | Eardrops: Polymyxin B/neomycin/ hydrocortisone; Alt: Ofloxacin drops | 7–10 days. |

*Continued*

TABLE 17-2

COMMON PEDIATRIC INFECTIONS: GUIDELINES FOR INITIAL MANAGEMENT—cont'd

| Infectious Syndrome | Usual Etiology | Suggested Empirical Therapy | Suggested Length of Therapy/Comments |
|---|---|---|---|
| **Parotitis** | *S. aureus* most common. Also: oral flora, gram-negative rods, viruses, or noninfectious causes | PO: Oxacillin or amoxicillin/clavulanic acid | Sialogogues, local heat, gentle massage of the gland from posterior to anterior, and hydration provide symptomatic relief. May consider test for HIV if chronic parotitis. |
| **Periorbital cellulitis** (preseptal) | Associated with sinusitis: See sinusitis<br>Associated with skin lesion: See cellulitis<br>Hematogenous (<2 yr): See bacteremia | IV: Oxacillin + cefotaxime<br>PO: Amoxicillin/clavulanic acid | 10–14 days. |
| **Pharyngitis** | GAS, Group C and G streptococci, viruses, mononucleosis | PO: Penicillin VK<br>IM: Benzathine penicillin G × 1 dose<br>Alt: Erythromycin, cephalexin | 10 days. TMP/SMX *not* effective. |
| **Pneumonia** | | | |
| Neonatal | *E. coli,* GBS, *S. aureus, Listeria monocytogenes, C. trachomatis* | Ampicillin + gentamicin or ampicillin + cefotaxime | 10–21 days. Blood cultures indicated. Effusions should be drained, Gram stain of fluid obtained. Vancomycin if MRSA prevalent. |
| 3 wk–4 mo | *C. trachomatis, S. pneumoniae*, viruses | Erythromycin; Alt: PO: Azithromycin, IV: Cefotaxime (if febrile) | 10 days. |
| Infant/child (6 wk–4 yr): Lobar | *S. pneumoniae* | PO: Amoxicillin; Alt: Clindamycin<br>IV: Ceftriaxone, cefotaxime | 7–10 days. |

| | | | |
|---|---|---|---|
| Infant/child (6 wk–4 yr): | | | |
| Atypical | *Bordetella pertussis* | Erythromycin (estolate preparation preferred), azithromycin, or clarithromycin | 14 days for erythromycin, 5 days for azithromycin, 7 days for clarithromycin Chemoprophylaxis indicated for close contacts. |
| | Respiratory viruses | No antibiotics indicated | |
| | Influenza | Zanamivir for flu A and B (>7 yr)<br>Oseltamivir for flu A and B (>1 yr)<br>Amantadine for flu A (>1 yr)<br>Rimantadine for flu A (>13 yr) | Reduces symptoms notably if given within 36 hr after onset of symptoms. |
| ≥4 yr: Lobar | *S. pneumoniae* | PO: Amoxicillin; Alt: Erythromycin<br>IV: Ceftriaxone, or cefotaxime + PO/IV macrolide | 7–10 days. Vancomycin or clindamycin if severe illness or features suggestive of *S. aureus*. |
| | | Clarithromycin | 10 days. |
| | | Azithromycin | 5 days. |
| ≥4 yr: Atypical | *Mycoplasma pneumoniae* or *Chlamydia pneumoniae* | Clarithromycin or azithromycin; Alt: Doxycycline or erythromycin | 14–21 days (5 days if using azithromycin). |
| | Influenza | Zanamivir or oseltamivir | Reduces symptoms notably if given within 36 hours after onset of symptoms. |
| **Postspinal fusion** | Staphylococcus or Streptococci spp.; likely GI or GU gram-negative organisms | Vancomycin, piperacillin/tazobactam, and gentamicin +/− rifampin | Consider suction irrigation to wound initially. Deep tissue culture of wound may direct treatment. Removal of instrumentation may be necessary. |
| **Septic arthritis** | | | |
| <5 yr | *S. aureus,* GBS, Hib, gram-negative bacteria | See osteomyelitis. | 3–4 wk IV. May switch to PO after response.<br>Aspiration of affected joint recommended. |
| >5 yr | *S. aureus,* GAS | | |
| Adolescent | Add *N. gonorrhoeae* | See Table 17-9. | |

*Continued*

TABLE 17-2

COMMON PEDIATRIC INFECTIONS: GUIDELINES FOR INITIAL MANAGEMENT—cont'd

| Infectious Syndrome | Usual Etiology | Suggested Empirical Therapy | Suggested Length of Therapy/Comments |
|---|---|---|---|
| **Sinusitis** | | | |
| Acute | *S. pneumoniae, H. influenzae, M. catarrhalis* | See otitis media. Seriously ill child: Vancomycin + cefotaxime or ceftriaxone | 10–14 days. Parenteral therapy generally reserved for complicated sinusitis. |
| Chronic | Add *S. aureus,* anaerobes | Amoxicillin/clavulanic acid or cefpodoxime | 21 days; 7 days after resolution of symptoms. |
| **UTI** | | | |
| Uncomplicated | *E. coli, Proteus, Staph. saprophyticus,* enterococci | PO: TMP/SMX, cefixime. IV: Cefotaxime *or* ampicillin and gentamicin | 7–14 days (cystitis vs. pyelonephritis and age-dependent). |
| Abnormal host/urinary tract | Add *Pseudomonas* | Ampicillin and gentamicin, piperacillin/tazobactam, or ticarcillin/clavulanic acid. | 14–21 days. Parenteral until afebrile for 24 hr. |
| **Ventriculoperitoneal shunt, infected** | *S. epidermidis, S. aureus,* Enterobacteriaceae | Vancomycin + cefotaxime or ceftriaxone. Add aminoglycoside if culture suggests Enterobacteriaceae. Consider adding rifampin. | 10–21 days, depending on organism and response. Shunt removal or revision may be necessary. |

TABLE 17-3

COMMON ETIOLOGIES OF CONGENITAL INFECTIONS AND THEIR ASSOCIATED CLINICAL FINDINGS

| Congenital Infection | Clinical Finding |
|---|---|
| Rubella | IUGR, cataracts, cardiac anomalies, deafness, "blueberry muffin" rash |
| Toxoplasma | Retinopathy, cerebral calcifications, hydrocephalus |
| CMV | Jaundice, hepatosplenomegaly, microcephaly, thrombocytopenia |
| Syphilis | Hepatosplenomegaly, bone abnormalities, rash |
| HSV | Rash, retinopathy, meningoencephalitis |

CMV, cytomegalovirus; HSV, herpes simplex virus; IUGR, intrauterine growth restriction.



**Table 17-3 helps differentiate possible infections based on clinical features. Initial evaluation of a neonate depends on level of suspicion and severity of clinical findings.[7] Consider head computed tomography or head ultrasound (intracerebral calcifications), long-bone films (metaphyseal abnormalities), ophthalmologic examination (keratoconjunctivitis and chorioretinitis), brainstem evoked responses for hearing evaluation, and blood, urine, and cerebrospinal fluid (CSF) evaluation (cultures, serology, cell counts) as part of initial investigation. (See Table 17-4 for specific diagnostic criteria and therapy for the most common intrauterine infections.)**

2. **Group B streptococcal (GBS) Infection (Fig. 17-4):**

a. **Presentation:**

(1) **Early-onset disease (<7 days old):** Respiratory distress, apnea, shock, pneumonia, and less often, meningitis.

(2) **Late-onset disease (1 week–3 months):** Bacteremia, meningitis, osteomyelitis, septic arthritis, and cellulitis.

b. **Maternal intrapartum antibiotic prophylaxis:** To prevent early-onset GBS, chemoprophylaxis regimen is penicillin G or ampicillin. For penicillin-allergic patients with low anaphylaxis risk, may use cefazolin; otherwise, use clindamycin or erythromycin. For resistant organisms or if susceptibility is unknown, use vancomycin. Appropriate prophylaxis is indicated for:

(1) Mothers of previous infants with invasive GBS disease.

(2) GBS bacteriuria during the current pregnancy.

(3) Positive GBS screening culture during pregnancy (unless a planned cesarean delivery is performed, in the absence of labor or amniotic membrane rupture).

(4) Unknown GBS status **and** delivery is <37 weeks' gestation, ≥18 hr rupture of amniotic membrane rupture, or intrapartum temperature of >100.4°F (>38.0°C)

TABLE 17-4

**DIAGNOSTIC CRITERIA AND THERAPY FOR COMMON INTRAUTERINE AND PERINATAL INFECTIONS**

| Disease | Diagnostic Criteria | Therapy |
|---|---|---|
| Cytomegalovirus (CMV) | CMV IgM from serum; CMV culture from urine, stool, respiratory tract secretions; or CSF or blood CMV PCR obtained within 3 wk of birth. | Treatment of symptomatic infants with ganciclovir may decrease hearing loss; efficacy data are limited. |
| Enterovirus | Cultures from throat, stool, rectal swab; CSF for culture and PCR. | IVIG |
| Hepatitis B | Check maternal HepBsAg status. If mother is positive for both HBsAg and HBeAg, the risk for chronic HBV infection is 70%–90% by age 6 mo in the absence of postexposure immunoprophylaxis.[8] | See Chapter 16 for initial management. To monitor success of efforts to prevent perinatal transmission of HBV, obtain HepBsAg and anti-HBs at age 9 to 18 mo after completion of HepB series (series should be at birth, 1 mo, and 6 mo). If HepBsAg is negative on follow-up, but anti-HBs concentration is <10 mIU/mL, infant should repeat vaccine series (0, 1, and 6 mo) with testing of anti-HBs 1 mo after third dose. |
| Hepatitis C | Check maternal anti-HCV or HCV RNA at time of delivery. If possible, check infant's HepC antibody status at age 18 mo. If symptomatic or earlier diagnosis needed, HCV PCR or HCV RNA can be checked at age 1–2 mo. | No therapy until HCV status ascertained at 1 yr of life. Treatment with interferon-α and ribavirin is under investigation in children. |
| Herpes simplex virus (HSV) | HSV culture of blood, urine, CSF, and skin vesicles; surface cultures from conjunctiva, nasopharynx, throat, and rectum. Positive surface cultures obtained from any of these sites >48 hr after birth indicate viral replication suggestive of infection rather than contamination after intrapartum exposure.[5] | Parenteral acyclovir 60 mg/kg/day divided q8hr for 14 days if only SEM disease; give 60 mg/kg/day for 21 days if CNS or disseminated disease. Infants with ocular involvement should also receive topical ophthalmologic drug (1%–2% trifluridine, 1% iododeoxyuridine, or 3% vidarabine). 45 mg/kg/day for disease beyond early infancy. |

CNS, central nervous system; CSF, cerebrospinal fluid; HCV, hepatitis C virus; HepBeAg, hepatitis B e antigen; HepBsAg, hepatitis B surface antigen; IgM, immunoglobulin M; IVIG, intravenous immune globulin; PCR, polymerase chain reaction.

*Continued*

TABLE 17-4

**DIAGNOSTIC CRITERIA AND THERAPY FOR COMMON INTRAUTERINE AND PERINATAL INFECTIONS—cont'd**

| Disease | Diagnostic Criteria | Therapy |
|---|---|---|
| HIV | See section II.E. | |
| Parvovirus | Parvovirus PCR and IgM antibody from serum. | Intrauterine blood transfusions may be indicated in selected cases. Infant treatment is supportive. |
| Rubella | Rubella virus can usually be obtained from nasal specimens. Throat swabs, blood, urine, and CSF can also yield virus. Check serum for rubella IgM.[5] Knowledge of maternal rubella immune status at onset of pregnancy is most helpful information. If checked late in pregnancy, infection early in pregnancy cannot be excluded. | Treatment is supportive. Postexposure prophylaxis with immunoglobulin not routinely recommended. Mothers with nonimmune status should be vaccinated in the immediate postpartum period, even if breast-feeding. Rubella declared eliminated from the United States in 2006. |
| Syphilis | See section II.C.4. | |
| Toxoplasmosis | *Prenatal diagnosis*: A definitive diagnosis can be made either by detecting the parasite in fetal blood or amniotic fluid or by documenting *Toxoplasmosis gondii* IgM or IgA antibody in fetal blood. *T gondii* DNA by PCR from amniotic fluid also can be valid.<br>*Postnatal diagnosis*: Attempts should be made to isolate *T. gondii* from placenta, umbilical cord, or assay for *T. gondii* by PCR from peripheral blood, CSF, and amniotic fluid. A positive IgM or IgA within first 6 mo of life or persistently positive IgG titers beyond first 1 yr of life can also be diagnostic. | Treatment indicated for chorioretinitis, meningitis, or significant organ damage. Treat with pyrimethamine in combination with sulfadiazine (supplemented with leucovorin) for 1 yr. |

*Continued*

TABLE 17-4

DIAGNOSTIC CRITERIA AND THERAPY FOR COMMON INTRAUTERINE AND PERINATAL INFECTIONS—cont'd

| Disease | Diagnostic Criteria | Therapy |
|---|---|---|
| Varicella (VZV) | Direct fluorescent antigen (DFA) from vesicle scraping is rapid and sensitive. VZV PCR from body fluid or tissue is also very sensitive. Virus may be cultured from vesicle base during first 3–4 days of eruption. It can be difficult to distinguish VZV from HSV lesions clinically. | *Maternal*: Acyclovir may be beneficial during pregnancy. VariZIG or IVIG after exposure for susceptible pregnant women is recommended. VariZIG is available under an investigational new drug protocol by calling 1-800-843-7477.[9]<br>*Infant*: Varizig or IVIG not indicated if the mother has zoster.[5] Acyclovir if neonate develops varicella. |

c. **Prophylaxis or treatment of neonatal GBS disease:** Penicillin G or ampicillin, plus an aminoglycoside (usually gentamicin). Duration of therapy depends on extent of disease. Alternative: cefotaxime.

3. **Clinical presentations of perinatal viral infections (see Table 17-4 for diagnoses and treatments):**

a. **VZV:** If a mother develops varicella from 5 days before to 2 days after delivery, varicella infection in the infant can be severe and even fatal. Neonates usually look well at birth, then develop vesicles between 3–10 days of life. Dissemination can result in pneumonitis, encephalitis, purpura fulminans, widespread bleeding, hypotension, and death. If mother develops varicella >5 days before delivery and infant's gestational age is >28 weeks, severity of disease tends to be milder secondary to transplacental transfer of antibody.[5]

b. **Herpes simplex virus:** Neonatal HSV infections are often severe, with high mortality and morbidity despite therapy. HSV infection can present as (1) **disseminated disease** with lung and severe liver disease, (2) **localized CNS infection,** or (3) **disease localized to skin, eye, and mouth (SEM).** Initial symptoms can occur any time in the first 4–5 weeks of life. Disseminated disease often occurs in the first week of life. CNS disease presents latest, often in the second or third week of life.[9]

c. **Enterovirus:** Neonates (usually <2 weeks old) who develop enterovirus infections can develop severe disease with major systemic manifestations (hepatic necrosis, myocarditis, encephalitis, pneumonia, necrotizing enterocolitis, and disseminated intravascular coagulation)

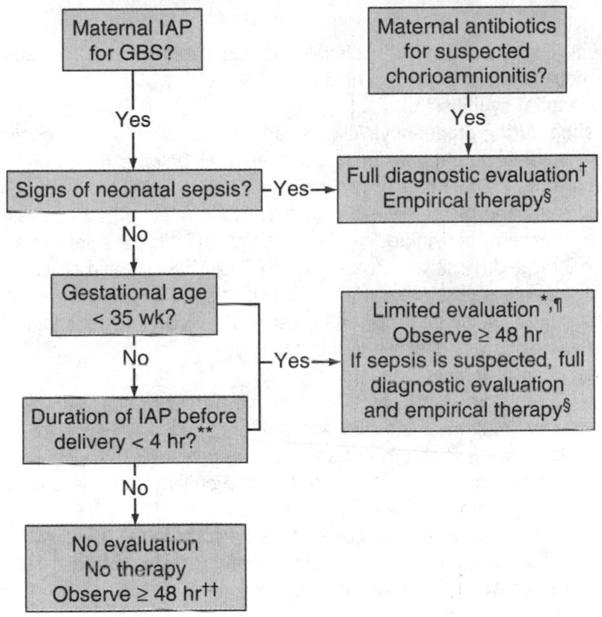


* If no maternal intrapartum prophylaxis for GBS was administered despite an indication being present, data are insufficient on which to recommend as a single management strategy.

† Includes complete blood cell count and differential, blood culture, and chest radiograph if respiratory abnormalities are present. When signs of sepsis are present, a lumbar puncture, if feasible, should be performed.

§ Duration of therapy varies depending on results of blood culture, cerebrospinal fluid findings, if obtained, and the clinical course of the infant. If laboratory results and clinical course do not indicate bacterial infection, duration may be as short as 48 hours.

¶ CBC with differential and blood culture.

** Applies only to penicillin, ampicillin, or cefazolin and assumes recommended dosing regimen.

†† A healthy-appearing infant who was ≥38 weeks' gestation at delivery and whose mother received ≥4 hours of intrapartum prophylaxis before delivery may be discharged home after 24 hours if other discharge criteria have been met and a person able to comply fully with instructions for home observation will be present. If any one of these conditions is not met, the infant should be observed in the hospital for at least 48 hours and until criteria for discharge are achieved.

FIG. 17-4

Empirical management of neonate born to a mother who received intrapartum antimicrobial prophylaxis (IAP) to prevent early-onset group B streptococcal disease. This algorithm is a suggested, but not exclusive, approach to management. *(From MMWR Recommendations and Reports 2002;51[RR-11]:1–22.)*

mimicking overwhelming bacterial infection. Death is typically caused by hepatic failure or myocarditis.

4. **Congenital syphilis:**[5]

a. **Testing during pregnancy:** All pregnant women should be screened with a nontreponemal antibody test **(Venereal Disease Research Laboratory [VDRL] test or rapid plasma reagin [RPR] test)** early in pregnancy and preferably again at delivery. In areas of high prevalence and in patients considered high risk, a test early in the third trimester is also indicated. Positive screening for RPR or VDRL should be confirmed with a treponemal antibody test (FTA). If there is evidence of infection, treatment is indicated, and serologies (RPR or VDRL titers) should be followed to assess effectiveness of therapy.

b. **Evaluation of infants:**

(1) No newborn should be discharged from the hospital without determining mother's serologic status for syphilis. Testing of cord blood or infant serum not adequate for screening.

(2) All infants of women diagnosed with syphilis should have a venous nontreponemal antibody test.

(3) An infant should be evaluated for congenital syphilis if born to a mother who has a positive nontreponemal test, confirmed by a positive treponemal test, and who has one or more of the following:

(a) No treatment, inadequate treatment, or undocumented treatment.

(b) Treatment with nonpenicillin regimen; e.g., erythromycin (a pregnant woman with syphilis and a penicillin allergy history should be treated with penicillin after desensitization).

(c) Treated <1 month before delivery.

(d) Appropriately treated but expected fourfold or more decrease in RPR or VDRL titers did not occur.

(e) Had insufficient serologic follow-up to ensure that she responded appropriately to treatment by demonstrating a fourfold or greater decrease in titers in 3 months after course of treatment.

(f) Maternal titer has increased fourfold, infant titer is at least fourfold greater than mother's, or the infant is symptomatic.

(4) Further evaluation of infants with the preceding conditions should include the following:

(a) Physical examination (e.g., rash [vesiculobullous], hepatomegaly, generalized lymphadenopathy, persistent rhinitis).

(b) Quantitative nontreponemal test on infant's serum (cord blood not adequate).

(c) Examine CSF for protein, cell count, and VDRL test. CSF VDRL is specific but *not* sensitive. (Do not perform RPR or FTA-ABS test [fluorescent treponemal antibody absorption] on CSF.)

TABLE 17-5

GUIDE FOR INTERPRETATION OF THE SYPHILIS SEROLOGY OF MOTHERS AND THEIR INFANTS

| Nontreponemal Test (e.g., VDRL, RPR, ART) | | Treponemal Test (e.g., MHA-TP, FTA-ABS) | | |
|---|---|---|---|---|
| **Mother** | **Infant** | **Mother** | **Infant** | **Interpretation*** |
| – | – | – | – | No syphilis or incubating syphilis in mother or infant. |
| + | + | – | – | No syphilis in mother or infant (false-positive nontreponemal test with passive transfer to infant). |
| + | + or – | + | + | Maternal syphilis with possible infant infection; mother treated for syphilis during pregnancy; or mother with latent syphilis and possible infection of infant.† |
| + | + | + | + | Recent or previous syphilis in the mother; possible infant infection. |
| – | – | + | + | Mother successfully treated for syphilis before or early in pregnancy; or mother with Lyme disease (i.e., false-positive serologic test result); infant syphilis unlikely. |

*Table presents a guide and not the definitive interpretation of serologic tests for syphilis in mothers and their newborns. Other factors that should be considered include the timing of maternal infection, the nature and timing of maternal treatment, quantitative maternal and infant titers, and serial determination of nontreponemal test titers in both mother and infant.
†Mothers with latent syphilis may have nonreactive nontreponemal tests.
ART, automated reagin test; MHA-TP, microhemagglutination test for *T. pallidum*.

Modified from Pickering LK (ed). 2006 Red Book: Report of the Committee on Infectious Diseases, 27th ed. Elk Grove Village, Ill, American Academy of Pediatrics, 2006, p 636

(d) Radiologic studies: Long bone films for diaphyseal periostitis, osteochondritis.
(e) If available, antitreponemal immunoglobulin M (IgM) through a testing method recognized by the Centers for Disease Control and Prevention (CDC) either as a standard or provisional method.
(f) Complete blood cell (CBC) count and platelet count.
(g) Other tests as clinically indicated (e.g., chest radiograph, liver function tests).

(5) Guide for interpretation of the syphilis serology of mothers and their infants[5] (Table 17-5).
(6) Treatment of neonates with proven or possible congenital syphilis (Table 17-6): Follow nontreponemal serologic tests at 3, 6, and 12 months after treatment.
(7) Treatment of syphilis (postneonatal) (Table 17-7).

TABLE 17-6

TREATMENT OF NEONATES (≤4 WEEKS OF AGE) WITH PROVEN OR POSSIBLE CONGENITAL SYPHILIS

| Clinical Status | Antimicrobial Therapy* |
|---|---|
| Proven or highly probable disease† | Aqueous crystalline penicillin G: 50,000 U/kg/dose IV q12hr for the first week, then q8hr for a total course of 10 days‡,§ |
| Asymptomatic, normal CSF and radiologic examination—maternal treatment history as follows: | |
| • None, inadequate penicillin treatment,‖ undocumented, failed, or reinfected | Aqueous crystalline penicillin G IV for 10–14 days‡,§ (see dosing for previous entry) *or* Clinical, serologic follow-up and benzathine penicillin G 50,000 U/kg IM, single dose¶ |
| • Adequate therapy given >1 mo before delivery, mother's response to treatment demonstrated by a fourfold decrease in titer of a nontreponemal serologic test, no evidence of reinfection or relapse | Clinical, serologic follow-up and benzathine penicillin G 50,000 U/kg IM, single dose¶ |

*See Formulary for further drug information.

†Proven or probable disease if: (1) Physical or radiologic evidence of active disease, (2) Infant's nontreponemal titer is at least four times higher than the mother's titer. (3) CSF VDRL is reactive or CSF cell count and/or protein is abnormal. (4) Positive antitreponemal IgM test. (5) Placenta or umbilical cord is positive for treponemal organisms using specific fluorescent antibody staining.

‡If >1 day of therapy is missed, the entire course should be restarted.

§Alternatively, some experts recommend procaine penicillin G 50,000 U/kg IM daily for 10–14 days, but CSF levels may be inadequate.

‖Mother's penicillin dose unknown, undocumented, inadequate, *or* lack of fourfold or greater decrease in nontreponemal antibody titer in mother.

¶Some experts recommend aqueous crystalline penicillin G as for proven or highly probable disease (see text). Other experts would follow the infant without giving antibiotic therapy if both clinical and serologic follow-up can be ensured.

Modified from Pickering LK (ed): 2006 Red Book: Report of the Committee on Infectious Diseases, 27th ed. Elk Grove Village, Ill, American Academy of Pediatrics, 2006, p 638.

## D. SELECTED SEXUALLY TRANSMITTED DISEASES

1. Pelvic inflammatory disease (PID) (Table 17-8).
2. Therapy for chlamydia, gonorrhea, and PID (Table 17-9).

## E. HUMAN IMMUNODEFICIENCY VIRUS (HIV) AND ACQUIRED IMMUNODEFICIENCY SYNDROME (AIDS)

For the most recent information on the diagnosis and management of children with HIV infection, check the recommendations at www.aidsinfo.nih.gov/.

1. **Counseling and testing:** Legal requirements vary by state. Counseling includes informed consent for testing, implications of positive test results, and prevention of transmission. All pregnant women should

TABLE 17-7

TREATMENT FOR SYPHILIS (POSTNEONATAL)

| Type or Stage | First-Line Drug and Dosage | Alternatives |
|---|---|---|
| Congenital syphilis (diagnosed >4 wk of age) | Aqueous crystalline penicillin G 50,000 U/kg/dose IV q4–6 hr × 10 days | Procaine penicillin G 50,000U/kg/day IM × 10 days |
| Early latent syphilis of <1 yr duration | Benzathine benzylpenicillin 50,000U/kg (maximum $2.4 \times 10^6$ U) IM × 1 dose (*Note*: Must examine CSF to exclude asymptomatic neurosyphilis in children) | Tetracycline 500 mg PO q6hr × 14 days (for >8 yr) ***or*** Doxycycline 4 mg/kg/24 hr (maximum 200 mg) PO q12hr × 14 days (for >8 yr) |
| Syphilis of >1 yr duration (late syphilis) | Benzathine benzylpenicillin 50,000 U/kg/dose (maximum $2.4 \times 10^6$ U) IM every wk × 3 successive wk | Tetracycline 500 mg PO q6hr × 28 days (for >8 yr) ***or*** Doxycycline 4 mg/kg/24 hr (maximum 200 mg) PO q12hr × 28 days (for >8 yr) |
| Neurosyphilis | Aqueous crystalline benzylpenicillin 200,000–300,000 U/kg/day IV q4–6 hr (maximum $4 \times 10^6$ U IV q4hr) × 10–14 days, may be followed by benzathine penicillin 50,000 U/kg/dose (maximum $2.4 \times 10^6$ U) IM every wk × 3 wk | Aqueous procaine benzylpenicillin $2.4 \times 10^6$ U IM q24hr × 10–14 days + probenecid 500 mg PO q6hr ×10–14 days; may be followed by benzathine penicillin 50,000 U/kg/ dose (maximum $2.4 \times 10^6$ U) IM every week × 3 wk. (If penicillin- allergic, especially if <9 yr, consider penicillin desensitization and administration in an appropriate setting. Also, patient should be managed in consultation with a specialist.) |

Modified from Pickering LK (ed): 2006 Red Book: Report of the Committee on Infectious Diseases, 27th ed. Elk Grove Village, Ill, American Academy of Pediatrics, 2006, p 640.



be offered counseling and testing, regardless of risk factors, so that they can make an informed decision regarding therapy aimed at reducing transmission to their infants. When maternal HIV status has not been determined before delivery, mother and/or newborn should undergo HIV antibody testing after counseling and consent of the mother (unless state law allows newborn testing without consent). Adolescents ≥13 years of age should be offered HIV testing at least once during adolescence and annually if sexually active (more frequently if high-risk behaviors). (See http://www.cdc.gov/mmwr/preview/mmwrhtml/rr5514a1.htm.)

TABLE 17-8

**DIAGNOSIS OF PELVIC INFLAMMATORY DISEASE**

| Etiology | Diagnostic Criteria | Diagnostic Techniques | Admission Criteria |
|---|---|---|---|
| *Neisseria gonorrhoeae*<br>*Chlamydia trachomatis*<br>Lower genital tract flora (*Haemophilus influenzae*, gram-negative rods, anaerobes, *Streptococcus agalactiae*) | Empirical treatment of PID should be initiated in sexually active young women and others at risk of sexually transmitted infections if uterine or adnexal tenderness or cervical motion tenderness are present without other identifiable cause.<br>Additional criteria:<br>1. Temperature ≥ 38.3°C<br>2. Abnormal cervical or vaginal discharge<br>3. Elevated erythrocyte sedimentation rate<br>4. Elevated C-reactive protein<br>5. Presence of white blood cells on saline microscopy of vaginal secretions<br>6. Laboratory confirmation of infection with *N. gonorrhoeae* or *C. trachomatis*<br>Other:<br>1. Endometriosis<br>2. Tubo-ovarian abscess | *Chlamydia trachomatis*<br>1. *Definitive:* Tissue culture (only acceptable method for evaluation of child abuse).<br>2. *Presumptive:* Antigen detection through fluorescent staining with DNA probe, enzyme immunoassay (EIA), or monoclonal antibody (DFA); nucleic acid amplification test (NAAT) may be used on urine or cervical samples; DNA probe not reliable on bloody specimens; serologies not available.<br>*Neisseria gonorrhoeae*<br>1. *Definitive:* Tissue culture (selective media with carbon dioxide incubation for transport).<br>2. *Presumptive:* Gram-negative intracellular diplococci on smear, or EIA or DNA probe of specimen; PCR or LCR may be used on urine or cervical sample. | Cannot exclude diagnosis of surgical abdomen (such as appendicitis)<br>Presence of tubo-ovarian abscess<br>Pregnancy<br>Immunodeficiency<br>Inability to tolerate or follow outpatient oral regimen<br>Failure to respond to oral antibiotic therapy<br>Clinical follow-up cannot be arranged (especially in adolescents) |

TABLE 17-9

THERAPY FOR CHLAMYDIA, GONORRHEA, AND PELVIC INFLAMMATORY DISEASE

| Type or Stage | First-Line Drug and Dosage | Alternatives |
|---|---|---|
| *CHLAMYDIA TRACHOMATIS* | | |
| Urethritis, cervicitis, or proctitis | Doxycycline 100 mg PO bid × 7 days (if >9 yr) ***or***<br>Azithromycin 1 g PO × 1 dose | Erythromycin base 500 mg PO qid × 7 days ***or***<br>Erythromycin ethylsuccinate 800 mg PO qid × 7 days ***or***<br>Ofloxacin 300 mg PO bid × 7 days (if >18 yr)<br>Levofloxacin 500 mg PO daily × 7 days |
| Infection in pregnancy | Erythromycin base 500 mg PO qid × 7 days ***or*** 250 mg PO qid × 14 days | Erythromycin ethylsuccinate 400 mg PO qid × 14 days ***or***<br>Azithromycin 1 g PO × 1 dose ***or*** amoxicillin 500 mg PO tid × 7 days (alternative but less effective regimen) |
| Neonatal ophthalmia | Erythromycin base or ethylsuccinate 50 mg/kg/24 hr PO or IV ÷ qid × 14 days | Topical treatment is ineffective. |
| Neonatal pneumonia | Erythromycin base or ethylsuccinate 50 mg/kg/24 hr PO or IV ÷ qid × 14 days | *Note*: Association between PO erythromycin and pyloric stenosis has been reported. |
| GONORRHEA* | | |
| **Newborns** | | |
| Sepsis, arthritis, meningitis, scalp abscess | Ceftriaxone 25–50 mg/kg/24 hr IV/IM q24hr × 7 days (10–14 days if meningitis) | — |
| Neonatal ophthalmia | Ceftriaxone 25–50 mg/kg (maximum 125 mg) IV/IM × 1 dose plus saline irrigation ***or***<br>Cefotaxime 100 mg/kg per dose IM/IV × 1 dose | All infants should receive silver nitrate, tetracycline, or erythromycin ointment instilled into each eye within 1 hr of birth. *Note*: All infants with gonococcal conjunctivitis should be evaluated for possible sepsis/disseminated disease and the need to be treated for a longer time. |

*Therapy should include treatment for presumed concomitant chlamydia infection.

From Centers for Disease Control and Prevention: Sexually transmitted diseases treatment guidelines. MMWR 2006;55(RR-56) and Updated recommended treatment regimens for gonoccocal infections and associated conditions. MMWR April 2007;55(14):332–336.

*Continued*

TABLE 17-9

THERAPY FOR CHLAMYDIA, GONORRHEA, AND PELVIC INFLAMMATORY DISEASE—cont'd

| Type or Stage | First-Line Drug and Dosage | Alternatives |
|---|---|---|
| GONORRHEA*—cont'd | | |
| **Prepubertal children who weigh <100 lb (45 kg)** | | |
| Uncomplicated urethritis, vulvovaginitis, proctitis, or pharyngitis | Ceftriaxone 125 mg IM × 1 dose | Spectinomycin 40 mg/kg (maximum 2 g) IM × 1 dose + erythromycin 50 mg/kg/day in 4 divided doses × 7 days ***or*** Azithromycin 20 mg/kg (max 1 g) × 1 dose |
| Bacteremia, peritonitis, or arthritis | Ceftriaxone 50 mg/kg/24 hr (maximum 1 g) IM/IV q24hr × 7–10 days and erythromycin, doxycycline, or azithromycin | — |
| **Children who weigh ≥100 lb (45 kg) and are ≥9 yr** | | |
| Uncomplicated endocervicitis, urethritis, or proctitis | Ceftriaxone 125 mg IM × 1 dose ***or*** Cefixime 400 mg PO × 1 dose ***or***<br>Spectinomycin 2 g IM × 1 dose ***or***<br>Ceftizoxime 500 mg IM × 1 dose ***or***<br>Doxycycline 100 mg PO bid × 7 days | Cefotaxime 500 mg IM × 1 dose ***or***<br>Cefoxitin 2 g IM × 1 dose with probenicid 1 g PO × 1 dose<br>Some evidence indicates that cefpodoxime 400 mg and cefuroxime axetil 1 g might be oral alternatives. |
| Pharyngitis | Ceftriaxone 125 mg IM × 1 dose | |
| Disseminated gonococcal infections | Ceftriaxone 1 g/24 hr IV/IM q24hr for 24–48 hr after clinical improvement, then switch to one of the following for at least 1 wk of therapy:<br>Cefixime 400 mg PO bid ***or***<br>Cefixime suspension 500 mg PO bid ***or***<br>Cefpodoxime 400 mg PO bid | Cefotaxime or ceftizoxime 1 g IV q8hr for 24–48 hr after clinical improvement, then switch to oral therapy for 1 wk<br>For persons allergic to β-lactam drugs: Spectinomycin 2 g IM q12hr × 7 days<br>Fluoroquinolones may be alternative treatment if antimicrobial susceptibility can be documented by culture. |

| | | |
|---|---|---|
| Epididymitis | Ceftriaxone 250 mg IM × 1 dose +<br>Doxycycline 100 mg PO bid × 10 days | If acute epididymitis most likely caused by enteric organisms, or with negative gonococcal culture: Ofloxacin 300 mg PO bid × 10 days or levofloxacin 500 mg PO q24hr × 10 days |
| Bacteremia or arthritis | Ceftriaxone 50 mg/kg/day (maximum dose 1 g) IM or IV q24hr × 10–14 days | — |
| **PELVIC INFLAMMATORY DISEASE (PID)** | | |
| Parenteral regimen | *Regimen A*<br>Cefotetan 2 g IV q12hr ***or***<br>Cefoxitin 2 g IV q6hr +<br>Doxycycline 100 mg IV/PO q12hr<br><br>*Regimen B*<br>Clindamycin 900 mg IV q8hr +<br>Gentamicin 2 mg/kg loading dose, then<br>Gentamicin 1.5 mg/kg IV q8hr maintenance dose | Ampicillin/sulbactam 3g IV q6h +<br>Doxycycline 100 mg PO/IV q12hr |
| Oral regimen | Ceftriaxone 250 mg IM × 1 dose +<br>Doxycycline 100 mg PO bid × 14 days +/–<br>Metronidazole 500 mg PO bid × 14 days ***or***<br>Cefoxitin 2 g IM × 1 dose and probenicid 1 g PO × 1 dose +<br>Doxycycline 100 mg PO bid × 14 days +/–<br>Metronidazole 500 mg PO bid × 14 days | Ceftizoxime or cefotaxime + Doxycycline 100 mg PO bid × 14 days +/– Metronidazole 500 mg PO bid × 14 days<br>If parenteral cephalosporin is not feasible, fluoroquinolones (levofloxacin 500 mg PO daily or ofloxacin 400 mg PO bid × 14 days) +/– metronidazole (500 mg PO bid × 14 days) may be considered if community prevalence and individual risk of gonorrhea are low. |

2. **Diagnosis of HIV in children:**

a. **Infected child:**

(1) A child <18 months of age is considered HIV infected if 2 separate blood samples (excluding cord blood) with a positive DNA PCR assay result (DNA PCR preferred but RNA PCR also used). Viral culture and p24 antigen detection are generally not used for diagnosis in the United States.

(2) Child >18 months of age is considered HIV infected if:

(a) HIV antibody positive by repeated reactive enzyme immunoassay (EIA) and confirmatory test (e.g., Western blot), *or*

(b) Meets the criteria for a child <18 months of age.

b. **Perinatally exposed child:** A child is considered exposed when he or she does not meet the aforementioned criteria, and

(1) Is HIV seropositive by EIA and confirmatory test (e.g., Western blot or IFA) and is <18 months of age at the time of the test, *or*

(2) Has unknown antibody status but was born to a mother known to be infected with HIV.

c. **Exclusion of HIV infection in a perinatally exposed child:**

(1) HIV can be reasonably excluded in an exposed asymptomatic infant with two negative HIV DNA or RNA PCR studies, one obtained at age 1 month or older and the other at age 4 months or older.

(2) HIV is definitively excluded if HIV antibody testing is negative at age 12–18 months in an asymptomatic nonbreast-feeding child with negative HIV DNA PCR studies (as in previous entry). An infant with 2 blood samples obtained after age 6 months at an interval of at least 1 month apart that are both negative for HIV antibody can also be considered uninfected.

3. **Pediatric HIV immunologic categories (Table 17-10).**

4. **Guidelines for prophylaxis against first episode of opportunistic infections (Table 17-11).**

TABLE 17-10

**1994 REVISED PEDIATRIC HIV CLASSIFICATION SYSTEM: IMMUNOLOGIC CATEGORIES BASED ON AGE-SPECIFIC CD4+ LYMPHOCYTE COUNT AND PERCENT**

| | Age of Child | | |
|---|---|---|---|
| Immunologic Category | <12 mo cells/μL (%) | 1–5 yr cells/μL (%) | 6–12 yr cells/μL (%) |
| 1. No suppression | ≥1500 (≥25) | ≥1000 (≥25) | ≥500 (≥25) |
| 2. Moderate suppression | 750–1499 (15–24) | 500–999 (15–24) | 200–499 (15–24) |
| 3. Severe suppression | <750 (<15) | <500 (<15) | <200 (<15) |

From Centers for Disease Control and Prevention: MMWR Recomm Rep 1994;43(RR–12):4.

TABLE 17-11

**PROPHYLAXIS FOR FIRST EPISODE OF OPPORTUNISTIC DISEASE IN HIV-INFECTED INFANTS AND CHILDREN**

| | | Preventive Regimens | |
|---|---|---|---|
| **Pathogen** | **Indication** | **First Choice** | **Alternatives** |
| **STRONGLY RECOMMENDED AS STANDARD OF CARE** | | | |
| *Pneumocystis jiroveci* (formerly *Pneumocystis carinii*) | HIV-infected or HIV-indeterminate infants 4–6 wk to 12 mo of age; HIV-infected children 1–5 yr with CD4+ count <500 µL or CD4+ percent <15%; HIV-infected children 6–12 yr with CD4+ count <200 µL or CD4+ percent <15% | TMP/SMX 150/750 mg/m²/day in two divided doses PO 3×/wk on consecutive days. Acceptable altemative dosage schedules: • Single dose PO 3×/wk on consecutive days. • Two divided doses PO every day. • Two divided doses PO 3×/wk on alternate days. | Aerosolized pentamidine (children ≥5 yr) 300 mg via Respirgard II inhaler monthly; dapsone (children ≥1 mo) 2 mg/kg (maximum 100 mg) PO every day or 4 mg/kg (maximum 200 mg) PO every week. Atovaquone (1–3 mo and >24 mo) 30 mg/kg daily; (4–24 mo) 45 mg/kg daily. |
| *Mycobacterium tuberculosis* | | | |
| Isoniazid-sensitive | Tuberculin skin test reaction ≥5 mm or prior positive TST result without treatment or contact with case of active tuberculosis | Isoniazid 10–15 mg/kg (maximum 300 mg) PO every day × 9 mo or 20–30 mg/kg (maximum 900 mg) PO biweekly × 9 mo. | Rifampin 10–20 mg/kg (maximum 600 mg) PO or IV every day × 4–6 mo. |
| Isoniazid-resistant | Same as for previous entry; high probability of exposure to isoniazid-resistant tuberculosis | Rifampin 10–20 mg/kg (maximum 600 mg) PO every day × 4–6 mo. | Uncertain. |
| Multidrug (isoniazid and rifampin)-resistant | Same as for previous entry; high probability of exposure to multidrug-resistant tuberculosis | Choice of drug requires consultation with public health authorities. | None. |

From 2002 USPHS/IDSA guidelines for prevention of opportunistic infections in persons infected with HIV. MMWR 2002;51(RR–08):42.

*Continued*

TABLE 17-11

**PROPHYLAXIS FOR FIRST EPISODE OF OPPORTUNISTIC DISEASE IN HIV-INFECTED INFANTS AND CHILDREN—cont'd**

| Pathogen | Indication | Preventive Regimens: First Choice | Preventive Regimens: Alternatives |
|---|---|---|---|
| **STRONGLY RECOMMENDED AS STANDARD OF CARE—cont'd** | | | |
| *Mycobacterium avium* complex | For children:<br><1 yr, CD4+ count <750/μL<br>1–2 yr, CD4+ count <500/μL<br>2–6 yr, CD4+ count <75/μL<br>≥6 yr, CD4+ count <50/μL | Clarithromycin 7.5 mg/kg (maximum 500 mg) PO bid *or* azithromycin 20 mg/kg (maximum 1200 mg) PO once weekly. | Azithromycin 5 mg/kg (max 250 mg) PO every day.<br>Children ≥6 yr: Rifabutin 300 mg PO every day. |
| Varicella zoster virus | Significant exposure to varicella with no history of chickenpox or shingles | VariZIG,[†] or, if unavailable, IVIG 400 mg/kg × 1 dose administered ≤96 hr after exposure, ideally within 48 hr. | None. |
| **GENERALLY RECOMMENDED** | | | |
| *Toxoplasma gondii** | IgG antibody to *Toxoplasma* and severe immunosuppression | TMP/SMX 150/750 mg/m²/day in 2 divided doses PO every day. | Dapsone (children ≥1 mo): 2 mg/kg or 15 mg/m² (maximum 25 mg) PO every day plus pyrimethamine 1 mg/kg PO every day plus leucovorin 5 mg PO daily every 3 days. Atovaquone can also be used. |
| Varicella zoster virus | HIV-infected children who are mildly or not symptomatic and not severely immunosuppressed | Varicella zoster vaccine. | None. |

*Protection against *Toxoplasma* is provided by the preferred anti-*Pneumocystis* regimens. Pyrimethamine alone probably provides little, if any, protection.

[†]VariZIG may be obtained 24 hours a day from FFF Enterprisas at 1-800-843-7479 or online at www.fffenterprises.com.

*Continued*

TABLE 17-11

PROPHYLAXIS FOR FIRST EPISODE OF OPPORTUNISTIC DISEASE IN HIV-INFECTED INFANTS AND CHILDREN—cont'd

| Pathogen | Indication | Preventive Regimens: First Choice | Preventive Regimens: Alternatives |
|---|---|---|---|
| Influenza virus | All patients (annually before flu season) | Inactivated split trivalent influenza virus vaccine. | Oseltamivir for children >13 yr (during influenza A or B outbreak); rimantidine or amantadine for children >1 yr (during influenza A outbreak). |
| **NOT RECOMMENDED FOR MOST PATIENTS; INDICATED FOR USE ONLY IN UNUSUAL CIRCUMSTANCES** | | | |
| *Cryptococcus neoformans* | Severe immunosuppression | Fluconazole 3–6 mg/kg PO every day. | Itraconazole 2–5 mg/kg PO q12–24hr. |
| *Histoplasma capsulatum* | Severe immunosuppression, endemic geographic area | Itraconazole 2–5 mg/kg PO q12–24hr. | None. |
| Cytomegalovirus (CMV)† | CMV antibody positivity and severe immunosuppression | Oral ganciclovir 30 mg/kg PO tid. | None. |

†Oral ganciclovir and perhaps valganciclovir result in reduced CMV shedding in CMV-infected children. Acyclovir is not protective against CMV.

HIV, human immunodeficiency virus; TMP/SMX, trimethoprim-sulfamethoxazole, VariZIG, human varicella immune globulin.

5. **Management of perinatal HIV exposure:** Recommendations provided are current at the time of publication; check the recent recommendations for most current therapy at www.http://aidsinfo.nih.gov/.

a. **Prevention of vertical transmission:** Use of antiretroviral therapy during pregnancy, during delivery, and in the newborn dramatically reduces HIV transmission. Bottle-feeding of formula is also recommended in the United States to reduce transmission through breast milk.

(1) **Pregnancy:** All HIV-infected women should be offered antiretroviral therapy for their own health, consistent with the standards of nonpregnant adults. Zidovudine (ZDV) should be included in the pregnant woman's regimen; ZDV given during pregnancy (initiated at 14–34 weeks' gestation) and then given to the infant at delivery and for 6 weeks postnatally significantly reduces vertical transmission of HIV (Table 17-12). Elective cesarean section (before onset of labor or membrane rupture) has been shown to decrease transmission in women not receiving antiretroviral therapy

TABLE 17-12

**TIME OF ZDV REGIMEN ADMINISTRATION AND RECOMMENDED REGIMEN**

| Stage of Labor | Recommended Regimen |
|---|---|
| Antepartum | Oral administration of 100 mg ZDV five times daily*, initiated at 14–34 weeks' gestation and continued throughout the pregnancy. |
| Intrapartum | During labor, IV administration of ZDV in a 1-hour initial dose of 2 mg/kg, followed by continuous infusion of 1 mg/kg/hr until delivery. |
| Postpartum | Oral administration of ZDV to the newborn (ZDV at 2 mg/kg/dose q6hr) for the first 6 weeks of life, beginning at 8–12 hr after birth.† |

*Oral ZDV administered as 200 mg tid or 300 mg bid is currently used in general clinical practice and is an acceptable alternative regimen to 100 mg PO five times daily.

†Intravenous dosage for full-term infants who cannot tolerate oral intake is 1.5 mg/kg IV q6hr. ZDV dosing for infants <35 weeks' gestation at birth is 1.5 mg/kg/dose IV or 2.0 mg/kg/dose PO q12hr, advancing to q8hr at 2 weeks of age if >30 weeks' gestation at birth or at 4 weeks of age if <30 weeks' gestation at birth.

and in those with high viral loads. Health care professionals who are treating HIV-infected pregnant women and their newborn infants should report all instances of prenatal exposure to antiretroviral drugs to the Antiretroviral Pregnancy Registry (1-800-258-4263 or www.apregistry.com).

(2) **Labor:** See Table 17-12 for ZDV regimen during labor. Invasive procedures such as fetal scalp electrode monitoring are generally avoided. Consider adding nevirapine (NVP) for high-risk situations such as high viral load in mother, no prenatal care, or break in infant's skin; in such cases, because of high risk of developing resistance to NVP even after a single dose, some experts offer mother a 1-week course of ZDV/3TC to reduce likelihood of maternal resistance to NVP.

(3) **Newborn:** See Table 17-12 for ZDV regimen in newborns. In high-risk situations in which the mother received intrapartum NVP >1 hr before delivery, give a single dose of 2 mg/kg PO to the neonate at 48–72 hr of life. In high-risk situations in which the mother did not receive intrapartum NVP or received it <1 hr before delivery, some experts give one dose of 2 mg/kg/dose PO immediately after birth, and a second dose at 48–72 hr of life. Monitor ZDV toxicity with periodic CBCs with differential count. Main toxicities are anemia and neutropenia.

b. **Ongoing management of indeterminate infants:**

(1) **Pneumocystis jiroveci (formerly *carinii*) pneumonia (PCP) prophylaxis** with trimethoprim-sulfamethoxazole (TMP/SMX) should be initiated for all HIV-exposed infants at 4–6 weeks of life. PCP prophylaxis should be continued until HIV infection is reasonably excluded. Dose is 75 mg/m2/dose TMP PO twice daily for 3 consecutive days per week. Alternatives: dapsone, atovaquone, or aerosolized pentamidine (for older children). (See Table 17-11 for PCP prophylaxis medications and dosing.)

(2) **HIV diagnostic tests (DNA PCR)** should be obtained in infants to determine infection status as follows: between birth and 2 weeks of life (cord blood should not be used), age 1–2 months, age 4–6 months. A positive test should be immediately repeated for confirmation of infection. If all tests are negative, the infant should be tested for HIV antibody at ages 12 and 18 months to document disappearance of the antibody.

(3) **Clinical monitoring:** Infants should be evaluated at routine well-child visits for signs and symptoms of HIV infection. In addition to HIV diagnostic tests, T-cell subsets and quantitative HIV RNA are obtained for HIV monitoring, and CBC with differential and chemistries are obtained for toxicity monitoring. Any suspicious clinical or laboratory findings merit careful and close follow-up. Avoid breast-feeding (in the United States).

**6. Management of HIV-infected infants and children:**

**Note** *Primary care physicians are encouraged to participate in the care and management of HIV-infected children in consultation with specialists who have expertise in the care of such children. Knowledge about antiretroviral therapy is changing, and in areas where enrollment into clinical trials is possible, it should be encouraged.*

a. **Criteria for initiation of antiretroviral therapy:**

(1) Initiation of antiretroviral therapy depends on virologic, immunologic, and clinical status.

(2) All HIV-infected infants (<12 months of age) regardless of immunologic, virologic, or clinical status, should usually be started on antiretroviral therapy.

(3) Antiretroviral therapy should be initiated in children with evidence of immune suppression, as indicated by CD4 lymphocyte absolute number or percentage in Immunologic Category 2 or 3 (see Table 17-10).

(4) Therapy should be initiated in any child with clinical symptoms related to HIV infection.

(5) For HIV-infected children >1 year of age, recommendations to initiate, consider, or defer therapy are based on significant HIV-related symptoms, degree of immunosuppression, and height of viral load.

b. **Antiretroviral regimen:** For most recent recommendations, refer to http://www.aidsinfo.nih.gov/. Data support the use of combination therapy for initial and ongoing therapy. If an infant is identified as HIV-infected while receiving ZDV prophylaxis, therapy should be changed to combination therapy.

c. **Clinical and laboratory monitoring in HIV-infected children:** Immune status, viral load, and evidence of HIV progression and drug toxicity should be monitored on a regular basis (about every 3 months). Careful attention to routine aspects of pediatric care, such as growth, development, and vaccines, is essential.

7. **Immunizations in HIV-infected or HIV-exposed infants and children:** **Perinatally exposed infants should receive all scheduled U.S. infant immunizations. Measles/mumps/rubella (MMR) and varicella vaccine can be given to selected HIV-infected children (see Chapter 16). HIV-infected children should receive PPS23 at age 2 and 5 years. Influenza vaccine should be given annually in the fall to all infected children ≥6 months of age as well as children ≥6 months of age who have HIV-infected household contacts.**

## F. TUBERCULOSIS

1. **Recommended tuberculosis testing:**

a. Tuberculin skin test (TST) recommendations (from 2006 Red Book):[5] Bacille Calmette-Guérin (BCG) immunization is not a contraindication to tuberculin skin testing.
   (1) Immediate testing:
      (a) Contacts of people with confirmed or suspected infectious tuberculosis (contact investigation).
      (b) Children with clinical or radiographic findings of tuberculosis.
      (c) Children immigrating from or with history of travel to TB-endemic areas (e.g., Asia, the Middle East, Africa, Latin America); children with close contacts from TB-endemic areas. (If the child is well, TST should be delayed for up to 10 weeks after return.)
   (2) Annual testing (initial TST is at the time of diagnosis or circumstance, beginning as early as age 3 months):
      (a) HIV-infected children.
      (b) Incarcerated adolescents.
      (c) Children without specific risk factors residing in high-prevalence areas (may vary within each region of country).

**Note** *For children without specific risk factors residing in low-prevalence communities, testing is not indicated since most result in false-positive tests.*

   (3) Children at increased risk for progression of infection to disease: Medical conditions such as diabetes mellitus, chronic renal failure, malnutrition, and congenital or acquired immunodeficiencies. Immunodeficiency itself may increase risk for progression to severe disease; if exposure is likely, immediate and periodic TST should be considered; TST should always be performed before initiation of immunosuppressive therapy.

b. Standard TST is the Mantoux test. Tine test (multipuncture test) is no longer recommended.
   (1) Inject 5 tuberculin units (5 TU) of purified protein derivative (0.1 mL) intradermally on the volar aspect of the forearm to form a 6- to 10-mm weal. Results of skin testing (in millimeters of

BOX 17-1

**DEFINITIONS OF POSITIVE TUBERCULIN SKIN TESTING[5]**

INDURATION ≥5 MM

Children in close contact with known or suspected contagious cases of tuberculosis

Children suspected to have tuberculosis based on clinical or radiographic findings

Children on immunosuppressive therapy or with immunosuppressive conditions (including HIV infection)

INDURATION ≥10 MM

Children at increased risk for dissemination based on young age (<4 yr) or with other medical conditions (cancer, diabetes mellitus, chronic renal failure, or malnutrition)

Children with increased exposure: those born in or whose parents were born in endemic countries; those with travel to endemic countries; those exposed to HIV-infected adults, homeless persons, illicit drug users, nursing home residents, incarcerated or institutionalized persons, migrant farm workers

INDURATION ≥15 MM

Children ≥4 yr of age without any risk factors

induration) should be read 48–72 hr later by qualified medical personnel.

(2) Definition of positive Mantoux test (regardless of whether BCG has been previously administered): Box 17-1.

2. **Drug therapy:**

a. Treatment of latent tuberculosis infection

(1) Indications:

(a) Children with positive tuberculin tests but no evidence of clinical disease.

(b) Recent contacts, especially HIV-infected children, of people with infectious tuberculosis, even if tuberculin test and clinical evidence are not indicative of disease.

(2) Recommendations (see Formulary for specific doses and Table 17-13).

b. Treatment for active tuberculosis disease. (For details, see 2006 Red Book.[5] See also Table 17-13.)

## G. SELECTED TICK-BORNE ILLNESSES (Table 17-14)

## H. FUNGAL AND YEAST INFECTIONS

1. **Place specimen (nail or skin scrapings, biopsy specimens, fluids from tissues or lesions) in 10% KOH on glass slide to look for hyphae, pseudohyphae.**
2. **Germ tube screen of yeast (3 hr) for *Candida albicans*: All germ tube-positive yeast are *C. albicans,* but not all *C. albicans* are germ tube-positive.**

TABLE 17-13

**RECOMMENDED TREATMENT REGIMENS FOR DRUG-SUSCEPTIBLE TUBERCULOSIS IN INFANTS, CHILDREN, AND ADOLESCENTS**

| Infection or Disease Category | Regimen | Remarks |
|---|---|---|
| **Latent tuberculosis infection** (positive skin test, no disease) | | |
| Isoniazid-susceptible | 9 mo of isoniazid q24hr | If daily therapy is not possible, DOT twice a wk may be used for 9 mo. |
| Isoniazid-resistant | 6 mo of rifampin q24hr | If daily therapy is not possible, DOT twice a wk may be used for 6 mo. |
| Isoniazid/rifampin-resistant* | Consultation with a tuberculosis specialist | For management of neonates born to mothers with evidence of tuberculosis infection, see *2006 Red Book,* pp. 694–695.[8] |
| **Pulmonary and extrapulmonary (except meningitis)** | 2 mo of isoniazid, rifampin, and pyrazinamide q24hr, followed by 4 mo of isoniazid and rifampin by DOT<br>9–12 mo of isoniazid and rifampin for drug-susceptible *M. bovis* | If possible drug resistance is a concern, another drug (ethambutol or an aminoglycoside) is added to the initial 3-drug therapy until drug susceptibilities are determined. DOT is highly desirable.<br>If hilar adenopathy only, a 6-mo course of isoniazid and rifampin is sufficient.<br>Drugs can be given 2 or 3 times/wk under DOT in the initial phase if nonadherence is likely. |
| **Meningitis** | 2 mo of isoniazid, rifampin, pyrazinamide, and an aminoglycoside or ethionamide q24hr, followed by 7–10 mo of isoniazid and rifampin q24hr or twice per wk (9–12 mo total)<br>At least 12 mo of therapy without pyrazinamide for drug-susceptible *M. bovis* | A fourth drug, such as an aminoglycoside, is given with initial therapy until drug susceptibility is known.<br>For patients who may have acquired tuberculosis in geographic areas where resistance to streptomycin is common, capreomycin(15–30 mg/kg/day) or kanamycin (15–30 mg/kg/day) may be used instead of streptomycin. |

*Duration of therapy is longer in HIV-infected persons, and additional drugs may be indicated.
DOT, directly observed therapy.

Modified from Pickering LK (ed): 2006 Red Book: Report of the Committee on Infectious Diseases, 27th ed. Elk Grove Village, Ill, American Academy of Pediatrics, 2006, p 686.

3. Common community-acquired fungal infections, etiology, and treatment (Table 17-15).

## I. EXPOSURES TO BLOOD-BORNE PATHOGENS AND POSTEXPOSURE PROPHYLAXIS (PEP)

1. **HIV:**[9,10,11]

a. **Occupational exposure:** Risk for occupational transmission of HIV:

(1) **Needle sticks:** Three infections for every 1000 exposures (0.3%). Risk is greater when the exposure involves a larger volume of blood and/or higher titer of HIV, as in a deep injury, visible blood on the device causing the injury, a device previously used in the source patient's vein or artery, or a source patient in the late stages of HIV infection.

(2) **Mucous membrane exposure:** One infection for every 1000 exposures (0.1%). The risk may be higher when the exposure involves a larger volume of blood and a higher titer of HIV, prolonged skin contact, extensive surface area of exposure, or skin integrity that is visibly compromised.

b. **Nonoccupational HIV exposure in children and adolescents:**[12]

(1) **Injury from needles of discarded syringes:** No confirmed reports of HIV acquisition from percutaneous injury by a needle found in the community. Risk for transmission from a "found needle" (i.e., a needle discarded in a public place) is low. However, if the needle or syringe is found to have visible blood and the source is known to be HIV-infected, PEP should be considered. Testing the syringe for HIV is not practical or reliable.

(2) **Repeated sexual encounters or a single episode of sexual abuse:** Risk is highest with unprotected receptive anal intercourse (0.5%–3.2%), intermediate with receptive vaginal intercourse (0.05%–0.15%), and lowest with insertive vaginal intercourse (0.03%–0.09%). If the exposure source has genital ulcer disease or another sexually transmitted infection or if there was tissue damage, the risk for HIV transmission is higher, increasing the benefit of PEP relative to the burden and risk for drug toxicity.

(3) **Human milk:**[13] In the United States, women who are HIV-infected should be counseled not to breast-feed. An infant who has a single exposure to human milk from a woman with HIV infection is estimated to have 100 times lower risk than that of other mucous membrane exposures, and PEP is likely not warranted.

(4) **Human bites:** Transmission is extremely rare even when saliva is contaminated with blood; saliva inhibits HIV infectivity, HIV is rarely isolated from saliva, and concentrations of HIV in saliva of HIV-infected persons is low even in the presence of periodontal disease.

c. **Prophylaxis:**

(1) Optimally, PEP should be initiated as soon as possible, preferably within 1–3 hr rather than days of exposure. The usual duration of PEP, if tolerated, is 28 days.

TABLE 17-14

SELECTED TICK-BORNE ILLNESSES

| Disease | Presentation | Transmission | Diagnosis | Treatment |
|---|---|---|---|---|
| Lyme disease | (1) *Early localized disease:* 3–32 days after tick bite. Erythema migrans (annular rash at site of bite, target lesion with clear or necrotic center), fever, headache, myalgia, malaise.<br>(2) *Early disseminated disease:* 3–10 wk after the tick bite. Secondary erythema migrans with multiple, smaller target lesions, cranioneuropathy (especially facial nerve palsy), systemic symptoms as previously listed, and lymphadenopathy; 1% may develop carditis with heart block or aseptic meningitis.<br>(3) *Late disease:* Intermittent, recurrent symptoms occur 2–12 mo from initial tick bite. Pauciarticular arthritis affecting large joints (7% of those untreated), peripheral neuropathy, encephalopathy. | Spirochete *Borrelia burgdorferi*.<br>Inoculation occurs by the bite of a deer tick, *Ixodes scapularis* or *Ixodes pacificus;* disseminates systemically through the blood and lymphatics.<br>Transmission of *B. burgdorferi* requires 24–48 hr of tick attachment.<br>Occurs commonly in New England and the Middle Atlantic, Upper Midwest, and Pacific Northwest. April to October is the peak season. | *Clinical exam:* Most cases of early Lyme disease can be diagnosed clinically by the characteristic erythema migrans rash or illness compatible with early or late disease (e.g., meningitis, facial palsy, arthritis).<br>*Laboratory markers:* Immunoassays for *B. burgdorferi*–specific immunoglobulin M (IgM), which begins at 3–4 wk and peaks at 6–8 wk after disease onset, and with *B. burgdorferi*–specific IgG, which rises wk to mo after symptoms appear and persists.<br>False-positive results of these assays occur as result of cross-reactivity with viral infections, other spirochetal infections, and autoimmune diseases.<br>Western blot assays should be used to confirm positive enzyme-linked immunosorbent assay (ELISA).<br>Lyme disease–specific antibodies can be isolated from CSF in patients with CNS involvement. | Therapy depends on stage of disease. Antibiotic prophylaxis not routinely recommended for ticks attached <24–48 hr.<br>For early localized disease, doxycycline for 14–21 days is treatment of choice for patients ≥8 yr of age. Amoxicillin recommended for younger children.<br>The following early disseminated and late-onset disease manifestations are treated by the same oral regimen as early disease, with treatment extended as indicated: multiple erythema migrans therapy for 21 days, isolated facial palsy treatment for 21–28 days, and arthritis treatment for 28 days.<br>Persistent or recurrent arthritis (>2 mo) and carditis may be treated with 14–21 days of ceftriaxone or 14–28 days of parenteral penicillin. Meningitis or encephalitis should be treated with ceftriaxone or parenteral penicillin for 14–28 days. |

| | | | | |
|---|---|---|---|---|
| Rocky Mountain spotted fever | Incubation period: 1–55 days.<br>Fever, headache, and a characteristic rash that usually occurs by day 6 of illness; initially erythematous and macular and progresses to maculopapular and petechial. The rash usually appears on wrists and ankles and spreads proximally. Palms and soles are often involved. Other symptoms: Myalgia, nausea, anorexia, abdominal pain, diarrhea.<br>*Laboratory manifestations:* Thrombocytopenia, hyponatremia, and anemia. White blood cell count usually normal.<br>Severe disease may manifest in CNS, cardiac, pulmonary, gastrointestinal tract, and renal involvement, disseminated intravascular involvement, and shock leading to death. | *Rickettsia rickettsii*, an obligate intracellular pathogen transmitted to humans by a tick bite.<br>Incidence highest between April and September. Most cases are reported in the south Atlantic, southeastern, and south central United States, although the disease is widespread in the United States and also occurs in Canada, Mexico, and Central and South America. | Diagnosis is by rickettsial group-specific serologic tests, which may be negative early in the illness. A fourfold or greater change between acute- and convalescent-phase serum specimens is diagnostic when determined by indirect immunofluorescence antibody (IFA) assay, enzyme immunoassay, or complement fixation, latex agglutination, indirect hemagglutination, or microagglutination tests.<br>Probable diagnosis can be established by a single serum titer of 1:64 or greater by IFA assay.<br>Culture of *R. rickettsii* is generally not attempted because of danger of transmission to laboratory personnel. *R. rickettsii* can be obtained by immunohistochemical staining of tissue specimens obtained before initiation of antimicrobial therapy. This method is highly specific but not sensitive. | Doxycycline is recommended drug for children of any age. Chloramphenicol is an alternative, although less favored because of serious side effects, the need to monitor levels, and lack of an oral preparation in the United States.<br>Treatment initiated on the basis of clinical features and epidemiologic considerations. Usually lasts 7–10 days and is continued until the patient is afebrile for ≥3 days and has demonstrated clinical improvement. |

*Continued*

TABLE 17-14

SELECTED TICK-BORNE ILLNESSES—cont'd

| Disease | Presentation | Transmission | Diagnosis | Treatment |
|---|---|---|---|---|
| Ehrlichiosis/ anaplasmosis | Caused by three distinct tick-borne pathogens: *Ehrlichia chaffeensis* (human monocytic ehrlichiosis, or HME), *Anaplasma phagocytophilum* (human granulocytotrophic anaplasmosis, or HGA), and *Ehrlichia ewingii*.<br>Systemic febrile illness with headache, chills, rigors, malaise, myalgia, arthralgia, nausea, vomiting, anorexia, or acute weight loss. Rash is variable in location and appearance. | *Ehrlichia* infections caused by HME and *E. ewingii* are associated with the bite of a lone star tick (*Amblyomma americanum*), although other tick species may be vectors. HGA is transmitted by the deer tick (*Ixodes scapularis*).<br>Mammalian reservoirs for agents of human ehrlichiosis include | Diagnosis confirmed by isolation of *Ehrlichia* organisms from blood or CSF, a fourfold or greater change in antibody titer by IFA assay between acute and convalescent serum specimens, PCR assay amplification of ehrlichial DNA from a clinical specimen, or detection of an intraleuko-cytoplasmic cluster of bacteria in conjunction with a single IFA titer ≥64.<br>PCR from acute-phase peripheral blood of patients with ehrlichiosis seems sensitive, specific, and promising for early diagnosis. | Doxycycline is drug of choice, 4.4 mg/kg/day q12hr IV or PO (maximum, 100 mg/dose).<br>Ehrlichiosis may be severe or fatal in untreated patients; treatment should therefore be initiated early. Failure to respond within the first 3 days should suggest infection with an agent other than *Ehrlichia* spp. Treatment should be continued for at least 3 days after defervescence for a minimum total course of 5–10 days. |

| | |
|---|---|
| *Laboratory manifestations*: Leukopenia, anemia, and hepatitis are common.<br>*More severe disease:* Pulmonary infiltrates, bone marrow hypoplasia, respiratory failure, encephalopathy, meningitis, disseminated intravascular coagulation, spontaneous hemorrhage, and renal failure. | white-tailed deer and white-footed mice.<br>Most HME infections occur in the southeastern and south central United States. Most cases of HGA are reported from the north central and northeastern United States.<br>Most human infections occur between April and September, with peak occurrence from May through July. |

TABLE 17-15

COMMON COMMUNITY-ACQUIRED FUNGAL INFECTIONS

| Disease | Usual Etiology | Suggested Therapy | Suggested Length of Therapy |
|---|---|---|---|
| Tinea capitis (ringworm of scalp) | *Trichophyton tonsurans*, *Microsporum canis* | Oral griseofulvin: Give with fatty foods. Fungal shedding decreased with1%–2.5% selenium sulfide shampoo<br>Alt: Terbinafine, itraconazole, or fluconazole | 4–6 wk or 2 wk after clinical resolution |
| Tinea corporis/ pedis (ringworm of body/feet) | *Trichophyton rubrum*, *Trichophyton mentagrophytes*, *Microsporum canis* | Topical antifungal (miconazole, clotrimazole)<br>Terbinafine | 4 wk<br>2 wk |
| Oral candidiasis (thrush) | *Candida albicans*, *Candida tropicalis* | Nystatin suspension or clotrimazole troches | 3 days after clinical resolution |
| Candidal skin infections (intertriginous) | *Candida albicans* | Topical nystatin, miconazole, clotrimazole | 3 days after clinical resolution |
| Tinea unguium (ringworm of nails) | *Trichophyton rubrum*, *Epidermophyton floccosum* | Oral terbinafine<br>Itraconazole<br>Fluconazole | 6 wk<br>3 mo<br>3–6 mo |

(2) A clinician with experience in treatment of individuals with HIV infection should be consulted whenever possible (without causing PEP initiation delay) before initiating therapy. Decision about need for PEP is based on HIV status of source, type, and severity of potential exposure and individual risk tolerance. PEP is generally composed of two-drug or three-drug regimens, frequently available in fixed-dose combination pills for older children and adults. No clear evidence of superior efficacy of a three-drug regimen over a two-drug regimen in preventing HIV infection after exposure, but many experts prefer to use three drugs; this practice must be balanced against the increased toxicity potential when additional drugs are used. Typical regimens include two nucleoside reverse transcriptase inhibitors (NRTIs) (e.g., zidovudine + lamivudine or, in adolescent/adults, tenofovir + emtricitabine), two NRTIs plus a protease inhibitor (PI) (e.g., lopinavir/ritonavir) or two NRTIs plus a non-nucleoside reverse transcriptase inhibitor (NNRTI) (e.g.,

efavirenz). Full descriptions of potential regimens can be found in CDC and AAP guidelines.

(3) Use of zidovudine alone as PEP is no longer recommended.

For most recent recommendations, refer to CDC and AAP guidelines. The CDC's postexposure prophylaxis hotline (open 24 hr/day) is 888-448-4911.

2. **Hepatitis B: Most readily transmitted of the blood-borne pathogens.** Recommendations for hepatitis B prophylaxis in nonimmune person after percutaneous exposure to blood that contains (or might contain) HBsAg include hepatitis B immune globulin and initiation of hepatitis B vaccine series. For details, see Chapter 16.
3. **Hepatitis C:** No preventive therapy available. Serologic testing and follow-up are important to document if infection occurs. Infections become chronic in the majority of patients.

## J. INFECTIOUS DISEASES IN INTERNATIONALLY ADOPTED CHILDREN

For more information, see American Academy of Pediatrics. Medical evaluation of internationally adopted children for infectious diseases. In *2006 Red Book,*[5] pp. 182–187.



## REFERENCES


1. Gilbert DN et al: The Sanford Guide to Antimicrobial Therapy, 37th ed. Sperryville, Va, Antimicrobial Therapy, 2007.
2. Mandell GL et al: Principles and Practice of Infectious Disease. New York, Churchill Livingstone, 1995.
3. Livermore DM: β-Lactamases in laboratory and clinical resistance. Clin Microbiol Rev 1995;8:557–584.
4. Wong CS et al: The risk of hemolytic-uremic syndrome after antibiotic treatment of *Escherichia coli* O157:H7 infections. NEJM 2000;342:1930–1936.
5. Pickering LK (ed): 2006 Red Book: Report of the Committee on Infectious Diseases, 27th ed. Elk Grove Village, Ill, American Academy of Pediatrics, 2006.
6. Behrman RE, Kliegman RM: Nelson Textbook of Pediatrics, 17th ed. Philadelphia, WB Saunders, 2004.
7. McMillan JA et al (eds): Oski's Pediatrics: Principles and Practice, 4th ed. Philadelphia, Lippincott Williams and Wilkins, 2006.
8. Wong VC et al: Prevention of the HBsAg carrier state in newborn infants of mothers who are chronic carriers of HBsAg and HBeAg by administration of hepatitis-B vaccine and hepatitis-B immunoglobulin: Double-blind randomised placebo-controlled study. Lancet 1984;1(8383):921–926.
9. Centers for Disease Control and Prevention: A new product (VariZIG) for postexposure prophylaxis of varicella available under an investigational drug application expanded access protocol. MMWR 2006;55:209–210.
10. Centers for Disease Control and Prevention: Updated U.S. Public Health Service guidelines for the management of occupational exposures to HIV and recommendations for postexposure prophylaxis. MMWR 2005;54(RR-09): 1–17.

11. Council of State and Territorial Epidemiologists, AIDS Program, Center for Infectious Diseases: Revision of the CDC surveillance case definition for acquired immunodeficiency syndrome. MMWR 1987;36(Suppl 1):1S–5S.
12. Havens P et al: Postexposure prophylaxis in children and adolescents for nonoccupational exposure to human immunodeficiency virus. Pediatrics 2003;111(6):1475–1489.
13. Siberry G et al: Management of infants born to HIV infected mothers. Hopkins HIV Rep 2003;15(6):7–12.

# Neonatology

*Nathaly M. Francisco Sweeney, MD, MPH*

18

## I. FETAL ASSESSMENT

### A. FETAL ANOMALY SCREENING

1. **Fetal karyotyping:**
   a. Chorionic villus sampling: Segment of placenta obtained either transcervically or transabdominally at 8–11 weeks' gestation. Detects chromosomal abnormalities and metabolic disorders but cannot detect neural tube defects or measure α-fetoprotein (AFP). Complications include pregnancy loss (0.5%–2%), maternal infection, increased risk for fetomaternal hemorrhage, and fetal limb and jaw malformation.
   b. Amniocentesis: 20–30 mL of amniotic fluid is withdrawn under ultrasound guidance after 16–18 weeks' gestation. Detects chromosomal abnormalities, metabolic disorders, and neural tube defects. Complications include pregnancy loss (<5/1000), chorioamnionitis (<1/1000), leakage of amniotic fluid (1/300), and fetal scarring or dimpling of the skin.
2. **Routine ultrasound: Performed at 18–20 weeks' gestation.**
3. **Maternal AFP (Box 18-1).**
4. **Amniotic fluid volume estimation and the amniotic fluid index (AFI) (Box 18-2).**

AFI calculated with ultrasound by adding together width of amniotic fluid pockets in 4 quadrants.

5. **Biophysical profile test (Table 18-1).**

### B. ESTIMATION OF GESTATIONAL AGE

1. **Last menstrual period (LMP): Nägele's rule, most accurate determination of gestational age.**

$$\text{Estimated due date} = (\text{LMP} - 3\ \text{months}) + 7\ \text{days}$$

2. **Ultrasound: Crown-rump length obtained between 6 and 12 weeks' gestation predicts gestational age ±3–4 days. After 12 weeks, the biparietal diameter is accurate within 10 days; beyond 26 weeks, accuracy diminishes to ±3 weeks.**
3. **Postmenstrual age: Gestational age + chronological age in weeks. Used in perinatal period during hospitalization.**

### C. EXPECTED BIRTH WEIGHT BY GESTATIONAL AGE (Table 18-2)

### D. INTRAPARTUM FETAL HEART RATE (FHR) MONITORING

1. **Normal baseline FHR:** 120–160 bpm. Mild bradycardia is 100–120 bpm. Severe bradycardia is <90 bpm.
2. **Normal beat-to-beat variability:** Deviation from baseline of >6 bpm. Absence of variability is <2 bpm from baseline and is a sign of potential fetal distress, particularly when combined with variable or late decelerations.

BOX 18-1

**MATERNAL α-FETOPROTEIN ASSOCIATIONS**

| ELEVATED (>2.5 MULTIPLES OF THE MEDIAN) | LOW (<0.75 MULTIPLES OF THE MEDIAN) |
|---|---|
| Incorrect gestational dating | Underestimation of gestational age |
| Neural tube defects | Intrauterine growth retardation |
| Anencephaly | Trisomy 13 |
| Multiple pregnancy | Trisomy 18 |
| Turner syndrome | Down syndrome |
| Omphalocele | |
| Cystic hygroma | |
| Epidermolysis bullosa | |
| Renal agenesis | |

BOX 18-2

**AMNIOTIC FLUID VOLUME ESTIMATION AND AMNIOTIC FLUID INDEX (AFI)**

| OLIGOHYDRAMNIOS (<500 mL)/(AFI 0–5) | POLYHYDRAMNIOS (>2L)/(AFI >25) |
|---|---|
| Renal and urologic anomalies: | GI anomalies: Gastroschisis, duodenal atresia, tracheoesophageal fistula, diaphragmatic hernia |
| Potter syndrome | CNS anomalies associated with impaired swallowing: Anencephaly, Werdnig-Hoffman syndrome, spinomuscular atrophy (SMA) |
| Lung hypoplasia | Chromosomal trisomies |
| Limb deformities | Maternal diabetes |
| Premature rupture of membranes | Cystic adenomatoid malformation of the lung |
| Placental insufficiency | |

3. **Accelerations: Associated with fetal movement, are benign, and indicate fetal well-being.**
4. **Decelerations**

a. Early decelerations: Begin with the onset of contractions. The heart rate reaches the nadir at the peak of the contraction and returns to baseline as the contraction ends. Occur secondary to changes in vagal tone after brief hypoxic episodes or head compression and are benign.

b. Variable decelerations: Represent umbilical cord compression and have no uniform temporal relationship to the onset of the contraction. They are considered severe when the heart rate drops to <60 bpm for about 60 sec with slow recovery to baseline.

c. Late decelerations: Occur after the peak of contraction, persist after the contraction stops, and show a slow return to baseline. Result from uteroplacental insufficiency and indicate fetal distress.

TABLE 18-1

THE BIOPHYSICAL PROFILE

| Biophysical Variable | Normal (Score = 2) | Abnormal (Score = 0) |
|---|---|---|
| Fetal breathing movements | 1 or more episodes of ≥20 sec within 30 min | Absent or no episode of ≥20 sec within 30 min |
| Gross body movements | 2 or more discrete body/limb movements within 30 min (episodes of active continuous movement considered as a single movement) | <2 episodes of body/limb movements within 30 min |
| Fetal tone | 1 or more episodes of active extension with return to flexion of fetal limb(s) or trunk (opening and closing of hand considered normal tone) | Slow extension with return to partial flexion, movement of limb in full extension, absent fetal movement, or partially open fetal hand |
| Reactive fetal heart rate | 2 or more episodes of acceleration of ≥15 bpm* and of >15 sec associated with fetal movement within 20 min | 1 or more episodes of acceleration of fetal heart rate or acceleration of <15 bpm within 20 min |
| Qualitative amniotic fluid volume | 1 or more pockets of fluid measuring ≥2 cm in vertical axis | Either no pockets or largest pocket <2 cm in vertical axis |

*bpm, beats per minute.

Adapted from Gearhart et al., Biophysical profile, ultrasound. Emedicine June 6, 2005. Available at www.emedicine.com.

TABLE 18-2

PREDICTED ENDOTRACHEAL TUBE SIZE AND EXPECTED BIRTH WEIGHT BY GESTATIONAL AGE*

| Gestational Age (wk) | Weight (g)* | ETT Size (mm) | ETT Depth of Insertion (cm from upper lip) |
|---|---|---|---|
| 24 | 700 | 2.5 | 7 |
| 26 | 900 | 2.5 | 7 |
| 28 | 1100 | 2.5–3.0 | 7 |
| 30 | 1350 | 3.0 | 7 |
| 32 | 1650 | 3.0 | 7 |
| 34 | 2100 | 3.5 | 8 |
| 36 | 2600 | 3.5 | 8 |
| 38 | 3000 | 3.5–4.0 | 9 |

*Weight is the 50th percentile for age.

ETT, endotracheal tube.

Data from Usher R, McLean F: Intrauterine growth of liveborn Caucasion infauts at sea level: Standards obtained from measurements in seven dimensions of infauts born between 25 and 44 week gestation. J Pediatr 1969;74:901–910, and Welty SE: Intrauterine guidelines for neonatal resuscitation and emergency cardiovascular care—International Consensus on Science. Pediatrics 2000;106(3):e29.

18 NEONATOLOGY

## II. NEWBORN RESUSCITATION

### A. NALS ALGORITHM FOR NEONATAL RESUSCITATION (Fig. 18-1)

For infants with meconium in the amniotic fluid, routine intrapartum oropharyngeal and nasopharyngeal **suctioning is not recommended.** If the infant is not vigorous, endotracheal intubation should be performed immediately after birth and suction should be applied to the endotracheal tube as it is withdrawn.[1]

### B. ENDOTRACHEAL TUBE SIZE AND DEPTH OF INSERTION (see Table 18-2)

### C. VENTILATORY SUPPORT (see Chapter 4)

### D. VASCULAR ACCESS (see Chapter 3 for umbilical venous catheter and umbilical artery catheter placement)

## III. NEWBORN ASSESSMENT

### A. VITAL SIGNS

Average heart rate and respiratory rate are 120–160 bpm and 40–60 breaths/min, respectively. Arterial blood pressure is related to birth weight and gestational age (see Chapter 7). Normal core temperature in the neonate is 36.5°–37.5°C rectally. (See Chapter 21 for height, weight, and head circumference growth charts in the premature infant.)

### B. APGAR SCORES (Table 18-3)

Apgar scores are assessed at 1 and 5 min and may be repeated at 5-min intervals for infants with 5-min scores <7.[2]

### C. NEW BALLARD GESTATIONAL AGE ESTIMATION

The Ballard score is most accurate when performed between age 12 and 20 hours.[3] Approximate gestational age is calculated based on the sum of the neuromuscular and physical maturity ratings (Fig. 18-2).

**1. Neuromuscular maturity:**

a. Posture: Observe infant quiet and supine. Score 0 for arms, legs extended; 1 for starting to flex hips and knees, arms extended; 2 for stronger flexion of legs, arms extended; 3 for arms slightly flexed, legs flexed and abducted; and 4 for full flexion of arms and legs.
b. Square window: Flex hand on forearm enough to obtain fullest possible flexion without wrist rotation. Measure angle between the hypothenar eminence and the ventral aspect of the forearm.
c. Arm recoil: With infant supine, flex forearms for 5 seconds, fully extend by pulling on hands, then release. Measure the angle of elbow flexion to which the arms recoil.
d. Popliteal angle: Hold infant supine with pelvis flat, thigh held in the knee-chest position. Extend leg by gentle pressure and measure the popliteal angle.
e. Scarf sign: With baby supine, pull infant's hand across the neck toward the opposite shoulder. Determine how far the elbow will go across.

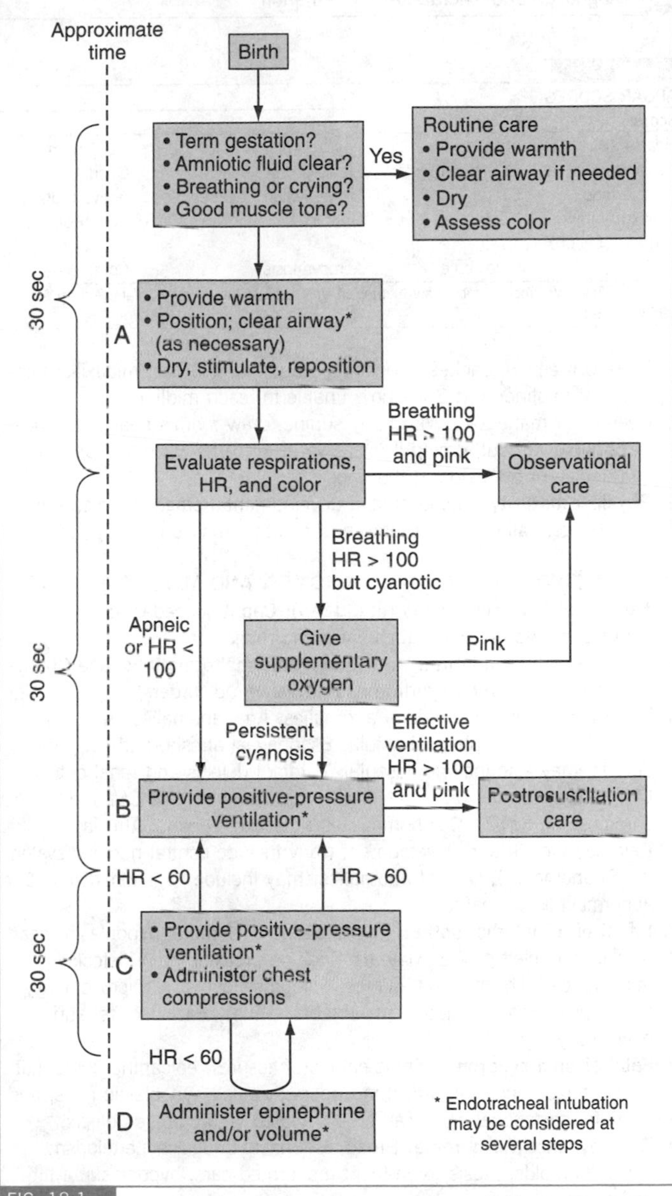


FIG. 18-1

Overview of resuscitation in the delivery room. *(2005 AHA Guidelines for Cardiopulmonary Resuscitation and Emergency Cardiovascular Care of Pediatric and Neonatal Patients: Neonatal Resuscitation Guidelines. Pediatrics 2006;117: e1029-e1038.)*

TABLE 18-3

APGAR SCORES

| Score | 0 | 1 | 2 |
|---|---|---|---|
| Heart rate | Absent | <100 bpm | >100 bpm |
| Respiratory effort | Absent, irregular | Slow, crying | Good |
| Muscle tone | Limp | Some flexion of extremities | Active motion |
| Reflex irritability (nose suction) | No response | Grimace | Cough or sneeze |
| Color | Blue, pale | Acrocyanosis | Completely pink |

Data from Apgar V: Proposal for a new method of evaluation of the newborn infant. Anesth Analg 1953;32:260.

Score 0 if elbow reaches opposite axillary line; 1 if past midaxillary line; 2 if past midline; and 3 if elbow unable to reach midline.

f. Heel-to-ear maneuver: With baby supine, draw foot as near to the head as possible without forcing it. Observe distance between foot and head and degree of extension at the knee.

2. **Physical maturity: Based on the developmental stage of eyes, ears, breasts, genitalia, skin, lanugo, and plantar creases (see Fig. 18-2).**

## D. SELECTED ANOMALIES, SYNDROMES, AND MALFORMATIONS

1. **Extradural fluid collections (Fig. 18-3): Caput succedaneum, cephalohematoma, and subgaleal hemorrhage.**
2. **Miscellaneous syndromes and teratogenic malformations** (see Chapter 13 for more common syndromes and genetic disorders).

a. **VATER association: V**ertebral anomalies, **A**nal anomalies and anal atresia, **T**racheoesophageal fistula, **E**sophageal atresia, and **R**adial defects. May also include vascular (cardiac) defects and renal defects.

b. **CHARGE syndrome** (associated with mutations in gene *CHD7* on chromosome 8q12): **C**oloboma, **H**eart disease, choanal **A**tresia, **R**etarded growth and development (may include central nervous system [CNS] anomalies), **G**enital anomalies (may include hypogonadism), **E**ar abnormalities or deafness.

c. **Infant of a diabetic mother:** Sacral agenesis, femoral hypoplasia, heart defects, and cleft palate. May also include preaxial radial defects, microtia, cleft lip, microphthalmos, holoprosencephaly, microcephaly, anencephaly, spina bifida, hemivertebra, urinary tract defects, and polydactyly.

d. **Fetal alcohol syndrome:** Short palpebral fissures, epicanthal folds, flat nasal bridge, long philtrum, thin upper lip, small hypoplastic nails, and small for gestational age. May be associated with cardiac defects.

e. **Fetal hydantoin syndrome:** Broad, low nasal bridge; hypertelorism, epicanthal folds, ptosis, prominent malformed ears, hypoplasia of fifth nail of toe or finger.

f. **Fetal valproate syndrome:** Neural tube defects, fused metopic suture, trigonocephaly, epicanthal folds, midface hypoplasia, anteverted nostrils, oral cleft, heart defects, hypospadias, clubfeet, and psychomotor retardation.

Neuromuscular maturity

| Neuromuscular maturity sign | Score −1 | 0 | 1 | 2 | 3 | 4 | 5 | Record score here |
|---|---|---|---|---|---|---|---|---|
| Posture | | | | | | | | |
| Square window (wrist) | > 90° | 90° | 60° | 45° | 30° | 0° | | |
| Arm recoil | | 180° | 140–180° | 110–140° | 90–110° | < 90° | | |
| Popliteal angle | 180° | 160° | 140° | 120° | 100° | 90° | < 90° | |
| Scarf sign | | | | | | | | |
| Heel to ear | | | | | | | | |

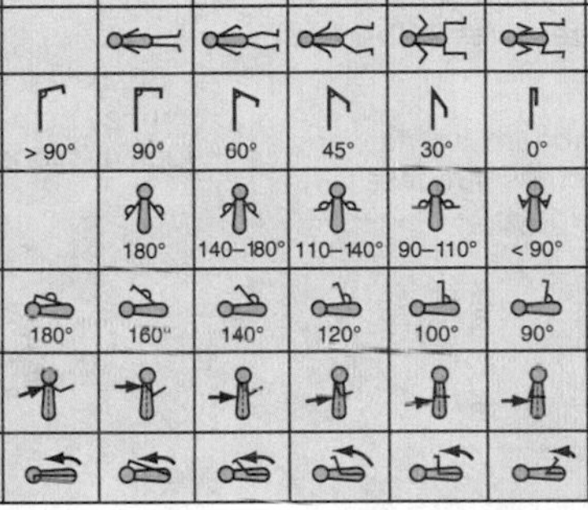

TOTAL NEUROMUSCULAR MATURITY SCORE

Physical maturity

| Physical maturity sign | Score −1 | 0 | 1 | 2 | 3 | 4 | 5 | Record score here |
|---|---|---|---|---|---|---|---|---|
| Skin | Sticky, friable, transparent | Gelatinous, red, translucent | Smooth, pink, visible veins | Superficial peeling and/or rash, few veins | Cracking, pale areas, rare veins | Parchment, deep cracking, no vessels | Leathery, cracked, wrinkled | |
| Lanugo | None | Sparse | Abundant | Thinning | Bald areas | Mostly bald | | |
| Plantar surface | Heel-toe 40–50 mm: −1 < 40 mm: −2 | > 50 mm, no crease | Faint red marks | Anterior transverse crease only | Creases anterior two thirds | Creases over entire sole | | |
| Breast | Imperceptible | Barely perceptible | Flat areola, no bud | Stippled areola, 1–2 mm bud | Raised areola, 3–4 mm bud | Full areola, 5–10 mm bud | | |
| Eye/ear | Lids fused: loosely: −1 tightly: −2 | Lids open, pinna flat, stays folded | Sl. curved pinna, soft, slow recoil | Well-curved pinna, soft but ready recoil | Formed and firm, instant recoil | Thick cartilage, ear stiff | | |
| Genitals (male) | Scrotum flat, smooth | Scrotum empty, faint rugae | Testes in upper canal, rare rugae | Testes descending, few rugae | Testes down, good rugae | Testes pendulous, deep rugae | | |
| Genitals (female) | Clitoris prominent and labia flat | Prominent clitoris and small labia minora | Prominent clitoris and enlarging minora | Majora and minora equally prominent | Majora large, minora small | Majora cover clitoris and minora | | |

TOTAL PHYSICAL MATURITY SCORE

Score

Neuromuscular______
Physical______
Total______

Maturity rating

| Score | −10 | −5 | 0 | 5 | 10 | 15 | 20 | 25 | 30 | 35 | 40 | 45 | 50 |
|---|---|---|---|---|---|---|---|---|---|---|---|---|---|
| Weeks | 20 | 22 | 24 | 26 | 28 | 30 | 32 | 34 | 36 | 38 | 40 | 42 | 44 |

Gestational age (weeks)

By dates______
By ultrasound______
By exam______

FIG. 18-2

Neuromuscular and physical maturity (New Ballard Score). *(Modified from Ballard JL et al: New Ballard Score, expanded to include extremely premature infants. J Pediatr 1991;119:417–423.)*

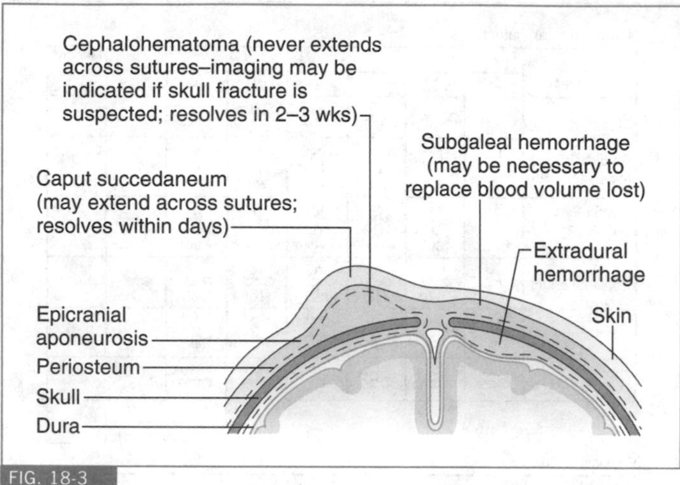


FIG. 18-3

Types of extradural fluid collections seen in newborn infants.

TABLE 18-4

INSENSIBLE WATER LOSS IN PRETERM INFANTS*

| Body Weight (g) | Insensible Water Loss (mL/kg/day) |
|---|---|
| <1000 | 60–70 |
| 1000–1250 | 60–65 |
| 1251–1500 | 30–45 |
| 1501–1750 | 15–30 |
| 1751–2000 | 15–20 |

*Estimates of insensible water loss at different body weights during the first few days of life.

Data from Veille JC: Clin Perinatol 1988;15:863.

## IV. FLUIDS, ELECTROLYTES, AND NUTRITION

### A. FLUIDS

1. **Insensible water loss in preterm infants (Table 18-4).**
2. **Water requirements of newborns (Table 18-5).**

### B. GLUCOSE

1. **Requirements:** Preterm neonates require about 5–6 mg/kg/min of glucose to maintain euglycemia (40–100 mg/dL).[4] Term neonates require about 3–5 mg/kg/min of glucose to maintain euglycemia. The formula to calculate rate of glucose infusion follows:

$$\text{glucose (mg/kg/min)} = (\%\ \text{glucose in solution} \times 10) \times (\text{rate of infusion per hour})/60 \times \text{weight (kg)}$$

TABLE 18-5

WATER REQUIREMENTS OF NEWBORNS

| | Water Requirements (mL/kg/24 hr) by Age | | |
|---|---|---|---|
| Birth Weight (g) | 1–2 days | 3–7 days | 7–30 days |
| <750 | 100–250 | 150–300 | 120–180 |
| 750–1000 | 80–150 | 100–150 | 120–180 |
| 1000–1500 | 60–100 | 80–150 | 120–180 |
| <1500 | 60–80 | 100–150 | 120–180 |

Data from Taeusch HW, Ballard RA (eds): Schaffer and Avery's Diseases of the Newborn, 7th ed. Philadelphia, WB Saunders, 1998.

2. **Management of hyperglycemia and hypoglycemia (Tables 18-6 and 18-7).**

## C. ELECTROLYTES, MINERALS, AND VITAMINS

1. **Electrolyte requirements (Table 18-8).**
2. **Mineral and vitamin requirements:**

a. Infants born at <34 weeks' gestation have higher calcium, phosphorus, sodium, iron, and vitamin D requirements and require breast-milk fortifier or special preterm formulas with iron. Fortifier should be added to breast milk only after the second week of life.

b. Iron: Enterally fed preterm infants require elemental iron supplementation of 2 mg/kg/day after age 4–8 weeks.

## D. NUTRITION

1. **Growth and caloric requirements:**

a. Preterm infants (healthy and thermoneutral environments):
 (1) Caloric requirements:
  (a) Maintaining weight: 50–75 kcal/kg/day.
  (b) Adequate growth: 115–130 kcal/kg/day (may be up to 150 kcal/kg/day for very low birth weight infants).
 (2) Growth (after 10 days of life): 15–20 g/kg/day.

b. Term infants:
 (1) Caloric requirements: 100–120 kcal/kg/day.
 (2) Growth (after 10 days of life): 10 g/kg/day.

2. **Total parenteral nutrition (see Chapter 21).**

# V. CYANOSIS IN THE NEWBORN

## A. DIFFERENTIAL DIAGNOSIS (Fig. 18-4)

## B. EVALUATION

1. **Physical examination:** Note central versus peripheral and persistent versus intermittent cyanosis, degree of respiratory effort, single versus split $S_2$, and presence or absence of a heart murmur. Acrocyanosis is often a normal finding in newborns.

TABLE 18-6

MANAGEMENT OF HYPERGLYCEMIA AND HYPOGLYCEMIA[5]

| | Hypoglycemia | Hyperglycemia |
|---|---|---|
| **Definition** | Serum glucose <40 mg/dLin term and preterm infants | Serum glucose >125 mg/dL in term infants, >150 mg/dL in preterm infants |
| **Differential diagnosis** | Insufficient glucose delivery<br>Decreased glycogen stores<br>Increased circulating insulin (infant of a diabetic mother, maternal drugs, Beckwith-Wiedemann syndrome, tumors)<br>Endocrine and metabolic disorders<br>Sepsis<br>Hypothermia<br>Polycythemia<br>Asphyxia<br>Shock | Excess glucose administration<br>Sepsis<br>Hypoxia<br>Hyperosmolar formula<br>Transient neonatal diabetes mellitus<br>Medications |
| **Evaluation** | Ensure venous sample confirms bedside testing<br>Assess for symptoms<br>Calculate glucose delivery to infant<br>Serum glucose<br>Complete blood count with differential<br>Blood cultures<br>Urinalysis<br>Urine cultures<br>Electrolytes<br>Lumbar puncture if warranted<br>Insulin and C-peptide levels if warranted | |
| **Management** | Change dextrose infusion rates gradually. Generally, it should not exceed 2 mg/kg/min in a 2-hr interval. (See Table 18-7 for further guidelines).<br>Monitor glucose levels every 30–60 min until normal values have been established. | Gradually decrease glucose infusion rate if receiving >5 mg/kg/min.<br>Monitor glucosuria. Consider insulin infusion for persistent hyperglycemia.<br>Consider consulting an endocrinologist. |

TABLE 18-7

**GUIDELINES FOR TREATMENT OF NEONATAL HYPOGLYCEMIA[5]**

| Plasma Glucose (mg/dL)—Venous Sample | Asymptomatic or Mildly Symptomatic | Symptomatic |
|---|---|---|
| 35–45 | Breast-feed or give formula or $D_5W$ by nipple/gavage | IV glucose ($D_{5-12.5}W$) at 4–6 mg/kg/min* |
| 25–34 | IV glucose ($D_{5-12.5}W$) at 6–8 mg/kg/min* | IV glucose ($D_{5-12.5}W$) at 6–8 mg/kg/min* |
| <25 | Mini-bolus of 2 mL/kg ($D_{10}W$) and continue at a rate to provide 6–8 mg/kg/min† | |

*Changes in infusion rates should not exceed 2 mg/kg/min per change.

†If blood glucose <25 mg/dL and IV access is not available, give glucagon, 0.1 mg/kg per dose (maximum, 1 mg/dose) IM or SC every 30 min. Not as effective in small-for-gestational-age or extremely premature infants.

Modified from Cornblath M: Neonatal hypoglycemia. In Donn SM, Fisher CW (eds): Risk Management Techniques in Perinatal and Neonatal Practice. Armonk, NY, Futura, 1996, pp 437–448.

TABLE 18-8

**ELECTROLYTE REQUIREMENTS**

| | Before 48 Hours of Life | After 48–72 Hours of Life |
|---|---|---|
| Sodium | None, unless serum sodium <135 mEq/L without evidence of volume overload | Term infants: 2–3 mEq/kg/day<br>Preterm infants: 3–5 mEq/kg/day |
| Potassium | None | 1–2.5 mEq/kg/day if adequate urine output is established and serum level <4.5 mEq/L |

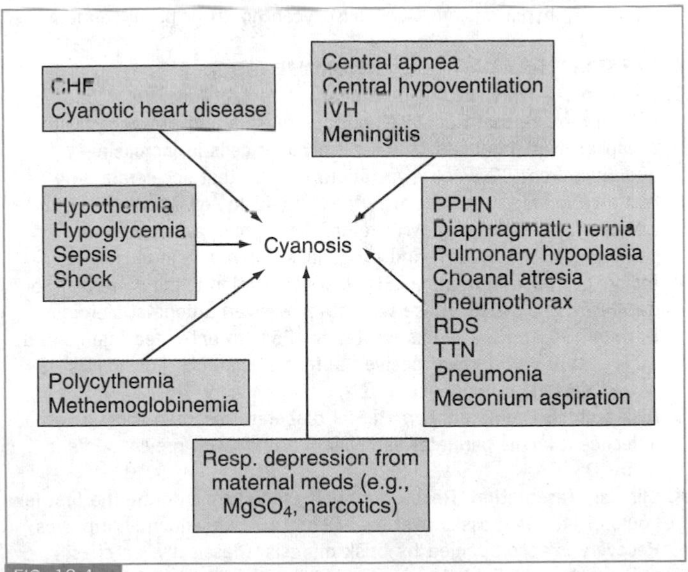


FIG. 18-4

Causes of cyanosis in the newborn.

18 NEONATOLOGY

2. **Clinical tests:** Oxygen challenge test (see Chapter 7), preductal and postductal arterial blood gas levels, or pulse oximetry to assess for right-to-left shunt, transillumination of chest for possible pneumothorax.
3. **Other data:** Complete blood count with differential, serum glucose, chest radiograph, electrocardiogram (ECG), echocardiography. Consider blood, urine, and cerebrospinal fluid cultures if sepsis is suspected, and methemoglobin level if cyanosis does not match degree of hypoxemia.

## VI. RESPIRATORY DISEASES

### A. GENERAL RESPIRATORY CONSIDERATIONS

1. **Exogenous surfactant therapy:**
   a. Indications: Respiratory distress syndrome in preterm infants, meconium aspiration, pneumonia, persistent pulmonary hypertension.
   b. Administration: Each preparation has specific dosing instructions. If the infant is ≤26 weeks' gestation, the first dose is typically given in the delivery room or as soon as stabilized; repeat dosing may follow at 6-hr intervals.
   c. Complications: Pneumothorax, pulmonary hemorrhage.
2. **Supplemental $O_2$:** Adjust inspired oxygen to maintain $O_2$ saturation between 88% and 92% until the retina is fully vascularized, between 94% and 98% if the retinas are mature, and >97% in cases of pulmonary hypertension. Consider oxygen hoods or nasal cannula.

### B. RESPIRATORY DISTRESS SYNDROME (RDS)

1. **Definition:** A deficiency of pulmonary surfactant (a phospholipid protein mixture that decreases surface tension and prevents alveolar collapse). It is produced by type II alveolar cells in increasing quantities from 32 weeks' gestation. Factors that accelerate lung maturity include maternal hypertension, sickle cell disease, narcotic addiction, intrauterine growth retardation, prolonged rupture of membranes, fetal stress, and exogenous antenatal steroids.
2. **Incidence:** 60% in infants <30 weeks' gestation without steroids, but decreases to 35% for those who have received antenatal steroids. Between 30 and 34 weeks' gestation, 25% in untreated infants and 10% in those who have received antenatal steroids. For infants >34 weeks' gestation, incidence is 5%.
3. **Risk factors:** Prematurity, maternal diabetes, cesarean section without antecedent labor, perinatal asphyxia, second twin, previous infant with RDS.
4. **Clinical presentation:** Respiratory distress worsens during the first few hours of life, progresses over 48–72 hr, and subsequently improves. Recovery is accompanied by brisk diuresis. Classically, on chest radiograph, lung fields have a "reticulogranular" pattern that may obscure the heart border.

5. **Management:**
a. Support ventilation and oxygenation.
b. Surfactant therapy.
6. **Intrauterine acceleration of fetal lung maturation:** Maternal administration of steroids antenatally has been shown to decrease neonatal morbidity and mortality. In particular, the risk for RDS is decreased in babies born >24 hours and <7 days after maternal steroid administration.

## C. PERSISTENT PULMONARY HYPERTENSION OF THE NEWBORN (PPHN)



1. **Etiology:** Idiopathic or secondary to conditions leading to increased pulmonary vascular resistance. Most commonly seen in term or post-term infants, infants born by cesarean section, and infants with a history of fetal distress and low Apgar scores. Usually presents within 12–24 hr of birth. Accounts for up to 2% of all neonatal admissions to the intensive care unit (ICU).
a. Vasoconstriction secondary to hypoxemia and acidosis (neonatal sepsis).
b. Interstitial pulmonary disease (meconium aspiration syndrome, pneumonia).
c. Hyperviscosity syndrome (polycythemia).
d. Pulmonary hypoplasia, either primary or secondary to congenital diaphragmatic hernia or renal agenesis.
2. **Diagnostic features:**
a. Severe hypoxemia ($Pa_{O_2}$ <35–45 mm Hg in 100% $O_2$) disproportionate to radiologic changes.
b. Structurally normal heart with right-to-left shunt at foramen ovale and/or ductus arteriosus; decreased postductal oxygen saturations compared with preductal values. (Difference of at least 7–15 mm Hg between preductal and postductal $Pa_{O_2}$ is significant.)
c. Must distinguish from cyanotic heart disease. Infants with heart disease will have an abnormal cardiac examination and show little to no improvement in oxygenation with increased fraction of inspired $O_2$ ($Fi_{O_2}$) and hyperventilation. See Chapter 7 for interpretation of oxygen challenge test.
3. **Principles of therapy:** There is no clear consensus on the management of PPHN; however, there are clear basic treatment goals.
a. **Improve alveolar oxygenation** with supplemental oxygen ($Fi_{O_2}$): Optimize oxygen-carrying capacity with blood transfusions as needed.
b. **Minimize pulmonary vasoconstriction.**
   (1) Minimal handling and limited invasive procedures. Sedation and occasionally paralysis of intubated neonates may be necessary.
   (2) Alkalosis: Metabolic (pH 7.45–7.55) or respiratory ($Pc_{O_2}$ in low 30s); may improve oxygenation, although they have not been noted to affect outcome. Avoid severe hypocarbia ($Pc_{O_2}$ <30), which can be associated with myocardial ischemia and decreased

cerebral blood flow. Hyperventilation may result in barotrauma, which predisposes to chronic lung disease. Consider high-frequency ventilation.

c. **Maintenance of systemic blood pressure and perfusion** with reversal of right-to-left shunt through volume expanders and/or inotropes.

d. **Consider pulmonary vasodilator therapy.**

(1) Inhaled nitric oxide (NO), a pulmonary vasodilator: A specific therapy shown to reduce pulmonary vascular resistance (PVR). It is blended with ventilatory gases and titrated to effect. Typical starting doses are 20 parts per million (ppm) titrated to effect. Unlikely to be efficacious >40 ppm. Complications include methemoglobinemia (reduce NO dose for methemoglobin >4%), $NO_2$ poisoning (reduce NO dose for $NO_2$ concentration >1–2 ppm).

(2) Prostaglandin $I_2$ (prostacyclin): A complex molecule made from arachidonic acid; is one of the major endogenous vasodilators in the lung. Normally produced by lung when lung vessels are in a constricted state, thereby relaxing them.

e. **Administer broad-spectrum antibiotics:** Sepsis is a common underlying cause of PPHN.

f. **Consider extracorporeal membrane oxygenation (ECMO):** If infant has severe cardiovascular instability, if oxygenation index (OI) is >40 for >3 hr, or if alveolar-arterial gradient (A-$ao_2$) is ≥610 for 8 hr (see Chapter 4 for the calculation of OI and A-$ao_2$. $Pao_2$ should be measured at a postductal site). Patients typically need to be >2000 g and >34 weeks' gestation, and should have head ultrasound and echocardiogram before going on ECMO.

4. **Mortality depends on underlying diagnosis: Mortality rates generally lower for RDS and meconium aspiration but higher in sepsis and diaphragmatic hernia.**

### D. SPONTANEOUS PNEUMOTHORAX

1. **Seen in 1%–2% of normal newborns.**
2. **Associated with underlying diseases such as RDS, meconium aspiration, and pneumonia.**
3. **Patient should be monitored in an ICU setting.**

## VII. APNEA AND BRADYCARDIA

### A. APNEA[6]

1. **Definition:** **Respiratory pause >20 sec, or a shorter pause associated with cyanosis, pallor, hypotonia, or bradycardia <100 bpm. In preterm infants, apneic episodes may be central (no diaphragmatic activity), obstructive (upper airway obstruction), or mixed central and obstructive. Common causes of apnea in the newborn are listed in Figure 18-5.**
2. **Incidence:** **Apnea of prematurity occurs in most infants born at <28 weeks' gestation, about 50% of infants born at 30–32 weeks'**

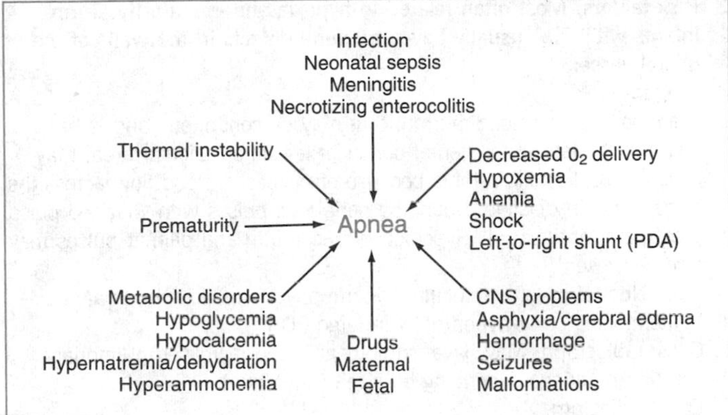


FIG. 18-5

Causes of apnea in the newborn. *(From Klaus MH, Fanaroff AA: Care of the High-Risk Neonate, 5th ed. Philadelphia, WB Saunders, 2001, p 268.)*



**gestation, and <7% of infants born at 34–35 weeks' gestation. It usually resolves by 34–36 weeks' postconceptual age, but may persist after term in infants born at <25 weeks' gestation.**

3. **Management:**
   a. Consider pathologic causes for apnea.
   b. Pharmacotherapy with theophylline, aminophylline, caffeine, or doxapram (see Formulary for dosage information).
   c. Continuous positive-airway pressure or mechanical ventilation (see Chapter 4 for details).

### B. BRADYCARDIA WITHOUT CENTRAL APNEA

Obstructive apnea, mechanical airway obstruction, gastroesophageal reflux, increased intracranial pressure (ICP), increased vagal tone (defecation, yawning, rectal stimulation, placement of nasogastric [NG] tube), electrolyte abnormalities, heart block.

## VIII. CARDIAC DISEASES

### A. PATENT DUCTUS ARTERIOSUS (PDA)

1. **Summary:** Failure of the ductus arteriosus to close in the first few days of life or reopening after functional closure. Typically results in left-to-right shunting of blood once PVR has decreased. If PVR remains high, blood may be shunted right to left, resulting in hypoxemia (see section VI.C).
2. **Incidence:** Up to 60% in preterm infants weighing <1500 g, higher in those <1000 g. Female-to-male ratio is 2:1. Obligatory PDA is found in 10% of infants with congenital heart disease.

**3. Risk factors:** **Most often related to hypoxia and immaturity. Term infants with PDA usually have structural defects in the walls of the ductal vessel.**

**4. Diagnosis:**

a. Examination: A systolic murmur that may be continuous and is best heard at the left upper sternal border or left infraclavicular area. May have apical diastolic rumble because of increased blood flow across the mitral valve in diastole. Bounding peripheral pulses with widened pulse pressure if large shunt. Hyperactive precordium and palmar pulses may also be present.

b. ECG: Normal or left ventricular hypertrophy in small to moderate PDA. Bilateral ventricular hypertrophy in large PDA.

c. Chest radiograph: May have cardiomegaly and increased pulmonary vascular markings depending on size of the shunt.

d. Echocardiogram.

**5. Management:**

a. Indomethacin: A prostaglandin synthetase inhibitor; 80% closure rate in preterm infants.

(1) For dosage information and contraindications, see Formulary. It should be used with great caution.

(2) Complications: Transient decrease in glomerular filtration rate and subsequent decreased urine output; transient gastrointestinal bleeding (not associated with an increased incidence of necrotizing enterocolitis [NEC]); and prolonged bleeding time and disturbed platelet function for 7–9 days independent of platelet number (not associated with increased incidence of intracranial hemorrhage). Spontaneous isolated intestinal perforations are seen with indomethacin use. Rates are higher with concomitant hydrocortisone use.

b. Surgical ligation of the duct.

### B. CYANOTIC HEART DISEASE

See Chapter 7.

## IX. HEMATOLOGIC DISEASES

### A. UNCONJUGATED HYPERBILIRUBINEMIA IN THE NEWBORN[7]

1. **Summary:** **During the first 3–4 days of life, infants' serum bilirubin increases from cord bilirubin levels of 1.5 mg/dL to 6.5 ± 2.5 mg/dL. The maximum rate of increase in bilirubin for otherwise normal infants with nonhemolytic hyperbilirubinemia is 5 mg/dL/24 hr, or 0.2 mg/dL/hr. Visible jaundice or a total bilirubin concentration >5 mg/dL on the first day of life is outside the normal range and suggests a potentially pathologic cause. Infants <37 weeks' gestation tend to have maximum serum indirect bilirubin levels 30%–50% higher compared with term infants. Treatment guidelines for preterm infants (Table 18-9) differ from those for term infants (Figs. 18-6 and 18-7).**

TABLE 18-9

GUIDELINES FOR USE OF PHOTOTHERAPY IN PRETERM INFANTS <1 WEEK OF AGE

| Weight (g) | Phototherapy (mg/dL) | Consider Exchange Transfusion (mg/dL) |
|---|---|---|
| 500–1000 | 5–7 | 12–15 |
| 1000–1500 | 7–10 | 15–18 |
| 1500–2500 | 10–15 | 18–20 |
| >2500 | >15 | >20 |



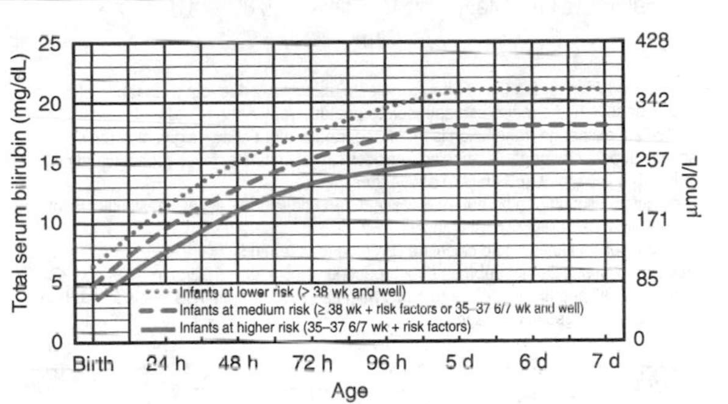


- Use total bilirubin. Do not subtract direct reacting or conjugated bilirubin.
- Risk factors: Isoimmune hemolytic disease, G6PD deficiency, asphyxia, significant lethargy, temperature instability, sepsis, acidosis, or albumin < 3.0 g/dL (if measured).
- For well infants 35–37 6/7 wk can adjust TSB levels for intervention around the medium risk line. It is an option to intervene at lower TSB levels for infants closer to 35 wks and at higher TSB levels for those closer to 37 6/7 wk.
- It is an option to provide conventional phototherapy in hospital or at home at TSB levels 2–3 mg/dL (35–50 mmol/L) below those shown, but home phototherapy should not be used in any infant with risk factors.

FIG. 18-6

Guidelines for phototherapy in infants born at 35 weeks' gestation or more.

2. **Evaluation:**

a. Maternal prenatal testing: ABO and Rh (D) typing and serum screen for isoimmune antibodies.

b. Infant or cord blood: Evaluation of blood smear, direct Coombs test, blood type, and Rh typing if mother has not had prenatal blood typing or she is blood type O or Rh negative.

3. **Management:**

a. Phototherapy:

(1) Preterm newborn (see Table 18-9): Bilirubin levels may significantly increase in the infant who is <36 weeks' gestation,

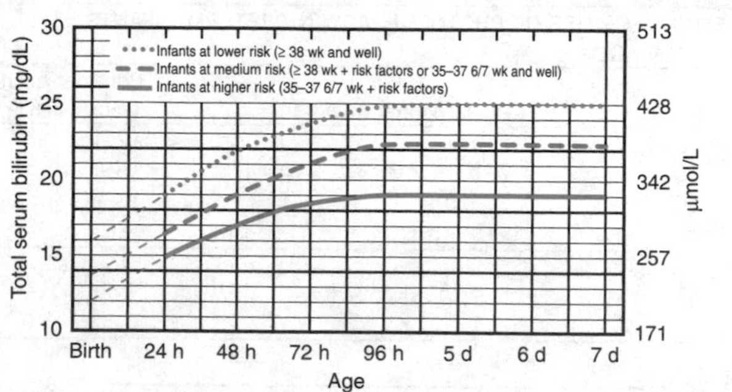


- The dashed lines for the first 24 hours indicate uncertainty due to a wide range of clinical circumstances and a range of responses to phototherapy.
- Immediate exchange transfusion is recommended if infant shows signs of acute bilirubin encephalopathy (hypertonia, arching, retrocollis, opisthotonos, fever, high-pitched cry) or if TBS is ≥ 5 mg/dL (85 μmol/L) above these lines.
- Risk factors: Isoimmune hemolytic disease, G6PD deficiency, asphyxia, significant lethargy, temperature instability, sepsis, acidosis.
- Measure serum albumin and calculate B/A ratio (see legend).
- Use total bilirubin. Do not subtract direct reacting or conjugated bilirubin.
- If infant is well and 35–37 6/7 wk (median risk) can individualize TSB levels for exchange based on actual gestational age.

FIG. 18-7

Guidelines for exchange transfusion in infants born at 35 weeks' gestation or more.

weighs <2500 g, and is breast-feeding. These infants may require phototherapy at lower bilirubin levels.

(2) Term newborn (see Fig. 18-6): Intensive phototherapy should produce a decline of the total serum bilirubin (TSB) level of 1–2 mg/dL within 4–6 hr. TSB level should continue to fall and remain below the threshold level for exchange transfusion. If this does not occur, it is considered a failure of phototherapy.

b. Neonatal exchange transfusion (see Table 18-9 and Fig. 18-7): To complete double-volume exchange, transfuse 160 mL/kg for full-term infant and 160–200 mL/kg for preterm infant. During the exchange, blood is removed through the umbilical artery catheter and an equal volume is infused through the venous catheter. If unable to pass an arterial catheter, use a single venous catheter. Exchange in 15-mL increments in vigorous full-term infants, smaller volumes for smaller, less stable infants. Withdraw and infuse blood 2–3 mL/kg/min to avoid mechanical trauma to patient and donor cells. Complications include emboli, thromboses, hemodynamic instability, electrolyte disturbances, coagulopathy, infection, and death.

**Note** *CBC, reticulocyte count, peripheral smear, bilirubin, $Ca^{2+}$, glucose, total protein, infant blood type, Coombs test, and newborn screen should be performed on a pre-exchange sample of blood because they are of no diagnostic value on postexchange blood. If indicated, save pre-exchange blood for serologic or chromosome studies.*

### B. CONJUGATED HYPERBILIRUBINEMIA

1. **Definition:** Direct bilirubin is >2.0 mg/dL and is >10% of the total serum bilirubin.
2. **Etiology:** Biliary obstruction/atresia, choledochal cyst, hyperalimentation, $\alpha_1$-antitrypsin deficiency, hepatitis, sepsis, infections (especially urinary tract infections), hypothyroidism, inborn errors of metabolism, cystic fibrosis, red blood cell abnormalities.
3. **Management:** Phenobarbital for infants not on full feeds, ursodiol for infants on full feeds.

### C. POLYCYTHEMIA

1. **Definition:** Venous hematocrit >65% confirmed on two consecutive samples. May be falsely elevated when sample obtained by heel stick. Arterial hematocrit samples may be lower and should not be used for the evaluation of polycythemia.
2. **Etiology:** Delayed cord clamping; twin-twin transfusion; maternal-fetal transfusion; intrauterine hypoxia; trisomy 13, 18, or 21; Beckwith-Wiedemann syndrome; maternal gestational diabetes; neonatal thyrotoxicosis; and congenital adrenal hyperplasia.
3. **Clinical findings:** Plethora, respiratory distress, cardiac failure, tachypnea, hypoglycemia, irritability, lethargy, seizures, apnea, jitteriness, poor feeding, thrombocytopenia, hyperbilirubinemia.
4. **Complications:** Hyperviscosity predisposes to venous thrombosis and CNS injury. Hypoglycemia may result from increased erythrocyte utilization of glucose.
5. **Management:** Partial exchange transfusion for symptomatic infants with isovolemic replacement of blood with isotonic fluid. Blood is exchanged in 10- to 20-mL increments to reduce hematocrit to <55. (See Chapter 14 to calculate the amount of blood to be exchanged. Use birth weight (kg) × 90 for estimated blood volume.)

## X. GASTROINTESTINAL DISEASES

### A. NECROTIZING ENTEROCOLITIS

1. **Definition:** Serious intestinal inflammation and injury thought to be secondary to bowel ischemia, immaturity, and infection.
2. **Incidence:** More common in preterm infants (3%–4% of infants <2000 g) and African-American infants. Occurs principally in infants who have been fed. There is no gender predominance.
3. **Risk factors:** Prematurity, asphyxia, hypotension, polycythemia-hyperviscosity syndrome, umbilical vessel catheterization, exchange

TABLE 18-10

**CONSIDERATIONS IN BILIOUS EMESIS**

| | Bilious Emesis | |
|---|---|---|
| **Pathophysiology** | **Proximal Intestinal Obstruction** | **Distal Intestinal Obstruction** |
| Differential diagnosis | Duodenal atresia<br>Annular pancreas<br>Malrotation with or without volvulus<br>Jejunal obstruction/atresia | Ileal atresia<br>Meconium ileus<br>Colonic atresia<br>Meconium plug—hypoplastic left colon syndrome<br>Hirschsprung disease |
| Physical exam | Abdominal distention not prominent | Abdominal distention |
| Diagnosis | Abdominal x-ray: "Double bubble"<br>Upper GI series | Abdominal x-ray: Dilated loops of bowel<br>Contrast enema<br>Sweat test<br>Mucosal rectal biopsy |

**transfusion, bacterial and viral pathogens, enteral feeds, PDA, congestive heart failure, cyanotic heart disease, RDS, intra-uterine cocaine exposure.**

4. **Clinical findings:**
   a. Systemic: Temperature instability, apnea, bradycardia, metabolic acidosis, hypotension, disseminated intravascular coagulation.
   b. Intestinal: Elevated pregavage residuals with abdominal distention, blood in stool, absent bowel sounds, and/or abdominal tenderness or mass. Elevated pregavage residuals in the absence of other clinical symptoms rarely raise suspicion of NEC.
   c. Radiologic: Ileus, intestinal pneumatosis, portal vein gas, ascites, pneumoperitoneum.
5. **Management: No food or water by mouth, NG tube decompression, maintain adequate hydration and perfusion, antibiotics for 7–14 days, surgical consultation. Surgery is performed for signs of perforation or necrotic bowel.**

### B. BILIOUS EMESIS (Table 18-10)

Must eliminate malrotation as an etiology because its complication is a surgical emergency.

### C. ABDOMINAL WALL DEFECTS

Omphalocele and gastroschisis (Table 18-11).

## XI. NEUROLOGIC DISEASES

### A. INTRAVENTRICULAR HEMORRHAGE (IVH)

1. **Definition: Intracranial hemorrhage usually arising in the germinal matrix and periventricular regions of the brain.**

TABLE 18-11

DIFFERENCES BETWEEN OMPHALOCELE AND GASTROSCHISIS

| | Omphalocele | Gastroschisis |
|---|---|---|
| Position | Central abdominal | Right paraumbilical |
| Hernia sac | Present | Absent |
| Umbilical ring | Absent | Present |
| Umbilical cord insertion | At the vertex of the sac | Normal |
| Herniation of other viscera | Common | Rare |
| Extraintestinal anomalies | Frequent | Rare |
| Intestinal infarction, atresia | Less frequent | More frequent |



2. **Incidence:** About 30%–40% of infants weighing <1500 g; 50%–60% of infants weighing <1000 g. Highest incidence in first 72 hours of life, 60% within 24 hours, 85% within 72 hours, <5% after 1 week postnatal age.
3. **Diagnosis and classification:** Ultrasonography is used in diagnosis and classification of IVH. Routine screening is indicated in infants <32 weeks' gestational age within the first week of life and should be repeated in the second week. The grade is based on the maximum amount of hemorrhage seen by age 2 weeks.
   a. Grade I: Hemorrhage in germinal matrix only.
   b. Grade II: IVH without ventricular dilatation.
   c. Grade III: IVH with ventricular dilatation (30%–45% incidence of motor and cognitive impairment).
   d. Grade IV: IVH with periventricular hemorrhagic infarct (60%–80% incidence of motor and cognitive impairment).
4. **Prophylaxis:** Maintain acid-base balance and avoid fluctuations in blood pressure. Indomethacin is considered for IVH prophylaxis in some newborns (<28 weeks' gestation, birth weight <1250 g) and is most efficacious if given in the first 6 hours of life (see Formulary for dosage information).
5. **Outcome:** Infants with grade III and IV hemorrhages have a higher incidence of neurodevelopmental disabilities and an increased risk for posthemorrhagic hydrocephalus.

## B. PERIVENTRICULAR LEUKOMALACIA

1. **Definition and ultrasound findings:** Ischemic necrosis of periventricular white matter characterized by CNS depression within first week and ultrasound findings of cysts with or without ventricular enlargement caused by cerebral atrophy.
2. **Incidence:** More common in preterm infants but also occurs in term infants; 3.2% in infants <1500 g.
3. **Etiology:** Primarily ischemia-reperfusion injury, hypoxia, acidosis, hypoglycemia, acute hypotension, low cerebral blood flow.
4. **Outcome:** Commonly associated with cerebral palsy with or without sensory and cognitive deficit.

## C. NEONATAL SEIZURES (see Chapter 20).

## D. NEONATAL ABSTINENCE SYNDROME

Onset of symptoms usually occurs within the first 24–72 hr of life (methadone may delay symptoms until 96 hours or later). The duration of symptoms may last 8 weeks and persist for 4 months. Box 18-3 shows signs and symptoms of opiate withdrawal.

## E. PERIPHERAL NERVE INJURIES (Table 18-12)

1. **Etiology:** Result from lateral traction on the shoulder (vertex deliveries) or the head (breech deliveries).
2. **Clinical features** (see Table 18-12).
3. **Management:** Evaluate for associated trauma (clavicular and humeral fractures, shoulder dislocation, facial nerve injury, and cord injuries). Treatment includes immobilization for 7–10 days. Full recovery is seen in 85%–95% of cases in the first year of life.

BOX 18-3

OPIATE WITHDRAWAL

| | Signs and Symptoms of Opiate Withdrawal |
|---|---|
| W | Wakefulness |
| I | Irritability, insomnia |
| T | Tremors, temperature variation, tachypnea, twitching (jitteriness) |
| H | Hyperactivity, high-pitched cry, hiccoughs, hyperreflexia, hypertonia |
| D | Diarrhea (explosive), diaphoresis, disorganized suck |
| R | Rubmarks, respiratory distress, rhinorrhea, regurgitation |
| A | Apnea, autonomic dysfunction |
| W | Weight loss |
| A | Alkalosis (respiratory) |
| L | Lacrimation (photophobia), lethargy |
| S | Seizures, sneezing, stuffy nose, sweating, sucking (nonproductive) |

TABLE 18-12

PLEXUS INJURIES

| Plexus Injury | Spinal Level Involved | Clinical Features |
|---|---|---|
| Erb-Duchenne palsy (90% of cases) | C5 to C6 Occasionally involves C4 | Adduction and internal rotation of the arm. Forearm is pronated. Wrist is flexed. Diaphragm paralysis may occur if C4 is involved. |
| Total palsy (8%–9% of cases) | C5 to T1 Occasionally involves C4 | Upper arm, lower arm, and hand are involved. Horner syndrome (ptosis, anhydrosis, and miosis) exists if T1 is involved. |
| Klumpke paralysis (<2% of cases) | C7 to T1 | Hand flaccid with little control. Horner syndrome if T1 is involved. |

## XII. RETINOPATHY OF PREMATURITY (ROP)[8]

### A. DEFINITION

Interruption of the normal progression of retinal vascularization.

### B. ETIOLOGY

Exposure of the immature retina to high oxygen concentrations can result in vasoconstriction and obliteration of the retinal capillary network, followed by vasoproliferation. Risk is greatest in the most immature infant.

### C. DIAGNOSIS

All infants born ≤32 weeks' gestation, and any infant born weighing 1500–2000 g or at >32 weeks' gestation with an unstable clinical course, including those requiring cardiorespiratory support, should have a dilated funduscopic examination (Table 18-13).





### D. CLASSIFICATION

1. **Stage:**
   a. Stage 1: Demarcation line separates avascular from vascularized retina.
   b. Stage 2: Ridge forms along demarcation line.
   c. Stage 3: Extraretinal fibrovascular proliferation tissue forms on ridge.
   d. Stage 4: Partial retinal detachment.
   e. Stage 5: Total retinal detachment.
2. **Zone** (Fig. 18-8).
3. **Plus disease: Increased venous dilatation and arteriolar tortuosity of the posterior retinal vessels; may be present at any stage.**
4. **Number of clock hours or 30-degree sectors involved.**

### E. MANAGEMENT[9]

1. **Type 1 ROP: Peripheral retinal ablation should be considered. Type 1 ROP is classified as:**
   a. Zone I, any stage ROP with plus disease.
   b. Zone I, stage 3 ROP with or without plus disease.
   c. Zone II, stage 2 or 3 ROP with plus disease.

TABLE 18-13

**TIMING OF FIRST RETINAL EXAMINATION BASED ON GESTATIONAL AGE AT BIRTH**

| Gestational Age at Birth (wk) | Recommended Age for Initial Exam—Postmenstrual Age (wk) |
|---|---|
| ≥27 | 31 |
| 28 | 32 |
| 29 | 33 |
| 30 | 34 |
| 31 | 35 |
| 32 | 36 |

Modified from American Academy of Pediatrics: Screening examination of premature infants for retionpathy of prematurity, AAP Policy statement. Pediatrics 2006;117(2):572–576.

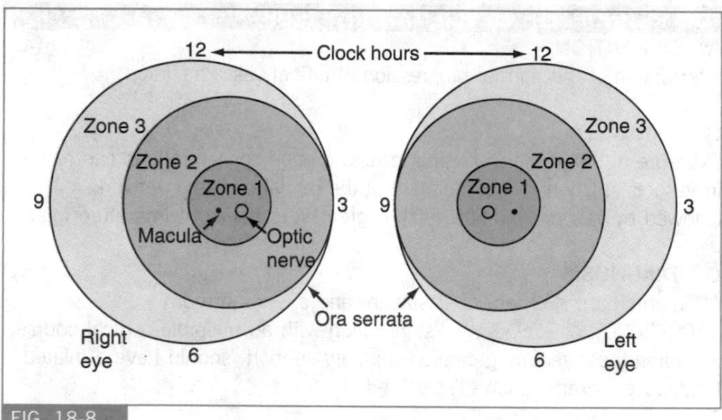


FIG. 18-8

Zones of the retina. *(From American Academy of Pediatries: Screening examination of premature infants for retinopathy of prematurity, AAP Policy Statement. Pediatrics 2006;117(2):572–576.)*

TABLE 18-14

**SUGGESTED SCHEDULE FOR FOLLOW-UP OPHTHALMOLOGIC EXAM IN RETINOPAHTY OF PREMATURITY**

| ≤1 week | 1–2 weeks | 2 weeks | 2–3 weeks |
|---|---|---|---|
| Stage 1 or 2 ROP: zone I<br>Stage 3 ROP: zone II | Immature vascularization: zone I, no ROP<br>Stage 2 ROP: zone II<br>Regressing ROP: zone I | Stage 1 ROP: zone II<br>Regressing ROP: zone II | Immature vascularization: zone II, no ROP<br>Stage 1 or 2 ROP: zone III<br>Regressing ROP: zone III |

*Note:* The presence of plus disease in Zone I or II indicates that peripheral ablation, rather than observation, is appropriate.

From American Academy of Pediatrics: Screening examination of premature infants for retinopathy of prematurity, AAP Policy statement: Pediatrics 2006;117(2):572–576.

2. **Type 2 ROP: Serial examinations instead of retinal ablation should be considered. Type 2 ROP is classified as:**
a. Zone I, stage 1 or 2 ROP without plus disease.
b. Zone II, stage 3 ROP without plus disease.
3. **Follow-up** (Table 18-14).

## XIII. CONGENITAL INFECTIONS

See Chapter 17.

## REFERENCES

1. Wiswell TE et al: Delivery room management of the apparently vigorous meconium-stained neonate: Results of the multicenter, international collaborative trial. Pediatrics 2000;105:1–7.

2. Apgar V: A proposal for new method of evaluation of the newborn infant. Anesth Analg 1953;32:260–267.
3. Ballard JL et al: New Ballard Score, expanded to include extremely premature infants. J Pediatr 1991;119:417–423.
4. Cornblath M: Neonatal hypoglycemia. In Donn SM, Fisher CW (eds): Risk Management Techniques in Perinatal and Neonatal Practice. Armonk, NY, Futura, 1996.
5. American Academy of Pediatrics: Clinical Practice Guideline. Pediatrics 2004;114:297–316.
6. Klaus MH, Fanaroff AA: Care of the High-Risk Neonate, 4th ed. Philadelphia, WB Saunders, 1993.
7. American Academy of Pediatrics: Subcommittee on Hyperbilirubinemia: Management of hyperbilirubinemia in the newborn infant 35 or more weeks of gestation. Pediatrics 2004;114(1):297–316. Erratum in Pediatrics 2004;114(4):1138.
8. Ben-Sira I et al: An international classification of retinopathy of prematurity. Pediatrics 1984;74:127–133.
9. Good WV: Early Treatment for Retinopathy of Prematurity Cooperative Group. Arch Ophthalmol 2003;121:1684–1694.

# Nephrology

*Jade M. Tan, MD*

19

## I. URINALYSIS, URINE DIPSTICK

Best if urine specimen is evaluated within 1 hr after voiding, ideally after the first morning void.

### A. COLOR

Normal urine: Varies in color from almost colorless to dark yellow or amber and is clear. Appears red or dark in the brick-dust phenomenon, due to precipitation of urates present in infant's urine.

### B. TURBIDITY

Cloudy urine: Can be normal; is most often the result of crystal formation at room temperature. Uric acid crystals form in acidic urine, and phosphate crystals form in alkaline urine. Cellular material and bacteria can also cause turbidity.

### C. SPECIFIC GRAVITY

1. **Normal findings:** Normal specific gravity is between 1.003 and 1.030.
2. **Measurement:** Measured in a refractometer and requires one drop of urine; is based on the principle that the refractive index (RI) of a solution is related to the content of dissolved solids present. RI varies with, but is not identical to, specific gravity. The refractometer measures RI but is calibrated for specific gravity. Glucose, abundant protein, and iodine containing contrast materials can give falsely high readings.

### D. PH

Estimated using indicator paper or dipstick. To improve accuracy, use a freshly voided specimen and pH meter. Levels can be inappropriately high with hypokalemia. Urine pH can also be used to assess various types of renal tubular acidosis (Table 19-1).

### E. PROTEIN

See Section VI.B and related figures.

1. **Normal values in a 24-hour urine collection:** <4 mg of protein/m²/hr; significant: 4–40 mg/m²/hr; nephrotic range: >40 mg/m²/hr.[1]
2. Assess completeness of 24-hour collection by simultaneously measuring urine creatinine (Cr): ≥15 mg/kg body weight in a 24-hour collection.

### F. SUGARS

1. **Normal urine:** Does not contain sugars. Glucosuria is suggestive but not diagnostic of diabetes mellitus or proximal renal tubular disease

TABLE 19-1

BIOCHEMICAL AND CLINICAL CHARACTERISTICS OF THE VARIOUS TYPES OF RENAL TUBULAR ACIDOSIS

| | Distal (Type 1) | Type 1 With $HCO_3^-$ Wasting | Proximal (Type 2) | Hyperkalemic (Type 4) |
|---|---|---|---|---|
| **AT SUBNORMAL ($HCO_3^-$)*** | | | | |
| Minimal urine pH | >5.5 | >5.5 | <5.5 | <5.5 |
| Urinary citrate excretion | ↓ | ↓ | ↑ | ? |
| Plasma $K^+$ concentration | Normal or ↓ | Normal or ↓ | Usually ↓ | ↑ |
| Urine anion gap† | Positive | Positive | Positive or ? negative | Positive |
| **AT NORMAL ($HCO_3^-$)** | | | | |
| Plasma $K^+$ concentration | Normal | Normal | Normal or ↓ | Normal or ↑ |
| Therapeutic alkali requirement (mEq/kg/day) | 1–3 | 5–10 | 5–20 | 1–5 |
| Nephrocalcinosis/ nephrolithiasis | Common | Common | Rare | Absent |

*Plasma bicarbonate concentration.

†Urine anion gap = $[Na^+] + [K^+] - [Cl^-]$ (based on urine electrolytes).

From Holliday MA et al: Pediatric Nephrology. Baltimore, Williams & Wilkins, 1994, p 650.

(see section IV.B). The presence of other reducing sugars can be confirmed by chromatography.

2. **Dipstick:** Easiest method, but only detects glucose. False-negative results occur with high levels of ascorbic acid (used as preservative in antibiotics) in urine.
3. **Clinitest tablet (Ames Co.):** Nonspecific test; changes color if urine is positive for reducing substances, including reducing sugars (glucose, fructose, galactose, pentoses, lactose), amino acids, ascorbic acid, chloral hydrate, chloramphenicol, Cr, cysteine, glucuronates, hippurate, homogentisic acid, isoniazid, acetoacetic acid, acetone, nitrofurantoin, oxalate, total parenteral nutrition, penicillin, salicylates, streptomycin, sulfonamides, tetracycline, and uric acid. Because sucrose is not a reducing sugar, it is not detected by Clinitest.

## G. KETONES

1. **Ketoacidosis:** Except for trace amounts, ketonuria suggests ketoacidosis, usually from diabetes mellitus or catabolism induced by inadequate intake. Neonatal ketoacidosis may occur with a metabolic defect, such as propionic acidemia, methylmalonic aciduria, or a glycogen storage disease.

TABLE 19-2

URINALYSIS FOR BILIRUBIN/UROBILINOGEN

| | Normal | Hemolytic Disease | Hepatic Disease | Biliary Obstruction |
|---|---|---|---|---|
| Urine urobilinogen | Normal | Increased | Increased | Decreased |
| Urine bilirubin | Negative | Negative | +/− | Positive |

2. **Dipstick:** Detects acetoacetic acid best, acetone less well; does not detect β-hydroxybutyrate. False-positive results may occur after phthalein administration or with phenylketonuria.
3. **Acetest tablet (Ames Co.):** Detects only acetoacetic acid and acetone.

### H. HEMOGLOBIN, MYOGLOBIN

Dipstick reads positive with intact red blood cells (RBCs), hemoglobin, and myoglobin and can detect as few as 3–4 RBCs per high-power field (hpf). False-positive results can occur with the presence of bacterial peroxidases, high ascorbic acid concentrations, and povidone-iodine (Betadine) (i.e., from fingers of medical staff).

### I. BILIRUBIN, UROBILINOGEN

Dipstick measures each individually.

1. **Urine bilirubin:** Will be positive with conjugated hyperbilirubinemia; in this form, bilirubin is water soluble and excreted by the kidney.
2. **Urobilinogen:** Will be increased in cases of hyperbilirubinemia in which there is no obstruction to enterohepatic circulation (Table 19-2).

## II. URINALYSIS, MICROSCOPY

### A. RBCs

1. **Normal values:** Centrifuged urine usually contains <5 RBCs/hpf. Significant hematuria is 5–10 RBCs/hpf and corresponds to a Chemstrip reading of 50 RBCs/hpf or Labstix reading *trace hemolyzed* or *small.* Microscopy is used to differentiate hemoglobinuria or myoglobinuria from hematuria (intact RBCs). Examination of RBC morphology by phase-contrast microscopy may help to localize source of bleeding. Dysmorphic, small RBCs suggest a glomerular origin; normal RBCs suggest lower tract bleeding.
2. **Differentiation between hemoglobinuria and myoglobinuria:**

a. History: Hemoglobinuria is seen with intravascular hemolysis or in hematuric urine that has been standing for extended period. Myoglobinuria is seen in crush injuries, vigorous exercise, major motor seizures, fever and malignant hyperthermia, electrocution, snake bites, ischemia, some muscle and metabolic disorders, and some infections such as influenza.

b. Laboratory studies: Clinical laboratories may use many techniques to measure hemoglobin or myoglobin directly. Other laboratory data may also be used to indirectly identify the source of urinary pigment. For example, in nephropathy from myoglobinuria, the blood urea nitrogen (BUN)/Cr ratio is low (Cr is released from damaged muscles), and the creatine kinase level is high.

3. **Suggested evaluation of persistent hematuria:** See section VI.A and related figures.

### B. SEDIMENT

Using light microscopy, unstained, centrifuged urine can be examined for formed elements, including casts, cells, and crystals.

### C. EPITHELIAL CELLS

Squamous epithelial cells (>10 per low-power field) are useful as an index of possible contamination by vaginal secretions in females or by foreskin in uncircumcised males.

### D. WHITE BLOOD CELLS (WBCs)

>5 WBCs/hpf of properly spun urine specimen is suggestive of a urinary tract infection (UTI). Sterile pyuria is rare in the pediatric population. If present, it is usually transient and accompanies systemic disorder (e.g., Kawasaki disease). May also be a sign of urolithiasis.

### E. BACTERIA, URINE GRAM STAIN

Gram stain is used to screen for UTIs. One organism per high-power field in uncentrifuged urine represents at least $10^5$ colonies/mL.

## III. EVALUATION AND MANAGEMENT OF UTIs[2,3]

AAP Recommendations:[4] (1) The presence of UTI should be considered in infants and young children 2 months to 2 years of age with unexplained fever. (2) If an infant or young child 2 months to 2 years of age with unexplained fever is assessed as being sufficiently ill to warrant immediate antimicrobial therapy, a urine specimen should be obtained by suprapubic aspiration or transurethral bladder catheterization. (3) If an infant or young child 2 months to 2 years of age with unexplained fever is assessed as not being so ill as to require immediate antimicrobial therapy, two options exist: (a) Obtain urine culture by suprapubic aspiration or catheterization. (b) Obtain urine specimen for urinalysis by most convenient method. If urinalysis suggests UTI, obtain urine culture by suprapubic aspiration or catheterization. If urinalysis does not suggest UTI, it is reasonable to follow clinical course without antimicrobial therapy, recognizing that a negative urinalysis does not rule out UTI. (4) Diagnosis of a UTI requires a culture of the urine.

**Note** *These recommendations are suggestions and vary from institution to institution and physician to physician. Use them together with the routinely practiced guidelines of your institution.*

## A. HISTORY

Voiding history (stool, urine) with stream characteristics in toilet-trained children, sexual intercourse, sexual abuse, circumcision, masturbation, pinworms, prolonged baths, bubble baths, evaluation of growth curve, recent antibiotic use, and family history of vesicoureteral reflux (VUR), recurrent UTIs, or chronic kidney disease.

## B. PHYSICAL EXAMINATION

Vital signs, especially blood pressure (BP); abdominal examination for flank masses, bowel distention, evidence of impaction; meatal stenosis or circumcision in males; vulvovaginitis or labial adhesions in females; neurologic examination of lower extremities; perineal sensation and reflexes; rectal and sacral examination (for anteriorly placed anus).

## C. LABORATORY STUDIES

Urinalysis with microscopic examination and urine culture (Table 19-3).

**Note** *All tests must be confirmed with a urine culture. Also helpful if available are the studies that follow.*

TABLE 19-3

URINALYSIS WITH MICROSCOPIC EXAMINATION AND URINE CULTURE

| Method of Collection | Colony Count (Pure Culture) | Probability of Infection (%) |
|---|---|---|
| Suprapubic aspiration | Gram-negative bacilli: Any number | >99 |
| | Gram-positive cocci: More than a few thousand | |
| Transurethral catheterization | >100,000 | 95 |
| | 10,000–100,000 | Infection likely |
| | 1000–10,000 | Suspicious; repeat |
| | <1000 | Infection unlikely |
| Clean-voided (boy) | >10,000 | Infection likely |
| Clean-voided (girl) | 3 specimens >100,000 | 95 |
| | 2 specimens >100,000 | 90 |
| | 1 specimen >100,000 | 80 |
| | 50,000–100,000 | Suspicious; repeat |
| | 10,000–50,000 | Symptomatic, suspicious; repeat |
| | 10,000–50,000 | Asymptomatic; infection unlikely |
| | <10,000 | Infection unlikely |

1. **Nitrite test:** Detects nitrites produced by the reduction of dietary nitrates by urinary gram-negative bacteria (especially *Escherichia coli* and *Klebsiella* and *Proteus* spp.). A positive test is virtually diagnostic of UTI. False-negative results can occur with inadequate dietary nitrates, insufficient time for bacterial proliferation, inability of bacteria to reduce nitrates to nitrites (many gram-positive organisms such as *Enterococcus* and *Mycobacterium* spp. and fungi), and large volumes of dilute urine.
2. **Leukocyte esterase test:** Detects esterases released from broken-down leukocytes, an indirect test for WBCs that may or may not be present with a UTI.
3. **BUN/Cr ratio.**

### D. CULTURE-POSITIVE UTI

Treatment: Based on urine culture and sensitivities if possible; for empirical therapy, see Chapter 17.

1. **Upper versus lower UTI: Differentiating pyelonephritis (upper UTI) from cystitis (lower UTI) is a clinical diagnosis suggested by the presence of fever, systemic symptoms, and costovertebral angle tenderness. Fever that persists for >48 hr after initiating appropriate antibiotics is suggestive of pyelonephritis. Although $^{99m}$Tc-dimercaptosuccinic acid (DMSA) is the "gold standard" to diagnose pyelonephritis, infants with febrile UTI are assumed to have pyelonephritis without diagnosis and are treated as such.**

a. Organisms: 75%–90% of pediatric UTIs are caused by E. coli. Other common pathogens include Klebsiella and Proteus spp., Staphylococcus saprophyticus, and S. aureus. Group B streptococci and other blood-borne pathogens are important in neonatal UTIs, whereas enterococcus and pseudomonal species are more prevalent in abnormal hosts (i.e., recurrent UTI, abnormal anatomy, neurogenic bladder, hospitalized patients, or those with frequent catheterizations).

b. Treatment considerations:

(1) Hospitalize all febrile children <4 weeks of age and treat with IV antibiotics due to risk for bacteremia and meningitis.

(2) Oral treatment is equally efficacious to 3 days of parenteral antibiotics followed by 11 days of oral antibiotics.

(3) American Academy of Pediatrics (AAP) recommends parenteral antibiotics for children who are toxic, dehydrated, and unable to tolerate oral medication due to vomiting or noncompliance. AAP also recommends 7–14 days of treatment for all UTIs.[4] Studies comparing duration are inconclusive, but experts recommend 7–10 days for uncomplicated cases and 14 days for toxic children and those with pyelonephritis (any febrile UTI).

c. Inadequate response to therapy: Repeat urine culture in children with expected response is controversial and thought to be unnecessary by AAP. A repeat culture, as well as renal ultrasound, to rule out abscess or obstruction is indicated in children with poor response to therapy. Repeat cultures should also be considered in patients with recurrent UTIs to rule out persistent bacteruria.

d. Antibiotic prophylaxis (Table 19-4): Low-dose antibiotic prophylaxis recommended in all children with diagnosed VUR and obstructive disease as well as in children pending evaluation with renal ultrasound and voiding cystourethrogram (VCUG). Prophylaxis in children with recurrent infections but normal anatomy is controversial and is based on individualized decisions.

2. **Imaging studies[4,5] (Fig. 19-1):**

a. **Indications:** Renal ultrasound and VCUG to rule out obstructive disease or VUR should be done in all male patients with their first UTI, all female patients <5 years of age, and all children with recurrent UTI. Infants and young children who do not demonstrate expected clinical response within 2 days of antimicrobial therapy should undergo ultrasound promptly and either VCUG or radionuclide cystography (RNC) at earliest convenient time. Infants and young children who have the expected response to antimicrobials should have a sonogram and either VCUG or RNC performed at earliest convenient time.

b. **Abdominal radiograph:** If indicated to check stool pattern and to rule out spinal dysraphism.

c. **Renal sonography:** A noninvasive, nonionizing evaluation for gross structural defects, obstructive lesions, positional abnormalities, and renal size and growth. Indications regarding appropriate use remain controversial.

d. **VCUG:** Performed when asymptomatic and cleared of bacteriuria. May be substituted with RNC, which has 1/100 the radiation exposure of VCUG and increased sensitivity for transient reflux. RNC does not visualize urethral anatomy, is not sensitive for low-grade reflux, and cannot grade reflux.

TABLE 19-4

ANTIBIOTIC PROPHYLAXIS

| Grade | Age (yr) | Scarring | Initial Treatment | Follow-up Treatment Considerations for Refractory Disease |
|---|---|---|---|---|
| I–II | Any | Yes/no | Antibiotic prophylaxis | No consensus |
| III–IV | 0–5 | Yes/no | Antibiotic prophylaxis | Surgery |
| III–IV | 6–10 | Yes/no | Unilateral: Antibiotic prophylaxis<br>Bilateral: Surgery | Surgery |
| V | <1 | Yes/no | Antibiotic prophylaxis | Surgery |
| V | 1–5 | No | Unilateral: Antibiotic prophylaxis | Surgery |
| V | 1–5 | No | Bilateral: Surgery | |
| V | 1–5 | Yes | Surgery | |
| V | 6–10 | Yes/no | Surgery | |

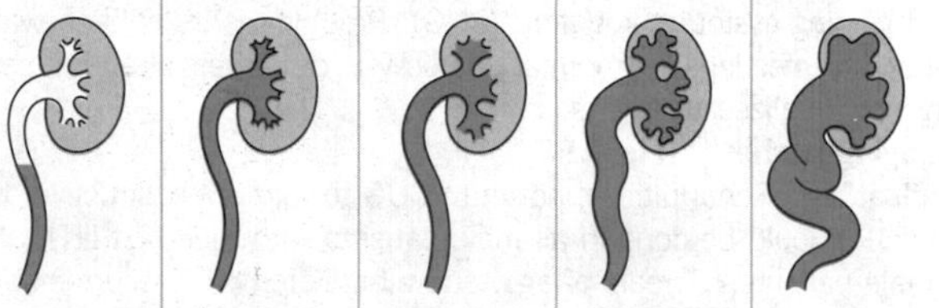

| Grade I | Grade II | Grade III | Grade IV | Grade V |
|---|---|---|---|---|
| Ureter only | Ureter, pelvis, calyces; no dilatation, normal calyceal fornices | Mild or moderate dilatation and/or tortuosity of ureter; mild or moderate dilatation of the pelvis, but no or slight blunting of the fornices | Moderate dilatation and/or tortuosity of the ureter; mild dilatation of renal pelvis and calyces; complete obliteration of sharp angle of fornices, but maintenance of papillary impressions in majority of calyces | Gross dilatation and tortuosity of ureter; gross dilatation of renal pelvis and calyces; papillary impressions are no longer visible in majority of calyces |

FIG. 19-1

International classification of vesicoureteral reflux. *(Modified from Rushton H: Urinary tract infections in children: Epidemiology, evaluation, and management. Pediatr Clin North Am 1997:44:5 and International Reflux Committee: Medical vs. surgical treatment of primary vesicoureteral reflux: Report of the International Reflux Study Committee. Pediatrics 1981;67:392.)*

e. **DMSA:** $^{99m}$Tc-DMSA scan can detect areas of decreased uptake that may represent acute pyelonephritis or renal scarring; does not differentiate between the two. Routine use not recommended; may be indicated in patients with an abnormal VCUG or renal sonography, in patients with history of asymptomatic bacteriuria and fever or prenatally diagnosed VUR, and in neonates and infants secondary to high incidence of hematologic spread and difficult examination. Repeat in 3–6 months if initial study is positive to evaluate for persistent infection and renal scarring.

f. **DTPA/MAG-3:** May also be used for indications given for DMSA use. Provides quantitative assessment of renal function and drainage of dilated collecting system, as in cases of hydronephrosis in the absence of VUR or ureteropelvic junction obstruction.

3. **Asymptomatic bacteriuria:** Defined as bacteria in urine on microscopy and Gram stain in an afebrile, asymptomatic patient without pyuria. Antibiotics not necessary if voiding habits and urinary tract are normal. Prophylaxis may be necessary in patients with bacteriuria and voiding dysfunction. DMSA may be helpful in differentiating pyelonephritis from fever and coincidental bacteriuria.
4. **Nonsurgical management of VUR:**[4,5] Amoxicillin recommended in first 2 months of life, otherwise trimethoprim-sulfamethoxazole or nitrofurantoin with urine cultures every 4 months and when febrile. No need to discontinue antibiotics before screening urine culture. Change antibiotic therapy if patient has breakthrough UTIs while on prophylactic regimen. Repeat VCUG in 12–18 months to determine whether VUR has resolved. Surgical correction is indicated in children >2 years of age with high-grade reflux (grades IV or V) and children with breakthrough pyelonephritis (especially with DMSA changes) while on prophylaxis.
5. **Referral to pediatric urology:** Consider referral in children with abnormal voiding function on imaging, neurogenic bladder, abnormal anatomy (grade 3 VUR or higher), recurrent UTI, or poor response to appropriate antibiotics.



## IV. RENAL FUNCTION TESTS

### A. TESTS OF GLOMERULAR FUNCTION

1. **Creatinine clearance (Ccr):**

a. Timed urine specimen: Standard measure of glomerular filtration rate (GFR); closely approximates inulin clearance in the normal range of GFR. When GFR is low, Ccr is greater than inulin clearance. Usually inaccurate in children with obstructive uropathy or problems with bladder emptying.

$$\text{Ccr (mL/min/1.73 m}^2\text{)} = (\text{U} \times [\text{V/P}]) \times 1.73/\text{BSA}$$

where U (mg/dL) = urinary creatinine concentration; V (mL/min) = total urine volume (mL) divided by the duration of the collection (min) (24 hours = 1440 min); P (mg/dL) = serum creatinine concentration (may average two levels) and BSA (m2) = body surface area.

b. Estimated GFR from plasma creatinine: Useful when a timed specimen cannot be collected; reasonable estimate of GFR for children with relatively normal renal function and body habitus. If habitus is markedly abnormal or precise measurement of GFR is needed, more standard methods of measuring GFR must be used.

$$\text{Estimated GFR (mL/min/1.73 m}^2\text{)} = \text{kL/Pcr}$$

where k = proportionality constant; L = height (cm); Pcr = plasma creatinine (mg/dL) (Table 19-5).

TABLE 19-5

PROPORTIONALITY CONSTANT FOR CALCULATING GLOMERULAR FILTRATION RATE

| Age | *k* Values |
|---|---|
| Low birth weight during first year of life | 0.33 |
| Term AGA during first year of life | 0.45 |
| Children and adolescent girls | 0.55 |
| Adolescent boys | 0.70 |

AGA, appropriate for gestational age.

From Schwartz GJ et al: The use of plasma creatinine concentration for estimating glomerular filtration rate in infants, children, and adolescents. Pediatr Clin North Am 1987;34:571.

TABLE 19-6

NORMAL VALUES OF GLOMERULAR FILTRATION RATE

| Age | GFR (Mean) (mL/min/1.73 m$^2$) | Range (mL/min/1.73 m$^2$) |
|---|---|---|
| Neonates <34 wk gestational age | | |
| 2–8 days | 11 | 11–15 |
| 4–28 days | 20 | 15–28 |
| 30–90 days | 50 | 40–65 |
| Neonates >34 wk gestational age | | |
| 2–8 days | 39 | 17–60 |
| 4–28 days | 47 | 26–68 |
| 30–90 days | 58 | 30–86 |
| 1–6 mo | 77 | 39–114 |
| 6–12 mo | 103 | 49–157 |
| 12–19 mo | 127 | 62–191 |
| 2 yr–adult | 127 | 89–165 |

From Holliday MA et al: Pediatric Nephrology. Baltimore, Williams & Wilkins, 1994, p 1306.

2. **Glomerular function as determined by nuclear medicine scans: Normal values of GFR (measured by inulin clearance) are shown in Table 19-6.**

## B. TESTS OF TUBULAR FUNCTION

### 1. Proximal tubule:

a. Proximal tubule reabsorption: Proximal tubule is responsible for reabsorption of electrolytes, glucose, and amino acids. Studies to determine proximal tubular function compare urine and blood levels of specific compounds, arriving at a percentage of tubular reabsorption (Tx):

$$Tx = 1 - [(Ux/Px)/(Ucr/Pcr)] \times 100\%$$

where Ux = concentration of compound in urine; Px = concentration of compound in plasma; Ucr = concentration of creatinine in urine; Pcr = concentration of creatinine in plasma. This formula can be used for amino acids, electrolytes, calcium, and phosphorus.

b. Calculation of fractional excretion of sodium (FENa) is derived from the previous equation:

$$FENa = [(UNa/PNa)/(UCr/PCr)] \times 100\%$$

FENa is usually <1% in prerenal azotemia or glomerulonephritis and is >1% (usually >3%) in acute tubular necrosis (ATN) or postrenal azotemia. Recent diuretic use may give inaccurate results.

c. Glucose reabsorption: Glucose threshold is plasma glucose concentration at which significant amounts of glucose appear in urine. Glucosuria must be interpreted in relation to simultaneously determined plasma glucose concentration. If plasma glucose concentration is <120 mg/dL, and glucose is present in urine, this implies incompetent tubular reabsorption of glucose and proximal renal tubular disease.

d. Bicarbonate reabsorption: Majority occurs in proximal tubule. Abnormalities in reabsorption lead to type 2 renal tubular acidosis (RTA; see Table 19-1).



**2. Distal tubule:**

a. Urine acidification: A urine acidification defect (distal RTA) should be suspected when random urine pH values are >6 in the presence of moderate systemic metabolic acidosis. Confirm acidification defects by simultaneous venous or arterial pH, plasma bicarbonate concentration, and pH meter (not dipstick) determination of the pH of fresh urine.

b. Urine concentration occurs in the distal tubule:[6] A random urine specific gravity of ≥1.023 indicates intact concentrating ability within limits of clinical testing; no further tests are indicated. A first-voided specimen after an overnight fast is adequate to test concentrating ability. (For more formal testing, see the water deprivation test in Chapter 10.)

c. Urine calcium: Hypercalciuria is seen usually with distal RTA, vitamin D intoxication, hyperparathyroidism, immobilization, excessive calcium intake, and use of steroids or loop diuretics. May be idiopathic (associated with hematuria and renal calculi). Diagnosis is as follows:

(1) 24-hour urine: Calcium >4 mg/kg/24 hr.

(2) Spot urine: Determine calcium to creatinine (Ca/Cr) ratio. Follow up abnormally elevated spot urine Ca/Cr ratio with a 24-hr urine calcium determination (Table 19-7).

TABLE 19-7

**AGE-ADJUSTED CALCIUM/CREATININE RATIOS**

| Age | $Ca^{2+}/Cr$ Ratio (mg/mg) (95th Percentile for Age) |
|---|---|
| <7 mo | 0.86 |
| 7–18 mo | 0.60 |
| 19 mo–6 yr | 0.42 |
| Adults | 0.22 |

From Sargent JD et al: Normal values for random urinary calcium to creatinine ratios in infancy. J Pediatr 1993;123:393.

## V. TUBULAR DISORDERS[7-12]

### A. RENAL TUBULAR ACIDOSIS

A group of transport defects in the reabsorption of bicarbonate ($HCO_3^-$) the excretion of hydrogen ions ($H^+$), or both, which results in abnormal urine acidification. Results in a persistent **nonanion gap metabolic acidosis accompanied by hyperchloremia.** The RTA syndromes often do not progress to renal failure but are instead characterized by a normal GFR. Clinical presentation is characterized by failure to thrive, polyuria, constipation, vomiting, and dehydration (see Table 19-1).

### B. TYPE 1 (DISTAL) RTA

1. **Etiology:** May be hereditary or secondary to a systemic disorder (e.g., obstructive uropathy, sickle cell nephropathy, toxins). The defect is in hydrogen ion secretion in the distal renal tubules, resulting in 15% of filtered sodium bicarbonate being lost in the urine.
2. **Laboratory findings:** Hyperchloremic metabolic acidosis, mild hypokalemia, and alkaline urine. Characteristically complicated by hypercalciuria progressing to nephrocalcinosis and nephrolithiasis (urine $Ca^{2+}$/Cr >0.21 mg/mg).
3. **Treatment:** 1–3 mEq/kg/day $NaHCO_3$ (Bicitra or Polycitra), a characteristic that distinguishes it from type 2 RTA.

### C. TYPE 2 (PROXIMAL) RTA

1. **Etiology:** May be hereditary (part of Fanconi syndrome) or a secondary process (tubular immaturity in premature infants). The defect is in the proximal tubule, caused by a lowering of the renal threshold for bicarbonate reabsorption (requires a lower serum pH to trigger bicarbonate reabsorption from the urine).
2. **Laboratory findings:** Hyperchloremic metabolic acidosis and hypokalemia.

### D. TYPE 3 (COMBINED PROXIMAL AND DISTAL) RTA

Infants with mild type 1 and mild type 2 defects were previously classified as type 3 RTA. Studies have shown that this is not a genetic entity itself; has resulted in reclassification as a subtype of type 1 RTA that occurs primarily in premature infants.

### E. TYPE 4 RTA (MINERALOCORTICOID DEFICIENCY, ALDOSTERONE DEPENDENT)

1. **Etiology:** Due to absolute mineralocorticoid deficiency or resistance (e.g., adrenal failure, congenital adrenal hyperplasia, diabetes mellitus, pseudohypoaldosteronism, interstitial nephritis).
2. **Laboratory findings:** Hyperchloremic acidosis and distinguishing hyperkalemia. Nephrocalcinosis is rare.

3. **Treatment:** 1–4 mEq/kg/day of Bicitra or Polycitra; potassium-sparing drugs are discontinued. Fludrocortisone (0.05–0.15 mg/m²/day) may be added, as well as potassium binders.

### F. FANCONI SYNDROME

A generalized dysfunction of the proximal tubule resulting not only in bicarbonate loss, but also in variable wasting of phosphate, glucose, and amino acids. May be hereditary, as in cystinosis and galactosemia, or acquired through toxin injury and other immunologic factors. Clinically characterized by rickets and impaired growth.

## VI. CLINICAL MANIFESTATIONS OF RENAL DISEASE



### A. HEMATURIA[1,7,8,13–17]

1. **Gross hematuria:** Bright red blood, clots in urine, or tea-colored urine.
2. **Microscopic hematuria:** >5 RBCs/hpf on more than two occasions. Significant or persistent hematuria: Three positive urinalyses, based on dipstick and microscopic examination, over a 2- to 3-week period.
3. **Etiology:** Gross hematuria occurs with kidney stones, trauma, and arteriovenous malformations. Can also occur with ATN and renal vein thrombosis. Asymptomatic hematuria alone, without proteinuria, is often not indicative of significant kidney disease; however, a number of glomerular diseases, including immunoglobulin A (IgA) nephropathy and Alport nephritis, can present with recurrent gross hematuria.
4. **Suggested evaluation of persistent hematuria** (Fig. 19-2):
   a. Examination of urine sediment, urine dipstick for protein, urine culture, sickle cell screen, urine Ca/Cr ratio, family history, medication history, and audiology screen if indicated.
   b. Serum electrolytes, BUN, serum Cr, serum total protein and albumin, complete blood count (CBC) with smear, immunoglobulins, and hepatitis serologies; consider testing for human immunodeficiency virus (HIV).
   c. ASO titers, C3, C4, and antinuclear antibodies (ANAs)
   d. Renal ultrasonography and other indicated radiologic studies.
5. **Management algorithm** (Fig. 19-3).

### B. PROTEINURIA[7–8]

1. **More likely than hematuria to indicate significant renal disease.** Protein can be found in the urine of healthy children, with a reasonable upper limit being 150 mg/24 hr (4 mg/m²/hr).
2. **Detection:** Commonly detected by dipstick with results of negative, trace, 1+ (~30 mg/dL), 2+ (~100 mg/dL), 3+ (~300 mg/dL), and 4+ (>2000 mg/dL). Dipstick is useful primarily for albuminuria; not an accurate measure of protein excretion. Persistent proteinuria should be precisely quantified by a timed 24-hr urine collection (Table 19-8). If unable to obtain, a timed urine excretion can be

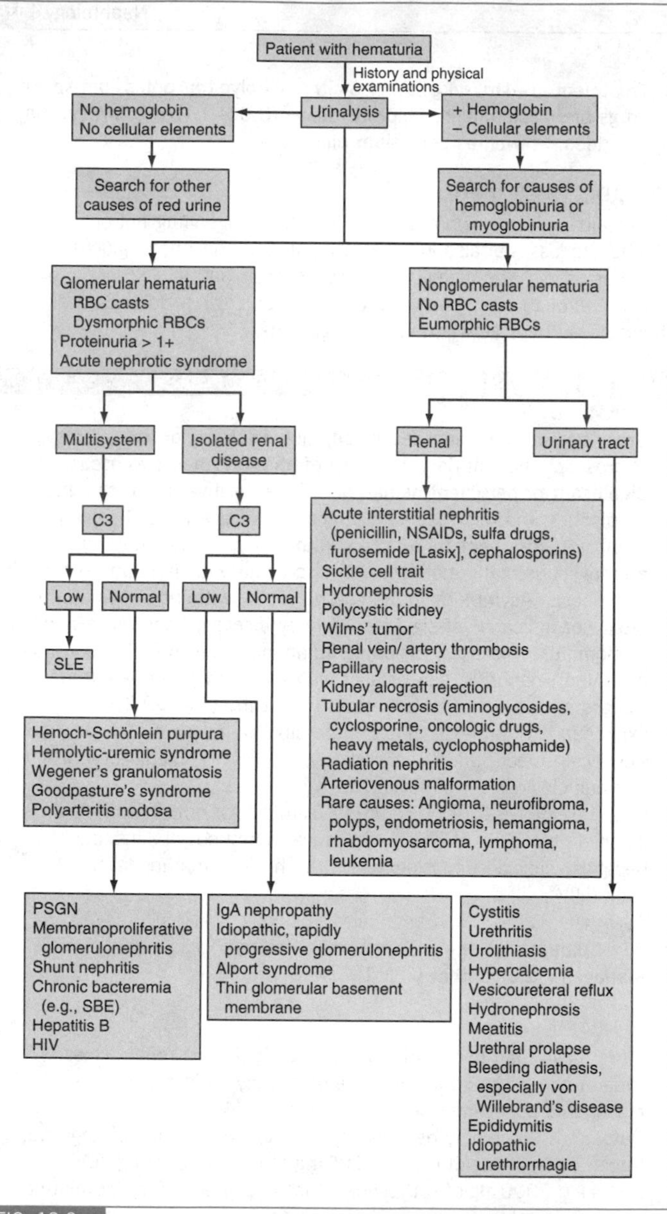


FIG. 19-2

A diagnostic strategy for hematuria. HIV, human immunodeficiency virus; NSAIDs, nonsteroidal anti-inflammatory drugs; PSGN, poststreptococcal glomerulonephritis; RBC, red blood cell; SBE, subacute bacterial endocarditis; SLE, systemic lupus erythematosus.

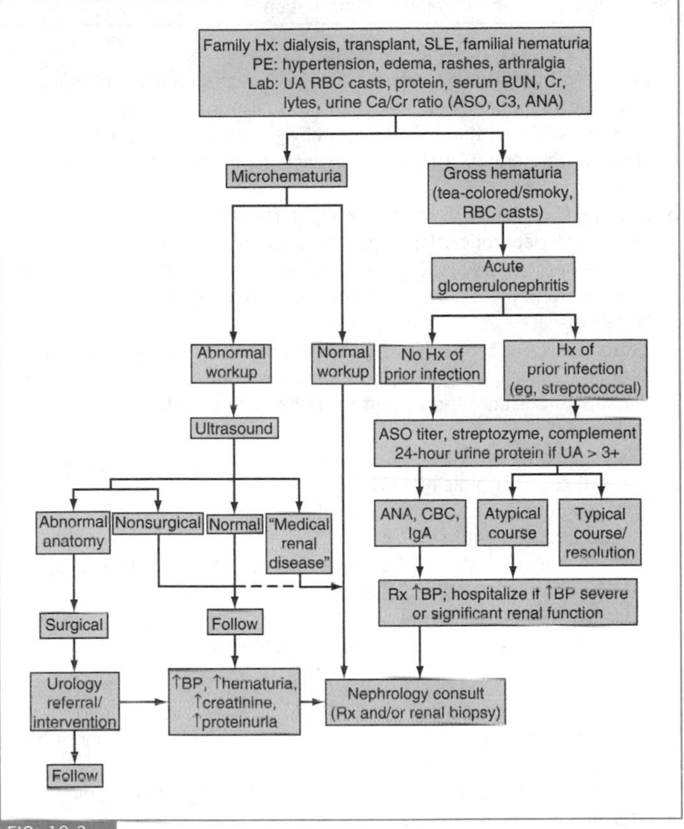


FIG. 19-3

Management algorithm for hematuria. *(Data from Hay WW et al: Current Pediatric Diagnosis and Treatment, 17th ed. Stamford, Conn, Appleton & Lange, 2005, p 709.)*



TABLE 19-8

**24-HOUR URINE PROTEIN EXCRETION IN CHILDREN OF DIFFERENT AGES (NORMAL RANGES)**

| Age | Protein Concentration (mg/L) | Protein Excretion (mg/24 hr) | Protein Excretion (mg/24 hr/m² BSA) |
|---|---|---|---|
| Premature (5–30 days) | 88–845 | 29 (14–60) | 182 (88–377) |
| Full-term | 94–455 | 32 (15–68) | 145 (68–309) |
| 2–12 mo | 70–315 | 38 (17–85) | 109 (48–244) |
| 2–4 yr | 45–217 | 49 (20–121) | 91 (37–223) |
| 4–10 yr | 50–223 | 71 (26–194) | 85 (31–234) |
| 10–16 yr | 45–391 | 83 (29–238) | 63 (22–181) |

BSA, body surface area.

From Cruz C, Spitzer A: When you find protein or blood in urine. Contemp Pediatr 1998;15(9):89.

estimated by the ratio of urine protein to creatinine concentrations in a first morning voided specimen (or spot urine). Ratios (mg/mg) <0.5 in children <2 years of age and <0.2 in older children are normal. A ratio >2 suggests nephrotic range proteinuria.

3. **Etiology (Fig. 19-4):** Can be usefully differentiated into nephrotic versus non-nephrotic. Non-nephrotic proteinuria, generally <40 mg/m$^2$/hr in adults, is rarely associated with edema. Significant non-nephrotic proteinuria is one of the earliest signs of chronic kidney disease.
4. **Evaluation (Fig. 19-5):** Not significant unless persistent and present in both supine and standing positions. When no protein is found in the supine position, the patient likely has benign orthostatic proteinuria.
   a. If proteinuria is significant (persistent and nonorthostatic), evaluation for potential cause of proteinuria is indicated.
   b. Evaluation of significant, non-nephrotic proteinuria: Comprehensive metabolic panel, serum Cr, albumin, C3, C4, and ANA; evaluation for hepatitis B and C; and renal sonogram to evaluate for structural causes. A 24-hr urine protein and creatinine should be obtained.
   c. If protein level is persistently >4 mg/m$^2$/hr or if this subgroup has worsening proteinuria, a renal biopsy is recommended.

## C. EDEMA[1]

Secondary to excessive accumulation of both $Na^+$ and water. Causes of generalized edema include the following:

1. **Inability to excrete $Na^+$ with or without water** (e.g., glomerular diseases resulting in decreased GFR, excess salt intake).
2. **Decreased oncotic pressure** (e.g., nephrotic syndrome, protein-losing enteropathy, hepatic failure, congestive heart failure [CHF]).
3. **Reduced cardiac output** (e.g., CHF, pericardial disease).
4. **Mineralocorticoid excess** (e.g., hyperreninemia, hyperaldosteronism).

## D. OLIGURIA[9]

Urine output <300 mL/m$^2$/24 hr, or <0.5 mL/kg/hr in children and <1.0 mL/kg/hr in infants. May be a normal physiologic response to water with or without salt depletion (prerenal state) or a reflection of renal failure that is associated with azotemia.

1. **BUN/Cr ratio (both in mg/dL):**[18]
   a. Normal ratio: 10–20; suggests intrinsic renal disease in the setting of oliguria.
   b. >20: Suggests dehydration, prerenal azotemia, or gastrointestinal bleeding.
   c. <5: Suggests liver disease, starvation, inborn error of metabolism.
2. **Laboratory differentiation of oliguria (Table 19-9).**

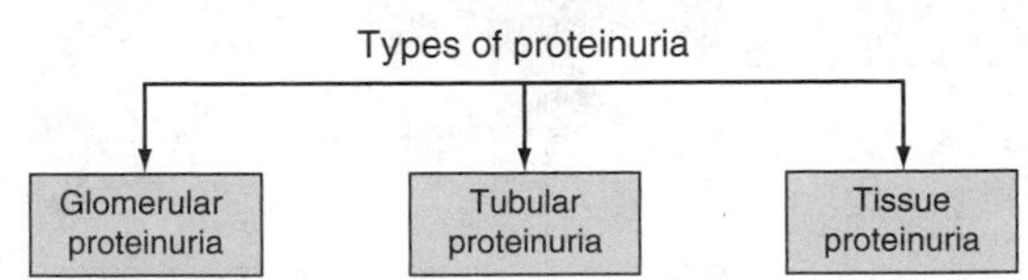


A. GLOMERULAR

1. Transient proteinuria: Most common in children. Associated with exercise, stress, dehydration, postural changes, cold exposure, fever, seizures, congestive heart failure, and vasoactive drugs. Serial urine tests should be negative for protein.

2. Orthostatic proteinuria: Common, not associated with renal pathology. Repeat measure of excreted urinary protein in recumbent position should be negative. Rarely exceeds 1 g/dy (see Table 19-8).

3. Proteinuria secondary to glomerulopathies

a. Primary glomerular disease: Minimal change disease, focal segmental glomerulonephritis, membranous glomerulonephritis, IgM nephropathy, IgA nephropathy.

b. Secondary glomerular disease: medications (e.g., NSAIDs, captopril, lithium), postinfectious (poststreptococcal, hepatitis B, chronic shunt infections, subacute bacterial endocarditis), infectious (bacterial, fungal, viral), neoplastic (solid tumors, leukemia), multisystem (systemic lupus erythematosus, Henoch-Schönlein purpura, sickle cell disease), reflux nephropathy, congenital nephrotic syndrome.

B. TUBULAR

1. Overload proteinuria: Occurs when excessive amount of low-molecular-weight proteins overwhelms the tubular reabsorption capacity (e.g., light chains: multiple myeloma; lysozyme: monocytic and myelocytic leukemias; myoglobin: rhabdomyolysis; hemoglobin: hemolysis).

2. Tubular dysfunction or disorders: Occurs when normal amounts of low-molecular-weight proteins (e.g., amino acids) are not adequately reabsorbed because of damaged or dysfunctional tubular cells (Fanconi syndrome, Lowe's syndrome, reflux nephropathy, cystinosis, drugs/heavy metals [mercury, lead, cadmium, outdated tetracyclines]), ischemic tubular injury, and renal hypoplasia/dysplasia.

C. TISSUE

1. Acute inflammation of urinary tract
2. Uroepithelial tumors

FIG. 19-4

Types of proteinuria. NSAIDs, nonsteroidal anti-inflammatory drugs.

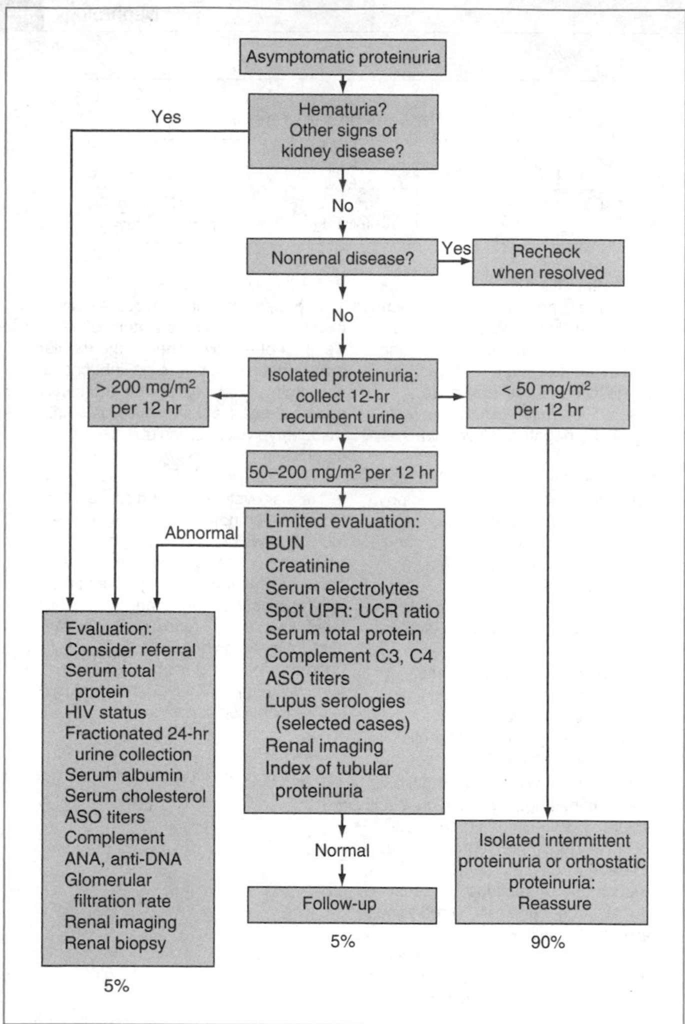


FIG. 19-5

Suggested evaluation of proteinuria in asymptomatic patients. *(From Cruz C, Spitzer A: When you find protein or blood in the urine. Contemp Pediatr 1998;15[9]:89.)*

TABLE 19-9

**LABORATORY DIFFERENTIATION OF OLIGURIA**

| Test | Prerenal | Renal |
|---|---|---|
| FENa | <1% | >3% |
| BUN/Cr ratio | >20:1 | <10:1 |
| Urine specific gravity | >1.015 | <1.010 |

BUN, blood urea nitrogen; Cr, creatinine; FENa, fractional excretion of sodium.

### E. POLYURIA[9]

Water conservation is dependent on antidiuretic hormone (ADH) and its effects on the distal renal tubules. Etiologies of polyuria include the following:

1. **Central diabetes insipidus:** ADH deficiency, may be idiopathic or acquired (through infection or pituitary trauma).
2. **Nephrogenic diabetes insipidus:** Unresponsive receptors; may be hereditary or acquired (through interstitial nephritis, sickle cell disease, or chronic renal insufficiency).
3. **Psychogenic polydipsia.**

## VII. GLOMERULAR DISEASES[8,9]



Injury to glomeruli results in either inflammatory or noninflammatory lesions. Many glomerular disorders involve both types of lesions.

### A. INFLAMMATORY (NEPHRITIC) LESIONS (CASTS)

Consist of necrotic areas that result in loss of large particles such as RBCs as well as edematous areas resulting in decreased filtration. Nephritic disorders clinically present with **fluid retention, hypertension, oliguria, and hematuria**. Classic example is poststreptococcal glomerulonephritis.

### B. NONINFLAMMATORY (NEPHROTIC) LESIONS (NO CASTS)

Result in leakage through the injured glomerular basement membrane. Nephrotic disorders, when uncomplicated, do not compromise filtration. Classic example is minimal-change nephrotic syndrome (MCNS).

### C. NEPHROTIC SYNDROME

The most severe form of proteinuria.[8,19] Classically characterized by **proteinuria (>40 mg/m²/hr), hypercholesterolemia (>200 mg/dL), hypoproteinemia (<2 g/dL), and edema**. Clinically, hypoalbuminemia with concomitant decrease in oncotic pressure results in generalized edema. The initial swelling occurs on the face (especially periorbital) as well as in the pretibial area. Prominent swelling of the scrotum and labia can also be seen. Decreased oncotic pressure also results in compromised splanchnic flow, leading to abdominal pain.

1. **Etiology: Exclusively a glomerular disorder that can be primary in the kidney or secondary to other systemic disorder resulting in injury.**
   a. Primary causes: Idiopathic (most common) and genetic disorders.
   b. Secondary causes: Infections (HIV; hepatitis B, C), drugs, and malignancy (leukemias, lymphomas).
   c. The three most common histologic causes: Account for >90% of cases; MCNS, focal segmental glomerulosclerosis, and membranoproliferative glomerulonephritis.[8,19]
2. **Factors suggesting a diagnosis other than idiopathic MCNS: Age <1 year or >11 years, positive family history, extrarenal disease (arthritis,**

rash, anemia), chronic disease, symptoms due to intravascular volume expansion (hypertension, pulmonary edema), renal failure, active urine sediment (RBC casts).

3. **Management of MCNS:[20]** Aims at restoring intravascular volume and encouraging diuresis to avoid fluid overload. A course of corticosteroid treatment without renal biopsy is recommended for children without atypical features; responsiveness to steroids is a better indicator than kidney histology of long-term prognosis for renal function. Renal biopsy often reserved for steroid-dependent and steroid-resistant nephritic syndrome. Complications: Infection and thromboembolic disease acutely, and potential for bone disease and cardiovascular disease in the long-term.
   a. **Steroid-responsive:** Roughly 95% of patients with MCNS and 20% with focal segmental glomerulosclerosis achieve remission with an 8-wk course of prednisone (60 mg/m$^2$ daily for 4 weeks followed by 40 mg/m$^2$ on alternate days for 4 weeks).
   b. **Frequently relapsing:** Defined as two or more relapses within 6 mos of initial response or four or more relapses in any 12-mo period. Steroid-dependent: defined as two consecutive relapses during tapering or within 14 days of cessation of steroids. Some patients can be managed with low-dose steroids given daily or on alternate days, but many still relapse. Second-line treatments for frequently relapsing and steroid-dependent nephrotic syndrome: Cyclophosphamide, chlorambucil, cyclosporine, or levamisole.
   c. **Steroid-resistant:** Often requires continued high-dose steroid treatment beyond 8 wks. Second-line agents, including calcineurin inhibitors, are often used, as well as high-dose pulse methylprednisolone, mostly in combination with an alkylating agent.

## VIII. ACUTE RENAL FAILURE

Sudden decline in renal function with increasing BUN/Cr ratio, with or without changes in urine output. Causative factors: Impaired renal perfusion, acute renal disease, renal ischemia, or obstructive uropathy.

### A. ETIOLOGY

Causes are generally subdivided into three categories:

1. **Prerenal: Most common etiology in children;** usually a result of dehydration, although other forms of impaired perfusion can be a cause.
2. **Renal:**
   a. Parenchymal disease through arterial or glomerular lesions.
   b. ATN: Diagnosis of exclusion; when no evidence of renal parenchymal disease is present and prerenal and postrenal causes have been eliminated if possible.
3. **Postrenal:** Obstruction of the urinary tract, found often in neonates with anatomic abnormalities.

### B. CLINICAL PRESENTATION

Pallor, decreased urine output, edema, hypertension, vomiting, and lethargy. The hallmark of early renal failure is oliguria.

### C. ACUTE TUBULAR NECROSIS

Clinically defined by three phases:

1. **Oliguric phase:** A period of severe oliguria that lasts about 10 days. If oliguria or anuria persists for longer than 3–6 weeks, renal recovery from ATN is highly unlikely.
2. **Diuretic phase:** Begins with an increase in urine output to passage of large volumes of isosthenuric urine containing sodium levels of 80–150 mEq/L.
3. **Recovery phase:** Signs and symptoms usually resolve rapidly, but polyuria may persist for days to weeks.

### D. TREATMENT CONSIDERATIONS

1. **Placement of indwelling catheter** to monitor urine output.
2. **Prerenal and postrenal factors should be excluded** and intravascular volume maintained with appropriate fluids in consultation with a pediatric nephrologist.

### E. COMPLICATIONS

Often dependent on clinical severity; usually includes fluid overload (hypertension, CHF, pulmonary edema), electrolyte disturbances (hyperkalemia), metabolic acidosis, hyperphosphatemia, and uremia.

## IX. ACUTE DIALYSIS

### A. INDICATIONS

1. **Indicated when metabolic or fluid derangements are not controlled by aggressive medical management alone.** Generally accepted criteria include the following, although a nephrologist should always be consulted:
   a. Volume overload with evidence of pulmonary edema or hypertension that is refractory to therapy.
   b. Hyperkalemia >6.0 mEq/L if hypercatabolic or >6.5 mEq/L despite conservative measures.
   c. Metabolic acidosis with pH <7.2 or $HCO_3^- < 10$.
   d. BUN >150; lower if rising rapidly.
   e. Neurologic symptoms secondary to uremia or electrolyte imbalance.
   f. Calcium and phosphorus imbalance (e.g., hypocalcemia with tetany or seizures in the presence of a very high serum phosphate level).
2. **Dialyzable toxin or poison** (e.g., lactate, ammonia, alcohol, barbiturates, ethylene glycol, isopropanol, methanol, salicylates, theophylline).

### B. TECHNIQUES[21]

1. **Peritoneal dialysis:** Requires catheter to access peritoneal cavity. May be used acutely or chronically, as in continuous ambulatory or continuous cycling peritoneal dialysis.
2. **Hemodialysis:** Requires placement of special vascular access devices. May be method of choice for certain toxins (e.g., ammonia, uric acid, poisons) or when there are contraindications to peritoneal dialysis.
3. **Continuous arteriovenous hemofiltration/hemodialysis (CAVH/D) and continuous venovenous hemofiltration/hemodialysis (CVVH/D):** Therapies with the primary goal of continuous generation of a plasma ultrafiltrate. Indications: Fluid management, renal failure with profound hemodynamic instability, electrolyte disturbances, and intoxication with substances that are freely filtered across the particular ultrafiltration membrane. Can be helpful in the management of oliguric patients who are in need of better nutritional support, postoperative cardiac patients, and patients with septicemia. Require special vascular access devices.

## X. CHRONIC RENAL FAILURE

Kidney damage for >3 mos, as defined by structural or functional abnormalities, with or without decreased GFR, or a GFR <60 mL/min/ 1.73 $m^2$ for >3 mos with or without kidney damage.

### A. ETIOLOGY

Close association with age at which renal failure is first detected. Chronic renal failure in children <5 years of age most commonly a result of anatomic abnormalities (i.e., hypoplasia, dysplasia, malformations), whereas older children predominantly have acquired glomerular diseases (e.g., glomerulonephritis, hemolytic-uremic syndrome) or hereditary disorders (e.g., Alport syndrome, cystic disease).

### B. COMPLICATIONS (Table 19-10)

## XI. CHRONIC HYPERTENSION

**Note** *For management of acute hypertension and normal BP parameters, see Chapters 4 and 7.*

### A. DEFINITION

For the definition of chronic hypertension, see Chapter 7.

1. **Normal BP:** Systolic and diastolic BP <90th percentile for age, gender, height, and weight.
2. **High-normal BP (prehypertension):** Average systolic and/or diastolic BP between the 90th and 95th percentiles for age, gender, height, and weight.

TABLE 19-10

**CLINICAL MANIFESTATIONS OF CHRONIC RENAL FAILURE**

| Manifestation | Mechanisms |
|---|---|
| Accumulation of nitrogenous waste products (azotemia) | Decline in GFR |
| Acidosis | Urinary bicarbonate wasting<br>Decreased ammonia excretion<br>Decreased acid excretion |
| Sodium wasting | Solute diuresis<br>Tubular damage<br>Function tubular adaptation for sodium excretion |
| Sodium retention | Nephrotic syndrome<br>CHF<br>Anuria<br>Excessive salt intake |
| Urinary concentrating defect | Nephron loss<br>Solute diuresis<br>Increased medullary blood flow |
| Hyperkalemia | Decline in GFR<br>Acidosis<br>Excessive potassium intake<br>Hypoaldosteronism |
| Renal osteodystrophy | Decreased intestinal calcium absorption<br>Impaired production of 1,25-dihydroxy vitamin D by the kidneys<br>Hypocalcemia and hyperphosphatemia<br>Secondary hyperparathyroidism |
| Growth retardation | Protein-calorie deficiency<br>Renal osteodystrophy<br>Acidosis<br>Anemia<br>Inhibitors of insulin-like growth factors<br>Unknown factors |
| Anemia | Decreased erythropoietin production<br>Low-grade hemolysis<br>Bleeding<br>Decreased erythrocyte survival<br>Inadequate iron intake<br>Inadequate folic acid intake<br>Inhibitors of erythropoiesis |
| Bleeding tendency | Thrombocytopenia<br>Defective platelet function |
| Infection | Defective granulocyte function |

Data from Brenner BM: Brenner and Rector's The Kidney, 6th ed. Philadelphia, WB Saunders, 2000.

*Continued*

TABLE 19-10

CLINICAL MANIFESTATIONS OF CHRONIC RENAL FAILURE—cont'd

| Manifestation | Mechanisms |
| --- | --- |
| Neurologic (fatigue, poor concentration, headache, drowsiness, loss of memory, slurred speech, muscle weakness and cramps, seizures, coma, peripheral neuropathy, asterixis) | Uremic factors<br>Aluminum toxicity |
| Gastrointestinal ulceration | Gastric acid hypersecretion; gastritis<br>Reflux<br>Decreased motility |
| Hypertension | Sodium and water overload<br>Excessive renin production |
| Hypertriglyceridemia | Diminished plasma lipoprotein lipase activity |
| Pericarditis and cardiomyopathy | Unknown |
| Glucose intolerance | Tissue insulin resistance |

3. **Significant hypertension:** Average of three separate systolic and/or diastolic BPs >95th percentile for age, gender, height, and weight.
4. **Severe hypertension:** Average of three systolic and/or diastolic BPs >99th percentile for age, gender, height, and weight.
5. **Measurement of BP in children**

a. Children ≥3 years of age should have BP measured at all routine and emergency visits. Children <3 years of age with risk factors, such as history of prematurity, low birth weight, congenital heart disease, kidney disease or family history of kidney disease, history of malignancy, or solid organ or bone marrow transplant, should have BP measured.

b. BP should be measured at least twice on each occasion at least 3–5 min after resting seated.

c. Appropriate cuff size is two thirds of upper arm length. Choose the larger size cuff if there is a choice between two cuffs.

## B. CAUSES OF HYPERTENSION IN NEONATES, INFANTS, AND CHILDREN (Table 19-11)

## C. EVALUATION OF CHRONIC HYPERTENSION[22–24]

1. **Rule out causes:** Rule out "factitious" causes of hypertension (improper cuff size or measurement technique [i.e., manual versus Dyna map]), "nonpathologic" causes of hypertension (i.e., fever, pain, anxiety, muscle spasm), and iatrogenic mechanisms (e.g., medications and excessive fluid administration).
2. **History and physical examination:** Headache, blurred vision, history of UTIs, family history of renal dysfunction or hypertension, pitting edema, dyspnea on exertion, jugular venous distention, or displaced point of maximal impulse.

TABLE 19-11

CAUSES OF HYPERTENSION BY AGE GROUP

| Age | Cause: Most Common | Cause: Less Common |
|---|---|---|
| Neonates/infants | Renal artery thrombosis after umbilical artery catheterization<br>Coarctation of the aorta<br>Renal artery stenosis | Bronchopulmonary dysplasia<br>Medications<br>Patent ductus arteriosus<br>Intraventricular hemorrhage |
| 1–10 yr | Renal parenchymal disease<br>Coarctation of aorta | Renal artery stenosis<br>Hypercalcemia<br>Neurofibromatosis<br>Neurogenic tumors<br>Pheochromocytoma<br>Mineralocorticoid increase<br>Hyperthyroidism<br>Transient hypertension<br>Induced by immobilization<br>Sleep apnea<br>Essential hypertension<br>Medications |
| 11 yr–adolescence | Renal parenchymal disease<br>Essential hypertension | All diagnoses listed in this table |

Modified from Sinaiko A: Hypertension in children. N Engl J Med 1996;335:26.



3. **Clinical evaluation of confirmed hypertension.**
   a. **Laboratory studies:** Urinalysis with microscopic evaluation, urine culture, serum electrolytes, CBC, Cr, BUN, calcium, uric acid, cholesterol, and plasma renin level.
   b. **Imaging:** Renal ultrasonography, including renal artery Doppler and other imaging studies as indicated (e.g., echocardiography, renal arteriography).
   c. Consider human chorionic gonadotropin, thyroid function tests, urine catecholamines, and plasma and urinary steroids. Consider polysomnography, fasting lipid profile, fasting glucose, and toxicology screen to evaluate for comorbidity. Consider echocardiogram and retinal examination to evaluate target-organ damage.
4. **Refer any patient with significant hypertension to a pediatric nephrologist.**

## D. TREATMENT OF HYPERTENSION

1. **Nonpharmacologic:** **Aerobic exercise, salt restriction, smoking cessation, and weight loss, indicated in patients with systolic BP and/or diastolic BP >90th percentile.**
2. **Pharmacologic:** Indications include significant hypertension (especially diastolic hypertension), secondary hypertension, symptomatic

hypertension, target-organ damage, diabetes mellitus, and persistent hypertension despite nonpharmacologic measures.

3. **Parental:** Acute hypertensive crisis.

## E. CLASSIFICATION OF HYPERTENSION IN CHILDREN AND ADOLESCENTS, WITH MEASUREMENT FREQUENCY AND THERAPY RECOMMENDATIONS (Table 19-12)

## F. ANTIHYPERTENSIVE DRUGS FOR OUTPATIENT MANAGEMENT OF HYPERTENSION IN CHILDREN, AGE 1–17 YEARS (Table 19-13)

TABLE 19-12

**CLASSIFICATION OF HYPERTENSION IN CHILDREN AND ADOLESCENTS AND THERAPY RECOMMENDATIONS**

| | SBP or DBP Percentile | Frequency of BP Measurement | Pharmacologic Therapy (in addition to lifestyle modifications) |
|---|---|---|---|
| Normal | <90th percentile | Recheck at next physical examination | None |
| Prehypertension | 90th to <95th percentile or if BP exceeds 120/80 mm Hg even if <90th percentile | Recheck in 6 mo | None unless compelling indications, such as chronic kidney disease, diabetes mellitus, heart failure, or LVH, exist |
| Stage 1 hypertension | 95th–99th percentile plus 5 mm Hg | Recheck in 1–2 wk, sooner if the patient is symptomatic; if persistently elevated on 2 additional occasions, evaluate or refer | Initiate therapy based on symptoms, secondary hypertension, end-organ damage, diabetes, persistent hypertension despite nonpharmacologic measures |
| Stage 2 hypertension | >99th percentile plus 5 mm Hg | Evaluate or refer within 1 wk or immediately if the patient is symptomatic | Initiate therapy |

DBP, diastolic blood pressure; LVH, left ventricular hypertrophy; SBP, systolic blood pressure.

Modified from National High Blood Pressure Education Program Working Group on High Blood Pressure in Children and Adolescents: The Fourth Report on the Diagnosis, Evaluation and Treatment of High Blood Pressure in Children and Adolescents. Pediatrics 2004;114(2):555–576.

TABLE 19-13

**ANTIHYPERTENSIVE DRUGS FOR OUTPATIENT MANAGEMENT OF HYPERTENSION IN CHILDREN, 1–17 YEARS OLD**

| Class | Drug | Comments |
|---|---|---|
| Angiotensin-converting enzyme (ACE) inhibitor | Benazepril<br>Captopril<br>Enalapril<br>Fosinopril<br>Lisinopril<br>Quinapril | Blocks angiotensin I to angiotensin II.<br>Decreases proteinuria while preserving renal function.<br>All ACE inhibitors are contraindicated in pregnancy.<br>Contraindicated in compromised renal perfusion.<br>Check serum potassium and creatinine periodically to monitor for hyperkalemia and azotemia. Elimination is dependent on creatinine clearance.<br>Cough and angioedema are reportedly less common with newer members of this class than with captopril. |
| Angiotensin-II receptor blocker (ARB) | Irbesartan<br>Losartan | All ARBs are contraindicated in pregnancy; females of childbearing age should use reliable contraception.<br>Check serum potassium and creatinine periodically to monitor for hyperkalemia and azotemia. |
| Alpha and beta blocker | Labetalol | Causes decreased peripheral resistance and decreased heart rate.<br>Extremely potent and can be used in hypertensive crisis.<br>Asthma and overt heart failure are contraindications.<br>Heart rate is dose-limiting.<br>May impair athletic performance.<br>Should not be used in insulin-dependent diabetics |
| Beta blocker | Atenolol<br>Bisopropol/HCTZ<br>Metoprolol<br>Propranolol | Decreases heart rate, cardiac output, and renin release.<br>Noncardioselective agents (i.e., propranolol) are contraindicated in asthma and heart failure.<br>Metoprolol and Atenolol are beta-1 selective.<br>Heart rate is dose-limiting.<br>May impair athletic performance.<br>Should not be used in insulin-dependent diabetics.<br>A sustained-release formulation of propranolol is available that is dosed once daily. |

Modified from National High Blood Pressure Education Program Working Group on High Blood Pressure in Children and Adolescents: The Fourth Report on the Diagnosis, Evaluation, and Treatment of high blood pressure in children and adolescents. Pediatrics 2004(2);114:568–569; Hospital for Sick Children: The HSC Handbook of Pediatrics, 9th ed. St. Louis, Mosby, 1997; Sinaiko A: Treatment of hypertension in children. Pediatr Nephrol 1994:8:603–609; and Khattak S et al: Efficacy of amlodipine in pediatric bone marrow transplant patients. Clin Pediatr 1998:37:31–35.

*Continued*

TABLE 19-13

**ANTIHYPERTENSIVE DRUGS FOR OUTPATIENT MANAGEMENT OF HYPERTENSION IN CHILDREN, 1–17 YEARS OLD—cont'd**

| Class | Drug | Comments |
|---|---|---|
| Calcium channel blocker | Amlodipine<br>Felodipine<br>Isradipine<br>Extended-release nifedipine | Acts on vascular smooth muscles.<br>Renal perfusion/function is minimally affected.<br>Ideal for post-renal-transplant hypertension.<br>Ideal in low renin/volume dependent hypertension.<br>Amlodipine and isradipine can be compounded into stable extemporaneous suspensions.<br>Felodipine and extended-release nifedipine tablets must be swallowed whole.<br>Isradipine is available in both immediate-release and sustained-release formulations.<br>May cause tachycardia. |
| Central alpha agonist | Clonidine | Stimulates brainstem α 2 receptors and peripheral adrenergic drive.<br>May cause dry mouth and/or sedation (↓ opiate withdrawal).<br>Effective in renal failure.<br>Transdermal preparation also available.<br>Sudden cessation of therapy can lead to severe rebound hypertension. |
| Diuretic | HCTZ<br>Budesonide<br>Chlorthalidone<br>Furosemide<br>Spironolactone<br>Triamterene<br>Amiloride | All patients treated with diuretics should have electrolytes monitored shortly after initiating therapy and periodically thereafter.<br>Useful as add-on therapy in patients being treated with drugs from other drug classes.<br>Thiazides are not effective when GFR <50% of normal. Side effects are hypokalemia, hypercalcemia, hyperuricemia, and hyperlipidemia.<br>Furosemide/bumetanide are useful in renal failure. Bumetanide has 40 times more diuretic activity than furosemide but varies with patient/route. Side effects are hyponatremia, hypokalemia, ototoxicity.<br>Potassium-sparing diuretics (i.e., spironolactone, triamterene, amiloride) are modest antihypertensives. They may cause severe hyperkalemia, especially if given with ACE inhibitor or ARB. |
| Peripheral alpha antagonist | Doxazosin<br>Prazosin<br>Terazosin | May cause hypotension and syncope, especially after first dose. |

TABLE 19-13

**ANTIHYPERTENSIVE DRUGS FOR OUTPATIENT MANAGEMENT OF HYPERTENSION IN CHILDREN, 1–17 YEARS OLD—cont'd**

| Class | Drug | Comments |
|---|---|---|
| Vasodilator | Hydralazine<br>Minoxidil | Directly acts on vascular smooth muscle and is very potent.<br>Tachycardia (reflex): and Na and water retention are common side effects.<br>Used in combination with diuretics or beta blockers.<br>Hydralazine can cause a lupus-like syndrome in slow acetylators.<br>Minoxidil is usually reserved for patients with hypertension resistant to multiple drugs. |



## REFERENCES


1. Norman ME: An office approach to hematuria and proteinuria. Pediatr Clin North Am 1987;34:545–559.
2. Chon CH et al: Pediatric urinary tract infections. Pediatr Clin North Am 2001;48:1441–1459.
3. Layton KL: Diagnosis and management of pediatric urinary tract infections. Clin Fam Pract 2003;5:367–382.
4. American Academy of Pediatrics, Committee on Quality Improvement, Subcommittee on Urinary Tract Infection: Practice parameter: The diagnosis, treatment, and evaluation of the initial urinary tract infection in febrile infants and young children. Pediatrics 1999;103(4):843–852.
5. Hoberman A et al: Oral versus initial intravenous therapy for urinary tract infections in young febrile children. Pediatrics 1999;104(1):79–86.
6. Edelmann CM Jr et al: A standardized test of renal concentrating capacity in children. Am J Dis Child 1967;114:639–644.
7. Behrman RE: Nelson Textbook of Pediatrics, 16th ed. Philadelphia, WB Saunders, 2000.
8. Sabella C et al: The Cleveland Clinic Intensive Review of Pediatrics. Philadelphia, Lippincott Williams & Wilkins, 2003.
9. Haynes TS: BIOTEST Study Aids. Ventura, Calif, Biotest Publishing, 2002.
10. Brenner BM: Brenner and Rector's The Kidney, 6th ed. Philadelphia, WB Saunders, 2000.
11. Rodriguez Soriano J: Frontiers in nephrology: Renal tubular acidosis. J Am Soc Nephrol 2002;13(8):2160–2170.
12. Hay WW et al: Current Pediatric Diagnosis and Treatment, 17th ed. Stamford, Conn, Appleton & Lange, 2005.
13. Roy S III: Hematuria. Pediatr Ann 1996;25(5):284–287.
14. Feld L et al: Hematuria: An integrated medical and surgical approach. Pediatr Clin North Am 1997;44:1191–1210.
15. Cilento B et al: Hematuria in children: A practical approach. Urol Clin North Am 1995;22:43–55.
16. Fitzwater D, Wyatt R: Hematuria. Pediatr Rev 1994;15:102–108.
17. Belman A: Vesicoureteral reflex. Pediatr Clin North Am 1997;44(5):1171–1190.

18. Greenhill A, Gruskin AB: Laboratory evaluation of renal function. Pediatr Clin North Am 1976;23:661–679.
19. Roth KS et al: Nephrotic syndrome: Pathogenesis and management. Pediatr Rev 2002;23(7):237–248.
20. Eddy A, Symons J: Nephrotic syndrome in childhood. Lancet 2003;362 (9384):629–639.
21. Rogers MC: Textbook of Pediatric Intensive Care. Baltimore, Williams & Wilkins, 1992.
22. Sinaiko A: Hypertension in children. NEJM 1996;335(26):1968–1973.
23. National High Blood Pressure Education Program Working Group on High Blood Pressure in Children and Adolescents: The Fourth Report on the Diagnosis, Evaluation, and Treatment of High Blood Pressure in Children and Adolescents. Pediatrics 2004;114(2):555–576.
24. Sadowski R, Falkner B: Hypertension in pediatric patients. Am J Kidney Dis 1996;27(3):305–315.

# Neurology

*Lisa Emrick, MD*

20

## I. NEUROLOGIC EXAMINATION[1]

Starts with a thorough history, with emphasis on onset, duration, and progression of symptoms. Must be evaluated relative to developmental norms.

### A. WEBSITE

Examples of developmentally appropriate neurologic examinations: http://library.med.utah.edu/pedineurologicexam/html/home_exam.html.

### B. MENTAL STATUS

Patient should be alert and oriented to time, person, place, and current situation. Assess attentiveness and behavior in infants.

### C. CRANIAL NERVES (Table 20-1)

### D. MOTOR

1. **Muscle bulk.**
2. **Tone:** High, low.
   a. Passive movements: Resting resistance to examiner's movement.
   b. Active movements: Regulation of power with defined movements (e.g., posture, gait, pull to stand).
   c. Infants who have low tone will slip when you hold them under their arms.
   d. Note anatomic distribution of abnormalities. Regional increase in tone (e.g., adducted thumbs, limited hand supination, equinus of feet) suggests central nervous system dysfunction. Note quality (e.g., rigid, spastic).
3. **Power, strength: Observe and describe activity (e.g., rising from the floor). Quantify (e.g., distance of standing broad jump, time to run 30 feet, time to climb stairs); see Box 20-1.**

### E. SENSORY (Fig. 20-1)

Primary disorders of sensation are rare in children, and reliable examination takes time. Sensory evaluation is most important when there is a specific question of anatomic localization. Compare side to side, distal to proximal positions within an extremity, and upper to lower extremities as appropriate to the question being asked.

1. **Spinal cord level: Best assessed with pinprick and temperature. If concerned about spinal cord impairment, ask about continence. Compare lower to upper, check both anterior and posterior trunk.**
2. **Intraspinal lesions:**
   a. Anterior pathways: pinprick and temperature.
   b. Posterior pathways: vibratory and joint position sense.
3. **Root/plexus/nerve impairment:** Pin sensibility, consult dermatomal/nerve maps (see Fig. 20-1).

TABLE 20-1

**CRANIAL NERVES**

| Function/Region | Cranial Nerve | Test/Observation |
|---|---|---|
| Olfactory | I | Smell (e.g., coffee, vanilla, peppermint) |
| Vision | II | Acuity, fields, fundus |
| Pupils | II, III | Sympathetics, size, reaction to light, accommodation |
| Eye movements and eyelids | III, IV, VI | Range and quality of eye movements, saccades, pursuits, nystagmus, ptosis |
| Sensation | V | Corneal reflexes, facial sensation |
| Muscles of mastication | V | Clench teeth |
| Facial strength | VII | Observe degree of expression of emotions, eye closure strength, smile, puff out cheeks, asymmetry forehead and lower face |
| Hearing | VIII | Localize sound, attend to finger rub, audiologic testing |
| Mouth, pharynx | VII, IX, X, XII | Swallowing, speech quality (labial, lingual, or palatal articulation deficits), symmetrical palatal elevation, tongue protrusion |
| Head control | XI | Lateral head movement, shoulder shrug |

BOX 20-1

**STRENGTH RATING SCALE**

0/5: No movement, i.e., no palpable tension at the tendon
1/5: Flicker of movement or less than full range of movement in a gravity-neutral plane
2/5: Movement in a gravity-neutral plane
3/5: Movement against gravity but not resistance
4/5: Subnormal strength against resistance
5/5: Normal strength against resistance

4. **Polyneuropathy: Large fiber (vibration and position sense) versus small fiber (pinprick and temperature). Compare distal to proximal sites in a limb, and lower to upper extremities.**

## F. TENDON REFLEXES

This assessment is most helpful in localizing other abnormalities, especially in the presence of weakness or asymmetry (Box 20-2 and Table 20-2).

1. **Clinical finding:**

a. Isolated abnormality of reflexes: Little significance in the setting of normal strength and coordination.
b. Brisk reflexes combined with weakness: Indicate upper motor neuron disorder.

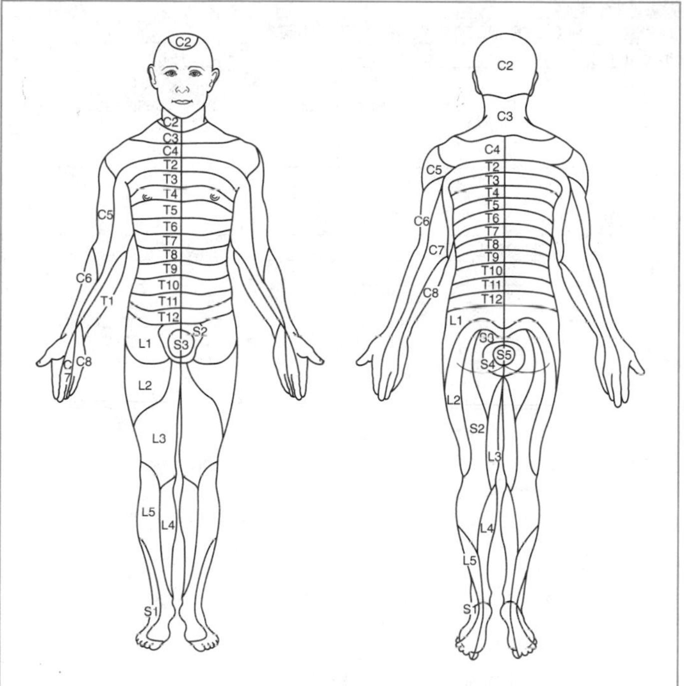


FIG 20-1

Dermatomes. *(From Athreya BH, Silverman BK: Pediatric Physical Diagnosis. Norwalk, Conn, Appleton-Century-Crofts, 1985, pp 238–239.)*



BOX 20-2

**REFLEX RATING SCALE**

| | |
|---|---|
| 0: | None |
| 1+: | Diminished (need use of clasped hands or gritting teeth in order to engage reflex) |
| 2+: | Normal |
| 3+: | Increased (reflexes cross neighboring joint or cross to other side) |
| 4+: | Hyperactive with clonus |

c. Absent reflexes: Suggest motor neuron, nerve, or muscle causes. In muscle disease, reflexes are usually diminished commensurate with power. Selective reflex dropout can help localize a spinal cord, root, or nerve lesion (Table 20-3). Compare side to side, upper extremities to lower extremities, and distal to proximal reflexes.

2. **Newborn reflexes age range and abnormal response:**

TABLE 20-2

UPPER AND LOWER MOTOR NEURON FINDINGS

| On Exam | Upper | Lower |
|---|---|---|
| Power | Decreased | Decreased |
| Reflexes | Increased | Decreased |
| Tone | Increased | Normal or decreased |
| Babinski | Present | Absent |

TABLE 20-3

MUSCLE STRETCH REFLEXES

| Reflex | Site |
|---|---|
| Biceps | C5, C6 |
| Brachioradialis | C5, C6 |
| Triceps | C7, C8 |
| Knee | L(2,3)4 |
| Ankle | L5–S2 |

a. Moro reflex: Abnormal if not present from 32 weeks' gestation to age 2 months or if still present at age 6 months.
b. Grasp reflex (palmar and plantar): Abnormal if not present from 32 weeks' gestation to age 2 months or if ever asymmetrical.
c. Extensor plantar response: Abnormal after age 8 to 12 months.
d. Tonic neck reflex: Abnormal after age 6 to 7 months or if ever asymmetrical.

### G. COORDINATION AND MOVEMENT

1. **Evaluate general coordination while watching activities (e.g., throwing a ball, dressing, writing, or drawing).**
2. **Tests for cerebellar function include rapid alternating and repetitive movements, finger to nose, heel to shin, orbiting, walking, and running. Note involuntary movements (e.g., tremor, dystonia, chorea, athetosis, tics, myoclonus) and conditions under which they are enhanced or suppressed. Note abnormal gait (e.g., waddling, wide based, tiptoed).**

## II. HEADACHES[2]

### A. EVALUATION OF HEADACHES

1. **Classification:** ***The International Classification of Headache Disorders*, 2nd ed., classifies headaches as primary versus secondary.**[3]

a. Primary headaches: Migraines, tension type, cluster or other trigeminal etiologies.
b. Secondary headaches: Caused by other underlying pathologies, such as trauma, substance use or withdrawal, vascular malformations, infection, mass effect, referred pain from teeth, sinuses, and/or eyes, or psychiatric. For the purpose of pediatric headache it is beneficial to differentiate headache based on onset and duration.

2. **History and physical examination: Differentiate between acute, acute recurrent, chronic nonprogressive, and chronic progressive (Boxes 20-3 and 20-4). See Box 20-5 for important information to gather during the history taking. Careful general, neurologic, and funduscopic examinations should be performed (Table 20-4; see also Table 20-5).**
3. **Studies:**
a. Strongest evidence for the use of neuroimaging is abnormal neurologic examination.
   (1) Variables that increase likelihood of a space-occupying lesion causing headache: Headache duration <1 month, absence of family history of migraine, abnormal neurologic examination, gait abnormalities, and occurrence of seizures.[4]
   (2) Computed tomography (CT) without contrast or magnetic resonance imaging (MRI): Obtain for focal neurologic findings, suspected increased intracranial pressure (ICP), atypical or progressive



BOX 20-3

**DIFFERENTIAL DIAGNOSIS OF ACUTE HEADACHE**

Evaluation of the first acute headache should exclude pathologic causes listed here before consideration of more common etiologies.

1. Increased intracranial pressure (ICP): Trauma, hemorrhage, tumor, hydrocephalus, pseudotumor cerebri, abscess, arachnoid cyst, cerebral edema
2. Decreased ICP: After ventriculoperitoneal shunt, lumbar puncture, cerebrospinal fluid leak from basilar skull fracture
3. Meningeal inflammation: Meningitis, leukemia, subarachnoid or subdural hemorrhage
4. Vascular: Vasculitis, arteriovenous malformation, hypertension, cerebrovascular accident
5. Bone, soft tissue: Referred pain from scalp, eyes, ears, sinuses, nose, teeth, pharynx, cervical spine, temporomandibular joint
6. Infection: Systemic infection, encephalitis, sinusitis, etc.
7. First migraine

BOX 20-4

**DIFFERENTIAL DIAGNOSIS OF RECURRENT OR CHRONIC HEADACHES**

1. Migraine (with or without aura)
2. Tension
3. Analgesic rebound
4. Caffeine withdrawal
5. Sleep deprivation (e.g., in children with sleep apnea) or chronic hypoxia
6. Tumor
7. Psychogenic: Conversion disorder, malingering
8. Cluster headache

BOX 20-5

**IMPORTANT HISTORICAL INFORMATION IN EVALUATING HEADACHE**

1. Age at onset
2. Associated trauma
3. Presence or absence of aura
4. Change in weight or other constitutional symptoms
5. Change in vision or any other neurologic symptom
6. Frequency, severity, and duration of headaches (ask about school absences)
7. Quality, site, and radiation of pain (focal occipital pain is concerning for secondary headaches)
8. Associated symptoms, such as weakness or tingling
9. Triggers and relieving and worsening factors (triggers: foods, environmental factors, etc.); presence of photophobia, phonophobia; worsens with activity; relieved by sleep, medications (NSAIDs, acetaminophen), remaining still
10. Family history of migraine
11. Changes and possible new stressors in school or at home

TABLE 20-4

**PHYSICAL AND NEUROLOGIC EXAMINATION OF THE CHILD WHO HAS HEADACHES[4]**

| Feature | Significance |
|---|---|
| Growth parameters | Chronic illness may affect linear growth.<br>Hypothalamic-pituitary dysfunction may disturb growth. |
| Head circumference | Increased intracranial pressure before fusion of the sutures may accelerate head growth. |
| Skin | Evidence of trauma or a neurocutaneous disorder. |
| Blood pressure | Hypertension. |
| Neurologic exam | Signs of increased intracranial pressure.<br>Focal abnormality. |
| Cranial bruits | May reflect an intracranial arteriovenous malformation. |

pattern, seizures, abrupt-onset severe headache (see Chapter 25 for advantages of each modality). Note that CT provides poor imaging of the posterior fossa.

b. Lumbar puncture (LP): Fever, infection, papilledema, sudden severe headache, headache worse when lying down and improves on standing (evaluate opening pressure with legs extended if concern for pseudotumor cerebri). Contraindicated in increased ICP or mass effect secondary to risk for herniation. **To correct the white blood cell (WBC) count in traumatic taps** in assessment of meningitis, allow 1 WBC for every 700 (500–1500) red blood cells (RBCs). Or follow this formula for true cerebrospinal fluid (CSF) WBCs:[5]

CSF WBC = (CSF WBC − serum WBC) × (CSF RBC/serum RBC)

4. **Warning signs:** Pain that awakens child from sleep, increases in morning with rising or with Valsalva maneuver; headache associated with emesis, neurologic signs, changes in chronic pattern, and altered mental status (e.g., change in mood, personality, and school performance). If subarachnoid hemorrhage (SAH) suspected, CT without contrast is preferred method of evaluation, then LP (if CT is negative) to rule out xanthochromia (develops about 12 hr after event). Send tubes 1 and 4 of CSF sample for cell counts and xanthochromia. Persistently high RBC count and xanthochromia if SAH exists. Significant decline of the RBC count between tubes 1 and 4 in the absence of xanthochromia suggests microtrauma from the LP.



**Note** *The classic headache secondary to SAH is acute, severe, continuous, and generalized—the "worst headache of my life."*

## B. MIGRAINE HEADACHE

1. **Characteristics as defined by the International Headache Society:** Chronic recurrent (at least two attacks with aura and five attacks with no aura); throbbing, pulsatile, or pressure-like in children; usually bifrontal in children, unilateral in adolescents and adults, lasting from 4–72 hr; relieved by sleep; many potential triggers (e.g., stress, caffeine, diet, menses, sleep disruption); hereditary predisposition. Associated symptoms include nausea, vomiting, abdominal pain, motion sickness in smaller children, photophobia, phonophobia, paresthesia, tinnitus, vertigo; rare associated symptoms include focal weakness, aphasia, ataxia, confusion.
2. **Classification:**
   a. With aura: "Classic," often frontotemporal, usually unilateral, may have associated neurologic complications. Aura is any preceding neurologic abnormality (e.g., visual aberrations, reversible sensory symptoms such as pins and needles or numbness or dysphasia).
   b. Without aura: "Common," often bifrontal.
3. **Associated reversible neurologic deficits (rare):** Paresthesia, visual-field cuts, aphasia, hemiplegia, ophthalmoplegia, vertigo, ataxia, confusion.
4. **Treatment:** Includes reassurance and education. The acute and chronic treatment of migraine headaches in the pediatric population is not well studied.
   a. Acute symptomatic:
      (1) For all ages: Dark and quiet room and sleep.
      (2) For <12 years of age: Nonsteroidal anti-inflammatory drugs (NSAIDs; i.e., naproxen, ketorolac) and less effective acetaminophen.

(3) For >12 years of age: Objective data support nasal sumatriptan. If nausea is a factor, antiemetics (metoclopramide). Other agents: Not enough evidence regarding efficacy of oral sumitriptan, rizatriptan, or zolmitriptan; or subcutaneous sumitriptan.

b. Chronic treatment (if >3 or 4 per month or if migraines interfere with daily functioning or school):
   (1) Avoid triggers and stress, improve general health with balanced diet restrictive of certain "migraine-causing" foods, suggest headache journal to help identify potential triggers. Encourage aerobic exercise and regular sleep.
   (2) Explore issues of secondary gain and role of pain in family's relationships. Offer counseling when appropriate; also consider biofeedback.
   (3) Consider medications. See Table 20-5 for summary of therapies, doses, and adverse effects.
   (4) The natural history of chronic headache includes spontaneous improvement. Delayed treatment may be indicated. No child should be on chronic therapy without re-evaluation. Avoid abortive medication overuse (>2–3 doses/wk), which can lead to rebound headache. Refer any child with focal deficits to a pediatric neurologist.

TABLE 20-5

PREVENTIVE THERAPIES FOR MIGRAINE[6]

| Therapies | Age (years) | Dose | Adverse Events |
|---|---|---|---|
| **ANTIEPILEPTIC MEDICATIONS** | | | |
| Divalproex sodium | 7–16 | 15–45 mg/kg/dose | Dizziness, drowsiness, weight gain, GI upset |
| | 9–17 | 500–1000 mg/dose | Dizziness, drowsiness increased appetite |
| Topiramate | 8–15 | 12.5–225 mg/dose | Cognitive changes, weight loss, sensory changes |
| Levetiracetam | 3–17 | 250–500 mg/dose | Somnolence, dizziness, irritability |
| **ANTIDEPRESSANT MEDICATION** | | | |
| Amitriptyline | 9–15<br>3–12 | 1 mg/kg/day<br>10 mg/day | Minimal to mild sedation |
| **ANTIHISTAMINE** | | | |
| Cyproheptadine | 3–12 | 4 mg/day | Sedation, increased appetite |
| **CALCIUM CHANNEL BLOCKER** | | | |
| Flunarizine* | 5–13 | 5 mg/day | Drowsiness, weight gain |

*Flunarizine-only therapy demonstrated efficacy in prospective randomized, double-blind trials. Other therapies have demonstrated some efficacy in uncontrolled studies.

## III. PAROXYSMAL EVENTS

### A. DIFFERENTIAL DIAGNOSIS OF RECURRENT EVENTS THAT MIMIC EPILEPSY IN CHILDHOOD (Table 20-6)

### B. SEIZURE DISORDERS[7,8]

1. **Definitions:**

a. **Seizure:** Paroxysmal synchronized discharge of cortical neurons, resulting in alteration of function (motor, sensory, cognitive).

TABLE 20-6

**DIFFERENTIAL DIAGNOSIS OF RECURRENT EVENTS THAT MIMIC EPILEPSY IN CHILDHOOD[7]**

| Event | Differentiation from Epilepsy |
|---|---|
| Pseudoseizure (psychogenic seizure) | No EEG changes except movement artifact during event; movements thrashing rather than clonic; brief/absent postictal period; most likely to occur in patient with epilepsy. |
| Paroxysmal vertigo (toddler) | Patient frightened and crying; no loss of awareness; staggers and falls, vomiting, dysarthria. |
| GER in infancy, childhood | Paroxysmal dystonic posturing associated with meals (Sandifer syndrome). |
| Breath-holding spells (18 mo–3 yr) | Loss of consciousness and generalized convulsions, always provoked by an event that makes child cry. |
| Syncope | Loss of consciousness with onset of dizziness and clouded or tunnel vision; slow collapse to floor; triggered by postural change, heat, emotion, etc. |
| Cardiogenic syncope | Abnormal ECG/Holter monitor finding (e.g., prolonged QT, atrioventricular block, other arrhythmias); exercise a possible trigger; episodic loss of consciousness without consistent convulsive movement. |
| Cough syncope | Prolonged cough spasm during sleep in asthmatic, leading to loss of consciousness, often with urinary incontinence. |
| Paroxysmal dyskinesias | May be precipitated by sudden movement or startle; not accompanied by change in alertness. |
| Shuddering attacks | Brief shivering spells with continued awareness. |
| Night terrors (4–6 yr) | Brief nocturnal episodes of terror without typical convulsive movements. |
| Rages (6–12 yr) | Provoked and goal-directed anger. |
| Tics/habit spasms | Involuntary, nonrhythmic, repetitive movements not associated with impaired consciousness; suppressible. |
| Narcolepsy | Sudden loss of tone secondary to cataplexy; emotional trigger; no postictal state or loss of consciousness; EEG with recurrent REM sleep attacks. |
| Migraine (confusional) | Headache or visual changes that may precede attack; family history of migraine; autonomic or sensory changes that can mimic focal seizure; EEG with regional area of slowing during attack |
| Myoclonus | Involuntary muscle jerking or twitch |

ECG, electrocardiography; EEG, electroencephalography; GER, gastroesophageal reflux; REM, rapid eye movement.

b. Epilepsy: Demonstrated tendency for recurrent seizures not precipitated by acute causes (i.e., not due to recurrent fever, metabolic disruption, trauma).
c. Status epilepticus: Prolonged or recurrent seizures lasting ≥30 min without the patient regaining consciousness. See Chapter 1 for treatment.

2. **Seizure etiology:** Can be due to diffuse brain dysfunction (e.g., fever, metabolic compromise, toxin or drugs, hypertension, idiopathic epilepsy) or to focal brain dysfunction (e.g., stroke, neoplasm, focal cortical dysgenesis, trauma, focal idiopathic epilepsy).
3. **Diagnosis:** History and physical examination attempt to establish etiology and seizure type (e.g., primary generalized or primary partial; Box 20-6), which generally determines treatment.

BOX 20-6

**INTERNATIONAL CLASSIFICATION OF EPILEPTIC SEIZURES**[8]

I. Partial seizures (seizures with focal onset)
   A. Simple partial seizures (consciousness unimpaired)
      1. With motor signs
      2. With somatosensory or special sensory symptoms
      3. With autonomic symptoms or signs
      4. With psychic symptoms (higher cerebral functions)
   B. Complex partial seizures (consciousness impaired)
      1. Starting as simple partial seizures
         (a) Without automatisms
         (b) With automatisms (such as lip smacking and drooling, dazed eyes look)
      2. With impairment of consciousness at onset
         (a) Without automatisms
         (b) With automatisms
   C. Partial seizures evolving into secondarily generalized seizures
II. Generalized seizures
   A. Absence seizures: Brief lapse in awareness without postictal impairment (atypical absence seizures may have the following: mild clonic, atonic, tonic, automatism, or autonomic components)
   B. Myoclonic seizures: Brief, repetitive, symmetrical muscle contractions
   C. Clonic seizures: Rhythmic jerking; flexor spasm of extremities
   D. Tonic seizures: Sustained muscle contraction
   E. Tonic-clonic seizures
   F. Atonic seizures: Abrupt loss of muscle tone
III. Unclassified epileptic seizures

**4. Studies: Evaluation of first afebrile seizure lasting <30 min and age >28 days of life.[9]**

a. Depend on clinical scenario, age of patient, and if patient's mental status has returned to baseline. Consider assessment of glucose, sodium, potassium, calcium, magnesium, phosphate, blood urea nitrogen, creatinine, complete blood count (CBC), toxicology screen, blood pressure (supine and upright), electroencephalography (EEG) with video monitoring, electrocardiography, head CT and/or MRI, LP, tilt-table test, and sleep study. If febrile, consider age-appropriate sepsis evaluation.

**Note** *If this is not the first seizure and if patient is receiving antiepileptic therapy, a change in seizure pattern should prompt a drug level (see Table 20-7 for therapeutic drug levels).*

b. Imaging: Although not required for diagnosis, MRI and CT can detect focal brain abnormalities that may predispose to focal seizures.
   (1) Head CT without contrast: Can detect mass lesions, acute hemorrhage, hydrocephalus, and calcifications secondary to congenital disease such as cytomegalovirus infection (head ultrasound may be used in early infancy and requires open fontanelles).
   (2) Brain MRI with contrast: Obtain in infants with epilepsy, children with recurrent partial seizures, focal neurologic deficits, or developmental delay. Not routinely indicated in the evaluation of a first-time seizure.

c. EEG: Recommended in all children with first nonfebrile seizures to classify if there is an epilepsy syndrome.[9] Controversial; routine interictal EEGs are frequently normal. Repeat EEGs, prolonged EEG monitoring with video, or studies done with sleep deprivation or photic stimulation may be more informative.

**5. Treatment:[9]**

a. If patient's first seizure, seizure was nonfocal, and patient has returned to baseline: No antiepileptic medication indicated. Overall recurrence of seizure varies from 14%–65%, with most recurrences occurring in the first 2 yr after initial event. EEG is most important indicator for evidence of risk for recurrence.

b. Educate parents and patient regarding how to live with epilepsy.[10] Review seizure first aid and cardiopulmonary resuscitation. Recommend that child participate in activities but have supervision during bathing or swimming. Individualize other restrictions. Know driver's license laws in the state. Advocate teacher and school awareness.

c. Pharmacotherapy (Table 20-7): Weigh risk for more seizures without therapy against risk for treatment side effects plus residual seizures

TABLE 20-7

COMMONLY USED ANTICONVULSANTS, IN ALPHABETICAL ORDER

| Anticonvulsant (Trade Name) | Typical Target Dosage (mg/kg/day) | Standard Therapeutic Levels (mg/dL) | Efficacy (Generalized/Partial) | Side Effects |
|---|---|---|---|---|
| Carbamazepine (Tegretol, Carbatrol) | 10–20 | 8–12 | P | Sedation, ataxia, diplopia, Stevens-Johnson syndrome, blood dyscrasias, hepatotoxicity, may worsen generalized seizures |
| Clonazepam (Klonopin) | 0.05–0.2 | N/A | G/P | Sedation, drooling, dependence |
| Ethosuximide (Zarontin) | 10–20 | 40–100 | G | Gastrointestinal upset |
| Felbamate (Felbatol) | 15–45 | 40–100 | G/P | Weight loss, hepatotoxicity, sleep disturbances, aplastic anemia (1:7900) |
| Gabapentin (Neurontin) | 20–40 | 3–18 | P | Weight gain, leg edema |
| Lamotrigine (Lamictal) | 5–15 | 3–18 | G/P | Rash (increased risk in combination with valproate) |
| Levetiracetam (Keppra) | 10–40 | 30–60 | P | Behavioral changes, irritability, rare psychosis |
| Oxcarbazepine (Trileptal) | 10–30 (3:2 ratio compared with carbamazepine) | MHD level (5–40) | P | Hyponatremia |
| Phenobarbital (Luminal) | 5–10 | 15–40 | P | Altered cognition, sedation |
| Phenytoin (Dilantin) | 5–10 | 10–20 | P | Hirsutism, gingival hyperplasia, teratogenicity, rash, purple-glove syndrome with infusion |
| Tiagabine (Gabitril) | 1–2 | N/A | P | Can worsen generalized seizures |
| Topiramate (Topamax) | 1–9 | 2–20 | G/P | Cognitive side effects, weight loss, renal stones, acidosis, glaucoma |
| Valproic acid (Depakote, Depakene) | 10–20 | 50–100 | G/P | Weight gain, alopecia, hepatotoxicity, pancreatitis, polycystic ovary disease |
| Zonisamide (Zonegran) | 5–10 | 20–40 | G/P | Renal stones, weight loss, hyphidrosis |

G, generalized; MHD, 10-Monohydroxy metabolite; P, partial.

Based on personal communication with Eric Kossoff, MD, Johns Hopkins Pediatric Neurology, July 2007.

despite therapy. Reserve pharmacotherapy for recurrent afebrile seizures. Monotherapy may reduce complications; polytherapy increases risk of complications and side effects more than efficacy.

d. Ketogenic diet:[11] High-fat, low-carbohydrate therapy used for intractable seizures. Urine ketones can be monitored, and side effects (e.g., acidosis with bicarbonate value as low as 10–15 mEq/L, kidney stones [6%], constipation), can occur.
e. Vagus nerve stimulation: Employs a subcutaneous, 5-cm, programmable device to periodically stimulate the vagus nerve.

### C. SPECIAL SEIZURE SYNDROMES

See Table 20-8 for seizure types, etiologies, evaluations, and treatments of many common seizure syndromes. See Figure 20-2 for febrile seizure evaluation guidelines.



## IV. HYDROCEPHALUS

### A. DIAGNOSIS

Assess increasing head circumference, misshapen skull, frontal bossing, bulging large anterior fontanelle, Increased ICP (sunset sign, increased tone/reflexes, vomiting, irritability, papilledema), and developmental delay. Obtain head CT if increase in head circumference crosses more than two percentile lines or if patient is symptomatic. Differentiate hydrocephalus from megalencephaly or hydrocephalus ex vacuo.

### B. TREATMENT[12]

1. **Medical:**

a. Emergently manage acute increase of ICP (see Chapter 4).
b. Slowly progressive hydrocephalus: Acetazolamide may be effective in children age 2 weeks to 10 months with slowly progressive communicating hydrocephalus (see Formulary for dosing).

2. **Surgical: CSF shunting.**

a. Shunt types: Ventriculoperitoneal shunts used most commonly. Ventriculoatrial and pleural shunts are associated with cardiac arrhythmias, pleural effusions, and higher rates of infection.
b. Shunt complications: Shunt dysfunction may be caused by infection, obstruction (clogging or kinking), disconnection, and migration of proximal and distal tips. Patient will develop signs of increased ICP with shunt malfunction.

### C. EVALUATION OF SHUNT INTEGRITY

Obtain head CT to evaluate shunt position, ventricular size, and evidence of increased ICP. Obtain shunt series (skull, neck, chest, and abdominal radiographs) to look for kinking or disconnection. Referral to a neurosurgeon is then warranted to test shunt function and for possible percutaneous shunt drainage.

TABLE 20-8

SPECIAL SEIZURE SYNDROMES

| Syndrome | Etiology | Evaluation |
|---|---|---|
| Febrile[13,14] | Unknown genetic predisposition, possible viral association | Workup cause of fever, no workup of seizure if at baseline |
| Atypical febrile[13,14] | Same as febrile | Workup cause of fever<br>Workup cause of seizure based on clinical scenario<br>LP strongly recommended if <12 mo; consider LP if age 12–18 mo |
| Neonatal seizures[15] | Underlying brain disorder, hypoxic-ischemic injury, intracranial hemorrhage or metabolic | Screen electrolyte and metabolic abnormalities, pyridoxine deficiency<br>Workup for sepsis<br>LP, ultrasound, CT or MRI<br>EEG |
| Infantile spasms | Symptomatic—67%; CNS malformation (acquired infantile brain injury, tuberous sclerosis, inborn errors of metabolism)<br>Cryptogenic—33% | EEG–hypsarrhythmia<br>MRI<br>Ketogenic diet |
| Benign rolandic epilepsy | Autosomal dominant inheritance | EEG–characteristic pattern |
| Juvenile myoclonic epilepsy | Unknown genetic predisposition | Clinical history, sleep-deprived EEG |

CT, computed tomography; EEG, electroencephalography; LP, lumbar puncture; MRI, magnetic resonance imaging.

## V. ATAXIA[16,17]

### A. DIFFERENTIAL DIAGNOSIS OF ACUTE OR RECURRENT ATAXIA (Box 20-7)

### B. DIFFERENTIAL DIAGNOSIS OF CHRONIC OR PROGRESSIVE ATAXIA (Box 20-8)

### C. EVALUATION

Depends on clinical scenario; consider CBC, electrolytes, blood and urine toxicology screens, brain imaging, LP, EEG, electromyelography, urine for vanillylmandelic acid and homovanillic acid, and imaging of the chest and abdomen if neuroblastoma is suspected.

| Treatment | Comment |
|---|---|
| None, diazepam prn<br>Antipyretics not indicated | Incidence 2%–5%, age 6 mo–5 yr<br>Risk of recurrence 30% after first seizure, 50% after second<br>Risk of epilepsy 2% vs. 1% general population |
| Same as febrile | Defined as >15 min, onset >24 hr after fever, focal seizure, >1 seizure, or abnormal neurologic exam |
| Treat underlying abnormality<br>Consider pyridoxine with or without EEG<br>Phenobarbital; may need additional agent<br>Topiramate or zonisamide | Occurs within first 28 days of life<br>May be myoclonic, tonic, or subtle blinking, chewing, bicycling, or apnea |
| Corticotropin, valproic acid, benzodiazepine, vigabatrin, topiramate, zonisamide<br>Consider ketogenic diet | Usual onset after age 2 mos, peak onset age 4–6 mos<br>Initiate treatment as soon as possible<br>Presents as head nodding with flexion and extension of the trunk and extremities |
| No treatment necessary<br>If frequent seizures, then carbamazepine | Age 3–13 yr, nighttime seizure<br>Clonic activity, grimacing, vocalizations<br>Most patients outgrow by adulthood |
| Levetiracetem, other AEDs for generalized seizure | |



## VI. STROKE[18]

### A. ETIOLOGY

Risk factors for childhood stroke: Include, but are not limited to, congenital heart disease (most common), arteriovenous ischemia secondary to infections (e.g., meningitis), coagulation disorders or hematologic disorders (most commonly sickle cell disease), head or neck trauma, and drugs.

### B. DIFFERENTIAL DIAGNOSIS (Box 20-9)

Should be considered in the differential diagnosis for any child who presents with acute-onset focal neurologic deficit, focal seizures with

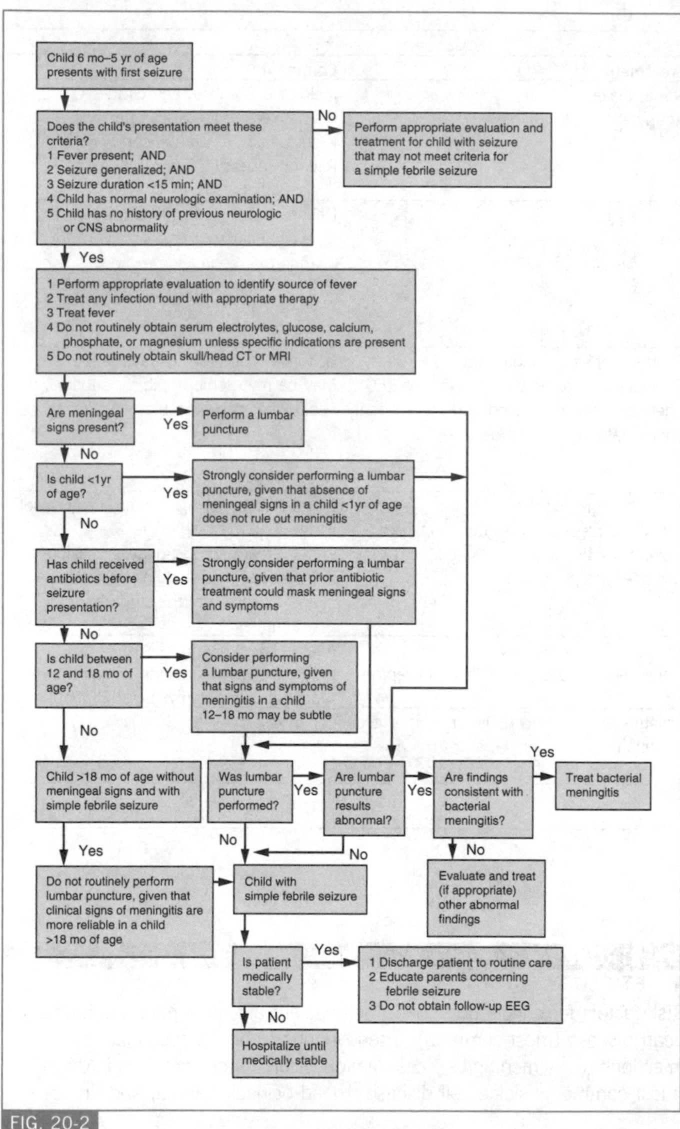


FIG. 20-2
Guidelines for febrile seizure evaluation.[13]

BOX 20-7

**DIFFERENTIAL DIAGNOSIS OF ACUTE OR RECURRENT ATAXIA**

1. Drug ingestion (e.g., phenytoin, carbamazepine, sedatives, hypnotics, and phencyclidine) or intoxication (e.g., alcohol, ethylene glycol, hydrocarbon fumes, lead, mercury, or thallium)
2. Postinfectious (cerebellitis [e.g., varicella], acute disseminated encephalomyelitis)
3. Head trauma
4. Basilar migraine
5. Benign paroxysmal vertigo (migraine equivalent)
6. Brain tumor or neuroblastoma (if accompanied by opsoclonus or myoclonus [i.e., "dancing eyes, dancing feet"])
7. Hydrocephalus
8. Infection (e.g., labyrinthitis, abscess)
9. Seizure (ictal or postictal)
10. Vascular events (e.g., cerebellar hemorrhage or stroke)
11. Miller-Fisher variant of Guillain-Barré syndrome (ataxia, ophthalmoplegia, and areflexia). Warning: If bulbar signs present, disease is likely progressive; patient may lose ability to protect airway and/or ability to breathe
12. Inherited ataxias
13. Inborn errors of metabolism (e.g., mitochondrial disorders, amino acidopathies, urea cycle defects) (See Chapter 13 for workup)
14. Conversion reaction
15. Multiple sclerosis

BOX 20-8

**DIFFERENTIAL DIAGNOSIS OF CHRONIC OR PROGRESSIVE ATAXIA**

1. Hydrocephalus
2. Hypothyroidism
3. Tumor or paraneoplastic syndrome
4. Low vitamin E levels (e.g., cystic fibrosis)
5. Wilson disease
6. Inborn errors of metabolism
7. Inherited ataxias (e.g., ataxia-telangiectasia, Friedreich ataxia)

BOX 20-9

**DIFFERENTIAL DIAGNOSIS OF CHILDHOOD STROKE**

1. Hemiplegic migraine
2. Focal seizure with postictal (Todd's) paralysis
3. Cervical spinal cord injury (deficits spare the face)
4. Ischemic stroke
5. Hemorrhagic stroke

Based on personal communication with Lori Jordan, MD, Johns Hopkins Pediatric Neurology, July 2007.

prolonged postictal paralysis, new-onset refractory focal status epilepticus, altered mental status, or unexplained encephalopathy.

### C. INITIAL WORKUP

1. **Acute diagnostic evaluation:** Urgent noncontrast head CT (to exclude hemorrhage) and initial laboratory studies, including CBC, comprehensive metabolic panel, prothrombin time, partial thromboplastin time, international normalization ratio, and type and screen (specifically in patients with sickle cell disease) and a urine toxicology screen.
2. **MRI with diffusion-weighted imaging and magnetic resonance angiography:** Urgency may vary from acute to within 24–48 hr.
3. **Less acute studies:** Echocardiogram, erythrocyte sedimentation rate, lipid panel, human immunodeficiency virus testing, and further evaluation for coagulation disorders, systemic lupus erythematosus, and other metabolic and rheumatologic diseases.

### D. MANAGEMENT

1. No evidence-based guidelines for evaluation or management of stroke in children.
2. **Supportive care:** Critical and should proceed rapidly and parallel with initial workup. Ensure airway patency, and provide supplemental oxygen to maintain $Sao_2$ >94%.
3. **Optimize cerebral perfusion pressure:** Adequate fluid volume and maintenance of median blood pressure for age. Treatment of hypertension is controversial. Unless blood pressure is extremely elevated, do not use acute antihypertensive therapy because hypertension may be a compensatory reaction to maintain cerebral perfusion.
4. **Neurologic status:** Monitor frequently. Aim for normoglycemia (blood glucose, 60–120 mg/dL). Treat hyperthermia with goal temperature <37°C. Treat seizures aggressively.
5. **Antiplatelet and anticoagulation therapy:** Controversial; consider on a case-by-case basis. Urgent consultation with a neurologist is indicated, along with transfer to a tertiary care center with expertise in childhood stroke.

## VII. WEB RESOURCES

www.childneurologysociety.org
http://aan.com/practice/guideline

## REFERENCES


1. Athreya BH, Silverman BK: Pediatric Physical Diagnosis. Norwalk, Conn, Appleton-Century-Crofts, 1985.
2. Forsyth R, Farrell K: Headache in childhood. Pediatr Rev 1999;20(2):39–45.

3. Olesen J: The International Classification of Headache Disorders, 2nd ed. J Neurol Neurosurg Psychiatry 2004;75(6):808–811.
4. Lewis DW: Practice parameter: Evaluation of children and adolescents with recurrent headaches. Neurology 2002;59:490–498.
5. Fishman RA: Cerebral Spinal Fluid in Diseases of the Nervous System. Philadelphia, WB Saunders, 1992, p 190.
6. Lewis D: Practice parameter: Pharmacological treatment of migraine headache in children and adolescents. Neurology 2004;63:2215–2224.
7. Murphy JV, Dehkharghani F: Diagnosis of childhood seizure disorder. Epilepsia 1994;35(Suppl 2):S7–S17.
8. Committee on Classification and Terminology of the International League against Epilepsy: Classification of epilepsia: Its applicability and practical value of different diagnostic categories. Epilepsia 1996;38(11):1051–1059.
9. Hirtz D et al: Practice parameter: Treatment of the child with a first unprovoked seizure. Neurology 2003;60:166–175.
10. Freeman J et al: Seizures and Epilepsy in Childhood: A Guide to Parents, 3rd ed. Baltimore, Johns Hopkins University Press, 2000.
11. Freeman J: The ketogenic diet: One decade later. Pediatrics 2007;119: 535–543.
12. Rogers M (ed): Textbook of Pediatric Intensive Care, 3rd ed. Baltimore, Williams & Wilkins, 1996.
13. American Academy of Pediatrics Subcommittee: Practice parameter: The neurodiagnostic evaluation of the child with a first simple febrile seizure. Pediatrics 1996;97(5):769–772.
14. Baumann RJ, Duffner PK: Treatment of children with simple febrile seizures: The AAP practice parameter. Pediatr Neurol 2000;23(1):11–17.
15. Scher MS: Seizures in the newborn infant: Diagnosis, treatment and outcomes. Clin Perinatol 1997;24(4):735–772.
16. Dinolfo EA: Evaluation of ataxia. Pediatr Rev 2001;22(5):177–178.
17. Ryan M: Acute ataxia in childhood. J Child Neurol 2003;18(5):309–316.
18. Ichord R: Treatment of pediatric neurologic disorders. In Singer H et al (eds): Treatment of Pediatric Neurologic Disorders. Boca Raton, Fla, Taylor & Francis Group, 2005.

# Nutrition and Growth

*Peter Claybour, MD, and*
*Jenifer Hampsey, MS, RD, CSP*

## I. ASSESSMENT OF NUTRITIONAL STATUS

### A. ELEMENTS OF NUTRITIONAL ASSESSMENT

1. **Anthropometric measurements** (weight, length/height, head circumference, body mass index [BMI], skin folds): Data are plotted on growth charts according to age and compared with a reference population.
2. **Clinical assessment** (general appearance, including hair, skin, oral mucosa, and gastrointestinal symptoms of nutritional deficiencies).
3. **Dietary evaluation** (feeding history, current intake).
4. **Physical activity and exercise.**
5. **Laboratory findings** (comparison with age-based norms).



### B. INDICATORS OF NUTRITIONAL STATUS[1] (Figs. 21-1 to 21-17)

1. **Growth:** Ideally, should be evaluated over time, but one measurement can be used for screening. Height (or length), weight, and weight for height should be plotted on a growth chart.
2. **BMI:** Defined as an index of healthy weight and as a predictor of morbidity and mortality risk. It is used to classify underweight and overweight individuals.[2] BMI should be determined and plotted for children ≥2 years of age. Use this formula to calculate BMI.

$$BMI = wt\ (kg)/[height\ (m^2)]$$

or

$$BMI = wt\ (lb)/[height\ (in^2)] \times 703$$

3. **BMI percentile:** BMI percentile is plotted on the CDC growth charts for children ≥2 years of age. Although not a direct measure of body fat, it is a reliable indicator of body fatness in most children and adolescents. Both the CDC and Institute of Medicine define BMI percentiles.[2,3]
4. **Interpretation of growth charts:**

a. **Stunting** Length or height for age <5th percentile.

b. **Underweight:**
   (1) Children <3 years: Weight for length <5th percentile.
   (2) Children ≥2 years: BMI for age <5th percentile.

c. **Risk for overweight:** Children >2 years, BMI for age 85th–95th percentile.

d. **Overweight:**
   (1) Children <3 years: Weight for length >95th percentile.
   (2) Children ≥2 years: BMI for age >95th percentile.

e. The Institute of Medicine recommends children ages 2–18 years with a BMI ≥30 kg/m² or ≥95th percentile BMI for age be considered obese.[3]

5. **Recommendations for management of overweight and obese children** (see Fig. 21-1).[4]
6. **Growth charts:** For boys and girls, including weight, height, head circumference, BMI, and height velocity (see Figs. 21-2 to 21-12). Growth charts can be downloaded from http://www.cdc.gov/nchs/about/major/nhanes/growthcharts/clinical_charts.htm.
7. **Growth charts for special populations:**
   a. Down syndrome: www.ndss.org, follow links to health and medical tools (Figs. 21-14 to 21-17).
   b. Turner syndrome: http://aappolicy.aappublications.org/cgi/content/full/pediatrics;111/3/692/F1.
   c. Achondroplasia: http://aappolicy.aappublications.org/cgi/content/full/pediatrics;116/3/771.
8. **Waist circumference and waist-height ratio:** Both waist circumference (WC) and waist-height ratio are indicators of visceral fat or abdominal obesity in children and adolescents age 2–19 years. Increased visceral adiposity measured by WC increases the risk of obesity-related morbidity and mortality. WC should be measured at the high point of the ileac crest when the individual is standing and at minimal respiration. Waist-height ratio is calculated as a ratio of waist circumference (cm) and height (cm).[5] See CDC waist circumference tables for individuals ages 2–19 years: www.cdc.gov/nchs/data/nhanes/t47.pdf.

## II. ESTIMATING ENERGY NEEDS

### A. DEFINITIONS OF ENERGY NEEDS[2]

1. **Basal metabolic rate (BMR):** Rate of energy expenditure after an overnight fast, resting comfortably, supine, awake, and motionless in a thermoneutral environment.
2. **Basal energy expenditure (BEE):** BMR over 24 hours.
3. **Thermic effect of food (TEF):** Increase in energy expenditure elicited by food consumption.
4. **Energy deposition:** Energy requirement for growth.
5. **Total energy expenditure (TEE):** Sum of BEE, TEF, physical activity, thermoregulation, and the energy expended in depositing new tissues and/or in producing milk.
6. **Physical activity level (PAL):** Ratio of total to basal daily energy expenditure (TEE/BEE). Describes and accounts for physical activity habits.
7. **Physical activity coefficient (PA):** The physical activity coefficient that correlates with PAL (Table 21-1) can be used to calculate estimated energy requirements (EER; see section II.B).

### B. ESTIMATED ENERGY REQUIREMENTS[2]

1. **EER:** Dietary energy intake that is predicted to maintain energy balance in a healthy individual. In children, it includes the needs associated with growth. For most healthy infants and children, the equations here can be used to determine energy needs.

a. For infants, children, and adolescents, EER (kcal/day) = TEE + energy deposition.
b. For most hospitalized patients, it can be assumed PAL = sedentary, PA = 1.

**2. EER equations (calculate calories/day):**

a. **Infants and young children:**
   (1) 0–3 months: EER = (89 × weight [kg] – 100) + 175
   (2) 4–6 months: EER = (89 × weight [kg] – 100) + 56
   (3) 7–12 months: EER = (89 × weight [kg] – 100) + 22
   (4) 13–35 months: EER = (89 × weight [kg] – 100) + 20

b. **Boys ages 3–18:**
   (1) 3–8 years: EER = 88.5 – 61.9 × age (yr) + PA × (26.7 × weight [kg] + 903 × height [m]) + 20
   (2) 9–18 years: EER = 88.5 – 61.9 × age (yr) + PA × (26.7 × weight [kg] + 903 × height [m]) + 25

c. **Girls ages 3–18:**
   (1) 3–8 years: EER = 135.3 – 30.8 × age (yr) + PA × (10 × weight [kg] + 934 × height [m]) + 20
   (2) 9–18 years: EER = 135.3 – 30.8 × age (yr) + PA × (10 × weight [kg] + 934 × height [m]) + 25

d. **Pregnancy (14–18 years):** EER = adolescent EER + pregnancy energy deposition:
   (1) First trimester = adolescent EER + 0 kcal
   (2) Second trimester = adolescent EER + 340 kcal
   (3) Third trimester = adolescent EER + 452 kcal

e. **Lactation (14–18 years):** EER = adolescent EER + milk energy output – weight loss:
   (1) First 6 months = adolescent EER + 500 – 170
   (2) Second 6 months = adolescent EER + 400 – 0

**3. Table 21-2[2] contains the estimated EER for healthy boys and girls of median weight (weight for age at 50th percentile) at both sedentary and active PAL levels.**

## C. EER UNDER STRESSED CONDITIONS[6]

**Calculation of BEE:** In many cases, there is little need to provide critically ill patients with more than their BEE. Ideally, energy expenditure should be measured in critically ill patients, but this requires expensive equipment and may not always be practical. Numerous prediction equations are available. The following equation is from the *Dietary Reference Intakes*:[6]

For Boys: BEE (kcal/d) = 68 – 43.3 × age (yr) + 712 × height (m) + 19.2 × weight (kg)

For Girls: BEE (kcal/d) = 189 – 17.6 × age (yr) + 625 × height (m) + 7.9 × weight (kg)

Appropriate changes should be made as indicated by real (not fluid) weight gain and signs and symptoms of overfeeding.

*Text continued on p. 577*

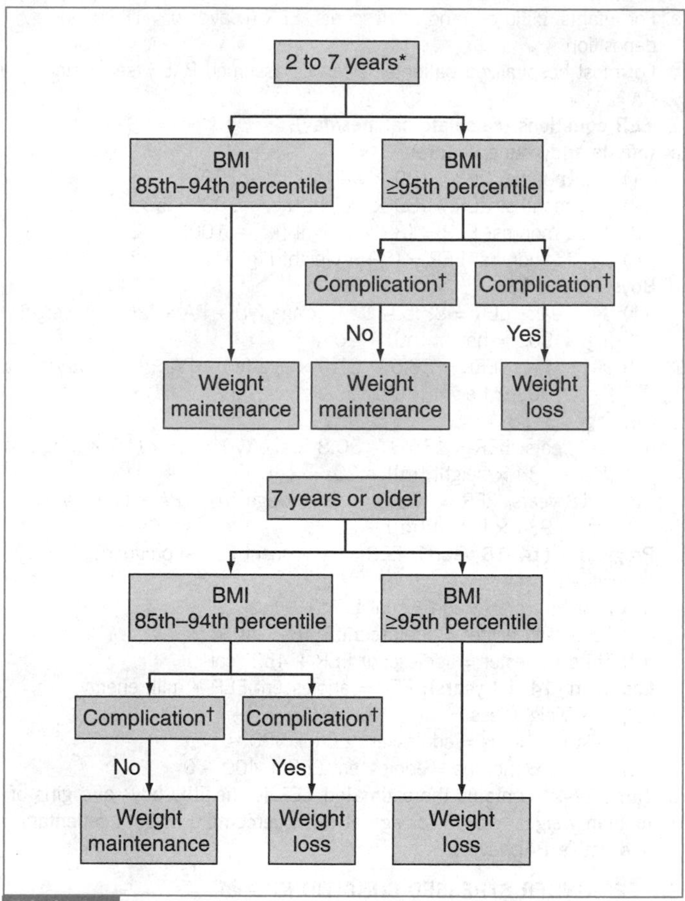


FIG. 21-1

Obesity decision tree. Recommendations for obesity management. Asterisk (*) indicates that children <2 years of age should be referred to a pediatric obesity center for treatment. Dagger (†) indicates complications such as mild hypertension, dyslipidemias, and insulin resistance. Patients with acute complications, such as pseudotumor cerebri, sleep apnea, obesity hypoventilation syndrome, or orthopedic problems, should be referred to a pediatric obesity center. Weight maintenance implies no change in weight while child grows in height. *(Modified from Barlow SE, Dietz WH: Obesity evaluation and treatment: Expert Committee recommendations—The Maternal and Child Health Bureau, Health Resources and Services Administration and the Department of Health and Human Services. Pediatrics 1998;102[3]:7.)*

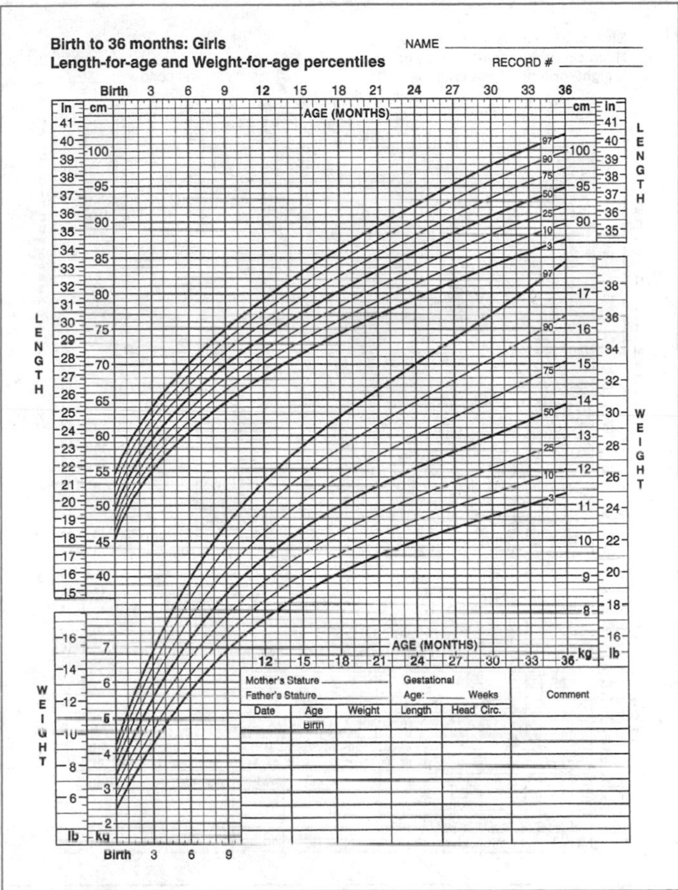


FIG. 21-2

Length and weight for girls, from birth to age 36 months. *(Developed by the National Center for Health Statistics in collaboration with the National Center for Chronic Disease Prevention and Health Promotion, 2000.)*

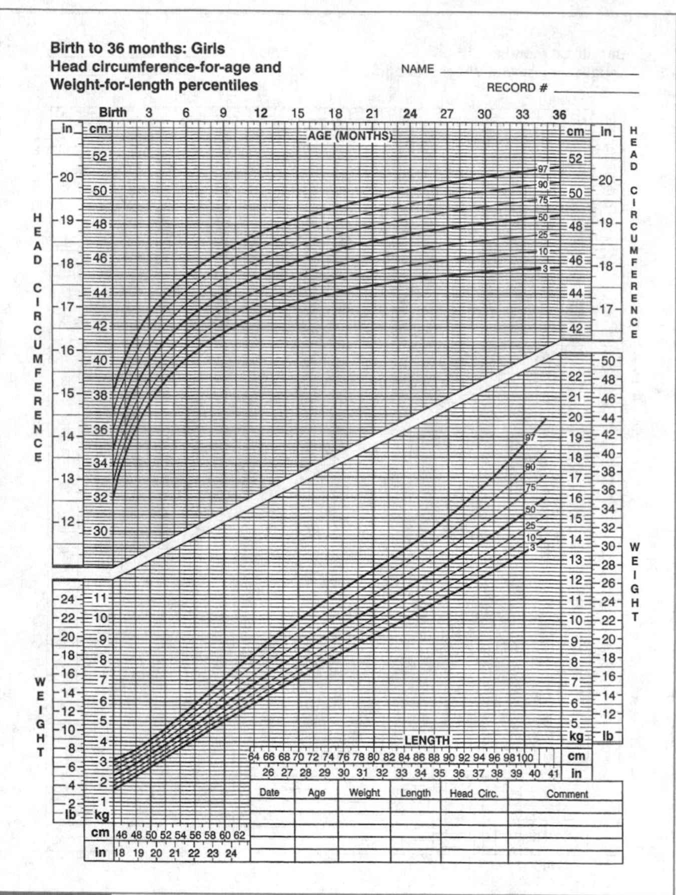


FIG. 21-3

Head circumference and length-to-weight ratio for girls, from birth to age 36 months. *(Developed by the National Center for Health Statistics in collaboration with the National Center for Chronic Disease Prevention and Health Promotion, 2000.)*

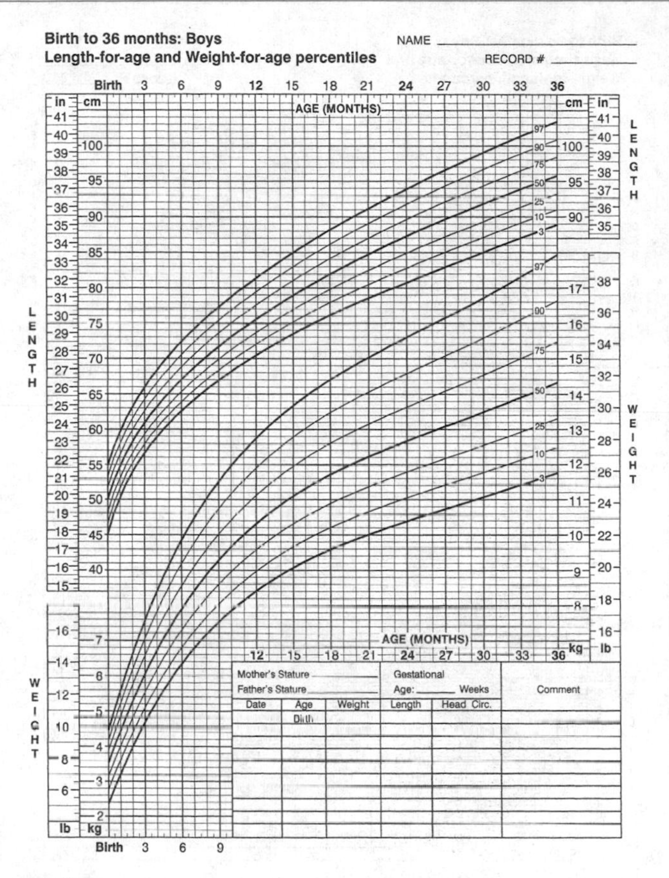


FIG. 21-4

Length and weight for boys, from birth to age 36 months. *(Developed by the National Center for Health Statistics in collaboration with the National Center for Chronic Disease Prevention and Health Promotion, 2000.)*

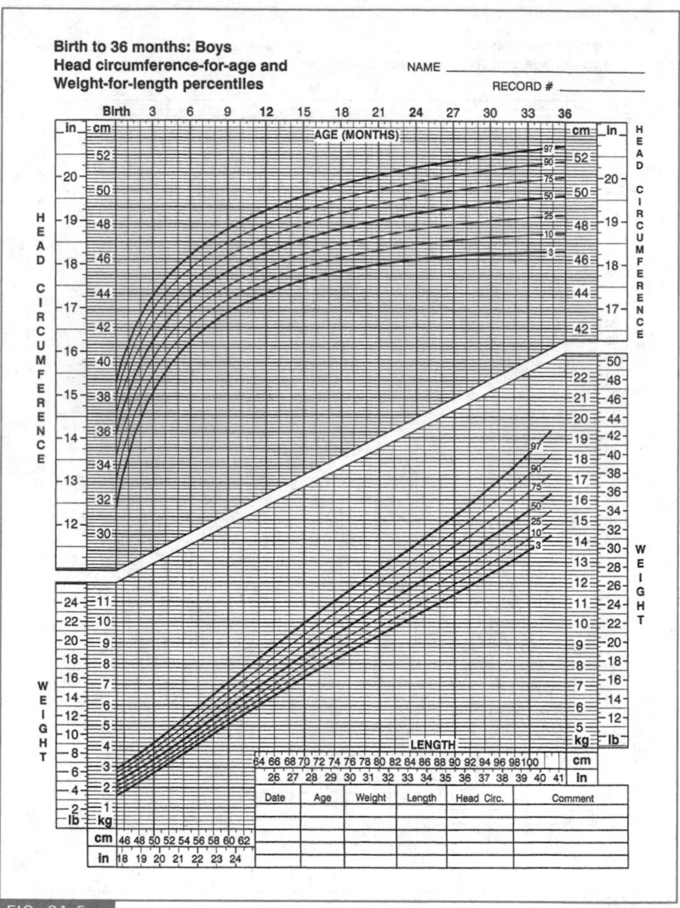


FIG. 21-5

Head circumference and length-to-weight ratio for boys, from birth to age 36 months. *(Developed by the National Center for Health Statistics in collaboration with the National Center for Chronic Disease Prevention and Health Promotion, 2000.)*

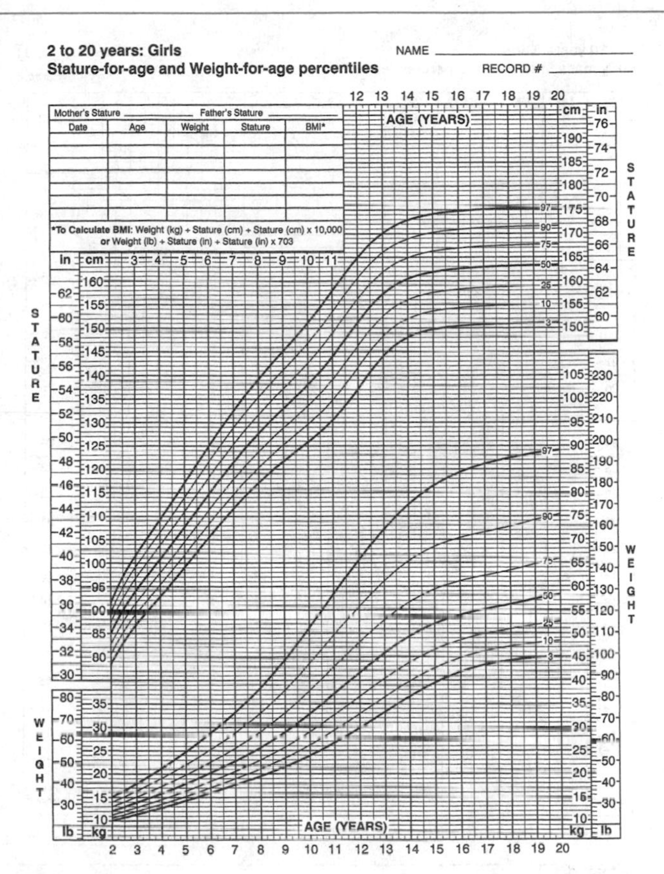


FIG. 21-6

Stature and weight for girls ages 2–20 years. *(Developed by the National Center for Health Statistics in collaboration with the National Center for Chronic Disease Prevention and Health Promotion, 2000.)*

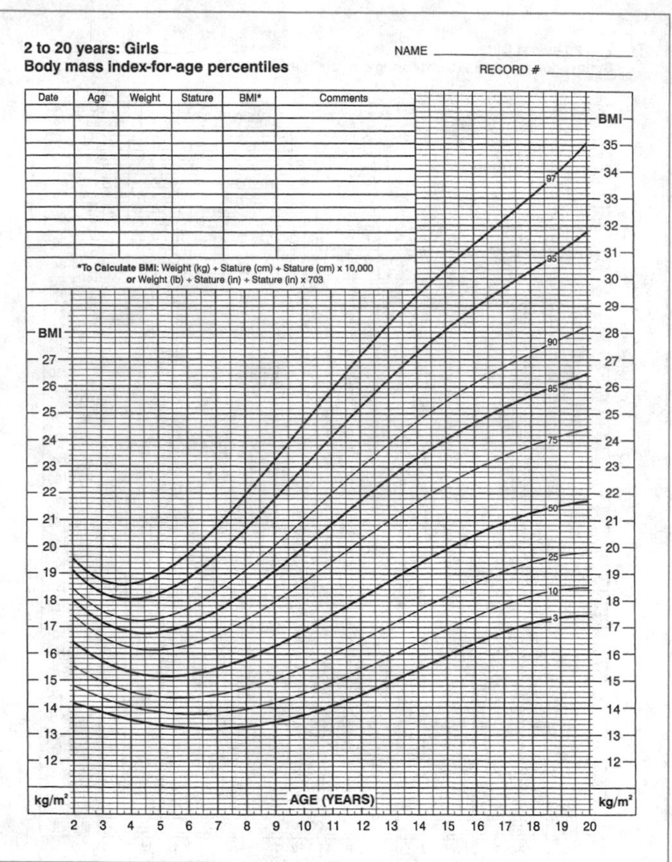


FIG. 21-7

Body mass index for girls ages 2–20 years. *(Developed by the National Center for Health Statistics in collaboration with the National Center for Chronic Disease Prevention and Health Promotion, 2000.)*

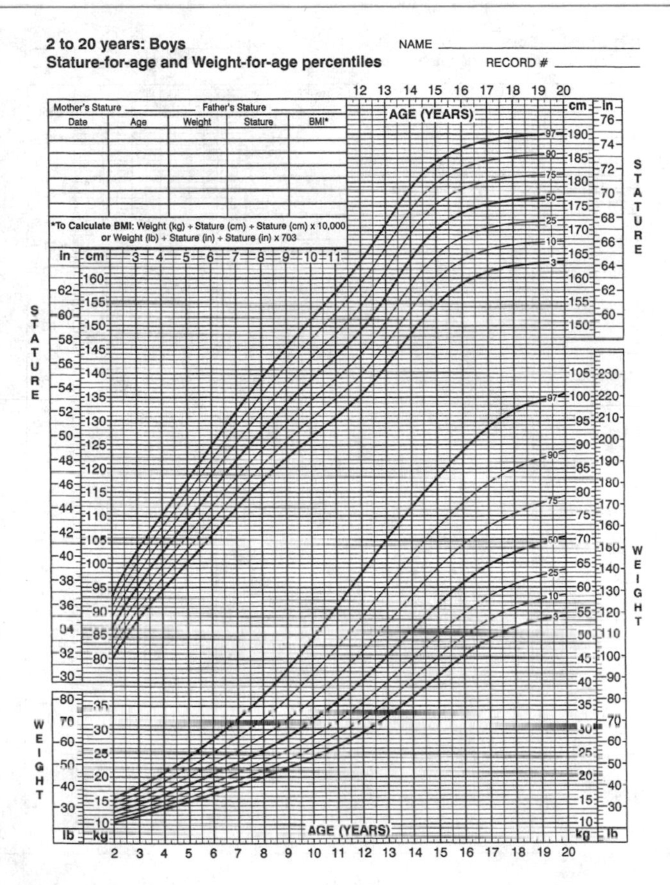


FIG. 21-8

Stature and weight for boys ages 2–20 years. *(Developed by the National Center for Health Statistics in collaboration with the National Center for Chronic Disease Prevention and Health Promotion, 2000.)*

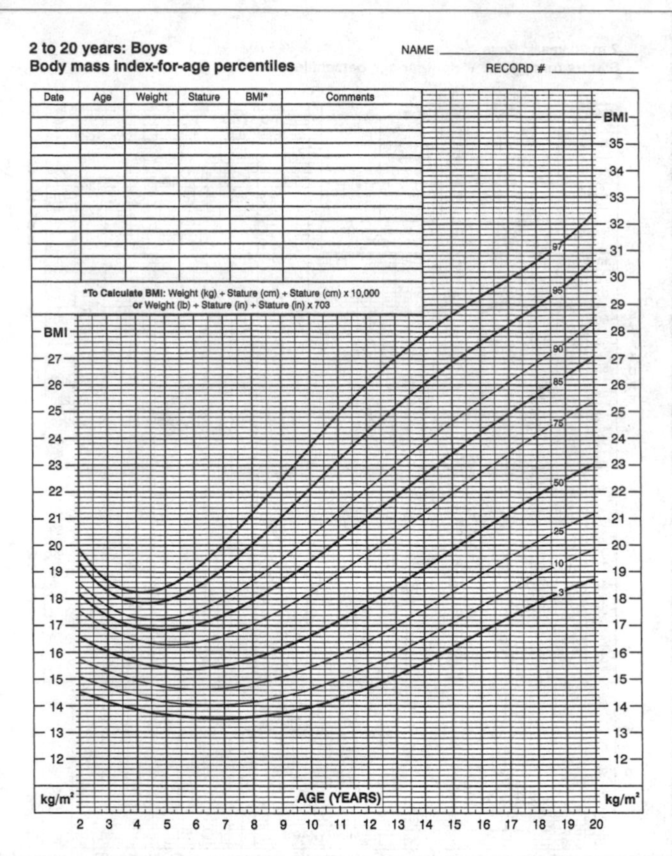


FIG. 21-9

Body mass index for boys ages 2–20 years. *(Developed by the National Center for Health Statistics in collaboration with the National Center for Chronic Disease Prevention and Health Promotion, 2000.)*

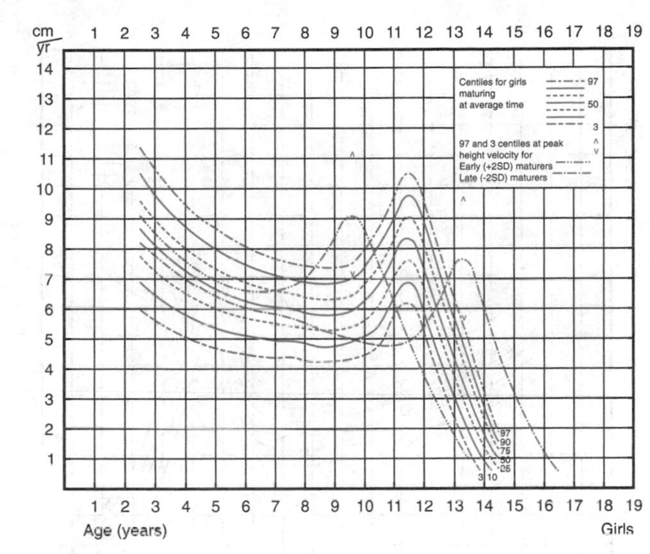


FIG. 21-10

Height velocity for girls ages 2–18 years. *(Modified from Tanner JM, Davis PS: Clinical longitudinal standards for height and height velocity in North American Children. J Pediatr 1985;107:317–329. Courtesy of Castlemead Publications, 1985. Distributed by Serono Laboratories.)*

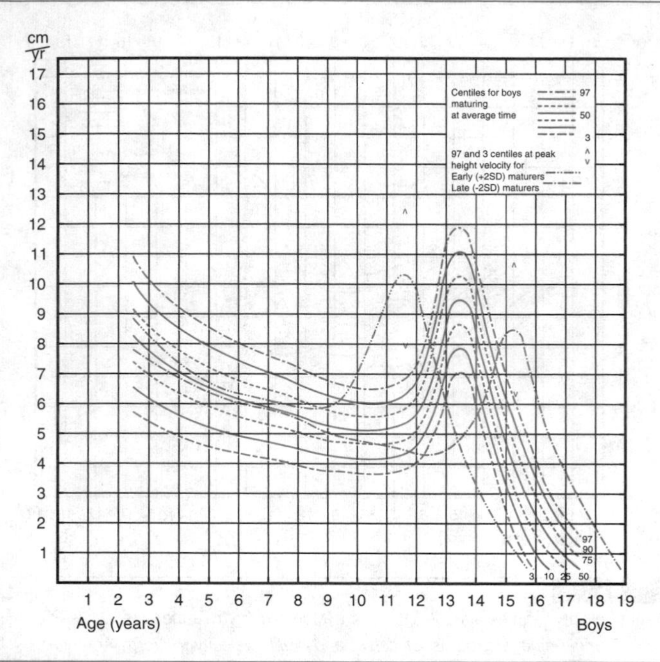


FIG. 21-11

Height velocity for boys ages 2–18 years. *(Modified from Tanner JM, Davis PS: Clinical longitudinal standards for height and height velocity in North American Children. [Data from Portland Health Institute, Inc., Portland, Oregon.] J Pediatr 1985;107:317–329. Courtesy of Castlemead Publications, 1985. Distributed by Serono Laboratories.)*

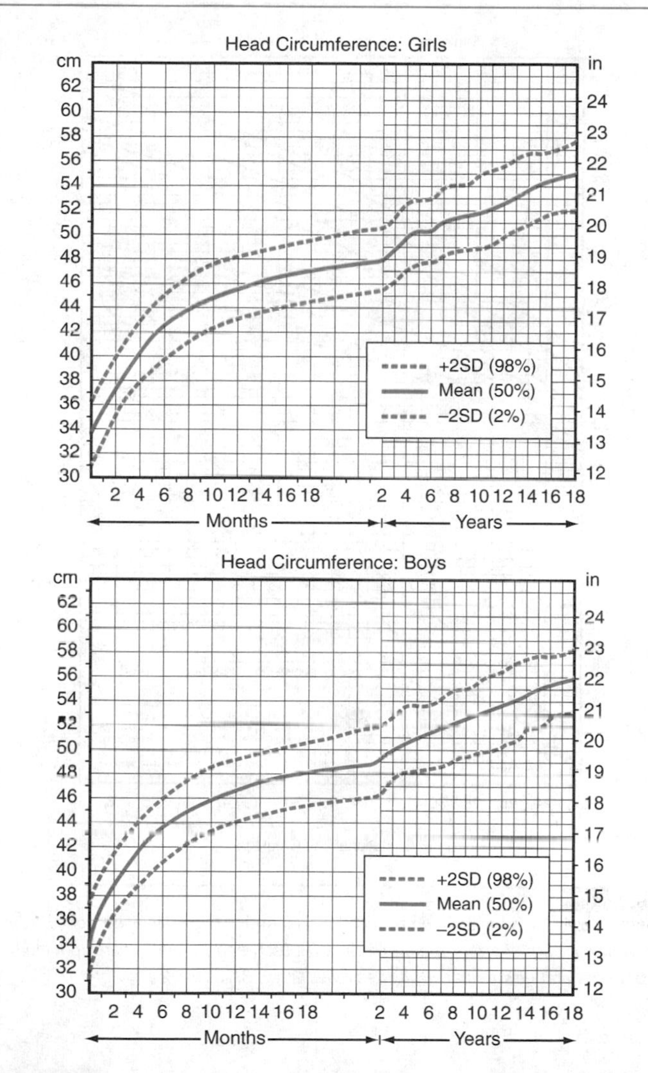


FIG. 21-12
Head circumference for girls and boys ages 2 to 18 years. *(Modified from Nelhaus G: J Pediatr 1968;48:106.)*

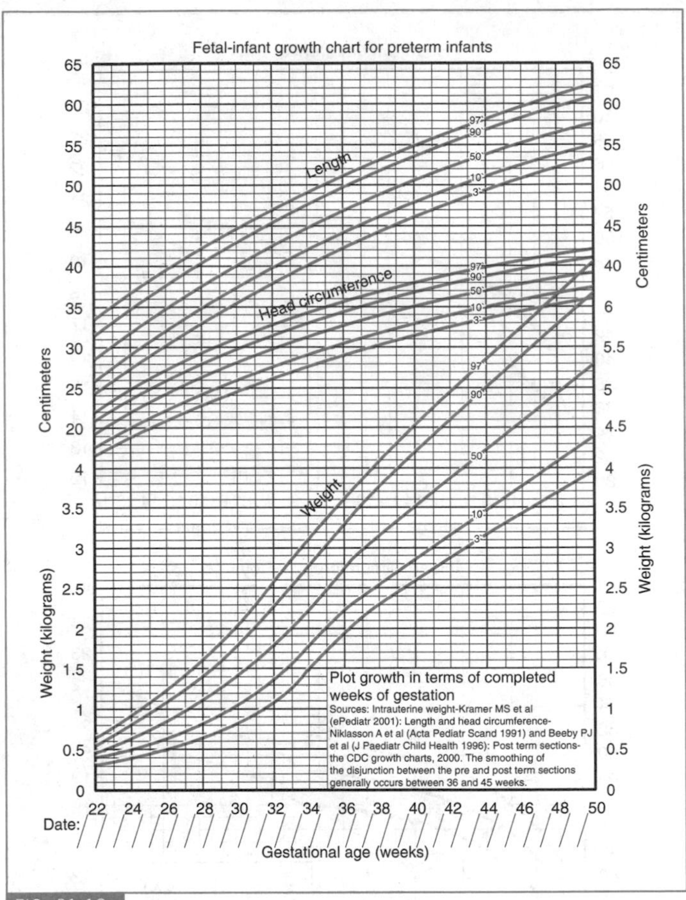


FIG. 21-13

Length, weight, and head circumference for preterm infants. *(Modified from Fenton TR: A new growth chart for preterm babies: Babson and Benda's chart updated with recent data and new format. BMC Pediatrics 2003;3:13, fig. 2.)*

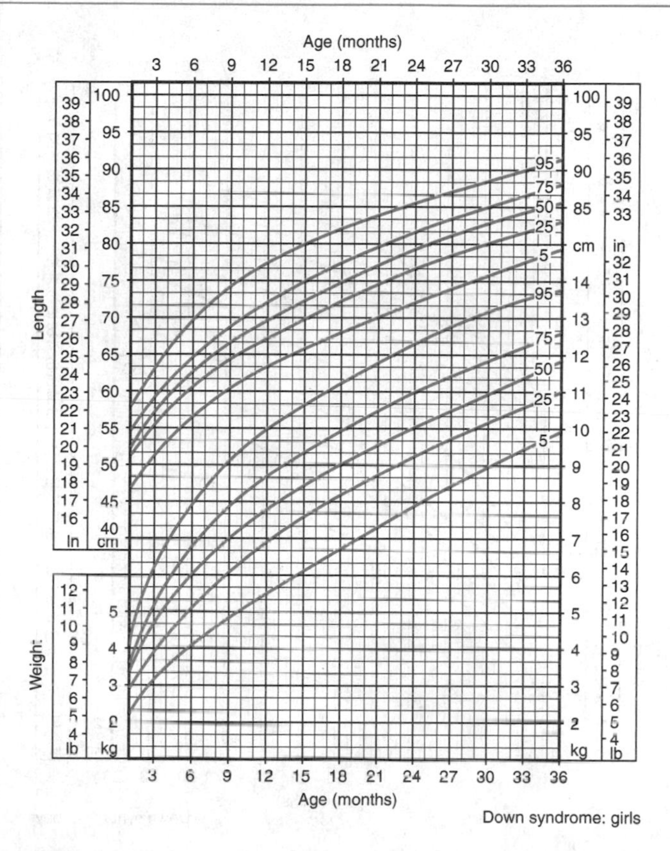


FIG. 21-14

Length and weight for girls with Down syndrome, from birth to ages 36 months. *(Modified from Cronk C et al: Growth charts for children with Down syndrome: 1 month to 18 years of age. Pediatrics 1988;81:102–110.)*

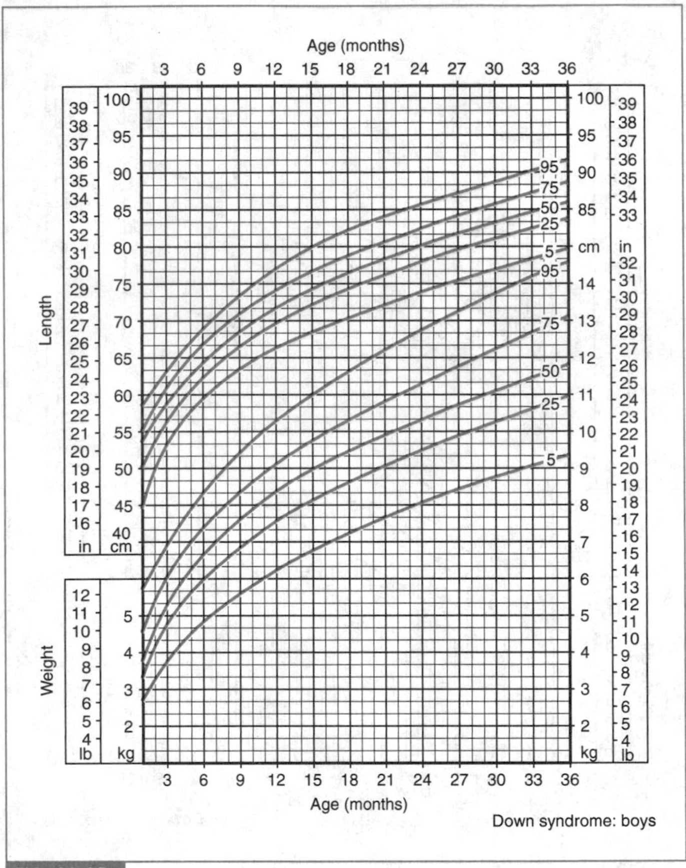


FIG. 21-15

Length and weight for boys with Down syndrome, from birth to ages 36 months. *(Modified from Cronk C et al: Growth charts for children with Down syndrome: 1 month to 18 years of age. Pediatrics 1988;81:102–110.)*

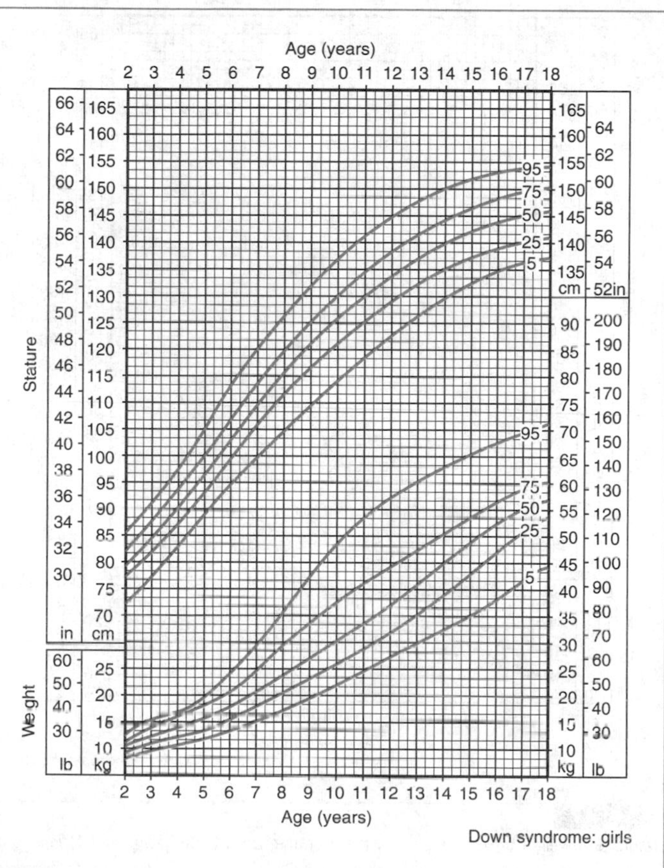


FIG. 21-16

Stature and weight for girls with Down syndrome, ages 2–18 years. *(Modified from Cronk C et al: Growth charts for children with Down syndrone: 1 month to 18 years of age. Pediatrics 1988;81:102–110.)*

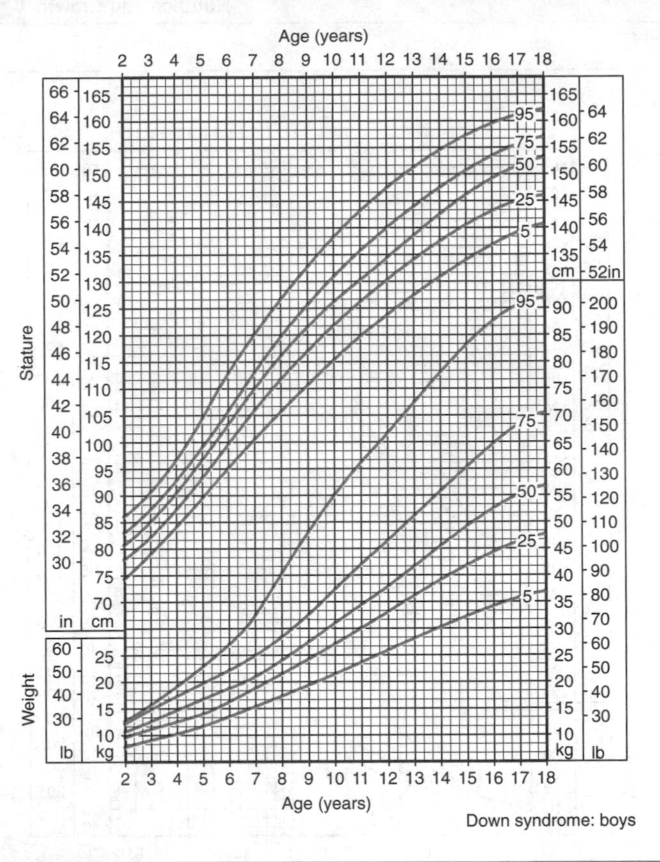


FIG. 21-17

Stature and weight for boys with Down syndrome, ages 2–18 years. *(Modified from Cronk C et al: Growth charts for children with Down syndrome: 1 month to 18 years of age. Pediatrics 1988;81:102–110.)*

TABLE 21-1

**PHYSICAL ACTIVITY COEFFICIENTS**

| | Sedentary Activity (Physical Activity Levels Required for Independent Living) | Low Active (30–45 min Sustained Daily Activity) | Active (60 min Sustained Daily Activity) | Very Active (≥90 min Sustained Daily Activity) |
|---|---|---|---|---|
| PAL | ≥1.0 or <1.4 | ≥1.4 or <1.6 | ≥1.6 or <1.9 | ≥1.9 or <2.5 |
| PA (boys ages 3–18) | 1.00 | 1.13 | 1.26 | 1.42 |
| PA (girls ages 3–18) | 1.00 | 1.16 | 1.31 | 1.56 |

TABLE 21-2

SAMPLE ESTIMATED ENERGY REQUIREMENTS FOR HEALTHY BOYS AND GIRLS OF MEDIAN WEIGHT AND HEIGHT*

| Age | Boys EER (kcal/kg/day) | Girls EER (kcal/kg/day) |
|---|---|---|
| 0–2 mo | 107 | 104 |
| 3 mo | 95 | 95 |
| 4–35 mo | 82 | 82 |

| | Boys | | | Girls | | |
|---|---|---|---|---|---|---|
| | Median Weight, Boys (kg) | Sedentary† (kcal/kg/d) | Active† (kcal/kg/d) | Median Weight, Girls (kg) | Sedentary† (kcal/kg/d) | Active† (kcal/kg/d) |
| 3 yr | 14.3 | 80 | 104 | 13.9 | 76 | 100 |
| 4 yr | 16.2 | 74 | 97 | 15.8 | 70 | 93 |
| 5 yr | 18.4 | 68 | 90 | 17.9 | 65 | 87 |
| 6 yr | 20.7 | 63 | 84 | 20.2 | 61 | 81 |
| 7 yr | 23.1 | 59 | 80 | 22.8 | 56 | 75 |
| 8 yr | 25.6 | 56 | 75 | 25.6 | 52 | 71 |
| 9 yr | 28.6 | 53 | 71 | 29.0 | 48 | 65 |
| 10 yr | 31.9 | 49 | 67 | 32.9 | 44 | 60 |
| 11 yr | 35.9 | 46 | 63 | 37.2 | 41 | 56 |
| 12 yr | 40.5 | 44 | 60 | 41.6 | 38 | 52 |
| 13 yr | 45.6 | 42 | 57 | 45.8 | 36 | 50 |
| 14 yr | 51.0 | 40 | 55 | 49.4 | 34 | 47 |
| 15 yr | 56.3 | 39 | 54 | 52.0 | 33 | 45 |
| 16 yr | 60.9 | 38 | 52 | 53.9 | 32 | 44 |
| 17 yr | 64.6 | 36 | 50 | 55.1 | 31 | 43 |
| 18 yr | 67.2 | 35 | 49 | 56.2 | 30 | 42 |

*Weight and height for age at 50th percentile.

†See definition of sedentary and active PAL for further information.

Data from Otten JJ et al (eds): Dietary Reference Intakes: The Essential Guide to Nutrient Requirements. Washington, DC, National Academies Press, 2006.

## D. CATCH-UP GROWTH REQUIREMENT FOR MALNOURISHED INFANTS AND CHILDREN (<3 YEARS OF AGE)[7]

1. **Growth failure** (also known as failure to thrive): Condition of undernutrition generally identified in the first 3 years of life. Can be described by the following growth scenarios: weight for age <5th percentile on the CDC growth charts, weight for length (or height) <5th percentile, or decreased growth velocity resulting in weight falling >2 major percentiles over 3–6 months.
2. **Catch-up growth:** Time period of accelerated growth as a result of caloric provision in excess of the dietary reference intakes (DRIs). Approximately 20%–30% more energy may be required to achieve catch-up growth in children. Protein needs also increase. This should continue until the previous growth percentiles are regained. Catch-up in linear growth may lag several months behind that in weight. Box 21-1 lists the steps for determining catch-up growth requirements.

BOX 21-1

**DETERMINING CATCH-UP GROWTH REQUIREMENTS**

1. Plot the child's height and weight on CDC growth charts.
2. Determine recommended calories needed for age (DRI; see section II.B for EER equations).
3. Determine the ideal weight (50th percentile) for child's height.*
4. Multiply the DRI calories by ideal body weight for height (kg).
5. Divide this value by the child's actual weight (kg).

For example, for a 12-month-old male whose weight is 7 kg and length is 72 cm, DRI for age would be 78 kcal/kg/day and ideal body weight for height is 9 kg (50th percentile weight for height). Thus, his catch-up growth requirement would be as follows:

$$\text{Catch-up growth requirements (kcal/kg/d)} =$$

$$\text{DRI kcal for age (kcals/kg/d)} \times \frac{\text{ideal weight for height (kg)}}{\text{actual weight (kg)}}$$

$$78 \text{ kcal/kg/day} \times (9 \text{ kg}/7 \text{ kg}) = 100 \text{ kcal/kg/day}$$

*The ideal weight can be 10th–85th percentile weight for height, depending on past growth trends; clinical judgment should be used.

**Note** *Aggressive refeeding in the severely malnourished child can result in metabolic alterations, vomiting, diarrhea, and circulatory decompensation known as refeeding syndrome (hypophosphatemia, hypokalemia, hypomagnesemia, and glucose and/or fluid intolerance).*[8]

## III. DIETARY REFERENCE INTAKES FOR INDIVIDUALS[6]

### A. DIETARY REFERENCE INTAKES (DRIs)

Reference values that are quantitative estimates of nutrient intakes and are measured in several ways, including the following:

1. **Estimated average requirement (EAR):** Daily nutrient intake level estimated to meet the requirement of half the healthy individuals in a particular life stage and gender group.
2. **Recommended dietary allowance (RDA):** EAR ±2 standard deviations. The daily nutrient intake level estimated to meet the requirement of 97%–98% of healthy individuals in a particular life stage and gender group.
3. **Adequate intake (AI):** Observed range of intakes in a healthy population used when there are not sufficient data to calculate the EAR and RDA.
4. **Tolerable upper intake level (UL):** Highest daily nutrient intake level that is likely to pose no risk for adverse health effects to almost all individuals in the general population.

## B. PROTEIN REQUIREMENTS (Table 21-3)[6]
## C. FAT REQUIREMENTS (Table 21-4)[6]
## D. VITAMIN REQUIREMENTS (Table 21-5)[6]
## E. MINERAL REQUIREMENTS (Table 21-6)[6]
## F. FIBER REQUIREMENTS (Table 21-7)[6]

TABLE 21-3

PROTEIN REQUIREMENTS (DRI VALUES)

| Age | RDA (g/kg/d) |
|---|---|
| 0–6 mo | 1.52 (AI)* |
| 7–12 mo | 1.2 |
| 1–3 yr | 1.05 |
| 4–8 yr | 0.95 |
| 9–13 yr | 0.95 |
| 14–18 yr | 0.85 |
| Pregnancy (second half) | 1.1 |
| Pregnancy (first half) | Unchanged |
| Lactation | 1.3 |

*If sufficient scientific evidence is not available to establish an RDA, an AI (Adequate Intake) is usually developed. For healthy breast-fed infants, the AI is the mean intake.

Data from Otten JJ et al (eds): Dietary Reference Intakes: The Essential Guide to Nutrient Requirements. Washington, DC, National Academies Press, 2006.

TABLE 21-4

FAT REQUIREMENTS: ADEQUATE INTAKE*

| Age | Total Fat (g/d) | Linoleic Acid (g/d) | α Linolenic Acid (g/d) |
|---|---|---|---|
| 0–6 mo | 31 | 4.4 (n-6 PUFA) | 0.5 (n-3 PUFA) |
| 7–12 mo | 30 | 4.6 (n-6 PUFA) | 0.5 (n-3 PUFA) |
| 1–3 yr | † | 7 | 0.7 |
| 4–8 yr | † | 10 | 0.9 |
| 9–13 yr, boys | † | 12 | 1.2 |
| 9–13 yr, girls | † | 10 | 1.0 |
| 14–18 yr, boys | † | 16 | 1.6 |
| 14–18 yr, girls | † | 11 | 1.1 |
| Pregnancy | † | 13 | 1.4 |
| Lactation | † | 13 | 1.3 |

*If sufficient scientific evidence is not available to establish an RDA, an AI is usually developed. For healthy breast-fed infants, the AI is the mean intake. The AI for other life stage and gender groups is believed to cover the needs of all healthy individuals in the group, but a lack of data or uncertainty in the data prevents being able to specify with confidence the percentage of individuals covered by this intake.

†No AI, EAR, or RDA established.

Data from Otten JJ et al (eds): Dietary Reference Intakes: The Essential Guide to Nutrient Requirements. Washington, DC, National Academies Press, 2006.

TABLE 21-5

DIETARY REFERENCE INTAKES: RECOMMENDED INTAKES—VITAMINS

| Life Stage | Vit. A* (IU) | Vit. C (mg/d) | Vit. D[†,‡] (IU) | Vit. E[§] (IU) | Vit. K (μg/d) | Thiamin (mg/d) | Riboflavin (mg/d) |
|---|---|---|---|---|---|---|---|
| **Infants** | | | | | | | |
| 0–6 mo | **1333** | 40** | 200 | 4** | 2.0** | 0.2** | 0.3** |
| 7–12 mo | **1666** | 50** | 200 | 5** | 2.5** | 0.3** | 0.4** |
| **Children** | | | | | | | |
| 1–3 yr | **1000** | **15** | 200 | **6** | 30** | **0.5** | **0.5** |
| 4–8 yr | **1333** | **25** | 200 | **7** | 55** | **0.6** | **0.6** |
| **Males** | | | | | | | |
| 9–13 yr | **2000** | **45** | 200 | **11** | 60** | **0.9** | **0.9** |
| 14–18 yr | **3000** | **75** | 200 | **15** | 75** | **1.2** | **1.3** |
| 19–30 yr | **3000** | **90** | 200 | **15** | 120** | **1.2** | **1.3** |
| **Females** | | | | | | | |
| 9–13 yr | **2000** | **45** | 200 | **11** | 60** | **0.9** | **0.9** |
| 14–18 yr | **2333** | **65** | 200 | **15** | 75** | **1.0** | **1.0** |
| 19–30 yr | **2333** | **75** | 200 | **15** | 90** | **1.1** | **1.1** |
| **Pregnancy** | | | | | | | |
| <18 yr | **2500** | **80** | 200 | **15** | 75** | **1.4** | **1.4** |
| 19–30 yr | **2567** | **85** | 200 | **15** | 90** | **1.4** | **1.4** |
| **Lactation** | | | | | | | |
| <18 yr | **4000** | **115** | 200 | **19** | 75** | **1.4** | **1.6** |
| 19–30 yr | **4333** | **120** | 200 | **19** | 90** | **1.4** | **1.6** |

*Note:* This table (taken from the DRI reports; see www.nap.edu) presents Recommended Dietary Allowances (RDAs) in **bold type** and Adequate Intakes (AIs) in regular type followed by a double asterisk (**), RDAs and AIs may both be used as goals for individual intake. RDAs are set to meet the needs of almost all (97%–98%) individuals in a group. For healthy breast-fed infants, the AI is the mean intake. The AI for other life stage and gender groups is believed to cover needs of all individuals in the group, but lack of data or uncertainty in the data prevent being able to specify with confidence the percentage of individuals covered by this intake.

*One IU = 0.3 μg retinol equivalent.

[†]One μg cholecalciferol = 40 IU vitamin D.

[‡]In the absence of adequate exposure to sunlight.

[§]One IU = 1 mg vitamin E.

[||]As niacin equivalents (NE). 1 mg of niacin = 60 mg of tryptophan; 0–6 months = preformed niacin (not NE).

| Niacin[‖] (mg/d) | Vit. $B_6$ (mg/d) | Folate[¶] (μg/d) | Vit. $B_{12}$ (μg/d) | Pantothenic Acid (mg/d) | Biotin (μg/d) | Choline[#] (mg/d) |
|---|---|---|---|---|---|---|
| 2** | 0.1** | 65* | 0.4** | 1.7** | 5** | 125** |
| 4** | 0.3** | 80** | 0.5** | 1.8** | 6** | 150** |
| **6** | **0.5** | **150** | 0.9 | 2** | 8** | 200** |
| **8** | **0.6** | **200** | 1.2 | 3** | 12** | 250** |
| **12** | **1.0** | **300** | 1.8 | 4** | 20** | 375** |
| **16** | **1.3** | **400** | 2.4 | 5** | 25** | 550** |
| **16** | **1.3** | **400** | 2.4 | 5** | 30** | 550** |
| **12** | **1.0** | **300** | 1.8 | 4** | 20** | 375** |
| **14** | **1.2** | **400** | 2.4 | 5** | 25** | 400** |
| **14** | **1.3** | **400** | 2.4 | 5** | 30** | 425** |
| **18** | **1.9** | **600** | 2.6 | 6** | 30** | 450** |
| **18** | **1.9** | **600** | 2.6 | 6** | 30** | 450** |
| **17** | **2.0** | **500** | 2.8 | 7** | 35** | 550** |
| **17** | **2.0** | **500** | 2.8 | 7** | 35** | 550* |

[¶]As dietary folate equivalents (DFE). 1 DFE = 1 μg food folate = 0.6 μg of folic acid from fortified food or as a supplement consumed with food = 0.5 μg of a supplement taken on an empty stomach. In view of evidence linking folate intake with neural tube defects in the fetus, it is recommended that all women capable of becoming pregnant consume 400 μg from supplements or fortified foods in addition to intake of food folate from a varied diet. It is assumed that women will continue consuming 400 μg from supplements or fortified food until their pregnancy is confirmed and they enter prenatal care, which ordinarily occurs after the end of the periconceptual period—the critical time for formation of the neural tube.

[#]Although AIs have been set for choline, there are few data to assess whether a dietary supply of choline is needed at all life stages, and it may be that the choline requirement can be met by endogenous synthesis at some of these stages.

Modified from Otten JJ et al (eds): Dietary Reference Intakes: The Essential Guide to Nutrient Requirements. Washington, DC, National Academies Press, 2006.

TABLE 21-6

**DIETARY REFERENCE INTAKES: RECOMMENDED INTAKES—ELEMENTS**

| Life Stage | Calcium (mg/d) | Chromium (μg/d) | Copper (μg/d) | Fluoride (mg/d) | Iodine (μg/d) | Iron (mg/d) |
|---|---|---|---|---|---|---|
| **Infants** | | | | | | |
| 0–6 mo | 210* | 0.2* | 200* | 0.01* | 110* | 0.27* |
| 7–12 mo | 270* | 5.5* | 220* | 0.5* | 130* | **11** |
| **Children** | | | | | | |
| 1–3 yr | 500* | 11* | **340** | 0.7* | **90** | **7** |
| 4–8 yr | 800* | 15* | **440** | 1.0* | **90** | **10** |
| **Males** | | | | | | |
| 9–13 yr | 1300* | 25* | **700** | 2* | **120** | **8** |
| 14–18 yr | 1300* | 35* | **890** | 3* | **150** | **11** |
| 19–30 yr | 1000* | 35* | **900** | 4* | **150** | **8** |
| **Females** | | | | | | |
| 9–13 yr | 1300* | 21* | **700** | 2* | **120** | **8** |
| 14–18 yr | 1300* | 24* | **890** | 3* | **150** | **15** |
| 19–30 yr | 1000* | 25* | **900** | 3* | **150** | **18** |
| **Pregnancy** | | | | | | |
| <18 yr | 1300* | 29* | **1000** | 3* | **220** | **27** |
| 19–30 yr | 1000* | 30* | **1000** | 3* | **220** | **27** |
| **Lactation** | | | | | | |
| <18 yr | 1300* | 44* | **1300** | 3* | **290** | **10** |
| 19–30 yr | 1000* | 45* | **1300** | 3* | **290** | **9** |

*Note:* This table presents Recommended Dietary Allowances (RDAs) in **bold type** and Adequate Intakes (AIs) in ordinary type followed by an asterisk (*). RDAs and AIs may both be used as goals for individual intake. RDAs are set to meet the needs of almost all (97%–98%) individuals in a group. For healthy breast-fed infants, the AI is the mean intake. The AI for other life stage and gender groups is believed to cover needs of all individuals in the group, but lack of data or uncertainty in the data prevent being able to specify with confidence the percentage of individuals covered by this intake.

TABLE 21-7

**FIBER REQUIREMENTS: ADEQUATE INTAKE***

| Age | Total Fiber (g/d) |
|---|---|
| 0–12 mo | Not determined |
| 1–3 yr | 19 |
| 4–8 yr | 25 |
| 9–13 yr, boys | 31 |
| 9–13 yr, girls | 26 |
| 14–18 yr, boys | 38 |
| 14–18 yr, girls | 26 |
| Pregnancy | 28 |
| Lactation | 29 |

*Adequate Intake (AI). If sufficient scientific evidence is not available to establish an RDA, an AI is usually developed. For healthy breast-fed infants, the AI is the mean intake. The AI for other life stages and gender groups is believed to cover the needs of all healthy individuals in the group, but a lack of data or uncertainty in the data prevents being able to specify with confidence the percentage of individuals covered by this intake.

Data from Otten JJ et al (eds): Dietary Reference Intakes: The Essential Guide to Nutrient Requirements. Washington, DC, National Academies Press, 2006.

| Magnesium (mg/d) | Manganese (mg/d) | Molybdenum (μg/d) | Phosphorus (mg/d) | Selenium (μg/d) | Zinc (mg/d) |
|---|---|---|---|---|---|
| 30* | 0.003* | 2* | 100* | 15* | 2* |
| 75* | 0.6* | 3* | 275* | 20* | **3** |
| | | | | | |
| **80** | 1.2* | **17** | **460** | **20** | **3** |
| **130** | 1.5* | **22** | **500** | **30** | **5** |
| | | | | | |
| **240** | 1.9* | **34** | **1250** | **40** | **8** |
| **410** | 2.2* | **43** | **1250** | **55** | **11** |
| **400** | 2.3* | **45** | **700** | **55** | **11** |
| | | | | | |
| **240** | 1.6* | **34** | **1250** | **40** | **8** |
| **360** | 1.6* | **43** | **1250** | **55** | **9** |
| **310** | 1.8* | **45** | **700** | **55** | **8** |
| | | | | | |
| **400** | 2.0* | **50** | **1250** | **60** | **13** |
| **350** | 2.0* | **50** | **700** | **60** | **11** |
| | | | | | |
| **360** | 2.6* | **50** | **1250** | **70** | **14** |
| **310** | 2.6* | **50** | **700** | **70** | **12** |

Modified from Otten JJ et al (eds): Dietary Reference Intakes: The Essential Guide to Nutrient Requirements. Washington, DC, National Academies Press, 2006.



## IV. VITAMIN-MINERAL SUPPLEMENTATION[9]

### A. VITAMIN D

200 IU per day is recommended for the following individuals:

1. **All breast-fed infants consuming <500 mL/day of vitamin D–fortified formula or milk.**
2. **All nonbreast-fed infants ingesting <200 mL/day of vitamin D–fortified formula or milk.**
3. **Children and adolescents who do not get regular sunlight exposure, do not ingest 500 mL/day of vitamin D–fortified milk, or do not take a daily multivitamin supplement containing at least 200 IU of vitamin D.**

Generally, an A, D, C multivitamin, such as Tri-Vi-Sol or Vi-Daylin ADC, can be used (Table 21-8).

### B. FLUORIDE

1. **Supplementation** not needed during the first 6 months of life. Thereafter, 0.25 mg/day is recommended for the exclusively breast-fed infant.
2. Consider the use of bottled water and home filtration systems. Most bottled water does not contain adequate amounts of fluoride. Some home water treatment systems can reduce fluoride levels.

TABLE 21-8

**INFANT MULTIVITAMIN DROPS ANALYSIS (PER ML)***

| Nutrient | Poly-Vi-Sol/(Flor) [w/iron], Multivitamin [with iron] | Tri-Vi-Sol/(Flor) [w/iron], Vi-Daylin A,D,C [w/iron] | ADEK[†‡] | Aquadek |
|---|---|---|---|---|
| Vitamin A (IU) | 1500 | 1500 | 3170 | 5751 |
| Vitamin D (IU) | 400 | 400 | 400 | 400 |
| Vitamin E (IU) | 5 | — | 40 | 50 |
| Vitamin C (mg) | 35 | 35 | 45 | 45 |
| Thiamin (mg) | 0.5 | — | 0.5 | 0.6 |
| Riboflavin (mg) | 0.6 | — | 0.6 | 0.6 |
| Niacin (mg) | 8 | — | 6 | 6 |
| Vitamin $B_6$ (mg) | 0.4 | — | 0.6 | 0.6 |
| Vitamin $B_{12}$ (μg) | 2[§] | — | 4 | — |
| Vitamin K (μg) | — | — | 100 | 400 |
| Iron (mg) | [10] | [10] | — | — |
| Fluoride (mg) | (0.25) | (0.25) | — | — |
| Zinc (mg) | | | 5 | 5 |

*Standard dose = 1 mL.

[†]Also contains biotin 15 μg; pantothenic acid 3 mg; 50% vitamin A as β-carotene.

[‡]Recommended for use in infants with fat malabsorption, such as cystic fibrosis, liver disease.

[§]Poly-Vi-Sol only.

**3. To avoid fluorosis, children should not use fluoridated toothpaste until age 2 years, and then only a small pea-sized amount up to age 6 years. See Formulary for complete fluoride recommendations (i.e., in areas where water is not fluoridated).**

## C. IRON

**1. Breast-fed infants:**

a. Full-term breast-fed infants: Approximately 1 mg/kg/day is recommended after age 4–6 months, preferably from iron-fortified cereal or elemental iron if sufficient cereal is not consumed.

b. Preterm or low-birth-weight breast-fed infants: Iron supplement of 2 mg/kg/day should be given after approximately age 2 months until age 12 months.

c. All infants younger than 12 months: Only iron-fortified formula should be used for weaning or supplementing breast milk.

**2. Formula-fed infants:**

a. Full-term formula-fed infants: Iron-fortified formula containing 4–12 mg/L of iron from birth to age 12 months.

b. Preterm formula-fed infants: An additional 1 mg/kg/day, administered either as iron drops or in a vitamin preparation with iron.

## D. EXAMPLES OF MULTIVITAMINS FOR CHILDREN (Table 21-9)

## V. ENTERAL NUTRITION

### A. MIXING INSTRUCTIONS FOR FULL-TERM STANDARD AND SOY-BASED INFANT FORMULAS (Table 21-10)

### B. COMMON CALORIC MODULARS FOR THE CHILD WHO NEEDS ADDITIONAL PROTEIN, CARBOHYDRATE, FAT, OR A COMBINATION (Table 21-11)

### C. ENTERAL FORMULAS, INCLUDING THEIR MAIN NUTRIENT COMPONENTS (Table 21-12A-C)

A comprehensive (but not complete) list. Most of these formulas are cow's milk–based and are designed for normal digestive tracts.

### D. CLINICAL CONDITIONS REQUIRING SPECIAL DIETS, AND SUGGESTED FORMULA(S) (Table 21-13A-C)

A comprehensive (but not complete) list of special clinical conditions (e.g., cow's milk allergy or intolerance) and the growing number of formulas designed for these conditions.

### E. COMMON ORAL REHYDRATION SOLUTIONS (Table 21-14)

## VI. PARENTERAL NUTRITION (PN)[10]

Necessary to adequately support the pediatric patient with insufficient enteral intake.

### A. SITUATIONS IN WHICH PN IS SUGGESTED

1. **Inability to feed enterally (e.g., extreme prematurity, tracheoesophageal fistulas).**
2. **When alimentation via gastrointestinal tract needs to be restricted (e.g., chylothorax/chylous ascites bowel, pseudo-obstruction).**
3. **GI dysfunction and/or malabsorption (e.g., short-gut syndrome, intestinal atresias, enteric fistulas, gastroschisis).**
4. **Increased losses or requirements (e.g., severe diarrhea, intractable vomiting, persistent or severe failure to thrive).**

### B. SUGGESTED FORMULATIONS FOR INITIATION AND ADVANCEMENT OF PN (Table 21-15)

Suggested glucose, protein, and fat during initiation, as well as recommendations for advancement and maximum allowable amounts.

### C. RECOMMENDED PARENTERAL FORMULATIONS (Table 21-16)

Based on age groups; includes recommendations for electrolytes, elements, and minerals.

### D. SUGGESTED MONITORING SCHEDULE FOR PATIENTS RECEIVING PARENTERAL NUTRITION (Table 21-17)

Important to monitor growth parameters as well as laboratory studies for these patients on periodic basis.

TABLE 21-9

MULTIVITAMIN TABLETS (ANALYSIS/TABLET)

| | Multivitamins | | | |
|---|---|---|---|---|
| Nutrient | Flintstones Original Bugs Bunny Generic Poly-Vi-Sol/(Flor) Vi-Daylin/(F) [w/iron] | Flintstones + Extra C Sunkist + Extra C Generic + C Bugs Bunny + Extra C | Centrum Jr | Flintstones Complete Generic Complete |
| Vitamin A (IU) | 2500 | 2500 | 5000 | 5000 |
| Vitamin D (IU) | 400 | 400 | 400 | 400 |
| Vitamin E (IU) | 15 | 15 | 30 | 30 |
| Vitamin K (μg) | — | — | 10 | — |
| Vitamin C (mg) | 60 | 250 | 60 | 60 |
| Thiamin (mg) | 1.05 | 1.05 | 1.5 | 1.5 |
| Riboflavin (mg) | 1.2 | 1.2 | 1.7 | 1.7 |
| Niacin (mg) | 13.5 | 13.5 | 20 | 20 |
| Vitamin $B_6$ (mg) | 1.05 | 1.06 | 2 | 2 |
| Folate (μg) | 300 | 300 | 400 | 400 |
| Vitamin $B_{12}$ (μg) | 4.5 | 4.5 | 6 | 6 |
| Biotin (μg) | — | — | 45 | 40 |
| Pantothenic acid (mg) | — | — | 10 | 10 |
| Calcium (mg) | — | — | 108 | 100 |
| Phosphorus (mg) | — | — | 50 | 100 |
| Iron (mg) | [10–15] | — | 18 | 18 |
| Iodine (μg) | — | — | 150 | 150 |
| Magnesium (mg) | — | — | 40 | 20 |
| Zinc (mg) | — | — | 15 | 15 |
| Copper (mg) | — | — | 2 | 2 |
| Manganese (mg) | — | — | 1 | — |
| Chromium (μg) | — | — | 20 | — |
| Molybdenum (μg) | — | — | 20 | — |
| Selenium (μg) | — | — | — | — |
| Fluoride (mg) | [0.25, 0.5, 1.0] | — | — | — |

*Vitamin A as palmitate and 60% β-carotene.

†Vitamin A: 3600 IU as retinol and 5400 IU as β-carotene.

‡Vitamin A as acetate and 50% β-carotene.

| Fat Malabsorption | | | Prenatal | | Powder |
|---|---|---|---|---|---|
| ADEK | SourceCF | Vitamax | StuartNatal Plus 3 | Obegyn Prenatal‖ | Phlexy-Vits (7 g Packet) |
| 9000* | 9000† | 5000‡ | 3000§ | 5000¶ | 2664 |
| 400 | 400 | 400 | 400 | 400 | 400 |
| 150 | 200 | 200 | 22 | 30 | 13.5 |
| 150 | 50 | 200 | — | — | 70 |
| 60 | 100 | 60 | 120 | 120 | 50 |
| 1.2 | 1.5 | 1.5 | 1.8 | 1.7 | 1.2 |
| 1.3 | 1.7 | 1.7 | 4 | 2 | 1.4 |
| 10 | 20 | 20 | — | 20 | 20 |
| 1.5 | 1.9 | 2 | 25 | 10 | 1.6 |
| 200 | 200 | 200 | 1 | 1 | 700 |
| 12 | 6 | 6 | 12 | 12 | 5 |
| 50 | 100 | 300 | — | 300 | 150 |
| 10 | 12 | 10 | — | — | 5 |
| | | | | | |
| — | — | — | 200 | 455 | 1000 |
| — | — | — | — | — | 775 |
| — | — | — | 27 | 18 | 15.1 |
| — | — | — | — | 0.15 | 150 |
| — | — | — | 25 | 150 | 300 |
| 7.5 | 10 | 7.5 | 25 | 25 | 11.1 |
| — | — | — | 2 | 2 | 1.5 |
| — | — | — | — | — | 1.5 |
| — | — | — | — | — | 30 |
| — | — | — | — | — | 70 |
| — | — | — | — | — | 75 |
| — | — | — | — | — | — |

§Vitamin A as β-carotene.
‖Contraindicated with kidney stones.
¶Vitamin A as 50% palmitate and 50% β-carotene.

21 NUTRITION AND GROWTH

TABLE 21-10

**PREPARATION OF INFANT FORMULAS FOR FULL-TERM STANDARD AND SOY FORMULAS***

| Formula Type | Caloric Concentration (kcal/oz) | Amount of Formula | Water (oz) |
|---|---|---|---|
| Liquid concentrates (40 kcal/oz) | 20 | 13 oz | 13 oz |
| | 24 | 13 oz | 8.5 oz |
| | 27 | 13 oz | 6.3 oz |
| | 30 | 13 oz | 4.3 oz |
| Powder (44 kcal/scoop) | 20 | 1 scoop | 2 oz |
| | 24 | 3 scoops | 5 oz |
| | 27 | 3 scoops | 4.25 oz |
| | 30 | 3 scoops | 4 oz |

*Does not apply to EnfaCare LIPIL, Neocate Infant, Neosure Advance, EleCare; Enfamil AR should not be concentrated greater than 24 kcal/oz. Use a packed measure for Nutramigen LIPIL and Pregestimil LIPIL; all others unpacked powder.

## VII. WEB RESOURCES

### A. PROFESSIONAL AND GOVERNMENTAL ORGANIZATIONS

The Centers for Disease Control and Prevention website has growth charts and nutrition information: www.cdc.gov.

The American Dietetic Association: www.eatright.org.

American Society for Parenteral and Enteral Nutrition: www.clinnutr.org.

### B. INFANT AND PEDIATRIC FORMULA COMPANY WEBSITES FOR OBTAINING COMPLETE AND UP-TO-DATE PRODUCT INFORMATION

www.meadjohnson.com (products include Enfamil, EnfaCare, Nutramigen, and Pregestimil)

www.nestle-nutrition.com (products include Carnation, Good Start, Nutren, and Peptamen)

www.abbottnutrition.com (products include Alimentum, EleCare, Ensure, NeoSure, PediaSure, and Similac)

www.pbmproducts.com (products include America's Store Brand and Bright Beginnings)

www.hormelhealthlabs.com (products include Pro-Peptide)

www.novartisnutrition.com (products include Boost, Peptinex, and Resource)

www.shsna.com (products include Ketocal, Neocate, and Pepdite)

*Text continued on p. 602*

TABLE 21-11

**COMMON CALORIC MODULARS***

| Component | Calories |
|---|---|
| **PROTEIN** | |
| Casec | 3.7 kcal/g (0.9 g protein)<br>17 kcal/tbsp (4 g protein) |
| Beneprotein | 25 kcal/scoop (6 g protein) |
| Complete Amino Acid Mix | 3.28 kcal/g (0.82 g protein) |
| **CARBOHYDRATE** | |
| Polycose | Powder: 3.8 kcal/g; 8 kcal/tsp<br>Liquid: 2.0 kcal/mL, 10 kcal/tsp |
| **FAT** | |
| MCT oil[†] | 7.7 kcal/mL |
| Vegetable oil | 8.3 kcal/mL |
| Microlipid | 4.5 kcal/mL |
| **FAT AND CARBOHYDRATE** | |
| Duocal | 42 kcal/tbsp (59% carbohydrates, 41% fat; 35% fat as MCT oil) |

*Use these caloric supplements when you want to increase protein or when you have reached the maximum concentration tolerated and wish to further increase caloric density.

[†]MCT oil is unnecessary unless there is fat malabsorption.

TABLE 21-12

**ENTERAL NUTRITION COMPONENTS (PER LITER)**

**A. INFANTS**

| | Kcal/oz | Protein (g) |
|---|---|---|
| **Human Milk** | | |
| Term | 20 | 11 |
| Preterm | 20 | 14 |
| **Human Milk and Fortifiers Analysis** | | |
| Enfamil HMF + preterm human milk (1 pkt/25 mL) | 24 | 26 |
| Similac HMF + preterm human milk (1 pkt/25 mL) | 24 | 23 |
| **Preterm Formulas** | | |
| Enfamil Premature LIPIL 20 | 20 | 20 |
| Enfamil Premature LIPIL 24 | 24 | 24 |
| NeoSure | 22 | 21 |
| EnfaCare LIPIL | 22 | 21 |
| Similac Special Care Advance 20 | 20 | 20 |
| Similac Special Care Advance 24 | 24 | 24 |
| Similac Special Care Advance 30 | 30 | 30 |
| **Cow's Milk–Based Formulas** | | |
| Bright Beginnings Milk Formula with DHA | 20 | 15 |
| Enfamil LIPIL | 20 | 14 |
| Enfamil AR LIPIL | 20 | 17 |
| Enfamil LactoFree LIPIL | 20 | 14 |
| Enfamil NextStep LIPIL | 20 | 18 |
| Evaporated milk (13 oz + 19 oz water + 2 T corn syrup) | 20 | 27 |
| Organic Milk–Based Infant Formula | 20 | 15 |
| Similac Advance | 20 | 14 |
| Similac Go & Grow Milk-Based Formula | 20 | 14 |
| Similac Sensitive | 20 | 14 |
| Similac Organic | 20 | 14 |
| Similac PM 60/40 | 20 | 15 |
| Similac with Iron | 20 | 14 |
| **Soy-Based Formulas** | | |
| Similac Sensitive R. S. | 20 | 14 |
| Good Start 2 Soy DHA & ARA | 20 | 19 |
| Bright Beginnings Soy Formula with DHA | 20 | 18 |
| Good Start Supreme Soy DHA & ARA | 20 | 17 |
| Isomil | 20 | 17 |
| Similac Go & Grow Soy-Based Formula | 20 | 17 |
| Isomil Advance | 20 | 17 |
| Isomil DF | 20 | 18 |
| NextStep ProSobee LIPIL | 20 | 22 |
| ProSobee LIPIL | 20 | 17 |
| **Casein, Extensively Hydrolyzed** | | |
| Alimentum | 20 | 19 |
| Nutramigen LIPIL | 20 | 19 |
| Pregestimil LIPIL | 20 | 19 |

| Fat (g) | Carbs (g) | Na (mEq) | K (mEq) | Ca (mg) | P (mg) | Fe (mg) | Osmolality |
|---|---|---|---|---|---|---|---|
| 39 | 72 | 8 | 14 | 279 | 143 | 0.3 | 286 |
| 39 | 66 | 11 | 15 | 248 | 128 | 1.2 | 290 |
| | | | | | | | |
| 49 | 70 | 18 | 22 | 1140 | 630 | 16 | 326 |
| 41 | 82 | 17 | 30 | 1381 | 777 | 4.6 | 385 |
| | | | | | | | |
| 34 | 74 | 17 | 17 | 1120 | 560 | 3.4 | 240 |
| 41 | 89 | 20 | 21 | 1340 | 670 | 4.1 | 300 |
| 41 | 75 | 11 | 27 | 781 | 461 | 13.4 | 250 |
| 39 | 77 | 11 | 20 | 890 | 490 | 13.3 | 260 |
| 37 | 70 | 13 | 22 | 1220 | 680 | 12.2 | 235 |
| 44 | 84 | 15 | 27 | 1460 | 810 | 14.6 | 280 |
| 67 | 78 | 19 | 34 | 1830 | 1010 | 18.3 | 325 |
| | | | | | | | |
| 35 | 71 | 7 | 14 | 420 | 280 | 12 | 360 |
| 36 | 74 | 8 | 19 | 530 | 290 | 12.2 | 300 |
| 34 | 74 | 12 | 19 | 530 | 360 | 12 | 230 |
| 36 | 74 | 9 | 19 | 560 | 310 | 12.2 | 200 |
| 36 | 71 | 10 | 23 | 1320 | 880 | 13.5 | 270 |
| 31 | 72 | 21 | 32 | 1066 | 832 | 0.8 | N/A |
| 36 | 71 | 7 | 14 | 422 | 281 | 12 | 274 |
| 37 | 73 | 7 | 18 | 528 | 284 | 12 | 300 |
| 37 | 72 | 7 | 18 | 1014 | 548 | 13.5 | 300 |
| 37 | 72 | 9 | 19 | 568 | 379 | 12.2 | 200 |
| 37 | 71 | 7 | 18 | 527 | 284 | 12.2 | 225 |
| 38 | 69 | 7 | 14 | 379 | 189 | 4.7 | 280 |
| 37 | 73 | 7 | 18 | 528 | 284 | 12.2 | 300 |
| | | | | | | | |
| 37 | 72 | 9 | 19 | 568 | 379 | 12 | 180 |
| 34 | 73 | 12 | 20 | 1273 | 710 | 13 | 173 |
| 35 | 69 | 9 | 18 | 599 | 420 | 12 | 162 |
| 34 | 75 | 12 | 20 | 429 | 241 | 10.1 | 180 |
| 37 | 70 | 13 | 19 | 710 | 507 | 12.2 | 200 |
| 37 | 70 | 13 | 19 | 1014 | 676 | 13.5 | 200 |
| 37 | 70 | 13 | 19 | 710 | 507 | 12.2 | 200 |
| 37 | 68 | 13 | 19 | 710 | 507 | 12.2 | 240 |
| 30 | 80 | 10 | 21 | 1320 | 880 | 13.5 | 230 |
| 36 | 72 | 10 | 21 | 710 | 470 | 12.2 | 170 |
| | | | | | | | |
| 37 | 69 | 13 | 20 | 710 | 507 | 12.2 | 370 |
| 36 | 70 | 14 | 19 | 640 | 350 | 12.2 | 300 |
| 38 | 69 | 14 | 19 | 640 | 350 | 12.2 | 250 |

*Continued*

TABLE 21-12

**ENTERAL NUTRITION COMPONENTS (PER LITER)—cont'd**

**A. INFANTS—cont'd**

| | Kcal/oz | Protein (g) |
|---|---|---|
| **Whey, Partially Hydrolyzed** | | |
| Good Start Supreme | 20 | 15 |
| Good Start Supreme DHA & ARA | 20 | 15 |
| Good Start Supreme DHA & ARA Natural Cultures | 20 | 15 |
| Good Start 2 Supreme DHA & ARA | 20 | 15 |
| **Whey and Casein, Partially Hydrolyzed** | | |
| Enfamil Gentlease LIPIL | 20 | 16 |
| **Amino Acid–Based Formulas** | | |
| EleCare | 20 | 20 |
| Neocate Infant (also w/DHA/ARA) | 20 | 21 |
| Nutramigen AA LIPIL | 20 | 19 |
| **Specialized Formulas** | | |
| 3232A | 13 | 19 |
| RCF | 20 | 20 |

**B. TODDLERS AND YOUNG CHILDREN AGES 1–10 YEARS**

| | Kcal/oz | Protein (g) |
|---|---|---|
| **Cow's Milk–Based Formulas** | | |
| Carnation Instant Breakfast Juice Drink | 30 | 40 |
| Carnation Instant Breakfast Ready-to-Drink | 23.8 | 41 |
| Compleat Pediatric | 30 | 38 |
| Cow's milk, 2% | 15 | 35 |
| Cow's milk, whole | 19 | 34 |
| KetoCal 4:1 | 43 | 30 |
| Kindercal Beverage, Vanilla | 32 | 30 |
| Kindercal TF, Vanilla | 32 | 30 |
| Monogen | 30 | 27 |
| Nutren Junior | 30 | 30 |
| Nutren Junior with Fiber | 30 | 30 |
| PediaSure Enteral | 30 | 30 |
| PediaSure Enteral with Fiber | 30 | 30 |
| PediaSure Vanilla | 30 | 30 |
| PediaSure with Fiber, Vanilla | 30 | 30 |
| Portagen | 30 | 32 |
| Resource Just for Kids | 30 | 30 |
| Resource Just for Kids with Fiber | 30 | 30 |
| Resource Just for Kids 1.5 Cal | 45 | 42 |
| Resource Just for Kids 1.5 Cal with Fiber | 45 | 42 |
| Bright Beginnings Pediatric Drink | 30 | 30 |
| **Soy-Based Formulas** | | |
| Bright Beginnings Soy Pediatric Drink | 30 | 30 |

| Fat (g) | Carbs (g) | Na (mEq) | K (mEq) | Ca (mg) | P (mg) | Fe (mg) | Osmolality |
|---|---|---|---|---|---|---|---|
| | | | | | | | |
| 34 | 75 | 8 | 19 | 429 | 241 | 10.1 | 250 |
| 34 | 75 | 8 | 19 | 429 | 241 | 10.1 | 250 |
| 34 | 75 | 8 | 19 | 429 | 241 | 10.1 | 250 |
| 34 | 75 | 8 | 19 | 1273 | 710 | 13.4 | 180 |
| | | | | | | | |
| 36 | 73 | 10 | 19 | 550 | 310 | 12.2 | 220 |
| | | | | | | | |
| 32 | 72 | 13 | 26 | 730 | 548 | 12 | 335 |
| 30 | 78 | 11 | 27 | 827 | 621 | 12.4 | 375 |
| 35 | 69 | 14 | 19 | 630 | 350 | 12 | 350 |
| | | | | | | | |
| 28 | 28 | 13 | 19 | 639 | 428 | 12.8 | 250 |
| 36 | 68 | 13 | 19 | 710 | 507 | 12.2 | 168 |

| Fat (g) | Carbs (g) | Na (mEq) | K (mEq) | Ca (mg) | P (mg) | Fe (mg) | Osmolality |
|---|---|---|---|---|---|---|---|
| | | | | | | | |
| 0.6 | 208 | 17 | 7 | 509 | 1018 | 9.2 | 990 |
| 16 | 108 | 25 | 26 | 1585 | 1585 | 14 | N/A |
| 39 | 130 | 33 | 41 | 1440 | 1000 | 13 | 380 |
| 20 | 50 | 22 | 41 | 1258 | 979 | 0.5 | N/A |
| 34 | 48 | 22 | 40 | 1226 | 956 | 0.5 | 285 |
| 144 | 6 | 26 | 55 | 1600 | 1300 | 22 | N/A |
| 44 | 135 | 16 | 34 | 1010 | 850 | 10.6 | 440 |
| 44 | 135 | 16 | 34 | 1010 | 850 | 10.6 | 345 |
| 28 | 163 | 21 | 22 | 617 | 480 | 10.1 | 370 |
| 50 | 110 | 20 | 34 | 1000 | 800 | 14 | 350 |
| 50 | 110 | 20 | 34 | 1000 | 800 | 14 | 350 |
| 40 | 133 | 17 | 34 | 970 | 844 | 14 | 335 |
| 40 | 138 | 17 | 34 | 970 | 844 | 14 | 345 |
| 50 | 110 | 17 | 34 | 970 | 802 | 14 | 430 |
| 50 | 114 | 17 | 34 | 970 | 802 | 14 | 440 |
| 44 | 105 | 22 | 29 | 855 | 646 | 17.1 | 350 |
| 50 | 110 | 26 | 55 | 1600 | 1300 | 22 | 390 |
| 50 | 110 | 26 | 55 | 1600 | 1300 | 22 | 390 |
| 75 | 165 | 30 | 33 | 1304 | 992 | 14 | 390 |
| 75 | 165 | 30 | 33 | 1304 | 992 | 14 | 405 |
| 50 | 110 | 17 | 34 | 970 | 802 | 14 | 350 |
| | | | | | | | |
| 50 | 110 | 17 | 40 | 970 | 902 | 14 | 350 |

*Continued*

TABLE 21-12

ENTERAL NUTRITION COMPONENTS (PER LITER)—cont'd

B. TODDLERS AND YOUNG CHILDREN AGES 1–10 YEARS—cont'd

| | Kcal/oz | Protein (g) |
|---|---|---|
| **Whey, Extensively Hydrolyzed** | | |
| Pediatric Peptinex DT | 30 | 30 |
| Peptamen Junior Fiber | 30 | 30 |
| Peptamen Junior with Prebio | 30 | 30 |
| Peptamen Junior, Unflavored | 30 | 30 |
| Vital Junior | 30 | 30 |
| **Soy and Pork, Extensively Hydrolyzed** | | |
| Pepdite Junior | 30 | 31 |
| **Amino Acid–Based Formulas** | | |
| EleCare (Unflavored and Vanilla) | 30 | 30 |
| EO28 Splash | 30 | 25 |
| Neocate Junior Flavored | 30 | 35 |
| Neocate Junior Unflavored | 30 | 33 |
| Neocate One + | 30 | 25 |
| Vivonex Pediatric | 24 | 24 |

C. OLDER CHILDREN AND ADULTS

| | Kcal/oz | Protein (g) |
|---|---|---|
| **Cow's Milk–Based Formulas** | | |
| Boost | 30 | 42 |
| Boost Breeze | 20 | 34 |
| Boost with Benefiber and FOS | 30 | 42 |
| Boost Diabetic | 32 | 58 |
| Boost High Protein | 30 | 61 |
| Boost Plus | 45 | 59 |
| Compleat | 32 | 48 |
| Crucial | 45 | 94 |
| Enlive | 38 | 42 |
| Ensure | 32 | 38 |
| Ensure Plus | 44 | 55 |
| Glucerna | 30 | 42 |
| Isocal | 32 | 34 |
| Isocal HN | 32 | 44 |
| Jevity 1 Cal | 32 | 44 |
| Jevity 1.2 Cal | 36 | 56 |
| Jevity 1.5 Cal | 45 | 64 |
| Nepro | 53 | 81 |
| Novasource Renal | 60 | 74 |
| Nutren 1.0 | 30 | 40 |
| Nutren Fiber | 30 | 40 |
| Nutren 1.5 | 45 | 60 |
| Nutren 2.0 | 60 | 80 |
| Nutren Glytrol | 30 | 45 |

| Fat (g) | Carbs (g) | Na (mEq) | K (mEq) | Ca (mg) | P (mg) | Fe (mg) | Osmolality |
|---|---|---|---|---|---|---|---|
| | | | | | | | |
| 39 | 138 | 30 | 26 | 1140 | 1000 | 14 | 290 |
| 38 | 137 | 20 | 34 | 1000 | 800 | 14 | 390 |
| 38 | 137 | 20 | 34 | 1000 | 800 | 14 | 365 |
| 38 | 138 | 20 | 34 | 1000 | 800 | 14 | 260 |
| 41 | 134 | 31 | 35 | 1055 | 844 | 13.9 | 390 |
| | | | | | | | |
| 50 | 106 | 18 | 35 | 1129 | 937 | 13.8 | 430 |
| | | | | | | | |
| 48 | 109 | 20 | 39 | 1096 | 822 | 18 | 551 |
| 35 | 146 | 9 | 24 | 620 | 620 | 7.7 | 820 |
| 47 | 110 | 19 | 36 | 1200 | 738 | 16 | 690 |
| 50 | 104 | 18 | 35 | 1130 | 697 | 15 | 590 |
| 35 | 146 | 9 | 24 | 620 | 620 | 7.7 | 610 |
| 24 | 130 | 17 | 31 | 970 | 800 | 10 | 360 |

| Fat (g) | Carbs (g) | Na (mEq) | K (mEq) | Ca (mg) | P (mg) | Fe (mg) | Osmolality |
|---|---|---|---|---|---|---|---|
| | | | | | | | |
| 18 | 173 | 24 | 43 | 1390 | 1310 | 19 | 610 |
| 0 | 131 | 9 | 25 | 630 | 1480 | 0 | 900 |
| 17 | 180 | 31 | 41 | 1270 | 1270 | 19 | 600 |
| 49 | 84 | 45 | 27 | 1160 | 928 | 15 | 400 |
| 23 | 139 | 31 | 41 | 1390 | 1310 | 19 | 650 |
| 58 | 190 | 31 | 41 | 1390 | 1310 | 19 | 670 |
| 40 | 120 | 43 | 44 | 760 | 760 | 14 | 340 |
| 68 | 134 | 51 | 48 | 1000 | 1000 | 18 | 490 |
| 0 | 270 | 11 | 4 | 250 | 83 | 11.3 | 825 |
| 25 | 169 | 37 | 40 | 1269 | 1058 | 19 | 600 |
| 212 | 47 | 44 | 44 | 1269 | 1269 | 19 | 680 |
| 54 | 96 | 41 | 40 | 705 | 705 | 13 | 355 |
| 44 | 135 | 23 | 34 | 630 | 530 | 9.5 | 270 |
| 45 | 124 | 40 | 41 | 850 | 850 | 15.2 | 270 |
| 35 | 155 | 40 | 40 | 910 | 760 | 14 | 300 |
| 39 | 172 | 59 | 47 | 1200 | 1200 | 18 | 450 |
| 50 | 216 | 61 | 55 | 1200 | 1200 | 18 | 525 |
| 96 | 167 | 46 | 27 | 1060 | 700 | 19 | 600 |
| 100 | 200 | 39 | 21 | 1300 | 650 | 18 | 700 |
| 38 | 127 | 38 | 32 | 668 | 668 | 12 | 315 |
| 38 | 127 | 38 | 32 | 668 | 668 | 12 | 330 |
| 68 | 169 | 51 | 48 | 1000 | 1000 | 18 | 430 |
| 104 | 196 | 57 | 49 | 1340 | 1340 | 24 | 745 |
| 48 | 100 | 32 | 36 | 720 | 720 | 12.8 | 280 |

*Continued*

TABLE 21-12

**ENTERAL NUTRITION COMPONENTS (PER LITER)—cont'd**

**C. OLDER CHILDREN AND ADULTS—cont'd**

| | Kcal/oz | Protein (g) |
|---|---|---|
| **Cow's Milk–Based Formulas—cont'd** | | |
| Nutren Renal | 60 | 70 |
| Optimental | 30 | 51 |
| Osmolite | 32 | 37 |
| Promote | 30 | 63 |
| Promote with Fiber | 30 | 63 |
| Pulmocare | 45 | 63 |
| Renalcal | 60 | 34 |
| Replete, Unflavored | 30 | 62 |
| Replete with Fiber (Unflavored) | 30 | 62 |
| Suplena | 53 | 45 |
| TraumaCal | 45 | 82 |
| Ultracal | 32 | 45 |
| **Soy-Based Formulas** | | |
| Fibersource | 36 | 43 |
| Isosource | 36 | 43 |
| Isosource HN | 36 | 53 |
| Isosource VHN | 30 | 62 |
| **Whey, Extensively Hydrolyzed** | | |
| Peptamen, Unflavored | 30 | 40 |
| Peptamen with Prebio | 30 | 40 |
| Peptamen 1.5, Unflavored | 45 | 68 |
| Peptinex 1.5 | 45 | 76 |
| Peptinex DT | 30 | 50 |
| **Amino Acid–Based Formulas** | | |
| Free Amino Acid Diet (f.a.a.) | 30 | 50 |
| Tolerex | 30 | 21 |
| Vivonex RTF | 30 | 50 |
| Vivonex Plus | 30 | 45 |
| Vivonex T.E.N. | 30 | 38 |

| Fat (g) | Carbs (g) | Na (mEq) | K (mEq) | Ca (mg) | P (mg) | Fe (mg) | Osmolality |
|---|---|---|---|---|---|---|---|
| | | | | | | | |
| 104 | 204 | 32 | 32 | 1400 | 700 | 24 | 650 |
| 28 | 139 | 46 | 45 | 1060 | 1060 | 13 | 540 |
| 35 | 151 | 28 | 26 | 535 | 535 | 9.6 | 300 |
| 26 | 130 | 44 | 51 | 1200 | 1200 | 18 | 340 |
| 28 | 138 | 57 | 54 | 1200 | 1200 | 18 | 380 |
| 93 | 106 | 57 | 50 | 1060 | 1060 | 19 | 475 |
| 82 | 290 | 0 | 0 | 0 | 0 | 0 | 600 |
| 34 | 113 | 38 | 39 | 1000 | 1000 | 18 | 300 |
| 34 | 113 | 38 | 39 | 1000 | 1000 | 18 | 310 |
| 96 | 202 | 34 | 29 | 1060 | 700 | 19 | 600 |
| 68 | 144 | 51 | 36 | 750 | 750 | 8.9 | 560 |
| 39 | 142 | 59 | 47 | 1000 | 1000 | 18 | 300 |
| | | | | | | | |
| 39 | 170 | 52 | 51 | 1000 | 940 | 15 | 490 |
| 39 | 170 | 48 | 49 | 1200 | 1100 | 15 | 490 |
| 39 | 160 | 48 | 49 | 1200 | 1200 | 15 | 490 |
| 29 | 130 | 60 | 46 | 800 | 800 | 14 | 300 |
| | | | | | | | |
| 39 | 127 | 24 | 39 | 800 | 700 | 18 | 270 |
| 39 | 127 | 24 | 39 | 800 | 700 | 18 | 300 |
| 56 | 188 | 44 | 48 | 1000 | 1000 | 27 | 550 |
| 42 | 206 | 83 | 38 | 1470 | 1470 | 17 | 550 |
| 17 | 164 | 48 | 31 | 670 | 670 | 12 | 460 |
| | | | | | | | |
| 11 | 176 | 24 | 39 | 800 | 700 | 18 | 850 |
| 2 | 230 | 20 | 30 | 560 | 560 | 10 | 550 |
| 12 | 175 | 29 | 31 | 670 | 670 | 12 | 630 |
| 67 | 190 | 27 | 27 | 560 | 560 | 10 | 650 |
| 3 | 210 | 26 | 24 | 500 | 500 | 9 | 630 |

TABLE 21-13

FORMULAS FOR SPECIAL CLINICAL CIRCUMSTANCES

| | |
|---|---|
| **A. INFANTS** | |
| **Preterm:** | |
| Predischarge | Enfamil Premature LIPIL |
| Postdischarge (through age 12 mo) | Similac Special Care Advance<br>Enfamil EnfaCare LIPIL<br>Similac NeoSure Advance |
| **Lactose intolerance** | Enfamil LactoFree LIPIL<br>Similac Sensitive |
| **Vegetarian, lactose intolerance, or galactosemia** | Bright Beginnings Soy Formula with DHA<br>Good Start Supreme Soy DHA & ARA<br>Good Start 2 Supreme Soy DHA & ARA (9–24 mo)<br>Isomil Advance<br>Similac Go & Grow Soy-Based Formula (9–24 mo)<br>NextStep ProSobee LIPIL (9–24 mo)<br>ProSobee LIPIL |
| **Protein (e.g., cow's milk) allergy/intolerance and/or fat malabsorption** | Alimentum Advance<br>EleCare<br>Neocate Infant (with DHA and ARA)<br>Nutramigen AA LIPIL<br>Nutramigen LIPIL<br>Pregestimil LIPIL |
| **Severe carbohydrate intolerance** | 3232A<br>RCF |
| **Requiring lower calcium and phosphorus** | Similac PM 60/40 |
| **B. TODDLERS AND YOUNG CHILDREN AGES 1–10 YR** | |
| **Vegetarian, lactose intolerance, or milk protein intolerance** | Bright Beginnings Soy Pediatric Drink |
| **Protein allergy/intolerance and/or fat malabsorption** | Pediatric Peptinex DT<br>Peptide Jr<br>Peptamen Junior (with and without Prebio)<br>Vivonex Pediatric<br>Vital jr.<br>EleCare (unflavored and vanilla)<br>Neocate Junior Unflavored and Tropical Fruit Flavored<br>EO28 Splash<br>Neocate One + |
| **Fat malabsorption, intestinal lymphatic obstruction, or chylothorax** | Portagen<br>Monogen |

TABLE 21-13

FORMULAS FOR SPECIAL CLINICAL CIRCUMSTANCES—cont'd

| B. TODDLERS AND YOUNG CHILDREN AGES 1–10 YR | |
|---|---|
| **Increased caloric needs** | Carnation Instant Breakfast Ready-to-Drink<br>Kindercal (also with fiber)<br>Nutren Junior (also with fiber)<br>PediaSure (also with fiber)<br>Resource Just for Kids (also with fiber)<br>Resource Just for Kids 1.5 (also with fiber)<br>Bright Beginnings Milk-Based Pediatric Drink |
| Requiring clear liquid diet | Carnation Instant Breakfast Juice Drink |
| **Intractable epilepsy** | KetoCal |
| **C. OLDER CHILDREN AND ADULTS** | |
| **Malabsorption of protein and/or fat** | Free Amino Acid Diet (f.a.a.)<br>Peptamen, Peptamen w/ Prebio, Peptamen 1.5<br>Peptinex DT<br>Tolerex<br>Vital HN<br>Vivonex Plus and Vivonex T.E.N. |
| **Critically ill and/or malabsorption** | Crucial<br>Optimental<br>Pulmocare<br>Ultracal |
| **Impaired glucose tolerance** | Glucerna<br>Glytrol |
| **Dialysis patients** | Magnacal Renal<br>Nepro<br>Nutren Renal |
| **Patients with acute renal failure not on dialysis** | Renalcal<br>Suplena |
| **Increased Caloric Needs with a normal GI tract** | Boost, Boost with fiber<br>Boost Plus, Boost High Protein<br>Carnation Instant Breakfast with whole milk<br>Ensure<br>Nutra/Shake |
| **Clear liquid diet** | Boost Breeze<br>Carnation Instant Breakfast Juice Drink<br>Enlive |
| **Patients with cystic fibrosis** | Scandishake with whole milk |

TABLE 21-14

**ORAL REHYDRATION SOLUTIONS**

| Solution | Kcal/mL (kcal/oz) | Carbohydrate (g/L) | Na (mEq/L) | K (mEq/L) | Osmolality (mOsm/kg $H_2O$) |
|---|---|---|---|---|---|
| CeraLyte-70 | 0.16 (4.9) | Rice digest 40 | 70 | 20 | 232 |
| CeraLyte-50 | 0.16 (4.9) | Rice digest, glucose 40 | 50 | 20 | 200 |
| Enfalyte | 0.12 (3.7) | Rice syrup solids 30 | 50 | 25 | 200 |
| Oral Rehydration Salts (WHO) | 0.06 (2) | Dextrose 20 | 90 | 20 | 330 |
| Pedialyte (unflavored) | 0.1 (3) | Dextrose 25 | 45 | 20 | 250 |

TABLE 21-15

**INITIATION AND ADVANCEMENT OF PARENTERAL NUTRITION***

| Nutrient | Initial Dose | Advancement | Maximum |
|---|---|---|---|
| Glucose | 5%–10% | 2.5%–5%/day | 12.5% peripheral<br>18 mg/kg/min (maximum rate of infusion) |
| Protein | 1 g/kg/day | 0.5–1 g/kg/day | 3 g/kg/day<br>10%–16% of calories |
| Fat[†] | 0.5–1 g/kg/day | 1 g/kg/day | 4 g/kg/day<br>0.17 g/kg/hr (maximum rate of infusion) |

*Acceptable osmolarity of parenteral nutrition through a peripheral line varies between 900 and 1050 osm/L by institution. An estimate of the osmolarity of parenteral nutrition can be obtained with the following formula: Estimated osmolarity = (dextrose concentration × 50) + (amino acid concentration × 100) + (mEq of electrolytes × 2). Consult individual pharmacy for hospital limitations.

[†]Essential fatty acid deficiency (EFAD) may occur in fat-free parenteral nutrition within 2–4 weeks in infant and children, and as early as 2–14 days in neonates. A minimum of 2%–4% of total caloric intake as linoleic acid and 0.25%–0.5% as linolenic acid is necessary to meet essential fatty acid requirements.

Modified from Baker RD et al: Pediatric Parenteral Nutrition. New York, Chapman and Hall, 1997, and Cox JH, Melbardis IM: Parenteral nutrition. In Samour PQ, King K (eds): Handbook of Pediatric Nutrition, 3rd ed. Boston, Jones and Bartlett Publishers, 2005.

TABLE 21-16

**PARENTERAL NUTRITION FORMULATION RECOMMENDATIONS**

| Component | Preterm | Term Infants | 1–3 yr | 4–6 yr | 7–10 yr | 11–18 yr |
|---|---|---|---|---|---|---|
| Energy (kcal/kg/day) | 85–105 | 90–108 | 75–90 | 65–80 | 55–70 | 30–55 |
| Protein (g/kg/day) | 2.5–4 | 2.5–3.5 | 1.5–2.5 | 1.5–2.5 | 1.5–2.5 | 0.8–2 |
| Sodium (mEq/kg/day) | 2–4 | 2–4 | 2–4 | 2–4 | 2–4 | 60–150 mEq/day |
| Potassium (mEq/kg/day) | 2–4 | 2–4 | 2–4 | 2–4 | 2–4 | 70–180 mEq/day |
| Calcium (mg/kg/day) | 50–60 | 20–40 | 10–20 | 10–20 | 10–20 | 200–800 mg/day |
| Phosphorus (mg/kg/day) | 30–45 | 30–45 | 15–40 | 15–40 | 15–40 | 280–900 mg/day |
| Magnesium (mEq/kg/day) | 0.5–1 | 0.25–1 | 0.25–0.5 | 0.25–0.5 | 0.25–0.5 | 8–24 mEq/day |
| Zinc (mcg/kg/day) | 325–400 | 100–250 | 100 | 100 | 50 | 2–5 mg/day |
| Copper (mcg/kg/day)* | 20 | 20 | 20 | 20 | 5–20 | 200–300 mcg/day |
| Manganese (mcg/kg/day)* | 1 | 1 | 1 | 1 | 1 | 40–50 mcg/day |
| Selenium (mcg/kg/day) | 2 | 2 | 2 | 2 | 1–2 | 40–60 mcg/day |

*Copper and manganese needs may be lowered in cholestasis.

Modified from Baker RD et al: Pediatric Parenteral Nutrition. New York, Chapman and Hall, 1997; Cox JH, Melbardis IM: Parenteral nutrition. In Samour PQ, King K (eds): Handbook of Pediatric Nutrition, 3rd ed. Boston, Jones and Bartlett Publishers, 2005; and American Society for Parenteral and Enteral Nutrition (ASPEN): Safe practices for parenteral nutrition. JPEN 2004;28(6):S39–S70.

TABLE 21-17

MONITORING SCHEDULE FOR PATIENTS RECEIVING PARENTERAL NUTRITION*

| Variable | Initial Period† | Later Period‡ |
|---|---|---|
| **GROWTH** | | |
| Weight | Daily | 2 times/wk |
| Height | Weekly (infants)<br>Monthly (children) | Monthly |
| Head circumference (infants) | Weekly | Monthly§ |
| **LABORATORY STUDIES** | | |
| Electrolytes and glucose | Daily until stable | Weekly |
| BUN/creatinine | 2 times/wk | Weekly |
| Albumin or prealbumin | Weekly | Weekly |
| $Ca^{2+}$, $Mg^{2+}$, P | 2 times/wk | Weekly |
| ALT, AST, ALP | Weekly | Weekly |
| Total and direct bilirubin | Weekly | Weekly |
| CBC | Weekly | Weekly |
| Triglycerides | With each increase | Weekly |
| Vitamins | — | As indicated |
| Trace minerals | — | As indicated |

*For patients on long-term parenteral nutrition, monitoring every 2–4 weeks is adequate in most cases.

†The period before nutritional goals are reached or during any period of instability.

‡When stability is reached, no changes in nutrient composition.

§Weekly in preterm infants.

ALP, alkaline phosphatase; ALT, alanine transaminase; AST, aspartate transaminase; BUN, blood urea nitrogen; CBC, complete blood count.

## REFERENCES


1. Centers for Disease Control and Prevention (CDC). Available at http://www.cdc.gov/growthcharts/. Accessed January 27, 2008.
2. Centers for Disease Control and Prevention (CDC). Available at http://www.cdc.gov/nccdphp/dnpa/bmi/index.htm. Accessed January 27, 2008.
3. Krebs NH et al: Assessment of child and adolescent overweight and obesity. Pediatrics 2007;120:S193–S228.
4. Barlow SE, Dietz WH: Obesity evaluation and treatment: Expert Committee recommendations. Pediatrics 1998;102(3):e29.
5. Li C et al: Recent trends in waist circumference and waist-height ratio among US children and adolescents. Pediatrics 2006;118:e1390–e1398.
6. Otten JJ et al. (eds): Dietary Reference Intakes: The Essential Guide to Nutrient Requirements. Washington, DC, National Academies Press, 2006.
7. Corrales KM, Utter SL: Growth failure. In Samour PQ, King K (eds): Handbook of Pediatric Nutrition. Boston, Jones and Bartlett Publishers, 2005.
8. Solomon SM, Kirby DF: The refeeding syndrome: A review. J Parenteral Enteral Nutr 1990;14:90–96.
9. Kleinman RE (ed), and the Committee on Nutrition of the AAP: Pediatric Nutrition Handbook, 5th ed. Chicago, American Academy of Pediatrics, 2004.
10. American Society for Parenteral and Enteral Nutrition (ASPEN): Safe practices for parenteral nutrition. JPEN 2004;28(6):S39–S70.

# Oncology

*Rachel Brennan, MD*

22

## I. WEBSITES: RESOURCES FOR PHYSICIANS, PATIENTS, AND FAMILIES

National Cancer Institute: Provides comprehensive information regarding individual types of pediatric malignancies (separate summaries for health care professionals and families) on their PDQ website: http://www.cancer.gov/cancertopics/pdq/pediatrictreatment

Oncology Link: Provides information regarding individual types of pediatric malignancies: www.Oncolink.org

## II. PRESENTING SIGNS AND SYMPTOMS OF PEDIATRIC MALIGNANCIES (Table 22-1)

**Note** *Common presenting signs and symptoms of many malignancies include weight loss, failure to thrive, anorexia, malaise, fever, pallor, and lymphadenopathy.*

## III. FEVER AND NEUTROPENIA[1,2]

See Figure 22-1.

## IV. ONCOLOGIC EMERGENCIES[1,3]

### A. TUMOR LYSIS SYNDROME

1. **Etiology: Lysis of tumor cells before or during early stages of chemotherapy (especially Burkitt lymphoma/leukemia, T-cell acute lymphocytic leukemia [ALL]); lymphoblasts have four times more intracellular phosphate than lymphocytes.**
2. **Presentation: Hyperuricemia, hypocalcemia, hyperkalemia, hyperphosphatemia. Can lead to acute renal failure.**
3. **Prevention and management:**

a. Hydration and alkalinization: $D_5W$ or $D_5\frac{1}{4}$ normal saline +25 to 50 mEq NaHCO3 (without K+) at two times the maintenance rate. Keeping urine specific gravity <1.010 and pH 7.0–7.5 reduces risk for urate crystal formation. Reduce NaHCO3 if pH >7.5 to avoid calcium phosphate precipitation.

b. Allopurinol (100 mg/m$^2$/dose) q8hr by mouth (PO), alternative dosing 10 mg/kg/day divided q8hr PO. May also use IV (200–400 mg/m$^2$/day in three divided doses; max dose = 600 mg/day). Consider rasburicase (recombinant urate oxidase, converts uric acid to allantoin; specific criteria for eligibility).

c. Check K+, Ca2+, phosphate, uric acid, and urinalysis frequently. Risk for calcium phosphate crystal formation and precipitation when Ca × Phosphate > 60 mg/dL.

d. Manage abnormal electrolytes as described in Chapter 11. See Chapter 19 for dialysis indications.

TABLE 22-1

COMMON SIGNS AND SYMPTOMS OF PEDIATRIC MALIGNANCIES

| Type of Malignancy | Signs/Symptoms | Initial Work-up |
|---|---|---|
| Leukemia | Limp, hepatomegaly, splenomegaly, petechiae/bruising, bone pain, anemia, thrombocytopenia | BMA, LP, laboratory studies |
| Lymphoma | Night sweats; pruritus; stridor; persistent respiratory symptoms; GI bleeding; back pain; hepatomegaly; splenomegaly; abdominal, head, neck, or chest mass | CT scans (chest/abdomen/pelvis), bone scan, LP, BMA, ferritin/LDH/uric acid/ESR |
| Wilms' tumor | Hypertension, abdominal mass, abdominal distention, hematuria | Imaging (CT chest/abdomen/pelvis), echocardiogram, abdominal ultrasound with Doppler |
| Neuroblastoma | Emesis; diarrhea; hypertension; opsoclonus-myoclonus; periorbital ecchymoses; Horner syndrome; stridor; persistent respiratory symptoms; abdominal, head, neck or chest mass; limp; blue subcutaneous nodules | Imaging (CT/MRI staging), BMA, echocardiogram, HVA/VMA |
| CNS tumors | Irritability, headache, emesis, seizure, cranial nerve palsies, visual changes, proptosis, ataxia | MRI of brain and spine, LP (cytopathology) |
| Testicular tumors | Abdominal pain or tenderness, scrotal swelling or mass | Imaging (CT chest/abdomen/pelvis), serum β-hCG, AFP, LDH, uric acid |
| Bone tumors | Limp, back pain, persistent limb pain, fracture | Imaging (CT chest, primary site), x-ray primary site, bone scan; bilateral BMA (Ewing's sarcoma) |
| Histiocytic disease | Polyuria, polydipsia, otorrhea, hepatomegaly, splenomegaly, cutaneous lesions, osteolytic lesions, pulmonary infiltrates, anemia, thrombocytopenia | LDH/ferritin/uric acid, skeletal survey, BMA, chest x-ray |
| Retinoblastoma | Leukocoria, asymmetrical red reflex, orbital inflammation, hyphema, pupil irregularity | Brain MRI, LP for CSF |

AFP, alpha fetoprotein; BMA, bone marrow aspirate; CSF, cerebrospinal fluid; CT, computed tomography; ESR, erythrocyte sedimentation rate; β-hCG, β-human chorionic gonadotropin; HVA/VMA, urine catecholamines; LDH, lactate dehydrogenase; LP, lumbar puncture; MRI, magnetic resonance imaging.

Data from Crist WM: Principles of diagnosis. In Behrman RE et al (eds): Nelson's Textbook of Pediatrics, 17th ed. Philadelphia, WB Saunders, 2004, pp 1684–1688, and Hogarty MD et al: Oncologic emergencies. In Fleisher G, Ludwig S (eds): Textbook of Pediatric Emergency Medicine. Philadelphia, Lippincott Williams & Wilkins, 2000, pp 1239–1253.

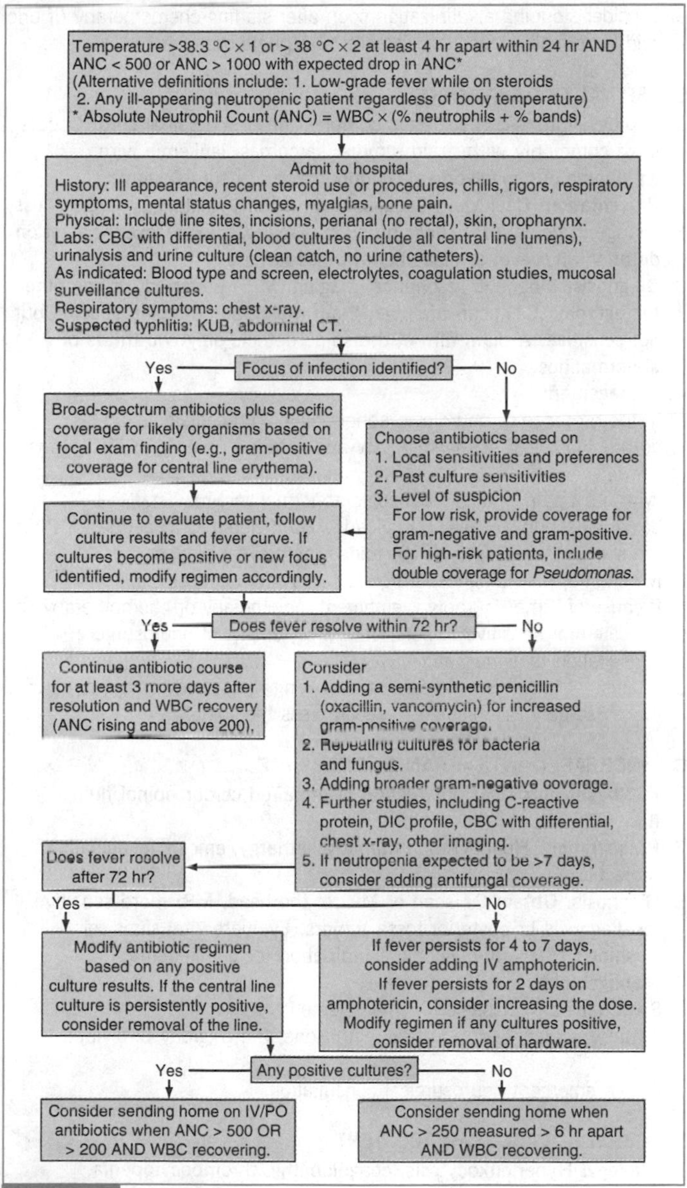

Temperature >38.3 °C × 1 or > 38 °C × 2 at least 4 hr apart within 24 hr AND ANC < 500 or ANC > 1000 with expected drop in ANC*
(Alternative definitions include: 1. Low-grade fever while on steroids
2. Any ill-appearing neutropenic patient regardless of body temperature)
* Absolute Neutrophil Count (ANC) = WBC × (% neutrophils + % bands)

↓

Admit to hospital
History: Ill appearance, recent steroid use or procedures, chills, rigors, respiratory symptoms, mental status changes, myalgias, bone pain.
Physical: Include line sites, incisions, perianal (no rectal), skin, oropharynx.
Labs: CBC with differential, blood cultures (include all central line lumens), urinalysis and urine culture (clean catch, no urine catheters).
As indicated: Blood type and screen, electrolytes, coagulation studies, mucosal surveillance cultures.
Respiratory symptoms: chest x-ray.
Suspected typhlitis: KUB, abdominal CT.

↓

Focus of infection identified?

- Yes → Broad-spectrum antibiotics plus specific coverage for likely organisms based on focal exam finding (e.g., gram-positive coverage for central line erythema).
- No → Choose antibiotics based on
  1. Local sensitivities and preferences
  2. Past culture sensitivities
  3. Level of suspicion
     For low risk, provide coverage for gram-negative and gram-positive.
     For high-risk patients, include double coverage for *Pseudomonas*.

↓

Continue to evaluate patient, follow culture results and fever curve. If cultures become positive or new focus identified, modify regimen accordingly.

↓

Does fever resolve within 72 hr?

- Yes → Continue antibiotic course for at least 3 more days after resolution and WBC recovery (ANC rising and above 200).
- No → Consider
  1. Adding a semi-synthetic penicillin (oxacillin, vancomycin) for increased gram-positive coverage.
  2. Repeating cultures for bacteria and fungus.
  3. Adding broader gram-negative coverage.
  4. Further studies, including C-reactive protein, DIC profile, CBC with differential, chest x-ray, other imaging.
  5. If neutropenia expected to be >7 days, consider adding antifungal coverage.

  ↓

  Does fever resolve after 72 hr?

  - Yes → Modify antibiotic regimen based on any positive culture results. If the central line culture is persistently positive, consider removal of the line.
  - No → If fever persists for 4 to 7 days, consider adding IV amphotericin. If fever persists for 2 days on amphotericin, consider increasing the dose. Modify regimen if any cultures positive, consider removal of hardware.

↓

Any positive cultures?

- Yes → Consider sending home on IV/PO antibiotics when ANC > 500 OR > 200 AND WBC recovering.
- No → Consider sending home when ANC > 250 measured > 6 hr apart AND WBC recovering.

FIG. 22-1

Fever and neutropenia.

e. Consider stopping alkalinization soon after starting chemotherapy (if uric acid is normal) to facilitate calcium phosphate excretion.

## B. SPINAL CORD COMPRESSION

1. **Etiology:** Intrinsic or extrinsic compression of the spinal cord. Occurs most commonly with brain tumors, sarcomas, leukemia with lymphomatous involvement, lymphoma, and neuroblastoma.
2. **Presentation:** Back pain (localized, radicular), weakness, sensory loss, change in bowel or bladder function. Prognosis for recovery based on duration and level of disability at presentation.
3. **Diagnosis:** Magnetic resonance imaging (MRI) preferred, or computed tomography (CT) scan of spine. Plain radiograph of spine specific but not sensitive. A plain film of the spine detects only two thirds of abnormalities.
4. **Management:**

a. In the presence of neurologic abnormalities, immediately start dexamethasone 1–2 mg/kg/day IV and obtain an emergent MRI of the spine.
b. With back pain and no neurologic abnormalities, may start dexamethasone, 0.25–0.5 mg/kg/day PO divided q6hr; perform MRI of the spine within 24 hours. Steroids may prevent diagnosis of lymphoma; plan diagnostic procedure as soon as possible.
c. If cause of tumor is known, emergent radiotherapy or chemotherapy indicated for sensitive tumors; otherwise, emergent neurosurgery consultation is warranted.
d. If cause of tumor is unknown or debulking may remove most or all of tumor, surgery is indicated to decompress the spine.

## C. INCREASED INTRACRANIAL PRESSURE

1. **Etiology:** Ventricular obstruction or impaired cerebrospinal fluid flow.
2. **Presentation:** Headaches, irritability, lethargy, emesis (especially if projectile).
3. **Diagnosis:** Obtain CT scan or MRI of the head. MRI more sensitive for diagnosis of posterior fossa tumors. Evaluate vital signs for Cushing's triad, funduscopic examination for papilledema.
4. **Management:**

a. See Chapter 4 for basic ICP management.
b. If tumor is identified, add dexamethasone, 2 mg/kg/day IV divided q6hr.
c. Obtain emergent neurosurgical consultation.

## D. CEREBROVASCULAR ACCIDENT

1. **Etiology:** Hyperleukocytosis, coagulopathy, thrombocytopenia, chemotherapy-related (e.g., L-asparaginase-induced hemorrhage or thrombosis, after methotrexate, or radiation-induced fibrosis).

2. **Diagnosis and management:**
a. Platelet transfusions, fresh-frozen plasma (FFP) as needed to replace factors (e.g., if depleted by L-asparaginase).
b. Brain CT scan with contrast, MRI, magnetic resonance angiography, or magnetic resonance venography if venous thrombosis is suspected.
c. Administer heparin acutely, followed by warfarin, for thromboses (if no venous hemorrhage observed on MRI).
d. Avoid L-asparaginase.
e. Leukapheresis for hyperleukocytosis.

## E. RESPIRATORY DISTRESS AND SUPERIOR VENA CAVA SYNDROME



1. **Etiology:** Hodgkin disease, non-Hodgkin lymphoma (e.g., lymphoblastic lymphoma), ALL (T-lineage), germ cell tumors.
2. **Presentation:** Orthopnea, headaches, facial swelling, dizziness, plethora.
3. **Diagnosis:** Chest radiograph. Consider CT or MRI scan to assess airway. Attempt diagnosis of malignancy (if not known) by least invasive method possible.
4. **Management:**
a. Control airway.
b. Biopsy (e.g., bone marrow, pleurocentesis, lymph-node biopsy) before therapy if patient can tolerate sedation or general anesthesia.
c. Empirical therapy: Radiotherapy, steroids, chemotherapy.

## F. TYPHLITIS (NEUTROPENIC ENTEROCOLITIS)

1. **Etiology:** Inflammation of bowel wall, usually localized to cecum. Occurs most often in association with prolonged neutropenia.
2. **Presentation:** Right lower quadrant abdominal pain, nausea, diarrhea, and fever (fever may be absent early in course; neutropenic patient with abdominal pain warrants evaluation for typhlitis and empiric antibacterial coverage). Risk for perforation.
3. **Diagnosis:**
a. Careful serial abdominal examinations.
b. X-ray may show pneumatosis intestinalis, bowel wall edema.
c. CT (non-contrast) most sensitive imaging; may reveal bowel wall thickening, pneumatosis intestinalis.
4. **Management:**
a. NPO, IV fluids; consider nasogastric decompression.
b. Broad anaerobic and gram-negative antibiotic coverage (consider coverage for *Clostridium difficile*).
c. Follow closely with surgery consult.

## G. HYPERLEUKOCYTOSIS

1. **Etiology:** In acute myeloid leukemia (AML) (especially M4 and M5), hyperleukocytosis occurs with a white blood cell (WBC) count as low

as 100,000/μL. It can occur in ALL/CML with a WBC count >300,000/μL.

2. **Presentation:** Hypoxia and dyspnea from pulmonary leukostasis, mental status changes, headaches, seizures, papilledema from leukostasis in cerebral vessels; occasionally, gastrointestinal (GI) bleeding, abdominal pain, renal failure, priapism, and tumor lysis syndrome.
3. **Management:**

a. Transfuse platelets as needed to keep count above 20,000/μL (reduce risk for intracranial hemorrhage).
b. Avoid red blood cell (RBC) transfusions because they will raise viscosity (keep hemoglobin ≤10 g/dL). If RBCs are required, consider partial exchange transfusion.
c. Hydration, alkalinization, and allopurinol should be initiated (as discussed in section IV.A).
d. Administer FFP and vitamin K if coagulopathy is present.
e. Before cytotoxic therapy, consider leukapheresis to lower WBC count if central nervous system (CNS) or pulmonary symptoms exist.

## V. COMMON COMPLICATIONS OF BONE MARROW TRANSPLANT[1]

### A. GRAFT-VERSUS-HOST DISEASE (GVHD)

1. **Etiology:** Primarily T-cell-mediated reaction to foreign antigen; occurs after hematopoietic cell transplant. Risk factors include human leukocyte antigen (HLA) disparity, radiation therapy, gender disparity, and increasing age.
2. **Presentation:** Acute GVHD usually occurs within 100 days after transplantation. Maculopapular skin rash develops, which can progress to bullous lesions and toxic epidermal necrolysis. Laboratory findings notable for abnormal liver enzymes, especially increased direct bilirubin and elevated alkaline phosphatase. Upper GI symptoms: Anorexia, dyspepsia, nausea, and vomiting. Lower GI symptoms: Abdominal cramping and diarrhea.
3. **Diagnosis:** Triad of classic rash, abdominal cramping with diarrhea, and rising bilirubin level suggestive of diagnosis. Tissue biopsy of skin or rectum provides histologic confirmation.
4. **Prevention and management:**

a. Prophylaxis: T-cell depletion of donor marrow or immunomodulation; commonly used adjuvants are methotrexate and prednisone.
b. Steroids are first-line treatment. Commonly used second-line agents include cyclosporine, tacrolimus, sirolimus, antithymocyte globulin, and mycophenolate mofetil. Psoralens plus ultraviolet A photopheresis (PUVA) is an alternative for skin GVHD. Pentostatin is useful in treating cutaneous and oral GVHD.
c. Chronic GVHD: Acute therapies are complemented by monoclonal antibodies, such as infliximab (anti-tumor necrosis factor-α).

### B. VENO-OCCLUSIVE DISEASE (SINUSOIDAL OBSTRUCTION SYNDROME)

1. **Etiology:** Occlusive fibrosis of terminal intrahepatic venules and sinusoids; occurs as a consequence of hematopoietic cell transplantation, hepatotoxic chemotherapy, and/or high-dose liver radiation. Typically occurs within 3 weeks of the insult. Incidence highest with unmatched, unrelated transplants and lowest with autologous transplantation.
2. **Presentation:** Hepatomegaly, right upper quadrant abdominal pain, jaundice, edema, ascites, and sudden weight gain.
3. **Diagnosis:** Liver ultrasound with Doppler, looking for reversal of portal venous flow, or MRI. Laboratory studies show elevated bilirubin and aminotransferases (ALT, AST). More severe disease will result in prolongation of prothrombin time and a decrease in factor VII levels. Portal-hepatic venous gradient: A useful but invasive measurement;. gradient >10 mm Hg is consistent with veno-occlusive disease.
4. **Prevention and management:**
   a. Prophylactic measures: Ursodeoxycholic acid, glutamine, and heparin; have not shown consistent benefit.
   b. Treatment: Primarily supportive with fluid and sodium restriction. Alteplase (tissue plasminogen activator) with or without heparin has been used but has a risk of hemorrhage. Defibrotide has shown promising results with little toxicity. Antithrombin infusion may benefit patients with low antithrombin levels. For severe disease, surgical intervention with transjugular intrahepatic portosystemic stent shunt is effective in reducing the portal-hepatic venous gradient. Liver transplantation is considered for the most severe cases.

22 ONCOLOGY

## VI. HEMATOLOGIC CARE AND COMPLICATIONS[1]

**Note** *Transfuse only irradiated packed RBC (PRBC)/platelets, cytomegalovirus (CMV) negative or leukofiltered PRBC/platelets for CMV-negative patients. Use leukofiltered PRBC/platelets for those who may undergo bone marrow transplantation (BMT) in the future to prevent alloimmunization, or for those who have had nonhemolytic febrile transfusion reactions.*

### A. ANEMIA

1. **Etiology:** Blood loss, chemotherapy, marrow infiltration, hemolysis.
2. **Management:**
   a. See Chapter 14 for specific details on PRBC transfusions
   b. Generally, PRBC transfusions in cancer patients are not recommended until hematocrit falls below 20%–22%, or if the patient is symptomatic.

### B. THROMBOCYTOPENIA

1. **Etiology:** Chemotherapy, marrow infiltration, consumptive coagulopathy, medications.

2. **Management:**
a. See Chapter 14 for specific details on platelet transfusions.
b. Generally, maintain platelet count above 10,000/μL unless patient is clinically bleeding or febrile, or before selected procedures (e.g., intramuscular injection). Consider maintaining platelet counts at higher levels for patients who have brain tumors, recent brain surgery, or history of a stroke.

### C. NEUTROPENIA

1. **Etiology:** Chemotherapy, marrow infiltration, radiation.
2. **Management:**
a. Broad-spectrum antibiotics with concomitant fever (see Fig. 22-1).
b. Granulocyte colony-stimulating factor (daily versus monthly dosing) to assist in recovery of neutrophils.
c. Rarely, use of neutrophil transfusion.

## VII. NAUSEA TREATMENT IN CANCER PATIENTS[1]

### A. ETIOLOGY

Usual cause is chemotherapy treatment. Also suspect opiate therapy, GI and CNS radiotherapy, obstructive abdominal process, CNS mass, certain antibiotics, or hypercalcemia.

### B. PRESENTATION

1. **Acute:** Emesis within 24 hr of starting chemotherapy; occurs in one third of patients despite treatment.
2. **Delayed:** Emesis occurring 24 hr after chemotherapy; increased risk for females, prior acute emesis, certain agents (e.g., cisplatin).
3. **Anticipatory:** Emesis prior to chemotherapy administration.

### C. THERAPY

Hydration plus one or more antinausea medications (see Formulary for dosing).

1. **Serotonin (5-$HT_3$) antagonists:** Ondansetron, dolasetron, granisetron, or palonosetron. Usually a first-line therapy. Patients may respond preferentially to one of these agents. Beware of QT prolongation, widening of QRS.
2. **Histamine-1 antagonist:** Diphenhydramine; also cyproheptadine (with anticholinergic side effect of appetite stimulation).
3. **Steroids:** Dexamethasone; especially helpful in patients with brain tumor. Synergy of unknown mechanism with 5-$HT_3$ antagonists.
4. **Benzodiazepines:** Lorazepam; used as an adjunct antiemetic agent.
5. **Metoclopramide:** Use diphenhydramine to reduce extrapyramidal symptoms (EPS).
6. **Phenothiazines:** Promethazine, chlorpromazine; use diphenhydramine to reduce EPS.

7. **Cannabinoids:** Dronabinol; can be helpful in resistant cases, especially in patients with large tumor burden. May also be used as an appetite stimulant in malnourished patients.
8. **Substance P and neurokinin-1 receptor antagonist:** Aprepitant.

## VIII. ANTIMICROBIAL PROPHYLAXIS IN ONCOLOGY PATIENTS (Table 22-2)

**Note** *Treatment length and dosage may vary per protocol.*

## IX. BEYOND CHILDHOOD CANCER: TREATING A CANCER SURVIVOR



### A. WEB RESOURCES

Long-term follow-up guidelines for survivors of childhood, adolescent and young adult cancers: http://www.survivorshipguidelines.org/

### B. UNDERSTAND THE TREATMENT REGIMEN

1. **Identify all components of therapy received: "Comprehensive treatment summary" from oncologist, summarizing:**
   a. Diagnosis: Site/stage, date, relapse.
   b. Chemotherapy: Cumulative doses, "high dose" versus "low dose" for methotrexate and cytarabine.
   c. Radiation: Locations, cumulative dose.
   d. Surgeries: Dates, sites, resection.
   e. BMT: Prep regimen, source of donor cells (including degree of HLA mismatch), GVHD, complications.
   f. Investigational treatments.
   g. Adverse drug reactions or allergies
2. **Follow-up any investigational treatments used.**
3. **Determine any potential problems by organ system, and devise plan for routine evaluation.**

TABLE 22-2

ANTIMICROBIAL PROPHYLAXIS IN ONCOLOGY PATIENTS

| Organism | Medication | Indication |
|---|---|---|
| *Pneumocystis jiroveci* | TMP-SMX, atovaquone, dapsone, or pentamidine | Chemotherapy and BMT per protocol (usually at least 6 mo after chemotherapy, 12 mo after BMT) |
| HSV | Acyclovir (dosing is different for zoster, varicella, and mucocutaneous HSV) | After BMT if patient or donor is HSV or CMV positive; recurrent zoster |
| *Candida albicans* | Fluconazole or voriconazole | After BMT (usual at least 28 days) |
| Gram-positive organisms | Penicillin | After BMT (usually at least 1 mo) |

BMT, bone marrow transplantation; CMV, cytomegalovirus; HSV, herpes simplex virus; TMP-SMX, trimethoprim-sulfamethoxazole.

### C. COMMON LATE EFFECTS[4] (Table 22-3)

1. **Immunocompromise:**

a. No utility in "getting vaccinations in" before chemotherapy or hematopoietic stem cell transplantation (HSCT).

b. After treatment is finished, time to full recovery of adaptive immune function is variable. Typically takes 3–6 months for patients treated with chemotherapy but no HSCT; for patients treated with HSCT, takes a minimum of several months and often >1 year.

c. Chronic GVHD: Functionally asplenic; no live-virus vaccinations, reimmunize against pneumococcus, *Haemophilus influenzae* type b, meningococcus.

d. Patients treated with chemotherapy, but no HSCT:

(1) Do not give vaccines during chemotherapy, including ALL maintenance, *except* inactivated influenza (safe but variable efficacy).

(2) Patients may lose protective titers based on age (increased risk in younger patients) and vaccine (likelihood of titer loss: HBV > MMR > DTaP > IPV).

(a) Age at diagnosis <18 months: Full catch-up of all vaccinations required.

(b) Age at diagnosis >18 months: May either check titers 3–6 months after chemotherapy is finished and give boosters as needed, or assume all protective titers were lost and give boosters for all immunizations.

e. Patients treated with HSCT:

(1) Consider these patients unimmunized and needing a full catchup immunization schedule.

(2) Do *not* give vaccines from the start of chemotherapy preparation to at least 6 months after HSCT (longer if patient has active GVHD or is taking immunosuppressive medications, such as cyclosporine).

f. Specific recommendations for vaccination after treatment (Table 22-4).

2. **Endocrine: Obesity, precocious puberty, growth hormone deficiency, hyperthyroidism/hypothyroidism.**

3. **Fertility:** **Ovarian and testicular dysfunction (hypogonadism, infertility), early menopause.**

4. **Neurocognitive/psychosocial:** **Due to cranial radiation, chemotherapy during development of young brain, psychosocial stressors of a life-threatening illness.**

a. Cognitive dysfunction, leukoencephalopathy, hearing/vision loss: Obtain full evaluation and refer early for intervention.

b. Peripheral neuropathy, seizures.

c. Depression/anxiety, post-traumatic stress.

d. Limitations in health care and insurance.

5. **Skeletal: Osteopenia/osteoporosis.**

TABLE 22-3

COMMONLY USED CHEMOTHERAPY AND SUGGESTED LONG-TERM FOLLOW-UP

| Type of Chemotherapy | Immediate Toxicity | Delayed/Late Toxicity | Suggested Follow-up |
|---|---|---|---|
| **Alkylators**<br>Busulfan<br>Cyclophosphamide | Seizures<br>Hemorrhagic cystitis, SIADH | Myelosuppression<br>Secondary MDS/AML | Complete blood counts<br>History, urinalysis |
| **Antimetabolites**<br>5-FU<br>6-MP<br>Methotrexate<br>Cytarabine | Neurologic changes<br>Hepatotoxicity<br>Nephrotoxicity, pneumonitis<br>High dose: conjunctivitis, fever | Hyperbilirubinemia<br>Dacrocystitis (5-FU)<br>Osteonecrosis/ osteoporosis | Routine exams, blood work<br>Bone density evaluation |
| **Asparaginase** | Liver damage, coagulopathy<br>Pancreatitis | Clots/complications of clots<br>Pancreatic insufficiency (diabetes mellitus) | Routine exams, blood work |
| **Intercalators**<br>Bleomycin<br>Anthracyclines<br>Platinum compounds | Fever within 24 hr<br>Cardiac arrhythmias<br>Nausea/vomiting, magnesium wasting | Pulmonary fibrosis<br>Cardiomyopathy<br>Renal insufficiency, ototoxicity, peripheral neuropathy | Chest x-ray, PFTs with $DL_{CO}$<br>Echocardiogram, ECG, lipid profile<br>Audiology, creatinine, blood pressure, urinalysis |
| **Kinase Inhibitor**<br>Imatinib | Myalgias, edema | Fatigue, pigmentation changes | Routine exam |
| **Microtubule Polymerization Inhibitors**<br>Vinblastine/vincristine | Constipation, peripheral neuropathy, hepatotoxicity | Peripheral neuropathy | Routine exam, blood work |
| **Topoisomerase Inhibitor**<br>Etoposide | Diarrhea | Secondary MDS/AML | Routine blood work |

AML, acute myeloid leukemia; $DL_{CO}$, carbon monoxide diffusing capacity; ECG, electrocardiography; 5-FU, 5-fluorouracil, MDS, myelodysplastic syndrome; PFTs, pulmonary function tests; 6-MP, 6-mercaptopurine.

Data adapted from Krishnan K:. Chemotherapy. In Pediatric Oncology Nuts and Bolts. Johns Hopkins Hospital, version 2005–06.

22 ONCOLOGY

TABLE 22-4

**IMMUNIZATIONS IN ONCOLOGY PATIENTS*[,5,6]**

| Vaccine | Treated with HSCT | Treated with Chemotherapy Only |
|---|---|---|
| Inactivated influenza | >6 mo after HSCT, then annually | Annually, including during therapy (questionable efficacy) |
| Other killed and component vaccines | >12 mo after HSCT† | >6 mo after chemotherapy‡ |
| MMR | >24 mo after HSCT, unless chronic GVHD | >6 mo after chemotherapy |
| VZV | *None* (no safety data) | >6 mo after chemotherapy |

*No recommendation for rotavirus vaccine at this time.

†Dose schedule: Td (if >7 yr) or DTap/DT if <7 yr, inactivated polio vaccine, and *Haemophilus influenzae* type b at 12, 14, and 24 mo after HSCT.

‡Consider checking titers in patients >18 mo of age and giving boosters as needed.

HSCT, hematopoetic stem cell transplant; MMR: measles, mumps, rubella; VZV: varicella zoster vaccination.

Data from Sung L et al: Practical vaccination guidelines for children with cancer. Pediatr Child Health 2001:6;379–383; CDC: Guidelines for preventing opportunistic infections among hematopoietic stem cell transplant recipients. MMWR Recommendations and Reports 2000;49(RR-10):1–128; and Pickering LK (ed): 2006 Red Book: Report of the Committee on Infectious Diseases, 27th ed. Elk Grove Village, Ill, American Academy of Pediatrics, 2006, pp 71–85.

6. **Cardiac:** Cardiomyopathy (anthracyclines), arrhythmias, atherosclerotic disease/coronary artery disease (radiation), valvular disease, pericardial complications (pericarditis).
7. **Secondary malignancies:** Secondary MDS/AML (etoposide, alkylators), brain tumors (cranial x-ray therapy), breast cancer (x-ray therapy for Hodgkin's disease).

## REFERENCES


1. Poplack D, Pizzo P: Principles and Practice of Pediatric Oncology, 5th ed. Philadelphia, Lippincott Williams and Wilkins, 2006.
2. Chanock SJ, Pizzo PA: Fever in the neutropenic host. Infect Dis Clin North Am 1996;10(4):777–796.
3. Kelly KM, Lange B: Oncologic emergencies. Pediatr Clin North Am. 1997;44(4):809–830.
4. Meck MM et al: Late effects in survivors of childhood cancer. Pediatr Rev2006;27(7):257–262.
5. Sung L et al: Practical vaccination guidelines for children with cancer. Pediatr Child Health 2001:6;379–383.
6. Pickering LK (ed): 2006 Red Book: Report of the Committee on Infectious Diseases, 27th ed. Elk Grove Village, Ill, American Academy of Pediatrics, 2006.

# Palliative Care

*Amy Valasek, MD*

23

## I. PALLIATIVE CARE

### A. DEFINITION[1–2]

Palliative care is the active total care of the child's body, mind, and spirit with the intent to prevent and relieve suffering. It supports the best quality of life for child and family beginning at diagnosis of a life-limiting condition and continuing regardless of whether or not the child receives treatment. Hospice care: A form of palliative care that focuses on the end of life and bereavement. Effective palliative care requires an interdisciplinary approach that works with child and family to determine goals of care.

### B. PALLIATIVE CARE TEAM COMPOSITION

1. **Child and family.**
2. **Physicians: Primary care physician, specialist attending physician, fellow, resident, intern.**
3. **Nurses: Primary nurse, charge nurse, home care nurse, hospice nurse.**
4. **Pain specialist and hospice palliative care specialist.**
5. **Social worker.**
6. **Child life specialist.**
7. **Pastoral care.**
8. **Patient care coordinator and case manager.**
9. **Bereavement coordinator.**
10. **Community resources: School, faith community, hospice program.**

## II. DECISION MAKING

### A. DECISION-MAKING TOOLS (DMT)[3]

1. **Provides consistent, reliable format for discussion and formulation of plan of care. Patients, families, and health care providers all participate in the process.**
2. **Four domains of DMT should be updated regularly, especially during "non-crisis" periods.**

a. Medical indications: Diagnosis, symptoms, risk/benefits of treatment, cure/relapse rate, complications.
b. Patient and family preferences: Information, decision making, desire for autonomy and privacy.
c. Quality of life: Important activities of child, important relationships, emotional/spiritual well-being.
d. Contextual issues: Identify family unit, home environment, financial barriers, legal issues, cultural and spiritual beliefs.

### B. CHILD PARTICIPATION

1. **Development of death concepts in children[4-7] (Table 23-1).**

TABLE 23-1

CONCEPTUALIZATION OF DEATH IN CHILDREN

| Age Range | Characteristics | Concepts of Death | Interventions |
|---|---|---|---|
| 0–2 yr | Achieve object permanence<br>May sense something is wrong | None | Provide maximal comfort with familiar persons and favorite toys. |
| 2–6 yr | Magical thoughts | Believes death is temporary<br>Does not personalize death<br>Believes death can be caused by thoughts | Minimize separation from parents; correct perceptions that the illness is punishment. |
| 6–12 yr | Concrete thoughts | Understands death can be personal<br>Interested in details of death | Be truthful, evaluate fears, provide concrete details if requested; allow participation in decision making. |
| 12–18 yr | Reality becomes objective<br>Capable of self-reflection | Searches for meaning, hope, purpose, and value of life | Be truthful, allow expression of strong feelings, allow participation in decision making. |

2. **Child's capacity to participate in health care decisions: Minor children can participate meaningfully in decision making if they demonstrate all of the following:**

a. Communicate understanding of the medical information.

b. State his/her preference.

c. Communicate understanding of the consequences of decisions.

### C. ADVANCE DIRECTIVE

1. **Adolescents age 18 years and older can name another adult to make health care decisions if they are unable to speak for themselves.**
2. **Health care team can help patients voice preferences for future health care decisions.**

## III. LEGACY AND MEMORY MAKING

### A. MEMORY MAKING

1. **Provide opportunities for the family to participate in memory making (e.g., create memory boxes/packets, lock of hair, foot/hand molds or prints, videos, photographs).**
2. **Older children may have specific wishes for funeral, memorial, or for distribution of personal belongings.**

### B. RITUALS

Allow for culturally important rituals to be performed by the family (e.g., Baptism, bathing, music, faith ceremonies or prayer).

## IV. DECISIONS TO LIMIT INTERVENTIONS

### A. DO NOT ATTEMPT RESUSCITATION (DNAR)

1. In the event of cardiorespiratory arrest, cardiopulmonary resuscitation (CPR) is automatically initiated in hospitals by health care team and in community settings by first responders. For patients with life-threatening conditions, CPR may not prolong or enhance quality of life, making it inconsistent with goals of care. Health care team should offer patients and families the option of forgoing CPR and other resuscitative interventions as part of overall care plan that emphasizes comfort and quality of living (Box 23-1).
2. If this option is desired, physician must write a specific order *not* to attempt CPR (e.g., "In the event of cardiopulmonary arrest, do not attempt resuscitation.") Orders must follow local emergency medical services (EMS) policies for patients at home.

### B. DO NOT ESCALATE TREATMENT

When escalation of treatment no longer supports goals of care, offer patients and families option to forgo treatment changes even as patient's condition worsens. Because death is expected, DNAR must also be discussed. Examples of such requests include the following:



BOX 23-1

**SAMPLE FROM STATE OF MARYLAND EMS/DNAR FORMS AND BRACELET AUTHORIZATION FORM**

The physician must sign the "Physician Certification and Order" and initial ONLY ONE of the two options on the form.

**Option A:**

**Maximum Efforts to Prevent Cardiac/Respiratory Arrest**

**DNAR if Arrest Occurs—No CPR**

**Option B:**

**Supportive Care Prior to Cardiac/Respiratory Arrest**

**DNAR if Arrest Occurs—No CPR**

**NOTE** If a valid EMS/DNAR Order is located after resuscitation has begun, EMS personnel may withdraw resuscitation.

**NOTE** Ambulance personnel cannot honor specific instructions in advance directives that do not conform to the care selections in the "Physician's Order" (e.g., wants intubation but no CPR).

1. Do not increase the dose of current medications, such as vasopressors.
2. Do not add new medications, such as antibiotics.
3. Do not initiate new interventions, such as dialysis or mechanical ventilation.
4. Initiate and increase interventions to treat pain and reduce suffering.

### C. DISCONTINUING CURRENT INTERVENTIONS

When death is expected regardless of intervention, especially if current interventions are prolonging the dying process, patient and families can be offered the option of discontinuing these interventions (e.g., "Discontinue blood products, monitors, mechanical ventilation, medically provided hydration or nutrition"). Because death is expected, DNAR must also be discussed.

## V. BODY, MIND, AND SPIRIT CHANGES AS DEATH APPROACHES[8]

### A. PHYSICAL CHANGES

1. Cardiac: Blood pressure lowers, heart rate increases, and pulse becomes weaker.
2. Circulation: Cool extremities; cyanosis of fingers, nails, lips; mottling of skin.
3. Gastrointestinal: Metabolism slows and there is gradual decrease in appetite. Liquids are preferred to solids. The body will become naturally dehydrated, and fevers may occur as death approaches. Provide relief with ice chips, moist mouth swabs, antipyretic per rectum.
4. Respiratory: Variable pattern of breathing (tachypnea followed by periods of apnea); congestion secondary to secretion build-up. Provide relief as follows:
   a. Turn patient every few hours, elevate head of bed, provide frequent mouth care, hyoscyamine as needed.
   b. Relief of air hunger: Morphine and lorazepam as needed, oxygen for comfort.
   c. **NOTE** Deep suctioning is not helpful.
5. Sensation changes: Senses become overactive; bright lights, noise, or television may be upsetting. Hearing is typically the last sense to diminish. Provide relief by dimming lights, reducing noise, and providing soft background music.
6. Sleep: Need for sleep increases as death approaches. Occasionally, the child exhibits "a surge of energy" to play, eat, socialize.

### B. EMOTIONAL CHANGES

Detachment from the outside world: Reduced need to socialize leads to pulling inward of thoughts, emotions, and fears. Listen and reassure family about decreased interactions.

### C. MENTAL CHANGES

Mental status: Confusion, restlessness, agitation, delirium. Provide relief by keeping child oriented to surroundings, surrounding him/her with family as a way to reinforce safety, speaking in calm tones; use lorazepam and haloperidol as needed.

### D. SPIRITUAL CHANGES

Spiritual: Child may call out or reach out for loved ones who are not physically present. Reassure the family that this is not unusual during the dying process.

## VI. LAST HOURS: MEDICATION AND MANAGEMENT[9] (Table 23-2)



TABLE 23-2

**COMMON MEDICATIONS USED FOR SYMPTOMATIC RELIEF IN PALLIATIVE CARE**

| Indication | Medication | Initial Regimen |
|---|---|---|
| Pain | Morphine | 0.3 mg/kg/dose PO, SL, PR q2–4hr*<br>0.1–0.2 mg/kg/dose IV q2–4hr*<br>**NOTE** *Morphine should be titrated to symptomatic relief.* |
| Dyspnea | Morphine | 0.1–0.25 mg/kg/dose PO, SL, PR q2–4hr<br>0.05–0.1 mg/kg/dose IV q2–4hr<br>2.5–5 mg/3 mL normal saline nebulizer q4hr<br>**NOTE** *Nebulized morphine can cause severe bronchospasm and worsen dyspnea. Nebulized fentanyl may be preferred.* |
| Agitation | Lorazepam | 0.05 mg/kg/dose PO, IV, SL, PR q4–8hr |
| | Haloperidol | 0.01–0.02 mg/kg/dose PO, SL, PR q8–12hr |
| Pruritus | Diphenhydramine | 0.5–1 mg/kg/dose PO, IV q6–8hr |
| Nausea and vomiting | Prochlorperazine | 0.1–0.15 mg/kg/dose PO, PR q6–8hr |
| | Ondansetron | 0.15 mg/kg/dose PO, IV q6–8hr |
| Seizures | Diazepam | 0.3–0.5 mg/kg/dose PR q2–4hr |
| | Lorazepam | 0.05–0.1 mg/kg/dose IV q2–4hr |
| Secretions | Hyoscyamine | 0.03–0.06 mg/dose PO, SL q4hr (if <2 yr)<br>0.06–0.12 mg/dose PO, SL q4hr (if 2–12 yr)<br>0.12–0.25 mg/dose PO, SL q4hr (if >12 yr) |

*Infants <6 mo should receive one third to one half the dose.

IV, intravenous; PO, oral; PR, rectal; SL, sublingual.

Adapted from Himelstein BP et al: Pediatric palliative care. NEJM 2004;350(17):1752–1762.

## VII. DEATH PRONOUNCEMENT[10]

Residents may be called to pronounce the death of a patient in the hospital. This important task should be carried out with competence, compassion, and respect.

### A. PREPARATION

1. **Know the child's name and gender.**
2. **Be prepared to answer simple pertinent questions from family and friends.**
3. **Consult with nursing for relevant information: Recent events, family response, and family dynamics.**
4. **Determine the need and call for interdisciplinary support: Social work, child life, pastoral care, bereavement coordinator.**

### B. ENTERING THE ROOM

1. **Enter quietly and respectfully along with the primary nurse.**
2. **Introduce yourself and identify your role:**

a. "I am Dr. ______, the doctor on call."
b. Determine the relationships of those in the room.
c. Inform the family of the purpose ("I am here to examine your child") and invite them to remain in the room.

### C. PROCEDURE FOR PRONOUNCEMENT

1. **Check ID bracelet and pulse.**
2. **Respectfully check response to tactile stimuli.**
3. **Check for spontaneous respirations.**
4. **Check for heart sounds.**
5. **Record the time of death.**
6. **Inform the family of death.**
7. **Offer to contact other family members.**

### D. DOCUMENT DEATH IN THE CHART

1. **Write date, time of death, and the provider pronouncing the death.**
2. **Document absence of pulse, respirations, and heart sounds.**
3. **Identify family members who were present and informed of death.**
4. **Document notification of attending physician.**

### E. DEATH CERTIFICATE

1. **Locate a copy of a sample death certificate for reference.**
2. **Use BLACK INK only and complete "Physician sections."**

a. **NOTE** Do *NOT* use abbreviations (i.e., spell out the month: January 31 and not 1/31).
b. **NOTE** Do *NOT* cross out or use white out; must begin again if mistakes are made.
c. **NOTE** Cardiopulmonary or respiratory arrest is *NOT* an acceptable primary cause of death.

### F. AUTOPSY CONSENT

**1. Obtain family consent if indicated.**

**2. Plan follow-up to contact and review autopsy results.**

## VIII. BEREAVEMENT[10]

### A. ETIQUETTE

Families want to know that their children are not forgotten. Sending condolence cards, attending funerals, and making contact weeks to months later are all appropriate physician activities that are deeply valued by bereaved families. Respectful listening and sharing of memories provide support during bereavement.



### B. AVAILABLE SERVICES

Be familiar with available services: Pastoral care, social work, bereavement coordinator, community support groups, counseling services, bereavement follow-up programs.



## REFERENCES

1. Sepulveda C: Palliative care: World Health's Organization global perspective. J Pain Symptom Manage 2002;24(2):91–96.
2. Nelson R: Palliative care for children: Policy statement. Pediatrics 2007;119(2):351–357.
3. Smith J et al: Life's toughest moments. In Jonsen A et al (eds): Clinical Ethics, 5th ed. New York, McGraw-Hill Press, 2002.
4. Sourkes BM: Armfuls of Time: The Psychological Experience of Children with Life-Threatening Illnesses. Pittsburgh, University of Pittsburgh Press, 1995.
5. Corr CA: Children's understanding of death: Striving to understand death. In Doka KJ (ed): Children Mourning, Mourning Children. Washington, DC, Hospice Foundation of America, 1995, pp 8–10.
6. Corr CA, Balk DE (eds): Handbook of Adolescent Death and Bereavement. New York, Springer, 1996.
7. Faulkner K: Children's understanding of death. In Armstrong-Dailey A, Zarbock S (eds): Hospice Care for Children, 2nd ed. New York, Oxford University Press, 2001, pp 9–22.
8. Sigrist D: Journey's End: A Guide to Understanding the Final Stages of the Dying Process. Rochester, NY, Genesee Region Home Care, 1995.
9. Himelstein BP et al: Pediatric palliative care. NEJM 2004;350(17):1752–1762.
10. Bailey A: The Palliative Response. Birmingham, Ala, Menasha Ridge Press, 2003.

# Pulmonology

*Fatimah S. Dawood, MD*

## I. WEBSITES

American Lung Association: www.lungusa.org
Cystic Fibrosis Foundation: www.cff.org
American Academy of Allergy, Asthma and Immunology: www.aaaai.org
National Asthma Education and Prevention Program www.nhlbi.nih.gov

## II. RESPIRATORY PHYSICAL EXAMINATION

### A. NORMAL RESPIRATORY RATES (Table 24-1)

### B. RESPIRATORY AUSCULTATION (Table 24-2)

24

## III. ASTHMA

### A. PATHOGENESIS

A chronic inflammatory disorder of the airways resulting in recurrent episodes of wheezing, breathlessness, chest tightness, and cough, particularly at night and in the early morning.[1] These episodes are usually associated with widespread yet variable airflow obstruction, reversible either spontaneously or with therapy. The inflammation also causes increased airway hyperreactivity to a variety of stimuli (viral infections, cold air, exercise, emotions, as well as environmental allergens and pollutants).

### B. CLINICAL MANIFESTATIONS

1. **Increased work of breathing: Tachypnea, retractions, accessory muscle use.**
2. **Wheezing: No audible wheezing may indicate very poor air movement and severe bronchospasm.**
3. **Hypoxia and hypoventilation.**

### C. TREATMENT

1. **Acute management and status asthmaticus; see Chapter 1.**
2. **Classification of asthma severity and initiation of therapy for children 0–4 years of age (**Fig. 24-1**). Stepwise approach to managing asthma for children 0–4 years of age (**Fig. 24-2**).**
3. **Classification of asthma severity, initiation of therapy, and stepwise approach to managing asthma for children ages 5–11 and children ages 12 or older (see the figures at the back of the book).**

### D. ASTHMA ACTION PLAN (www.nationalasthma.org.au/publications/action)

An important educational and therapeutic tool for patients. Patients should leave all visits with a copy of their individual plan.

## IV. ACUTE RESPIRATORY ILLNESS

### A. UPPER AIRWAY OBSTRUCTION (see Chapter 1)

### B. BRONCHIOLITIS[2,3]

TABLE 24-1

**NORMAL RESPIRATORY RATES IN CHILDREN**

| Age (yr) | Respiratory Rate (breaths/min) |
|---|---|
| 0–1* | 24–38 |
| 1–3 | 22–30 |
| 4–6 | 20–24 |
| 7–9 | 18–24 |
| 10–14 | 16–22 |
| 14–18 | 14–20 |

*Slightly higher respiratory rates (i.e., 40–50 breaths/min) in the neonatal period may be normal in the absence of other signs and symptoms.

Data from Bardella IJ: Pediatric advanced life support: A review of the AHA recommendations. Am Fam Phys 1999;60(6):1743–1750.

TABLE 24-2

**RESPIRATORY AUSCULTATION**

| Sound | Description | Possible Causes |
|---|---|---|
| Crackles (rales) | Intermittent, scratchy, bubbly noises<br>Heard predominantly on inspiration<br>Produced by reopening of airways closed on previous expiration | Bronchiolitis, pulmonary edema<br>Pneumonia |
| Wheezes | Continuous, high-pitched, musical sound | Asthma, bronchiolitis, foreign body |
| Rhonchi | Continuous, low-pitched, nonmusical sound | Pneumonia, cystic fibrosis |
| Stridor | High-pitched, harsh, blowing sound<br>Heard predominantly on inspiration | Croup, laryngomalacia, subglottic stenosis, allergic reaction, vocal cord dysfunction |

**1. Definition: Lower respiratory tract infection common in infants; characterized by acute inflammation, edema, and necrosis of airway epithelium leading to increased mucus production and bronchospasm.**

a. Most common cause: Respiratory syncytial virus (RSV).

b. Other causes: Parainfluenza, adenovirus, *Mycoplasma*, metapneumovirus.

**2. Clinical manifestations: Variable and dynamic course ranging from transient apnea and mucus plugging to progressive lower airway disease.**

a. Initial symptoms: Clear rhinorrhea, diminished appetite, fever.

b. Later symptoms: Tachypnea, wheezing, dyspnea, irritability.

c. Radiographic findings: Hyperinflation and patchy atelectasis.

**3. Treatment: Mainstay of treatment is supportive care.**

a. Supplemental oxygen therapy.

b. Bronchodilators:

(1) Should not be used routinely in bronchiolitis.

CLASSIFYING ASTHMA SEVERITY AND INITIATING TREATMENT IN CHILDREN 0–4 YEARS OF AGE

Assessing severity and initiating therapy in children who are not currently taking long-term control medication

<table>
<tr><th colspan="2" rowspan="3">Components of severity</th><th colspan="4">Classification of asthma severity (0–4 years of age)</th></tr>
<tr><th rowspan="2">Intermittent</th><th colspan="3">Persistent</th></tr>
<tr><th>Mild</th><th>Moderate</th><th>Severe</th></tr>
<tr><td rowspan="4">Impairment</td><td>Symptoms</td><td>≤2 days/week</td><td>>2 days/week but not daily</td><td>Daily</td><td>Throughout the day</td></tr>
<tr><td>Nighttime awakenings</td><td>0</td><td>1–2×/month</td><td>3–4×/month</td><td>>1×/week</td></tr>
<tr><td>Short-acting beta$_2$-agonist use for symptom control (not prevention of EIB)</td><td>≤2 days/week</td><td>>2 days/week but not daily</td><td>Daily</td><td>Several times per day</td></tr>
<tr><td>Interference with normal activity</td><td>None</td><td>Minor limitation</td><td>Some limitation</td><td>Extremely limited</td></tr>
<tr><td rowspan="2">Risk</td><td rowspan="2">Exacerbations requiring oral systemic corticosteroids</td><td>0–1/year</td><td colspan="3">≥2 exacerbations in 6 months requiring oral systemic corticosteroids, or ≥4 wheezing episodes/1 year lasting >1 day AND risk factors for persistent asthma</td></tr>
<tr><td colspan="4">← Consider severity and interval since last exacerbation. Frequency and severity → may fluctuate over time.<br>Exacerbations of any severity may occur in patients in any severity category.</td></tr>
<tr><td colspan="2" rowspan="2">Recommended step for initiating therapy<br>(See Fig. 24-2 for treatment steps.)</td><td>Step 1</td><td>Step 2</td><td colspan="2">Step 3 and consider short course of oral systemic corticosteroids</td></tr>
<tr><td colspan="4">In 2–6 weeks, depending on severity, evaluate level of asthma control that is achieved. If no clear benefit is observed in 4–6 weeks, consider adjusting therapy or alternative diagnoses.</td></tr>
</table>

Key: EIB, exercise-induced bronchospasm

**Notes**

- The stepwise approach is meant to assist, not replace, the clinical decision making required to meet individual patient needs.
- Level of severity is determined by both impairment and risk. Assess impairment domain by patient's/caregiver's recall of previous 2–4 weeks. Symptom assessment for longer periods should reflect a global assessment such as inquiring whether the patient's asthma is better or worse since the last visit. Assign severity to the most severe category in which any feature occurs.
- At present, there are inadequate data to correspond frequencies of exacerbations with different levels of asthma severity. For treatment purposes, patients who had ≥2 exacerbations requiring oral systemic corticosteroids in the past 6 months, or ≥4 wheezing episodes in the past year, and who have risk factors for persistent asthma may be considered the same as patients who have persistent asthma, even in the absence of impairment levels consistent with persistent asthma.

FIG. 24-1

Guidelines for classifying asthma severity and initiating treatment in infants and young children (0–4 years of age). *(Adapted from NAEPP—Expert Panel Report 3: Guidelines for the diagnosis and management of asthma, August 2007. Available at www.nhlbi.nih.gov/guidelines/asthma/asthgdln.htm.)*

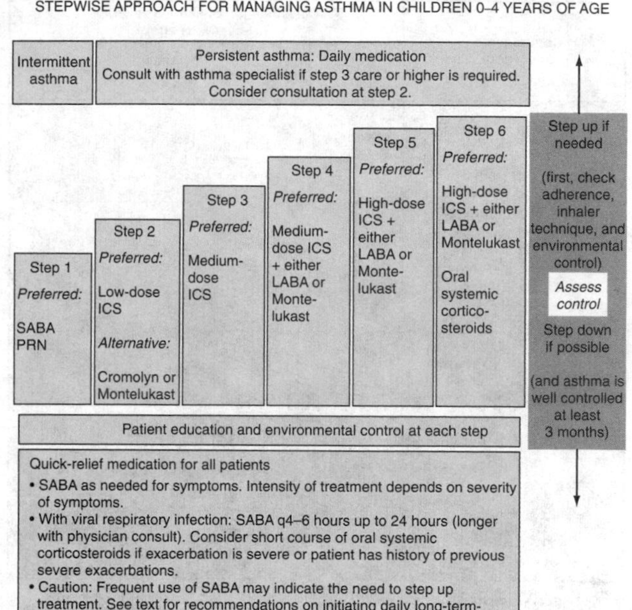

STEPWISE APPROACH FOR MANAGING ASTHMA IN CHILDREN 0–4 YEARS OF AGE
Intermittent asthma
Persistent asthma: Daily medication
Consult with asthma specialist if step 3 care or higher is required.
Consider consultation at step 2.
Step 1
Preferred:
SABA PRN
Step 2
Preferred:
Low-dose ICS
Alternative:
Cromolyn or Montelukast
Step 3
Preferred:
Medium-dose ICS
Step 4
Preferred:
Medium-dose ICS + either LABA or Montelukast
Step 5
Preferred:
High-dose ICS + either LABA or Montelukast
Step 6
Preferred:
High-dose ICS + either LABA or Montelukast
Oral systemic corticosteroids
Step up if needed
(first, check adherence, inhaler technique, and environmental control)
Assess control
Step down if possible
(and asthma is well controlled at least 3 months)
Patient education and environmental control at each step
Quick-relief medication for all patients
• SABA as needed for symptoms. Intensity of treatment depends on severity of symptoms.
• With viral respiratory infection: SABA q4–6 hours up to 24 hours (longer with physician consult). Consider short course of oral systemic corticosteroids if exacerbation is severe or patient has history of previous severe exacerbations.
• Caution: Frequent use of SABA may indicate the need to step up treatment. See text for recommendations on initiating daily long-term-control therapy.


Key: **Alphabetical order is used when more than one treatment option is listed within either preferred or alternative therapy**. ICS, inhaled corticosteroid; LABA, long-acting inhaled beta$_2$-agonist; SABA, short-acting inhaled beta$_2$-agonist

Notes:

- The stepwise approach is meant to assist, not replace, the clinical decision making required to meet individual patient needs.
- If alternative treatment is used and response is inadequate, discontinue it and use the preferred treatment before stepping up.
- If clear benefit is not observed within 4–6 weeks and patient/family medication technique and adherence are satisfactory, consider adjusting therapy or alternative diagnosis.
- Studies on children 0–4 years of age are limited. Step 2 preferred therapy is based on Evidence A. All other recommendations are based on expert opinion and extrapolation from studies in older children.

FIG. 24-2

Stepwise approach for managing asthma in infants and young children (0–4 years of age). *(Adapted from NAEPP—Expert Panel Report 3: Guidelines for the diagnosis and management of asthma, August 2007. Available at www.nhlbi.nih.gov/guidelines/asthma/asthgdln.htm.)*

(2) A trial of alpha- or beta-adrenergic medication is an option; should be continued only if there is documented improved clinical response.

c. Corticosteroids: Should not be used routinely in bronchiolitis.

d. Hospitalization: Should be considered based on clinical presentation. Strongly consider hospitalization for patients <12 weeks of age, with a history of prematurity, underlying cardiopulmonary disease, or immunodeficiency.

**4. Prevention: See Chapter 16.**

## C. APPARENT LIFE-THREATENING EVENT (ALTE)[4]

**1. Definition: Events that are frightening to the observer, and include some combination of obstructive or central apnea, color change (usually cyanosis and/or pallor), a marked change in muscle tone (usually extreme limpness), choking, or gagging. In some cases the observer fears the infant has died or would have died without significant intervention.**

**2. Causes (Box 24-1).**

**3. Work-up/treatment: Full history and physical examination guide the work-up. Treatment is tailored to diagnosis and prevention of further events.**

## D. SUDDEN INFANT DEATH SYNDROME (SIDS)[4]

**1. Definition: Sudden death of an infant under age 1 year, which remains unexplained after a thorough case investigation, including performance of complete autopsy, examination of death scene, and review of clinical history.**

**2. Incidence: 0.56 per 1,000, 2–3 times higher in African American and Native American populations.**

**3. Risk factors (Box 24-2).**

**4. Prevention: Infants under 6 months of age should not leave hospital or clinic setting without a review of SIDS risk factors.**

a. Babies should be placed on their backs to sleep with no head covering; very light covering with low room temperatures.

b. Feet-to-foot: Infants should lie at the foot of the bed on their back so that they cannot roll or crawl underneath the covers. Covers should be tucked in so the infant cannot pull the cover over his or her head.

c. Pillows increase risk. Infants should lie on a mattress designed for infant sleep.

d. Infants should live and sleep in a smoke-free zone.

e. Infants co-sleeping with others in the same bed are at increased risk of death if they sleep with parents who drink, smoke, or take drugs to sleep, sleep with multiple people, if they are covered with quilts or comforters, and if they are <14 weeks of age.

f. Infants should sleep in the same room with the parents in a safe infant bed or bassinet for the first few months of life.

g. Pacifiers (dummies, comforters) are protective against SIDS and should be used in bottle-fed infants or after breast-feeding is well established for the first year of life.

BOX 24-1

**DIFFERENTIAL DIAGNOSIS OF ALTE**

| |
|---|
| **Gastroenterologic (33%)** |
| Gastroesophageal reflux disease |
| Gastroenteritis |
| Esophageal dysfunction |
| Surgical abdomen |
| Dysphagias |
| **Neurologic (15%)** |
| Seizure |
| Central apnea/hypoventilation |
| Meningitis/encephalitis |
| Hydrocephalus |
| Brain tumor |
| Neuromuscular disorders |
| Vasovagal reaction |
| **Idiopathic Apnea of Infancy (23%)** |
| **Respiratory (11%)** |
| Respiratory syncytial virus |
| Pertussis |
| Aspiration |
| Respiratory tract infection |
| Reactive airway disease |
| Foreign body |
| **Otolaryngologic (4%)** |
| Laryngomalacia |
| Subglottic and/or laryngeal stenosis |
| Obstructive sleep apnea |
| **Cardiovascular (1%)** |
| Congenital heart disease |
| Cardiomyopathy |
| Cardiac arrhythmias/prolonged QT syndrome |
| Myocarditis |
| **Metabolic/Endocrine** |
| Inborn error of metabolism |
| Hypoglycemia |
| Electrolyte disturbance |
| **Infectious** |
| Sepsis |
| Urinary tract infection |

Modified from DeWolfe CC: Apparent life-threatening event: A review. Pediatr Clin North Am. 2005;52:4.

*Continued*

**BOX 24-1**

**DIFFERENTIAL DIAGNOSIS OF ALTE—cont'd**

**Other Diagnosis**

Child maltreatment syndrome
Shaken baby syndrome
Breath-holding spell
Choking
Drug or toxin reaction
Anemia
Unintentional smothering
Periodic breathing
Munchhausen-by-proxy syndrome

**BOX 24-2**

**RISK FACTORS ASSOCIATED WITH SIDS[4]**

Premature birth
Low birth weight
Young maternal age
High maternal parity
African American race
Recent infection
Congenital abnormalities
Cigarette smoke exposure
Overbundling
Sleeping in prone position
Sleeping on soft bedding or sofa
Unemployment
Some co-sleeping situations
Crowded conditions

## V. CYSTIC FIBROSIS (CF)

An autosomal recessive disorder in which most patients have chronic obstructive pulmonary disease, pancreatic exocrine insufficiency, and abnormally high sweat electrolyte concentrations.[5]

### A. CLINICAL MANIFESTATIONS OF CYSTIC FIBROSIS BY SYSTEM (Table 24-3)

### B. DIAGNOSTIC TESTING

1. **Newborn screening:** Many states have adopted universal newborn screening for CF by measuring infants' immunoreactive trypsinogen (IRT) levels. If infant has abnormally elevated IRT, measure again at 2 weeks of age. If another abnormally elevated result, infant should undergo sweat chloride testing.
2. **Sweat chloride test[6]:**

TABLE 24-3

MAJOR CLINICAL MANIFESTATIONS OF CYSTIC FIBROSIS BY ORGAN SYSTEM

| | |
|---|---|
| Respiratory | Chronic productive cough, hemoptysis<br>Bronchiectasis, bronchitis, pneumonia<br>Sinusitis<br>Nasal polyposis |
| Gastrointestinal | Meconium ileus<br>Rectal prolapse<br>Pancreatic insufficiency<br>Distal intestinal obstruction syndrome (DIOS)<br>Fat-soluble vitamin deficiency (A, D, E, K) |
| Genitourinary | Infertility (male) and decreased fertility (female)<br>Absence of vas deferens |
| Miscellaneous | Increased sweat electrolytes<br>Hypokalemic alkalosis<br>Digital clubbing<br>Pulmonary hypertrophic osteoarthropathy<br>Failure to thrive |

a. Values:
   (1) Normal (1 week to adult): <40 mmol/L.
   (2) Patients with CF: >60 mmol/L (mmol/L = mEq/L).
b. Sweat obtained through quantitative pilocarpine iontophoresis (>75 mg must be collected).
c. Results of 40–60 mmol/L require repeat testing or other tests for CF, including genetic analysis.
d. Normal levels (false-negative results): May be found in patients with CF in presence of edema and hypoproteinemia or inadequate sweat rate.
e. Elevated chloride levels: May be from CF, untreated adrenal insufficiency, glycogen storage disease type I, fucosidosis, hypothyroidism, nephrogenic diabetes insipidus, ectodermal dysplasia, malnutrition, mucopolysaccharidosis, panhypopituitarism, or poor testing technique.

## VI. SLEEP-DISORDERED BREATHING (SDB)[7]

A "disorder of breathing during sleep characterized by prolonged increased upper airway resistance, partial upper airway obstruction, or complete obstruction that disrupts pulmonary ventilation, oxygenation, or sleep quality."[8] Encompasses a spectrum of disordered breathing from snoring to complete upper airway obstruction with accompanying hypoxemia and obstructive hypoventilation. Complications from SDB include growth impairment, behavior problems, neurocognitive impairment, cor pulmonale, and disturbed sleep. Also referred to as sleep apnea or obstructive sleep apnea.

### A. SYMPTOMS

1. Snoring sometimes accompanied by intermittent pauses in breathing, snorts, or gasps.
2. Increased respiratory effort during sleep.
3. Disturbed or restless sleep; may be accompanied by increased arousals and awakenings.
4. Daytime cognitive and/or behavioral problems. Young children rarely present with daytime sleepiness. The absence of daytime symptoms does not rule out SDB.

### B. RISK FACTORS

1. Adenotonsillar hypertrophy.
2. Obesity.
3. Craniofacial or laryngeal anomalies.
4. Central nervous system disease, including brainstem dysfunction or compression, cerebral palsy, and neuromuscular disease.
5. Cigarette smoke exposure.

### C. WORKUP FOR SDB[8]

1. Screen for snoring during routine well-child care.
2. Refer to specialist for nocturnal polysomnography (sleep study) for patients with history of snoring, risk factors, and/or daytime symptoms.
3. Nocturnal polysomnography: Quantitates abnormalities in ventilation and sleep. Does not evaluate for daytime symptoms and has not been clearly demonstrated to identify children at risk for adverse clinical events. Abnormal result is useful, but normal results do not rule out SDB.

### D. TREATMENT OPTIONS FOR SDB[8]

1. Tonsillectomy and adenoidectomy.
2. Continuous positive airway pressure or bilevel positive airway pressure.
   a. Initiation often requires assistance from psychologists and developmental specialists.
   b. Requires follow-up by physician with sleep expertise for pressure titration mask adjustment and monitoring craniofacial development.
   c. Prolonged use of tight-fitting mask may alter the growth and shape of midface region.
3. Weight loss in obese children.
4. Treatment of upper respiratory allergies.

## VII. PULMONARY FUNCTION TESTS (PFTS)

Provide objective and reproducible measurements of airway function and lung volumes. Used to characterize disease, assess severity, and follow response to therapy.

TABLE 24-4

PREDICTED AVERAGE PEAK EXPIRATORY FLOW RATES FOR NORMAL CHILDREN

| Height Inches (cm) | PEFR (L/min) | Height Inches (cm) | PEFR (L/min) |
|---|---|---|---|
| 43 (109) | 147 | 56 (142) | 320 |
| 44 (112) | 160 | 57 (145) | 334 |
| 45 (114) | 173 | 58 (147) | 347 |
| 46 (117) | 187 | 59 (150) | 360 |
| 47 (119) | 200 | 60 (152) | 373 |
| 48 (122) | 214 | 61 (155) | 387 |
| 49 (124) | 227 | 62 (157) | 400 |
| 50 (127) | 240 | 63 (160) | 413 |
| 51 (130) | 254 | 64 (163) | 427 |
| 52 (132) | 267 | 65 (165) | 440 |
| 53 (135) | 280 | 66 (168) | 454 |
| 54 (137) | 293 | 67 (170) | 467 |
| 55 (140) | 307 | | |

PEFR, peak expiratory flow rate.

Data from Voter KZ: Diagnostic tests of lung function. Pediatr Rev 1996;17(2):53–63.

## A. PEAK EXPIRATORY FLOW RATE (PEFR)

Maximum flow rate generated during a forced expiratory maneuver.

1. **Useful in following the course of asthma and response to therapy; can compare a patient's PEFR to the previous "personal best" and the normal predicted value (Table 24-4).**
2. **Normal predicted values vary across different racial groups; best indicator of patient condition is comparison with their own personal best. PEFRs are effort dependent and insensitive to small airway function.**

## B. SPIROMETRY (FOR CHILDREN ≥6 YEARS OF AGE)

Plot of airflow versus time. Measurements are made from a rapid, forceful, and complete expiration from total lung capacity (TLC) to residual volume (RV). Usually performed before and after bronchodilation to assess response to therapy or after bronchial challenge to assess airway hyperreactivity.

1. **Forced vital capacity (FVC):** Maximum volume of air exhaled from the lungs after a maximum inspiration. Bedside measurement of vital capacity with a handheld spirometer can be useful in confirming or predicting hypoventilation associated with muscle weakness. FVC <15 mL/kg may be an indication for ventilatory support.
2. **Forced expiratory volume in 1 second ($FEV_1$):** Volume exhaled during the first second of an FVC maneuver. Single best measure of airway function.
3. **Forced expiratory flow ($FEF_{25-75}$):** Mean rate of airflow over the middle half of the FVC between 25% and 75% of FVC. Sensitive to medium and small airway obstruction.

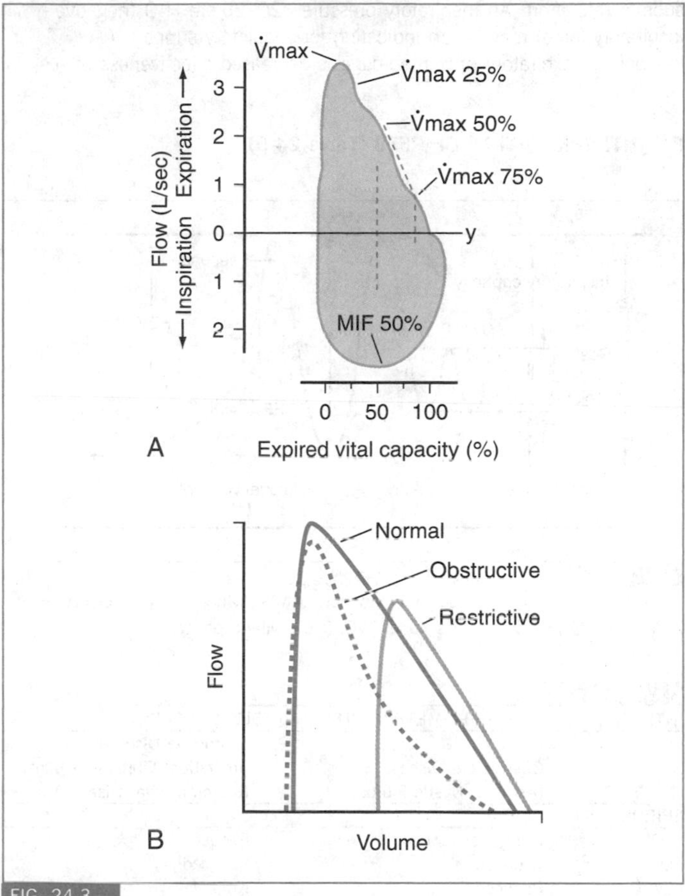


FIG. 24-3

**A,** Normal flow-volume curve. **B,** Worsening intrathoracic airway obstruction as in asthma or cystic fibrosis. *(**B,** Data from Baum GL, Wolinsky E: Textbook of Pulmonary Diseases, 5th ed. Boston, Little, Brown, 1994.)*

## C. FLOW-VOLUME CURVES

The plot of airflow versus lung volume. Useful in characterizing different patterns of airway obstruction (Fig. 24-3).

## D. LUNG VOLUMES (Fig. 24-4)

## E. MAXIMAL INSPIRATORY AND EXPIRATORY PRESSURES

Obtained by asking patient to inhale and exhale against a fixed obstruction. Low pressures suggest a neuromuscular problem or submaximal effort. An inspiratory pressure <20–25 cm $H_2O$ (negative inspiratory force) may be an indication for ventilatory support. A low positive expiratory pressure suggests decreased effectiveness of coughing.

## F. INTERPRETATION OF PFTS (Table 24-5)

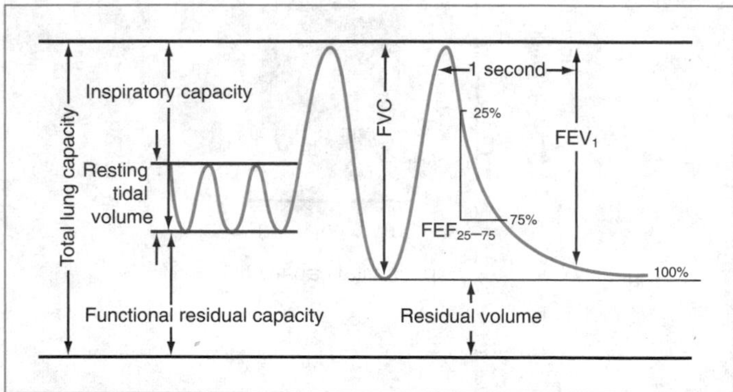


FIG. 24-4

Lung volumes. $FEF_{25-75}$, forced expiratory flow between 25% and 75% of FVC; $FEV_1$, forced expiratory volume in 1 second; FVC, forced vital capacity.

TABLE 24-5

**INTERPRETATION OF SPIROMETRY AND LUNG VOLUME READINGS**

| | Obstructive Disease (Asthma, Cystic Fibrosis) | Restrictive Disease (Interstitial Fibrosis, Scoliosis, Neuromuscular Disease) |
|---|---|---|
| **SPIROMETRY** | | |
| FVC* | Normal or reduced | Reduced |
| $FEV_1$* | Reduced | Reduced§ |
| $FEV_1$/FVC† | Reduced | Normal |
| $FEF_{25-75}$ | Reduced | Normal or reduced§ |
| PEFR* | Normal or reduced | Normal or reduced§ |
| **LUNG VOLUMES** | | |
| TLC* | Normal or increased | Reduced |
| RV* | Increased | Reduced |
| RV/TLC‡ | Increased | Unchanged |
| FRC | Increased | Reduced |

*Normal range: ±20% of predicted.
†Normal range: >85%.
‡Normal range: 20 ± 10%.
§Reduced proportional to FVC.
$FEF_{25-50}$, forced expiratory flow between 25% and 75% of FVC; $FEV_1$, forced expiratory volume in 1 second; FRC, functional residual capacity; FVC, forced vital capacity; PEFR, peak expiratory flow rate; RV, residual volume; TLC, total lung capacity.

## VIII. PULMONARY GAS EXCHANGE

### A. ARTERIAL BLOOD GASES

Measurement of arterial blood gases (ABGs) is used to assess oxygenation ($Pao_2$), ventilation (V), $Paco_2$, and acid-base status (pH and $HCO_3^-$). See Chapter 27 for normal mean ABG values.

### B. VENOUS BLOOD GASES

Measurement of venous blood gas (VBGs) through peripheral venous samples is strongly affected by the local circulatory and metabolic environment. It can be used to assess acid-base status. $Pvco_2$ averages 6–8 mm Hg higher than $Paco_2$, and venous pH is slightly lower than arterial pH.

### C. CAPILLARY BLOOD GASES

Correlation of capillary blood gas (CBGs) with arterial sampling is generally best for pH, moderate for $Pco_2$, and worst for $Po_2$.

### D. ANALYSIS OF ACID-BASE DISTURBANCES[9,10] (Fig. 24-5)

1. **Pure respiratory acidosis (or alkalosis):** 10 mm Hg rise (fall) in $Paco_2$ results in an average 0.08 fall (rise) in pH.
2. **Pure metabolic acidosis (or alkalosis):** 10 mEq/L fall (rise) in $HCO_3^-$ results in an average 0.15 fall (rise) in pH.
3. **Determine primary disturbance; then assess for mixed disorder by calculating expected compensatory response (Table 24-6).**

### E. PULSE OXIMETRY[11,12]

1. **Arterial oxygen saturation ($Sao_2$):** Noninvasive indirect method of measuring $Sao_2$ Uses light absorption characteristics of oxygenated and deoxygenated hemoglobin to estimate $O_2$ saturation.
2. **Oxyhemoglobin dissociation curve (Fig. 24-6):** Relates $Sao_2$ to $Pao_2$. Increased hemoglobin affinity for oxygen (shift to the left) occurs with alkalemia, hypothermia, hypocapnia, decreased 2,3-diphosphoglycerate (2,3-DPG), increased fetal hemoglobin, and anemia. Decreased hemoglobin affinity for oxygen (shift to the right) occurs with acidemia, hyperthermia, hypercapnia, and increased 2,3-DPG.
3. **Important uses of pulse oximetry:**

a. Rapid and continuous assessment of oxygenation in acutely ill patients.
b. Monitoring of patients requiring oxygen therapy.
c. Assessment of oxygen requirements during feeding, sleep, and exercise.
d. Home monitoring of physiologic effects of apnea and bradycardia.

4. **Limitations of pulse oximetry:**

a. Measures saturation ($Sao_2$) and not $O_2$ delivery to tissues. A marginally low saturation may be clinically significant in an anemic patient because a normal $Sao_2$ does not ensure a normal $O_2$-carrying capacity (see oxygen content calculation in Chapter 4).

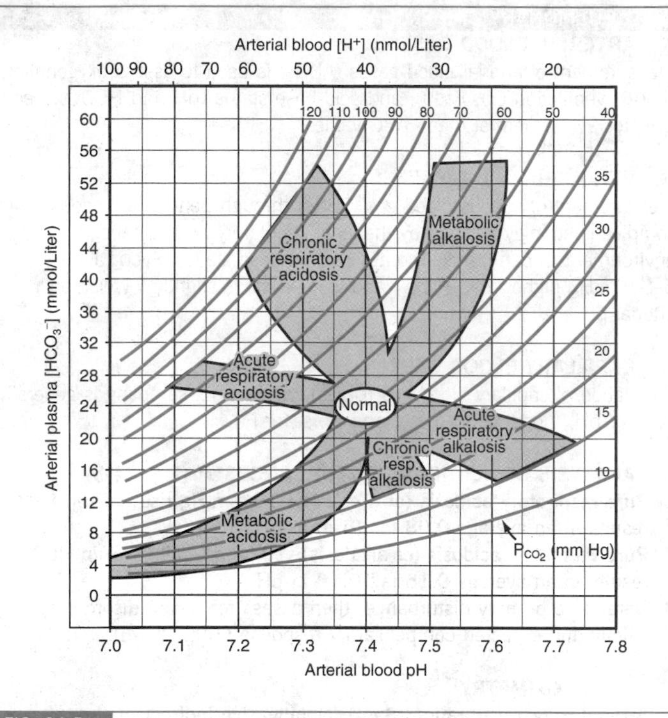


FIG. 24-5

Interpretation of arterial blood gases. *(Modified from Siggaard-Anderson O: The Acid-Base Status of the Blood, 4th ed. Copenhagen, Munksgaard, 1976.)*

TABLE 24-6

**CALCULATION OF EXPECTED COMPENSATORY RESPONSE**

| Disturbance | Primary Change | pH | Expected Compensatory Response |
|---|---|---|---|
| Acute respiratory acidosis | ↑ $Paco_2$ | ↓ pH | ↑ $HCO_3^-$ by 1 mEq/L for each 10 mm Hg rise in $Paco_2$ |
| Acute respiratory alkalosis | ↓ $Paco_2$ | ↑ pH | ↓ $HCO_3^-$ by 1–3 mEq/L for each 10 mm Hg fall in $Paco_2$ |
| Chronic respiratory acidosis | ↑ $Paco_2$ | ↓ pH | ↑ $HCO_3^-$ by 4 mEq/L for each 10 mm Hg rise in $Paco_2$ |
| Chronic respiratory alkalosis | ↓ $Paco_2$ | ↑ pH | ↓ $HCO_3^-$ by 2–5 mEq/L for each 10 mm Hg fall in $Paco_2$ |
| Metabolic acidosis | ↓ $HCO_3^-$ | ↓ pH | ↓ $Paco_2$ by 1–1.5 times fall in $HCO_3^-$ |
| Metabolic alkalosis | ↑ $HCO_3^-$ | ↑ pH | ↑ $Paco_2$ by 0.25–1 times rise in $HCO_3^-$ |

Data from Schrier RW: Renal and Electrolyte Disorders, 3rd ed. Boston, Little, Brown, 1986.

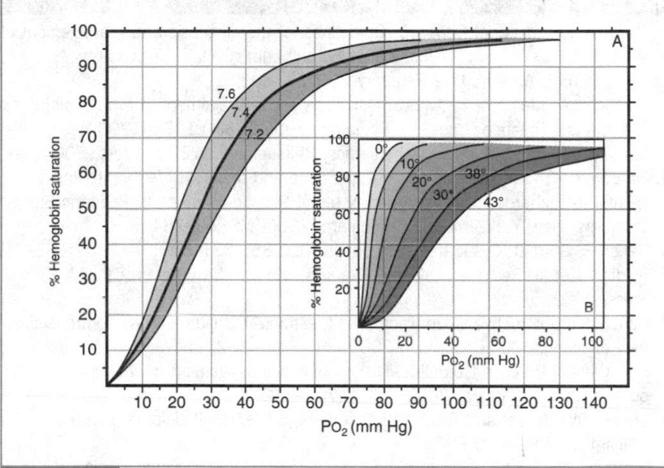


FIG. 24-6

Oxyhemoglobin dissociation curve. **A,** Curve shifts to the left as pH increases. **B,** Curve shifts to the left as temperature decreases. *(Data from Lanbertsten CJ: Transport of oxygen, $CO_2$, and inert gases by the blood. In Mountcastle VB [ed]: Medical Physiology, 14th ed. St. Louis, Mosby, 1980.)*

b. Unreliable when detection of pulse signal is poor as a result of physiologic conditions (hypothermia, hypovolemia, shock) or movement artifact. Oximeter's pulse rate should match patient's heart rate to ensure accurate measurement.
c. Insensitive to hyperoxia because of the sigmoid shape of the oxyhemoglobin curve.
d. $Sao_2$ is artificially increased by carboxyhemoglobin levels >1%–2% (e.g., in chronic smokers or with smoke inhalation).
e. $Sao_2$ is artificially decreased by patient motion, intravenous dyes, such as methylene blue and indocyanine green, and opaque nail polish.
f. $Sao_2$ is artificially decreased by methemoglobin levels >1%; electrosurgical interference or xenon arc surgical lamps may alter accuracy of pulse oximeter readings.
g. $Sao_2$ reading often does not correlate with $Pao_2$ in sickle cell disease.[13]

## F. CAPNOGRAPHY

Measures $CO_2$ concentration of expired gas by infrared spectroscopy or mass spectroscopy. End-tidal $CO_2$ ($ETco_2$) correlates with $Paco_2$ (usually within 5 mm Hg in healthy subjects). Capnography can be used for demonstrating proper placement of an endotracheal tube, continuous monitoring of $CO_2$ trends in ventilated patients, and monitoring ventilation during polysomnography.

## REFERENCES

1. NAEPP—Expert Panel Report 3: Guidelines for the diagnosis and management of asthma, August 2007. Available at www.nhlbi.nih.gov/guidelines/asthma/asthgdln.htm. Accessed 22 February 2007.
2. American Academy of Pediatrics: Diagnosis and management of bronchiolitis: AAP Clinical Practice Guideline. Pediatrics 2006;118(4):1774–1793.
3. Berham: Nelson's Textbook of Pediatrics. Philadelphia, WB Saunders, 2004.
4. Halbower AC: Sudden infant death syndrome and apparent life-threatening events. In Richardson M, Friedman N (eds): Clinician's Guide to Pediatric Sleep Disorders. New York, Informa Healthcare, 2006. pp 269–284.
5. Ratjen F, Gerd D: Cystic fibrosis. Lancet 2003;361:681–689.
6. Soldin SJ et al: Pediatric Reference Ranges, 4th ed. Washington, DC, AACC Press, 2003.
7. Carroll JL: Obstructive sleep-disordered breathing in children: New controversies, new directions. Clin Chest Med 2003;24(2):261–282.
8. AAP Clinical Practice Guideline: Diagnosis and management of childhood obstructive sleep apnea. 2002;109(4):704–712.
9. Schrier RW: Renal and Electrolyte Disorders, 6th ed. Philadelphia, Lippincott, Williams and Wilkins, 2002.
10. Brenner BM, Rector FC (eds): The Kidney, vol. 1, 7th ed. Philadelphia, WB Saunders, 2003.
11. Murray CB, Loughlin GM: Making the most of pulse oximetry. Contemp Pediatr 1995;12(7):45–62.
12. Lanbertsten CJ: Transport of oxygen, $CO_2$, and inert gases by the blood. In Mountcastle VB (ed): Medical Physiology, 14th ed. St. Louis, Mosby, 1980.
13. Comber JT, Lopez BL: Examination of pulse oximetry in sickle cell anemia patients presenting to the emergency department in acute vasoocclusive crisis. Am J Emerg Med 1996;14(1):16–18.

# Radiology

*John Holcroft, MD*

## I. HEAD[1]

Most intracranial processes, malformations, and tumors are best imaged with magnetic resonance imaging (MRI). MRI is useful for neurodegenerative and demyelination disorders, diffuse axonal injury, neurocutaneous syndromes, structural lesions in focal seizure disorders, and vascular lesions. Compared with computed tomography (CT), MRI is more useful in detecting lesions in the posterior fossa.



### A. GERMINAL MATRIX HEMORRHAGE

Premature infants should undergo head ultrasonography (US) to detect intraventricular hemorrhage and periventricular leukomalacia and to screen for hydrocephalus and congenital abnormalities.

### B. CONGENITAL MALFORMATIONS

Once detected on US, malformations are further defined with MRI.

### C. CONGENITAL INFECTIONS

1. **Congenital infections such as herpes simplex virus (HSV): Best imaged on MRI.**
2. **Calcifications consistent with toxoplasmosis and cytomegalovirus (CMV) infection: CT may detect these. Calcifications in toxoplasmosis have a predilection for the basal ganglia and tend to be more diffuse than those of CMV, which primarily affects the periventricular region.**

### D. HEAD TRAUMA

1. **Best imaged by non-contrast CT to reveal skull fractures and subdural and epidural hematomas. A head CT should be part of a physical abuse workup.**
2. **Skull radiography: Of limited value.**
3. **Multiple hemorrhages of various ages: Best detected with MRI.**

### E. VENTRICULOPERITONEAL SHUNT MALFUNCTION

Initial imaging includes head CT to determine ventricle size. If signs of shunt malfunction are noted, radiographs of the length of the shunt (a shunt series) should follow to look for kinks or disconnections.

### F. CRANIOSYNOSTOSIS

Suture examination is best done initially with radiographs of the skull. If there are changes consistent with craniosynostosis, three-dimensional CT reconstructions should then be obtained.

## II. EYES: ORBITAL CELLULITIS

Best imaged with contrast CT with orbital cuts. To determine whether an infection is preseptal or postseptal, a line is drawn from the medial to the lateral bony walls of the orbit on transverse cuts.

## III. SPINE

### A. CERVICAL SPINE TRAUMA[2,3]

1. After immobilization in a collar, lateral and anteroposterior (AP) radiographs of the cervical spine (C-spine) should be performed in all children who have sustained significant head trauma or deceleration injury or in those who have undergone unwitnessed trauma. The seventh cervical vertebral body and the C7–T1 junction must be visualized. C-spine injuries are most common from the occiput to C3 in children (especially subluxation at the atlanto-occipital joint or atlantoaxial joint in infants and toddlers) and in the lower C-spine in older children and adults.
2. Flexion-extension films may be helpful, especially in patients with Down syndrome, who are at risk for atlantoaxial subluxation.
3. Odontoid views may be helpful in older children with suspected occipitocervical injury (e.g., whiplash).

### B. READING C-SPINE FILMS[2,3]

The following ABCDDS (or ABCDs) mnemonic is useful:

1. **Alignment:** The anterior vertebral body line, posterior vertebral body line, facet line, and spinous process line should each form a continuous line with smooth contour and no step-offs.
2. **Bones:** Assess each bone looking for chips or fractures.
3. **Count:** Must see C7 body in its entirety.
4. **Dens:** Examine for chips or fractures.
5. **Disk spaces:** Should see consistent distance between each vertebral body.
6. **Soft tissue:** Assess for swelling, particularly in the prevertebral area.

### C. SCIWORA[2,3]

1. Spinal cord injury without radiographic abnormality (SCIWORA): A functional C-spine injury that cannot be excluded by abnormality on a radiograph; thought to be attributable to the increased mobility of a child's spine. Should be suspected in the setting of normal C-spine images when clinical signs or symptoms (e.g., point tenderness, focal neurologic symptoms) suggest C-spine injury.
2. If neurologic symptoms persist despite normal C-spine and flexion-extension views, MRI is indicated to rule out swelling, contusion, or intramedullary hemorrhage of the cord.

### D. SPINAL DYSRAPHISM (e.g., myelocele, myelomeningocele)

Initial imaging: Radiographs. Most often screened for with US. Complications are followed by MRI.

### E. SCOLIOSIS

Best evaluated by erect AP spine radiograph. PA views can be used in postpubertal girls to decrease breast radiation dose.

## IV. AIRWAY[2]

### A. LATERAL RADIOGRAPH

1. Lateral radiograph of the upper airway is the most useful film for evaluating a child with stridor. If possible, should be obtained on inspiration.
2. A radiologic workup should always include AP and lateral radiographs of the chest, with inclusion of the upper airway on the AP chest radiograph. Diagnosis is based on airway radiologic examination in conjunction with clinical presentation (Table 25-1; Figs. 25-1 and 25-2).

### B. VASCULAR RINGS

1. Vascular rings and other masses that extrinsically obstruct the lower airways can be imaged with contrast-enhanced CT or MRI.
2. Tracheomalacia and intrinsic masses can be studied with bronchoscopy.

### C. FOREIGN BODIES

1. **Lower airway foreign bodies:** In the absence of a radiopaque foreign body, radiologic findings include air trapping, hyperinflation, atelectasis, consolidation, pneumothorax, and pneumomediastinum. Further studies should include expiratory films (in a cooperative patient), bilateral decubitus chest films (in an uncooperative patient), or airway fluoroscopy.

TABLE 25-1

DIAGNOSIS OF DISEASES BASED ON AIRWAY RADIOLOGIC EXAMINATION

| Diagnosis | Findings on Airway Films |
|---|---|
| Croup | AP and lateral films with subglottic narrowing ("steeple sign") |
| Epiglottitis | Enlarged, indistinct epiglottis on lateral film ("thumb print sign") |
| Vascular ring | AP and lateral films with narrowing; double or right aortic arch |
| Retropharyngeal abscess or pharyngeal mass | Soft tissue air or persistent enlargement of prevertebral soft tissues; more than half of a vertebral body above C3 and one vertebral body below C3 |
| Immunodeficiency | Absence of adenoidal and tonsillar tissue after age 6 mo |

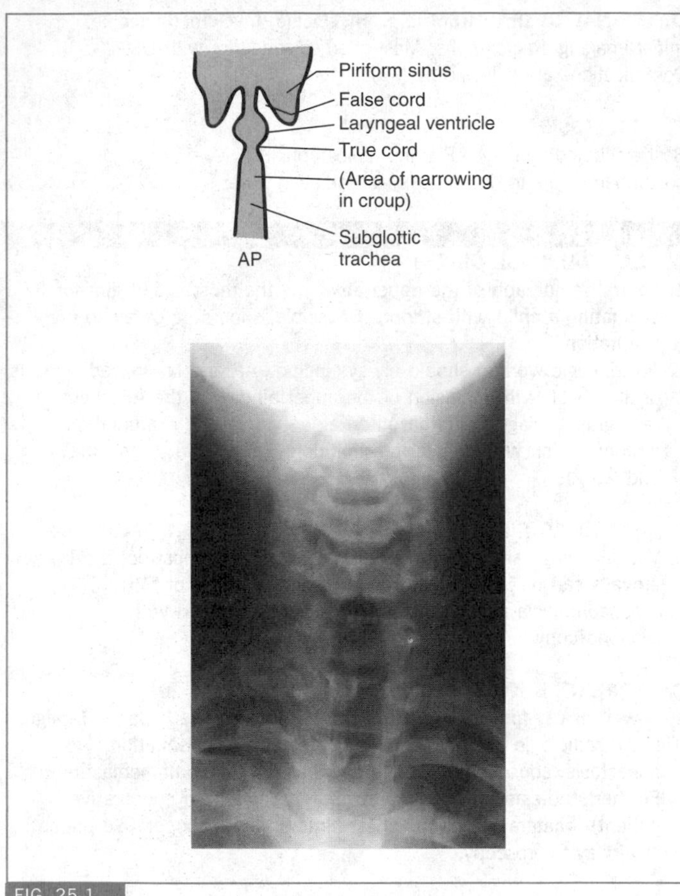


FIG. 25-1
Anteroposterior (AP) neck film with normal anatomy on AP airway view.

2. **Esophageal foreign bodies:** Usually lodged at one of three locations: the thoracic inlet, the level of the aortic arch and left mainstem bronchus, or the gastroesophageal junction. Evaluation should include the following:
   a. Lateral airway film (include nasopharynx).
   b. AP film of the chest and abdomen (including the supraclavicular region).
   c. Contrast study of the esophagus if other films are normal. If perforation is suspected, use nonionic, water-soluble contrast.

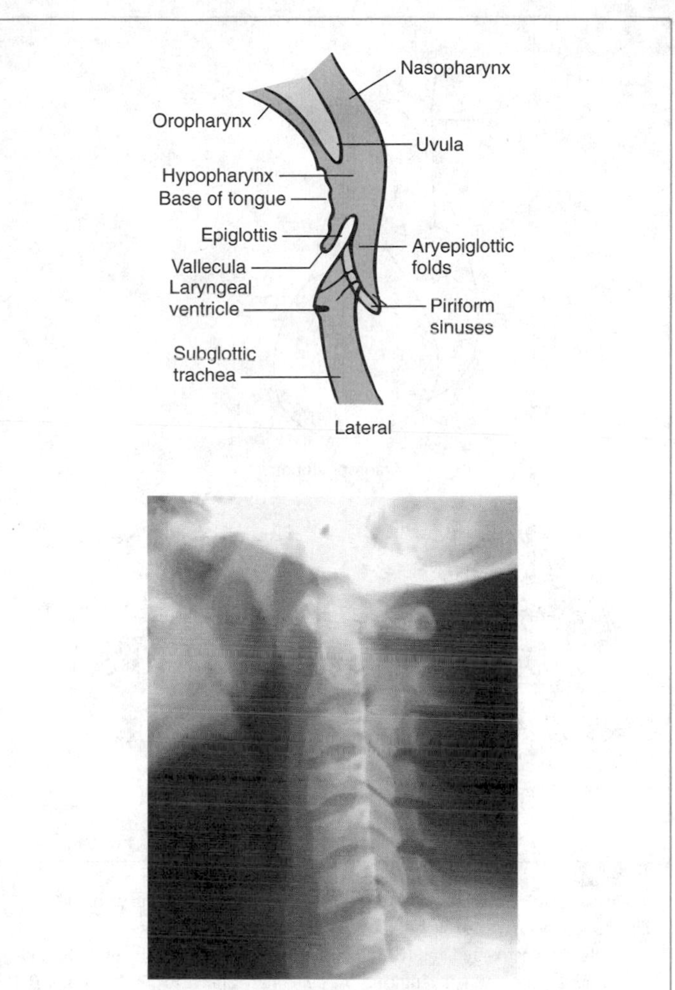


FIG. 25-2

Lateral neck film with normal anatomy on lateral airway view.

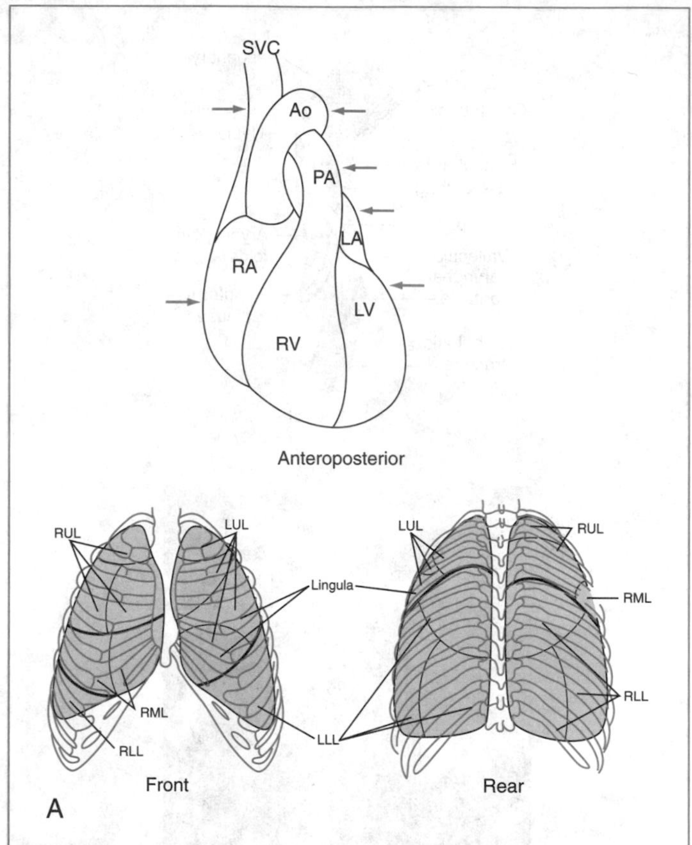


FIG. 25-3A

**A,** Lung and cardiac anatomy on an AP chest radiograph. Divisions within lobes indicate segments matched with x-rays. *Arrows* indicate contours seen on anteroposterior chest x-ray films (**B**). Ao, aorta; LA, left atrium; LLL, left lower lobe; LUL, left upper lobe; LV, left ventricle; PA, pulmonary artery; RA, right atrium; RLL, right lower lobe; RML, right middle lobe; RUL, right upper lobe; RV, right ventricle; SVC, superior vena cava. *(Heart diagram modified from Kirks DR et al: Practical Pediatric Imaging: Diagnostic Radiology of Infants and Children, 3rd ed. Philadelphia, Lippincott-Raven, 1998.)*

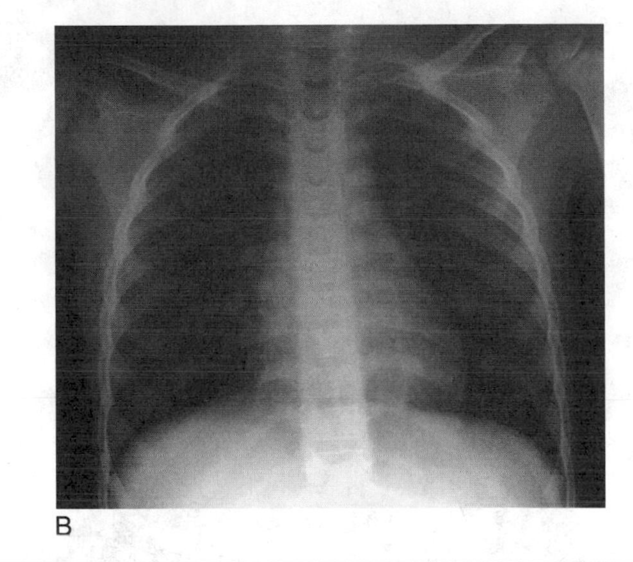

FIG. 25-3B



## V. CHEST[2,3]

### A. POSTEROANTERIOR AND LATERAL RADIOGRAPHS

First images obtained when studying the chest (Figs. 25-3 and 25-4).

### B. PNEUMONIA

1. Lobar or segmental consolidation: More typical of bacterial infections.
2. Hyperinflation, bilateral patchy or streaky densities, and peribronchial thickening. More typical of nonbacterial disease.

### C. ATELECTASIS VERSUS INFILTRATE

1. **Atelectasis:** When air is removed from the lung, the tissue collapses, resulting in volume loss on chest radiographs. If severe enough, the mediastinum and/or diaphragm are pulled toward the lesion. Air may still remain in larger bronchi, creating air bronchograms on radiograph. Collapse and re-expansion can occur quickly.
2. **Infiltrate:** A fluid (blood, pus, edema) that invades one of the compartments of the lung (bronchoalveolar air space or peribronchial interstitial space) is seen as a density on a radiograph. When alveolar air is displaced by fluid, but air remains in the bronchi, the classic pneumonic infiltrate with air bronchograms is seen. When infiltrate is interstitial, its borders are more vague, and bronchial walls may be thickened. Typically, infiltrates resolve in 2–6 weeks.

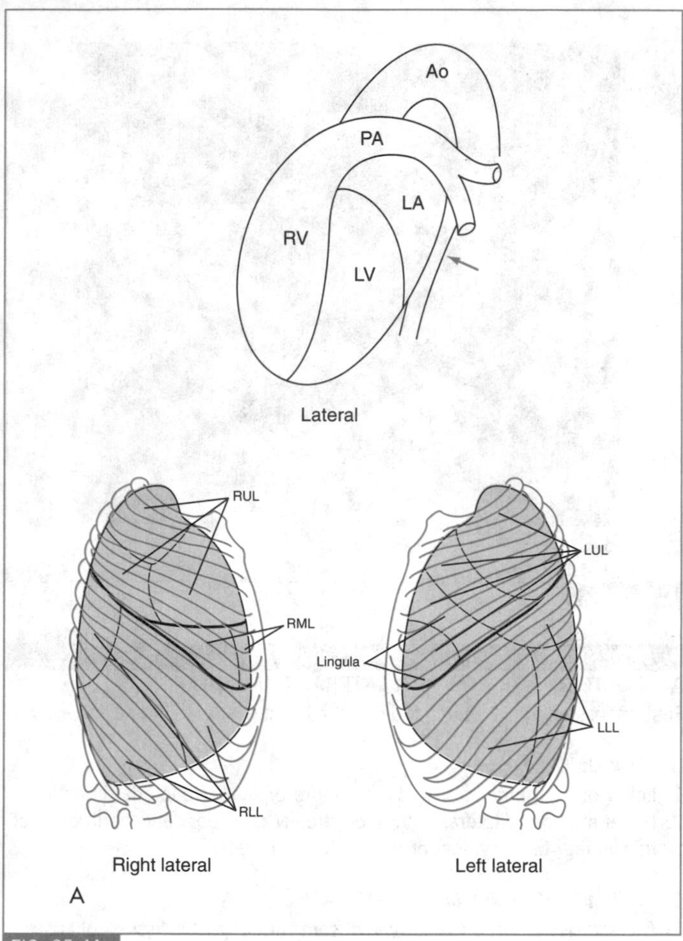


FIG. 25-4A

**A,** Lung and cardiac anatomy on lateral chest radiograph. Divisions within lobes indicate segments matched with x-rays. *Arrow* indicates contours seen on lateral chest x-ray films (**B**). Ao, aorta; LA, left atrium; LLL, left lower lobe; LUL, left upper lobe; LV, left ventricle; PA, pulmonary artery; RLL, right lower lobe; RML, right middle lobe; RUL, right upper lobe; RV, right ventricle. *(Heart diagram modified from Kirks DR et al: Practical Pediatric Imaging: Diagnostic Radiology of Infants and Children, 3rd ed. Philadelphia, Lippincott-Raven, 1998.)*

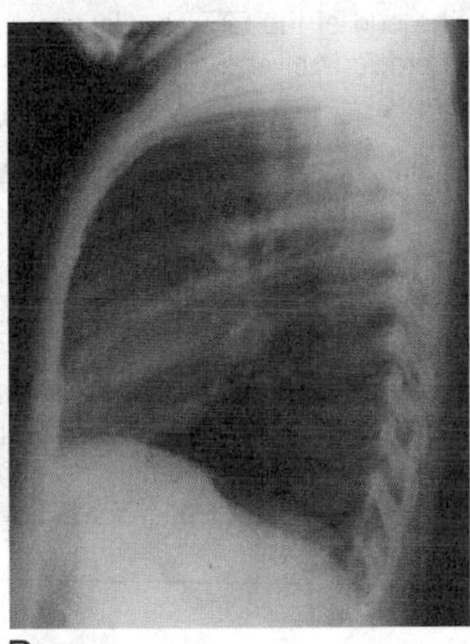


FIG. 25-4B



## D. PARAPNEUMONIC EFFUSIONS AND EMPYEMA

Initially, PA and lateral radiographs are obtained. Lateral decubitus radiographs may also be helpful, followed by either US or contrast-enhanced CT to determine if effusion is loculated, and to mark area for percutaneous drainage.

## E. PARENCHYMAL FINDINGS

1. **Lung abscess, cavitary necrosis, and lung contusions: Best imaged with contrast-enhanced CT.**
2. **Pneumatocele and fungal infections: Use non-contrast CT.**

## F. MEDIASTINAL MASSES

Mediastinal masses (thymus, lymphoma, bronchogenic cyst, neuroblastoma, neurofibroma) are initially imaged with plain films, followed by contrast-enhanced CT or MRI.

## G. CENTRAL LINE PLACEMENT

On chest radiograph, central venous catheters entering from the neck or arm are ideally placed with catheter tip at the junction of the superior vena cava and the right atrium. Some extension into the right atrium is acceptable, but if the catheter is noted to curve to the patient's left on PA film, the catheter may be positioned in the right ventricle. Catheters inserted below the diaphragm should be placed with tip at the level of the diaphragm.

### H. ENDOTRACHEAL TUBE (ETT) PLACEMENT

On chest radiograph, the end of the ETT should rest approximately midway between the thoracic inlet and the carina. The lung fields should show symmetrical aeration.

## VI. HEART AND VESSELS[2]

### A. CONGENITAL HEART DISEASE

Most often and clearly defined by echocardiography, but evaluation of an initial PA and lateral chest radiograph may yield important clues:

1. **Position of the aortic arch:** Left or right.
2. **Situs:** Noting the position of the apex, stomach bubble, and liver.
3. **Heart size:** With particular attention paid to the lateral chest radiograph.
4. **Pulmonary vascularity:** Increased or decreased flow in arteries and veins.

### B. VESSELS

1. Moving blood is detected by ultrasonographic frequency shifts.
2. Color Doppler flow imaging: Can be used to evaluate deep-vein thrombosis, vascular patency, intracranial blood flow (including transcranial Doppler to screen for ischemic brain injury risk in sickle cell disease), cardiac shunt flow, transplant vascularity, veno-occlusive disease of the liver, and testicular perfusion in testicular torsion.
3. Power Doppler is particularly sensitive in detecting slow flow in small vessels (e.g., infant testes).

### C. VESSEL ABNORMALITIES

Can be studied with echocardiography/US, CT, and MRI, which can detect coarctation of the aorta, aortic stenosis, pulmonary artery and vein abnormalities, vascular rings, arteriovenous malformations and hemangiomas, aneurysms, and postoperative complications such as thrombosis and stenosis.

## VII. ABDOMEN[2,3]

### A. NEONATAL ENTEROCOLITIS

Clinically diagnosed and followed by abdominal radiographs, which may show focal dilation, featureless loops, pneumatosis, and portal venous gas.

### B. ESOPHAGEAL ATRESIA AND TRACHEOESOPHAGEAL FISTULA (TEF)

Studied initially with radiographs of the chest, which may reveal the air-distended esophageal atretic pouch, the nasogastric tube curled up in this pouch, or excessive dilation of stomach as a result of fistula communication.

## C. HIGH INTESTINAL OBSTRUCTION

1. Diagnosed with upper gastrointestinal (UGI) series: Contrast is ingested, and esophagus, stomach, and duodenum are visualized. Causes: Esophageal webs and rings, masses, duodenal atresia or webs, annular pancreas, midgut volvulus, and Ladd bands.
2. UGI can also help evaluate hiatal hernias, varices, gastric outlet obstruction, motility problems, ulcerations, and reflux.
3. During UGI, identification of the duodenojejunal junction (the ligament of Treitz) helps to diagnose malrotation. Normally, the junction is to the left of spine, at or above level of duodenal bulb.



## D. PYLORIC STENOSIS

1. US: Directly visualizes the muscle; the preferred examination. Normally, pylorus is <17 mm in length and its muscular wall <4 mm in width.
2. Radiographs: Show gastric distention.
3. UGI: Delayed gastric emptying and a narrow pyloric channel will be evident.

## E. BOWEL OBSTRUCTION

1. Determination of large or small bowel obstruction: Often aided by supine radiograph, prone radiograph, and either upright, supine cross-table lateral, or left lateral decubitus film to look for free air and air-fluid levels. Causes of obstruction: Adhesions, appendicitis, incarcerated inguinal hernias, Meckel diverticulum, and intussusception.
2. US: Can be helpful in thin patients as well as in female patients who have ovarian pathology in their differential for abdominal pain.
3. CT with intravenous, oral, or rectal contrast is more useful with an obese patient or when looking for perforated appendicitis or abscess.
4. Contrast enemas with dilute, water-soluble agents can also be useful in lower intestinal obstruction in the newborn.

## F. INTUSSUSCEPTION

1. On abdominal radiographs, particularly the prone view, findings include minimal gas in right abdomen and ascending colon.
2. Both US and CT will show alternating rings. Air insufflation is preferred, but contrast enema with fluoroscopic guidance can also reduce an intussusception. These methods are contraindicated if perforation is suspected.

## G. MECKEL DIVERTICULUM

Suggested by painless lower GI bleeding; diagnosed by nuclear scintigraphy using $^{99m}$Tc-pertechnetate.

### H. ABDOMINAL TRAUMA

CT of abdomen and pelvis to detect solid organ injury, vascular extravasation, free fluid, bowel wall thickening, and organ laceration.

### I. BILIARY ATRESIA

1. **In neonates with jaundice, US initially to distinguish biliary atresia from hepatitis. The gallbladder will be small or absent with biliary atresia.**
2. **Hepatobiliary scintigraphy with $^{99m}$Tc iminodiacetate (HIDA) reveals the absence of radionuclide in the GI tract with biliary atresia.**

### J. NASODUODENAL TUBE PLACEMENT

Visualize tube on a plain abdominal AP film passing through the stomach, crossing the midline and penetrating the duodenal bulb (where tip of tube will just begin to point inferiorly). If it remains unclear if tube is in duodenum or coiled in stomach, a lateral film is indicated.

## VIII. GENITOURINARY TRACT[2]

### A. URINARY TRACT INFECTION

1. **Initial febrile UTIs in children <5 years of age require imaging to look for congenital anomalies (e.g., posterior urethral valves, ureterocele), vesicoureteral reflux, baseline renal measurements, and damage to the cortex of the kidneys.**
2. **Workup first includes US to diagnose hydronephrosis, ureteropelvic junction obstruction, posterior urethral valves, multicystic dysplastic kidneys, chronic pyelonephritis, renal fusion (horseshoe kidney), and renal cysts.**
3. **Voiding cystourethrogram (VCUG) can then be done to diagnose vesicoureteral reflux; abnormalities of bladder or urethral function and anatomy, including ureterocele; and posterior urethral valves.**
4. **Occasionally, dimercaptosuccinic acid (DMSA) scan is useful in following renal cortical scarring and pyelonephritis.**

### B. UTERINE AND OVARIAN PATHOLOGY

Transvaginal or transabdominal US should be performed in women whose clinical picture is suspicious for ovarian torsion, tubo-ovarian abscess (TOA), or ectopic pregnancy.

## IX. EXTREMITIES[2]

### A. TRAUMA

Adequate evaluation requires AP and lateral radiograph. Restricting the film to include only area of interest improves the resolution (i.e., for a thumb injury, ask for an image of the thumb, not the hand). Comparison films of the uninvolved extremity not necessary, but may be helpful, such as in evaluation of joint effusions (particularly the hip), suspected osteomyelitis, or pyarthrosis and/or the evaluation of subtle fractures, especially in areas of multiple ossification centers such as the elbow. See Chapter 4 for the Salter-Harris classification of growth-plate injury. Avulsion injuries tend to occur at the knee and pelvis.

### B. STRESS FRACTURES

1. Occur most often at the tibia, fibula, metatarsals, and calcaneus.
2. Radiography will show a band of sclerosis and new bone formation.
3. Skeletal scintigraphy and CT can be used to make the diagnosis.



### C. OSTEOMYELITIS

1. Tends to occur at the metaphysis of long bones and within flat bones.
2. Radiography will show deep soft-tissue swelling and bony changes (may take 10 days to appear).
3. Skeletal scintigraphy and MRI will often be positive before radiographic changes are noticeable.



### D. HIP DISORDERS

Developmental dysplasia of the hip (congenital hip dislocation) is imaged initially with US. Once the femoral heads ossify, radiographs are more helpful. Legg-Calvé-Perthes disease (avascular necrosis of the femoral head) can be imaged with AP and frog-leg lateral hip films as well as MRI and bone scintigraphy. Slipped capital femoral epiphysis will show displacement of the femoral head on frog-leg lateral and AP radiographs.

### E. BONE AGE

Obtain a PA view of the left hand and wrist.

### F. SKELETAL SURVEY

1. In cases of suspected child abuse; should include lateral skull film with C-spine film, AP chest film (bone technique), oblique views of the ribs, AP view of the pelvis, abdominal film (bone technique) with the lateral thoracic and lumbar spine, and AP long-bone films.
2. Classic findings: Multiple metaphyseal injuries (especially corner and "bucket-handle" fractures) and other fractures of various ages. Suspicion should also be raised by fracture at unusual sites, such as posterior rib fractures or solitary spiral and transverse fractures of the long bones with an inconsistent history of trauma.

## X. RADIATION EXPOSURE

### A. CONSIDERATIONS UNIQUE TO THE PEDIATRIC POPULATION

Increased radiosensitivity of the thyroid, breast tissue, and gonads; lack of size-based radiation dosing; and a longer lifespan in which to manifest radiation-related cancer when compared with adults.

### B. CT EXAMINATIONS

Increasing in number, particularly in children. Compose largest amount of medical radiation exposure; CT scan of chest is approximately equivalent to 68 chest x-rays.[4]

### C. ALARA (*AS LOW AS REASONABLY ACHIEVABLE*)

To limit the side effects, the principle ALARA is used. To practice ALARA, first employ judicious use of CT; consider ultrasound or MRI if possible. Second, if CT is necessary, adjust technique to limit exposure: Set scanner specifically for each patient based on size and body area to be investigated, limit examination to relevant areas (e.g., do not include pelvis if only abdomen is needed), and avoid multiple scans (pre- and post-contrast images) as able.

## REFERENCES

1. Kirks DR et al: Practical Pediatric Imaging: Diagnostic Radiology of Infants and Children, 3rd ed. Philadelphia, Lippincott-Raven, 1998.
2. Kuhn JP et al: Caffey's Pediatric Diagnostic Imaging, 10th ed. St. Louis, Mosby, 2003.
3. Donnelly LF: Fundamentals of Pediatric Radiology. Philadelphia, WB Saunders, 2001.
4. Frush DP et al: Computed tomography and radiation risks: What pediatric health care providers should know. Pediatrics 2003;112:951–957.

# Rheumatology

*Keith A. Sikora, MD*

## I. LABORATORY STUDIES

Most laboratory studies used in diagnosis of rheumatic diseases are nonspecific for rheumatic diseases if considered alone; they must be put into the context of the full clinical picture. However, once a diagnosis is established, these can be used to follow the clinical course of rheumatic diseases, indicating flares or remission of disease state.

### A. ACUTE PHASE REACTANTS

26

General markers that can indicate presence of inflammation when elevated. Elevation is nonspecific; can result from trauma, infection, rheumatic diseases, and even some cancers.[1] Measures of acute phase reactants include erythrocyte sedimentation rate (ESR), C-reactive protein (CRP), platelet count, ferritin, haptoglobin, fibrinogen, serum amyloid A, and complement.[1,2]

1. **ESR: A measure of the rate of fall of red blood cells in anticoagulated blood within a vertical tube; reflects level of rouleaux formation caused by acute phase reactants.**[1]
   a. Can be falsely lowered in afibrinogenemia, anemia, and sickle cells; these states will interfere with rouleaux formation.[2]
   b. Levels can vary depending on age, ethnicity, gender, and freshness of blood sample.[1]
   c. Following levels over time can help in monitoring the state of rheumatic diseases such as systemic lupus erythematosus (SLE) and juvenile rheumatoid arthritis (JRA).
2. **CRP: An acute phase reactant synthesized by liver; assists in clearance of certain bacteria and damaged cells via activation of complement, mediates acute inflammation by alteration of cytokine release, and possibly prevents autoimmunity by binding to and masking autoantigens.**[3]
   a. Can increase and decrease rapidly because of its short half-life; about 18 hours.[1]
   b. More stable than ESR after being drawn from patient.
   c. Elevations are nonspecific, indicating only presence of inflammation.[1]
      (1) Most active phases of rheumatic diseases can result in an elevation to 1–10 mg/dL.
      (2) Levels of >10 mg/dL can be suspicious for a bacterial infection; can also occur in the presence of a systemic vasculitis.

### B. AUTOANTIBODIES (Table 26-1)

1. **Positive predictive value of any autoantibody depends on clinical context;** hence, antibody studies are useful for confirming a clinical suspicion, but are not useful as diagnostic tests in nonsuspicious clinical settings.

TABLE 26-1

**AUTOANTIBODIES AND THEIR ASSOCIATED DISEASE STATES**

| Autoantibody | Disease State(s) |
|---|---|
| ANCA-cytoplasmic/PR3* | Wegener's granulomatosis<br>Sometimes in microscopic polyangiitis and Churg-Strauss syndrome |
| ANCA-perinuclear/MPO* | Microscopic polyangiitis, pauci-immune rapidly progressive glomerulonephritis<br>Sometimes in inflammatory bowel disease, Churg-Strauss syndrome, Goodpasture's syndrome, a minority of Wegener's granulomatosis |
| Anti-Jo-1 | Dermatomyositis<br>Polymyositis |
| Anti-Ro | Neonatal lupus syndrome<br>Sjögren syndrome<br>Systemic lupus erythematosus |
| Anti-La | Neonatal lupus syndrome<br>Sjögren syndrome<br>Systemic lupus erythematosus |
| Anti-microsomal | Chronic active hepatitis<br>Systemic lupus erythematosus |
| Anti-centromere | CREST syndrome<br>Variant scleroderma |
| Anti-mitochondrial | Primary biliary cirrhosis<br>Systemic lupus erythematosus |
| Anti-phospholipids (anticardiolipin, lupus anticoagulant, anti-glycoprotein I) | Primary antiphospholipid syndrome<br>Systemic lupus erythematosus |
| Anti-RNP | Mixed connective tissue disease<br>Polymyositis<br>Scleroderma<br>Sjögren syndrome<br>Systemic lupus erythematosus |
| Anti–double-stranded DNA | Systemic lupus erythematosus |
| Anti-histone | Drug-induced systemic lupus erythematosus |
| Anti-Smith | Systemic lupus erythematosus |
| Anti-thyroid | Systemic lupus erythematosus<br>Thyroiditis |

*ANCA (antineutrophil cytoplasmic antibodies) are measured by indirect immunofluorescence (cytoplasmic-ANCA [c-ANCA] or perinuclear-ANCA [p-ANCA]) or ELISA methods (Proteinase 3 [PR3] or myeloperoxidase [MPO]).

Data from Behrman R, Kliegman R: Nelson Essentials of Pediatrics, 4th ed., Philadelphia, WB Saunders, 2002; Egner W: The use of laboratory tests in the diagnosis of SLE. J Clin Pathol 2000;53:424–432; Bosch X et al: Antineutrophil cytoplasmic antibodies. Lancet 2006;368:404–418; Harris E et al: Kelley's Textbook of Rheumatology, 7th ed. Philadelphia, WB Saunders, 2004; Gross W et al: Diagnosis and evaluation of vasculitis. Rheumatology 2000;39:245–252.

2. **A general autoantibody screen is useful in evaluation of a child with a possible rheumatologic disorder: Antinuclear antibody (ANA) screen. If positive, consider ordering individual autoantibodies: anti-dsDNA (double-stranded DNA), anti-Ro (Robert: SS-A), anti-La (Lane: SS-B), anti-RNP (ribonucleoprotein), and anti-Sm (Smith).**
3. **ANA screen is a nonspecific test for rheumatic disease.**[1,4] Anti-dsDNA and anti-Sm, for example, are highly specific for SLE.
   a. Usually performed semiquanitatively via indirect immunofluorescence (IIF) using patient's serum and a standardized human cell line. The pattern of IIF reported may suggest specific ANAs, but is not diagnostic.
   b. Approximately 60%–70% of children with an autoimmune disease have a positive ANA, but it can be seen in about 15%–35% of normal persons.
   c. Can also be positive in nonrheumatic diseases, such as neoplastic diseases, as well as transiently with infections, including mononucleosis, endocarditis, hepatitis, and malaria.
   d. Whether or not ANA is positive can be of great importance in pauciarticular JRA, where it connotes an increased risk of uveitis.
4. **Antineutrophil cytoplasmic antibodies (ANCA):**[5]
   a. Tests that suggest the presence of a vasculitis without immune complex deposition (pauci-immune vasculitis).
   b. Can be detected by two methods:
      (1) c-ANCA and p-ANCA; refer to groups of autoantibodies that produce a cytoplasmic or perinuclear pattern, respectively, on immunostaining neutrophils via IIF.
      (2) Most clinically relevant c-ANCA is anti-proteinase-3 (PR3); most clinically relevant p-ANCA is anti-myeloperoxidase (MPO). These autoantibodies can be quantitated via enzyme linked immunosorbent assay (ELISA). Clinical significance of other ANCA is unknown.
   c. c-ANCA IIF pattern: Mostly seen in Wegener's granulomatosis; also occasionally in microscopic polyangiitis (MPA) and Churg-Strauss syndrome.
   d. p-ANCA IIF pattern: Mostly seen in MPA and pauci-immune rapidly progressive glomerulonephritis, but may also be seen in Goodpasture's syndrome, Churg-Strauss syndrome, inflammatory bowel disease, and in a minority of Wegener's granulomatosis cases.

## C. RHEUMATOID FACTOR (RF)[1,6]

Immunoglobulin M antibodies to the Fc portion of immunoglobulin G:

1. **Positive RF, like ANA, is not specific for a rheumatic disease, nor does a negative test rule out a rheumatic disease.**
2. **Only about 5% of patients with JRA will be RF positive:** Those who are positive are almost always female with late-onset disease and have multiple joints involved (polyarthritis); denotes a more progressive disease if not treated aggressively.

3. **RF test should not be ordered to confirm a diagnosis of JRA:** Has almost no diagnostic utility in JRA, but has prognostic importance in a subset of previously diagnosed polyarticular JRA patients.
4. **Positive RF can occur in multiple states:**
   a. Rheumatic diseases such as SLE, mixed cryoglobulinemia, JRA, mixed connective tissue disease, and Henoch-Schönlein purpura.
   b. Numerous infections, such as hepatitis B, bacterial endocarditis, tuberculosis, and congenital TORCH infections.
5. **Anti-cyclic citrullinated peptide (anti-CCP) antibodies:** Currently being explored as an RF adjunct.[7–9]
   a. Although pediatric studies are few, anti-CCP has been shown to have a high sensitivity and specificity for adult rheumatoid arthritis (RA).
   b. May predict future development of RA in RF-negative patients who have undifferentiated arthritis, and a more progressive disease in established RA patients, thus allowing for earlier and/or aggressive treatment.
   c. Anti-CCP positive JRA patients are usually also RF positive; thus are females with late-onset polyarthritis.[9]
   d. Should not be routinely ordered in a general pediatric setting until its clinical significance becomes established.

## D. COMPLEMENT

Complement system is composed of multiple proteins important in the inflammatory processes involved in fighting infections. Any process that causes inflammatory response can affect complement proteins by increasing their synthesis or increasing their consumption.

1. **Total hemolytic complement level ($CH_{50}$): General measure of complement; also an acute phase reactant.**
   a. Increased in the acute phase response of numerous states that cause inflammation.
   b. Useful screening test for homozygous complement deficiency states.[10]
   c. Typically decreased in SLE.
2. **The two complement proteins primarily followed in rheumatic diseases are C3 and C4 because the immunoassays that measure them are the ones that are most widely available.[10] Because levels can be increased or decreased in rheumatic diseases, depending on where one is in the active phase of the disease as well as disease severity, it is more important to follow the complement trend over time rather than an isolated result.**
3. **Decreased levels of complement proteins:**[1,10]
   a. Indicator of immune complex formation, which can occur in the presence of active SLE as well as some vasculitides, and in multiple infections, including gram-negative sepsis, hepatitis, and pneumococcal infections. Decreased levels typically signify more severe SLE, particularly in regard to renal disease.
   b. Severe hepatic failure: Synthesis of complement proteins occurs primarily in the liver.

c. Congenital complement deficiency, which can predispose to the development of an autoimmune disease.

4. **Increased levels of complement proteins:**[10]

a. During the active phase of most rheumatic diseases, including SLE, JRA, and dermatomyositis.

b. Can be seen in multiple infections as part of the acute phase response, including hepatitis and pneumococcal pneumonia.

## E. URINALYSIS

In many rheumatic diseases, it is important to obtain a complete urinalysis to look for evidence of renal involvement: proteinuria, hematuria, and casts. See Chapter 19 for further details regarding urinalysis.



## F. SERUM MUSCLE ENZYMES[2]

Can be elevated in certain rheumatic diseases that cause muscle inflammation or destruction, such as dermatomyositis. Include aspartate transaminase (AST), lactate dehydrogenase (LDH), aldolase, and creatine kinase (CK).



**Note** *Patients with chronic, ongoing myositis may have an elevated CK-MB fraction (that is noncardiac in origin) when measuring serum CK levels.*

## G. JOINT FLUID ANALYSIS (Table 26-2)[11]

Evaluation of joint fluid in the presence of an effusion, especially in monoarticular disease, is important. Although an effusion can be seen in rheumatic diseases, it can also be present in other disease processes such as septic arthritis.

TABLE 26-2

JOINT FLUID ANALYSIS

| Disorder | Cells/μL | Glucose* |
|---|---|---|
| Trauma | RBCs > > WBCs; usually <2000 WBCs | Normal |
| Reactive arthritis | 3000–10,000 WBCs; mostly mononuclear | Normal |
| Juvenile rheumatoid arthritis and other inflammatory arthritides | 5000–80,000 WBCs, occasionally > 80,000 WBCs; mostly neutrophils | Usually normal or slightly low |
| Septic arthritis | >60,000 WBCs; >90% neutrophils | Low to normal |
| Lyme arthritis | 15,000–100,000 WBCs; variable cell types | Low to normal |

*Normal value is 75% or more of serum glucose value.

RBCs, red blood cells; WBCs, white blood cells.

Data from Hay W et al: Current Pediatric Diagnosis and Treatment, 17th ed. New York, Lange Medical/McGraw-Hill, 2005.

## II. JUVENILE RHEUMATOID ARTHRITIS (JRA)[1,2,10] OR JUVENILE IDIOPATHIC ARTHRITIS (JIA)[12]

Diagnosing a child with arthritis (defined as joint swelling or limitation/tenderness upon range of motion)[12] can be challenging; child may not present with joint pain or swelling, but with a variety of other symptoms, such as morning stiffness, walking with a limp, refusal to walk, irritability, poor growth, or limb discrepancy.

**Note** *When evaluating a child with a history of constant extremity pain (including nighttime awakenings due to pain), low white blood cell count, and low-normal platelets, consider malignancy such as acute lymphocytic leukemia, even without blasts seen on peripheral smear, as part of the differential diagnosis.*[13]

### A. CLASSICAL DIVISIONS

Based on clinical course over the first 6 months of illness in children <16 years of age with arthritis present for at least 6 weeks.[1,2] Multiple classification systems: American College of Rheumatology (ACR) and International League of Associations for Rheumatology (ILAR) are most widely used.[12] The divisions used here are based on the ACR.

1. **Pauciarticular JRA.**
2. **Polyarticular JRA.**
3. **Systemic-onset JRA.**

### B. PAUCIARTICULAR JRA (OLIGOARTHRITIS)

Most common type of JRA, accounting for approximately 60% of cases.[2,10] Characterized by involvement of ≤4 joints during the first 6 months of illness. On initial presentation, all pauciarticular cases should be evaluated for Lyme disease, especially if knee or other large joint is involved. Two major subtypes of pauciarticular JRA:

1. **Type I: Female-predominant subtype, with a >4 : 1 female-to-male ratio:**
   a. Age of onset: Peaks around preschool age.
   b. Presentation: Insidious onset, worse in morning, swollen > > tender joint(s) (knees, wrists, ankles, and elbows).
   c. Laboratory studies: Positive ANA in >50% of patients, with RF, anti-Sm, anti-Ro/La, anti-dsDNA being negative.
   d. Prognosis: Very good if treated appropriately. May affect >4 joints after the initial 6-month period in some individuals.[14]
   e. Major morbidities: Uveitis (~20% of patients) and leg-length discrepancy. There should be no other systemic involvement.
2. **Type II: Male-predominant subtype, with a >20 : 1 male-to-female ratio:**
   a. Traditionally referred to as a seronegative spondyloarthropathy, but referred to as *enthesitis-related arthritis* in the ILAR classification.[12]
   b. Age of onset: After age 6 years.

c. Presentation: Joint involvement starting commonly in lower extremities in an asymmetrical fashion. Hips also commonly involved; this is rare in the female-predominant subtype. Sacroiliac and intervertebral joints can become involved in adolescence.
d. Family history: Patient may have a first-degree relative with history of ankylosing spondylitis, enthesitis-related arthritis, sacroiliitis with inflammatory bowel disease, Reiter syndrome, or acute anterior uveitis.[12]
e. Laboratory studies: Usually include a negative ANA and RF. HLA-B27 is usually positive, but not always.
f. Major morbidities: Unlike the female-predominant subtype, associated uveitis is usually acute (symptomatic) rather than chronic in nature.



## C. POLYARTICULAR JRA

Accounts for approximately 30% of cases of JRA.[2,10] Characterized by involvement of ≥5 joints during the first 6 months of the illness. Like pauciarticular JRA, can be divided into two subtypes. There is an approximately 5:1 female-to-male ratio. Articular involvement may be unremitting, requiring rehabilitation or orthopedic surgery. Associated with mild systemic manifestations, such as fever and malaise.

1. **Seronegative for RF: most common subtype:**
a. Age of onset: Usually <10 years, with a peak onset of 1–3 years of age.
b. Laboratory studies: Approximately 25% are ANA positive.
c. Prognosis: Usually more favorable disease course than RF seropositive subtype; also responds better to nonsteroidal anti-inflammatory drug (NSAID) therapy

2. **Seropositive for RF:**
a. Age of onset: Usually older than 10 years.
b. Laboratory studies: Approximately 50% of patients are ANA positive.
c. Prognosis: Less favorable disease course than the RF-seronegative subtype, requiring more advanced therapies, such as methotrexate, glucocorticoids, etanercept, infliximab, and adalimumab. Usually by end of first year of illness, if left under-treated, joint destruction will be evident on radiographic films.

## D. SYSTEMIC-ONSET JRA

Accounts for approximately 10% of cases of JRA.[2,10] No gender predominance or peak age of onset.

1. **Presentation:** **Differentiated from other types of JRA due to predominance of extra-articular manifestations, such as fever, serositis, and evanescent rash, which can precede onset of articular symptoms and signs by months or longer.**
2. **Fever:** **Usually "quotidian" (spikes once daily, followed by a short period of relative hypothermia); must be present for at least 3 days.[12]**

3. **Laboratory studies:** Usually include a negative ANA, negative RF, leukocytosis, thrombocytosis, and elevated ESR and/or CRP demonstrating the systemic inflammation. (See section II.D.4 for labs that pertain to macrophage activation syndrome.)
4. **Prognosis:** Variable. Pericarditis, pleuropericarditis, macrophage activation syndrome (uncontrolled activation of T cells and macrophages with cytokine overproduction leading to unremitting fever, lymphadenopathy, hepatosplenomegaly, pancytopenia, increased liver function tests, hypertriglyceridemia, hyperferritinemia, disseminated intravascular coagulation, and neurologic symptoms[15]), and secondary amyloidosis are potentially serious manifestations of systemic-onset JRA.[16]

## E. PSORIATIC ARTHRITIS (PsA)[17–19]

Traditionally referred to as a seronegative spondyloarthropathy; ILAR classification considers PsA to be a subtype of JIA.[12]

1. **History of psoriasis not required for diagnosis, but patients will usually have a first-degree relative with psoriasis, or may develop skin findings months or years after onset of arthritis.**
2. **Presentation:** Mostly an oligoarthritis, but may be a polyarthritis or an axial arthritis. Patient may also have sacroiliitis, inflammatory spinal pain/stiffness, synovitis, enthesitis, or dactylitis (swelling beyond joint margins, producing a "sausage digit") of toes or fingers. Fingernails may show onycholysis or pitting.
3. **Laboratory studies:** RF is usually negative.
4. **Prognosis:** If left untreated, will result in a deforming combination of erosions and ankylosis within joints of digits.
5. **Major morbidities:** Patients may also develop chronic uveitis and should be screened by an ophthalmologist regularly.

## F. TREATMENT OF ARTHRITIS

1. **Pharmacologic agents:**[1,2,10,20]

a. NSAIDs: Usual initial treatment; examples include valdecoxib and naproxen.
b. Corticosteroids: Can be systemic or intra-articular.
c. Disease-modifying and cytotoxic drugs: Cyclosporine, hydroxychloroquine, sulfasalazine, and methotrexate.
d. Biologic immunomodulators: Tumor necrosis factor (TNF) inhibitors (etanercept, infliximab, and adalimumab), rituximab (anti-CD20), and anakinra (IL-1 receptor antagonist).

2. **Vaccines: Children with a rheumatologic disease should follow regular immunization schedule with a few noted exceptions.**

a. Live-virus vaccines contraindicated in children receiving immunosuppressive therapy; typically, vaccinations with live-virus vaccines should be postponed until at least 3 months after discontinuation of the immunosuppressive agent.[20]

b. Varicella vaccine: Give before starting immunosuppressive therapies if patient not previously vaccinated or has not previously had a documented case of varicella.
c. Influenza vaccine: Given to any patient receiving immunosuppressive therapies[1,20]; if <8 years of age when receiving first influenza vaccine, patient requires two injections 1 month apart to help ensure appropriate coverage.
d. Children with hypocomplementemia as part of their rheumatologic condition are at risk for infections with encapsulated bacteria; might benefit from vaccination with pneumococcal and meningococcal vaccines.[20]

3. **Prevention or minimization of osteopenia: Adequate calcium and vitamin D intake and weight-bearing activities.[1,10,21]**
4. **Physical and occupational therapy: Important in maintaining range of motion of a joint and strength of associated muscle groups as well as in decreasing pain and preventing joint deformity and contractures.[1,10]**
5. **Orthopedic surgery: Necessary in some cases for pain control, improvement in function, or contractures.[1,10]**



## G. UVEITIS

Due to insidious and asymptomatic development of uveitis, routine pediatric ophthalmology screening is required for children with JRA. First ophthalmologic examination should be within 1 month after initial diagnosis and then as detailed in Table 26-3, which assumes an inactive disease state.[22] If arthritis is active, patient should receive ophthalmologic examination every 3 months, regardless of ANA status.

TABLE 26-3

FREQUENCY OF OPHTHALMOLOGIC EXAMINATION IN PATIENTS WITH JRA*

| Type | ANA Status | Age of Onset (years) | Duration of Disease (years) | Eye Exam Frequency (months) |
|---|---|---|---|---|
| Oligoarthritis or | + | <6 | <4 | 3 |
| polyarthritis | + | <6 | >4 | 6 |
| | + | <6 | >7 | 12 |
| | + | >6 | <4 | 6 |
| | + | >6 | >4 | 12 |
| | – | <6 | <4 | 3 |
| | – | <6 | >4 | 6 |
| | – | >6 | N/A | 12 |
| Systemic disease | N/A | N/A | N/A | 12 |

*For JRA patients without known eye disease. If eye disease is known, allow ophthalmologist to determine frequency of visits.

Adapted from Cassidy J et al: Ophthalmologic examinations in children with juvenile rheumatoid arthritis. Pediatrics 2006;117:1843–1845.

### H. "GROWING PAINS"

1. **A diagnosis of exclusion:** Not JRA or any other rheumatologic disease, but a benign process. No evidence it is even caused by growth.
2. **Presentation:** Patient will awaken at night intermittently (not a nightly occurrence) and will complain of throbbing extremity pain. Usually after a day full of exercise or activity. Patient will not have a fever, and joint or extremity will display no swelling, erythema, or warmth on examination.
3. **Treatment:** Unlike other types of musculoskeletal pain, patient will welcome touching and massaging of painful extremity. Pain will usually resolve on holding, rocking, or massaging child. Also give patient and parental reassurance.

## III. REACTIVE ARTHRITIS[2]

### A. DEFINITION

A diverse group of inflammatory arthritides, which follow a bacterial or viral infection particularly involving the respiratory, gastrointestinal (GI), and genitourinary tracts.

1. **Onset:** Infection typically precedes development of arthritis by 1–4 weeks, with approximately 80% of cases being preceded by gastroenteritis.
2. **Some precipitating organisms:** *Mycoplasma, Chlamydia, Yersinia, Salmonella, Shigella, Campylobacter*, Epstein-Barr virus (EBV), parvovirus B19, and enteroviruses.
3. **Presentation:** Sometimes accompanied by constitutional signs and symptoms, including fever, weight loss, and fatigue, as well as dermatologic and ophthalmologic findings. For example, Reiter syndrome is reactive arthritis in the presence of conjunctivitis and urethritis.
4. **Strong association between HLA-B27 and susceptibility to developing reactive arthritis following an infection with a bacterial arthritogenic organism.** Approximately 50%–65% frequency of HLA-B27 seen in reactive arthritis.
5. **Laboratory studies:** May demonstrate evidence of systemic inflammation, including leukocytosis, thrombocytosis, and elevated ESR and CRP. Autoantibodies typically absent. Stool cultures, serum *Chlamydia pneumoniae* and *Mycoplasma* titres, and urinary *Chlamydia* DNA probe can be helpful in determining the organism involved. Negative stool culture does not exclude diagnosis of a reactive arthritis secondary to an enteric organism. Enterovirus, EBV, and parvovirus B19 antibody titers may be drawn looking for a viral cause. Joint fluid analysis may be helpful to distinguish a septic arthritis from a reactive arthritis, especially because, in the case of *Salmonella*, either a septic or reactive arthritis can develop.

6. **Prognosis:** Arthritis can last weeks to months, with eventual remission versus development of recurrent episodes.

## B. PHARMACOLOGY

See section II.F for treatment options.

# IV. SYSTEMIC LUPUS ERYTHEMATOSUS (SLE)

A multisystem inflammatory disease related to deposition of immune complexes in tissues.

## A. AMERICAN COLLEGE OF RHEUMATOLOGY CLASSIFICATION CRITERIA

Meet 4 or more of the 11 criteria (Table 26-4). These criteria are not strict *diagnostic* criteria, but *classification* criteria for research purposes. Do not exclude the possibility of an SLE diagnosis for a pediatric patient who does not fully meet these criteria. The majority of pediatric patients with "incomplete" SLE (<4 criteria) will likely completely fulfill these criteria in subsequent years. Furthermore, use caution when applying them to pediatric and international/multiethnic patients; there are few studies that validate the ACR criteria for these populations.[24,25]

## B. EPIDEMIOLOGY

1. **Females most commonly affected; onset usually at age 9–15 years (median age, 12 years).**[24]
2. **African Americans more commonly affected than whites.**[1]

## C. CLINICAL FEATURES

1. **Most common signs and symptoms for initial presentation: Hematologic** (positive direct Coombs, hemolytic anemia, leukopenia, thrombocytopenia), **cutaneous** (malar rash, discoid lesions, vasculitis, urticaria), **and musculoskeletal** (arthralgia and nonerosive arthritis mostly affecting knees, fingers, and wrists/ankles).[24]
2. **Renal involvement:** Leading cause of death; more common in childhood-onset than adult-onset SLE.[11] Monitor complete urinalysis, anti-dsDNA, C3 and C4, serum creatinine, and blood pressure on a routine basis.
3. **Atypical presentation is more common in childhood-onset SLE than in adult-onset SLE.**[24]

## D. LABORATORY STUDIES[1,11,24]

1. **Complete blood count (CBC) with differential and direct Coombs:** Look for hematologic abnormalities (cytopenias).
2. **ESR or CRP:** May be increased with active disease; CRP levels do not likely correlate with disease activity.[26]
3. **Urinalysis and serum creatinine:** To evaluate for renal involvement.

TABLE 26-4

**THE 1982 REVISED CRITERIA FOR CLASSIFICATION OF SYSTEMIC LUPUS ERYTHEMATOSUS**

| Criterion* | Definition |
|---|---|
| 1. Malar rash | Fixed erythema, flat or raised, over the malar eminences, tending to spare the nasolabial folds. |
| 2. Discoid rash | Erythematous, raised patches with adherent keratotic scaling and follicular plugging; atrophic scarring may occur in older lesions. |
| 3. Photosensitivity | Skin rash as a result of unusual reaction to sunlight, by patient history or physician observation. |
| 4. Oral ulcers | Oral or nasopharyngeal ulceration, usually painless, observed by physician. |
| 5. Arthritis | Nonerosive arthritis involving 2 or more peripheral joints, characterized by tenderness, swelling, or effusion. |
| 6. Serositis | (a) Pleuritis: Convincing history of pleuritic pain or rubbing heard by a physician or evidence of pleural effusion<br>*or*<br>(b) Pericarditis: Documented by ECG or rub or evidence of pericardial effusion. |
| 7. Renal disorder | (a) Persistent proteinuria >0.5 g/day or >3+ if quantitation not performed<br>*or*<br>(b) Cellular casts: May be red cell, hemoglobin, granular, tubular, or mixed. |
| 8. Neurologic disorder | (a) Seizures: In the absence of offending drugs or known metabolic derangements (e.g., uremia, ketoacidosis, or electrolyte imbalance)<br>*or*<br>(b) Psychosis: In the absence of offending drugs or known metabolic derangements (e.g., uremia, ketoacidosis, or electrolyte imbalance). |
| 9. Hematologic disorder | (a) Hemolytic anemia: With reticulocytosis<br>*or*<br>(b) Leukopenia: <4000/μL total on 2 or more occasions<br>*or*<br>(c) Lymphopenia: <1500/μL on 2 or more occasions<br>*or*<br>(d) Thrombocytopenia: <100,000/μL in the absence of offending drugs. |

*The proposed classification is based on 11 criteria. For the purpose of identifying patients in clinical studies, a person shall be said to have systemic lupus erythematosus if 4 or more of the 11 criteria are present, serially or simultaneously, during any interval of observation.

Data from American College of Rheumatology website, which was adapted from Tan E et al: The 1982 revised criteria for the classification of systemic lupus erythematosus. Arthritis Rheum 1982;25:1271–1277.

*Continued*

TABLE 26-4

THE 1982 REVISED CRITERIA FOR CLASSIFICATION OF SYSTEMIC LUPUS ERYTHEMATOSUS—cont'd

| Criterion | Definition |
|---|---|
| 10. Immunologic disorder | (a) Positive LE cell preparation *or* (b) Anti-DNA: Antibody to native DNA in abnormal titer *or* (c) Anti-Sm: Presence of antibody to Sm nuclear antigen *or* (d) False-positive serologic test for syphilis known to be positive for at least 6 months and confirmed by *Treponema pallidum* immobilization or fluorescent treponemal antibody absorption test. |
| 11. Antinuclear antibody | An abnormal titer of antinuclear antibody by immunofluorescence or an equivalent assay at any point in time and in the absence of drugs known to be associated with "drug-induced lupus" syndrome. |



4. **Low complement levels (C3 and C4): Serial levels most useful; congenital complement deficiencies may also be seen in SLE, especially in males with SLE. Decreasing complement levels may indicate renal disease.**
5. **Autoantibodies (see Table 26-1):**[1]

a. Most people with positive ANAs do not have SLE, but almost all people with SLE have positive ANAs.[1]
b. Anti-dsDNA can be seen in about 60% of patients with SLE and is highly specific for SLE; titers rise/fall depending on disease activity and usually increase during development of lupus nephritis. Not associated with discoid or subacute cutaneous lupus.[4]
c. Anti-Sm is highly specific for SLE; seen in about 10%–30% of patients with SLE.

## E. DRUG-INDUCED SLE[1]

Can be caused by multiple inciting drugs, including (but not limited to) hydralazine, minocycline, doxycycline, procainamide, isoniazid, chlorpromazine, phenytoin, and carbamazepine; usually resolves with discontinuation of drug. Of note, it is often associated with anti-histone antibodies.

## F. NEONATAL SLE[1]

Maternal autoantibodies, including anti-Ro (anti-SS-A) and anti-La (anti-SS-B) (also seen in Sjögren syndrome), cross the placenta, manifesting as discoid lesions with exposure to ultraviolet lights; may also present as thrombocytopenia, hemolytic anemia, or congenital heart block (associated with anti-Ro). Inflammatory features of neonatal lupus will resolve within 6 months as maternal autoantibodies are cleared, but congenital heart block is permanent and usually requires placement of a pacemaker.

## V. VASCULITIS

### A. DEFINITION

Inflammation of a blood vessel wall. Systemic vasculitis syndromes, although rare, are a concern in childhood. Clinical presentation of a vasculitic condition can be quite variable, from a fever of unknown origin to a rash to multisystem failure. There are no definitive laboratory tests to diagnose a vasculitis, with the exception of biopsy, which is not always possible. After complete history and physical examination, initial laboratory tests should include CBC, basic metabolic panel, liver function tests, acute phase reactants, stool guiac, and complete urinalysis. Magnetic resonance angiography may also be helpful, but a negative test does not rule out disease. Standard for diagnosing small-vessel vasculitis is biopsy; angiography required for definitive diagnosis of medium-to-large vessel vasculitis.

### B. HENOCH-SCHÖNLEIN PURPURA (HSP)

1. **Pathophysiology: Most common small-vessel vasculitis in children; characterized by nonthrombocytopenic palpable purpura, migratory polyarthritis and polyarthralgia, abdominal pain, and glomerulonephritis with immunoglobulin A (IgA) deposition.**[1,2,27]
2. **Epidemiology: Occurs more frequently in males than females; typical age of onset 2–7 years. History of an upper respiratory infection a few weeks preceding onset in one half to two thirds of cases.**
3. **Presentation:**[2,27,28]

a. Palpable purpura:
   (1) Most common and frequently presenting feature.
   (2) Evolution of rash starts with urticarial lesions with progression to a maculopapular rash followed by purpuric lesions.
   (3) Distribution typically involves ankles, buttocks, and elbows, beginning on lower extremities but can involve the entire body.
   (4) New lesions can appear for 2–4 weeks.

b. Migratory polyarthritis and/or polyarthralgias:
   (1) Presenting feature in one fourth of cases: Very tender and painful periarticular joint swelling.
   (2) No joint effusion present.
   (3) Ankles and knees most commonly affected.
   (4) Usually transient with no permanent deformities.

c. Abdominal pain:
   (1) Colicky in nature.
   (2) Secondary to hemorrhage and edema of the small intestine, which can result in intussusception in about 2% of cases (usually ileoileal).

(3) Stool can be guiac positive without obvious signs of intestinal bleeding.

d. Glomerulonephritis:

(1) Renal involvement can occur in one fourth to one half of cases, but may develop months after onset of rash or even prior to development of rash.

(2) Biopsy: Typically consistent with IgA nephropathy, but crescentic glomerulonephritis may also be seen.

(3) More common in male patients, those with GI bleeding, factor VIII activity <80%, and in patients >4 years of age.[29]

e. Other features: Dorsal edema of the feet.

4. **Laboratory studies:**[2,27]

a. Normal to elevated platelet count.

b. Normal platelet function tests and bleeding time.

c. Normal coagulation studies.

d. Urinalysis: May demonstrate proteinuria and hematuria, but casts are uncommon.

e. IgA levels: May be elevated, especially in the acute phase of the disease.

f. Stool guiac: May be positive.

g. ASO titer: may be elevated.

h. Throat culture: May be positive for group A β-hemolytic streptococcus, which requires treatment with antibiotics.

5. **Treatment:**[27]

a. Maintain adequate hydration.

b. Monitoring vital signs due to GI bleeding and renal involvement.

c. Analgesia for joint pain.

d. Possibly steroids, especially if GI and renal systems involved.

e. Prolonged immunosuppression may be needed for renal disease.

6. **Prognosis:** Typically self-limited course, but may reoccur in a minority (10%–20%) of cases.

## C. TAKAYASU ARTERITIS[30,31]

1. **Pathophysiology:** Vasculitis of aorta and its major branches, leading to aneurysms, thrombosis, and stenosis.
2. **Epidemiology:** Third most common vasculitis in children; seen mostly in females of childbearing age, with about 15% being <16 years of age.
3. **Presentation:** Most common findings include hypertension (88%), cardiomegaly (74%), high ESR (61%), and fever (40%). Asymmetrical blood pressures or absent pulses may also be seen.
4. **Diagnosis:** Angiographic findings include stenosis (mainly of abdominal aorta) and aneurysms.

## D. CHILDHOOD POLYARTERITIS NODOSA[32–34]

1. **Pathophysiology:** Vasculitis characterized by transmural necrosis of mostly medium-sized vessels. Likely due to immune-complex deposition.

2. **Epidemiology:** Very rare in childhood; mean age at diagnosis is 9 years.
3. **Presentation/diagnosis:** Must have biopsy showing necrotizing arteritis of small or mid-sized artery or angiographic abnormalities (if magnetic resonance angiogram is negative) and two of seven criteria
   a. Cutaneous findings (livedo reticularis, tender subcutaneous nodules, purpura).
   b. Arthralgias or myalgias.
   c. Systemic hypertension.
   d. Mononeuropathy multiplex (e.g., foot drop) or polyneuropathy.
   e. Abnormal urinalysis or renal dysfunction.
   f. Testicular pain/tenderness.
   g. Any other symptom suggestive of a vasculitis (abdominal pain, dyspnea, hemoptysis, seizure, symptoms of stroke, headache, angina).
4. **May have constitutional signs or symptoms:** Fatigue, weight loss, and/or fever.
5. **Laboratory studies:** Increased ESR and/or CRP. ANCA almost always negative. May be associated with hepatitis B antigenemia.

## E. CUTANEOUS POLYARTERITIS NODOSA [32–34]

1. **Presentation:** Skin lesions include maculopapular rash, subcutaneous nodules, livedo reticularis, panniculitis, or ischemic finger/toe lesions with arthralgias or myalgias. No organ involvement, but may have constitutional signs or symptoms.
2. **Laboratory studies:** Increased ESR and/or CRP. ANCA almost always negative.
3. **Often associated with streptococcal or other upper respiratory infection.**

## F. MICROSCOPIC POLYANGIITIS[32–34]

1. **Pathophysiology:** Necrotizing pauci-immune vasculitis affecting mostly small vessels, with glomerulonephritis as a major component.
2. **Presentation:** Constitutional symptoms, skin lesions, and pulmonary capillaritis sometimes seen.
3. **Laboratory studies:** Patients almost always p-ANCA positive.
4. **Often associated with streptococcal or other upper respiratory infection.**

## G. WEGENER'S GRANULOMATOSIS[35–37]

1. **Pathophysiology:** Necrotizing granulomatous vasculitis of small and medium-sized vessels that primarily affects upper and lower respiratory tracts as well as the kidneys, but may affect any organ system.[35]
2. **Epidemiology:** Most common granulomatous vasculitis of childhood. About 15% of all cases diagnosed before age 19 years.[31]

3. **Presentation:**
a. Upper airway disease: 60%–90% of patients. Symptoms: Rhinitis, sinusitis, hoarseness, epistaxis, nasal perforation, saddle-nose deformity, otitis, hearing loss, any other form of nasopharyngeal ulceration.
b. Pulmonary disease: 70%–90% of patients. Symptoms: Cough, dyspnea, wheezing/stridor, and hemoptysis. Subglottic stenosis may be seen. Chest CT will most commonly show nodules, ground-glass opacification, and air-space opacification.[36]
c. Glomerulonephritis: 50%–100% of patients. Usually asymptomatic. The airway disease usually drives patients to seek medical attention.
d. Other systems: Ocular involvement (scleritis, uveitis, optic neuritis, retro-orbital pseudotumor, peri-orbital mass with proptosis) in 10%–50% of patients. CNS involvement: cranial nerve (CN) palsies and meningitis. Arthritis/arthralgias; vasculitic rashes.

4. **Laboratory studies: Acute phase reactants usually increased. c-ANCA usually positive.**
5. **Diagnosis: EULAR/PReS (European) criteria require three out of the following six criteria:[37]**
a. Abnormal urinalysis: Hematuria or proteinuria.
b. Granulomatous inflammation on biopsy.
c. Nasal sinus inflammation.
d. Subglottic, tracheal, or endobronchial stenosis.
e. Abnormal chest x-ray or CT.
f. Positive PR3-ANCA or c-ANCA staining.

### H. BEHÇET'S DISEASE[2,38,39]

1. **Epidemiology: Mean age of onset is 30 years, with 10% of cases beginning in childhood. In one study, mean age of childhood-onset disease was 8.4 years, with mean age of diagnosis 13 years.[39] Seen mostly in patients of Middle Eastern, Japanese, or Turkish heritage.**
2. **Presentation:**
a. Oral and genital painful aphthous ulcers: Oral ulcers almost always present; genital ulcers present in about 85% of cases.
b. Ophthalmologic: Uveitis, conjunctivitis, retinal vasculitis, other eye disturbances.
c. Dermatologic: Erythema nodosum, papulopustules, other types of rashes.
d. Neurologic: Encephalitis, aseptic meningitis, peripheral nerve disturbances, increased intracranial pressure, psychiatric disturbances.
e. Arthralgias, positive pathergy reaction: Papular/pustular formation within 48 hours after large-bore needle injury to skin.

## VI. GRANULOMATOUS DISEASE

### A. DIFFERENTIAL DIAGNOSIS[40]

Includes, but is not limited to, infectious causes (tuberculosis, atypical mycobacterium including leprosy, histoplasmosis, coccidioidomycosis, brucellosis, chlamydia, tularemia, treponemal organisms, leishmaniasis, and toxoplasmosis), environmental exposures (hypersensitivity pneumonitis, berylliosis, silicosis, other metals [aluminum and titanium], and talc), malignancy, foreign bodies, medications, and immune dysregulation (Wegener's granulomatosis, primary biliary cirrhosis, Churg-Strauss syndrome, sarcoidosis, Takayasu arteritis, Crohn disease, and chronic granulomatous disease).

## B. SARCOIDOSIS[40-44]

1. **Pathophysiology: Multisystem infiltrative noncaseating granulomatous disease of unknown etiology.**
2. **Epidemiology: Very rare before puberty; primarily affects whites. After and during puberty, African Americans predominate. Incidence increases with age, peaking between ages 20 and 40 years. Males and females affected equally.**
3. **Two forms of pediatric sarcoidosis:**

a. Before puberty (usually <4 years of age): May be familial. Dominated by skin, musculoskeletal, and eye involvement.
b. During or after puberty: Very similar to adult disease. Dominated by lung, lymphatic, eye, and systemic involvement.

4. **Presentation: Mostly dictated by location of granulomas.**

a. General: Weight loss, fever, anorexia, and fatigue.
b. Musculoskeletal: Usually only seen in young children. Tenosynovitis and polyarthritis, mostly of wrists, knees, and ankles.[41]
c. Pulmonary: Dyspnea on exertion, chest pain, chronic dry cough, wheezing or stridor, bilateral hilar lymphadenopathy with or without parenchymal disease on chest x-ray or CT, and restrictive lung pattern and impaired gas exchange on pulmonary function tests.
d. Ophthalmologic: Bilateral uveitis (anterior, posterior, or pan-uveitis), band keratopathy, synechiae, iris nodules, cataracts, glaucoma, chorioretinitis, conjunctivitis, and papilledema.
e. Dermatologic: Erythema nodosum, plaques, maculopapules, and subcutaneous nodules.
f. Lymphatic: Hilar, mediastinal, and mobile, nontender peripheral lymphadenopathy.
g. Neurologic: Headache, seizures, CN (VI, VII, VIII) palsies (independent of increased intracranial pressure), pseudotumor cerebri, hypothalamic dysfunction (short stature, diabetes insipidus), obstructive hydrocephalus, and hemiparesis. CN VII palsy is the most common neurologic manifestation in adolescent and adult form.[42] MRI may show mass lesion(s), periventricular white matter lesions, and nodular or diffuse leptomeningeal enhancement.[43]
h. Cardiovascular: Arrhythmia, valvular disease, vasculitis of any size vessel.
i. Renal: Renal failure (due to hypercalcemia or parenchymal infiltration) and nephrolithiasis.

j. GI: Hepatosplenomegaly, elevated transaminases, and hyperbilirubinemia due to parenchymal and biliary tree infiltration, and parotitis.

5. **Laboratory studies:** Usually nonspecific. Hypercalcemia (from granuloma-produced vitamin D) in about 30% of patients; elevated serum angiotensin-converting enzyme in 60%–80% of patients.
6. **Basic evaluation:** Thorough history and physical examination, chest x-ray (chest CT may be more sensitive), complete metabolic panel, pulmonary function testing, electrocardiogram, and ophthalmologic (slit-lamp) examination.
7. **Diagnosis:** Biopsy demonstrating noncaseating granulomas in absence of other known cause.



## VII. JUVENILE DERMATOMYOSITIS[1,2,11,45–47]

### A. EPIDEMIOLOGY

A rare disease involving small-vessel vasculitis of the skin and muscles. One study found the incidence to be 3.2 cases per million children per year, with a female-to-male ratio of 2.3 : 1.[45] Peak age of onset for juvenile form is 5–14 years. In one British study, mean age at diagnosis was 7.7 years.[46]

### B. PRESENTATION

1. Constitutional: Fever, fatigue, and weight loss.
2. Musculoskeletal: Symmetrical proximal muscle pain or weakness involving shoulder and pelvic girdles.
3. Dermatologic: Heliotropic rash involving upper eyelids (or malar rash), a thickened, erythematous, and scaly rash on the extensor surfaces of elbows, knees, metacarpophalangeal and proximal interphalangeal joints (Gottron papules). In up to 40% of patients, dystrophic cutaneous calcifications may be present (although not likely on diagnosis).
4. Respiratory: Small subset of patients may report dysphagia or dyspnea/tachypnea (respiratory muscle weakness may produce a restrictive lung disease pattern). These symptoms denote a more severe disease and likely a poorer prognosis.
5. Other: Periorbital edema, nail-fold capillary abnormalities, including dilatation, aneurysms, and dropout. In some patients, these capillary changes may be seen along rim of eyelids.

### C. LABORATORY STUDIES

Significant for elevated muscle enzymes; AST, ALT, CK, LDH, and aldolase. Very small fraction of patients may have normal muscle enzymes at initial diagnosis.[47] Child can be ANA positive; acute phase reactants (ESR and CRP) frequently not elevated.[46]

### D. DIAGNOSIS

Muscle biopsy is the current standard for definitive diagnosis. MRI may be helpful in locating an optimal area for muscle biopsy. T1-weighted images may show fibrosis, atrophy, and fatty infiltration; T2-weighted images may demonstrate active myositis.

## E. COMPARED TO ADULT FORM

Unlike adult-onset dermatomyositis, juvenile form not associated with underlying malignancy.

## REFERENCES


1. Behrman R, Kliegman R: Nelson Essentials of Pediatrics, 4th ed. Philadelphia, WB Saunders, 2002.
2. Cassidy J, Petty R: Textbook of Pediatric Rheumatology, 5th ed. Philadelphia, WB Saunders, 2005.
3. Marnell L et al: C-reactive protein: Ligands, receptors and role in inflammation. Clin Immunol 2005;117:104–111.
4. Egner W: The use of laboratory tests in diagnosis of SLE. J Clin Pathol 2000;53:424–432.
5. Bosch X et al: Antineutrophil cytoplasmic antibodies. Lancet 2006;368:404–418.
6. Eichenfield A et al: Utility of rheumatoid factor in the diagnosis of juvenile rheumatoid arthritis. Pediatrics 1986;78:480–484.
7. van Venrooij W et al: Autoantibodies to citrullinated antigens in (early) rheumatoid arthritis. Autoimmun Rev 2006;6:37–41.
8. Kudo-Tanaka E et al: Autoantibodies to cyclic citrullinated peptide 2 (CCP2) are superior to other potential diagnostic biomarkers for predicting rheumatoid arthritis in early undifferentiated arthritis. Clin Rheumatol 2007; e-pub.
9. Kasapcopur O et al: Diagnostic accuracy of anti-cyclic citrullinated peptide antibodies in juvenile idiopathic arthritis. Ann Rheum Dis 2004;63:1687–1689.
10. Harris E et al: Kelley's Textbook of Rheumatology, 7th ed. Philadelphia, WB Saunders, 2004.
11. Hay W et al: Current Pediatric Diagnosis & Treatment, 17th ed. New York, Lange Medical/McGraw-Hill, 2005.
12. Petty R et al: International League of Associations for Rheumatology classification of juvenile idiopathic arthritis: Second revision, Edmonton, 2001. J Rheum 2004;31:390–392.
13. Jones O et al: A multicenter case-control study on predictive factors distinguishing childhood leukemia from juvenile rheumatoid arthritis. Pediatrics 2006;117:840–844.
14. Al-Matar M et al: The early pattern of joint involvement predicts disease progression in children with oligoarticular (pauciarticular) juvenile rheumatoid arthritis. Arthritis Rheum 2002;46:2708–2715.
15. Ravelli A: Macrophage activation syndrome. Curr Opin Rheum 2002;14:548–552.
16. Borchers A et al: Juvenile idiopathic arthritis. Autoimmun Rev 2006;5: 279–298.
17. Helliwell P et al: Classification and diagnostic criteria for psoriatic arthritis. Ann Rheum Dis 2005;64:3–8.
18. Southwood T et al: Psoriatic arthritis in children. Arthritis Rheum 1989;25:1991–1994.
19. Stoll M et al: Patients with juvenile psoriatic arthritis comprise two distinct populations. Arthritis Rheum 2006;54:3564–3572.

20. Milojevic D, Ilowite N: Treatment of rheumatic diseases in children: Special considerations. Rheum Dis Clin North Am 2002;28:461–482.
21. Lovell D et al: A randomized controlled trial of calcium supplementation to increase bone mineral density in children with juvenile rheumatoid arthritis. Arthritis Rheum 2006;54:2235–2242.
22. Cassidy J et al: Ophthalmologic examinations in children with juvenile rheumatoid arthritis. Pediatrics 2006;117(5):1843–1845.
23. Tan E et al: The 1982 revised criteria for the classification of systemic lupus erythematosus. Arthritis Rheum 1982;25:1271–1277.
24. Bader-Meunier B et al: Initial presentation of childhood-onset systemic lupus erythematosus: A French multicenter study. J Pediatr 2005;146: 648–653.
25. Petri M, Magder L: Classification criteria for systemic lupus erythematosus: A review. Lupus 2004;13:829–837.
26. Williams R et al: Studies of serum C-reactive protein in systemic lupus erythematosus. J Rheumatol 2005;32:454–461.
27. Sundel R, Szer I: Vasculitis in childhood. Rheum Dis Clin North Am 2002;28(3):625–654.
28. Gross W et al: Diagnosis and evaluation of vasculitis. Rheumatology 2000;39:245–252.
29. Sano H et al: Risk factors of renal involvement and significant proteinuria in Henoch-Schönlein purpura. Eur J Pediatr 2002;161:196–201.
30. Ting T, Hashkes P: Update on childhood vasculitides. Curr Opin Rheum 2004;16:560–565.
31. Kim S, Dedeoglu F: Update on pediatric vasculitis. Curr Opin Pediatr 2005;17:695–702.
32. Ozen S et al: Juvenile polyarteritis: Results of a multicenter survey of 110 children. J Pediatr 2004;145:517–522.
33. Dillon M, Ozen S: A new international classification of childhood vasculitis. Pediatr Nephrol 2006;21:1219–1222.
34. Dillon M: Childhood vasculitis. Lupus 1998;7:259–265.
35. Frosch M, Foell D: Wegener granulomatosis in childhood and adolescence. Eur J Pediatr 2004;163:425–434.
36. Levine D et al: Chest CT findings in pediatric Wegener's granulomatosis. Pediatr Radiol 2007;37:57–62.
37. Ozen S et al: EULAR/PReS endorsed consensus criteria for the classification of childhood vasculitides. Ann Rheum Dis 2006;65:936–941.
38. Borlu M et al: Clinical features of Behçet's disease in children. Int J Derm 2006;45:713–716.
39. Kone-Paut I et al: Clinical features of Behçet's disease in children: An international collaborative study of 86 cases. J Pediatr 1998;132: 721–725.
40. Newman L et al: Sarcoidosis. NEJM 1997;336:1224–1234.
41. Lindsley C, Petty R: Overview and report on international registry of sarcoid arthritis in children. Curr Rheumatol Rep 2000;2:343–348.
42. Baumann R, Robertson W: Neurosarcoid presents differently in children than in adults. Pediatrics 2003;112:e480–e486.
43. Nowak D, Widenka D: Neurosarcoidosis: A review of its intracranial manifestation. J Neurol 2001;248:363–372.
44. Shetty A, Gedalia A: Sarcoidosis in children. Curr Probl Pediatr 2000;30:153–176.

45. Mendez E et al: US incidence of juvenile dermatomyositis, 1995–1998: Results from the National Institute of Arthritis and Musculoskeletal and Skin Diseases Registry. Arthritis Rheum 2003;49:300–305.
46. McCann L et al: The Juvenile Dermatomyositis National Registry and Repository (UK and Ireland)—clinical characteristics of children recruited within the first 5 years. Rheumatology 2006;45:1255–1260.
47. Ravelli A et al: Clinical assessment in juvenile dermatomyositis. Autoimmunity 2006;39(3):197–203.

# PART III

# Reference

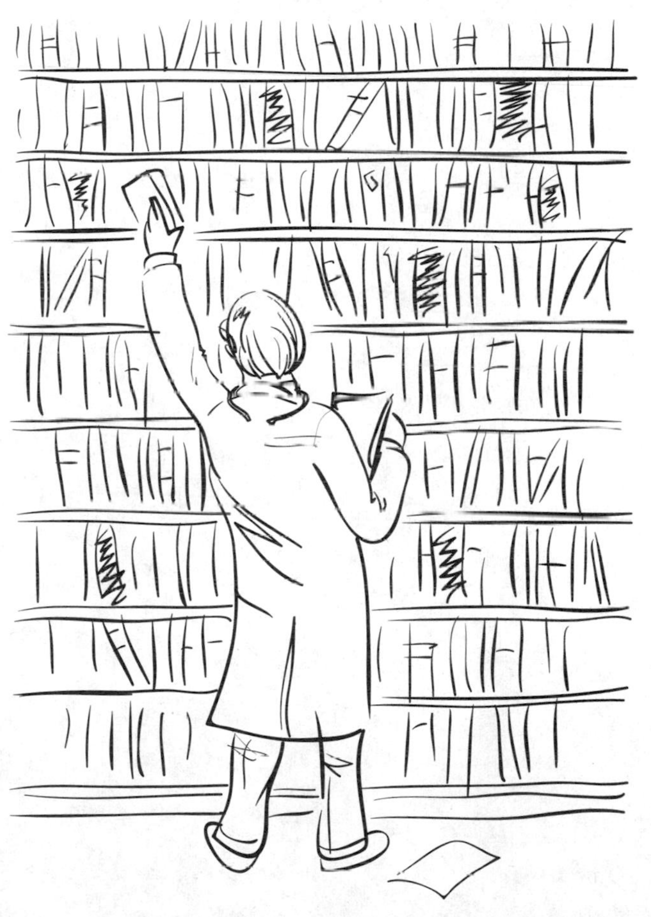

# Blood Chemistries and Body Fluids

*Jason W. Custer, MD*

27

These values are compiled from the published literature[1–6] and from the Johns Hopkins Hospital Department of Laboratory Medicine. Normal values vary with analytic method used. Consult your laboratory for its analytic method and range of normal values and for less commonly used parameters, which are beyond the scope of this text. Additional normal laboratory values may be found in Chapters 10, 14, and 15.

## I. REFERENCE VALUES (Table 27-1)

## II. EVALUATION OF BODY FLUIDS

### A. EVALUATION OF TRANSUDATE VERSUS EXUDATE (Table 27-2)

### B. EVALUATION OF CEREBROSPINAL FLUID (Table 27-3)

### C. EVALUATION OF SYNOVIAL FLUID (Table 27-4)

## III. CONVERSION FORMULAS

### A. TEMPERATURE

1. **To convert degrees Celsius to degrees Fahrenheit:**

$$([9/5] \times \text{Temperature}) + 32$$

2. **To convert degrees Fahrenheit to degrees Celsius:**

$$(\text{Temperature} - 32) \times (5/9)$$

### B. LENGTH AND WEIGHT

1. **Length:** To convert inches to centimeters, multiply by 2.54.
2. **Weight:** To convert pounds to kilograms, divide by 2.2.

*Text continued on p. 688*

TABLE 27-1

REFERENCE VALUES[1–6]

| | Conventional Units | SI Units |
|---|---|---|
| **ACID PHOSPHATASE** | | |
| (Major sources: Prostate and erythrocytes) | | |
| Newborn | 7.4–19.4 U/L | 7.4–19.4 U/L |
| 2–13 yr | 6.4–15.2 U/L | 6.4–15.2 U/L |
| Adult male | 0.5–11.0 U/L | 0.5–11.0 U/L |
| Adult female | 0.2–9.5 U/L | 0.2–9.5 U/L |
| **ALANINE AMINOTRANSFERASE (ALT)** | | |
| (Major sources: Liver, skeletal muscle, and myocardium) | | |
| Neonate/infant | 13–45 U/L | 13–45 U/L |
| Adult male | 10–40 U/L | 10–40 U/L |
| Adult female | 7–35 U/L | 7–35 U/L |
| **ALBUMIN** | | |
| (See Proteins) | | |
| **ALDOLASE** | | |
| (Major sources: Skeletal muscle and myocardium) | | |
| 10–24 mo | 3.4–11.8 U/L | 3.4–11.8 U/L |
| 2–16 yr | 1.2–8.8 U/L | 1.2–8.8 U/L |
| Adult | 1.7–4.9 U/L | 1.7–4.9 U/L |
| **ALKALINE PHOSPHATASE** | | |
| (Major sources: Liver, bone, intestinal mucosa, placenta, and kidney) | | |
| Infant | 150–420 U/L | 150–420 U/L |
| 2–10 yr | 100–320 U/L | 100–320 U/L |
| Adolescent male | 100–390 U/L | 100–390 U/L |
| Adolescent female | 100–320 U/L | 100–320 U/L |
| Adult | 30–120 U/L | 30–120 U/L |
| **AMMONIA** | | |
| (Heparinized venous specimen on ice analyzed within 30 min) | | |
| Newborn | 90–150 μg/dL | 64–107 μmol/L |
| 0–2 wk | 79–129 μg/dL | 56–92 μmol/L |
| >1 mo | 29–70 μg/dL | 21–50 μmol/L |
| Adult | 0–50 μg/dL | 0–35.7 μmol/L |
| **AMYLASE** | | |
| (Major sources: Pancreas, salivary glands, and ovaries) | | |
| Newborn | 5–65 U/L | 5–65 U/L |
| Adult | 27–131 U/L | 27–131 U/L |
| **ANTINUCLEAR ANTIBODY (ANA)** | | |
| Not significant | <1:80 | |
| Likely significant | >1:320 | |
| **Patterns with clinical correlation:** | | |
| Centromere: CREST | | |
| Nucleolar: Scleroderma | | |
| Homogeneous: SLE | | |

TABLE 27-1
REFERENCE VALUES—cont'd

| | Conventional Units | SI Units |
|---|---|---|
| **ANTISTREPTOLYSIN O TITER** | | |
| (Fourfold rise in paired serial specimens is significant) | | |
| Preschool | <1:85 | |
| School age | <1:170 | |
| Older adult | <1:85 | |
| **Note:** Alternatively, values up to 200 Todd units are normal. | | |
| **ASPARTATE AMINOTRANSFERASE (AST)** | | |
| (Major sources: Liver, skeletal muscle, kidney, myocardium, and erythrocytes) | | |
| Newborn | 25–75 U/L | 25–75 U/L |
| Infant | 15–60 U/L | 15–60 U/L |
| 1–3 yr | 20–60 U/L | 20–60 U/L |
| 4–6 yr | 15–50 U/L | 15–50 U/L |
| 7–9 yr | 15–40 U/L | 15–40 U/L |
| 10–11 yr | 10–60 U/L | 10–60 U/L |
| 12–19 yr | 15–45 U/L | 15–45 U/L |
| **BICARBONATE** | | |
| Newborn | 17–24 mEq/L | 17–24 mmol/L |
| 2 mo–2 yr | 16–24 mEq/L | 16–24 mmol/L |
| >2 yr | 22–26 mEq/L | 22–26 mmol/L |
| **BILIRUBIN (TOTAL)** | | |
| **Cord:** | | |
| Preterm | <2 mg/dL | <34 µmol/L |
| Term | <2 mg/dL | <34 µmol/L |
| **0–1 days:** | | |
| Preterm | <8 mg/dL | <137 µmol/L |
| Term | <8.7 mg/dL | <149 µmol/L |
| **1–2 days:** | | |
| Preterm | <12 mg/dL | <205 µmol/L |
| Term | <11.5 mg/dL | <197 µmol/L |
| **3–5 days:** | | |
| Preterm | <16 mg/dL | <274 µmol/L |
| Term | <12 mg/dL | <205 µmol/L |
| **Older infant:** | | |
| Preterm | <2 mg/dL | <34 µmol/L |
| Term | <1.2 mg/dL | <21 µmol/L |
| **Adult** | 0.3–1.2 mg/dL | 5–21 µmol/L |
| **BILIRUBIN (CONJUGATED)** | | |
| Neonate | <0.6 mg/dL | <10 µmol/L |
| Infants/children | <0.2 mg/dL | <3.4 µmol/L |

*Continued*

TABLE 27-1

**REFERENCE VALUES—cont'd**

**BLOOD GAS, ARTERIAL (BREATHING ROOM AIR)[7]**

| | pH | $Pa_{O_2}$ (mm Hg) | $Pa_{CO_2}$ (mm Hg) | $HCO_3^-$ (mEq/L) |
|---|---|---|---|---|
| Newborn (birth) | 7.26–7.29 | 60 | 55 | 19 |
| Newborn (>24 hr) | 7.37 | 70 | 33 | 20 |
| Infant (1–24 mo) | 7.40 | 90 | 34 | 20 |
| Child (7–19 yr) | 7.39 | 96 | 37 | 22 |
| Adult (>19 yr) | 7.35–7.45 | 90–110 | 35–45 | 22–26 |

*Note:* Venous blood gases can be used to assess acid-base status, not oxygenation. $P_{CO_2}$ averages 6–8 mm Hg higher than $Pa_{CO_2}$, and pH is slightly lower. Peripheral venous samples are strongly affected by the local circulatory and metabolic environment. Capillary blood gases correlate best with arterial pH and moderately well with $Pa_{CO_2}$.

| | Conventional Units | SI Units |
|---|---|---|
| **CALCIUM (TOTAL)** | | |
| Preterm | 6.2–11 mg/dL | 1.6–2.8 mmol/L |
| Full term <10 days | 7.6–10.4 mg/dL | 1.9–2.6 mmol/L |
| 10 days–24 mo | 9.0–11.0 mg/dL | 2.3–2.8 mmol/L |
| 2–12 yr | 8.8–10.8 mg/dL | 2.2–2.7 mmol/L |
| Adult | 8.6–10 mg/dL | 2.2–2.5 mmol/L |
| **CALCIUM (IONIZED)** | | |
| Newborn <36 hr | 4.20–5.48 mg/dL | 1.05–1.37 mmol/L |
| Newborn 36–84 hr | 4.40–5.68 mg/dL | 1.10–1.42 mmol/L |
| 1–18 yr | 4.80–5.52 mg/dL | 1.20–1.38 mmol/L |
| Adult | 4.64–5.28 mg/dL | 1.16–1.32 mmol/L |
| **CARBON DIOXIDE ($CO_2$ CONTENT)** | | |
| Cord blood | 14–22 mEq/L | 14–22 mmol/L |
| Newborn | 13–22 mEq/L | 13–22 mmol/L |
| Premature, 1 wk | 14–27 mEq/L | 14–27 mmol/L |
| Infant/child | 20–28 mEq/L | 20–28 mmol/L |
| Adult | 22–28 mEq/L | 22–28 mmol/L |
| **CARBON MONOXIDE (CARBOXYHEMOGLOBIN)** | | |
| Nonsmoker | 0.5%–1.5% of total hemoglobin | |
| Smoker | 4%–9% of total hemoglobin | |
| Toxic | 20%–50% of total hemoglobin | |
| Lethal | >50% of total hemoglobin | |

| | Conventional Units | SI Units |
|---|---|---|
| **CHLORIDE (SERUM)** | | |
| Newborn | 98–113 mEq/L | 98–113 mmol/L |
| Child/adult | 98–107 mEq/L | 98–107 mmol/L |
| **CHOLESTEROL** | | |
| (See Lipids) | | |
| **C-REACTIVE PROTEIN** | 0–0.5 mg/dL | |

TABLE 27-1
REFERENCE VALUES—cont'd

| | Conventional Units | SI Units |
|---|---|---|
| **CREATINE KINASE (CREATINE PHOSPHOKINASE)** | | |
| (Major sources: Myocardium, skeletal muscle, smooth muscle, and brain) | | |
| Newborn | 10–200 U/L | 10–200 U/L |
| Adult male | 15–105 U/L | 15–105 U/L |
| Adult female | 10–80 U/L | 10–80 U/L |
| **CREATININE (SERUM)** | | |
| Cord | 0.6–1.2 mg/dL | 53–106 μmol/L |
| Newborn | 0.3–1.0 mg/dL | 27–88 μmol/L |
| Infant | 0.2–0.4 mg/dL | 18–35 μmol/L |
| Child | 0.3–0.7 mg/dL | 27–62 μmol/L |
| Adolescent | 0.5–1.0 mg/dL | 44–88 μmol/L |
| Adult male | 0.7–1.3 mg/dL | 62–115 μmol/L |
| Adult female | 0.6–1.1 mg/dL | 53–97 μmol/L |
| **ERYTHROCYTE SEDIMENTATION RATE (ESR)** | | |
| Term neonate | 0–4 mm/hr | |
| Child | 4–20 mm/hr | |
| Adult male | 1–15 mm/hr | |
| Adult female | 4–25 mm/hr | |
| **FERRITIN** | | |
| Newborn | 25–200 ng/mL | 56–450 pmol/L |
| 1 mo | 200–600 ng/mL | 450–1350 pmol/L |
| 2–5 mo | 50–200 ng/mL | 112–450 pmol/L |
| 6 mo–15 yr | 7–140 ng/mL | 16–315 pmol/L |
| Adult male | 20–250 ng/mL | 45–562 pmol/L |
| Adult female | 10–120 ng/mL | 22–270 pmol/L |
| **FIBRINOGEN** | | |
| (See Chapter 14) | | |
| **FOLATE (SERUM)** | | |
| Newborn | 5–65 ng/mL | 11–147 nmol/L |
| Infant | 15–55 ng/mL | 34–125 nmol/L |
| 2–16 yr | 5–21 ng/mL | 11–48 nmol/L |
| >16 yr | 3–20 ng/mL | 7–45 nmol/L |
| **FOLATE (RBC)** | | |
| Newborn | 150–200 ng/mL | 340–453 nmol/L |
| Infant | 75–1000 ng/mL | 170–2265 nmol/L |
| 2–16 yr | >160 ng/mL | >362 nmol/L |
| >16 yr | 140–628 ng/mL | 317–1422 nmol/L |
| **GALACTOSE** | | |
| Newborn | 0–20 mg/dL | 0–1.11 mmol/L |
| Older child | <5 mg/dL | <0.28 mmol/L |

*Continued*

TABLE 27-1

**REFERENCE VALUES—cont'd**

| | Conventional Units | SI Units |
|---|---|---|
| **GAMMA-GLUTAMYL TRANSFERASE (GGT)** | | |
| (Major sources: Liver [biliary tree] and kidney) | | |
| Cord | 19–270 U/L | 19–270 U/L |
| Preterm | 56–233 U/L | 56–233 U/L |
| 0–3 wk | 0–130 U/L | 0–130 U/L |
| 3 wk–3 mo | 4–120 U/L | 4–120 U/L |
| 3–12 mo boy | 5–65 U/L | 5–65 U/L |
| 3–12 mo girl | 5–35 U/L | 5–35 U/L |
| 1–15 yr | 0–23 U/L | 0–23 U/L |
| Adult male | 11–50 U/L | 11–50 U/L |
| Adult female | 7–32 U/L | 7–32 U/L |
| **GLUCOSE (SERUM)** | | |
| Preterm | 20–60 mg/dL | 1.1–3.3 mmol/L |
| Newborn, <1 day | 40–60 mg/dL | 2.2–3.3 mmol/L |
| Newborn, >1 day | 50–80 mg/dL | 2.8–4.5 mmol/L |
| Child | 60–100 mg/dL | 3.3–5.6 mmol/L |
| >16 yr | 74–106 mg/dL | 4.1–5.9 mmol/L |
| **HAPTOGLOBIN** | | |
| Newborn | 5–48 mg/dL | 50–480 mg/L |
| >30 days | 26–185 mg/dL | 260–1850 mg/L |
| **HEMOGLOBIN $A_{1C}$** | 5.0%–7.5% of total hemoglobin | |
| **HEMOGLOBIN F (MEAN [SD] % TOTAL HEMOGLOBIN)** | | |
| 1 day | 77.0 (7.3) | |
| 5 days | 76.8 (5.8) | |
| 3 wk | 70.0 (7.3) | |
| 6–9 wk | 52.9 (11) | |
| 3–4 mo | 23.2 (16) | |
| 6 mo | 4.7 (2.2) | |
| 8–11 mo | 1.6 (1.0) | |
| Adult | <2.0 | |
| **IRON** | | |
| Newborn | 100–250 μg/dL | 17.9–44.8 μmol/L |
| Infant | 40–100 μg/dL | 7.2–17.9 μmol/L |
| Child | 50–120 μg/dL | 9.0–21.5 μmol/L |
| Adult male | 65–175 μg/dL | 11.6–31.3 μmol/L |
| Adult female | 50–170 μg/dL | 9.0–30.4 μmol/L |
| **KETONES (SERUM)** | | |
| Quantitative | 0.5–3.0 mg/dL | 5–30 mg/L |
| **LACTATE** | | |
| Capillary blood: | | |
| Newborn | <27 mg/dL | 0.0–3.0 mmol/L |
| Child | 5–20 mg/dL | 0.56–2.25 mmol/L |
| Venous | 5–20 mg/dL | 0.5–2.2 mmol/L |
| Arterial | 5–14 mg/dL | 0.5–1.6 mmol/L |

TABLE 27-1
REFERENCE VALUES—cont'd

| | Conventional Units | SI Units |
|---|---|---|
| **LACTATE DEHYDROGENASE (AT 37°C)** | | |
| (Major sources: Myocardium, liver, skeletal muscle, erythrocytes, platelets, and lymph nodes) | | |
| 0–4 days | 290–775 U/L | 290–775 U/L |
| 4–10 days | 545–2000 U/L | 545–2000 U/L |
| 10 days–24 mo | 180–430 U/L | 180–430 U/L |
| 24 mo–12 yr | 110–295 U/L | 110–295 U/L |
| >12 yr | 100–190 U/L | 100–190 U/L |
| **LEAD** | | |
| Child | <10 µg/dL | <0.48 µmol/L |
| **LIPASE** | | |
| 0–90 days | 10–85 U/L | 10–85 U/L |
| 3–12 mo | 9–128 U/L | 9–128 U/L |
| 1–11 yr | 10–150 U/L | 10–150 U/L |
| >11 yr | 10–220 U/L | 10–220 U/L |

| | Cholesterol (mg/dL) | | | LDL (mg/dL) | | | HDL (mg/dL) |
|---|---|---|---|---|---|---|---|
| | Desirable | Borderline | High | Desirable | Borderline | High | Desirable |
| **LIPIDS[8]** | | | | | | | |
| Child/adolescent | <170 | 170–199 | >200 | <110 | 110–129 | >130 | 45 |
| Adult | <200 | 200–239 | >240 | <100 | 100–159 | >160 | 45 |

| | Conventional Units | SI Units |
|---|---|---|
| **MAGNESIUM** | 1.3–2.0 mEq/L | 0.65–1.0 mmol/L |
| **METHEMOGLOBIN** | <1.5% of total hemoglobin | |
| **OSMOLALITY** | 275–295 mOsm/kg | 275–295 mmol/kg |
| **PHENYLALANINE** | | |
| Preterm | 2.0–7.5 mg/dL | 121–454 µmol/L |
| Newborn | 1.2–3.4 mg/dL | 73–206 µmol/L |
| Adult | 0.8–1.8 mg/dL | 48–109 µmol/L |
| **PHOSPHORUS** | | |
| Newborn | 4.5–9.0 mg/dL | 1.45–2.91 mmol/L |
| 10 days–24 mo | 4.5–6.7 mg/dL | 1.45–2.16 mmol/L |
| 24 mo–12 yr | 4.5–5.5 mg/dL | 1.45–1.78 mmol/L |
| >12 yr | 2.7–4.5 mg/dL | 0.87–1.45 mmol/L |
| **PORCELAIN[9]** | 9.0–25.04 mg/dL | 5.0–31.03 mmol/L |
| **POTASSIUM** | | |
| Newborn | 3.7–5.9 mEq/L | 3.7–5.9 mmol/L |
| Infant | 4.1–5.3 mEq/L | 4.1–5.3 mmol/L |
| Child | 3.4–4.7 mEq/L | 3.4–4.7 mmol/L |
| Adult | 3.5–5.1 mEq/L | 3.5–5.1 mmol/L |

*Continued*

TABLE 27-1

**REFERENCE VALUES—cont'd**

| | Conventional Units | SI Units |
|---|---|---|
| **PREALBUMIN** | | |
| Newborn | 7–39 mg/dL | |
| 1–6 mo | 8–34 mg/dL | |
| 6 mo–4 yr | 2–36 mg/dL | |
| 4–6 yr | 12–30 mg/dL | |
| 6–19 yr | 12–42 mg/dL | |

**PROTEIN ELECTROPHORESIS (g/dL)**

| Age | Total Protein | Albumin | α-1 | α-2 | β | γ |
|---|---|---|---|---|---|---|
| Cord | 4.8–8.0 | 2.2–4.0 | 0.3–0.7 | 0.4–0.9 | 0.4–1.6 | 0.8–1.6 |
| Newborn | 4.4–7.6 | 3.2–4.8 | 0.1–0.3 | 0.2–0.3 | 0.3–0.6 | 0.6–1.2 |
| 1 day–1 mo | 4.4–7.6 | 2.5–5.5 | 0.1–0.3 | 0.3–1.0 | 0.2–1.1 | 0.4–1.3 |
| 1–3 mo | 3.6–7.4 | 2.1–4.8 | 0.1–0.4 | 0.3–1.1 | 0.3–1.1 | 0.2–1.1 |
| 4–6 mo | 4.2–7.4 | 2.8–5.0 | 0.1–0.4 | 0.3–0.8 | 0.3–0.8 | 0.1–0.9 |
| 7–12 mo | 5.1–7.5 | 3.2–5.7 | 0.1–0.6 | 0.3–1.5 | 0.4–1.0 | 0.2–1.2 |
| 13–24 mo | 3.7–7.5 | 1.9–5.0 | 0.1–0.6 | 0.4–1.4 | 0.4–1.4 | 0.4–1.6 |
| 25–36 mo | 5.3–8.1 | 3.3–5.8 | 0.1–0.3 | 0.4–1.1 | 0.3–1.2 | 0.4–1.5 |
| 3–5 yr | 4.9–8.1 | 2.9–5.8 | 0.1–0.4 | 0.4–1.0 | 0.5–1.0 | 0.4–1.7 |
| 6–8 yr | 6.0–7.9 | 3.3–5.0 | 0.1–0.5 | 0.5–0.8 | 0.5–0.9 | 0.7–2.0 |
| 9–11 yr | 6.0–7.9 | 3.2–5.0 | 0.1–0.4 | 0.7–0.9 | 0.6–1.0 | 0.8–2.0 |
| 12–16 yr | 6.0–7.9 | 3.2–5.1 | 0.1–0.4 | 0.5–1.1 | 0.5–1.1 | 0.6–2.0 |
| Adult | 6.0–8.0 | 3.1–5.4 | 0.1–0.4 | 0.4–1.1 | 0.5–1.2 | 0.7–1.7 |

| | Conventional Units | SI Units |
|---|---|---|
| **PYRUVATE** | 0.3–0.9 mg/dL | 0.03–0.10 mmol/L |
| **RHEUMATOID FACTOR** | <30 U/mL | |
| **SODIUM** | | |
| Preterm | 130–140 mEq/L | 130–140 mmol/L |
| Older infant/chid | 133–146 mEq/L | 133–146 mmol/L |
| **TOTAL IRON-BINDING CAPACITY (TIBC)** | | |
| Infant | 100–400 μg/dL | 17.9–71.6 μmol/L |
| Adult | 250–425 μg/dL | 44.8–76.1 μmol/L |
| **TOTAL PROTEIN** (See Proteins) | | |
| **TRANSAMINASE (SGOT)** (See Aspartate aminotransferase [AST]) | | |
| **TRANSAMINASE (SGPT)** (See Alanine aminotransferase [ALT]) | | |
| **TRANSFERRIN** | | |
| Newborn | 130–275 mg/dL | 1.30–2.75 g/L |
| 3 mo–10 yr | 203–360 mg/dL | 2.03–3.6 g/L |
| Adult | 215–380 mg/dL | 2.15–3.8 g/L |

TABLE 27-1

**REFERENCE VALUES—cont'd**

**TOTAL TRIGLYCERIDE[10]**

| | 5th | Mean | 75th | 90th | 95th |
|---|---|---|---|---|---|
| Cord | 14 mg/dL | 34 mg/dL | | | 84 mg/dL |
| 1–4 yr: | | | | | |
| Male | 29 mg/dL | 56 mg/dL | 68 mg/dL | 85 mg/dL | 99 mg/dL |
| Female | 34 mg/dL | 64 mg/dL | 74 mg/dL | 95 mg/dL | 112 mg/dL |
| 5–9 yr: | | | | | |
| Male | 28 mg/dL | 52 mg/dL | 58 mg/dL | 70 mg/dL | 85 mg/dL |
| Female | 32 mg/dL | 64 mg/dL | 74 mg/dL | 103 mg/dL | 126 mg/dL |
| 10–14 yr: | | | | | |
| Male | 33 mg/dL | 63 mg/dL | 74 mg/dL | 94 mg/dL | 111 mg/dL |
| Female | 39 mg/dL | 72 mg/dL | 85 mg/dL | 104 mg/dL | 120 mg/dL |
| 15–19 yr: | | | | | |
| Male | 38 mg/dL | 78 mg/dL | 88 mg/dL | 125 mg/dL | 143 mg/dL |
| Female | 36 mg/dL | 73 mg/dL | 85 mg/dL | 112 mg/dL | 126 mg/dL |

| | Conventional Units | SI Units |
|---|---|---|
| **TROPONIN-I** | 0–0.1 μg/L | |
| **UREA NITROGEN** | | |
| Premature (<1 wk) | 3–25 mg/dL | 1.1–8.9 mmol/L |
| Newborn | 4–12 mg/dL | 1.4–4.3 mmol/L |
| Infant/child | 5–18 mg/dL | 1.8–6.4 mmol/L |
| Adult | 6–20 mg/dL | 2.1–7.1 mmol/L |
| **URIC ACID** | | |
| 0–2 yr | 2.4–6.4 mg/dL | 0.14–0.38 mmol/L |
| 2–12 yr | 2.4–5.9 mg/dL | 0.14–0.35 mmol/L |
| 12–14 yr | 2.4–6.4 mg/dL | 0.14–0.38 mmol/L |
| Adult male | 3.5–7.2 mg/dL | 0.20–0.43 mmol/L |
| Adult female | 2.4–6.4 mg/dL | 0.14–0.38 mmol/L |
| **VITAMIN A (RETINOL)** | | |
| Preterm | 13–46 μg/dL | 0.46–1.61 μmol/L |
| Full term | 18–50 μg/dL | 0.63–1.75 μmol/L |
| 1–6 yr | 20–43 μg/dL | 0.7–1.5 μmol/L |
| 7–12 yr | 20–49 μg/dL | 0.9–1.7 μmol/L |
| 13–19 yr | 26–72 μg/dL | 0.9–2.5 μmol/L |
| **VITAMIN $B_1$ (THIAMINE)** | 5.3–7.9 μg/dL | 0.16–0.23 μmol/L |
| **VITAMIN $B_2$ (RIBOFLAVIN)** | 4–24 μg/dL | 106–638 nmol/L |
| **VITAMIN $B_{12}$ (COBALAMIN)** | | |
| Newborn | 160–1300 pg/mL | 118–959 pmol/L |
| Child/adult | 200–835 pg/mL | 148–616 pmol/L |
| **VITAMIN C (ASCORBIC ACID)** | 0.4–1.5 mg/dL | 23–85 μmol/L |
| **VITAMIN $D_3$ (1,25-DIHYDROXY-VITAMIN D)** | 16–65 pg/mL | 42–169 pmol/L |
| **VITAMIN E** | | |
| <11 yr | 3–15 mg/L | 7.0–35 μmol/L |
| >11 yr | 5–20 mg/L | 11.6–46.4 μmol/L |
| **ZINC** | 70–120 mcg/dL | 10.7–18.4 mmol/L |

TABLE 27-2

**EVALUATION OF TRANSUDATE VS. EXUDATE (PLEURAL, PERICARDIAL, OR PERITONEAL FLUID)**

| Measurement* | Transudate | Exudate† |
|---|---|---|
| Specific gravity | <1.016 | >1.016 |
| Protein (g/dL) | <3.0 | >3.0 |
| Fluid : serum ratio | <0.5 | >0.5 |
| LDH (IU) | <200 | >200 |
| Fluid : serum ratio (isoenzymes not useful) | <0.6 | >0.6 |
| WBCs‡ | <1000/μL | >1000/μL |
| RBCs | <10,000 | Variable |
| Glucose | Same as serum | Less than serum |
| pH§ | 7.4–7.5 | <7.4 |

*Note*: Amylase >5000 U/mL or pleural fluid : serum ratio >1 suggests pancreatitis.
*Always obtain serum for glucose, LDH, protein, amylase, and so forth.
†All of the following criteria do not have to be met for consideration as an exudate.
‡In peritoneal fluid, WBC count >800/μL suggests peritonitis.
§Collect anaerobically in a heparinized syringe.
LDH, lactate dehydrogenase; RBCs, red blood cells; WBCs, white blood cells.

TABLE 27-3

**EVALUATION OF CEREBROSPINAL FLUID**

| | WBC Count/μL | Mean % PMNs |
|---|---|---|
| Preterm | 0–25 | 57% |
| Term (0–30 days)[11] | 7.3 ± 13.9 (0–130) | 61%–84% |
| Child | 0–7 | 5% |
| | **Conventional Units** | **SI Units** |
| **GLUCOSE** | | |
| Preterm | 24–63 mg/dL | 1.3–3.5 mmol/L |
| Term[11] | 51.2 ± 12.9 mg/dL | |
| Child | 40–80 mg/dL | 2.2–4.4 mmol/L |
| **CSF GLUCOSE/BLOOD GLUCOSE** | | |
| Preterm | 55%–105% | |
| Term | 44%–128% | |
| Child | 50% | |
| **LACTIC ACID DEHYDROGENASE** | 5–30 U/L (or about 10% of serum value) | |
| **MYELIN BASIC PROTEIN** | <4 ng/mL | |
| **OPENING PRESSURE (LATERAL RECUMBENT POSITION)** | | |
| Newborn | 8–11 cm $H_2O$ | |
| Infant/child | <20 cm $H_2O$ | |
| Respiratory variations | 0.5–1 cm $H_2O$ | |
| **PROTEIN** | | |
| Preterm | 65–150 mg/dL | 0.65–1.5 g/L |
| Term[11] | 64.2 ± 24.2 mg/dL | |
| Child | 5–40 mg/dL | 0.05–0.40 g/L |

CSF, cerebrospinal fluid; PMNs, polymorphonuclear lymphocytes; WBC, white blood cell.

Modified from Oski FA: Principles and Practice of Pediatrics, 3rd ed. Philadelphia, JB Lippincott, 1999.

TABLE 27-4

CHARACTERISTICS OF SYNOVIAL FLUID IN THE RHEUMATIC DISEASES

| Group | Condition | Synovial Complement | Color/Clarity | Viscosity | Mucin Clot | WBC Count | PMN (%) | Miscellaneous Findings |
|---|---|---|---|---|---|---|---|---|
| Noninflammatory | Normal | N | Yellow Clear | ↑↑ | G | <200 | <25 | |
| | Traumatic arthritis | N | Xanthochromic Turbid | ↑ | F–G | <2000 | <25 | Debris |
| | Osteoarthritis | N | Yellow Clear | ↑ | F–G | 1000 | <25 | |
| Inflammatory | Systemic lupus erythematosus | ↓ | Yellow Clear | N | N | 5000 | 10 | Lupus cells |
| | Rheumatic fever | N–↑ | Yellow Cloudy | ↓ | F | 5000 | 10–50 | |
| | Juvenile rheumatoid arthritis | N–↓ | Yellow Cloudy | ↓ | Poor | 15,000–20,000 | 75 | |
| | Reiter's syndrome | ↑ | Yellow Opaque | ↓ | Poor | 20,000 | 80 | Reiter's cells |
| Pyogenic | Tuberculous arthritis | N–↑ | Yellow-white Cloudy | ↓ | Poor | 25,000 | 50–60 | Acid-fast bacteria |
| | Septic arthritis | ↑ | Serosanguinous Turbid | ↓ | Poor | 50,000–300,000 | >75 | Low glucose, bacteria |

F, fair; G, good; H, high; N, normal; PMN, polymorphonuclear leukocyte; VH, very high; WBC, white blood cell; ↓, decreased; ↑, increased.

From Cassidy JT, Petty RE: Textbook of Pediatric Rheumatology, 5th ed. Philadelphia, WB Saunders, 2005.

## REFERENCES


1. Meites S (ed): Pediatric Clinical Chemistry, 2nd and 3rd eds. Washington, DC, American Association for Clinical Chemistry, 1981.
2. Burtis CA, Ashwood ER: Tietz Textbook of Clinical Chemistry, 3rd ed. Philadelphia, WB Saunders, 1999.
3. Soldin SJ et al: Pediatric Reference Intervals, 5th ed. Washington, DC, AACC Press, 2005.
4. Lundberg GD: SI unit implementation: The next step. JAMA 1988;260:73–76.
5. Wallach J: Interpretation of Diagnostic Tests. Boston, Little, Brown, 1992.
6. Beers MH: The Merck Manual of Diagnosis and Therapy, 18th ed. Rahway, NJ, Merck Research Laboratories, 2006.
7. Rogers M: Textbook of Pediatric Intensive Care, 3rd ed. Baltimore, Williams & Wilkins, 1996.
8. Summary of NCEP ATP II and ATP III reports: Highlights of the report of the expert panel on blood and cholesterol levels in children and adolescents, 1991, U.S. Department of Health and Human Services. JAMA 1993;269:3009–3014; and JAMA 2001;285:2486–2497.
9. Custer JW, Rau RE: Surviving Pediatric Chief Residency at Hopkins: Work Hard, Play Hard. Baltimore, Johns Hopkins University Press, 2007–2008.
10. Behrman RE et al: Nelson Textbook of Pediatrics, 17th ed. Philadelphia, WB Saunders, 2004.
11. Ahmed A et al: Cerebrospinal fluid values in the term neonate. Pediatr Infect Dis J 1996;15(4):298–303.

# Biostatistics and Evidence-Based Medicine

*Rachel E. Rau, MD*

28

## I. WEBSITES

Welch Medical Library, evidence-based medicine: www.welch.jhu.edu/internet/ebr.html.
Pediatric Critical Care Medicine: www.pedsccm.org.
TRIP Database for evidence-based medicine: www.tripdatabase.com.
The Cochrane Library: www.thecochranelibrary.com.
Agency for Healthcare Research and Quality: National Guideline Clearinghouse: www.guideline.gov.
PubMed: www.ncbi.nlm.nih.gov/entrez/.

## II. BIOSTATISTICS FOR MEDICAL LITERATURE

### A. STUDY DESIGN COMPARISON (Table 28-1)

### B. MEASUREMENTS IN CLINICAL STUDIES (Table 28-2)

1. **Prevalence:**
a. Proportion of study population who have a disease (at one point or period in time).
b. Number of old cases and new cases divided by total population.
c. In cross-sectional studies (see Table 28-2):

$$(A + B)/(A + B + C + D)$$

2. **Incidence:**
a. Number of people in study population who newly develop an outcome (disease) per total study population per given time period.
b. Number of new cases divided by the total population over a given time period.
c. For cohort studies and clinical trials (see Table 28-2):

$$(A + B)/(A + B + C + D)$$

3. **Relative risk (RR):**
a. Ratio of incidence of disease among people with risk factor to incidence of disease among people without risk factor.
b. For cohort studies or clinical trials (see Table 28-2):

$$[A/(A + C)]/[B/(B + D)]$$

c. Values:
(1) RR = 1: No effect of exposure (or treatment) on outcome (or disease).
(2) RR < 1: Exposure or treatment protective against disease.
(3) RR > 1: Exposure/treatment increases probability of outcome/disease.

TABLE 28-1

**STUDY DESIGN COMPARISON**

| Design Type | Definition | Advantages | Disadvantages |
|---|---|---|---|
| Case-control (often called retrospective) | Define diseased subjects (cases) and nondiseased subjects (controls); compare proportion of cases with exposure (risk factor) with proportion of controls with exposure (risk factor). | Good for rare diseases<br>Small sample size<br>Shorter study times (not followed over time)<br>Less expensive | Highest potential for biases (recall, selection, and others)<br>Weak evidence for causality<br>No prevalence, PPV, NPV |
| Cohort (usually prospective; occasionally retrospective) | In study population, define exposed group (with risk factor) and nonexposed group (without risk factor).<br>Over time, compare proportion of exposed group with outcome (disease) with proportion of nonexposed group with outcome (disease). | Defines incidence<br>Stronger evidence for causality<br>Decreases biases (sampling, measurement, reporting) | Expensive<br>Long study times<br>May not be feasible for rare diseases/ outcomes<br>Factors related to exposure and outcome may falsely alter effect of exposure on outcome (confounding) |
| Cross-sectional | In study population, concurrently measure outcome (disease) and risk factor.<br>Compare proportion of diseased group with risk factor with proportion of nondiseased group with risk factor. | Defines prevalence<br>Short time to complete | Selection bias<br>Weak evidence for causality |
| Clinical trial (experiment) | In study population, assign (randomly) subjects to receive treatment or receive no treatment.<br>Compare rate of outcome (e.g., disease cure) between treatment and nontreatment groups. | Randomized, blinded trial is gold standard<br>Randomization reduces confounding<br>Best evidence for causality | Expensive<br>Risks of experimental treatments in humans<br>Longer study time<br>Bad for rare outcomes/diseases |

NPV, negative predictive value; PPV, positive predictive value.

TABLE 28-2

GRID FOR CALCULATIONS IN CLINICAL STUDIES

| | Exposure or Risk Factor or Treatment | |
|---|---|---|
| Disease or Outcome | Positive | Negative |
| Positive | A | B |
| Negative | C | D |

4. **Odds ratio (OR):**
a. For case-control studies, ratio of odds of having risk factor in people with disease (A/B) to odds of having risk factor in people without disease (C/D) (see Table 28-2):

$$(A/B)/(C/D) = (A \times D)/(B \times C)$$

b. Good estimate of RR if disease is rare.
 (1) OR = 1: No risk factor–disease association.
 (2) OR > 1: Suggests risk factor associated with disease.
 (3) OR < 1: Suggests risk factor protective against disease.
5. **α (Significance level of statistical test):**
a. Probability of finding a statistical association by chance alone when there truly is no association (type I error).
b. Often set at 0.05; low α especially important when interpreting finding of an association.
6. **Power (of a statistical test):**
a. β = Probability of finding no statistical association when there truly is one (type II error).
b. Power = 1 − β = Probability of finding a statistical association when there truly is one.
c. Power often set at 0.80; high power especially important when interpreting a finding of no association.
7. **Sample size:** **Approximate number of subjects required in a clinical study to achieve a sufficiently high power and sufficiently low α to obtain a clinically relevant result.**
8. ***p* value:**
a. Probability of a finding by chance alone.
b. If *p* value is less than preset α level (often 0.05), finding is interpreted as unlikely to be due to chance simply from sampling.
9. **Confidence interval (95%): 95% probability that the reported interval contains the true value.**

## C. MEASUREMENTS FOR EVALUATING A CLINICAL TEST (Table 28-3)

1. **Sensitivity (Sens):**
a. Proportion of all diseased who have positive test (see Table 28-3):

$$A/(A + C)$$

TABLE 28-3

GRID FOR EVALUATING A CLINICAL TEST

| | Disease Status | |
|---|---|---|
| **Test Result** | **Positive** | **Negative** |
| Positive | A (true positive) | B (false positive) |
| Negative | C (false negative) | D (true negative) |

b. Use highly sensitive test to help exclude a disease. (Low false-negative rate. This is good for screening.)

**2. Specificity (Spec):**

a. Proportion of all nondiseased who have a negative test (see Table 28-3):

$$D/(B + D)$$

b. Use highly specific test to help confirm a disease. (Low false-positive rate.)

**3. Positive predictive value (PPV):**

a. Proportion of all those with positive tests who truly have disease (see Table 28-3):

$$A/(A + B)$$

b. Increased PPV with higher disease prevalence and higher specificity (and, to a lesser degree, higher sensitivity).

**4. Negative predictive value (NPV):**

a. Proportion of all those with negative tests who truly do not have disease (see Table 28-3):

$$D/(C + D)$$

b. Increased NPV with lower prevalence (rarer disease) and higher sensitivity.

**5. Likelihood ratio (LR):**

a. LR positive: Ability of positive test result to confirm diseased status:

$$\text{LR positive} = (\text{Sens})/(1 - \text{Spec})$$

b. LR negative: Ability of negative test result to confirm nondiseased status:

$$\text{LR negative} = (\text{Spec})/(1 - \text{Sens})$$

$$[\text{Alternative LR negative} = (1 - \text{Sens})/\text{Spec}]$$

c. Good tests have LR $\geq 10$. (Good tests have LR $\leq 0.1$ if using alternative LR-negative formula.) Physical examination findings often have LR of about 2.

d. LR should not be affected by disease prevalence. Can be used to calculate increase in probability of disease from baseline prevalence with positive test (LR positive) and decrease in probability of disease from baseline prevalence with negative test (using alternative LR negative) for any level of disease prevalence (Fig. 28-1).

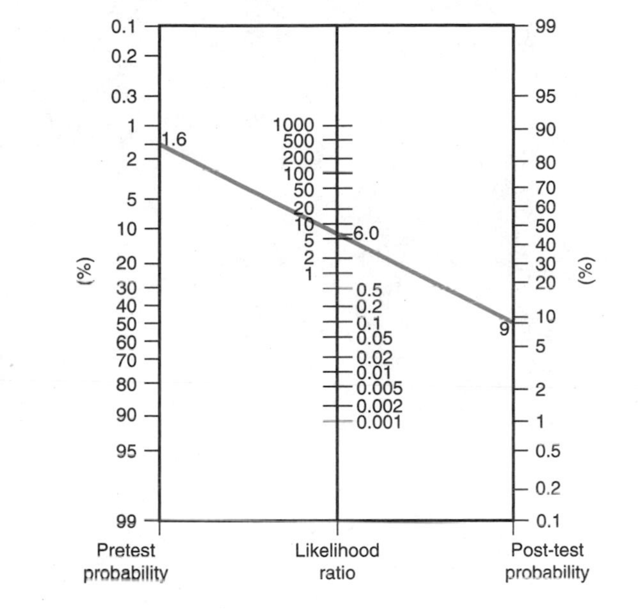


FIG. 28-1

Nomogram for calculating the change in probability by applying tests with known likelihood ratios (LRs). For example, the prevalence (i.e., pretest probability) of occult bacteremia in a well-appearing 3- to 36-month-old with temperature ≥39°C without source is 1.6%. LR positive for WBC >20 × $10^9$/L is 6.0. For infants, then, with a WBC >20 × $10^9$/L, you can use the nomogram to determine the increased probability from the positive test. Anchor a straight edge at 1.6% on the left pretest probability column and direct the straight edge through the central column at the LR of 6.0. The straight edge will intersect the right column with your answer to give a post-test probability of about 9%. It is then up to you to decide the clinical importance of a 9% probability of bacteremia. *(Data from Fagan TJ: Letter: Nomogram for Bayes theorem. NEJM 1975;293:257; Lee GM, Harper MB: Risk of bacteremia for febrile young children in the post-Haemophilus influenzae type b era. Arch Pediatr Adolesc Med 1998;152:624–628.)*

# PART IV

# Formulary

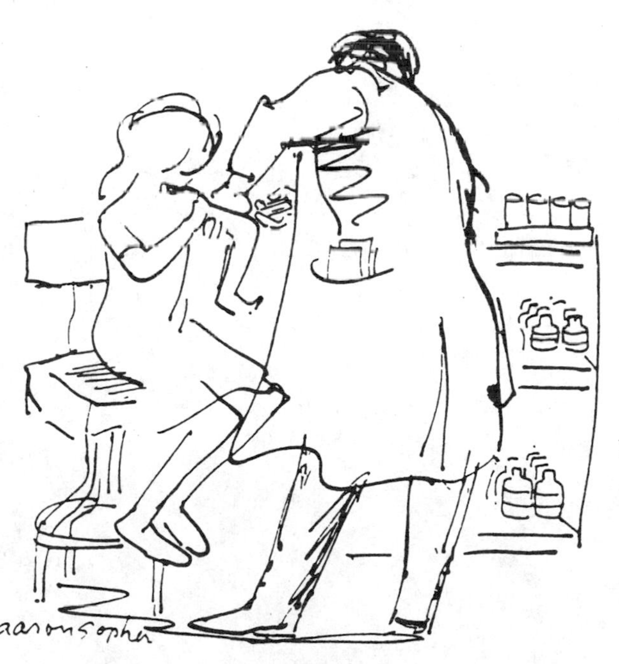

# Drug Doses

*Carlton Lee, PharmD, MPH, Jason W. Custer, MD, and Rachel E. Rau, MD*

## I. NOTE TO READER

The authors have made every attempt to check dosages and medical content for accuracy. Because of the incomplete data on pediatric dosing, many drug dosages will be modified after the publication of this text. We recommend that the reader check product information and published literature for changes in dosing, especially for newer medicines.

29

## II. SAMPLE ENTRY

**Pregnancy:** Refer to explanation of pregnancy categories (on facing page).
**Breast:** Refer to explanation of breast-feeding categories (on facing page).
**Kidney:** Indicates need for caution or need for dose adjustment in renal impairment (see also Chapter 31).
**Liver:** Indicates need for caution or need for dose adjustment in hepatic impairment.

**How supplied**

### ACETAZOLAMIDE ← Generic name

Yes Yes 1 C

Diamox and others ← Trade name and other names
***Carbonic anhydrase inhibitor, diuretic*** ← Drug category

**Tabs:** 125, 250 mg
**Oral suspension:** 25 mg/mL ← Mortar and pestle: Indicates need for extemporaneous compounding by a pharmacist
**Capsules (sustained release):** 500 mg
**Injection (sodium):** 500 mg/5 mL
Contains 2.05 mEq Na/500 mg drug

***Diuretic (PO, IV):***
***Child:*** 5 mg/kg/dose QD–QOD
***Adult:*** 250–375 mg/dose QD–QOD

***Glaucoma:***
***Child:***
***PO:*** 8–30 mg/kg/24 hr ÷ Q6–8 hr
***IM/IV:*** 20–40 mg/kg/24 hr ÷ Q6 hr
***Adult:***
***PO (simple chronic; open-angle):*** 1000 mg/24 hr ÷ Q6 hr
***IV (acute secondary; closed-angle):*** For rapid decrease in intraocular pressure, administer 500 mg/dose IV.
***Seizures:*** 8–30 mg/kg/24 hr ÷ Q6–12 hr PO
**Max. dose:** 1 g/24 hr
***Urine alkalinization:*** 5 mg/kg/dose PO repeated BID–TID over 24 hr
***Management of hydrocephalus (see remarks):*** Start with 20 mg/kg/24 hr ÷ Q8 hr PO/IV; may increase to 100 mg/kg/24 hr up to a **max. dose** of 2 g/24 hr.

Drug dosing

**Contraindicated** in hepatic failure, severe renal failure (GFR < 10 mL/min), and hypersensitiivity to sulfonamides.

$T_{1/2}$: 2–6 hr; **do not use** sustained-release capsules in seizures; IM injection may be painful; bicarbonate replacement therapy may be required during long-term use (see *Citrate* or *Sodium Bicarbonate*).

Possible side effects (more likely with long-term therapy) include GI irritation, paresthesias, sedation, hypokalemia, acidosis, reduced urate secretion, aplastic anemia, polyuria, and development of renal calculi.

May increase toxicity of cyclosporine. Aspirin may increase toxicity of acetazolamide. May decrease the effects of salicylates, lithium, and phenobarbital. False-positive urinary protein may occur with several assays. **Adjust dose in renal failure (see Chapter 31).**

Brief remarks about side effects, drug interactions, precautions, therapeutic monitoring, and other relevant information

## III. EXPLANATION OF BREAST-FEEDING CATEGORIES

See sample entry.

**1** Compatible
**2** Use with caution
**3** Unknown with concerns
**X** Contraindicated
**?** Safety not established

## IV. EXPLANATION OF PREGNANCY CATEGORIES

**A** Adequate studies in pregnant women have not demonstrated a risk to the fetus in the first trimester of pregnancy, and there is no evidence of risk in later trimesters.

**B** Animal studies have not demonstrated a risk to the fetus, but there are no adequate studies in pregnant women; or animal studies have shown an adverse effect, but adequate studies in pregnant women have not demonstrated a risk to the fetus during the first trimester of pregnancy, and there is no evidence of risk in later trimesters.

**C** Animal studies have shown an adverse effect on the fetus, but there are no adequate studies in humans; or there are no animal reproduction studies and no adequate studies in humans.

**D** There is evidence of human fetal risk, but the potential benefits from the use of the drug in pregnant women may be acceptable despite its potential risks.

**X** Studies in animals or humans demonstrate fetal abnormalities or adverse reaction; reports indicate evidence of fetal risk. The risk of use in pregnant women clearly outweighs any possible benefit.

## V. DRUG INDEX

| Trade Name | Generic Name |
|---|---|
| 1,25-Dihydroxycholecalciferol | Calcitriol |
| 2-PAM* | Pralidoxime Chloride |
| 3TC* | Lamivudine |
| 5-Aminosalicylic Acid | Mesalamine |
| 5-ASA | Mesalamine |
| 5-FC* | Flucytosine |
| 5-Fluorocytosine* | Flucytosine |
| 8-Arginine Vasopressin* | Vasopressin |
| 9-Fluorohydrocortisone* | Fludrocortisone Acetate |
| A-200 | Pyrethrins |
| Abelcet | Amphotericin B Lipid Complex |
| Accolate | Zafirlukast |
| AccuNeb (prediluted nebulized solution) | Albuterol |
| Accutane | Isotretinoin |
| Acetadote | Acetylcysteine |
| Acticin | Permethrin |

*Common abbreviation or other name (not recommended for use when writing a prescription).

| Trade Name | Generic Name |
|---|---|
| Actigall | Ursodiol |
| Actiq | Fentanyl |
| Activase | Alteplase |
| Acular, Acular LS, Acular PF | Ketorolac |
| Aczone | Dapsone |
| Adalat CC | Nifedipine |
| Adderall, Adderall XR | Dextroamphetamine + Amphetamine |
| Adenocard | Adenosine |
| Adrenaline | Epinephrine HCL |
| Advair Diskus, Advair HFA | Fluticasone Propionate and Salmeterol |
| Advil, Children's Advil | Ibuprofen |
| Aerobid, Aerobid-M | Flunisolide |
| Aerospan | Flunisolide |
| Afrin | Oxymetazoline |
| Aftate | Tolnaftate |
| Akarpine | Pilocarpine HCL |
| AK-Poly-Bac Ophthalmic | Bacitracin + Polymyxin B |
| AK-Spore H.C. Otic | Polymyxin B Sulfate, Neomycin Sulfate, Hydrocortisone |
| AK-Sulf | Sulfacetamide Sodium Ophthalmic |
| AKTob | Tobramycin |
| AK-Tracin Ophthalmic | Bacitracin |
| Alacol Oral Drops, Alacol Syrup | Brompheniramine with Phenylephrine |
| Albuminar | Albumin, Human |
| Albutein | Albumin, Human |
| Aldactone | Spironolactone |
| Alenaze-D NR | Brompheniramine with Phenylephrine |
| Aleve [OTC] | Naproxen/Naproxen Sodium |
| Allegra, Allegra ODT | Fexofenadine |
| Allegra-D 12 Hour, Allegra-D 24 Hour | Fexofenadine + Pseudoephedrine |
| Allergen Ear Drops | Antipyrine and Benzocaine |
| Alloprim | Allopurinol |
| Almacone, Almacone II Double Strength | Aluminum Hydroxide with Magnesium Hydroxide |
| AlternaGEL | Aluminum Hydroxide |
| Alu-Tab | Aluminum Hydroxide |
| AmBisome | Amphotericin B, Liposomal |
| Amicar | Aminocaproic Acid |
| Amikin | Amikacin Sulfate |
| Aminoxin | Pyridoxine |
| Amnesteem | Isotretinoin |
| Amoxil | Amoxicillin |
| Amphadase | Hyaluronidase |
| Amphocin | Amphotericin B |
| Amphojel | Aluminum Hydroxide |
| Anacin | Aspirin |
| Anaprox | Naproxen Sodium |
| Ancef | Cefazolin |
| Ancobon | Flucytosine |

| Trade Name | Generic Name |
|---|---|
| Anectine | Succinylcholine |
| Antilirium | Physostigmine Salicylate |
| Antiminth | Pyrantel Pamoate |
| Antizol | Fomepizole |
| Anzemet | Dolasetron |
| Apresoline | Hydralazine Hydrochloride |
| Aquachloral Supprettes | Chloral Hydrate |
| Aquasol A | Vitamin A |
| Aquasol E | Vitamin E |
| Aquavit-E | Vitamin E |
| Aralen | Chloroquine HCL/Phosphate |
| Aranesp | Darbepoetin Alfa |
| Aristospan | Triamcinolone |
| ASA* | Aspirin |
| Asacol | Mesalamine |
| Asmanex Twisthaler | Mometasone Furoate |
| Aspirin Free Anacin | Acetaminophen |
| Astelin | Azelastine |
| Ativan | Lorazepam |
| AtroPen | Atropine Sulfate |
| Atrovent | Ipratropium Bromide |
| Augmentin, Augmentin ES-600, Augmentin XR | Amoxicillin–Clavulanic Acid |
| Auralgan (available in Canada) | Antipyrine and Benzocaine |
| Auro Ear Drops | Carbamide Peroxide |
| Aventyl | Nortriptyline Hydrochloride |
| Avita | Tretinoin |
| Azactam | Aztreonam |
| Azasan | Azathioprine |
| Azasite | Azithromycin |
| Azmacort | Triamcinolone |
| Azo-Standard [OTC] | Phenazopyridine HCL |
| Azulfidine, Azulfidine EN-tabs | Sulfasalazine |
| Baciguent Topical | Bacitracin |
| Bactrim | Sulfamethoxazole and Trimethoprim |
| Bactroban, Bactroban Nasal | Mupirocin |
| BAL* | Dimercaprol |
| Beconase AQ | Beclomethasone Dipropionate |
| Benadryl | Diphenhydramine |
| Benzac AC Wash 2½, 5, 10; Benzac 5, 10 | Benzoyl Peroxide |
| Beta-Val | Betamethasone |
| Biaxin, Biaxin XL | Clarithromycin |
| Bicillin C-R, Bicillin C-R 900/300 | Penicillin G Preparations—Penicillin G Benzathine and Penicillin G Procaine |
| Bicillin L-A | Penicillin G Preparations—Benzathine |
| Biocef | Cephalexin |

*Common abbreviation or other name (not recommended for use when writing a prescription).

| Trade Name | Generic Name |
|---|---|
| Bleph 10 | Sulfacetamide Sodium Ophthalmic |
| Brethine | Terbutaline |
| Brevibloc | Esmolol HCL |
| Brevoxyl Creamy Wash | Benzoyl Peroxide |
| British Anti-Lewisite | Dimercaprol |
| Bufferin | Aspirin |
| Bumex | Bumetanide |
| Buminate | Albumin, Human |
| Cafcit | Caffeine Citrate |
| Cafergot | Ergotamine Tartrate + Caffeine |
| Calan, Calan SR | Verapamil |
| Calciferol | Ergocalciferol |
| Calcijex | Calcitriol |
| Calcionate | Calcium Glubionate |
| Calciquid | Calcium Glubionate |
| Cal-Citrate | Calcium Citrate |
| Calcium Disodium Versenate | Edetate (EDTA) Calcium Disodium |
| Cal-G | Calcium Glubionate |
| Cal-Lac | Calcium Lactate |
| Camphorated opium tincture | Paregoric |
| Canasa | Mesalamine |
| Cancidas | Caspofungin |
| Cankaid | Carbamide Peroxide |
| Capoten | Captopril |
| Carafate | Sucralfate |
| Carbatrol | Carbamazepine |
| Carbinox | Carbinoxamine |
| Cardene, Cardene SR | Nicardipine |
| Cardizem, Cardizem SR, Cardizem CD, Cardizem LA | Diltiazem |
| Carnitor | Carnitine |
| Catapres, Catapres TTS | Clonidine |
| Cathflo Activase | Alteplase |
| Ceclor, Ceclor CD | Cefaclor |
| Cecon | Ascorbic Acid |
| Cedax | Ceftibuten |
| Cefizox | Ceftizoxime |
| Cefobid | Cefoperazone |
| Cefotan | Cefotetan |
| Ceftin | Cefuroxime Axetil |
| Cefzil | Cefprozil |
| Celestone | Betamethasone |
| CellCept | Mycophenolate Mofetil |
| Cephulac | Lactulose |
| Ceptaz | Ceftazidime |
| Cerebyx | Fosphenytoin |
| Chemet | Succimer |
| Chibroxin | Norfloxacin |
| Chloromycetin | Chloramphenicol |

| Trade Name | Generic Name |
|---|---|
| Chlor-Trimeton | Chlorpheniramine Maleate |
| Cholestyramine Light | Cholestyramine |
| Chronulac | Lactulose |
| Ciloxan Ophthalmic | Ciprofloxacin |
| Cipro, Cipro XR | Ciprofloxacin |
| Citracel | Calcium Citrate |
| Claforan | Cefotaxime |
| Claravis | Isotretinoin |
| Clarinex, Clarinex RediTabs | Desloratadine |
| Claritin, Claritin Children's Allergy, Claritin RediTabs | Loratadine |
| Claritin-D 12 Hour, Claritin-D 24 Hour | Loratadine + Pseudoephedrine |
| Cleocin-T, Cleocin | Clindamycin |
| Cogentin | Benztropine Mesylate |
| Colace | Docusate |
| CoLyte | Polyethylene Glycol—Electrolyte Solution |
| Compazine | Prochlorperazine |
| Concerta | Methylphenidate HCL |
| Copegus | Ribavirin |
| Cordarone | Amiodarone HCL |
| Cordron-D NR, Cordron-D | Carbinoxamine + Pseudoephedrine |
| Cortef | Hydrocortisone |
| Cortifoam | Hydrocortisone |
| Cortisporin Otic | Polymyxin B Sulfate, Neomycin Sulfate, Hydrocortisone |
| Co-Trimoxazole | Sulfamethoxazole and Trimethoprim |
| Coumadin | Warfarin |
| Covera-HS | Verapamil |
| Cozaar | Losartan |
| Crolom | Cromolyn |
| Cruex | Clotrimazole |
| Cuprimine | Penicillamine |
| Curosurf | Surfactant, Pulmonary/Poractant Alfa |
| Cutivate | Fluticasone Propionate |
| Cyanoject | Cyanocobalamin/Vitamin $B_{12}$ |
| Cyclogyl | Cyclopentolate |
| Cyclomydril | Cyclopentolate with Phenylephrine |
| Cyomin | Cyanocobalamin/Vitamin $B_{12}$ |
| Cytovene | Ganciclovir |
| Dantrium | Dantrolene |
| Daraprim | Pyrimethamine |
| Daytrana | Methylphenidate HCL |
| DDAVP* | Desmopressin Acetate |
| DDS* | Dapsone |
| Debrox | Carbamide Peroxide |
| Decadron | Dexamethasone |
| Deltasone | Prednisone |
| Demerol | Meperidine HCL |

*Common abbreviation or other name (not recommended for use when writing a prescription).

| Trade Name | Generic Name |
|---|---|
| Deodorized Tincture of Opium | Opium Tincture |
| Depacon | Valproic Acid |
| Depakene | Valproic Acid |
| Depakote, Depakote ER | Divalproex Sodium |
| Depen | Penicillamine |
| Depo-Medrol | Methylprednisolone |
| Depo-Provera | Medroxyprogesterone |
| Depo-Sub Q Provera 104 | Medroxyprogesterone |
| Desferal | Deferoxamine Mesylate |
| Desquam-E 5, Desquam-E 10 | Benzoyl Peroxide |
| Desyrel (previously available as) | Trazodone |
| Dexedrine Spansules | Dextroamphetamine |
| DexFerrum | Iron—Injectable Preparations (iron dextran) |
| DextroStat | Dextroamphetamine |
| Di-5-ASA* | Olsalazine |
| Dialume | Aluminum Hydroxide |
| Diaminodiphenylsulfone | Dapsone |
| Diamox | Acetazolamide |
| Diastat, Diastat AcuDial | Diazepam |
| Diflucan | Fluconazole |
| Digibind, DigiFab | Digoxin Immune Fab (Ovine) |
| Digitek | Digoxin |
| Dilacor XR | Diltiazem |
| Dilantin, Dilantin Infatab | Phenytoin |
| Dilaudid, Dilaudid-HP | Hydromorphone HCL |
| Di-mesalazine | Olsalazine |
| Dimetapp Children's Cold and Allergy | Brompheniramine with Phenylephrine |
| Dipentum | Olsalazine |
| Diprolene, Diprolene AF | Betamethasone |
| Diprosone | Betamethasone |
| DisperMox | Amoxicillin |
| Ditropan, Ditropan XL | Oxybutynin Chloride |
| Diurigen | Chlorothiazide |
| Diuril | Chlorothiazide |
| DMSA (dimercaptosuccinic acid)* | Succimer |
| Dobutrex (previously available as) | Dobutamine |
| Dolophine | Methadone HCL |
| Dopram | Doxapram HCL |
| Doxidan | Bisacodyl |
| Dramamine, Children's Dramamine | Dimenhydrinate |
| Drisdol | Ergocalciferol |
| Dulcolax | Bisacodyl |
| Duraclon | Clonidine |
| Duragesic | Fentanyl |
| Duramist 12-Hour Nasal | Oxymetazoline |
| Duricef | Cefadroxil |
| Dycill | Dicloxacillin Sodium |

*Common abbreviation or other name (not recommended for use when writing a prescription).

| Trade Name | Generic Name |
|---|---|
| Dyrenium | Triamterene |
| EC-Naprosyn | Naproxen |
| Efidac 24 | Chlorpheniramine Maleate |
| Efidac/24-Pseudoephedrine | Pseudoephedrine |
| Elavil | Amitriptyline |
| Elidel | Pimecrolimus |
| Elimite | Permethrin |
| Elitek | Rasburicase |
| Elixophyllin | Theophylline |
| Elocon | Mometasone Furoate |
| EMLA | Lidocaine and Prilocaine |
| E-Mycin | Erythromycin Preparations |
| Enbrel | Etanercept |
| Endocet | Oxycodone and Acetaminophen |
| Enlon | Edrophonium Chloride |
| Enuloase | Lactulose |
| Epi-pen | Epinephrine HCL |
| Epitol | Carbamazepine |
| Epivir, Epivir HBV | Lamivudine |
| Epogen | Epoetin Alfa |
| Epsom Salts | Magnesium Sulfate |
| Ergomar | Ergotamine Tartrate |
| Ery-Ped | Erythromycin Preparations |
| Erythrocin | Erythromycin Preparations |
| Erythropoietin | Epoetin Alfa |
| Eryzole | Erythromycin Ethylsuccinate and Acetylsulfisoxazole |
| Famvir | Famciclovir |
| Fansidar | Pyrimethamine + Sulfadoxine |
| Felbatol | Felbamate |
| Fentora | Fentanyl |
| Feosol | Iron—Oral Preparations |
| Fergon | Iron—Oral Preparations |
| Fer-In-Sol | Iron—Oral Preparations |
| Ferrlecit | Iron—Injectable Preparations (ferric gluconate) |
| Feverall | Acetaminophen |
| Fiberall | Psyllium |
| FIV-ASA | Mesalamine |
| FK506 | Tacrolimus |
| Flagyl, Flagyl ER | Metronidazole |
| Fleet Babylax | Glycerin |
| Fleet Laxative, Fleet Bisacodyl | Bisacodyl |
| Fleet Mineral Oil | Mineral Oil |
| Fleet, Fleet Phospho-Soda | Sodium Phosphate |
| Fletcher's Castoria | Senna/Sennosides |
| Flonase HFA | Fluticasone Propionate |
| Florinef Acetate | Fludrocortisone Acetate |
| Flovent Diskus | Fluticasone Propionate |
| Floxin, Floxin Otic | Ofloxacin |

| Trade Name | Generic Name |
|---|---|
| Flumadine | Rimantadine |
| Fluohydrisone | Fludrocortisone Acetate |
| Fluoritab | Fluoride |
| Folvite | Folic Acid |
| Foradil Aerolizer | Formoterol |
| Fortamet | Metformin |
| Fortaz | Ceftazidime |
| Fortical Nasal Spray | Calcitonin—Salmon |
| Foscavir | Foscarnet |
| Fulvicin U/F, Fulvicin P/G | Griseofulvin |
| Fungizone | Amphotericin B |
| Furadantin | Nitrofurantoin |
| Gabarone | Gabapentin |
| Gabitril | Tiagabine |
| Galzin | Zinc Salts |
| Gamma Benzene Hexachloride* | Lindane |
| Gantrisin | Sulfisoxazole |
| Garamycin | Gentamicin |
| Gastrocrom | Cromolyn |
| Gas-X | Simethicone |
| Gengraf | Cyclosporine Modified |
| GlucaGen, Glucagon Emergency Kit | Glucagon HCL |
| Glucophage, Glucophage XR | Metformin |
| Gly-Oxide | Carbamide Peroxide |
| GoLYTELY | Polyethylene Glycol—Electrolyte Solution |
| Grifulvin V | Griseofulvin |
| Grisactin | Griseofulvin |
| Gris-PEG | Griseofulvin |
| Gyne-Lotrimin 3, Gyne-Lotrimin | Clotrimazole |
| H.P. Acthar Gel | Corticotropin |
| Haldol, Haldol Decanoate 50, Haldol Decanoate 100 | Haloperidol |
| Hexadrol | Dexamethasone |
| Humatin | Paromomycin Sulfate |
| Hydase | Hyaluronidase |
| Hydrodiuril | Hydrochlorothiazide |
| Hydro-Tussin CBX | Carbinoxamine + Pseudoephedrine |
| Hylenex | Hyaluronidase |
| Imitrex | Sumatriptan Succinate |
| Imodium, Imodium AD | Loperamide |
| Imuran | Azathioprine |
| Inapsine | Droperidol |
| Inderal | Propranolol |
| Indocin, Indocin SR, Indocin I.V. | Indomethacin |
| Infasurf | Surfactant, Pulmonary/Calfactant |
| INFeD | Iron—Injectable Preparations (iron dextran) |

*Common abbreviation or other name (not recommended for use when writing a prescription).

| Trade Name | Generic Name |
|---|---|
| INH* | Isoniazid |
| Intal | Cromolyn |
| Intropin (previously available as) | Dopamine |
| Invanz | Ertapenem |
| Iosat | Potassium Iodide |
| Iquix | Levofloxacin |
| Isoptin, Isoptin SR | Verapamil |
| Isopto Carpine | Pilocarpine HCL |
| Isopto Hyoscine | Scopolamine Hydrobromide |
| Isuprel | Isoproterenol |
| Kantrex | Kanamycin |
| Kaopectate, Kaopectate Children's | Bismuth Subsalicylate |
| Kayexalate | Sodium Polystyrene Sulfonate |
| Keflex | Cephalexin |
| Kemstro | Baclofen |
| Kenalog | Triamcinolone |
| Keppra | Levetiracetam |
| Ketalar | Ketamine |
| Kionex | Sodium Polystyrene Sulfonate |
| Klonopin | Clonazepam |
| Kondremul | Mineral Oil |
| Konsyl | Psyllium |
| K-PHOS Neutral, K-PHOS M.F., K-PHOS No. 2 | Phosphorus Supplements |
| Kytril | Granisetron |
| Lamictal | Lamotrigine |
| Laniazid | Isoniazid |
| Lanoxin, Lanoxicaps | Digoxin |
| Lariam | Mefloquine HCl |
| Lasix | Furosemide |
| Lax-Pills | Senna/Sennosides |
| L-Carnitine | Carnitine |
| Levaquin | Levofloxacin |
| Levocarnitine | Carnitine |
| Levophed | Norepinephrine Bitartrate |
| Levothroid | Levothyroxine ($T_4$) |
| Levoxyl | Levothyroxine ($T_4$) |
| Lialda | Mesalamine |
| Lidoderm | Lidocaine |
| Lioresal | Baclofen |
| Liquid Pred | Prednisone |
| Lithobid | Lithium |
| L-M-X | Lidocaine |
| Lopressor, Toprol-XL | Metoprolol |
| Lotrimin AF | Clotrimazole |
| Lotrimin AF | Miconazole |
| Lovenox | Enoxaparin |

*Common abbreviation or other name (not recommended for use when writing a prescription).

| Trade Name | Generic Name |
|---|---|
| Luminal | Phenobarbital |
| Luride | Fluoride |
| Maalox | Aluminum Hydroxide with Magnesium Hydroxide |
| Macrobid | Nitrofurantoin |
| Macrodantin | Nitrofurantoin |
| Mag-200, Mag-Ox 400, Uro-Mag | Magnesium Oxide |
| Marinol | Dronabinol |
| Maxidex | Dexamethasone |
| Maxipime | Cefepime |
| Maxivate | Betamethasone |
| Maxolon | Metoclopramide |
| Medrol, Medrol Dosepack | Methylprednisolone |
| Mefoxin | Cefoxitin |
| Mephyton | Phytonadione (Vitamin $K_1$) |
| Mepron | Atovaquone |
| Merrem | Meropenem |
| Mestinon | Pyridostigmine Bromide |
| Metadate ER | Methylphenidate HCL |
| Metamucil | Psyllium |
| Methadose | Methadone HCL |
| Methylin, Methylin ER | Methylphenidate HCL |
| MetroCream | Metronidazole |
| MetroGel, MetroGel-Vaginal | Metronidazole |
| MetroLotion | Metronidazole |
| Miacalcin, Miacalcin Nasal Spray | Calcitonin—Salmon |
| Micatin | Miconazole |
| MicroNefrin, Nephron, S-2 Inhalant | Epinephrine, Racemic |
| Milk of Magnesia | Magnesium Hydroxide |
| Minocin, Dynacin, Arestin | Minocycline |
| Mintezol | Thiabendazole |
| Mintox | Aluminum Hydroxide with Magnesium Hydroxide |
| MiraLax | Polyethylene Glycol—Electrolyte Solution |
| Monistat | Miconazole |
| Motrin, Children's Motrin | Ibuprofen |
| MS Contin | Morphine Sulfate |
| Mucomyst | Acetylcysteine |
| Mucosol | Acetylcysteine |
| Murine Ear | Carbamide Peroxide |
| Myambutol | Ethambutol HCL |
| Mycamine | Micafungin Sodium |
| Mycelex, Mycelex-7 | Clotrimazole |
| Mycifradin | Neomycin Sulfate |
| Mycobutin | Rifabutin |
| Mycostatin | Nystatin |
| Myfortic | Mycophenolate Sodium |
| Mylanta Gas | Simethicone |

| Trade Name | Generic Name |
|---|---|
| Mylanta, Mylanta Extra Strength | Aluminum Hydroxide with Magnesium Hydroxide |
| Mylicon | Simethicone |
| Mysoline | Primidone |
| Nallpen | Nafcillin |
| Naprelan | Naproxen Sodium |
| Naprosyn | Naproxen |
| Narcan | Naloxone |
| Nasacort HFA, Nasacort AQ | Triamcinolone |
| Nasalcrom | Cromolyn |
| Nasarel | Flunisolide |
| Nascobal | Cyanocobalamin (Vitamin $B_{12}$) |
| Nasonex | Mometasone Furoate |
| Nebcin | Tobramycin |
| NebuPent | Pentamidine Isethionate |
| Nembutal | Pentobarbital |
| NeoBenz Micro | Benzoyl Peroxide |
| Neo-fradin | Neomycin Sulfate |
| NeoProfen | Ibuprofen |
| Neoral | Cyclosporine Microemulsion |
| Neosporin, Neosporin Ophthalmic | Neomycin/Polymyxin B/Bacitracin |
| Neosporin GU Irrigant | Neomycin/Polymyxin |
| Neo-synephrine | Phenylephrine HCL |
| Neo-synephrine 12-Hour Nasal | Oxymetazoline |
| Neo-Tabs | Neomycin Sulfate |
| Nephron | Epinephrine, Racemic |
| Neupogen, G-CSF | Filgrastim |
| Neurontin | Gabapentin |
| Neut | Sodium Bicarbonate |
| NeutraPhos, NeutraPhos-K | Phosphorus Supplements |
| Nexium | Esomeprazole |
| Niacor | Niacin (Vitamin $B_3$) |
| Niaspan | Niacin (Vitamin $B_3$) |
| Nicotinic acid | Niacin (Vitamin $B_3$) |
| Nifediac CC | Nifedipine |
| Niferex | Iron—Oral Preparations |
| Nilstat | Nystatin |
| Nipride | Nitroprusside |
| Nitro-Bid | Nitroglycerin |
| Nitro-Dur | Nitroglycerin |
| Nitro-Mist | Nitroglycerin |
| Nitropress (previously available as) | Nitroprusside |
| Nitrostat | Nitroglycerin |
| Nitro-Time | Nitroglycerin |
| Nix | Permethrin |
| Nizoral, Nizoral A-D | Ketoconazole |
| Norcuron | Vecuronium Bromide |
| Noriate | Metronidazole |
| Normal Serum Albumin (Human) | Albumin, Human |

| Trade Name | Generic Name |
|---|---|
| Normodyne | Labetalol |
| Noroxin | Norfloxacin |
| Norvasc | Amlodipine |
| Nostrilla | Oxymetazoline |
| NuLYTELY | Polyethylene Glycol—Electrolyte Solution |
| Nutr-E-sol | Vitamin E/Alpha-Tocopherol |
| NVP* | Nevirapine |
| Nydrazid | Isoniazid |
| OCL* | Polyethylene Glycol—Electrolyte Solution |
| Ocuflox | Ofloxacin |
| Ocusulf-10 | Sulfacetamide Sodium Ophthalmic |
| Omnicef | Cefdinir |
| Omnipaque 140, Omnipaque 240, Omnipaque 300, and Omnipaque 350 | Iohexol |
| Omnipen | Ampicillin |
| Opticrom | Cromolyn |
| Optivar | Azelastine |
| Orajel Perioseptic | Carbamide Peroxide |
| Oramorph SR | Morphine Sulfate |
| Orapred, Orapred ODT | Prednisolone |
| Orasone | Prednisone |
| Orazinc | Zinc Salts |
| Os-Cal | Calcium Carbonate |
| Osmitrol | Mannitol |
| OsmoPrep | Sodium Phosphate |
| Oxy-5, Oxy-10 | Benzoyl Peroxide |
| OxyContin | Oxycodone |
| Oxytrol | Oxybutynin Chloride |
| Pacerone | Amiodarone HCL |
| Plasbumin | Albumin, Human |
| Palgic | Carbinoxamine |
| Palmitate-A 5000 | Vitamin A |
| Pamelor | Nortriptyline Hydrochloride |
| Pamix | Pyrantel Pamoate |
| Panadol | Acetaminophen |
| Patanol | Olopatadine |
| Pathocil | Dicloxacillin Sodium |
| Paxil, Paxil CR | Paroxetine |
| Pediaflor | Fluoride |
| Pediamycin | Erythromycin Preparations |
| Pediapred | Prednisolone |
| Pediazole | Erythromycin Ethylsuccinate and Acetylsulfisoxazole |
| PediOtic | Polymyxin B Sulfate, Neomycin Sulfate, Hydrocortisone |
| Pentam 300 | Pentamidine Isethionate |
| Pentasa | Mesalamine |

*Common abbreviation or other name (not recommended for use when writing a prescription).

| Trade Name | Generic Name |
|---|---|
| Pentothal | Thiopental Sodium |
| Pepcid, Pepcid AC [OTC], Pepcid Complete [OTC], Pepcid RPD | Famotidine |
| Pepto-Bismol | Bismuth Subsalicylate |
| Percocet | Oxycodone and Acetaminophen |
| Percodan | Oxycodone and Aspirin |
| Perdiem Fiber Therapy | Psyllium |
| Perforomist | Formoterol |
| Periactin (previously available as) | Cyproheptadine |
| Periostat | Doxycycline |
| Pexeva | Paroxetine |
| $PGE_1$* | Alprostadil |
| Pfizerpen | Penicillin G Preparations—Aqueous Potassium and Sodium |
| Phazyme | Simethicone |
| Phenergan | Promethazine |
| Phenytek | Phenytoin |
| PhosLo | Calcium Acetate |
| Pilocar | Pilocarpine HCL |
| Pima | Potassium Iodide |
| Pin-Rid | Pyrantel Pamoate |
| Pin-X | Pyrantel Pamoate |
| Pipracil | Piperacillin |
| Pitressin | Vasopressin |
| Plaquenil | Hydroxychloroquine |
| Polymox | Amoxicillin |
| Polysporin Ophthalmic | Bacitracin + Polymyxin B |
| Polysporin Topical | Bacitracin + Polymyxin B |
| Polytrim Ophthalmic Solution | Polymyxin B Sulfate and Trimethoprim Sulfate |
| Posture | Calcium Phosphate, Tribasic |
| Potassium Phosphate | Phosphorus Supplements |
| Prelone | Prednisolone |
| Prevacid | Lansoprazole |
| Prevalite | Cholestyramine |
| Prilosec, Prilosec OTC | Omeprazole |
| Primacor | Milrinone |
| Primaxin IV, Primaxin IM | Imipenem and Cilastatin |
| Principen | Ampicillin |
| Prinivil | Lisinopril |
| Procanbid | Procainamide |
| Procardia, Procardia XL | Nifedipine |
| Procrit | Epoetin Alfa |
| Proglycem | Diazoxide |
| Prograf | Tacrolimus |
| Pronestyl | Procainamide |
| Pronto | Pyrethrins |
| Prostaglandin E1 | Alprostadil |

*Common abbreviation or other name (not recommended for use when writing a prescription).

| Trade Name | Generic Name |
|---|---|
| Prostigmin | Neostigmine |
| Prostin VR Pediatric | Alprostadil |
| Protonix | Pantoprazole |
| Protopam | Pralidoxime Chloride |
| Protopic | Tacrolimus |
| Protostat | Metronidazole |
| Proventil, Proventil HFA | Albuterol |
| Provera | Medroxyprogesterone |
| Prozac, Prozac Weekly | Fluoxetine Hydrochloride |
| Pseudo Carb Pediatric | Carbinoxamine + Pseudoephedrine |
| PTU* | Propylthiouracil |
| Pulmicort Respules, Pulmicort Turbuhaler, Pulmicort Flexhaler | Budesonide |
| Pulmozyme | Dornase Alfa/Dnase |
| Pyrazinoic Acid Amide | Pyrazinamide |
| Pyridium | Phenazopyridine HCL |
| Pyrinyl | Pyrethrins |
| Quelicin | Succinylcholine |
| Questran, Questran Light | Cholestyramine |
| Quineprox | Hydroxychloroquine |
| Quinidex | Quinidine |
| Quixin | Levofloxacin |
| QVAR* | Beclomethasone Dipropionate |
| Raniclor | Cefaclor |
| Rapamune | Sirolimus |
| Rebetol | Ribavirin |
| Reese's Pinworm | Pyrantel Pamoate |
| Regitine | Phentolamine Mesylate |
| Reglan | Metoclopramide |
| Renova | Tretinoin |
| Resectisol | Mannitol |
| Retin-A, Retin-A Micro | Tretinoin |
| Retrovir, AZT* | Zidovudine |
| Revatio | Sildenafil |
| Reversol | Edrophonium Chloride |
| R-Gene 10 | Arginine Chloride |
| Rhinocort Aqua Nasal Spray | Budesonide |
| RID | Pyrethrins |
| Rifadin | Rifampin |
| Rimactane | Rifampin |
| Riomet | Metformin |
| Risperdal, Risperdal M-Tab, Risperdal Consta | Risperidone |
| Ritalin, Ritalin SR, Ritalin LA | Methylphenidate HCL |
| Robaspheres | Ribavirin |
| Robinul | Glycopyrrolate |
| Rocaltrol | Calcitriol |
| Rocephin | Ceftriaxone |

*Common abbreviation or other name (not recommended for use when writing a prescription).

| Trade Name | Generic Name |
|---|---|
| Rogaine, Men's Rogaine Extra Strength (previously available as) | Minoxidil |
| Romazicon | Flumazenil |
| Rowasa | Mesalamine |
| Roxanol | Morphine Sulfate |
| Roxicet | Oxycodone and Acetaminophen |
| Roxicodone | Oxycodone |
| Roxilox | Oxycodone and Acetaminophen |
| Roxiprin | Oxycodone and Aspirin |
| RuLox Plus | Aluminum Hydroxide with Magnesium Hydroxide |
| S-2 Inhalant | Epinephrine, Racemic |
| Salagen | Pilocarpine HCL |
| Salicylazosulfapyridine | Sulfasalazine |
| Sal-Tropine | Atropine Sulfate |
| Sandimmune | Cyclosporine |
| Sandostatin, Sandostatin LAR Depot | Octreotide Acetate |
| Sani-Supp | Glycerin |
| Sarafem | Fluoxetine Hydrochloride |
| SAS* | Sulfasalazine |
| Scopace | Scopolamine Hydrobromide |
| Selsun | Selenium Sulfide |
| Senna-Gen | Senna/Sennosides |
| Senokot | Senna/Sennosides |
| Septra | Sulfamethoxazole and Trimethoprim |
| Serevent Diskus | Salmeterol |
| Serutan | Psyllium |
| Sildec | Carbinoxamine + Pseudoephedrine |
| Silvadene | Silver Sulfadiazine |
| Singulair | Montelukast |
| Slo-Niacin | Niacin (Vitamin $B_3$) |
| Slow FE | Iron—Oral Preparations |
| Sodium Phosphate | Phosphorus Supplements |
| Solu-cortef | Hydrocortisone |
| Solu-Medrol | Methylprednisolone |
| Soluspan | Betamethasone |
| Sotret | Isotretinoin |
| Sporanox | Itraconazole |
| SPS | Sodium Polystyrene Sulfonate |
| SSD Cream, SSD AF Cream | Silver Sulfadiazine |
| SSKI | Potassium Iodide |
| Stimate | Desmopressin Acetate |
| Strattera | Atomoxetine |
| Streptase | Streptokinase |
| Sublimaze | Fentanyl |
| Sudafed | Pseudoephedrine |
| Sulfatrim | Sulfamethoxazole and Trimethoprim |
| Sumycin | Tetracycline HCL |

*Common abbreviation or other name (not recommended for use when writing a prescription).

| Trade Name | Generic Name |
|---|---|
| Sunkist Vitamin C | Ascorbic Acid |
| Suprax | Cefixime |
| Surfak | Docusate |
| Survanta | Surfactant, Pulmonary/Beractant |
| Symbicort | Budesonide and Formoterol |
| Symmetrel | Amantadine Hydrochloride |
| Synagis | Palivizumab |
| Synercid | Quinupristin and Dalfopristin |
| Synthroid | Levothyroxine ($T_4$) |
| Tagamet, Tagamet HB [OTC] | Cimetidine |
| Tambocor | Flecainide Acetate |
| Tamiflu | Oseltamivir Phosphate |
| Tapazole | Methimazole |
| Tazicef | Ceftazidime |
| Tazidime | Ceftazidime |
| Tegretol, Tegretol-XR | Carbamazepine |
| Tempra | Acetaminophen |
| Tenormin | Atenolol |
| Tensilon | Edrophonium Chloride |
| Tetrahydrocannabinol | Dronabinol |
| THC* | Dronabinol |
| Theo-24 | Theophylline |
| TheoCap | Theophylline |
| Theochron | Theophylline |
| Therazene | Silver Sulfadiazine |
| Thiamilate | Thiamine |
| Thorazine | Chlorpromazine |
| ThyroSave | Potassium Iodide |
| ThyroShield | Potassium Iodide |
| Tiazac | Diltiazem |
| Ticar | Ticarcillin |
| Tigan | Trimethobenzamide HCL |
| Timentin | Ticarcillin and Clavulanate |
| Tinactin | Tolnaftate |
| Tisit | Pyrethrins |
| TMP-SMX | Sulfamethoxazole and Trimethoprim |
| TOBI | Tobramycin |
| Tobrex | Tobramycin |
| Tofranil, Tofranil-PM | Imipramine |
| Topamax | Topiramate |
| Toprol-XL | Metoprolol |
| Totacillin | Ampicillin |
| tPA* | Alteplase |
| Trandate | Labetalol |
| Transderm Scop | Scopolamine Hydrobromide |
| Triaz | Benzoyl Peroxide |
| Trileptal | Oxcarbazepine |

*Common abbreviation or other name (not recommended for use when writing a prescription).

| Trade Name | Generic Name |
|---|---|
| Trilisate | Choline Magnesium Trisalicylate |
| TriLyte | Polyethylene Glycol—Electrolyte Solution |
| Trimethoprim-Sulfamethoxazole | Sulfamethoxazole and Trimethoprim |
| Trimox | Amoxicillin |
| Tums | Calcium Carbonate |
| Tylenol | Acetaminophen |
| Tylenol #1, #2, #3, #4 | Codeine and Acetaminophen |
| Tylox | Oxycodone and Acetaminophen |
| Unasyn | Ampicillin/Sulbactam |
| Unipen | Nafcillin |
| Uniphyl | Theophylline |
| Urecholine | Bethanechol Chloride |
| Uro-KP-Neutral | Phosphorus Supplements |
| Urolene Blue | Methylene Blue |
| Urso 250, Urso Forte | Ursodiol |
| Valcyte | Valganciclovir |
| Valium | Diazepam |
| Valtrex | Valacyclovir |
| Vancocin | Vancomycin |
| Vantin | Cefpodoxime Proxetil |
| VariZig | Varicella-Zoster Immune Globulin (Human) |
| Vasotec | Enalapril Maleate |
| Vasotec IV | Enalaprilat |
| Veetids | Penicillin V Potassium |
| Velosef | Cephradine |
| Venofer | Iron—Injectable Preparations (iron sucrose) |
| Ventolin HFA | Albuterol |
| Verelan, Verelan PM | Verapamil |
| Vermox | Mebendazole |
| Versed (previously available as) | Midazolam |
| VFEND | Voriconazole |
| Viagra | Sildenafil |
| Vibramycin | Doxycycline |
| Viramune, NVP* | Nevirapine |
| Virazole | Ribavirin |
| Visicol | Sodium Phosphate |
| Visine LR | Oxymetazoline |
| Vistaril | Hydroxyzine |
| Vistide | Cidofovir |
| Vitamin $B_1$ | Thiamine |
| Vitamin $B_2$ | Riboflavin |
| Vitamin $B_3$ | Niacin (Vitamin $B_3$) |
| Vitamin $B_6$ | Pyridoxine |
| Vitamin $B_{12}$ | Cyanocobalamin (Vitamin $B_{12}$) |
| Vitamin C | Ascorbic Acid |

*Common abbreviation or other name (not recommended for use when writing a prescription).

| Trade Name | Generic Name |
|---|---|
| Vitrase | Hyaluronidase |
| VoSpire ER | Albuterol |
| VZIG | Varicella-Zoster Immune Globulin (Human) |
| WinRho-SDF | $Rh_O$ (D) Immune Globulin Intravenous (Human) |
| Wycillin | Penicillin G Preparations—Procaine |
| Wymox | Amoxicillin |
| Xopenex, Xopenex HFA | Levalbuterol |
| Xylocaine | Lidocaine |
| Zantac, Zantac 75 [OTC], Zantac 150 Maximum Strength [OTC] | Ranitidine HCL |
| Zarontin | Ethosuximide |
| Zaroxolyn | Metolazone |
| Zegrid | Omeprazole |
| Zemuron | Rocuronium |
| Zestril | Lisinopril |
| Zinacef (IV) | Cefuroxime |
| Zincate | Zinc Salts |
| Zithromax, Zithromax TRI-PAK, Zithromax | Azithromycin |
| Zoderm | Benzoyl Peroxide |
| Zofran | Ondansetron |
| Zolicef | Cefazolin |
| Zoloft | Sertraline HCL |
| Zonegran | Zonisamide |
| ZORprin | Aspirin |
| Zosyn | Piperacillin with Tazobactam |
| Zovirax | Acyclovir |
| Z-PAK, Zmax | Azithromycin |
| Zyloprim | Allopurinol |
| Zyrtec, Children's Zyrtec | Cetirizine |
| Zyrtec-D 12 Hour | Cetirizine + Pseudoephedrine |
| Zyvox | Linezolid |

## VI. DRUG DOSES

### ACETAMINOPHEN

Tylenol, Tempra, Panadol, Feverall, Asprin Free Anacin, and many others

***Analgesic, antipyretic***

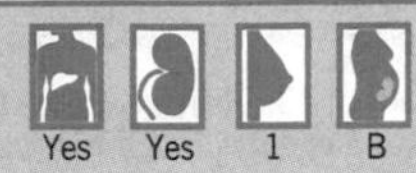


**Tabs [OTC]:** 325, 500, 650 mg
**Chewable tabs [OTC]:** 80, 160 mg; some may contain phenylalanine
**Infant drops, solution/suspension [OTC]:** 80 mg/0.8 mL
**Child suspension/syrup [OTC]:** 160 mg/5 mL
**Oral liquid [OTC]:** 160, 166.7 mg/5 mL; may contain 7% alcohol
**Elixir [OTC]:** 160 mg/5 mL
**Caplet [OTC]:** 160, 500, 650 mg
**Extended-release caplet/geltab [OTC]:** 650 mg
**Gelcap [OTC]:** 500 mg
**Capsules [OTC]:** 500 mg
**Dispersible tabs (Tylenol Children's Meltaways) [OTC]:** 80 mg
**Suppositories [OTC]:** 80, 120, 325, 650 mg
(Combination product with Codeine, see *Codeine and Acetaminophen*)

***Neonate:*** 10–15 mg/kg/dose PO/PR Q6 8 hr. Some advocate loading doses of 20–25 mg/kg/dose for PO dosing or 30 mg/kg/dose for PR dosing.
***Pediatric:*** 10–15 mg/kg/dose PO/PR Q4–6 hr; **max. dose:** 90 mg/kg/24 hr. For rectal dosing, some may advocate a 40–45 mg/kg/dose loading dose.

***Dosing by weight (preferred) or age (PO/PR Q4–6 hr):***

| Weight (lb) | Weight (kg) | Age | Dosage (mg) |
|---|---|---|---|
| 6–11 | 2.7–5 | 0–3 mo | 40 |
| 12–17 | 5.1–7.7 | 4–11 mo | 80 |
| 18–23 | 7.8–10.5 | 1–2 yr | 120 |
| 24–35 | 10.6–15.9 | 2–3 yr | 160 |
| 36–47 | 16–21.4 | 4–5 yr | 240 |
| 48–59 | 21.5–26.8 | 6–8 yr | 320 |
| 60–71 | 26.9 32.3 | 9–10 yr | 400 |
| 72–95 | 32.4–43.2 | 11 yr | 480 |

***Adult:*** 325–650 mg/dose
**Max. dose:** 4 g/24 hr, 5 doses/24 hr

Does not possess anti-inflammatory activity. **Use with caution** in patients with known G6PD deficiency.

$T_{1/2}$: 1–3 hr, 2–5 hr in neonates; metabolized in the liver; see Chapter 2, Table 2-3 for management of overdosage.

Some preparations contain alcohol (7%–10%) and/or phenylalanine; all suspensions should be shaken before use.

May decrease the activity of lamotrigine and increase the activity of zidovudine. Rifampin and anticholinergic agents (e.g., scopolamine) may decrease the effect of acetaminophen. Increased risk for hepatotoxicity may occur with barbiturates, carbamazepine, phenytoin, carmustine (with high acetaminophen doses), and chronic alcohol use. **Adjust dose in renal failure (see Chapter 31).**

For explanation of icons, see p. 698.

## ACETAZOLAMIDE

Diamox and others

***Carbonic anhydrase inhibitor, diuretic***

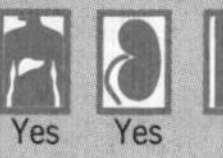 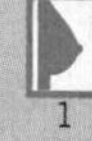 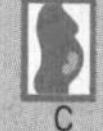

Yes Yes 1 C

**Tabs:** 125, 250 mg
**Oral suspension:** 25 mg/mL
**Capsules (sustained release):** 500 mg
**Injection (sodium):** 500 mg/5 mL
Contains 2.05 mEq Na/500 mg drug

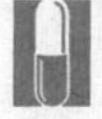

***Diuretic (PO, IV):***
***Child:*** 5 mg/kg/dose QD–QOD
***Adult:*** 250–375 mg/dose QD–QOD

***Glaucoma***
***Child:***
***PO:*** 8–30 mg/kg/24 hr ÷ Q6–8 hr
***IM/IV:*** 20–40 mg/kg/24 hr ÷ Q6 hr
***Adult:***
***PO (simple chronic; open angle):*** 1000 mg/24 hr ÷ Q6 hr
***IV (acute secondary; closed angle):*** For rapid decrease in intraocular pressure, administer 500 mg/dose IV.

***Seizures:*** 8–30 mg/kg/24 hr ÷ Q6–12 hr PO
**Max. dose:** 1 g/24 hr
***Urine alkalinization:*** 5 mg/kg/dose PO repeated BID–TID over 24 hr
***Management of hydrocephalus (see remarks):*** Start with 20 mg/kg/24 hr ÷ Q8 hr PO/IV; may increase to 100 mg/kg/24 hr up to a **max. dose** of 2 g/24 hr.

**Contraindicated** in hepatic failure, severe renal failure (GFR < 10 mL/min), and hypersensitivity to sulfonamides.

$T_{1/2}$: 2–6 hr; **do not use** sustained-release capsules in seizures; IM injection may be painful; bicarbonate replacement therapy may be required during long-term use (see *Citrate* or *Sodium Bicarbonate*).

Possible side effects (more likely with long-term therapy) include GI irritation, paresthesias, sedation, hypokalemia, acidosis, reduced urate secretion, aplastic anemia, polyuria, and development of renal calculi.

May increase toxicity of cyclosporine. Aspirin may increase toxicity of acetazolamide. May decrease the effects of salicylates, lithium, and phenobarbital. False-positive urinary protein may occur with several assays. **Adjust dose in renal failure (see Chapter 31).**

## ACETYLCYSTEINE

Mucomyst, Mucosol, Acetadote

***Mucolytic, antidote for acetaminophen toxicity***

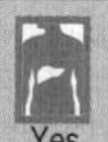 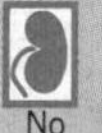 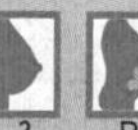 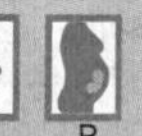

Yes No ? B

**Solution:** 100 mg/mL (10%) or 200 mg/mL (20%) (4, 10, 30 mL); contains EDTA
**Injectable (Acetadote):** 200 mg/mL (20%) (30 mL); contains EDTA 0.5 mg/mL

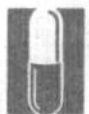

**For acetaminophen poisoning, see Chapter 2, Table 2-3.**
***Nebulizer:***
***Infant:*** 1–2 mL of 20% solution (diluted with equal volume of $H_2O$, or sterile saline to equal 10%), or 2–4 mL of 10% solution; administered TID–QID

*Continued*

ACETYLCYSTEINE *continued*

***Child:*** 3–5 mL of 20% solution (diluted with equal volume of $H_2O$, or sterile saline to equal 10%), or 6–10 mL of 10% solution; administer TID-QID

***Adolescent:*** 5–10 mL of 10% or 20% solution; administer TID-QID

***Distal intestinal obstruction syndrome in Cystic Fibrosis:***

***Adolescent and adult:*** 10 mL of 20% solution (diluted in a sweet drink) PO QID with 100 mL of 10% solution PR as an enema QD-QID

**Use with caution** in asthma. For nebulized use, give inhaled bronchodilator 10–15 min before use and follow with postural drainage and/or suctioning after acetylcysteine administration. Prior hydration is essential for distal intestinal obstruction syndrome treatment.

May induce bronchospasm, stomatitis, drowsiness, rhinorrhea, nausea, vomiting, and hemoptysis.

For IV use, elimination $T_{1/2}$ is longer in newborns (11 hr) than in adults (5.6 hr). $T_{1/2}$ is increased by 80% in patients with severe liver damage (Child-Pugh score of 7–13) and biliary cirrhosis (Child-Pugh score of 5–7).

## ACTH

See *Corticotropin*

## ACYCLOVIR

Zovirax and various generics

***Antiviral***

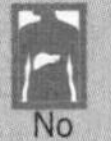
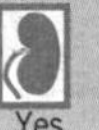
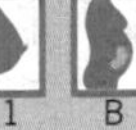
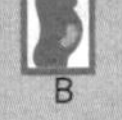

No Yes 1 B

**Capsules:** 200 mg
**Tabs:** 400, 800 mg
**Oral suspension:** 200 mg/5 mL; may contain parabens
**Ointment:** 5% (15 g)
**Cream:** 5% (2 g)
**Injection in powder (with sodium):** 500, 1000 mg
**Injection in solution (with sodium):** 50 mg/mL
Contains 4.2 mEq Na/1 g drug

**IMMUNOCOMPETENT:**

***Neonatal (HSV and HSV encephalitis):***

***<35 wk postconceptional age:*** 40 mg/kg/24 hr ÷ Q12 hr IV × 14–21 days

***≥35 wk postconceptional age:*** 60 mg/kg/24 hr ÷ Q8 hr IV × 14–21 days

***Mucocutaneous HSV (including genital):***

***Initial infection:***

***IV:*** 15 mg/kg/24 hr or 750 mg/m²/24 hr ÷ Q8 hr × 5–7 days

***PO:*** 1200 mg/24 hr ÷ Q8 hr × 7–10 days with a **max. dose** in children at 80 mg/kg/24 hr ÷ Q6–8 hr

***Recurrence:***

***PO:*** 1200 mg/24 hr ÷ Q8 hr or 1600 mg/24 hr ÷ Q12 hr × 5 days with a **max. dose** in children at 80 mg/kg/24 hr ÷ Q6–8 hr

***Chronic suppressive therapy:***

***PO:*** 800–1000 mg/24 hr ÷ 2–5 times/24 hr for up to 1 yr with a **max. dose** in children at 80 mg/kg/24 hr ÷ Q6–8 hr

*Continued*

For explanation of icons, see p. 698.

ACYCLOVIR *continued*

***IMMUNOCOMPETENT (cont'd):***

***Zoster:***

***IV:*** 30 mg/kg/24 hr or 1500 mg/m²/24 hr ÷ Q8 hr × 7–10 days

***PO:*** 4000 mg/24 hr ÷ 5 times/24 hr × 5–7 days for patients ≥ 12 yr

***Varicella:***

***IV:*** 30 mg/kg/24 hr or 1500 mg/m²/24 hr ÷ Q8 hr × 7–10 days

***PO:*** 80 mg/kg/24 hr ÷ QID × 5 days (begin treatment at earliest signs/symptoms); **max. dose:** 3200 mg/24 hr

**Max. dose** of oral acyclovir in children = 80 mg/kg/24 hr

**IMMUNOCOMPROMISED:**

***HSV:***

***IV:*** 750–1500 mg/m²/24 hr ÷ Q8 hr × 7–14 days

***PO:*** 1000 mg/24 hr ÷ 3–5 times/24 hr × 7–14 days

***HSV prophylaxis:***

***IV:*** 750 mg/m²/24 hr ÷ Q8 hr during risk period

***PO:*** 600–1000 mg/24 hr ÷ 3–5 times/24 hr during risk period

***Varicella or zoster:***

***IV:*** 1500 mg/m²/24 hr ÷ Q8 hr × 7–10 days

***PO:*** 250–600 mg/m²/dose 4–5 times/24 hr

***CMV prophylaxis:***

***IV:*** 1500 mg/m²/24 hr ÷ Q8 hr during risk period

***PO:*** 800–3200 mg/24 hr ÷ Q6–24 hr during risk period

**Max. dose** of oral acyclovir in children = 80 mg/kg/24 hr

***TOPICAL:*** Apply 0.5 inch ribbon of 5% ointment for 4 inch square surface area 6 times a day × 7 days.

See most recent edition of the AAP *Red Book* for further details. **Use with caution** in patients with pre-existing neurologic or **renal impairment (adjust dose; see Chapter 31)** or dehydration. Adequate hydration and slow (1 hr) IV administration are essential to prevent crystallization in renal tubules. **Do not use** topical product on the eye or for the prevention of recurrent HSV infections. Oral absorption is unpredictable (15%–30%). Use ideal body weight for obese patients when calculating dosages. Resistant strains of HSV and VZV have been reported in immunocompromised patients (e.g., advanced HIV infection).

Can cause renal impairment; has been infrequently associated with headache, vertigo, insomnia, encephalopathy, GI tract irritation, elevated liver function tests, rash, urticaria, arthralgia, fever, and adverse hematologic effects. Probenecid decreases acyclovir renal clearance. Acyclovir may increase the concentration of tenofovir, and meperidine and its metabolite (normeperidine).

## ADENOSINE

Adenocard

***Antiarrhythmic***

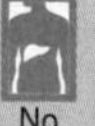
No
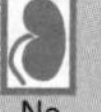
No
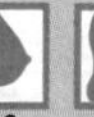
?
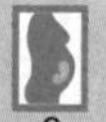
C

**Injection:** 3 mg/mL (2, 4 mL); preservative-free

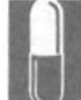

***Supraventricular tachycardia:***

***Child:*** 0.1–0.2 mg/kg rapid IV push over 1–2 seconds; may increase dose by 0.05 mg/kg increments every 2 min to **max.** of 0.25 mg/kg (up to 12 mg), or until termination of SVT. **Max. single dose:** 12 mg

***Adolescent and adult ≥ 50 kg:*** 6 mg rapid IV push over 1–2 seconds; if no response after 1–2 min, give 12 mg rapid IV push. May repeat a second 12 mg dose after 1–2 min if required. **Max. single dose:** 12 mg.

*Continued*

ADENOSINE *continued*

**Contraindicated** in 2nd and 3rd degree AV block or sick-sinus syndrome unless pacemaker placed. **Use with caution** in combination with digoxin (enhanced depressant effects on SA and AV nodes).

Follow each dose with NS flush. $T_{1/2}$: <10 seconds.

May precipitate bronchoconstriction, especially in asthmatics. Side effects include transient asystole, facial flushing, headache, shortness of breath, dyspnea, nausea, chest pain, and lightheadedness.

Carbamazepine and dipyridamole may increase the effects/toxicity of adenosine. Methylxanthines (e.g., caffeine and theophylline) may decrease the effects of adenosine.

## ALBUMIN, HUMAN

Albuminar, Albutein, Buminate, Plasbumin, Normal Serum Albumin (Human), and others

***Blood product derivative, plasma volume expander***

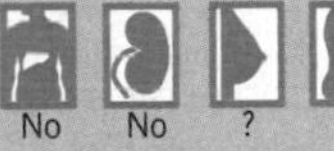

No No ? C

**Injection:** 5% (50 mg/mL) (50, 250, 500, mL) ; 25% (250 mg/mL) (20, 50, 100 mL); both concentrations contain 130–160 mEq Na/L

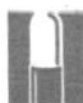

***Hypoproteinemia:***

***Child:*** 0.5–1 g/kg/dose IV over 30–120 min; repeat Q1–2 days PRN
***Adult:*** 25 g/dose IV over 30–120 min; repeat Q1–2 days PRN

***Hypovolemia:***

***Child:*** 0.5–1 g/kg/dose IV rapid infusion
***Adult:*** 25 g/dose IV rapid infusion; may repeat PRN

**Max. dose:** 6 g/kg/24 hr or 250 g/48 hr

**Contraindicated** in cases of CHF or severe anemia; rapid infusion may cause fluid overload; hypersensitivity reactions may occur; may cause rapid increase in serum sodium levels.

**Caution:** 25% concentration **contraindicated** in preterm infants due to risk of IVH. For infusion, use 5 micron filter or larger. Both 5% and 25% products are isotonic but differ in oncotic effects. Dilutions of the 25% product should be made with $D_5W$ or NS; **avoid sterile water.**

## ALBUTEROL

Proventil, VoSpire ER (sustained-release tabs), Proventil HFA (aerosol inhaler), Ventolin HFA (aerosol inhaler), AccuNeb (prediluted nebulized solution), and many others

***Beta-2-adrenergic agonist***

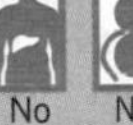

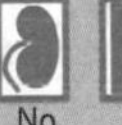

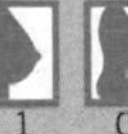

No No 1 C

**Tabs:** 2, 4 mg
**Sustained-release tabs:** 4, 8 mg
**Oral solution:** 2 mg/5 mL (473 mL)
**Aerosol inhaler:** 90 mcg/actuation (200 actuations/inhaler) (17 g)
**Nebulization solution:** 0.5% (5 mg/mL) (20 mL)
**Prediluted nebulized solution:** 0.63 mg in 3 mL NS, 1.25 mg in 3 mL NS, and 2.5 mg in 3 mL NS (0.083%)

*Continued*

For explanation of icons, see p. 698.

ALBUTEROL *continued*

***Inhalations (nonacute use):***
***Aerosol (MDI):*** 1–2 puffs (90–180 mcg) Q4–6 hr PRN
***Nebulization:***
- ***<1 yr:*** 0.05–0.15 mg/kg/dose Q4–6 hr
- ***1–5 yr:*** 1.25–2.5 mg/dose Q4–6 hr
- ***5–12 yr:*** 2.5 mg/dose Q4–6 hr
- ***>12 yr:*** 2.5–5 mg/dose Q4–8 hr

***For use in acute exacerbations more aggressive dosing may be employed.***
***Oral:***
- ***2–6 yr:*** 0.3 mg/kg/24 hr PO ÷ TID; **max. dose:** 12 mg/24 hr
- ***6–12 yr:*** 6 mg/24 hr PO ÷ TID; **max. dose:** 24 mg/24 hr
- ***>12 yr and adult:*** 2–4 mg/dose PO TID-QID; **max. dose:** 32 mg/24 hr

Inhaled doses may be given more frequently than indicated. In such cases, consider cardiac monitoring and monitoring of serum potassium. Systemic effects are dose related. Please verify the concentration of the nebulization solution used.

Use of oral dosage form is discouraged due to increased side effects and decreased efficacy compared to inhaled formulations.

Possible side effects include tachycardia, palpitations, tremor, insomnia, nervousness, nausea, and headache.

The use of tube spacers or chambers may enhance efficacy of the metered dose inhalers and have been proven to be just as effective and sometimes safer than nebulizers. Proventil HFA and Ventolin HFA are CFC-free metered dose inhalers. MDIs containing CFCs will be discontinued on Dec. 31, 2008.

## ALLOPURINOL

Zyloprim, Alloprim, and others
***Uric acid lowering agent, xanthine oxidase inhibitor***

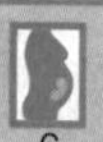

Yes Yes 1 C

**Tabs:** 100, 300 mg
**Oral suspension:** 20 mg/mL
**Injection (Alloprim):** 500 mg
Contains ~1.45 mEq Na/500 mg drug

**For use in tumor lysis syndrome, see Chapter 22.**
***Child:***
- ***Oral:*** 10 mg/kg/24 hr PO ÷ BID-QID; **max. dose:** 800 mg/24 hr
- ***Injectable:*** 200 mg/m²/24 hr IV ÷ Q6–12 hr; **max. dose:** 600 mg/24 hr

***Adult:***
- ***Oral:*** 200–800 mg/24 hr PO ÷ BID-TID
- ***Injectable:*** 200–400 mg/m²/24 hr IV ÷ Q6–12 hr; **max. dose:** 600 mg/24 hr

**Adjust dose in renal failure (see Chapter 31).** Must maintain adequate urine output and alkaline urine.

Drug interactions: increases serum theophylline level; may increase the incidence of rash with ampicillin and amoxicillin; increase risk of toxicity with azathioprine, didanosine and mercaptopurine; and increased risk of hypersensitivity reactions with ACE inhibitors and thiazide diuretics.

Side effects include rash, neuritis, hepatotoxicity, GI disturbance, bone marrow suppression, and drowsiness.

IV dosage form is very alkaline and must be **diluted to a minimum concentration** of 6 mg/mL and infused over 30 min.

## ALPROSTADIL

Prostin VR Pediatric, Prostaglandin $E_1$, $PGE_1$

***Prostaglandin $E_1$, vasodilator***

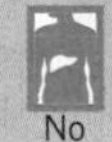
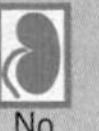
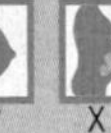

No No ? X

**Injection:** 500 mcg/mL (1 mL); contains dehydrated alcohol

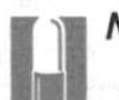

***Neonate:***

***Initial:*** 0.05–0.1 mcg/kg/min. Advance to 0.2 mcg/kg/min if necessary.

***Maintenance:*** When increase in $PaO_2$ is noted, decrease immediately to lowest effective dose. Usual dosage range: 0.01–0.4 mcg/kg/min; doses above 0.4 mcg/kg/min not likely to produce additional benefit.

***To prepare infusion:*** See the inside front cover.

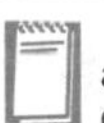

For palliation only. Continuous vital sign monitoring essential. May cause apnea (10%–12%), fever, seizures, flushing, bradycardia, hypotension, diarrhea, gastric outlet obstruction, and reversible cortical proliferation of long bones (with prolonged use). Decreases platelet aggregation.

## ALTEPLASE

Activase, Cathflo Activase, tPA

***Thrombolytic agent, tissue plasminogen activator***

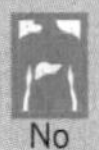
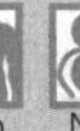
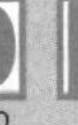
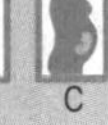

No No ? C

**Injection:**

**Cathflo Activase:** 2 mg

**Activase:** 50 mg (29 million unit), 100 mg (58 million unit)

Contains L-arginine and polysorbate 80

***Occluded IV catheter:***

***Aspiration method:*** Use 1 mg/1 mL concentration as follows:

| Age/Weight | Single-Lumen CVL | Double-Lumen CVL | Subcutaneous Port |
|---|---|---|---|
| <10 kg | 0.5 mg, dilute with normal saline to required volume to fill line | 0.5 mg each lumen, dilute with normal saline to required volume to fill line | 0.5 mg, dilute with normal saline to 3 mL |
| ≥10 kg | 1–2 mg, use required amount to fill lumen (**max:** 2 mg) | 1–2 mg each lumen, use required amount to fill lumen (**max:** 2 mg) and treat one lumen at a time | 2 mg, dilute with normal saline to 3 mL |

CVL, central venous line.

Instill into catheter over 1–2 min and leave in place for 2 hr before attempting blood withdrawal. After 2 hr, attempts to withdraw blood may be made every 2 hr for 3

*Continued*

FORMULARY

For explanation of icons, see p. 698.

ALTEPLASE *continued*

attempts. Dose may be repeated once in 24 hr using a longer catheter dwell time of 3–4 hr. After 3–4 hr (repeat dose), attempts to withdraw blood may be made every 2 hr for 3 attempts. **DO NOT** infuse into patient.

***Systemic thrombolytic therapy (use in consultation with a hematologist):*** 0.1–0.6 mg/kg/hr × 6 hr has been recommended (*Chest* 2004;126:645S-687S). The length of continuous infusion is variable as patients may respond to longer or shorter courses of therapy.

---

Current use in the pediatric population is limited. May cause bleeding, rash and increase prothrombin time.

**THROMBOLYTIC USE:** History of stroke, transient ischemic attacks, other neurologic disase and hypertension are **contraindications** for adults but considered relative **contraindications** for children. Monitor fibrinogen, thrombin clotting time, PT, and aPTT when used as a thrombolytic.

Newborns have reduced plasminogen levels (~50% of adult values) which decrease the thrombolytic effects of alteplase. Plasminogen supplementation may be necessary.

## ALUMINUM HYDROXIDE

Amphojel, Alu-Tab, Dialume, AlternaGEL, and various generics

***Antacid, phosphate binder***

No Yes ? C

**Tabs [OTC]:** 500, 600 mg
**Caps [OTC]:** 500 mg
**Oral suspension [OTC]:** 320 mg, 450 mg, 600 mg, 675 mg/5 mL (180, 360, 480 mL)
Each tablet, capsule, and 5 mL suspension contains <0.13 mEq Na.

---

***(mL volume dosages are based on the 320 mg/5 mL oral suspension concentration)***

***Peptic ulcer:***
- ***Child:*** 5–15 mL PO Q3–6 hr or 1–3 hr PC and HS
- ***Adult:*** 15–45 mL PO Q3–6 hr or 1–3 hr PC and HS

***Prophylaxis against GI bleeding:***
- ***Neonate:*** 1 mL/kg/dose PO Q4 hr PRN
- ***Infant:*** 2–5 mL PO Q1–2 hr
- ***Child:*** 5–15 mL PO Q1–2 hr
- ***Adult:*** 30–60 mL PO Q1–2 hr

***Hyperphosphatemia:***
- ***Child:*** 50–150 mg/kg/24 hr ÷ Q4–6 hr PO
- ***Adult:*** 30–40 mL TID-QID PO between meals and QHS

---

**Use with caution** in patients with renal failure and upper GI hemorrhage.

Interferes with the absorption of several orally administered medications, including digoxin, ethambutol, indomethacin, isoniazid, tetracyclines, quinolones (e.g., ciprofloxacin), and iron. Generally, **do not** take oral medications within 1–2 hr of taking aluminum dose unless specified.

May cause constipation, decreased bowel motility, encephalopathy, and phosphorus depletion.

## ALUMINUM HYDROXIDE WITH MAGNESIUM HYDROXIDE

Maalox, Mylanta, Mylanta Extra Strength, Almacone, Almacone II Double Strength, RuLox Plus, Mintox, and many others

***Antacid***

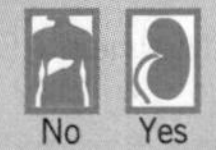
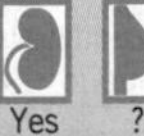
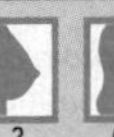
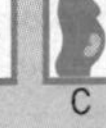

No Yes ? C

**Chewable tabs [OTC]:** ($Al(OH)_3$: $Mg(OH)_2$)
Mintox: 200 mg: 200 mg; contains saccharin
Almacone: 200 mg: 200 mg + simethicone 20 mg
Each tablet contains 0.03–0.06 mEq Na.

**Oral suspension [OTC]:**
Maalox, Mylanta, and Almacone: Each 5 mL contains 200 mg AlOH, 200 mg MgOH, and 20 mg simethicone (150, 360, 720 mL).
Mylanta Extra Strength, and Almacone II Double Strength: Each 5 mL contains 400 mg AlOH, 400 mg MgOH, and 40 mg simethicone (360, 480 mL).
RuLox Plus: Each 5 mL contains 500 mg AlOH, 450 mg MgOH, and 40 mg simethicone (355 mL).
Many other combinations exist.
Contains 0.03–0.06 mEq Na/5 mL

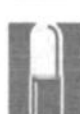

Same as for aluminum hydroxide preparations. **Do not use** combination product for hyperphosphatemia.

May have laxative effect. May cause hypokalemia. **Use with caution** in patients with renal insufficiency (magnesium), gastric outlet obstruction.

Interferes with the absorption of the benzodiazepines, chloroquine, digoxin, phenytoin, quinolones (e.g., ciprofloxacin), tetracyclines, and iron. Generally, **do not** take oral mediations within 1–2 hr of taking antacid dose unless specified.

## AMANTADINE HYDROCHLORIDE

Symmetrel and others

***Antiviral agent***

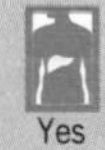
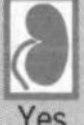
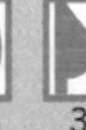
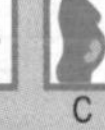
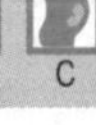

Yes Yes 3 C

**Capsule:** 100 mg
**Tabs:** 100 mg
**Syrup:** 50 mg/5 mL (480 mL); may contain parabens

***Influenza A prophylaxis and treatment (for treatment, it is best to initiate therapy immediately after the onset of symptoms; within 2 days):***

***1–9 yr:*** 5 mg/kg/24 hr PO ÷ QD-BID; **max. dose:** 150 mg/24 hr

***>9 yr:***

***<40 kg:*** 5 mg/kg/24 hr PO ÷ QD-BID; **max. dose:** 200 mg/24 hr

***≥40 kg:*** 200 mg/24 hr ÷ QD-BID

***Alternative dosing for influenza A prophylaxis:***

***Child >20 kg and adult:*** 100 mg/24 hr PO ÷ QD-BID

***Prophylaxis (duration of therapy):***

***Single exposure:*** At least 10 days

***Repeated/uncontrolled exposure:*** Up to 90 days

Use with influenza A vaccine when possible.

*Continued*

For explanation of icons, see p. 698.

AMANTADINE HYDROCHLORIDE *continued*

***Symptomatic treatment (duration of therapy):***
Continue for 24–48 hr after disappearance of symptoms.

**Do not use** in the first trimester of pregnancy. **Use with caution** in patients with liver disease, seizures, renal disease, congestive heart failure, peripheral edema, orthostatic hypotension, history of recurrent eczematoid rash, and in those receiving CNS stimulants. **Adjust dose in patients with renal insufficiency (see Chapter 31).** Individuals immunized with live attenuated influenza vaccine should not receive amantadine prophylaxis for 14 days after the vaccine.

May cause dizziness, anxiety, depression, mental status change, rash (livedo reticularis), nausea, orthostatic hypotension, edema, CHF, and urinary retention. Neuroleptic malignant syndrome has been reported with abrupt dose reduction or discontinuation (especially if patient is receiving neuroleptics).

## AMIKACIN SULFATE

Amikin

***Antibiotic, aminoglycoside***

No
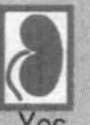

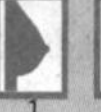

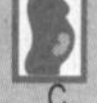


**Injection:** 50, 250 mg/mL; may contain sodium bisulfite

***Neonate:*** See the following table.

| Post-conceptional Age (wk) | Postnatal Age (days) | Dose (mg/kg/dose) | Interval (hr) |
|---|---|---|---|
| ≤29* | 0–7 | 18 | 48 |
| | 8–28 | 15 | 36 |
| | >28 | 15 | 24 |
| 30–33 | 0–7 | 18 | 36 |
| | >7 | 15 | 24 |
| 34–37 | 0–7 | 15 | 24 |
| | >7 | 15 | 18–24 |
| ≥38 | 0–7 | 15 | 24 |
| | >7 | 15 | 12–18 |

*Or significant asphyxia, PDA, indomethicin use, poor cardiac output, reduced renal function.

***Infant and child:*** 15–22.5 mg/kg/24 hr ÷ Q8 hr IV/IM; infants and patients requiring higher doses (see remarks) may receive initial doses of 30 mg/kg/24 hr ÷ Q8 hr IV/IM
***Adult:*** 15 mg/kg/24 hr ÷ Q8–12 hr IV/IM
**Initial max. dose:** 1.5 g/24 hr; then monitor levels

**Use with caution** in pre-existing renal, vestibular or auditory impairment; concomitant anesthesia or neuromuscular blockers, neurotoxic; concomitant neurotoxic, ototoxic, or nephrotoxic drugs; sulfite sensitivity; and dehydration. **Adjust dose in renal failure (see Chapter 31).** Rapidly eliminated in patients

*Continued*

AMIKACIN SULFATE *continued*

with cystic fibrosis, burns, and in febrile neutropenic patients. CNS penetration is poor beyond early infancy.

Therapeutic levels: peak, 20–30 mg/L; trough 5–10 mg/L. Recommended serum sampling time at steady-state: trough within 30 min prior to the third consecutive dose and peak 30–60 min after the administration of the third consecutive dose.

Peak levels of 25–30 mg/L have been recommended for CNS, pulmonary, bone, life-threatening infections and in febrile neutropenic patients. Longer dosing intervals may be necessary for neonates receiving indomethacin for PDAs and for all patients with poor cardiac output.

May cause ototoxicity, nephrotoxicity, neuromuscular blockade, and rash. Loop diuretics may potentiate the ototoxicity of all aminoglycoside antibiotics.

## AMINOCAPROIC ACID

Amicar and other generics

***Hemostatic agent***

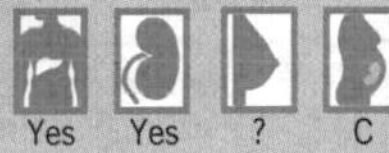

Yes Yes ? C

**Tabs:** 500, 1000 mg
**Oral liquid/syrup:** 250 mg/mL (480 mL); may contain 0.2% methylparaben and 0.05% propylparaben
**Injection:** 250 mg/mL (20 mL); contains 0.9% benzyl alcohol

***Child:***

***Loading dose:*** 100–200 mg/kg IV/PO
***Maintenance:*** 100 mg/kg/dose Q4–6 hr; **max. dose:** 30 g/24 hr

**Contraindications:** DIC, hematuria. **Use with caution** in patients with cardiac, renal, or hepatic disease. Should not be given with Factor IX Complex concentrates or Anti-Inhibitor Coagulant concentrates because of risk for thrombosis. Dose should be reduced by 75% in oliguria or end-stage renal disease. Hypercoagulation may be produced when given in conjunction with oral contraceptives.

May cause nausea, diarrhea, malaise, weakness, headache, decreased platelet function, hypotension, and false increase in urine amino acids. Elevation of serum potassium may occur, especially in patients with renal impairment.

## AMINOPHYLLINE

Various generic products

***Bronchodilator, methylxanthine***

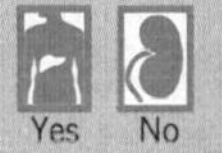
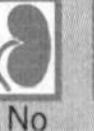
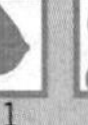
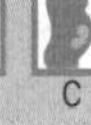

Yes No 1 C

**Tabs:** 100, 200 mg (79% theophylline)
**Injection:** 25 mg/mL (79% theophylline)
**Note:** Pharmacy may dilute IV dosage forms to enhance accuracy of neonatal dosing.

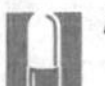

***PO:***

***Infant:*** (see *Theophylline* and convert to mg of Aminophylline)
***1–9 yr:*** 27 mg/kg/24 hr ÷ Q4–6 hr
***9–12 yr:*** 20 mg/kg/24 hr ÷ Q6 hr
***12–16 yr:*** 16 mg/kg/24 hr ÷ Q6 hr
***Adult:*** 12.5 mg/kg/24 hr ÷ Q6 hr

*Continued*

For explanation of icons, see p. 698.

AMINOPHYLLINE *continued*

***Neonatal apnea:***

***Loading dose:*** 5–6 mg/kg IV or PO

***Maintenance dose:*** 1–2 mg/kg/dose Q6–8 hr, IV or PO

***IV loading:*** 6 mg/kg IV over 20 min (each 1.2 mg/kg dose raises the serum theophylline concentration 2 mg/L)

***IV maintenance:*** Continuous IV drip:

***Neonate:*** 0.2 mg/kg/hr

***6 wk–6 mo:*** 0.5 mg/kg/hr

***6 mo–1 yr:*** 0.6–0.7 mg/kg/hr

***1–9 yr:*** 1–1.2 mg/kg/hr

***9–12 yr and young adult smoker:*** 0.9 mg/kg/hr

***>12 yr healthy nonsmoker:*** 0.7 mg/kg/hr

These total daily doses may also be administered IV ÷ Q4–6 hr.

Consider mg of theophylline available when dosing aminophylline.

Monitoring serum levels is essential especially in infants and young children. Intermittent dosing for infants and children 1–5 yr may require Q4 hr dosing regimen due to enhanced drug clearance. Side effects: restlessness, GI upset, headache, tachycardia, seizures (may occur in absence of other side effects with toxic levels).

Therapeutic level (theophylline): for asthma, 10–20 mg/L; for neonatal apnea, 6–13 mg/L.

Recommended Guidelines for obtaining levels:

IV bolus: 30 min after infusion

IV continuous: 12–24 hr after initiation of infusion

PO liquid, immediate-release tab:

*Peak:* 1 hr post dose

*Trough:* just before dose

PO sustained release:

*Peak:* 4 hr post dose

*Trough:* just before dose

Ideally, obtain levels after steady-state has been achieved (after at least one day of therapy). Liver impairment, cardiac failure, and sustained high fever may increase theophylline levels. See *Theophylline* for drug interactions.

Use in breast-feeding may cause irritability in infant.

## AMIODARONE HCL

Cordarone, Pacerone, and various generics

***Antiarrhythmic, Class III***

Yes No 3 D

**Tabs:** 100, 200, 400 mg

**Oral suspension:** 5 mg/mL

**Injection:** 50 mg/mL (3 mL) (contains 20.2 mg/mL benzyl alcohol and 100 mg/mL polysorbate 80 or Tween 80)

Contains 37% iodine by weight

***See the algorithms on the inside front cover for arrest dosing.***

***Child PO:***

***<11 yr:*** 600–800 mg/1.73 $m^2$/24 hr ÷ Q12–24 hr × 4–14 days and/or until adequate control achieved; then reduce to 200–400 mg/1.73 $m^2$/24 hr.

*Continued*

AMIODARONE HCL *continued*

≥***1 yr:*** 10–15 mg/kg/24 hr ÷ Q12–24 hr × 4–14 days and/or until adequate control achieved, then reduce to 5 mg/kg/24 hr ÷ Q12–24 hr if effective.

***Child IV (limited data):***

5 mg/kg over 30 min followed by a continuous infusion starting at 5 micrograms (mcg)/kg/min; infusion may be increased up to a **max. dose** of 15 mcg/kg/min or 20 mg/kg/24 hr.

***Adult PO:***

***Loading dose:*** 800–1600 mg QD for 1–3 wk

***Maintenance:*** 600–800 mg QD × 1 mo, then 200–400 mg QD

***Use lowest effective dose to minimize adverse reactions.***

***Adult IV:***

***Loading dose:*** 150 mg over 10 min (15 mg/min) followed by 360 mg over 6 hr (1 mg/min); followed by a maintenance dose of 0.5 mg/min. Supplemental boluses of 150 mg over 10 min may be given for breakthrough VF or hemodynamically unstable VT, and the maintenance infusion may be increased to suppress the arrhythmia. **Max. dose:** 2.1 g/24 hr.

---

Used in the resuscitation algorithm for ventricular fibrillation/pulseless ventricular tachycardia **(see the inside front cover for arrest dosing and the figures at the back of the book for the PALS algorithm).** Overall use of this drug may be limited to its potentially life-threatening side effects and the difficulties associated with managing its use.

**Contraindicated** in severe sinus node dysfunction, marked sinus bradycardia, second- and third-degree AV block. **Use with caution** in hepatic impairment.

Long elimination half-life (40–55 days). Major metabolite is active.

Increases cyclosporine, digoxin, phenytoin, tacrolimus, warfarin, calcium channel blockers, theophylline, and quinidine levels. Amiodarone is a CYP 450 3A3/4 substrate and inhibits CYP 3A3/4, 2C9, and 2D6.

Proposed therapeutic level with chronic oral use: 1–2.5 mg/L.

Asymptomatic corneal microdeposits should appear in all patients. Alters liver enzymes, thyroid function. Pulmonary fibrosis reported in adults. May cause worsening of preexisting arrhythmias with bradycardia and AV block. May also cause hypotension, anorexia, nausea, vomiting, dizziness, paresthesias, ataxia, tremor, SIADH, and hypothyroidism or hyperthyroidism.

Intravenous continuous infusion concentration for peripheral administration **should not exceed** 2 mg/mL and **must be** diluted with $D_5W$. The intravenous dosage form can leach out plasticizers such as DEHP. It is recommended to reduce the potential exposure to plasticizers in pregnant women and children at the toddler stages of development and younger by using alternative methods of IV drug administration. The preservative-free intravenous product is available as an orphan/compassionate use drug from Academic Pharmaceuticals, Inc. at (847) 735-1170.

Oral administration should be consistent with regards to meals because food increases the rate and extent of oral absorption.

For explanation of icons, see p. 698.

## AMITRIPTYLINE

Elavil and others

***Antidepressant, tricyclic***

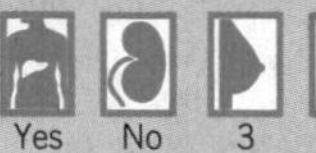

Yes No 3 C

**Tabs:** 10, 25, 50, 75, 100, 150 mg

***Antidepressant:***

***Child:*** Start with 1 mg/kg/24 hr ÷ TID PO for 3 days; then increase to 1.5 mg/kg/24 hr. Dose may be gradually increased to a **max. dose** of 5 mg/kg/24 hr if needed. Monitor ECG, BP, and heart rate for doses > 3 mg/kg/24 hr.

***Adolescent:*** 10 mg TID PO with 20 mg QHS; dose may be gradually increased up to a **max. dose** of 200 mg/24 hr if needed.

***Adult:*** 40–100 mg/24 hr ÷ QHS-BID PO; dose may be gradually increased up to 300 mg/24 hr if needed; gradually decrease dose to lowest effective dose when symptoms are controlled.

***Augment analgesia for chronic pain:***

***Initial:*** 0.1 mg/kg/dose QHS PO; increase as needed and tolerated over 2–3 wk to 0.5–2 mg/kg/dose QHS

***Migrane prophylaxis:***

***Child:*** Initial 0.1–0.25 mg/kg/dose QHS PO; increase as needed and tolerated every 2 wk by 0.1–0.25 mg/kg/dose up to a **max. dose** of 2 mg/kg/24 hr or 75 mg/24 hr. For doses > 1 mg/kg/24 hr, divide daily dose BID and monitor ECG.

***Adult:*** 25–50 mg/dose QHS PO

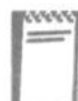

**Contraindicated** in narrow-angle glaucoma, seizures, severe cardiac disorders, and patients who received MAO inhibitors within 14 days. **See Chapter 2 for management of toxic ingestion.**

$T_{1/2}$ = 9–25 hr in adults. Maximum antidepressant effects may not occur for 2 wk or more after initiation of therapy. **Do not abruptly discontinue therapy in patients receiving high doses for prolonged periods.**

Therapeutic levels (sum of amitripylline and nortriptyline): 100–250 ng/mL. Recommended serum sampling time: obtain a single level 8 hr or more after an oral dose (following 4–5 days of continuous dosing). Amitriptyline is a substrate for CYP 450 1A2, 2C9, 2C19, 2D6, and 3A3/4.

Side effects include sedation, urinary retention, constipation, dry mouth, dizziness, drowsiness, liver enzyme elevation and arrhythmia. May discolor urine (blue/green). QHS dosing during first weeks of therapy will reduce sedation. Monitor ECG, BP, CBC at start of therapy and with dose changes. Decrease dose if PR interval reaches 0.22 sec, QRS reaches 130% of baseline, HR rises above 140/min, or if BP is more than 140/90. Tricyclics may cause mania. For antidepressant use, monitor for clinical worsening of depression and suicidal ideation/behavior following the initiation of therapy or after dose changes.

## AMLODIPINE

Norvasc

***Calcium channel blocker, antihypertensive***

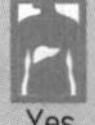 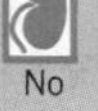 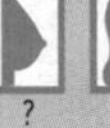 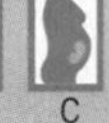

Yes No ? C

**Tabs:** 2.5, 5, 10 mg

**Oral suspension:** 1 mg/mL

*Continued*

AMLODIPINE *continued*

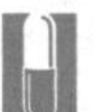

***Child:***

***Hypertension:*** Start with 0.1 mg/kg/dose (**max. dose:** 5 mg) PO QD-BID; dosage may be gradually increased to a **max. dose** of 0.6 mg/kg/24 hr up to 20 mg/24 hr.

***Adult:***

***Hypertension:*** 5–10 mg/dose QD PO; use 2.5 mg/dose QD PO in patients with hepatic insufficiency.

**Max. dose:** 10 mg/24 hr

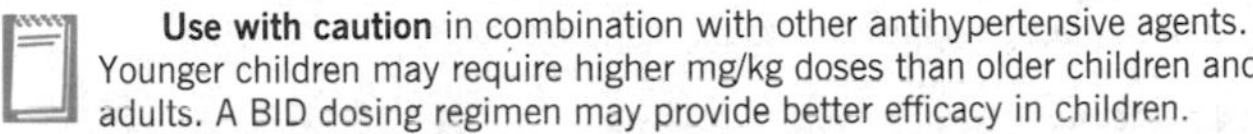

**Use with caution** in combination with other antihypertensive agents. Younger children may require higher mg/kg doses than older children and adults. A BID dosing regimen may provide better efficacy in children.

Reduce dose in hepatic insufficiency. Allow 5-7 days of continuous initial dose therapy before making dosage adjustments because of the drug's gradual onset of action and lengthy elimination half-life. Amlodipine is a substrate for CYP 450 3A4 and should be used with **caution** with 3A4 inhibitors such as protease inhibitors and azole antifungals (e.g., fluconazole and ketoconazole).

Dose-related side effects include edema, dizziness, flushing, fatigue, and palpitations. Other side effects include headache, nausea, abdominal pain, and somnolence.

## AMMONIUM CHLORIDE

***Diuretic, urinary acidifying agent***

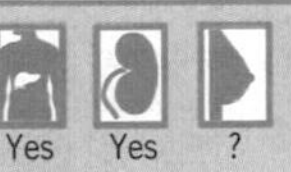

Yes Yes ? C

**Injection:** 5 mEq/mL (26.75%) (20 mL); contains EDTA
1 mEq = 53 mg

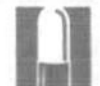

***Urinary acidification:***

***Child:*** 75 mg/kg/24 hr ÷ Q6 hr IV; **max. dose:** 6 g/24 hr

***Adult:*** 1.5 g/dose Q6 hr IV

***Drug administration:*** Dilute to concentration ≤ 0.4 mEq/mL. Infusion **not to exceed** 50 mg/kg/hr or 1 mEq/kg/hr.

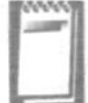

**Contraindicated** in hepatic or renal insufficiency and primary respiratory acidosis. **Use with caution** in infants.

May produce acidosis, hyperammonemia, and GI irritation. Monitor serum chloride level, acid/base status, and serum ammonia.

## AMOXICILLIN

Amoxil, Trimox, Wymox, Polymox, DisperMox, and others

***Antibiotic, aminopenicillin***

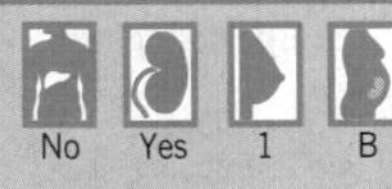

No Yes 1 B

**Drops:** 50 mg/mL (15, 30 mL)
**Oral suspension:** 125, 250 mg/5 mL (80, 100, 150 mL); and 200, 400 mg/5 mL (50, 75, 100 mL)
**Caps:** 250, 500 mg
**Tablets:** 500, 875 mg
**Chewable tabs:** 125, 200, 250, 400 mg

*Continued*

For explanation of icons, see p. 698.

AMOXICILLIN *continued*

**Tablets for oral suspension (DisperMox):** 200, 400 mg; contains phenylalanine

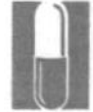

***Neonate – ≤3 mo:*** 20–30 mg/kg/24 hr ÷ Q12 hr PO
***Child:***
***Standard dose:*** 25–50 mg/kg/24 hr ÷ Q8–12 hr PO
***High dose (resistant* S. pneumoniae):** 80–90 mg/kg/24 hr ÷ BID PO
***Adult:***
***Mild/moderate infections:*** 250 mg/dose Q8 hr PO OR 500 mg/dose Q12 hr PO
***Severe infections:*** 500 mg/dose Q8 hr PO OR 875 mg/dose Q12 hr PO
**Max. dose:** 2–3 g/24 hr
***Recurrent otitis media prophylaxis:*** 20 mg/kg/dose QHS PO
***SBE prophylaxis:*** See Chapter 7.
***Early Lyme disease:***
***Child:*** 50 mg/kg/24 hr ÷ Q8 hr PO × 14–21 days; **max. dose:** 1.5 g/24 hr
***Adult:*** 500 mg/dose Q8 hr PO × 14–21 days

Renal elimination. **Adjust dose in renal failure (see Chapter 31).** Serum levels about twice those achieved with equal dose of ampicillin. Fewer GI effects, but otherwise similar to ampicillin. Side effects: rash and diarrhea.

High-dose regimen increasingly useful in respiratory infections, acute otitis media, and sinusitis, owing to increasing incidence of penicillin-resistant pneumococci. Chewable tablets and DisperMox may contain phenylalanine and should not be used by phenyketonurics.

DisperMox oral suspension is prepared by swirling/stirring each tablet thoroughly in approximately 10 mL of water only. **Do not** chew or swallow (whole tablets) DisperMox.

## AMOXICILLIN–CLAVULANIC ACID

Augmentin, Augmentin ES-600, Augmentin XR, and various generic products
***Antibiotic, aminopenicillin with beta-lactamase inhibitor***

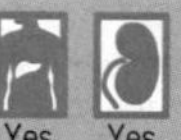
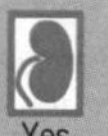
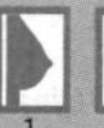
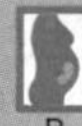


**Tabs:**
**For TID dosing:** 250, 500 mg (with 125 mg clavulanate)
**For BID dosing:** 875 mg amoxicillin (with 125 mg clavulanate); Augmentin XR: 1 g amoxicillin (with 62.5 mg clavulanate)
**Chewable tabs:**
**For TID dosing:** 125, 250 mg amoxicillin (31.25 and 62.5 mg clavulanate, respectively); contains saccharin
**For BID dosing:** 200, 400 mg amoxicillin (28.5 and 57 mg clavulanate, respectively); contains saccharin and aspartame
**Oral suspension:**
**For TID dosing:** 125, 250 mg amoxicillin/5 mL (31.25 and 62.5 mg clavulanate/5 mL, respectively) (75, 100, 150 mL); contains saccharin
**For BID dosing:** 200, 400 mg amoxicillin/5 mL (28.5 and 57 mg clavulanate/5 mL, respectively) (50, 75, 100 mL); 600 mg amoxicillin/5 mL (Augmentin ES-600; contains 42.9 mg clavulanate/5 mL) (50, 75, 100, 150 mL); contains saccharin and/or aspartame
Contains 0.63 mEq $K^+$ per 125 mg clavulanate (Augmentin ES-600 contains 0.23 mEq $K^+$ per 42.9 mg clavulanate)

*Continued*

AMOXICILLIN–CLAVULANIC ACID *continued*

***Dosage based on amoxicillin component.***
***Child < 3 mo:*** 30 mg/kg/24 hr ÷ Q12 hr PO (recommended dosage form is 125 mg/5 mL suspension)
***Child ≥ 3 mo:***
 ***TID dosing (see remarks):***
  20–40 mg/kg/24 hr ÷ Q8 hr PO
 ***BID dosing (see remarks):***
  25–45 mg/kg/24 hr ÷ Q12 hr PO
 ***Augmentin ES-600:***
  ***≥3 mo and <40 kg:*** 90 mg/kg/24 hr ÷ Q12 hr PO × 10 days
***Adult:*** 250–500 mg/dose Q8 hr PO or 875 mg/dose Q12 hr PO for more severe and respiratory infections
 ***Augmentin XR:***
  ***≥16 yr and adult:*** 2 g Q12 hr PO × 10 days for acute bacterial sinusitis or × 7–10 days for community-acquired pneumonia

Clavulanic acid extends the activity of amoxicillin to include beta-lactamase producing strains of *H. influenzae, M. catarrhalis, N. gonorrhoeae,* some *S. aureus* and may increase the risk for diarrhea. See *Amoxicillin* for additional remarks. **Adjust dose in renal failure (see Chapter 31). Contraindicated** in patients with a history of cholestatic jaundice/hepatic dysfunction associated with amoxicillin–clavulanic acid. Augmentin XR is **contraindicated** in patients with CrCl < 30 mL/min.

The BID dosing schedule is associated with less diarrhea. For BID dosing, the 875 mg, 1 g tablets, the 200 mg, 400 mg chewable tablets or the 200 mg/5 mL, 400 mg/5 mL, 600 mg/5 mL suspensions should be used. These BID dosage forms contain phenylalanine and **should not be used** by phenyketonurics. For TID dosing, the 250 mg, 500 mg tablets, the 125 mg, 250 mg chewable tablets or the 125 mg/5 mL, 250 mg/5 mL suspensions should be used.

Higher doses of 80–90 mg/kg/24 hr (amoxicillin component) have been recommended for resistant strains of *S. pneumoniae* in acute otitis media (use BID formulations containing 7:1 ratio of amoxicillin to clavulanic acid or Augmentin ES-600).

The 250 or 500 mg tablets **cannot** be substituted for Augmentin XR.

## AMPHOTERICIN B

Fungizone, Amphocin
***Antifungal, polyene***

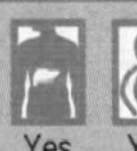
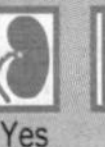
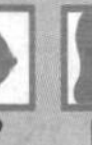

Yes Yes ? B

**Injection:** 50 mg vials

***IV:*** mix with $D_5W$ to concentration 0.1 mg/mL (peripheral administration) or 0.25 mg/mL (central line only). pH >4.2. Infuse over 2–6 hr.
***Optional test dose:*** 0.1 mg/kg/dose IV up to **max. dose** of 1 mg (followed by remaining initial dose).
***Initial dose:*** 0.5–1 mg/kg/24 hr; if test dose NOT used, infuse first dose over 6 hr and monitor frequently during the first several hr.
***Increment:*** Increase as tolerated by 0.25–0.5 mg/kg/24 hr QD or QOD
***Usual maintenance:***
 ***QD dosing:*** 0.5–1 mg/kg/24 hr QD
 ***QOD dosing:*** 1.5 mg/kg/dose QOD

*Continued*

For explanation of icons, see p. 698.

AMPHOTERICIN B *continued*

**Max. dose:** 1.5 mg/kg/24 hr

***Intrathecal:*** 25–100 mcg Q48–72 hr. Increase to 500 mcg as tolerated.

***Bladder irrigation for urinary tract mycosis:*** 5–15 mg in 100 mL sterile water for irrigation at 100–300 mL/24 hr. Instill solution into bladder, clamp catheter for 1–2 hr, then drain; repeat TID-QID for 2–5 days.

---

Monitor renal, hepatic, electrolyte, and hematologic status closely. Hypercalciuria, hypokalemia, hypomagnesemia, RTA, renal failure, acute hepatic failure, hypotension, and phlebitis may occur. **For dosing information in renal failure, see Chapter 31.**

Common infusion-related reactions include fever, chills, headache, hypotension, nausea, vomiting; may premedicate with acetaminophen and diphenhydramine 30 min before and 4 hr after infusion. Meperidine useful for chills. Hydrocortisone, 1 mg/mg ampho (**max.:** 25 mg) added to bottle may help prevent immediate adverse reactions.

Salt loading with 10–15 mL/kg of NS infused prior to each dose may minimize the risk of nephrotoxicity.

## AMPHOTERICIN B LIPID COMPLEX

Abelcet

***Antifungal, polyene***

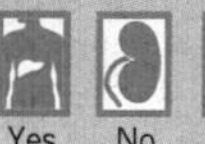
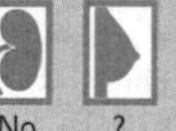
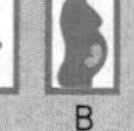

Yes No ? B

**Injection:** 5 mg/mL (10, 20 mL)
(formulated as a 1:1 molar ratio of amphotericin B to lipid complex comprised of dimyristoylphosphatidylcholine and dimyristoylphosphatidylglycerol)

---

***IV:*** 2.5–5 mg/kg/24 hr QD

For viseral leishmaniasis that failed to respond to or relapsed after treatment with antimony compound, a dosage of 1–3 mg/kg/24 hr QD × 5 days has been used.

Mix with $D_5W$ to concentration 1 mg/mL or 2 mg/mL for fluid restricted patients.

***Infusion rate:*** 2.5 mg/kg/hr; shake the infusion bag every 2 hr if total infusion time exceeds 2 hr. **Do not use** an in-line filter.

---

Monitor renal, hepatic, electrolyte, and hematologic status closely. Thrombocytopenia, anemia, leukopenia, hypokalemia, hypomagnesemia, diarrhea, respiratory failure, skin rash, and increases in liver enzymes and bilirubin may occur.

Highest concentrations achieved in spleen, lung, and liver from human autopsy data from one heart transplant patient. CNS/CSF levels are lower than amphotericin B, liposomal (AmBisome). In animal models, concentrations are higher in the liver, spleen, and lungs but the same in the kidneys when compared to conventional amphotericin B. Pharmacokinetics in renal and hepatic impairment have not been studied.

Common infusion-related reactions include fever, chills, rigors, nausea, vomiting, hypotension, and headache; may premedicate with acetaminophen, diphenhydramine and meperidine (see *Amphotericin B* remarks).

## AMPHOTERICIN B, LIPOSOMAL

AmBisome

***Antifungal, polyene***

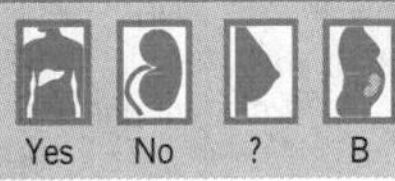


**Injection:** 50 mg (vials); contains sucrose
(formulated in liposomes composed of hydrogenated soy phosphatidylcholine, cholesterol, distearoylphosphatidylglycerol, and alpha-tocopherol)

***Systemic fungal infections:*** 3–5 mg/kg/24 hr IV QD; an upper dosage limit of 10 mg/kg/24 hr has been suggested based on pharmacokinetic endpoints and risk for hypokalemia. However, dosages as high as 15 mg/kg/24 hr have been used. Dosages as high as 10 mg/kg/24 hr have been used in patients with aspergillus.
***Empiric therapy for febrile neutropenia:*** 3 mg/kg/24 hr IV QD
***Cryptococcal meningitis in HIV:*** 6 mg/kg/24 hr IV QD
Mix with $D_5W$ to concentration 1–2 mg/mL (0.2–0.5 mg/mL may be used for infants and small children).
***Infusion rate:*** Administer dose over 2 hr; infusion may be reduced to 1 hr if well tolerated.

Monitor renal, hepatic, electrolyte, and hematologic status closely. Thrombocytopenia, tachycardia, hypokalemia, hypomagnesemia, hypocalcemia, hyperglycemia, diarrhea, dyspnea, skin rash, low back pain, and increases in liver enzymes and bilirubin may occur. Safety and effectiveness in neonates have not been established.

When compared to conventional amphotericin B, higher concentrations found in the liver and spleen; and similar concentrations found in the lungs and kidney. CNS/CSF concentrations are higher than other amphotericin B products. Pharmacokinetics in renal and hepatic impairment have not been studied.

Common infusion-related reactions include fever, chills, rigors, nausea, vomiting, hypotension, and headache; may premedicate with acetaminophen, diphenhydramine and meperidine (see *Amphotericin B* remarks).

## AMPICILLIN

Omnipen, Principen, Totacillin, and others

***Antibiotic, aminopenicillin***

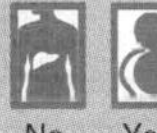

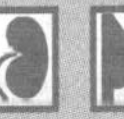

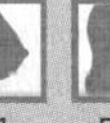

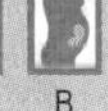


**Oral suspension:** 125 mg/5 mL (100, 150, 200 mL), 250 mg/5 mL (100, 200 mL)
**Caps:** 250, 500 mg
**Injection:** 250, 500 mg; 1, 2, 10 g
Contains 3 mEq Na/1 g IV drug

***Neonate (IM/IV):***
- ***<7 days:***
  - ***<2 kg:*** 50–100 mg/kg/24 hr ÷ Q12 hr
  - ***≥2 kg:*** 75–150 mg/kg/24 hr ÷ Q8 hr
  - ***Group B streptococcal meningitis:*** 200–300 mg/kg/24 hr ÷ Q8 hr
- ***≥7 days:***
  - ***<1.2 kg:*** 50–100 mg/kg/24 hr ÷ Q12 hr
  - ***1.2–2 kg:*** 75–150 mg/kg/24 hr ÷ Q8 hr
  - ***>2 kg:*** 100–200 mg/kg/24 hr ÷ Q6 hr
  - ***Group B streptococcal meningitis:*** 300 mg/kg/24 hr ÷ Q4–6 hr

*Continued*

For explanation of icons, see p. 698.

AMPICILLIN *continued*

***Infant/child:***

***Mild-moderate infections:***

***IM/IV:*** 100–200 mg/kg/24 hr ÷ Q6 hr

***PO:*** 50–100 mg/kg/24 hr ÷ Q6 hr; **max. PO dose:** 2–3 g/24 hr

***Severe infections:*** 200–400 mg/kg/24 hr ÷ Q4–6 hr IM/IV

***Adult:***

***IM/IV:*** 500–3000 mg Q4–6 hr

***PO:*** 250–500 mg Q6 hr

**Max. IV/IM dose:** 12 g/24 hr

***SBE prophylaxis:*** See Chapter 7.

Use higher doses to treat CNS disease. CSF penetration occurs only with inflammed meninges. **Adjust dose in renal failure (see Chapter 31).**

Produces the same side effects as penicillin, with cross-reactivity. Rash commonly seen at 5–10 days and rash may occur with concurrent EBV infection or allopurinol use. May cause interstitial nephritis, diarrhea, and pseudomembranous enterocolitis. Chloroquine reduces ampicillin's absorption.

## AMPICILLIN AND SULBACTAM

Unasyn

***Antibiotic, aminopenicillin with beta-lactamase inhibitor***

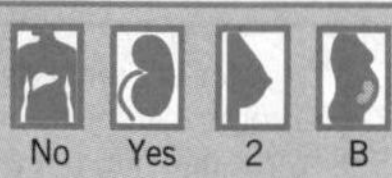


**Injection:**

1.5 g = ampicillin 1 g + sulbactam 0.5 g

3 g = ampicillin 2 g + sulbactam 1 g

Contains 5 mEq Na per 1.5 g drug combination

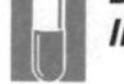

***Dosage based on ampicillin component:***

***Infant ≥ 1 mo:***

***Mild/moderate infections:*** 100–150 mg/kg/24 hr ÷ Q6 hr IM/IV

***Meningitis/severe infections:*** 200–300 mg/kg/24 hr ÷ Q6 hr IM/IV

***Child:***

***Mild/moderate infections:*** 100–200 mg/kg/24 hr ÷ Q6 hr IM/IV

***Meningitis/severe infections:*** 200–400 mg/kg/24 hr ÷ Q4–6 hr IM/IV

***Adult:*** 1–2 g Q6–8 hr IM/IV

**Max. dose:** 8 g ampicillin/24 hr

Similar spectrum of antibacterial activitiy to ampicillin with the added coverage of beta-lactamase producing organisms. Total sulbactam dose **should not exceed** 4 g/24 hr.

**Adjust dose in renal failure (see Chapter 31).** Similar CSF distribution and side effects to ampicillin.

## ANTIPYRINE AND BENZOCAINE

Allergen Ear Drops, Antipyrine and Benzocaine Otic, Autoguard Otic, Auralgan (available in Canada) and others

***Otic analgesic, cerumenolytic***

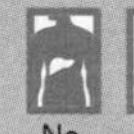 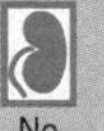 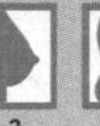

No No ? C

**Otic solution:** Antipyrine 5.4%, benzocaine 1.4% (15 mL); may contain oxyquinoline sulfate

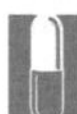

***Otic analgesia:*** Fill external ear canal (2–4 drops) Q1–2 hr PRN. After instillation of the solution, a cotton pledget should be moistened with the solution and inserted into the meatus.

***Cerumenolytic:*** Fill external ear canal (2–4 drops) TID–QID for 2–3 days.

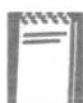

Benzocaine sensitivity may develop and not intended for prolonged use. **Contraindicated** if tympanic membrane perforated or PE tubes in place. Local reactions (e.g., burning, stinging) and hypersensitivity reactions may occur. Risk of benzocaine-induced methemoglobinemia may be increased in infants ≤ 3 mo of age.

## ARGININE CHLORIDE

R-Gene 10

***Metabolic alkalosis agent, urea cycle disorder treatment agent, growth hormone diagnostic agent***

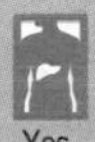 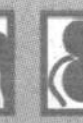 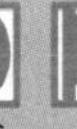 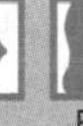 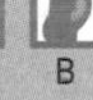

Yes Yes ? B

**Injection:** 10% (100 mg/mL) arginine hydrochloride, contains 47.5 mEq chloride per 100 mL (300 mL)
**Osmolality:** 950 mOsmol/L

***Used as a secondary alternative agent for patients that are unresponsive or unable to receive sodium chloride and potassium chloride.***

***Correction of hypochloremia:*** Arginine chloride dose in milliequivalents (mEq) = 0.2 × patient's weight (kg) × [103 − patient's serum chloride in mEq/L]. Administer ½ to ⅔ of the calculated dose and re-assess.

***Drug administration:*** **Do not exceed** an infusion rate of 1 g/kg/hr (4.75 mEq/kg/hr). Drug may be administered without further dilution but should be diluted to reduce risk of tissue irritation.

**Contraindicated** in renal or hepatic failure. **Use with extreme caution** as overdosages may result in hyperchloremic metabolic acidosis, cerebral edema and death. Arginine hydrochloride is metabolized to nitrogen-containing products for renal excretion. Excess arginine increases the production of nitric oxide (NO) to cause vasodilation/hypotension. Monitor acid/base status closely. Hyperglycemia, hyperkalemia, GI disturbances, IV extravasation, headache and flushing may occur.

In addition to being used for chloride supplementation, arginine is used in urea cycle disorder therapy (increases arginine levels and prevents breakdown of endogenous proteins) and as a diagnostic agent for growth hormone (stimulates pituitary release of growth hormone).

For explanation of icons, see p. 698.

## ASCORBIC ACID

Vitamin C, Cecon, Sunkist Vitamin C, and many others

***Water soluble vitamin***

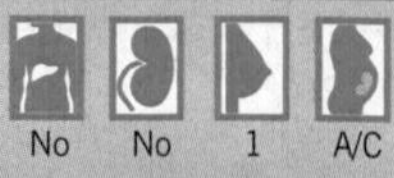


**Tabs [OTC]:** 100, 250, 500 mg, 1, 1.5 g
**Chewable tabs (Sunkist Vitamin C) [OTC]:** 60, 100, 200, 250, 500 mg; some may contain aspartame
**Tabs (timed release) [OTC]:** 0.5, 1, 1.5 g
**Caps [OTC]:** 500 mg
**Extended-release caps [OTC]:** 250, 500 mg
**Injection:** 500 mg/mL; may contain sodium hydrosulfite
**Oral solution (Cecon) [OTC]:** 100 mg/mL (50 mL with dropper)
**Oral liquid [OTC]:** 500 mg/5 mL (120, 480 mL)
**Lozenges [OTC]:** 25 mg (20s); contains 5 mg Na
**Crystals [OTC]:** 1 g per ¼ teaspoonful (170 g, 1000 g)
Some products may contain approximately 5 mEq Na/1 g drug and/or calcium.

***Scurvy (PO/IM/IV/SC):***
***Child:*** 100–300 mg/24 hr ÷ QD-BID for at least 2 wk
***Adult:*** 100–250 mg QD-BID for at least 2 wk
***U.S. Recommended Daily Allowance (RDA):***
***See Chapter 21.***

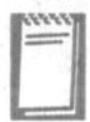

Adverse reactions: nausea, vomiting, heartburn, flushing, headache, faintness, dizziness, hyperoxaluria. Use high doses with **caution** in G6PD patients. May cause false-negative and false-positive urine glucose determinations with glucose oxidase and cupric sulfate tests, respectively.

Oral dosing is preferred with or without food. IM route is the preferred parenteral route. Protect the injectable dosage form from light.

Pregancy category changes to "C" if used in doses above the U.S. RDA.

## ASPIRIN

ASA, Anacin, Bufferin, ZORprin, and various trade names

***Nonsteroidal anti-inflammatory agent, antiplatelet agent, analgesic***

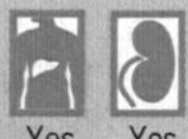

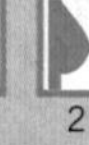

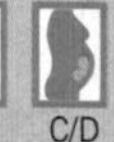


**Tabs [OTC]:** 325, 500 mg
**Tabs, enteric-coated [OTC]:** 81, 165, 325, 500, 650 mg
**Tabs, time-release:**
**OTC:** 81, 650 mg
**Prescription (ZORprin):** 800 mg
**Tabs, buffered [OTC]:** 325, 500 mg; may contain magnesium, aluminum, and/or calcium
**Tabs, chewable [OTC]:** 81 mg
**Gum [OTC]:** 227.5 mg
**Suppository [OTC]:** 120, 200, 300, 600 mg

*Continued*

ASPIRIN *continued*

***Analgesic/antipyretic:*** 10–15 mg/kg/dose PO/PR Q4–6 hr up to total of 60–80 mg/kg/24 hr
**Max. dose:** 4 g/24 hr
***Anti-inflammatory:*** 60–100 mg/kg/24 hr PO ÷ Q6–8 hr
***Kawasaki disease:*** 80–100 mg/kg/24 hr PO ÷ QID during febrile phase until defervesces then decrease to 3–5 mg/kg/24 hr PO QAM. Continue for at least 8 wk or until both platelet count and ESR are normal.

**Do not use** in children <16 yr for treatment of varicella or flu-like symptoms (risk for Reye's syndrome), in combination with other nonsteroidal anti-inflammatory drugs, or in severe renal failure. **Use with caution** in bleeding disorders, renal dysfunction, gastritis, and gout. May cause GI upset, allergic reactions, liver toxicity, and decreased platelet aggregation. **See Chapter 2 for management of overdose.**

Drug interactions: may increase effects of methotrexate, valproic acid, and warfarin which may lead to toxicity (protein displacement). Buffered dosage forms may decrease absorption of ketoconazole and tetracycline. GI bleeds have been reported with concurrent use of SSRIs (e.g., fluoxetine, paroxetine, sertraline).

Therapeutic levels: antipyretic/analgesic: 30–50 mg/L; anti-inflammatory: 150–300 mg/L. Tinnitus may occur at levels of 200–400 mg/L. Recommended serum sampling time at steady-state: Obtain trough level just prior to dose following 1–2 days of continuous dosing. Peak levels obtained 2 hr (for nonsustained-release dosage forms) after a dose may be useful for monitoring toxicity.

Pregnancy category changes to "D" if full-dose aspirin is used during the third trimester. **Adjust dose in renal failure (see Chapter 31).**

## ATENOLOL
Tenormin
***Beta-1 selective adrenergic blocker***

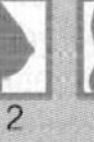
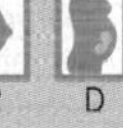
No Yes 2 D

**Injection:** 0.5 mg/mL (10 mL)
**Tab:** 25, 50, 100 mg
**Oral suspension:** 2 mg/mL

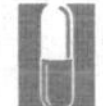
***Child and adolescent:*** 0.5–1 mg/kg/dose PO QD; **max. dose:** 2 mg/kg/24 hr up to 100 mg/24 hr.
***Adult:***
***PO:*** 25–100 mg/dose PO QD; **max. dose:** 200 mg/24 hr
***After myocardial infarction:*** 5 mg IV × 1 over 5 min and then repeat in 10 min if initial dose tolerated. Then start 50 mg/dose PO Q12 hr × 2 doses 10 min after last IV dose followed by 100 mg/24 hr PO ÷ QD–BID × 6–9 days. Discontinue atenolol if bradycardia or hypotension requiring treatment or any other untoward effects occur.

**Contraindicated** in pulmonary edema, cardiogenic shock. May cause bradycardia, hypotension, second- or third-degree AV block, dizziness, fatigue, lethargy, and headache. **Use with caution** in diabetes and asthma. Wheezing and dyspnea have occurred when daily dosage exceeds 100 mg/24 hr. Postmarketing evaluation reports a temporal relationship for causing elevated LFTs and/or bilirubin, hallucinations, psoriatic rash, thrombocytopenia, visual disturbances, and dry mouth. **Avoid** abrupt withdrawal of the drug. Does not cross the blood-brain

*Continued*

For explanation of icons, see p. 698.

ATENOLOL *continued*

barrier; lower incidence of CNS side effects compared to propranolol. Neonates born to mothers receiving atenolol during labor or while breast-feeding may be at risk for hypoglycemia.

**Adjust dose in renal impairment (see Chapter 31).** IV administration rate **not to exceed** 1 mg/min.

## ATOMOXETINE

Strattera

***Norepinephrine reuptake inhibitor, attention deficit hyperactivity disorder agent***

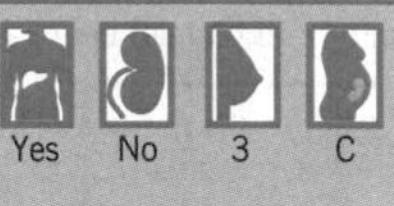


**Capsules:** 10, 18, 25, 40, 60, 80, 100 mg

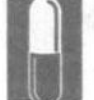

***≤70 kg (child ≥ 6 yr and adolescent):***

Start with 0.5 mg/kg/24 hr PO QAM and increase after a minimum of 3 days to approximately 1.2 mg/kg/24 hr PO ÷ QAM or BID (morning and late afternoon/early evening). **Max. daily dose:** 1.4 mg/kg/24 hr or 100 mg, whichever is less.

***If used with a strong CYP 450 2D6 inhibitor (e.g., fluoxetine, paroxetine, quinidine):*** Maintain above initial dose for 4 wk and increase to a **max.** of 1.2 mg/kg/24 hr if symptoms do not improve and initial dose is tolerated.

***>70 kg (child, adolescent, and adult):***

Start with 40 mg PO QAM and increase after a minimum of 3 days to about 80 mg/24 hr PO ÷ QAM or BID (morning and late afternoon/early evening). After 2–4 wk, dose may be increased to a **max.** of 100 mg/24 hr.

***If used with a strong CYP 450 2D6 inhibitor (e.g., fluoxetine, paroxetine, quinidine):*** Maintain above initial dose for 4 wk and increase to 80 mg/24 hr if symptoms do not improve and initial dose is tolerated.

**Contraindicated** in patients with narrow angle glaucoma. **Do not** administer with or within 2 wk after discontinuing an MAO inhibitor; fatal reactions have been reported. **Use with caution** in hypertension, tachycardia, cardiovascular or cerebrovascular diseases, or with concurrent albuterol therapy. Increased risk of suicidal thinking has been reported; closely monitor for clinical worsening, agitation, irritability, suicidal thinking or behaviors, and unusual changes in behavior when initiating (first few mo) or at times of dose changes (increases or decreases). Atomoxetine is a CYP 450 2D6 substrate.

Doses > 1.2 mg/kg/24 hr in patients ≤ 70 kg have not been shown to be of additional benefit. Reduce dose (initial and target doses) by 50% and 75% for patients with moderate (Child-Pugh Class B) and severe (Child-Pugh Class C) hepatic insufficiency, respectively.

Major side effects include GI discomfort, vomiting, fatigue, anorexia, dizziness, and mood swings. Hypersensitivity reactions, aggression, irritability, and severe liver injury have also been reported. Consider interrrupting therapy in patients who are not growing or gaining weight satisfactorily.

Doses may be administered with or without food. Atomoxetine can be discontinued without tapering.

A

## ATOVAQUONE
Mepron
***Antiprotozoal***

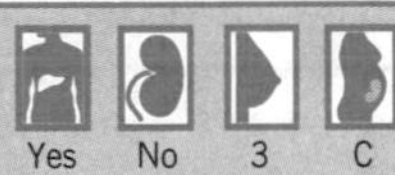
Yes No 3 C

**Oral suspension:** 750 mg/5 mL (210 mL); contains benzyl alcohol

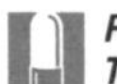

***Pneumocystis jiroveci (formerly carinii) pneumonia (PCP):***
***Treatment (21 day course):***
***Child:*** 30–40 mg/kg/24 hr PO ÷ BID with fatty foods; **max. dose:** 1500 mg/24 hr. Infants 3–24 mo may require higher doses of 45 mg/kg/24 hr.
***≥13 yr and adult:*** 750 mg/dose PO BID
***Prophylaxis (first episode and recurrence):***
***Child 1–3 mo or > 24 mo:*** 30 mg/kg/24 hr PO QD; **max. dose:** 1500 mg/24 hr
***Child 4–24 mo:*** 45 mg/kg/24 hr PO QD: **max. dose:** 1500 mg/24 hr
***≥13 yr and adult:*** 1500 mg/dose PO QD
***Toxoplasma gondii:***
***Child:***
***First episode prophylaxis:*** Use PCP prophylaxis dosages.
***Adult:***
***Treatment:*** 1500 mg/dose PO BID ± sulfadiazine 1000–1500 mg PO Q6 hr.
***First episode prophylaxis:*** 1500 mg/dose PO QD ± pyrimethamine 25 mg PO QD PLUS leucovorin 10 mg PO QD.
***Recurrence prophylaxis:*** 750 mg/dose PO Q6–12 hr ± pyrimethamine 25 mg PO QD PLUS leucovorin 10 mg PO QD.

**Not recommended** in the treatment of severe PCP due to the lack of clinical data. Patients with GI disorders or severe vomiting and who cannot tolerate oral therapy should consider alternative IV therapies. Rash, pruritus, sweating, GI symptoms, LFT elevation, dizziness, headache, insomnia, anxiety, cough and fever are common. Anemia has been reported.

Metoclopramide, rifampin, rifabutin and tetracycline may decrease atovaquone levels. Shake oral suspension well before dispensing all doses. Take all doses with high-fat foods to maximize absorption.

## ATROPINE SULFATE
Sal-Tropine, AtroPen, and many other generic products
***Anticholinergic agent***

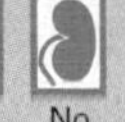
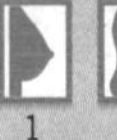
No No 1 C

**Tabs (Sal-Tropine):** 0.4 mg
**Injection:** 0.05, 0.1, 0.3, 0.4, 0.5, 0.8, 1 mg/mL
**Injection (auto-injector):**
**AtroPen 0.5 mg:** Delivers a single 0.5 mg (0.7 mL) dose (blue colored pen)
**AtroPen 1 mg:** Delivers a single 1 mg (0.7 mL) dose (dark red colored pen)
**AtroPen 2 mg:** Delivers a single 2 mg (0.7 mL) dose (green colored pen)
**Ointment (ophthalmic):** 1% (1, 3.5 g)
**Solution (ophthalmic):** 0.5%, 1%, 2% (1, 2, 5, 15 mL)

*Continued*


For explanation of icons, see p. 698.

ATROPINE SULFATE *continued*

***Pre-anesthesia dose (30-60 min pre operation):***
***Child:*** 0.01 mg/kg/dose SC/IV/IM, **max. dose:** 0.4 mg/dose; **min. dose:** 0.1 mg/dose; may repeat Q4–6 hr
***Adult:*** 0.5 mg/dose SC/IV/IM
***Cardiopulmonary resuscitation (see remarks):***
***Child:*** 0.02 mg/kg/dose IV Q5 min × 2–3 doses PRN; **min. dose:** 0.1 mg; **max. single dose:** 0.5 mg in children, 1 mg in adolescents; **max. total dose:** 1 mg children, 2 mg adolescents
***Adult:*** 0.5–1 mg/dose IV Q5 min; **max. total dose:** 2 mg
***Bronchospasm:*** 0.025–0.05 mg/kg/dose in 2.5 mL NS; **max. dose:** 2.5 mg/dose Q6–8 hr via nebulizer
***Nerve agent and insecticide poisoning for muscarinic symptoms (organophosphate or carbamate poisoning):***
***IV/IM/ET:*** see Chapter 2.
***AtroPen device (IM route):*** Inject as soon as exposure is known or suspected. Give one dose for mild symptoms and two additional doses (total 3 doses) in rapid succession 10 min after the first dose for severe symptoms as follows:
***Child 6 mo–4 yr (15–40 lb):*** 0.5 mg
***Child 4–10 yr (40–90 lb):*** 1 mg
***Child > 10 yr and adult (≥90 lb):*** 2 mg
***Ophthalmic (uveitis):***
***Child:*** (0.5% solution) 1–2 drops in each eye QD-TID
***Adult:*** (1% solution) 1–2 drops in each eye QD-QID

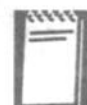

**Contraindicated** in glaucoma, obstructive uropathy, tachycardia, and thyrotoxicosis. **Use with caution** in patients sensitive to sulfites.

Doses < 0.1 mg have been associated with paradoxical bradycardia. Side effects include: dry mouth, blurred vision, fever, tachycardia, constipation, urinary retention, CNS signs (dizziness, hallucinations, restlessness, fatigue, headache).

In case of bradycardia, may give via endotracheal tube (dilute with NS to volume of 1–2 mL) or intraosseous (IO) route. Use injectable solution for nebulized use; can be mixed with albuterol for simultaneous administration.

## AURALGAN

See *Antipyrine and Benzocaine*

## AZATHIOPRINE

Imuran, Azasan, and others
***Immunosuppressant***

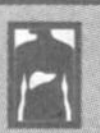
Yes
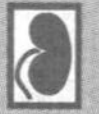
Yes
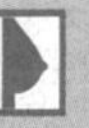
3
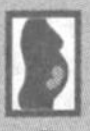
D

**Oral suspension:** 50 mg/mL
**Tabs:**
**Imuran:** 50 mg
**Azasan:** 75, 100 mg
**Injection:** 100 mg (20 mL)

*Continued*

AZATHIOPRINE *continued*

***Immunosuppression:***
***Initial:*** 3–5 mg/kg/24 hr IV/PO QD
***Maintenance:*** 1–3 mg/kg/24 hr IV/PO QD

Toxicity: bone marrow suppression, rash, stomatitis, hepatotoxicity, alopecia, arthralgias, and GI disturbances. Use ¼–⅓ dose when given with allopurinol. Severe anemia has been reported when used in combination with captopril or enalapril. Monitor CBC, platelets, total bilirubin, alkaline phosphatase, BUN, and creatinine. **Adjust dose in renal failure (see Chapter 31).**

Administer oral doses with food to minimize GI discomfort.

## AZELASTINE

Astelin, Optivar

***Antihistamine***

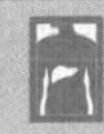 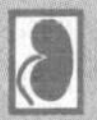  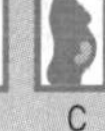

Yes Yes ? C

**Nasal spray (Astelin):** 1% (137 mcg/spray), 200 actuations (30 mL )
**Ophthalmic drops (Optivar):** 0.05% (0.5 mg/mL) (6 mL)

***Seasonal allergic rhinitis:***
***Child 5–11 yr:*** 1 spray each nostril BID
***≥12 yr and adult:*** 2 sprays each nostril BID
***Ophthalmic:***
***≥3 yr and adult:*** Instill 1 drop into each affected eye BID

**Use with caution** in asthmatics. Reduced dosages have been recommended in patients with renal and hepatic dysfunction. Optivar **should not be used** to treat contact lens related irritation. Soft contact lens users should wait at least 10 min after dose instillation before they insert their lenses.

Drowsiness may occur despite the nasal route of administration (**avoid** concurrent use of alcohol or CNS depressants). Bitter taste, nasal burning, pharyngitis, weight gain, fatigue, and epistaxis may also occur with nasal route. Eye burning and stinging have been reported in about 30% of patients receiving the ophthalmic dosage form.

## AZITHROMYCIN

Zithromax, Zithromax TRI-PAK, Zithromax Z-PAK, Zmax (extended-release oral suspension), Azasite

***Antibiotic, macrolide***

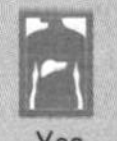 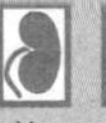 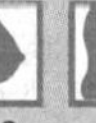

Yes Yes 2 B

**Tablets:** 250, 500, 600 mg
**TRI-PAK:** 500 mg (3s as unit dose pack)
**Z-PAK:** 250 mg (6s as unit dose pack)
**Oral suspension:** 100 mg/5 mL (15 mL), 200 mg/5 mL (15, 22.5, 30 mL)
**Oral Powder (Sachet):** 1 g (3s, 10s)
**Extended-release oral suspension (microspheres):**
**Zmax:** 2 g reconstituted with 60 mL of water
**Injection:** 500 mg; contains 9.92 mEq Na/1 g drug
**Ophthalmic solution (Azasite):** 1% (2.5 mL)

*Continued*

For explanation of icons, see p. 698.

AZITHROMYCIN *continued*

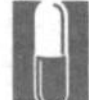

***Child:***
***Otitis media (≥6 mo):***
***5 day regimen:*** 10 mg/kg PO day 1 (**max. dose:** 500 mg), followed by 5 mg/kg/24 hr PO QD (**max. dose:** 250 mg/24 hr) on days 2–5
***3 day regimen:*** 10 mg/kg/24 hr PO QD × 3 days (**max. dose:** 500 mg/24 hr)
***1 day regimen (see remarks):*** 30 mg/kg/24 hr PO ×1 (**max. dose:** 1500 mg/24 hr)
***Community-acquired pneumonia (≥6 mo):*** Use the otitis media 5 day regimen
***Pharyngitis/tonsillitis (2–15 yr):*** 12 mg/kg/24 hr PO QD × 5 days (**max. dose:** 500 mg/24 hr)
***M. avium complex in HIV (see www.aidsinfo.nih.gov/guidelines for most current recommendations):***
***Prophylaxis for first episode:*** 20 mg/kg/dose PO Q7 days (**max. dose:** 1200 mg/dose); alternatively, 5 mg/kg/24 hr PO QD (**max. dose:** 250 mg/dose) with or without rifabutin
***Prophylaxis for recurrence:*** 5 mg/kg/24 hr PO QD (**max. dose:** 250 mg/dose), plus ethambutol 15 mg/kg/24 hr (**max. dose:** 900 mg/24 hr) PO QD with or without rifabutin 5 mg/kg/24 hr (**max. dose:** 300 mg/24 hr)
***Treatment:*** 10–12 mg/kg/24 hr PO QD (**max. dose:** 500 mg/24 hr) × 1 mo or longer, plus ethambutol 15–25 mg/kg/24 hr (**max. dose:** 1 g/24 hr) PO QD with or without rifabutin 10–20 mg/kg/24 hr (**max. dose:** 300 mg/24 hr)
***Anti-inflammatory agent in cystic fibrosis:***
***25–39 kg:*** 250 mg PO every Monday, Wednesday, and Friday.
***≥40 kg:*** 500 mg PO every Monday, Wednesday, and Friday.

***Adolescent and adult:***
***Pharyngitis, tonsillitis, skin, and soft tissue infection:*** 500 mg PO day 1, then 250 mg/24 hr PO on days 2–5
***Mild/moderate bacterial COPD exacerbation:*** above 5 day dosing regimen OR 500 mg PO QD × 3 days
***Community acquired pneumonia:***
***Tablets:*** 500 mg PO day 1, then 250 mg/24 hr PO on days 2–5
***Extended-release oral suspension (Zmax):*** Single dose 2 g PO
***IV and tablet regimen:*** 500 mg IV QD × 2 days followed by 500 mg PO QD to complete a 7–10 day regimen (IV and PO)
***Sinusitis:***
***Tablets:*** 500 mg PO QD × 3 days
***Extended-release oral suspension (Zmax):*** Single dose 2 g PO
***Uncomplicated chlamydial cervicitis or urethritis:*** Single 1 g dose PO
***Gonococcal cervicitis or urethritis:*** Single 2 g dose PO
***Acute PID (chlamydia):*** 500 mg IV QD × 1–2 days followed by 250 mg PO QD to complete a 7 day regimen (IV and PO).
***M. avium complex in HIV (see www.aidsinfo.nih.gov/guidelines for most recent recommendations):***
***Prophylaxis for first episode:*** 1200 mg PO Q 7 days with or without rifabutin 300 mg PO QD
***Prophylaxis for recurrence:*** 500 mg PO QD, plus ethambutol 15 mg/kg/dose PO QD, with or without rifabutin 300 mg PO QD
***Treatment:*** 500–600 mg PO QD with ethambutol 15 mg/kg/dose PO QD with or without rifabutin 300 mg PO QD.
***Anti-inflammatory agent in cystic fibrosis:*** Use same dosing used in children.

*Continued*

AZITHROMYCIN *continued*

***Ophthalmic:***

***≥1 yr and adult:*** Instill one drop into the affected eye(s) BID, 8–12 hr apart, × 2 days, followed by one drop QD for the next 5 days.

---

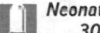

**Contraindicated** in hypersensitivity to macrolides. **Use with caution** in impaired hepatic function, GFR < 10 mL/min (limited data), and prolonged QT intervals. Extended-release oral suspension (Zmax) is currently not approved in children. Can cause increase in hepatic enzymes, cholestatic jaundice, GI discomfort, and pain at injection site (IV use). Compared to other macrolides, less risk for drug interactions. Nelfinavir may increase azithromycin levels; monitor for liver enzyme abnormalities and hearing impairment. Vomiting, diarrhea and nausea have been reported at higher frequency in otitis media with 1 day dosing regimen. CNS penetration is poor.

Aluminum- and magnesium-containing antacids decrease absorption. Oral dosage forms may be administered with or without food. Intravenous administration is over 1–3 hr; **do not** give as a bolus or IM injection.

Ophthalmic use: **Do not** wear contact lenses. Eye irritation is the most common side effect.

## AZTREONAM

Azactam

***Antibiotic, monobactam***

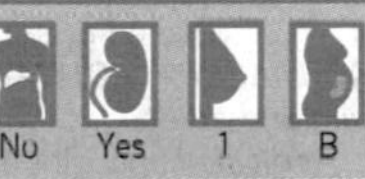


**Injection:** 0.5, 1, 2 g

**Frozen Injection:** 1 g/50 mL 3.4% dextrose, 2 g/50 mL 1.4% dextrose (iso-osmotic solutions)

Each 1 g drug contains approximately 780 mg L-Arginine.

---

***Neonate:***

***30 mg/kg/dose:***

***<1.2 kg and 0–4 wk age:*** Q12 hr IV/IM

***1.2–2 kg and 0–7 days:*** Q12 hr IV/IM

***1.2–2 kg and >7 days:*** Q8 hr IV/IM

***>2 kg and 0–7 days:*** Q8 hr IV/IM

***>2 kg and >7 days:*** Q6 hr IV/IM

***Child:*** 90–120 mg/kg/24 hr ÷ Q6–8 hr IV/IM

***Cystic fibrosis:*** 150–200 mg/kg/24 hr ÷ Q6–8 hr IV/IM

***Adult:***

***Moderate infections:*** 1–2 g/dose Q8–12 hr IV/IM

***Severe infections:*** 2 g/dose Q6–8 hr IV/IM

**Max. dose:** 8 g/24 hr

---

Typically indicated in multidrug resistant aerobic gram-negative infections when beta-lactam therapy is **contraindicated**. Well-absorbed IM. **Use with caution** in arginase deficiency. Low cross-allergenicity between aztreonam and other beta-lactams. Adverse reactions: thrombophlebitis, eosinophilia, leukopenia, neutropenia, thrombocytopenia, elevation of liver enzymes, hypotension, seizures, and confusion. Good CNS penetration. **Adjust dose in renal failure (see Chapter 31).**



For explanation of icons, see p. 698.

## BACITRACIN ± POLYMYXIN B

AK-Tracin Ophthalmic, Baciguent Topical, and others
In combination with polymyxin B: AK-Poly-Bac Ophthalmic, Polysporin Ophthalmic, Polysporin Topical and others
***Antibiotic, topical***

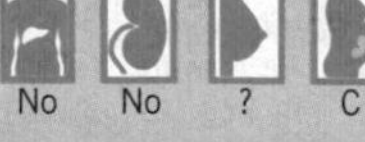


**BACITRACIN:**
Ophthalmic ointment: 500 units/g (3.5, 3.75 g)
Topical ointment: 500 units/g (0.9, 15, 30, 120, 454 g)
**BACITRACIN IN COMBINATION WITH POLYMYXIN B:**
Ophthalmic ointment: 500 units bacitracin + 10,000 units polymyxin B/g (3.5 g)
Topical ointment: 500 units bacitracin + 10,000 units polymyxin B/g (0.9, 15, 30 g)
Topical powder: 500 units bacitracin + 10,000 units polymyxin B/g (10 g)

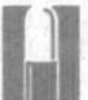

***BACITRACIN***
***Child and adult:***
***Topical:*** Apply to affected area 1–5 times/24 hr.
***Ophthalmic:*** Apply 0.25–0.5 inch ribbon into the conjunctival sac of the infected eye(s) Q3–12 hr; frequency depends on severity of infection.
***BACITRACIN + POLYMYXIN B***
***Child and adult:***
***Topical:*** Apply ointment or powder to affected area QD–TID
***Ophthalmic:*** Apply 0.25–0.5 inch ribbon into the conjunctival sac of the infected eye(s) Q3–12 hr; frequency depends on severity of infection.

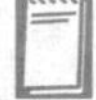

Hypersensitivity reactions to bacitracin and/or polymyxin B can occur. **Do not use** topical ointment for the eyes. Side effects may include rash, itching, burning, and edema. Ophthalmic dosage form may cause temporary blurred vision and retard corneal healing. For neomycin containing products, see *Neomycin/Polymyxin B/± Bacitracin.*

## BACLOFEN

Lioresal, Kemstro, and various
***Centrally acting skeletal muscle relaxant***

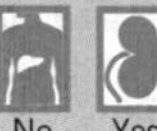
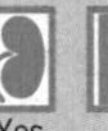
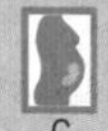
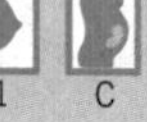


**Tabs:** 10, 20 mg
**Disintegrating oral tabs (Kemstro):** 10, 20 mg; contains phenylalanine
**Oral suspension:** 5, 10 mg/mL
**Intrathecal injection:** 50 mcg/mL (1 mL), 0.5 mg/mL (20 mL), 2 mg/mL (5 mL); preservative-free

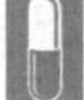

***Dosage increments are made at 3-day intervals until desired effect or*** **max. dose is achieved.**
***Child PO:***
***≥2 yr:*** 10–15 mg/24 hr ÷ Q8 hr
**Max. dose: <8 yr:** 40 mg/24 hr
**Max. dose: ≥8 yr:** 60 mg/24 hr
***Adult PO:***
5 mg TID; **max. dose:** 80 mg/24 hr

*Continued*

BACLOFEN *continued*

***Intrathecal continuous infusion maintenance therapy (not well established):***

*<12 yr:* Average dose of 274 mcg/24 hr (range: 24–1199 mcg/24 hr) has been reported.

*≥12 yr and adult:* Most required 300–800 mcg/24 hr (range: 12–2003 mcg/24 hr with limited experience at doses > 1000 mcg/24 hr).

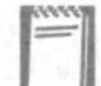

**Avoid** abrupt withdrawal of drug. **Use with caution** in patients with seizure disorder, impaired renal function. Approximately 70%–80% of the drug is excreted in the urine unchanged. Administer oral doses with food or milk.

Adverse effects: Drowsiness, fatigue, nausea, vertigo, psychiatric disturbances, rash, urinary frequency, and hypotonia. **Avoid** abrupt withdrawal of intrathecal therapy to prevent potential life-threatening events.

## BECLOMETHASONE DIPROPIONATE

QVAR, Beconase AQ

***Corticosteroid***

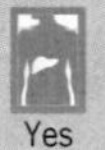
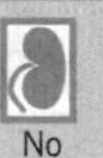
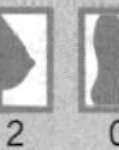
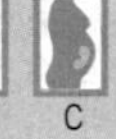

Yes No 2 C

**Inhalation, oral:**

**QVAR:** 40 mcg/inhalation (100 inhalations, 7.3 g), 80 mcg/inhalation (100 inhalations, 7.3 g); CFC-free product (HFA)

**Inhalation, nasal:**

**Beconase AQ:** 42 mcg/inhalation (200 metered doses, 25 g)

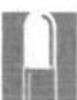

***Oral inhalation (QVAR):***

*5–11 yr:* 40 mcg BID; **max. dose:** 80 mcg BID

*≥12 yr and adult:*

*Corticosteroid naïve:* 40–80 mcg BID; **max. dose:** 320 mcg BID

*Previous corticosteroid use:* 40–160 mcg BID; **max. dose:** 320 mcg BID

***Nasal inhalation (Beconase AQ):***

*6–12 yr:* Start with 1 spray each nostril BID, may increase to 2 sprays each nostril BID if needed. Once symptoms are controlled, decrease dose to 1 spray each nostril BID.

*>12 yr and adult:* 1–2 spray(s) each nostril BID

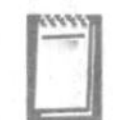

**Not recommended** for children <5 yr with oral inhalation and <6 yr with the nasal administration due to unknown safety and efficacy. Dose should be titrated to lowest effective dose. **Avoid** using higher than recommended doses.

CYP 450 3A4 inhibitors (e.g., ketoconazole, erythromycin, and protease inhibitors) or significant hepatic impairment may increase systemic exposure of beclomethasone.

Monitor for hypothalamic, pituitary, adrenal, or growth suppression, and hypercortism. Rinse mouth and gargle with water after oral inhalation; may cause thrush. Consider using with tube spacers for oral inhalation.

For explanation of icons, see p. 698.

## BENZOYL PEROXIDE

Benzac AC Wash 2½, 5, 10; Benzac 5, 10; Brevoxyl Creamy Wash, Desquam-E 5, Desquam-E 10, NeoBenz Micro, Oxy-5, Oxy-10, Triaz, Zoderm, and many other names

***Topical acne product***

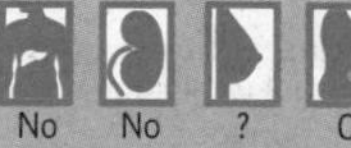


**Liquid wash:** 2.5% (240 mL), 5% (120, 150, 240 mL), 10% (120, 150, 240 mL)
**Liquid cream wash:** 4% (170 g), 8% (170 g)
**Bar:** 5% [OTC] (113 g), 10% [OTC] (106, 113 g)
**Lotion:** 3% (170, 340 g), 4% (297 g), 5% [OTC] (30 mL), 6% (170, 340 g), 8% (297 g), 10% [OTC] (30 mL, 85, 170, 340 g)
**Cleanser:** 4.5% (400 mL), 6.5% (400 mL), 8.5% (400 mL)
**Cleanser/Mask:** [OTC] 3.5% (125 mL)
**Cream:** 3.5% (45 g), 4.5% (125 mL), 5% [OTC] (18 g), 5.5% (45 g), 6.5% (125 mL), 8.5% (45 g, 125 mL), 10% [OTC] (18, 28 g)
**Gel:** 2.5% (45, 60, 90, 113 g), 3% (42.5 g), 4% (42.5, 90 g), 4.5% (125 mL), 5% [OTC] (42.5, 60, 85, 90, 113.4 g), 6% (42.5%), 7% (45, 90 g), 8% (42.5, 90 g), 8.5% (125 mL), 9% (42.5 g), 10% (45, 60, 90, 113.4 g)
**Note:** Some preparations may contain alcohol.
**Combination product with erythromycin (Benzamycin and others):**
  **Gel:** 30 mg erythromycin and 50 mg benzoyl peroxide per g (0.8, 23.3, 46 g); some preparations may contain 20% alcohol
**Combination product with clindamycin (BenzaClin, Duac):**
  **Gel:** 10 mg clindamycin and 50 mg benzoyl peroxide per g (25, 45 g); some preparations may contain methylparaben

---

***Child and adult:***

***Cleanser, liquid wash, or bar:*** Wet affected area prior to application. Apply and wash QD–BID; rinse thoroughly and pat dry. Modify dose frequency or concentration to control the amount of drying or peeling.

***Lotion, cream, or gel:*** Cleanse skin and apply small amounts over affected areas QD initially; increase frequency to BID–TID if needed. Modify dose frequency or concentration to control drying or peeling.

***Combination products:***

***Benzamycin and BenzaClin:*** Apply BID (morning and evening) to affected areas after washing and drying skin.

***Duac:*** Apply QHS to affected areas after washing and drying skin.

---

**Contraindicated** in known history of hypersensitivity to product's components (benzoyl peroxide, clindamycin, or erythromycin). **Avoid** contact with mucous membranes and eyes. May cause skin irritation, stinging, dryness, peeling, erythema, edema, and contact dermatitis. Concurrent use with tretinoin (Retin-A) will increase risk of skin irritation. Products containing clindamycin and erythromycin should not be used in combination. Any single application resulting in excessive stinging or burning may be removed with mild soap and water. Lotion, cream, and gel dosage forms should be applied to dry skin.

## BENZTROPINE MESYLATE

Cogentin and various generics

***Anticholinergic agent, drug-induced dystonic reaction antidote, anti-Parkinson's agent***

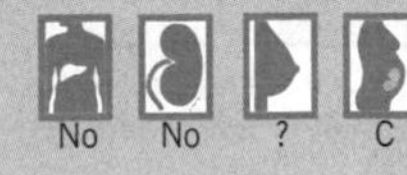


**Injection:** 1 mg/mL (2 mL)
**Tabs:** 0.5, 1, 2 mg

***Drug-induced extrapyramidal symptoms:***
*>3 yr:* 0.02–0.05 mg/kg/dose QD–BID PO/IM/IV
*Adult:* 1–4 mg/dose QD–BID PO/IM/IV

**Contraindicated** in myasthenia gravis, GI/GU obstruction, untreated narrow-angle glaucoma, and peptic ulcer. Use IV route **only** when PO and IM routes are not feasible. May cause anti-cholinergic side effects, especially constipation and dry mouth. Drug interactions include: potentiation of CNS depressant effects when used with CNS depressants; enhance CNS side effects of amantadine; and inhibit the response of neuroleptics.

Onset of action: 15 min for IV/IM and 1 hr for PO.
Oral doses should be administered with food to decrease GI upset.

## BERACTANT

See *Surfactant, Pulmonary/Beractant*

## BETAMETHASONE

Beta-Val, Celestone, Celestone Soluspan, Diprolene, Diprolene AF, Diprosone, Maxivate, and others

***Corticosteroid***

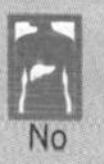
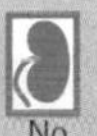
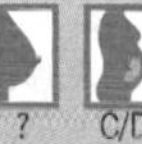
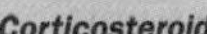


**Betamethasone base (Celestone):**
Oral solution: 0.6 mg/5 mL (120 mL); contains alcohol

**Na Phosphate and Acetate (Celestone Soluspan):**
Injection suspension: 6 mg/mL (3 mg/mL Na phosphate + 3 mg/mL betamethasone acetate) (5 mL)

**Dipropionate (Diprosone, Maxivate, and others):**
Topical aerosol: 0.1% (85 g) with 10% isopropyl alcohol
Topical cream: 0.05% (15, 45 g)
Topical lotion: 0.05% (20, 30, 60 mL); may contain 46.8% alcohol
Topical ointment: 0.05% (15, 45 g)

**Valerate (Beta-Val and others):**
Topical cream: 0.05%, 0.1% (15, 45 g)
Topical foam: 1.2 mg/g (100 g); may contain 60.4% ethanol, cetyl alcohol, stearyl alcohol
Topical lotion: 0.1% (60 mL); may contain 47.5% isopropyl alcohol
Topical ointment: 0.1% (15, 45 g)

**Dipropionate augmented (Diprolene, Diprolene AF, and others):**
Topical cream: 0.05% (15, 45, 50 g); contains propylene glycol
Topical gel: 0.05% (15, 45, 50 g); contains propylene glycol
Topical lotion: 0.05% (30, 60 mL); contains 30% isopropyl alcohol
Topical ointment: 0.05% (15, 45, 50 g); contains propylene glycol

*Continued*

For explanation of icons, see p. 698.

BETAMETHASONE *continued*

***All dosages should be adjusted based on patient response and severity of condition.***

***Anti-inflammatory:***

***Child:***

***Oral:*** 0.0175–0.25 mg/kg/24 hr or 0.5–7.5 mg/m²/24 hr ÷ Q6–8 hr

***IM:*** 0.0175–0.125 mg/kg/24 hr or 0.5–7.5 mg/m²/24 hr ÷ Q6–12 hr

***Adolescent and adult:***

***Oral:*** 2.4–4.8 mg/24 hr ÷ Q6–12 hr; may range from 0.6–7.2 mg/24 hr depending on disease being treated

***IM:*** 0.5–9 mg/24 hr ÷ Q12–24 hr

***Topical (see remarks):***

***Valerate and dipropionate forms:***

***Child and adult:*** Apply to affected areas QD–BID

***Dipropionate augmented forms:***

***≥13 yr–adult:*** Apply to affected areas QD–BID

**Max. dose:** 14 days and

***Cream and ointment:*** 45 g/wk

***Gel:*** 50 g/wk

***Lotion:*** 50 mL/wk

**Use with caution** in hypothyroidism, cirrhosis, and ulcerative colitis. See Chapter 30 for relative steroid potencies and doses based on body surface area. Betamethasone is inadequate when used alone for adrenocortical insufficiency because its minimal mineralocorticoid properties. Like all steroids, may cause hypertension, pseudotumor cerebri, acne, Cushing's syndrome, adrenal axis suppression, GI bleeding, hyperglycemia, and osteoporosis.

Na phosphate and acetate injectable suspension recommended for IM, intra-articular, intrasynovial intralesional, soft tissue use only; but **not** for IV use. **Topical betamethasone dipropionate augmented (Diprolene and Diprolene AF) is not recommended in children ≤ 12 yr owing to the higher risk for adrenal suppression.**

Used in premature labor to stimulate fetal lung maturation. Pregnancy category changes to "D" if used in first trimester.

## BETHANECHOL CHLORIDE

Urecholine and other brand names

***Cholinergic agent***

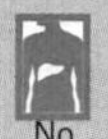

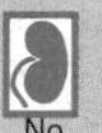

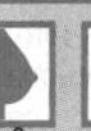

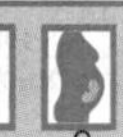


**Tabs:** 5, 10, 25, 50 mg

**Oral suspension:** 1, 5 mg/mL

***Child:***

***Abdominal distention/urinary retention:*** 0.6 mg/kg/24 hr ÷ Q6–8 hr PO

***Gastroesophageal reflux:*** 0.1–0.2 mg/kg/dose 30 min–1 hr before meals and QHS PO; **max. dose:** 4 doses/24 hr

***Adult:***

***Urinary retention:*** 10–50 mg Q6–12 hr PO

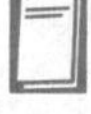

**Contraindicated** in asthma, mechanical GI or GU obstruction, peptic ulcer disease, hyperthyroidism, cardiac disease, and seizure disorder. May cause hypotension, nausea, bronchospasm, salivation, flushing, and abdominal cramps. **Warning: Severe hypotension may occur when given with ganglionic blockers (e.g., trimethaphan). Atropine is the antidote.**

## BICITRA

See *Citrate Mixtures*

## BISACODYL

Dulcolax, Fleet Laxative, Fleet Bisacodyl, Doxidan, and various other names

***Laxative, stimulant***

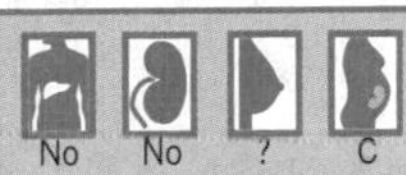


**Tabs (enteric-coated):** 5 mg
**Suppository:** 10 mg
**Enema (Fleet Bisacodyl):** 10 mg/30 mL (37.5 mL)
**Delayed-release tabs (Doxidan):** 5 mg

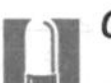

*Oral:*
- *Child (3–12 yr):* 0.3 mg/kg/24 hr or 5–10 mg to be given 6 hr before desired effect; **max. dose:** 30 mg/24 hr
- *Adult (>12 yr):* 5–15 mg to be given 6 hr before desired effect; **max. dose:** 30 mg/24 hr

*Rectal suppository (as a single dose):*
- *<2 yr:* 5 mg
- *2–11 yr:* 5–10 mg
- *>11 yr and adult:* 10 mg

*Rectal enema (as a single dose):*
- *≥ 12 yr and adult:* 30 mL

**Do not** chew or crush tablets (swallow whole); **do not** give within 1 hr of antacids or milk. **Do not use** in newborn period. May cause abdominal cramps, nausea, vomiting, and rectal irritation. Oral usually effective within 6–10 hr; rectal usually effective within 15–60 min.

## BISMUTH SUBSALICYLATE

Pepto-Bismol, Kaopectate, Kaopectate Children's, and others

***Antidiarrheal, gastrointestinal ulcer agent***

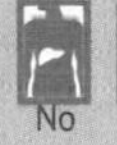

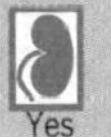

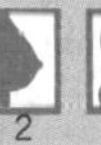

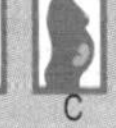


**Liquid [OTC]:** 130 mg/15 mL (240 mL), 262 mg/15 mL (120, 240, 360, 480 mL), 524 mg/15mL (120, 240, 360 mL)
**Kaopectate Children's [OTC]:** 87 mg/5 mL (180 mL)
**Caplet [OTC]:** 262 mg
**Chewable tabs [OTC]:** 262 mg
Contains 102 mg salicylate per 262 mg tablet; or 129 mg salicylate per 15 mL of the 262 mg/15 mL suspension

*Diarrhea:*
- *Child:* 100 mg/kg/24 hr ÷ 5 equal doses for 5 days; **max. dose:** 4.19 g/24 hr
- *Dosage by age:* Give following dose Q30 min to 1 hr PRN up to a **max. dose** of 8 doses/24 hr:
  - *3–5 yr:* 87.3 mg (⅓ tablet or 5 mL of 262 mg/15 mL)
  - *6–8 yr:* 174.7 mg (⅔ tablet or 10 mL of 262 mg/15 mL)

*Continued*

FORMULARY

For explanation of icons, see p. 698.

BISMUTH SUBSALICYLATE *continued*

***Diarrhea (cont'd):***

***9–11 yr:*** 262 mg (1 tablet or 15 mL of 262 mg/15 mL)

***≥12 yr–adult:*** 524 mg (2 tablets or 30 mL of 262 mg/15 mL)

***H. pylori gastric infection*** (in combination with ampicillin and metronidazole or with tetracycline and metronidazole for adults; doses not well established for children):

***<10 yr:*** 262 mg PO QID × 6 wk

***≥10 yr –adult:*** 524 mg PO QID × 6 wk

---

Generally **not recommended** in children <16 yr with chicken pox or flu-like symptoms (risk for Reye's syndrome), in combination with other nonsteroidal anti-inflammatory drugs, or in severe renal failure. **Use with caution** in bleeding disorders, renal dysfunction, gastritis, and gout. May cause darkening of tongue and/or black stools, GI upset, impaction, and decreased platelet aggregation.

Drug combination appears to have antisecretory and antimicrobial effects with some anti-inflammatory effects. Absorption of bismuth is negligible, whereas approximately 80% of the salicylate is absorbed. Decreases absorption of tetracycline.

## BROMPHENIRAMINE WITH PHENYLEPHRINE

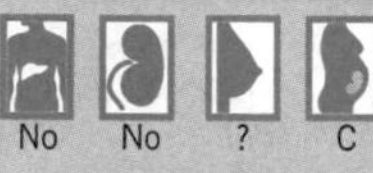


Alacol Oral Drops, Alacol Syrup, Alenaze -D NR, Dimetapp Children's Cold and Allergy, and others

***Antihistamine + decongestant***

**Drops (Alacol Oral Drops):** Brompheniramine 0.4 mg + phenylephrine 1 mg/1 mL (30 mL)
**Elixir (Dimetapp Children's Cold and Allergy) [OTC]:** Brompheniramine 1 mg + phenylephrine 2.5 mg/5 mL (237 mL)
**Syrup (Alacol Syrup):** Brompheniramine 2 mg + phenylephrine 5 mg/5 mL (473 mL)
**Liquid (Alenzae-D NR):** Brompheniramine 2 mg + phenylephrine 7.5 mg/5 mL (473 mL)
**Chewable tab (Dimetapp Children's Cold and Allergy) [OTC]:** Brompheniramine 1 mg + phenylephrine 2.5 mg

---

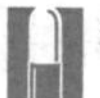

***All doses based on brompheniramine component.***

***2–<6 yr:*** 1 mg Q4 hr PO up to a **max. dose** of 6 mg/24 hr

***6–12 yr:*** 2 mg Q4 hr PO up to a **max. dose** of 12 mg/24 hr

***≥12 yr:*** 4 mg Q4 hr PO up to a **max. dose** of 24 mg/24 hr

***Alternatively, dosing based on specific dosage forms/products. CAUTION:* These products are available in different concentrations.**

***Oral, drops (Alacol Oral Drops):***

***2–<6 yr:*** 2.5 mL Q4 hr PO up to a **max. dose** of 15 mL/24 hr

***Oral, elixir (Dimetapp Children's Cold and Allergy):***

***6–<12 yr:*** 10 mL Q4 hr PO up to a **max. dose** of 60 mL/24 hr

***≥ 12 yr:*** 20 mL Q4 hr PO up to a **max. dose** of 120 mL/24 hr

***Oral, syrup (Alacol Syrup):***

***2–<6 yr:*** 2.5 mL Q4 hr PO up to a **max. dose** of 15 mL/24 hr

***6–12 yr:*** 5 mL Q4 hr PO up to a **max. dose** of 30 mL/24 hr

***≥12 yr:*** 10 mL Q4 hr PO up to a **max. dose** of 60 mL/24 hr

***Oral, liquid (Alenzae-D NR):***

***2–<6 yr:*** 1.25 mL Q6 hr PO up to a **max. dose** of 7.5 mL/24 hr

***6–12 yr:*** 2.5 mL Q6 hr PO up to a **max. dose** of 15 mL/24 hr

***≥12 yr:*** 5 mL Q6 hr PO up to a **max. dose** of 30 mL/24 hr

*Continued*

BROMPHENIRAMINE WITH PHENYLEPHRINE *continued*

***Oral, chewable tab (Dimetapp Children's Cold and Allergy):***
***6–12 yr:*** Chew 2 tablets Q4 hr PO; **max. dose:** 6 doses/24 hr

Generally **not recommended** for treating URIs for infants. No proven benefit for infants and young children with URIs. Over the counter (OTC or nonprescription) use of this product is **not recommended** for children less than 6 yr old due to reports of serious adverse effects (cardiac and respiratory distress, convulsions, and hallucinations) and fatalities (from unintentional overdosages, including combined use of other OTC products containing the same active ingredients).

**Contraindicated** with use of MAO inhibitors; concurrent use and within 14 days after discontinuing MAO inhibitor. **Use with caution** in narrow-angle glaucoma, bladder neck obstruction, asthma, pyloroduodenal obstruction, symptomatic prostatic hypertrophy, hypertension, coronary artery disease, diabetes mellitus, and thyroid disease. Discontinue use 48 hr prior to allergy skin testing. May cause drowsiness, fatigue, CNS excitation, xerostomia, blurred vision, and wheezing.

## BUDESONIDE

Pulmicort Respules, Pulmicort Turbuhaler, Pulmicort Flexhaler, Rhinocort Aqua Nasal Spray
***Corticosteroid***

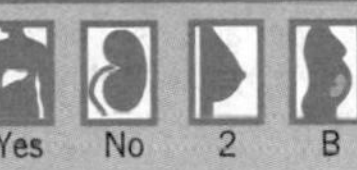


**Nasal spray (Rinocort Aqua):** 32 mcg/actuation (8.6 g, delivers approx. 120 sprays)
**Nebulized inhalation suspension (Pulmicort Respules):** 0.25 mg/2 mL, 0.5 mg/2 mL (30s)
**Oral inhaler:**
**Pulmicort Turbuhaler Inhalation powder:** 200 mcg/metered dose (104 mg, delivers approx. 200 doses)
**Pulmicort Flexhaler inhalation powder:** 90 mcg/metered dose (165 mg, delivers 60 doses), 180 mcg/metered dose (225 mg, delivers 120 doses); contains lactose

***Nebulized inhalation suspension:***
***Child 1–8 yr:***
***No prior steroid use:*** 0.5 mg/24 hr ÷ QD–BID; **max. dose:** 0.5 mg/24 hr
***Prior inhaled steroid use:*** 0.5 mg/24 hr ÷ QD–BID; **max. dose:** 1 mg/24 hr
***Prior oral steroid use:*** 1 mg/24 hr ÷ QD–BID; **max. dose:** 1 mg/24 hr

***Oral inhalation:***
***Pulmicort Turbuhaler:***
***Child ≥ 6 yr:*** Start at 1 inhalation (200 mcg) BID and increase, as needed, up to a **max. dose** of 4 inhalations/24 hr.
***Adult:***
***No prior steroid use:*** 1–2 inhalations (200–400 mcg) BID; **max. dose:** 4 inhalations/24 hr
***Prior inhaled steriod use:*** Start at 1–2 inhalations (200–400 mcg) BID and increase, as needed, up to a **max. dose** of 8 inhalations/24 hr.
***Prior oral steroid use:*** Start at 2–4 (400–800 mcg) inhalations BID; **max. dose:** 8 inhalations/24 hr.
***Pulmicort Flexhaler:***
***Child ≥ 6 yr:*** Start at 180 mcg BID; **max. dose:** 720 mcg/24 hr.
***Adult:*** Start at 180–360 mcg BID; **max. dose:** 1440 mcg/24 hr.

*Continued*

For explanation of icons, see p. 698.

BUDESONIDE *continued*

***Nasal inhalation (≥6 yr and adult):***

***Rhinocart Aqua:*** (initial): 1 spray in each nostril QD. Increase dose as needed up to **max. dose.**

**Max. nasal dose:** 6–11 yr: 128 mcg/24 hr (4 sprays/24 hr); ≥12 yr and adult: 256 mcg/24 hr (8 sprays/24 hr)

Reduce maintenance dose to as low as possible to control symptoms. May cause pharyngitis, cough, epistaxis, nasal irritation, and HPA-axis suppression. Rinse mouth after each use via the oral inhalation route. Nebulized budesonide has been shown effective in mild to moderate croup at doses of 2 mg × 1. Ref: *N Engl J Med* 331(5):285.

CYP 450 3A4 inhibitors (e.g., ketoconazole, erythromycin, and protease inhibitors) or significant hepatic impairment may increase systemic exposure of budesonide.

Onset of action for oral inhalation and nebulized suspension is within 1 day and 2–8 days, respectively, with peak effects at 1–2 wk and 4–6 wk, respectively. The therapeutic ratio between the Flexhaler and Turbuhaler product has not been established.

For nasal use, onset of action is seen after 1 day with peak effects after 3–7 days of therapy. Discontinue therapy if no improvement in nasal symptoms after 3 wk of continuous therapy.

## BUDESONIDE AND FORMOTEROL

Symbicort

***Corticosteroid and long-acting beta-2-adrenergic agonist***

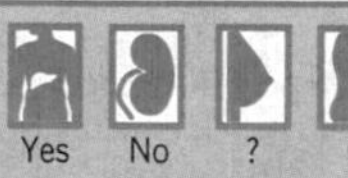


**Aerosol inhaler:**

**80 mcg budesonide + 4.5 mcg formoterol fumarate dihydrate (6.9 g delivers 60 inhalations, 10.2 g delivers about 120 inhalations)**

**160 mcg budesonide + 4.5 mcg formoterol fumarate dihydrate (6 g delivers 60 inhalations, 10.2 g delivers about 120 inhalations)**

***≥12 yr and adult:***

***No prior inhaled steroid use:*** Start with 2 inhalations BID of 80 mcg budesonide + 4.5 mcg formoterol OR 160 mcg budesonide + 4.5 mcg formoterol, depending on severity.

***Prior low to medium doses of inhaled steroid use:*** Start with two inhalations BID of 80 mcg budesonide + 4.5 mcg formoterol.

***Prior medium to high doses of inhaled steroid use:*** Start with two inhalations BID of 160 mcg budesonide + 4.5 mcg formoterol.

**Max. dose:** 2 inhalations of 160 mcg budesonide + 4.5 mcg formoterol BID

See *Budesonide* and *Formoterol* for remarks. Should be used only for patients not adequately controlled on other asthma-controller medications (e.g., low-to-medium dose inhaled corticosteroids) or whose disease severity requires the use of two maintenance therapies. Titrate to the lowest effective strength after asthma is adequately controlled. Proper patient educaion including dosage administration technique is essential; see patient package insert for detailed instructions. Rinse mouth after each use.

C
FORMULARY

## BUMETANIDE

Bumex and other generic injectable dosage forms
***Loop diuretic***

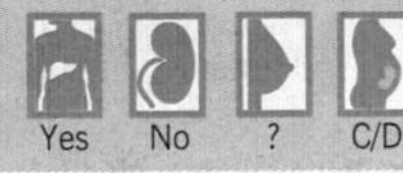


**Tabs:** 0.5, 1, 2 mg
**Injection:** 0.25 mg/mL (some preparations may contain 1% benzyl alcohol)

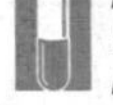

***Neonate and infant (see remarks):*** PO/IM/IV
***≤6 mo:*** 0.01–0.05 mg/kg/dose QD–QOD
***Infant and child:*** PO/IM/IV
***>6 mo:*** 0.015–0.1 mg/kg/dose QD–QOD; **max. dose:** 10 mg/24 hr
***Adult:***
***PO:*** 0.5–2 mg/dose QD-BID
***IM/IV:*** 0.5–1 mg over 1–2 min. May give additional doses Q2–3 hr PRN
**Usual max. dose** (PO/IM/IV): 10 mg/24 hr

Cross-allergenicity may occur in patients allergic to sulfonamides. Dosage reduction may be necessary in patients with hepatic dysfunction. Administer oral doses with food.

Side effects include cramps, dizziness, hypotension, headache, electrolyte losses (hypokalemia, hypocalcemia, hyponatremia, hypochloremia), and encephalopathy. May also lead to metabolic alkalosis.

Drug elimination has been reported to be slower in neonates with respiratory disorders compared to neonates without. May displace bilirubin in critically ill neonates. **Maximal** diuretic effect for infants ≤ 6 mo has been reported at 0.04 mg/kg/dose with greater efficacy seen at lower dosages.

Pregnancy category changes to "D" if used in pregnancy-induced hypertension.

## CAFFEINE CITRATE

Cafcit and others
***Methylxanthine, respiratory stimulant***

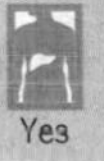
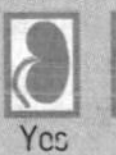
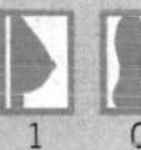


**Injection:** 20 mg/mL (3 mL)
**Oral liquid:** 20 mg/mL (3 mL), also available as powder for compounding 
20 mg/mL caffeine citrate salt = 10 mg/mL caffeine base

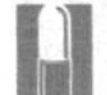

***Doses expressed in mg of caffeine citrate.***
***Neonatal apnea:***
***Loading dose:*** 10–20 mg/kg IV/PO × 1
***Maintenance dose:*** 5–10 mg/kg/dose PO/IV QD, to begin 24 hr after loading dose

**Avoid use** in symptomatic cardiac arrhythmias. **Do not use** caffeine benzoate formulation since it has been associated with kernicterus in neonates. **Use with caution** in impaired renal or hepatic function.

Therapeutic levels: 5–25 mg/L. Cardiovascular, neurologic, or GI toxicity reported at serum levels > 50 mg/L. Recommended serum sampling time: obtain trough level within 30 min prior to a dose. Steady-state is typically achieved 3 wk after the initiation of therapy. Levels obtained prior to steady-state are useful for preventing toxicity.

For explanation of icons, see p. 698.

## CALCITONIN—SALMON

Miacalcin, Miacalcin Nasal Spray, Fortical Nasal Spray

***Hypercalcemia antidote, antiosteoporotic***

No No ? C

**Injection:** 200 U/mL (2 mL); contains phenol
**Nasal spray:** 200 U/metered dose (3.7 mL, provides at least 30 doses); may contain benzyl alcohol

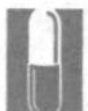

***Ostegenesis imperfecta (see remarks):***
***6 mo–15 yr:*** 2 U/kg/dose IM/SC 3 times per wk with oral calcium supplements

***Hypercalcemia (see remarks):***
***Adult:*** Start with 4 U/kg/dose IM/SC Q12 hr; if response is unsatisfactory after 1 or 2 days, increase dose to 8 U/kg/dose Q12 hr. If response remains unsatisfactory after 2 more days, increase to a **max. dose** of 8 U/kg/dose Q6 hr.

***Paget's disease:***
***Adult:***
***IM/SC (see remarks):*** Start with 100 U QD initially, followed by a usual maintenance dose of 50 U QD **or** 50–100 U Q1–3 days.
***Intranasal:*** 1–2 sprays (200–400 U) QD

**Contraindicated** in patients sensitive to salmon protein or gelatin. A skin test is recommended prior to starting IM/SC therapy due to hypersensitivity risk. Prepare a 10 U/mL dilution with normal saline and administer 0.1 mL intradermally as a skin test (observe for 15 min for wheal or significant erythemia).

Nausea, abdominal pain, flushing, and inflammation at the injection site has been reported with IM/SC route of administration. Nasal irritation (alternate nostrils to reduce risk), rhinitis, epistaxis may occur with use of the nasal spray. Periodic nasal examinations are recommended with intranasal use. If the injection volume exceeds 2 mL, use IM route and multiple sites of injection.

## CALCITRIOL

1,25-dihydroxycholecalciferol, Rocaltrol, Calcijex, and others

***Active form vitamin D, fat soluble***

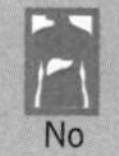 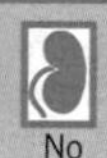  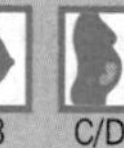

No No 3 C/D

**Caps:** 0.25, 0.5 mcg
**Oral solution:** 1 mcg/mL (15 mL)
**Injection:** (Calcijex and others) 1, 2 mcg/mL (1 mL); contains EDTA

***Renal failure (see remarks):***
***Child:***
***Oral:*** Suggested dose range 0.01–0.05 mcg/kg/24 hr. Titrate in 0.005–0.01 mcg/kg/24 hr increments Q4–8 wk based on clinical response.
***IV:*** 0.01–0.05 mcg/kg/dose given 3 times per wk

***Adult:***
***Oral initial:*** 0.25 mcg/dose PO QD–QOD
***Oral increment:*** 0.25 mcg/dose PO Q4–8 wk. Usual dose is 0.5–1 mcg/24 hr.
***IV:*** 0.5 mcg/24 hr given 3 times per wk. Usual dose is 0.5–3 mcg/24 hr given 3 times per wk

*Continued*

CALCITRIOL *continued*

***Hypoparathyroidism:***

***Child > 1 yr and adult:*** Initial dose of 0.25 mcg/dose PO QD. May increase daily dosage by 0.25 mcg at 2- to 4-wk intervals. Usual maintenance dosage as follows:

***<1 yr:*** 0.04–0.08 mcg/kg/dose PO QD
***1–5 yr:*** 0.25–0.75 mcg/dose PO QD
***>6 yr and adult:*** 0.5–2 mcg/dose PO QD

---

Most potent vitamin D metabolite available. Monitor serum calcium and phosphorus; and PTH in dialysis patients. **Avoid** concomitant use of $Mg^{2+}$-containing antacids. IV dosing applies if patient undergoing hemodialysis. A mean weekly IV dose of 1–1.4 mcg has been reported in 13- to 18-yr-old patients with ESRD.

**Contraindicated** in patients with hypercalcemia, vitamin D toxicity. Side effects include: weakness, headache, vomiting, constipation, hypotonia, polydipsia, polyuria, myalgia, metastatic calcification, etc. Allergic reactions, including anaphylaxis, have been reported.

Pregnancy category changes to "D" if used in doses above the recommended daily allowance.

## CALCIUM ACETATE

PhosLo; 25% Elemental Ca

***Calcium supplement, phosphorus-lowering agent***

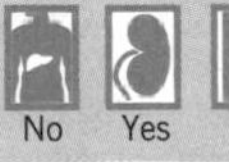
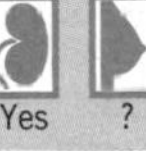
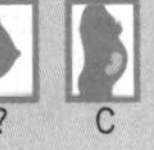

No Yes ? C

**Tabs:** 667 mg (169 mg elemental Ca)
**Capsules:** 333.5 mg (84.5 mg elemental Ca), 667 mg (169 mg elemental Ca)
**Gelcaps:** 667 mg (169 mg elemental Ca)
Contains polyethylene glycol 8000
Each 1 g of salt contains 12.7 mEq (250 mg) elemental Ca.

---

***Doses expressed in mg of calcium acetate.***

***Hyperphosphatemia:***

***Adult:*** Start with 1334 mg PO with each meal. Dosage may be increased gradually to bring serum phosphorus levels below 6 mg/dL, as long as hypercalcemia does not occur. Most patients require 2001–2668 mg PO with each meal.

---

**Contraindicated** in ventricular fibrillation. **Use with caution** in renal impairment as hypercalcemia may develop in end-stage renal failure. Nausea and hypercalcemia may occur. Approximately 40% of dose is systemically absorbed under fasting conditions and up to 30% in nonfasting conditions. May reduce absorption of tetracycline, iron, and effectiveness of polystyrene sulfonate. May potentiate effects of digoxin.

Administer with meals and plenty of fluids for use as a phosphorus lowering agent.

For explanation of icons, see p. 698.

## CALCIUM CARBONATE

Tums, Os-Cal, and many others; 40% Elemental Ca

***Calcium supplement, antacid***

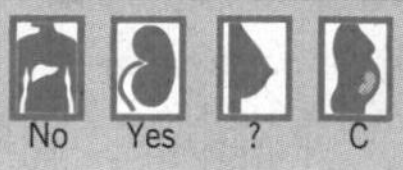


**Tab, chewable [OTC]:** 400, 420, 500, 750, 850, 1000, 1250 mg
**Tab [OTC]:** 500, 600, 650, 1250, 1500 mg
**Oral suspension [OTC]:** 1250 mg/5 mL
**Caps [OTC]:** 364, 1250 mg
**Gum [OTC]:** 300, 450, 500 mg; may contain phenylalanine
**Powder [OTC]:** 454 g
Each 1 g of salt contains 20 mEq elemental Ca (400 mg elemental Ca).

***Hypocalcemia (Doses expressed in mg of elemental calcium. To convert to mg of salt, divide elemental dose by 0.4):***

*Neonate:* 50–150 mg/kg/24 hr ÷ Q4–6 hr PO; **max. dose:** 1 g/24 hr
*Child:* 45–65 mg/kg/24 hr PO ÷ QID
*Adult:* 1–2 g/24 hr PO ÷ TID-QID

***Antacid (Doses expressed in mg of calcium carbonate):***

*2–5 yr:* 400 mg PO as symptoms occur; **max. dose:** 1200 mg/24 hr
*6–11 yr:* 800 mg PO as symptoms occur; **max. dose:** 2400 mg/24 hr
*>11 yr and adult:* 1000–3000 mg as symptoms occur; **max. dose:** 7500 mg/24 hr.

See *Calcium Acetate* for **contraindications, precautions,** and drug interactions. Side effects: constipation, hypercalcemia, hypophosphatemia, hypomagnesemia, nausea, vomiting, headache, and confusion. Some products may contain trace amounts of sodium. Administer with plenty of fluids. For use as a phosphorus lowering agent, administer with meals.

## CALCIUM CHLORIDE

Various generics; 27% Elemental Ca

***Calcium supplement***

No Yes ? C

**Injection:** 100 mg/mL (10%) (1.36 mEq Ca/mL); 1 g of salt contains 13.6 mEq (273 mg) elemental Ca
Each 1 g of salt contains 13.5 mEq (270 mg) elemental Ca.

***Doses expressed in mg of CaCl***
***Cardiac arrest:***
*Infant/child:* 20 mg/kg/dose IV Q10 min PRN
*Adult:* 500–1000 mg/dose IV Q10 min PRN or 2–4 mg/kg/dose Q10 min PRN

***MAX. IV ADMINISTRATION RATES:***

*IV push:* **Do not exceed** 100 mg/min.
*IV infusion:* **Do not exceed** 45–90 mg/kg/hr with a **max.** concentration of 20 mg/mL.

**Contraindicated** in ventricular fibrillation. **Not recommended** for asystole and electromechanical dissociation. **Use with caution** in renal impairment as hypercalcemia may develop in end-stage renal failure. May potentiate effects of digoxin.

Use IV with **extreme caution.** Extravasation may lead to necrosis. Hyaluronidase may be helpful for extravasation. Central-line administration is preferred IV route of administration. **Do not use** scalp veins. **Do not administer** IM or SC route.

*Continued*

CALCIUM CHLORIDE *continued*

Rapid IV infusion associated with bradycardia, hypotension, and peripheral vasodilation. May cause hyperchloremic acidosis.

## CALCIUM CITRATE

Cal-Citrate, Citracal, and others; 21% Elemental Ca

***Calcium supplement***

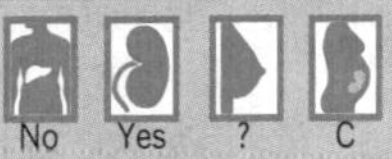


**Tabs [OTC]:** 950 mg (200 mg elemental Ca), 1150 mg calcium citrate (250 mg elemental Ca)

**Effervescent tabs [OTC]:**

**As elemental calcium:** 500 mg; contains phenylalanine

**Caps [OTC]:**

**As elemental calcium:** 180, 225 mg

**Granules [OTC]:**

**As elemental calcium:** 760 mg/teaspoonful (454 g)

Each 1 g of salt contains 10.6 mEq (211 mg) elemental Ca.

***Doses expressed as mg of elemental calcium. To convert to mg of salt, divide elemental dose by 0.21.***

***Hypocalcemia:***

***Neonate:*** 50–150 mg/kg/24 hr ÷ Q4–6 hr PO; **max. dose:** 1 g/24 hr

***Child:*** 45–65 mg/kg/24 hr PO ÷ QID

***Adult:*** 1–2 g/24 hr PO ÷ TID–QID

See *Calcium Acetate* for **contraindications, precautions,** and drug interactions. Side effects: constipation, hypercalcemia, hypophosphatemia, hypomagnesemia, nausea, vomiting, headache, and confusion.

Administer with meals for use as a phosphorus lowering agent or with use of the granule dosage form. For hypocalcemia, may administer without regard to food and take plenty of fluids.

## CALCIUM GLUBIONATE

Calcionate, Calciquid and others; 6.4% Elemental Ca

***Calcium supplement***

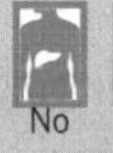
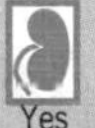
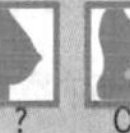


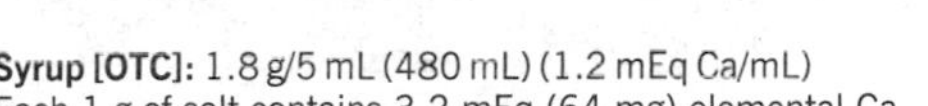

**Syrup [OTC]:** 1.8 g/5 mL (480 mL) (1.2 mEq Ca/mL)

Each 1 g of salt contains 3.2 mEq (64 mg) elemental Ca.

***Doses expressed in mg calcium glubionate.***

***Neonatal hypocalcemia:*** 1200 mg/kg/24 hr PO ÷ Q4–6 hr

***Maintenance:***

***Infant/child:*** 600–2000 mg/kg/24 hr PO ÷ QID; **max. dose:** 9 g/24 hr

***Adult:*** 6–18 g/24 hr PO ÷ QID

See *Calcium Acetate* for **contraindications, precautions,** and drug interactions. Side effects include GI irritation, dizziness, and headache. High osmotic load of syrup (20% sucrose) may cause diarrhea.

Best absorbed when given before meals. Absorption inhibited by high phosphate load.

For explanation of icons, see p. 698.

## CALCIUM GLUCONATE

Cal-G and various generics; 9% Elemental Ca

***Calcium supplement***

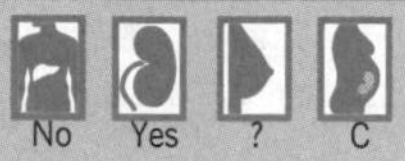


**Tabs [OTC]:** 500, 650, 975 mg
**Powder for oral suspension [OTC]:** 3852.2 mg (346.7 mg elemental Ca)/15 mL (454 g)
**Caps (Cal-G) [OTC]:** 700 mg
**Injection:** 100 mg/mL (10%) (0.45 mEq $Ca^{2+}$/mL)
Each 1 g of salt contains 4.5 mEq (90 mg) elemental Ca.

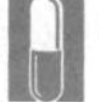

***Doses expressed in mg calcium gluconate.***
***Maintenance/hypocalcemia:***
***Neonate:*** IV: 200–800 mg/kg/24 hr ÷ Q6 hr
***Infant:***
***IV:*** 200–500 mg/kg/24 hr ÷ Q6 hr
***PO:*** 400–800 mg/kg/24 hr ÷ Q6 hr
***Child:*** 200–500 mg/kg/24 hr IV or PO ÷ Q6 hr
***Adult:*** 2–15 g/24 hr IV or PO ÷ Q6 hr
***For cardiac arrest:***
***Infant and child:*** 100 mg/kg/dose IV Q10 min
***Adult:*** 500–800 mg/dose IV Q10 min
**Max. dose:** 3 g/dose
***MAX. IV ADMINISTRATION RATES:***
***IV push:*** **Do not exceed** 100 mg/min
***IV infusion:*** **Do not exceed** 120–240 mg/kg/hr with a **max. concentration** of 50 mg/mL

**Contraindicated** in ventricular fibrillation. **Use with caution** in renal impairment as hypercalcemia may develop in end-stage renal failure. **Avoid** peripheral infusion as extravasation may cause tissue necrosis. IV infusion associated with hypotension and bradycardia. Also associated with arrythmias in digitalized patients. May reduce absorption of tetracycline, iron, and effectiveness of polystyrene sulfonate with oral route of administration.

May precipitate when used with bicarbonate. **Do not use** scalp veins. **Do not administer** IM or SC.

## CALCIUM LACTATE

Cal-Lac and various generics; 13% Elemental Ca

***Calcium supplement***

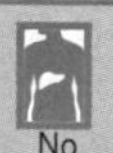
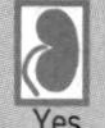
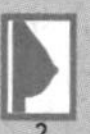
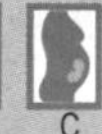


**Tabs [OTC]:** 650, 769.2 mg
**Caps (Cal-Lac) [OTC]:** 500 mg
Each 1 g salt contains 6.5 mEq (130 mg) elemental Ca.

***Doses expressed in mg of calcium lactate.***
***Hypocalcemia:***
***Infant:*** 400–500 mg/kg/24 hr PO ÷ Q4–6 hr
***Child:*** 500 mg/kg/24 hr PO ÷ Q6–8 hr
***Adult:*** 1.5–3 g PO Q8 hr
**Max. dose:** 9 g/24 hr

*Continued*

CALCIUM LACTATE *continued*

See *Calcium Acetate* for **contraindications, precautions,** and drug interactions. May cause constipation, headache, and hypercalcemia.

Give with or following meals and with plenty of fluids. **Do not** dissolve tablets in milk.

## CALCIUM PHOSPHATE, TRIBASIC

Posture; 39% Elemental Ca

***Calcium supplement***

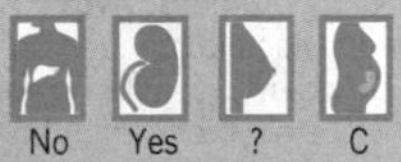


**Tabs [OTC]:** 600 mg elemental calcium

**Note:** Pharmacy may crush tablets into a powder to enhance drug delivery for children unable to swallow tablets and to accommodate smaller doses.

Each 1 g of salt contains 19.3 mEq (390 mg) elemental Ca and 280 mg elemental phosphorus.

***Doses expressed as mg of elemental calcium.***

***Hypocalcemia:***

***Neonate:*** 20–80 mg/kg/24 hr ÷ Q4–6 hr PO; **max. dose:** 1 g/24 hr

***Child:*** 45–65 mg/kg/24 hr PO ÷ Q6 hr

***Adult:*** 1–2 g/24 hr PO ÷ Q6–8 hr

**Contraindicated** in ventricular fibrillation. **Use with caution** in renal impairment as hypercalcemia may develop in end-stage renal failure (**avoid** use in dialysis with hypercalcemia), history of kidney stones and parathyroid disorders. May cause constipation, GI disturbances and hypercalcemia. See *Calcium Acetate* for drug interactions.

Give with or following meals and with plenty of fluids.

## CALFACTANT

See *Surfactant, Pulmonary/Calfactant*

## CAPTOPRIL

Capoten and various generics

***Angiotensin converting enzyme inhibitor, anti-hypertensive***

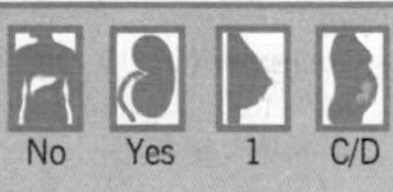


**Tabs:** 12.5, 25, 50, 100 mg

**Oral suspension:** 0.75, 1 mg/mL

***Neonate:*** 0.01–0.05 mg/kg/dose PO Q8–12 hr.

***Infant < 6 mo:*** Initially 0.01–0.5 mg/kg/dose PO BID–TID; titrate upward if needed; **max. dose:** 6 mg/kg/24 hr.

***Child:*** Initially 0.3–0.5 mg/kg/dose PO BID–TID; titrate upward if needed; **max. dose:** 6 mg/kg/24 hr up to 450 mg/24 hr.

***Adolescent and adult:*** Initially 12.5–25 mg/dose PO BID–TID; increase weekly if necessary by 25 mg/dose to **max. dose:** 450 mg/24 hr. Usual dosage range: 25–100 mg/24 hr ÷ BID.

*Continued*

For explanation of icons, see p. 698.

CAPTOPRIL *continued*

Onset within 15–30 min of administration. Peak effect within 1–2 hr. **Adjust dose with renal failure (see Chapter 31).** Should be administered on an empty stomach 1 hr before or 2 hr after meals. Titrate to minimal effective dose.

**Use with caution** in collagen vascular disease and concomitant potassium sparing diuretics. **Avoid use** with dialysis with high-flux membranes since anaphylactoid reactions have been reported. May cause rash, proteinuria, neutropenia, cough, angioedema (head, neck and intestinal), hyperkalemia, hypotension, or diminution of taste perception (with long term use). Known to decrease aldosterone and increase renin production. Captopril is a CYP 450 2D6 substrate.

Pregnancy category is a "C" during the first trimester but changes to a "D" for the second and third trimesters (fetal injury and death have been reported). Despite the pregnancy category, an increased risk for major congenital malformations has been reported with use of ACE inhibitors during the first trimester. Captopril should be discontinued as soon as possible when pregnancy is detected.

## CARBAMAZEPINE

Epitol, Tegretol, Tegretol-XR, Carbatrol, and various generics

***Anticonvulsant***

Yes Yes 2 D

**Tabs:** 200 mg
**Chewable tabs:** 100 mg
**Extended-release tabs (Tegretol-XR):** 100, 200, 400 mg
**Extended-release caps (Carbatrol):** 100, 200, 300 mg
**Oral suspension:** 100 mg/5 mL (450 mL)

***See remarks regarding dosing intervals and dosage forms.***

***<6 yr:***
***Initial:*** 10–20 mg/kg/24 hr PO ÷ BID-TID (QID for suspension)
***Increment:*** Q5–7 days up to **max. dose** of 35 mg/kg/24 hr PO

***6–12 yr:***
***Initial:*** 10 mg/kg/24 hr PO ÷ BID up to **max. dose:** 100 mg/dose BID
***Increment:*** 100 mg/24 hr at 1 wk intervals (÷ TID-QID) until desired response is obtained
***Maintenance:*** 20–30 mg/kg/24 hr PO ÷ BID-QID; usual maintenance dose is 400–800 mg/24 hr; **max. dose:** 1000 mg/24 hr

***>12 yr and adult:***
***Initial:*** 200 mg PO BID
***Increment:*** 200 mg/24 hr at 1 wk intervals (÷ BID-QID) until desired response is obtained
***Maintenance:*** 800–1200 mg/24 hr PO ÷ BID-QID

**Max. dose:**
***Child 12–15 yr:*** 1000 mg/24 hr
***Child > 15 yr:*** 1200 mg/24 hr
***Adult:*** 1.6–2.4 g/24 hr

**Contraindicated** for patients taking MAO inhibitors or who are sensitive to tricyclic antidepressants. Should not be used in combination with clozapine due to increased risk for bone marrow suppression and agranulocytosis.

*Continued*

CARBAMAZEPINE *continued*

Erythromycin, diltiazem, verapamil, cefixime, cimetidine, itraconazole, and INH may increase serum levels. Carbamazepine may decrease activity of warfarin, doxycycline, oral contraceptives, cyclosporine, theophylline, phenytoin, benzodiazepines, ethosuximide, and valproic acid. Carbamazepine is a CYP 450 3A3/4 substrate and inducer of CYP 450 1A2, 2C, and 3A3/4.

Suggested dosing intervals for specific dosage forms: extended-release tabs or caps (BID); chewable and immediate-release tablets (BID–TID); suspension (QID). Doses may be administered with food. **Do not** crush or chew extended-release dosage forms. Shake bottle well prior to dispensing oral suspension dosage form and **do not** administer simultaneously with other liquid medicines or diluents.

Drug metabolism typically increases after the first mo of therapy due to hepatic autoinduction.

Therapeutic blood levels: 4–12 mg/L. Recommended serum sampling time: obtain trough level within 30 min prior to an oral dose. Steady-state is typically achieved 1 mo following the initiation of therapy (following enzymatic autoinduction). Levels obtained prior to steady-state are useful for preventing toxicity. Blood levels of 7–10 mg/L have been recommended for bipolar disorders.

Side effects include sedation, dizziness, diplopia, aplastic anemia, neutropenia, urinary retention, nausea, SIADH, and Stevens-Johnson syndrome. Suicidal behavior or ideation have been reported. Pretreatment CBCs and LFTs are suggested. Patient should be monitored for hematologic and hepatic toxicity. **Adjust dose in renal impairment (see Chapter 31).**

See Chapter 2 for management of ingestions.

## CARBAMIDE PEROXIDE

Debrox, Murine Ear, Auro Ear Drops, Cankaid, Gly-Oxide, Orajel Perioseptic, and others
***Cerumenolytic, topical oral analgesic***

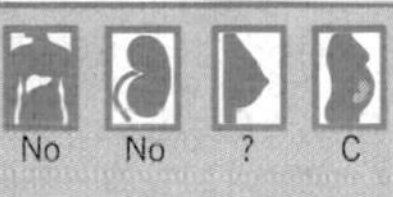


**Otic solution (OTC):** 6.5% (15, 30 mL); may contain propylene glycol or alcohol
**Oral liquid (OTC):** 10% (Cankaid, Gly-Oxide) (15, 60 mL), 15% (Orajel Perioseptic) (240 mL)

***Cerumenolytic:***

***<12 yr:*** Tilt head sideways and instill 1–5 drops (according to patient size) into affected ear and keep drops in ear for several min. Remove wax by gently flushing the ear with warm water, using a soft rubber bulb ear syringe. Dose may be repeated BID PRN for up to 4 days.

***≥12 yr:*** Following the same instructions for <12 yr; instill 5–10 drops into affected ear BID PRN for **up to** 4 days.

***Oral analgesic (see remarks):***

***Liquid:***

***≥3 yr (able to follow instructions):*** Instill several drops to affected area and expectorate after 2–3 min OR place 10 drops on tongue and mix with saliva, swish for several min and expectorate. Administer QID, after meals and QHS, for **up to** 7 days.

**Contraindicated** if tympanic membrane perforated; following otic surgery; ear discharge, drainage, pain, irritation or rash; or PE tubes in place. Tip of applicator should not enter ear canal when used as a cerumenolytic.

Prolonged use of the oral product may result in fungal overgrowth. **Do not** rinse the mouth or drink for at least 5 min when using oral preparation.

For explanation of icons, see p. 698.

## CARBINOXAMINE ± PSEUDOEPHEDRINE

Palgic, Carbinox
In combination with pseudoephedrine: Sildec, Cordron-D NR, Pseudo Carb Pediatric, Cordron-D, and Hydro-Tussin CBX
***Antihistamine with decongestant***

No Yes ? C

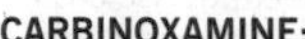

**CARBINOXAMINE:**
Liquid (Palgic, Carbinox): 4 mg/5 mL (473 mL)
Tabs (Palgic): 4 mg

**CARBINOXAMINE + PSEUDOEPHEDRINE:**
Oral drops (Sildec): Carbinoxamine 1 mg + pseudoephedrine 15 mg/1 mL (30 mL)
Oral liquid:
Cordron-D NR and Pseudo Carb Pediatric: Carbinoxamine 2 mg + pseudoephedrine 12.5 mg/5 mL (118, 473 mL)
Cordron-D: Carbinoxamine 2 mg + pseudoephedrine 17.5 mg/5 mL (473 mL)
Hydro-Tussin CBX: Carbinoxamine 2 mg + pseudoephedrine 25 mg/5 mL (30 mL)

***Child (PO):*** carbinoxamine at 0.2–0.4 mg/kg/24 hr and pseudoephedrine (with combination product) at 4 mg/kg/24 hr; alternative oral dosing of Palgic (carbinoxamine) by age (**do not exceed** 0.4 mg/kg/24 hr):
***2–3 yr:*** 2 mg TID–QID
***3–6 yr:*** 2–4 mg TID–QID
***≥6 yr:*** 4–6 mg TID–QID
***Adult:*** 4–8 mg TID–QID

Additional dosing information for combination products:

| Age | Oral Drops* | Oral Syrup† |
|---|---|---|
| 1–3 mo | 0.25 mL QID | |
| >3–6 mo | 0.5 mL QID | |
| >6–9 mo | 0.75 mL QID | |
| >9–18 mo | 1 mL QID | |
| >18 mo–6 yr | | 2.5 mL QID |
| ≥6 yr and adult | | 5 mL QID |

*1 mg carbinoxamine + 15 mg pseudoephedrine/1 mL.
†2 mg carbinoxamine + 15 mg pseudoephedrine/5 mL.

Generally **not recommended** for treating URIs for infants. No proven benefit for infants and young children with URIs. The FDA does **not recommend** use in children < 2 yr because of reports of increased fatalities.

**Contraindicated** in acute asthma, hypersensitivity with other ethanolamine antihistamines, MAO inhibitors, severe hypertension, narrow-angle glaucoma, severe coronary artery disease, and urinary retention. **Be aware of the corresponding amount of pseudoephedrine** if using combination product (see *Pseudoephedrine* for additional remarks).

May cause drowsiness, vertigo, dry mucous membranes, and headache. Contact dermatitis and CNS excitation have been reported.

**CARNITINE**

Levocarnitine, Carnitor, L-Carnitine

***Nutritional supplement, amino acid***

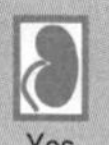
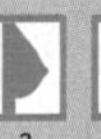

No Yes ? B

**Tabs:** 330, 500 mg
**Caps:** 250 mg
**Oral solution:** 100 mg/mL (118 mL)
**Injection:** 200 mg/mL (5 mL) (preservative free)

***Primary carnitine deficiency:***

***Oral:***

***Child:*** 50–100 mg/kg/24 hr PO ÷ Q8–12 hr; increase slowly as needed and tolerated to **max. dose** of 3 g/24 hr

***Adult:*** 330 mg to 1 g/dose BID–TID PO

***IV:***

***Child and adult:*** 50 mg/kg as loading dose; may follow with 50 mg/kg/24 hr IV infusion; maintenance: 50 mg/kg/24 hr ÷ Q4–6 hr; increase to **max. dose** of 300 mg/kg/24 hr if needed.

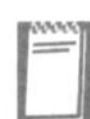

May cause nausea, vomiting, abdominal cramps, diarrhea, and body odor. Seizures have been reported in patients with or without a history of seizures. Safety in end-stage renal disease (ESRD) has not been established.

High doses to severely compromised renal function or ESRD on dialysis may result in accumulation of potentially toxic metabolites (trimethylamine and trimethylamine-N-oxide).

Give bolus IV infusion over 2–3 min.

**CASPOFUNGIN**

Cancidas

***Antifungal, echinocandin***

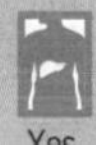
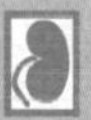
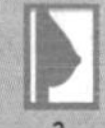
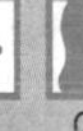
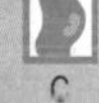

Yes No ? C

**Injection:** 50, 70 mg; contains sucrose (39 mg in 50 mg vial and 54 mg in 70 mg vial)

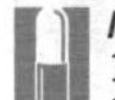

***Neonate (dosage used in case studies, but pharmacokinetic studies are limited):*** 1 mg/kg/dose IV QD × 2, then 2 mg/kg/dose IV QD.

***Child (pharmacokinetic data in 2–17 yr with oncological fever and neutropenia, see remarks):*** 50 mg/m²/dose IV QD; **max. dose:** 50 mg/dose

***Adolescent and adult (see remarks):***

***Loading dose:*** 70 mg IV × 1

***Maintenance dose:***

***Usual:*** 50 mg IV QD. If tolerated and response is inadequate, may increase to 70 mg IV QD.

***Hepatic insufficiency (Child-Pugh score 7 to 9):*** 35 mg IV QD

***Concomitant rifampin:*** 70 mg IV QD

**Use with caution** in hepatic impairment and concomitant enzyme inducing drugs. Higher maintenance doses (70 mg QD in adults) may be necessary for concomitant use of enzyme inducers such as carbamazepine, dexamethasone, phenytoin, nevirapine, or efavirenz. May cause fever, facial swelling, rash, nausea/vomiting, headache, infusion site phlebitis, and LFT elevation.

Use with cyclosporine may cause transient increase in LFTs and caspofungin level elevations. May decrease tacrolimus levels.

*Continued*

For explanation of icons, see p. 698.

CASPOFUNGIN *continued*

Administer doses by slow IV infusion over 1 hr. **Do not** mix or co-infuse with other medications and **avoid** using dextrose-containing diluents (e.g., $D_5W$).

## CEFACLOR

Ceclor, Ceclor CD, Raniclor, and others

***Antibiotic, cephalosporin (second generation)***

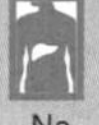 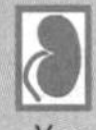 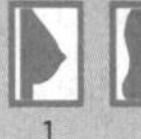 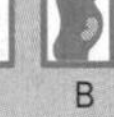

No Yes 1 B

**Caps:** 250, 500 mg
**Extended-release tabs (Ceclor CD):** 375, 500 mg
**Chewable tabs (Raniclor):** 125, 187, 250, 375 mg; contains phenylalanine
**Oral suspension:** 125 mg/5 mL (75, 150 mL); 187 mg/5 mL (50, 100 mL); 250 mg/5 mL (75, 150 mL); 375 mg/5 mL (50 , 100 mL)

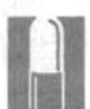

***Child > 1 mo old (use regular-release dosage forms):*** 20–40 mg/kg/24 hr PO ÷ Q8 hr; **max. dose:** 2 g/24 hr (Q12 hr dosage interval optional in otitis media or pharyngitis)
***Adult:*** 250–500 mg/dose PO Q8 hr; **max. dose:** 4 g/24 hr
***Extended-release tablets:*** 375–500 mg/dose PO Q12 hr

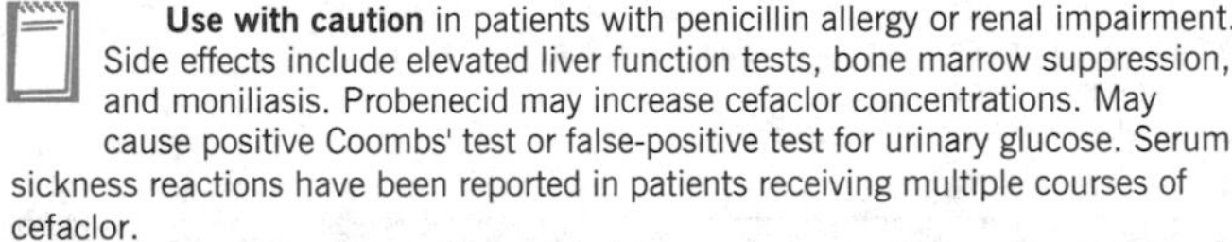

**Use with caution** in patients with penicillin allergy or renal impairment. Side effects include elevated liver function tests, bone marrow suppression, and moniliasis. Probenecid may increase cefaclor concentrations. May cause positive Coombs' test or false-positive test for urinary glucose. Serum sickness reactions have been reported in patients receiving multiple courses of cefaclor.

**Do not** crush, cut, or chew extended-release tablets. Doses should be given on an empty stomach. Extended-release tablets **not recommended** for children. **Adjust dose in renal failure (see Chapter 31).**

## CEFADROXIL

Duricef and others

***Antibiotic, cephalosporin (first generation)***

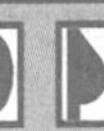 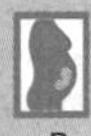 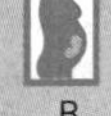

No Yes 1 B

**Suspension:** 125, 250, 500 mg/5 mL (50, 75, 100 mL)
**Tabs:** 1 g
**Caps:** 500 mg

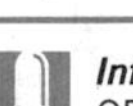

***Infant and child:*** 30 mg/kg/24 hr PO ÷ Q12 hr (daily dose may be administered QD for group A beta-hemolytic streptococci pharyngitis/tonsillitis); **max. dose:** 2 g/24 hr
***Adolescent and adult:*** 1–2 g/24 hr PO ÷ Q12–24 hr (administer Q12 hr for complicated UTIs); **max. dose:** 2 g/24 hr

See *Cephalexin* for **precautions** and interactions. Rash, nausea, vomiting, and diarrhea are common. Transient neutropenia and vaginitis have been reported. **Adjust dose in renal failure (see Chapter 31).**

## CEFAZOLIN

Ancef, Zolicef, and others

***Antibiotic, cephalosporin (first generation)***

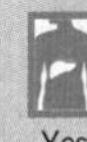 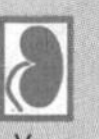 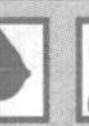 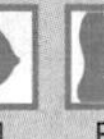

Yes Yes 1 B

**Injection:** 0.5, 1, 5, 10, 20 g
**Frozen injection:** 1 g/50 mL 5% dextrose (iso-osmotic solutions)
Contains 2.1 mEq Na/g drug

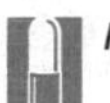

***Neonate IM, IV:***

***Postnatal age ≤ 7 days:*** 40 mg/kg/24 hr ÷ Q12 hr
***Postnatal age >7 days:***
***≤2000 g:*** 40 mg/kg/24 hr ÷ Q12 hr
***>2000 g:*** 60 mg/kg/24 hr ÷ Q8 hr

***Infant >1 mo/child:*** 50–100 mg/kg/24 hr ÷ Q8 hr IV/IM; **max. dose:** 6 g/24 hr
***Adult:*** 2–6 g/24 hr ÷ Q6–8 hr IV/IM; **max. dose:** 12 g/24 hr

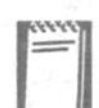

**Use with caution** in renal impairment or in penicillin-allergic patients. Does not penetrate well into CSF. May cause phlebitis, leukopenia, thrombocytopenia, transient liver enzyme elevation, false-positive urine reducing substance (Clinitest) and Coombs' test. **Adjust dose in renal failure (see Chapter 31).**

## CEFDINIR

Omnicef

***Antibiotic, cephalosporin (third generation)***

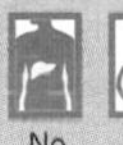 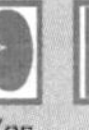 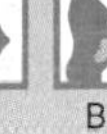 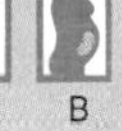

No Yes 1 B

**Caps:** 300 mg
**Oral suspension:** 125 mg/5 mL (60, 100 mL)

***6 mo–12 yr:***

***Otitis media, sinusitis, pharyngitis/tonsillitis:*** 14 mg/kg/24 hr PO ÷ Q12–24 hr; **max. dose:** 600 mg/24 hr
***Uncomplicated skin infections:*** 14 mg/kg/24 hr PO ÷ Q12 hr; **max. dose:** 600 mg/24 hr

***≥13 yr and adult:***

***Bronchitis, sinusitis, pharyngitis/tonsillitis:*** 600 mg/24 hr PO ÷ Q12–24 hr
***Community-acquired pneumonia, uncomplicated skin infections:*** 600 mg/24 hr PO ÷ Q12 hr

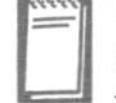

**Use with caution** in penicillin-allergic patients or in presence of renal impairment. Good gram-positive cocci activity. May cause diarrhea and false-positive urine reducing substance (Clinitest) and Coombs' test. Eosinophilia and abnormal liver function tests have been reported with higher than usual doses.

Once daily dosing has not been evaluated in pneumonia and skin infections. Probenecid increases serum cefdinir levels. **Avoid** concomitant administration with iron and iron-containing vitamins and antacids containing aluminum or magnesium (space by 2 hr apart) to reduce the risk for decreasing antibiotic's absorption. Doses may be taken without regard to food. **Adjust dose in renal failure (see Chapter 31).**

For explanation of icons, see p. 698.

## CEFEPIME

Maxipime

***Antibiotic, cephalosporin (fourth generation)***

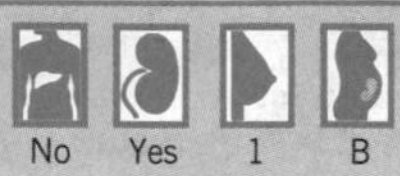


**Injection:** 0.5, 1, 2 g
Each 1 g drug contains 725 mg L-Arginine.

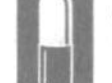

***Neonate:***

***<14 days:*** 60 mg/kg/24 hr ÷ Q12 hr IV/IM

***≥14 days:*** 100 mg/kg/24 hr ÷ Q12 hr IV/IM. For meningitis or *Pseudomonas* infections, use 150 mg/kg/24 hr ÷ Q8 hr IV/IM

***Child ≥ 2 mo:*** 100 mg/kg/24 hr ÷ Q12 hr IV/IM

***Meningitis, fever, and neutropenia, or serious infections:*** 150 mg/kg/24 hr ÷ Q8 hr IV/IM

**Max. dose:** 6 g/24 hr

***Cystic fibrosis:*** 150 mg/kg/24 hr ÷ Q8 hr IV/IM, up to a **max. dose** of 6 g/24 hr.

***Adult:*** 1–4 g/24 hr ÷ Q12 hr IV/IM

***Severe infections:*** 6 g/24 hr ÷ Q8 hr IV/IM

**Max. dose:** 6 g/24 hr

**Use with caution** in patients with penicillin allergy or renal impairment. Good activity against *P. aeruginosa* and other gram-negative bacteria plus most gram-positives (*S. aureus*). May cause thrombophlebitis, gastrointestinal discomfort, transient increases in liver enzymes, false-positive urine reducing substance (Clinitest) and Coombs' test. Probenecid increases serum cefepime levels. Encephalopathy, myoclonus, seizures, transient leukopenia, neutropenia, agranulocytosis and thrombocytopenia have been reported. **Adjust dose in renal failure (see Chapter 31).**

## CEFIXIME

Suprax

***Antibiotic, cephalosporin (third generation)***

No Yes 1 B

**Oral suspension:** 100 mg/5 mL (50, 75 mL)

***Infant (>6 mo) and child:*** 8 mg/kg/24 hr ÷ Q12–24 hr PO; **max. dose:** 400 mg/24 hr

***Acute UTI:*** 16 mg/kg/24 hr ÷ Q12 hr on day 1, followed by 8 mg/kg/24 hr Q24 hr PO × 13 days; **max. dose:** 400 mg/24 hr

***Adolescent and adult:*** 400 mg/24 hr ÷ Q12–24 hr PO

***Uncomplicated cervical, urethral, or rectal infections due to N. gonorrhoeae:*** 400 mg × 1 PO

**Use with caution** in patients with penicillin allergy or renal failure. Adverse reactions include diarrhea, abdominal pain, nausea, and headaches. **Do not use** tablets for the treatment of otitis media due to reduced bioavailability. Probenecid increases serum cefixime levels. May increase carbamazepine serum concentrations. May cause false-positive urine reducing substance (Clinitest), Coombs' test, and nitroprusside test for ketones. **Adjust dose in renal failure (see Chapter 31).**

## CEFOPERAZONE

Cefobid

***Antibiotic, cephalosporin (third generation)***

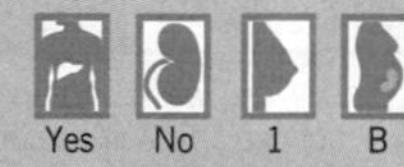


**Injection:** 1, 2, 10 g
Contains 1.5 mEq Na/g drug

***Infant and child:*** 100–150 mg/kg/24 hr ÷ Q8–12 hr IV/IM; **max. dose:** 12 g/24 hr
***Adult (see remarks):*** 2–4 g/24 hr ÷ Q12 hr IV/IM.
**Max. doses:**
***Usual:*** 12 g/24 hr
***Hepatic disease and/or biliary obstruction:*** 4 g/24 hr
***Mixed hepatic and renal impairment:*** 1–2 g/24 hr

**Use with caution** in penicillin-allergic patients or in patients with hepatic failure or biliary obstruction. Drug is extensively excreted in bile. May cause disulfiram-like reaction with ethanol, and false-positive urine reducing substance (Clinitest) and Coombs' test. Bleeding and bruising may occur especially in patients with vitamin K deficiency. Does not penetrate well into CSF.

Doses up to 16 g/24 hr administered by continuous IV infusion have been used in immunocompromised adults without complications (steady-state serum level of 150 mcg/mL).

## CEFOTAXIME

Claforan

***Antibiotic, cephalosporin (third generation)***

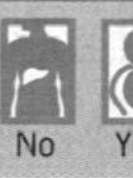
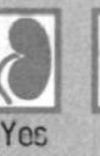
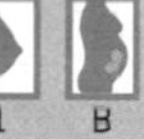


**Injection:** 0.5, 1, 2, 10 g
**Frozen injection:** 1 g/50 mL 3.4% dextrose, 2 g/50 mL 1.4% dextrose (iso-osmotic solutions)
Contains 2.2 mEq Na/g drug

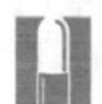

***Neonate:*** IV/IM:
***Postnatal age ≤ 7 days:***
***<2000 g:*** 100 mg/kg/24 hr ÷ Q12 hr
***≥2000 g:*** 100–150 mg/kg/24 hr ÷ Q8–12 hr
***Postnatal age >7 days:***
***<1200 g:*** 100 mg/kg/24 hr ÷ Q12 hr
***1200–2000 g:*** 150 mg/kg/24 hr ÷ Q8 hr
***>2000 g:*** 150–200 mg/kg/24 hr ÷ Q6–8 hr

***Infant and child (1 mo–12 yr and <50 kg):*** 100–200 mg/kg/24 hr ÷ Q6–8 hr IV/IM. Higher doses of 150–225 mg/kg/24 hr ÷ Q6–8 hr have been recommended for infections outside the CSF due to penicillin-resistant pneumococci.
***Meningitis:*** 200 mg/kg/24 hr ÷ Q6 hr IV/IM. Higher doses of 225–300 mg/kg/24 hr ÷ Q6–8 hr, in combination with vancomycin (60 mg/kg/24 hr), have been recommended for meningitis due to penicillin-resistant pneumococci.
**Max. dose:** 12 g/24 hr

***Child (> 12 yr or ≥ 50 kg) and adult:*** 1–2 g/dose Q6–8 hr IV/IM
***Severe infection:*** 2 g/dose Q4–6 hr IV/IM
**Max. dose:** 12 g/24 hr
***Uncomplicated gonorrhea:*** 0.5–1 g × 1 IM

*Continued*

For explanation of icons, see p. 698.

CEFOTAXIME *continued*

**Use with caution** in penicillin allergy and renal impairment (reduce dosage). Toxicities similar to other cephalosporins: allergy, neutropenia, thrombocytopenia, eosinophilia, false-positive urine reducing substance (Clinitest) and Coombs' test, elevated BUN, creatinine, and liver enzymes. Probenecid increases serum cefotaxime levels.

Good CNS penetration. **Adjust dose in renal failure (see Chapter 31).**

## CEFOTETAN

Cefotan

***Antibiotic, cephalosporin (second generation)***

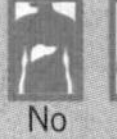
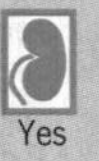
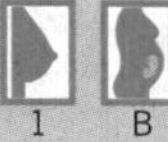

No Yes 1 B

**Injection:** 1, 2, 10 g
**Frozen injection:** 1 g/50 mL 3.8% dextrose, 2 g/50 mL 2.2% dextrose (iso-osmotic solutions)
Contains 3.5 mEq Na/g drug

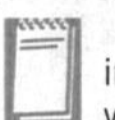

***Infant and child (limited data):*** 40–80 mg/kg/24 hr ÷ Q12 hr IV/IM
***Adolescent and adult:*** 2–6 g/24 hr ÷ Q12 hr IV/IM
***PID:*** 2 g Q12 hr IV × 24–48 hr after clinical improvement with doxycycline 100 mg Q12 hr PO/IV × 14 days
**Max. dose** (all ages): 6 g/24 hr

**Use with caution** in penicillin-allergic patients or in presence of renal impairment. Has good anaerobic activity. May cause disulfiram-like reaction with ethanol, increase effects/toxicities of anticoagulants, false-positive urine reducing substance (Clinitest), and false elevations of serum and urine creatinine (Jaffe method). Hemolytic anemia has been reported. CSF penetration is poor. **Adjust dose in renal failure (see Chapter 31).**

## CEFOXITIN

Mefoxin

***Antibiotic, cephalosporin (second generation)***

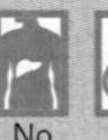
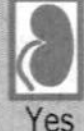
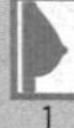
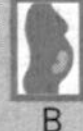

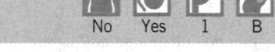

No Yes 1 B

**Injection:** 1, 2, 10 g
**Frozen injection:** 1 g/50 mL 4% dextrose, 2 g/50 mL 2.2% dextrose (iso-osmotic solutions)
Contains 2.3 mEq Na/g drug

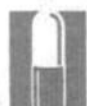

***Neonate:*** 90–100 mg/kg/24 hr ÷ Q8 hr IM/IV
***Infant (> 3 mo) and child:***
***Mild/moderate infections:*** 80–100 mg/kg/24 hr ÷ Q6–8 hr IM/IV
***Severe infections:*** 100–160 mg/kg/24 hr ÷ Q4–6 hr IM/IV
***Adult:*** 4–12 g/24 hr ÷ Q6–8 hr IM/IV
***PID:*** 2 g IV Q6h × 24–48 hr after clinical improvement with doxycycline 100 mg Q12 hr PO/IV × 14 days
**Max. dose** (all ages): 12 g/24 hr

**Use with caution** in penicillin-allergic patients or in presence of renal impairment. Has good anaerobic activity but poor CSF penetration. Probenecid

*Continued*

CEFOXITIN *continued*

increases serum cefoxitin levels. May cause false-positive urine reducing substance (Clinitest and other copper reduction method tests), and false elevations of serum and urine creatinine (Jaffe and KDA methods).

**Adjust dose in renal failure (see Chapter 31).**

## CEFPODOXIME PROXETIL

Vantin

***Antibiotic, cephalosporin (third generation)***

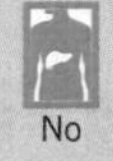
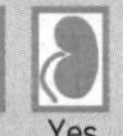
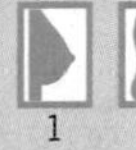
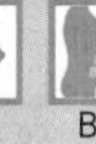
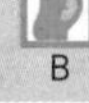

No Yes 1 B

**Tabs:** 100, 200 mg
**Oral suspension:** 50, 100 mg/5 mL (50, 75, 100 mL)

***2 mo–12 yr:***
***Otitis media:*** 10 mg/kg/24 hr PO ÷ Q12–24 hr; **max. dose:** 400 mg/24 hr
***Pharyngitis/tonsillitis:*** 10 mg/kg/24 hr PO ÷ Q12 hr; **max. dose:** 200 mg/24 hr
***Acute maxillary sinusitis:*** 10 mg/kg/24 hr PO ÷ Q12 hr; **max. dose:** 400 mg/24 hr
***≥13 yr–adult:*** 200–800 mg/24 hr PO ÷ Q12 hr
***Uncomplicated gonorrhea:*** 200 mg PO × 1

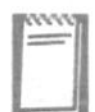

**Use with caution** in penicillin-allergic patients or in presence of renal impairment. May cause diarrhea, nausea, vomiting, vaginal candidiasis, and false-positive Coombs' test.

Tablets should be administered with food to enhance absorption. Suspension may be administered without regard to food. High doses of antacids or $H_2$ blockers may reduce absorption. Probenecid increases serum cefpodoxime levels.

**Adjust dose in renal failure (see Chapter 31).**

## CEFPROZIL

Cefzil and others

***Antibiotic, cephalosporin (second generation)***

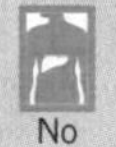
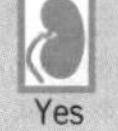
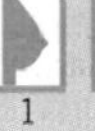
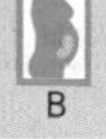

No Yes 1 B

**Tabs:** 250, 500 mg
**Oral suspension:** 125 mg/5 mL, 250 mg/5 mL (50, 75, 100 mL) (contains aspartame and phenylalanine)

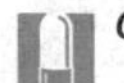

***Otitis media:***
***6 mo–12 yr:*** 30 mg/kg/24 hr PO ÷ Q12 hr
***Pharyngitis/tonsillitis:***
***2–12 yr:*** 15 mg/kg/24 hr PO ÷ Q12 hr
***Acute sinusitis:***
***6 mo–12 yr:*** 15–30 mg/kg/24 hr PO ÷ Q12–24 hr
***Uncomplicated skin infections:***
***2–12 yr:*** 20 mg/kg/24 hr PO ÷ Q24 hr
***Other:***
***≥13 yr and adult:*** 500–1000 mg/24 hr PO ÷ Q12–24 hr
**Max. dose** (all ages): 1 g/24 hr

*Continued*

For explanation of icons, see p. 698.

CEFPROZIL *continued*

**Use with caution** in penicillin-allergic patients or in presence of renal impairment. Oral suspension contains aspartame and phenylalanine and should not be used by phenyketonurics. May cause nausea, vomiting, diarrhea, liver enzyme elevations, false-positive urine reducing substance (Clinitest and other copper reduction method tests) and Coombs' test. Probenecid increases serum cefprozil levels. Absorption is not affected by food. **Adjust dose in renal failure (see Chapter 31).**

## CEFTAZIDIME

Fortaz, Tazidime, Tazicef, Ceptaz (arginine salt)
***Antibiotic, cephalosporin (third generation)***

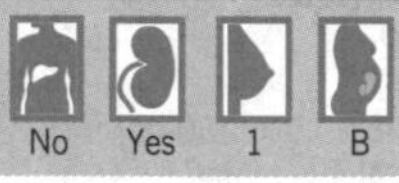


**Injection.:** 0.5, 1, 2, 6, 10 g
**Frozen injection:** 1g/50 mL 4.4% dextrose, 2 g/50 mL 3.2% dextrose (iso-osmotic solutions)
(Fortaz, Tazicef, Tazidime contains 2.3 mEq Na/g drug)
(Ceptaz contains 349 mg L-arginine/g drug)

***Neonate:*** IV/IM:
- ***Postnatal age ≤ 7 days:***
  - ***<2000 kg:*** 100 mg/kg/24 hr ÷ Q12 hr
  - ***≥2000 kg:*** 100–150 mg/kg/24 hr ÷ Q8–12 hr
- ***Postnatal age >7 days:***
  - ***<1200 g:*** 100 mg/kg/24 hr ÷ Q12 hr
  - ***≥1200 g:*** 150 mg/kg/24 hr ÷ Q8 hr

***Infant and child:*** 90–150 mg/kg/24 hr ÷ Q8 hr IV/IM; **max. dose:** 6 g/24 hr
- ***Cystic fibrosis and meningitis:*** 150 mg/kg/24 hr ÷ Q8 hr IV/IM; **max. dose:** 6 g/24 hr

***Adult:*** 2–6 g/24 hr ÷ Q8–12 hr IV/IM; **max. dose:** 6 g/24 hr

**Use with caution** in penicillin-allergic patients or in presence of renal impairment. Good *Pseudomonas* coverage and CSF penetration. May cause rash, liver enzyme elevations, false-positive urine reducing substance (Clinitest and other copper reduction method tests) and Coombs' test. Probenecid increases serum ceftazidime levels. **Adjust dose in renal failure (see Chapter 31).**

## CEFTIBUTEN

Cedax
***Antibiotic, cephalosporin (third generation)***

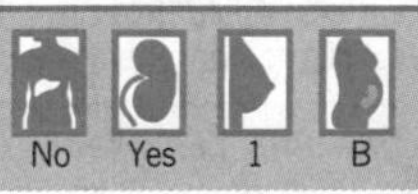


**Oral suspension:** 90 mg/5 mL (30, 60, 90, 120 mL)
**Caps:** 400 mg

***Child:***
- ***Otitis media and pharyngitis/tonsillitis:*** 9 mg/kg/24 hr PO QD; **max. dose:** 400 mg/24 hr

***≥12 yr:*** 400 mg PO QD; **max. dose:** 400 mg/24 hr

*Continued*

CEFTIBUTEN *continued*

**Use with caution** in penicillin-allergic patients or in presence of renal impairment. May cause GI symptoms and elevations in eosinophils and BUN. Gastric acid lowering medictions (e.g., ranitidine and omeprazole) may enhance bioavailability of ceftibutin.

Oral suspension should be administered 2 hr before or 1 hr after a meal. **Adjust dose in renal failure (see Chapter 31).**

## CEFTIZOXIME

Cefizox

***Antibiotic, cephalosporin (third generation)***

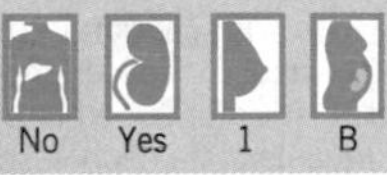

No Yes 1 B

**Injection:** 0.5, 1, 2, 10 g
**Frozen injection:** 1 g/50 mL 3.8% dextrose, 2 g/50 mL 1.9% dextrose (iso-osmotic solutions)
Contains 2.6 mEq Na/g drug

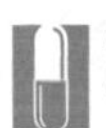

***Infant > 1 mo and < 6 mo:*** 100–200 mg/kg/24 hr ÷ Q6–8 hr IV/IM
***Infant ≥ 6 mo and child:*** 150–200 mg/kg/24 hr ÷ Q6–8 hr IV/IM; **max. dose:** 12 g/24 hr
***Adult:*** 2–12 g/24 hr ÷ Q8–12 hr IV/IM; **max. dose:** 12 g/24 hr
***Uncomplicated gonorrhea:*** 1 g IM × 1

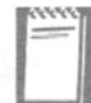

**Use with caution** in penicillin-allergic patients or in presence of renal impairment. May cause liver enzyme elevation, false-positive urine reducing substances (Clinitest, Benedict's solution) and interfere with serum and urine creatinine assays (Jaffe method). Good CNS penetration. Probenecid increases serum ceftizoxime levels. **Adjust dose in renal failure (see Chapter 31).**

## CEFTRIAXONE

Rocephin

***Antibiotic, cephalosporin (third generation)***

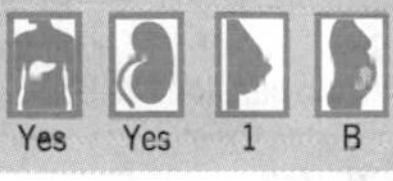

Yes Yes 1 B

**Injection:** 0.25, 0.5, 1, 2, 10 g
**Frozen injection:** 1 g/50 mL 3.8% dextrose, 2 g/50 mL 2.4% dextrose (iso-osmotic solutions)
**Intramuscular kit with 1% lidocaine diluent:** 0.5, 1 g
Contains 3.6 mEq Na/g drug

***Neonate:***
***Gonococcal ophthalmia or prophylaxis:*** 25–50 mg/kg/dose IM/IV × 1; **max. dose:** 125 mg/dose
***Infant and child:*** 50–75 mg/kg/24 hr ÷ Q12–24 hr IM/IV; **max. dose:** 2 g/24 hr . Higher doses of 80–100 mg/kg/24 hr ÷ Q12–24 hr (**max. dose:** 2 g/dose and 4 g/24 hr) has been recommended for infections outside the CSF due to penicillin-resistant pneumococci.
***Meningitis (including penicillin resistant pneumococci):*** 100 mg/kg/24 hr IM/IV ÷ Q12 hr; **max. dose:** 2 g/dose and 4 g/24 hr
***Acute otitis media:*** 50 mg/kg IM × 1; **max. dose:** 1 g

*Continued*

For explanation of icons, see p. 698.

CEFTRIAXONE *continued*

***Adult:*** 1–2 g/dose Q12–24 hr IV/IM; **max. dose:** 2 g/dose and 4 g/24 hr
***Uncomplicated gonorrhea or chancroid:*** 250 mg IM × 1

**Contraindicated** in neonates with hyperbilirubinemia. **Do not** administer with calcium-containing solutions or products (mixed or administered simultaneously via different lines) in newborns because of risk of precipitation of ceftriaxone-calcium salt. Cases of fatal reactions with calcium-ceftriaxone precipitates in lung and kidneys in term and pre-term neonates have been reported.

**Use with caution** in penicillin allergy; patients with gallbladder, biliary tract, liver, or pancreatic disease; presence of renal impairment; or in neonates with continuous dosing (risk for hyperbilirubinemia). In neonates, consider using an alternative third-generation cephalosporin with similar activity. Unlike other cephalosporins, ceftriaxone is significantly cleared by the biliary route (35%–45%).

Rash, injection site pain, diarrhea, and transient increase in liver enzymes are common. May cause reversible cholelithiasis, sludging in gallbladder, and jaundice. May interfere with serum and urine creatinine assays (Jaffe method) and cause false-positive urinary protein and urinary reducing substances (Clinitest).

For IM injections, dilute drug with either sterile water for injection or 1% lidocaine to a concentration of 250 or 350 mg/mL (250 mg/mL has lower incidence of injection site reactions). See *Lidocaine* for additional remarks.

## CEFUROXIME (IV, IM)/CEFUROXIME AXETIL (PO)

IV: Zinacef; PO: Ceftin
***Antibiotic, cephalosporin (second generation)***

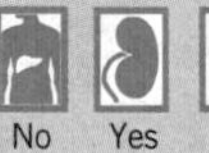
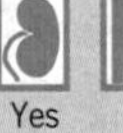
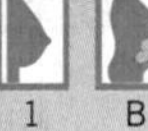

No Yes 1 B

**Injection:** 0.75, 1.5, 7.5 g
**Frozen injection:** 750 mg/50 mL 2.8% dextrose, 1.5 g/50 mL water (iso-osmotic solutions)
Injectable dosage forms contain 2.4 mEq Na/g drug
**Tabs:** 125, 250, 500 mg
**Oral suspension:** 125, 250 mg/5 mL (50, 100 mL)

***IM/IV:***
***Neonate:*** 20–100 mg/kg/24 hr ÷ Q12 hr
***Infant (> 3 mo)/child:*** 75–150 mg/kg/24 hr ÷ Q8 hr
***Adult:*** 750–1500 mg/dose Q8 hr
**Max. dose:** 9 g/24 hr

***PO:***
***Child (3 mo–12 yr):***
***Pharyngitis and tonsillitis:***
***Oral suspension:*** 20 mg/kg/24 hr ÷ Q12 hr; **max. dose:** 500 mg/24 hr
***Tab:*** 125 mg Q12 hr
***Otitis media, impetigo, and maxillary sinusitis:***
***Oral suspension:*** 30 mg/kg/24 hr ÷ Q12 hr; **max. dose:** 1 g/24 hr
***Tab:*** 250 mg Q12 hr
***Adult:*** 250–500 mg BID
**Max. dose:** 1 g/24 hr

**Use with caution** in penicillin-allergic patients or in presence of renal impairment. May cause GI discomfort; thrombophlebitis at the infusion site; false-positive urine reducing substance (Clinitest and other copper reduction method tests) and Coombs' test; and may interfere with serum and urine

*Continued*

CEFUROXIME (IV, IM)/CEFUROXIME AXETIL (PO) *continued*

creatinine determinations by the alkaline picrate method. **Not recommended** for meningitis.

Tablets and oral suspension are **NOT** bioequivalent and are **NOT** substitutable on a mg/mg basis. Administer suspension with food. Concurrent use of antacids, $H_2$ blockers, and proton pump inhibitors may decrease oral absorption. **Adjust dose in renal failure (see Chapter 31).**

## CEPHALEXIN

Keflex, Biocef, and others

***Antibiotic, cephalosporin (first generation)***

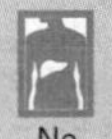
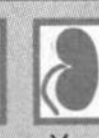
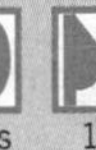
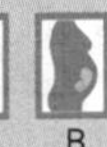
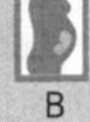

No Yes 1 B

**Caps and tabs:** 250, 500 mg
**Oral suspension:** 125 mg/5 mL, 250 mg/5 mL (100, 200 mL)

***Infant and child:*** 25–100 mg/kg/24 hr PO ÷ Q6 hr. Less frequent dosing (Q8–12 hr) can be used for uncomplicated infections. Total daily dose may be divided Q12 hr for streptococcal pharyngitis (>1 yr) and skin/skin structure infections.
***Adult:*** 1–4 g/24 hr PO ÷ Q6 hr
**Max. dose:** 4 g/24 hr

Some cross-reactivity with penicillins. **Use with caution** in renal insufficiency. May cause GI discomfort, false-positive urine reducing substance (Clinitest and other copper reduction method tests) and Coombs' test; false elevation of serum theophylline levels (HPLC method); and false urinary protein test. Probenecid increases serum cephalexin levels and concomitant administration with cholestyramine may reduce cephalexin absorption. May increase the effects of metformin.

Administer doses on an empty stomach; 2 hr prior or 1 hr after meals. **Adjust dose in renal failure (see Chapter 31).**

## CEPHRADINE

Velosef and others

***Antibiotic, cephalosporin (first generation)***

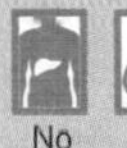
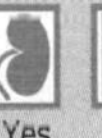
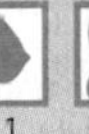
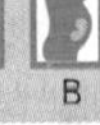

No Yes 1 B

**Oral suspension:** 125 mg/5 mL, 250 mg/5 mL (100, 200 mL)
**Caps:** 250, 500 mg

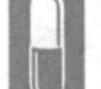

***Infant (≥ 9 mo) and child:*** 25–50 mg/kg/24 hr PO ÷ Q6–12 hr
***Adult:*** 1–4 g/24 hr PO ÷ Q6–12 hr
**Max. dose:** 4 g/24 hr

**Use with caution** in penicillin-allergic patients and in renal insufficiency. Does not penetrate well into CSF. May cause GI discomfort; rash; transient eosinophilia; interfere with serum and urine creatinine assays (Jaffe and KDA methods); theophylline assays (HPLC method); and cause false-positive urinary protein and urinary reducing substances (Clinitest). Probenecid increases serum cephradine levels.

**Adjust dose in renal failure (see Chapter 31).**

For explanation of icons, see p. 698.

## CETIRIZINE ± PSEUDOEPHEDRINE

Zyrtec, Children's Zyrtec
In combination with
pseudoephedrine: Zyrtec-D 12 Hour
***Antihistamine, less-sedating***

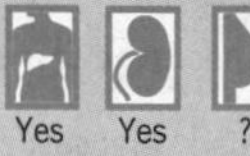
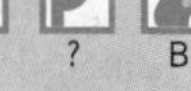

Yes Yes ? B

**Syrup (OTC):** 5 mg/5 mL (120, 473 mL)
**Tabs:** 5 mg 10 mg (OTC)
**Chewable tabs (OTC):** 5, 10 mg
**In combination with pseudoephedrine (PE):**
**Extended-release tabs (Zyrtec-D 12 Hour; OTC):** 5 mg cetirizine + 120 mg PE

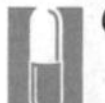

***Cetirizine (see remarks for dosing in hepatic impairment):***
***6 mo and <2 yr:*** 2.5 mg PO QD; dose may be increased for children 12–23 mo to a **max. dose** of 2.5 mg PO Q12 hr.
***2–5 yr:*** Initial dose: 2.5 mg PO QD; if needed, may increase dose to a **max. dose** of 5 mg/24hr.
***≥6 yr–adult:*** 5–10 mg PO QD
***Cetirizine in combination with pseudoephedrine (PE):***
***≥12 yr and adult:***
***Zyrtec-D 12 Hour:*** 1 tablet PO BID

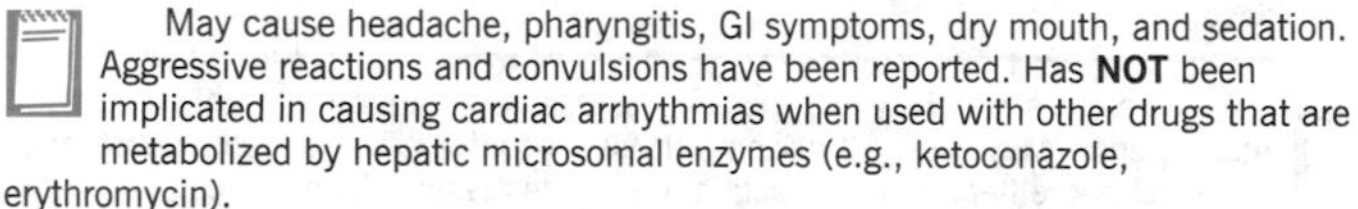

May cause headache, pharyngitis, GI symptoms, dry mouth, and sedation. Aggressive reactions and convulsions have been reported. Has **NOT** been implicated in causing cardiac arrhythmias when used with other drugs that are metabolized by hepatic microsomal enzymes (e.g., ketoconazole, erythromycin).

In hepatic impairment, the following doses have been recommended:
**<6 yr:** Use is **not recommended.**
**6 yr–adult:** 5 mg PO QD

Doses may be administered regardless of food. For Zyrtec-D 12 Hour, see *Pseudoephedrine* for additional remarks. **Dosage adjustment is recommended in renal impairment (see Chapter 31).**

## CHARCOAL, ACTIVATED

See Chapter 2

## CHLORAL HYDRATE

Aquachloral Supprettes and others
***Sedative, hypnotic***

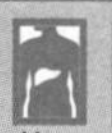
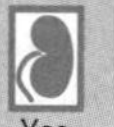
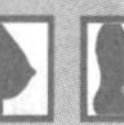
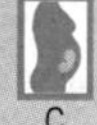

Yes Yes 1 C

**Caps:** 500 mg
**Syrup:** 250, 500 mg/5 mL
**Suppository (Aquachloral Supprettes):** 325, 500, 650 mg; may contain tartrazine

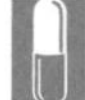

***Child:***
***Sedative:*** 25–50 mg/kg/24 hr PO/PR ÷ Q6–8 hr; **max. dose:** 500 mg/dose
***Sedation for procedures:*** 50–75 mg/kg/dose PO/PR 30–60 min prior to procedure; may repeat in 30 min if needed to up to a total **max. dose** of 120 mg/kg or 1 g total for infants and 2 g total for children

*Continued*

CHLORAL HYDRATE *continued*

***Adult:***

***Sedative:*** 250 mg/dose TID PO/PR
***Hypnotic:*** 500–1000 mg/dose PO/PR; **max. dose:** 2 g/24 hr

**Contraindicated** in patients with hepatic or renal disease. **Use with caution** in combination with IV furosemide (vasodilation) or warfarin (potentiates warfarin). May cause GI irritation, paradoxical excitement, hypotension, and myocardial/respiratory depression. Chronic administration in neonates can lead to accumulation of active metabolites. Requires same monitoring as other sedatives.

Not analgesic. Peak effects occur within 30–60 min. **Do not exceed** 2 wk of chronic use. **Avoid** use in moderate/severe renal failure. Sudden withdrawal may cause delirium tremens.

**For additional information, see Chapter 6.**

## CHLORAMPHENICOL

Chloromycetin and others
***Antibiotic***

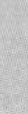
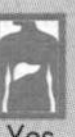
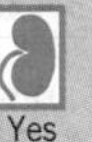
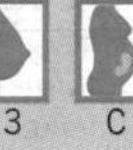

Yes Yes 3 C

**Injection:** 1 g
Contains 2.25 mEq Na/g drug

***Neonate IV:***

***Loading dose:*** 20 mg/kg
***Maintenance dose (first dose should be given 12 hr after loading dose):***
- ***≤7 days:*** 25 mg/kg/24 hr QD
- ***>7 days:***
  - ***≤2 kg:*** 25 mg/kg/24 hr QD
  - ***>2 kg:*** 50 mg/kg/24 hr ÷ Q12 hr

***Infant/child/adult:*** 50–75 mg/kg/24 hr IV ÷ Q6 hr
***Meningitis:*** 75–100 mg/kg/24 hr IV ÷ Q6 hr
**Max. dose:** 4 g/24 hr

Dose recommendations are just guidelines for therapy; monitoring of blood levels is essential in neonates and infants. Follow hematologic status for dose related or idiosyncratic marrow suppression. "Gray baby" syndrome may be seen with levels >50 mg/L. **Use with caution** in G6PD deficiency, renal or hepatic dysfunction, and neonates.

Concomitant use of phenobarbital and rifampin may lower chloramphenicol serum levels. Phenytoin may increase chloramphenicol serum levels. Chloramphenicol may increase the effects/toxicity of phenytoin, chlorpropamide, cyclosporine, tacrolimus, and oral anticoagulants; and decrease absorption of vitamin $B_{12}$. Chloramphenicol is an inhibitor of CYP 450 2C9.

Therapeutic levels: 15–25 mg/L for meningitis; 10–20 mg/L for other infections. Trough: 5–15 mg/L for meningitis; 5–10 mg/L for other infections. Recommended serum sampling time: trough (IV/PO) within 30 min prior to next dose; peak (IV) 30 min after the end of infusion; peak (PO) 2 hr after oral administration. Time to achieve steady-state: 2–3 days for newborns; 12–24 hr for children and adults. **NOTE:** Higher serum levels may be achieved using the oral, rather than the IV route.

For explanation of icons, see p. 698.

## CHLOROQUINE HCL/PHOSPHATE

Aralen and others

***Amebicide, antimalarial***

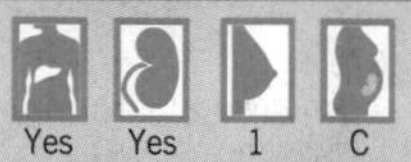


**Tabs:** 250, 500 mg as phosphate (150, 300 mg base, respectively)
**Oral suspension:** 16.67 mg/mL as phosphate (10 mg/mL base), 15 mg/mL as phosphate (9 mg/mL base)
**Injection:** 50 mg/mL as HCL (40 mg/mL base) (5 mL)

***Doses expressed in mg of chloroquine base.***
***Malaria prophylaxis (start 1 wk prior to exposure and continue for 4 wk after leaving edemic area):***
*Child:* 5 mg/kg/dose PO Q wk; **max. dose:** 300 mg/dose
*Adult:* 300 mg/dose PO Q wk
***Malaria treatment (chloroquine sensitive strains):***
***For treatment for malaria, consult with ID specialist or see the latest edition of the AAP* Red Book*. For IV use, consider safer alternatives such as quinidine or quinine.***
*Child:* 10 mg/kg/dose (**max. dose:** 600 mg/dose) PO × 1; followed by 5 mg/kg/dose (**max. dose:** 300 mg/dose) 6 hr later and then once daily for 2 days.
*Adult:* 600 mg/dose PO × 1; followed by 300 mg/dose 6 hr later and then once daily for 2 days.

**Use with caution** in liver disease, preexisting auditory damage or seizures, G6PD deficiency, psoriasis, porphyria or concomitant hepatotoxic drugs. May cause nausea, vomiting, ECG abnormalities, prolonged QT interval, blurred vision, retinal and corneal changes, headaches, confusion, skeletal muscle weakness, and hair depigmentation.

Antacids, ampicillin, and kaolin may decrease the absorption of chloroquine (allow 4 hr interval between chloroquine). Cimetidine may increase effects/toxicity of chloroquine. May increase serum cyclosporine levels. **Adjust dose in renal failure (see Chapter 31).**

## CHLOROTHIAZIDE

Diuril, Diurigen, and others

***Thiazide diuretic***

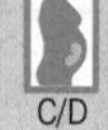

Yes Yes 1 C/D

**Tabs:** 250, 500 mg
**Oral suspension:** 250 mg/5 mL (237 mL); contains 0.5% alcohol, 0.12% methylparaben, 0.02% propylparaben, and 0.1% benzoic acid
**Injection:** 500 mg; contains 5 mEq Na/1g drug

***<6 mo:*** 20–40 mg/kg/24 hr ÷ Q12 hr PO/IV; alternatively, lower IV doses of 2–8 mg/kg/24 hr ÷ Q12 hr may be used.
***≥6 mo:*** 20 mg/kg/24 hr ÷ Q12 hr PO/IV; alternatively, lower IV doses of 4 mg/kg/24 hr ÷ Q12–24 hr may be used.
**Max. PO dose:**
***≤2 yr:*** 375 mg/24 hr
***2–12 yr:*** 1 g/24 hr
***Adult:*** 500–2000 mg/24 hr ÷ Q12–24 hr PO/IV; alternative IV dosing, some may respond to intermittent dosing on alternate days or on 3–5 days each wk.

*Continued*

CHLOROTHIAZIDE *continued*

**Use with caution** in liver and severe renal disease. May increase serum calcium, bilirubin, glucose, and uric acid. May cause alkalosis, pancreatitis, dizziness, hypokalemia, and hypomagnesemia.

**Avoid** IM or subcutaneous administration.

Pregnancy category changes to "D" if used in pregnancy-induced hypertension.

## CHLORPHENIRAMINE MALEATE/ DEXCHLORPHENIRAMINE MALEATE

Chlorpheniramine: Chlor-Trimeton, Efidac 24, and others

Dexchlorpheniramine: Various generics

***Antihistamine***

No No ? B

**CHLORPHENIRAMINE MALEATE:**

Tabs [OTC]: 4 mg
Caplets: 8 mg
Chewable tab [OTC]: 2 mg
Sustained-release caps: 8, 12 mg
Sustained-release tabs [OTC]: 8, 12 mg
Combined immediate- and sustained-release tab (Efidac 24) [OTC]: 16 mg (4 mg immediate and 12 mg sustained)
Syrup [OTC]: 2 mg/5 mL (473 mL); contains 5% alcohol
Oral suspension: 4 mg/5 mL (118 mL), 8 mg/5 mL (473 mL); contains methylparaben

**DEXCHLORPHENIRAMINE MALEATE:**

Sustained-release tabs: 4, 6 mg
Syrup: 2mg/5 mL (473 mL); contains alcohol

***CHLORPHENIRAMINE MALEATE DOSING:***

***Child:*** 0.35 mg/kg/24 hr PO ÷ Q4–6 hr or dose based on age as follows:
***2–5 yr:*** 1 mg/dose PO Q4–6 hr; **max. dose:** 6 mg/24 hr
***6–11 yr:*** 2 mg/dose PO Q4–6 hr; **max. dose** 12 mg/24 hr
***Sustained-release (6–12 yr):*** 8 mg/dose PO Q12 hr
***≥12 yr–adult:*** 4 mg/dose Q4–6 hr PO; **max. dose:** 24 mg/24 hr
***Sustained-release:*** 8 or 12 mg PO Q 12 hr
***Efidac 24:*** 16 mg PO Q24 hr; **max. dose:** 16 mg/24 hr

***DEXCHLORPHENIRAMINE MALEATE DOSING:***

***2–5 yr:*** 0.5 mg/dose PO Q4–6hr; **max. dose:** 3 mg/24 hr
***6–11 yr:*** 1 mg/dose PO Q4–6 hr; **max. dose:** 6 mg/24 hr
***Sustained-release:*** 4 mg PO QHS
***≥12 yr–adult:*** 2 mg/dose PO Q4–6hr; **max. dose:** 12 mg/24 hr
***Sustained-release:*** 4 or 6 mg PO QHS or Q8–10 hr; **max. dose:** 12 mg/24 hr

**Use with caution** in asthma. May cause sedation, dry mouth, blurred vision, urinary retention, polyuria, and disturbed coordination. Young children may be paradoxically excited.

**Note:** Dexchlorpheniramine maleate doses are 50% of chlorpheniramine maleate and do not possess any significant advantages over other antihistamines.

Doses may be administered PRN. Administer doses with food. Sustained-release forms are **NOT recommended** in children < 6 yr and should **NOT** be crushed, chewed, or dissolved.

For explanation of icons, see p. 698.

## CHLORPROMAZINE

Thorazine and others

***Antiemetic, antipsychotic, phenothiazine derivative***

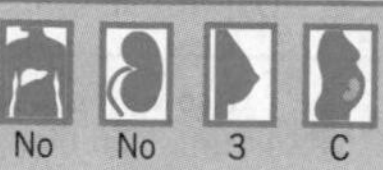


**Tabs:** 10, 25, 50, 100, 200 mg
**Extended-release caps:** 30, 75, 150 mg
**Suppository:** 100 mg
**Injection:** 25 mg/mL (contains 2% benzyl alcohol)

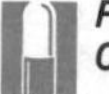

***Psychosis:***
***Child >6 mo:***
***IM/IV:*** 2.5–4 mg/kg/24 hr ÷ Q6–8 hr
***PO:*** 2.5–6 mg/kg/24 hr ÷ Q4–6 hr
***PR:*** 1 mg/kg/dose Q6–8 hr
**Max. IM/IV dose:**
***<5 yr:*** 40 mg/24 hr
***5–12 yr:*** 75 mg/24 hr
***Adult:***
***IM/IV:*** Initial: 25 mg; repeat with 25–50 mg/dose, if needed, Q1–4 hr up to a **max. dose** of 400 mg/dose Q4–6 hr
***PO:*** 10–25 mg/dose Q4–6 hr; **max. dose:** 2 g/24 hr

***Antiemetic:***
***Child (≥ 6 mo):***
***IV/IM:*** 0.55 mg/kg/dose Q6–8 hr PRN
**Max. IM/IV dose:**
***<5 yr:*** 40 mg/24 hr
***5–12 yr:*** 75 mg/24 hr
***PO:*** 0.55 mg/kg/dose Q4–6 hr PRN
***PR:*** 1.1 mg/kg/dose Q6–8 hr PRN
***Adult:***
***IV/IM:*** 25–50 mg/dose Q4–6 hr PRN
***PO:*** 10–25 mg/dose Q4–6 hr PRN
***PR:*** 50–100 mg/dose Q6–8 hr PRN

Adverse effects include drowsiness, jaundice, lowered seizure threshold, extrapyramidal/anticholinergic symptoms, hypotension (more with IV), arrhythmias, agranulocytosis, and neuroleptic malignant syndrome. May potentiate effect of narcotics, sedatives, and other drugs. Monitor BP closely. ECG changes include prolonged PR interval, flattened T waves, and ST depression. **Do not administer** oral liquid dosage form **simultaneously** with carbamazepine oral suspension because an orange rubbery precipitate may form.

## CHOLESTYRAMINE

Questran, Questran Light, Cholestyramine Light, Prevalite, and others

***Antilipemic, binding resin***

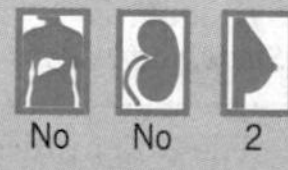


**Powder for oral suspension:**
Questran and others: 4 g anhydrous resin per 9 g powder (9, 378 g)
Questran Light: 4 g anhydrous resin per 6.4 g powder with aspartame (6.4, 268 g)

*Continued*

CHOLESTYRAMINE *continued*

Cholestyramine Light: 4 g anhydrous resin per 5.7 g powder with aspartame (5.7, 210, 231, 239 g)
Prevalite: 4 g anhydrous resin per 5.5 g powder with aspartame (5.5, 231 g)

***All doses based in terms of anhydrous resin. Titrate dose based on response and tolerance.***
***Child:*** 240 mg/kg/24 hr ÷ TID; doses normally **do not exceed** 8 g/24 hr (higher doses does not provide additional benefit). Give PO as slurry in water, juice, or milk before meals.
***Adult:*** 3–4 g of cholestyramine BID-QID
**Max. dose:** 32 g/24 hr

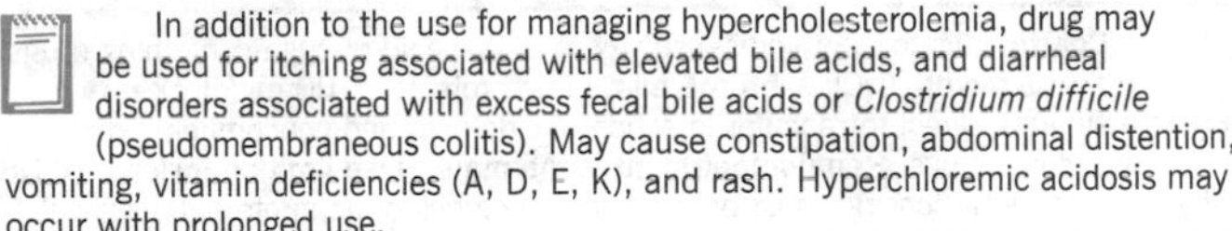

In addition to the use for managing hypercholesterolemia, drug may be used for itching associated with elevated bile acids, and diarrheal disorders associated with excess fecal bile acids or *Clostridium difficile* (pseudomembraneous colitis). May cause constipation, abdominal distention, vomiting, vitamin deficiencies (A, D, E, K), and rash. Hyperchloremic acidosis may occur with prolonged use.

Give other oral medications 4–6 hr after cholestyramine or 1 hr before dose to avoid decreased absorption.

## CHOLINE MAGNESIUM TRISALICYLATE

Trilisate and others
***Nonsteroidal anti-inflammatory agent***

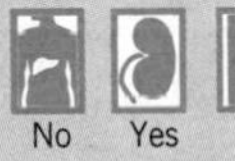
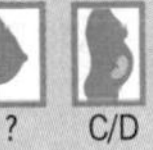

No Yes ? C/D

**Combination of choline salicylate and magnesium salicylate** (1:1.24 ratio, respectively); strengths expressed in terms of mg salicylate.

**Tabs:** 500, 750, 1000 mg
**Oral liquid:** 500 mg/5 mL (237 mL)

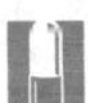

***Dose based on total salicylate content.***
***Child:*** 30–60 mg/kg/24 hr PO ÷ TID-QID
***Adult:*** 500 mg–1.5 g/dose PO QD-TID

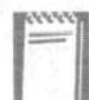

**Avoid use** in patients with suspected varicella or influenza due to concerns of Reye's syndrome. **Use with caution** in severe renal failure because of risk for hypermagnesemia, or in peptic ulcer disease. Less GI irritation than aspirin and other NSAIDs. No antiplatelet effects.

Pregnancy category changes to "D" if used during the third trimester.

Therapeutic salicylate levels, see *Aspirin*; 500 mg choline magnesium trisalicylate is equivalent to 650 mg aspirin.

## CIDOFOVIR

Vistide
***Antiviral***

No Yes 3 C

**Injection:** 75 mg/mL (5 mL); preservative free

*Continued*

For explanation of icons, see p. 698.

CIDOFOVIR *continued*

***Safety and efficacy has not been established in children.***
***CMV retinitis:***
***Induction:*** 5 mg/kg IV × 1 with probenecid and hydration
***Maintenance:*** 3 mg/kg IV Q7 days with probenecid and hydration
***Adenovirus infection after bone marrow transplant (limited data; see remarks):***
5 mg/kg/dose IV once weekly × 3, followed by 5 mg/kg/dose IV once every 2 wk. Administer oral probenecid 1–1.25 g/m$^2$/dose (rounded to the nearest 250 mg interval) 3 hr prior to and 1 hr and 8 hr after each dose of cidofovir. Also give IV normal saline at three times maintenance fluid 1 hr prior to and 1 hr after cidofovir, followed by 2 times maintenance fluid for an additional 2 hr.

**Contraindicated** in hypersensitivity to probenecid or sulfa-containing drugs; sCr > 1.5 mg/dL, CrCl ≤ 55 mL/min, urine protein ≥ 100 mg/dL (2+ proteinuria), direct intraocular injection of cidofovir, and concomitent nephrotoxic drugs. **Renal impairment is the major dose-limiting toxicity.** IV NS prehydration and probenecid must be used to reduce risk of nephrotoxicity. May also cause nausea, vomiting, headache, rash, metabolic acidosis, uveitis, decreased intraocular pressure, and neutropenia.

Reduce dose to 3 mg/kg if sCr increases 0.3–0.4 mg/dL from baseline. Discontinue therapy if sCr increases > 0.5 mg/dL from baseline or development of > 3+ proteinuria.

Administer doses via IV infusion over 1 hr at a concentration ≤ 8 mg/mL.

## CIMETIDINE

Tagamet, Tagamet HB [OTC], and many others
***Histamine-2-antagonist***

Yes Yes 2 B

**Tabs:** 200 (OTC), 300, 400, 800 mg
**Oral solution:** 300 mg/5 mL (240, 480 mL); may contain 2.8% alcohol
**Injection:** 150 mg/mL; may contain benzyl alcohol
**Pre-mixed injection:** 300 mg in 50 mL normal saline

***Neonate:*** 5–20 mg/kg/24 hr IM/PO/IV ÷ Q6–12 hr
***Infant:*** 10–20 mg/kg/24 hr IM/PO/IV ÷ Q6–12 hr
***Child:*** 20–40 mg/kg/24 hr IM/PO/IV ÷ Q6 hr
***Adult:***
***PO:*** 300 mg/dose QID or 400 mg/dose BID or 800 mg/dose QHS
***IV/IM:*** 300 mg/dose Q6 hr; **max. dose:** 2400 mg/24 hr
***Continuous IV infusion:*** 150 mg IV × 1 followed by 37.5 mg/hr; infusions have ranged from 40–600 mg/hr with a mean rate of 160 mg/hr
***Ulcer prophylaxis:*** 400–800 mg PO QHS

Diarrhea, rash, myalgia, confusion, neutropenia, gynecomastia, elevated liver function tests, or dizziness may occur. **Use with caution** in hepatic and renal impairment **(adjust dose in renal failure; see Chapter 31).**

Inhibits CYP 450 1A2, 2C9, 2C19, 2D6, 3A3/4, and 2C18 isoenzymes, therefore increases levels and effects of many hepatically metabolized drugs (i.e., theophylline, phenytoin, lidocaine, diazepam, warfarin). Cimetidine may decrease the absorption of iron, ketoconazole, and tetracyclines.

## CIPROFLOXACIN

Cipro, Cipro XR, Ciloxan ophthalmic, Ciprodex, Cipro HC Otic, and others

***Antibiotic, quinolone***

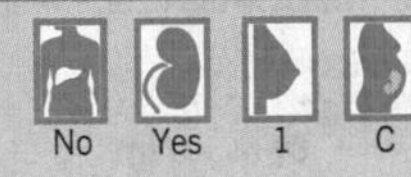


**Tabs:** 100, 250, 500, 750 mg
**Extended-release tabs (Cipro XR):** 500, 1000 mg
**Oral suspension:** 500 mg/5 mL (100 mL)
**Injection:** 10 mg/mL (20, 40 mL)
**Pre-mixed injection:** 200 mg/100 mL 5% dextrose, 400 mg/100 mL 5% dextrose (iso-osmotic solutions)
**Ophthalmic solution:** 3.5 mg/mL (2.5, 5, 10 mL)
**Ophthalmic ointment:** 3.3 mg/g (3.5 g)
**Otitic suspension:**
  **With dexamethasone (Ciprodex):** 3 mg/mL ciprofloxacin + 1 mg/mL dexamethasone (7.5 mL); contains benzalkonium chloride
  **With hydrocortisone (Cipro HC Otic):** 2 mg/mL ciprofloxacin + 10 mg/mL hydrocortisone (10 mL); contains benzyl alcohol

---

***Child:***
  ***PO:*** 20–30 mg/kg/24 hr ÷ Q12 hr; **max. dose:** 1.5 g/24 hr
  ***IV:*** 20–30 mg/kg/24 hr ÷ Q12 hr; **max. dose:** 800 mg/24 hr
***Complicated UTI or pyelonephritis:***
  ***PO:*** 20–40 mg/kg/24 hr ÷ Q12 hr; **max. dose:** 1.5 g/24 hr
  ***IV:*** 18–30 mg/kg/24 hr ÷ Q8 hr; **max. dose:** 1.2 g/24 hr
***Cystic fibrosis:***
  ***PO:*** 40 mg/kg/24 hr ÷ Q12 hr; **max. dose:** 2 g/24 hr
  ***IV:*** 30 mg/kg/24 hr ÷ Q8 hr; **max. dose:** 1.2 g/24 hr
***Anthrax (see remarks):***
  ***Inhalational/systemic/cutaneous:*** Start with 20–30 mg/kg/24 hr ÷ Q12 hr IV (**max. dose:** 800 mg/24 hr) and convert to oral dosing with clinical improvement at 20–30 mg/kg/24 hr ÷ Q12 hr PO (**max. dose:** 1 g/24 hr). Duration of therapy: 60 days (IV and PO combined)
  ***Post exposure prophylaxis:*** 20–30 mg/kg/24 hr ÷ Q12 hr PO × 60 days; **max. dose:** 1 g/24 hr

***Adult:***
  ***PO:***
    ***Immediate release:*** 250–750 mg/dose Q12 hr
    ***Extended release (Cipro XR):***
      ***Uncomplicated UTI/Cystitis:*** 500 mg/dose Q24 hr
      ***Complicated UTI/Uncomplicated pyelonephritis:*** 1000 mg/dose Q24 hr
  ***IV:*** 200–400 mg/dose Q12 hr
  ***Anthrax (see remarks):***
    ***Inhalational/systemic/cutaneous:*** Start with 400 mg/dose Q12 hr IV and convert to oral dosing with clinical improvement at 500 mg/dose Q12 hr PO. Duration of therapy: 60 days (IV and PO combined)
    ***Post exposure prophylaxis:*** 500 mg/dose Q12 hr PO × 60 days.

***Ophthalmic solution:*** 1–2 drops Q2 hr while awake × 2 days, then 1–2 gtts Q4 hr while awake × 5 days
***Ophthalmic ointment:*** Apply 0.5 inch ribbon TID × 2, then BID × 5 days
***Otic:***
  ***Ciprodex:***
    ***Acute otitis media with tympanostomy tubes or acute otitis externa, ≥ 6 mo and adults:*** 4 drops to affected ear(s) BID × 7 days

*Continued*

For explanation of icons, see p. 698.

CIPROFLOXACIN *continued*

***Otic (cont'd):***

***Cipro HC Otic:***

***Otitis externa, > 1 yr and adults:*** 3 drops to affected ear(s) BID × 7 days

Can cause GI upset, renal failure, and seizures. GI symptoms, headache, restlessness, and rash are common side effects. **Use with caution** in children < 18 yr. Like other quinolones, tendon rupture can occur during or after therapy. **Do not use** otic suspension with perforated tympanic membranes and with viral infections of the external ear canal.

Combinational antimicrobial therapy is recommended for anthrax. For penicillin susceptible strains, consider changing to high-dose amoxicillin (25–35 mg/kg/dose TID PO). See www.bt.cdc.gov for the latest information.

Inhibits CYP 450 1A2. Ciprofloxacin can increase effects and/or toxicity of theophylline, warfarin, tizanidine (excessive sedation and dangerous hypotension) and cyclosporine.

**Do not administer** antacids or other divalent salts with or within 2–4 hr of oral ciprofloxacin dose. **Adjust dose in renal failure (see Chapter 31).**

## CITRATE MIXTURES

***Alkalinizing agent, electrolyte supplement***

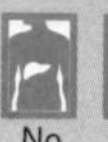
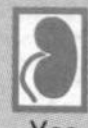
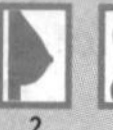
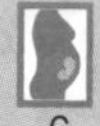

No Yes ? C

**Each mL contains (mEq):**

| | Na | K | Citrate or $HCO_3$ |
|---|---|---|---|
| Polycitra or Cytra-3 (120, 480 mL) | 1 | 1 | 2 |
| Polycitra-LC* or Cytra-LC* (120, 480 mL) | 1 | 1 | 2 |
| Polycitra-K or Cytra-K (120, 480 mL) | 0 | 2 | 2 |
| Bicitra,† Cytra-2, or Sodium Citrate/Citric Acid† (15, 30, 120, 480 mL) | 1 | 0 | 1 |
| Oracit (15, 30, 500 mL) | 1 | 0 | 1 |

*LC, low calorie (contains no sucrose, sorbitol, glycerin).
†Sugar-free.

***Dilute dose in water or juice.***

***All mEq doses based on citrate.***

***Infant and child:*** 5–15 mL/dose Q6–8 hr (after meals and before bedtime) PO or 2–3 mEq/kg/24 hr PO ÷ Q6–8 hr

***Adult:*** 15–30 mL/dose Q6–8 hr (after meals and before bedtime) PO or 100–200 mEq/24 hr PO ÷ Q6–8 hr

**Contraindicated** in severe renal impairment and acute dehydration. **Use with caution** in patients already receiving potassium supplements or who are sodium restricted. May have laxative effect and cause hypocalemia and metabolic alkalosis.

Adjust dose to maintain desired pH. 1 mEq of citrate is equivalent to 1 mEq $HCO_3$ in patients with normal hepatic function.

C
FORMULARY

## CLARITHROMYCIN

Biaxin, Biaxin XL
***Antibiotic, macrolide***

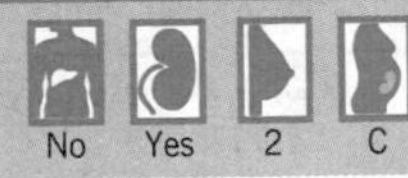


**Film tablets:** 250, 500 mg
**Extended-release tablets (Biaxin XL):** 500 mg
**Granules for oral suspension:** 125, 250 mg/5 mL (50, 100 mL)

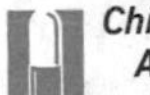

***Child:***
***Acute otitis media, pharyngitis/tonsillitis, pneumonia, acute maxillary sinusitis, or uncomplicated skin infections:*** 15 mg/kg/24 hr PO ÷ Q12 hr
***M. avium complex:***
***Prophylaxis (1st episode and recurrence):*** 15 mg/kg/24 hr PO ÷ Q12 hr
***Treatment:*** 15 mg/kg/24 hr PO ÷ Q12 hr with other antimycobacterial drugs
**Max. dose:** 1 g/24 hr

***Adult:***
***Pharyngitis/tonsillitis, acute maxillary sinusitis, bronchitis, pneumonia, or uncomplicated skin infections:***
***Immediate release:*** 250–500 mg/dose Q12 hr PO
***Extended release (Biaxin XL):*** 1000 mg Q24 hr PO (currently not indicated for pharyngiis/tonsillitis or uncomplicated skin infections)
***M. avium complex:***
***Prophylaxis (1st episode and recurrence):*** 500 mg/dose Q12 hr PO
***Treatment:*** 500 mg Q12 hr PO with other antimycobacterial drugs

**Contraindicated** in patients allergic to erythromycin. As with other macrolides, clarithromycin has been associated with QT prolongation and ventricular arrhythmias, including ventricular tachycardia and torsades de pointes. May cause cardiac arrhythmias in patients also receiving cisapride. Side effects: diarrhea, nausea, abnormal taste, dyspepsia, abdominal discomfort (less than erythromycin but greater than azithromycin), and headache. Rare cases of anaphylaxis, Stevens Johnson syndrome, and toxic epidermal necrolysis have been reported. May increase effects/toxicity of carbamazepine, theophylline, cyclosporine, digoxin, ergot alkaloids, fluconazole, tacrolimus, triazolam, and warfarin. Substrate and inhibitor of CYP 450 3A4, and inhibits CYP 1A2.

**Adjust dose in renal failure (see Chapter 31).** Doses, regardless of dosage form, may be administered with food.

## CLINDAMYCIN

Cleocin-T, Cleocin, and others
***Antibiotic, lincomycin derivative***

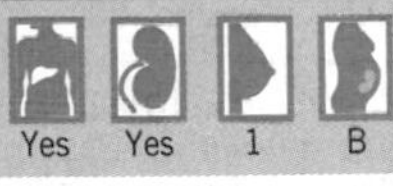


**Caps:** 75, 150, 300 mg
**Oral solution:** 75 mg/5 mL (100 mL)
**Injection:** 150 mg/mL (contains 9.45 mg/mL benzyl alcohol)
**Solution, topical (Cleocin-T):** 1% (1, 30, 60 mL); may contain 50% isopropyl alcohol
**Gel, topical (Cleocin-T):** 1% (7.5, 30, 42, 60, 77 g); may contain methylparaben
**Lotion, topical (Cleocin-T):** 1% (60 mL); may contain methylparaben
**Foam, topical:** 1% (50 g); contains 58% ethanol
**Vaginal cream:** 2% (40 g); may contain benzyl alcohol
**Vaginal suppository:** 100 mg (3s)

*Continued*

For explanation of icons, see p. 698.

CLINDAMYCIN *continued*

***Neonate:*** IV/ IM: 5 mg/kg/dose

***≤7 days:***

***≤2 kg:*** Q12 hr

***>2 kg:*** Q8 hr

***>7 days:***

***<1.2 kg:*** Q12 hr

***1.2–2 kg:*** Q8 hr

***>2 kg:*** Q6 hr

***Child:***

***PO:*** 10–30 mg/kg/24 hr ÷ Q6–8 hr

***IM/IV:*** 25–40 mg/kg/24 hr ÷ Q6–8 hr

***Adult:***

***PO:*** 150–450 mg/dose Q6–8 hr; **max. dose:** 1.8 g/24 hr

***IM/IV:*** 1200–1800 mg/24 hr IM/IV ÷ Q6–12 hr; **max. dose:** 4.8 g/24 hr

***Topical:*** Apply to affected area BID.

***Bacterial vaginosis:***

***Suppositories:*** 100 mg/dose QHS × 3 days

***Vaginal cream (2%):*** 1 applicator dose (5 g) QHS for 3 or 7 days in nonpregnant patients and for 7 days in pregnant patients in second and third trimester.

Not indicated in meningitis; CSF penetration is poor.

Pseudomembranous colitis may occur up to several wk after cessation of therapy. May cause diarrhea, rash, Stevens-Johnson syndrome, granulocytopenia, thrombocytopenia, or sterile abscess at injection site.

Clindamycin may increase the neuromuscular blocking effects of tubocurarine, pancuronium. **Do not exceed** IV infusion rate of 30 mg/min because hypotension, cardiac arrest has been reported with rapid infusions.

Dosage reduction may be required in severe renal or hepatic disease but not necessary in mild/moderate conditions. Oral liquid preparation is not palatable; consider use of oral capsules as a sprinkle onto applesauce or pudding.

## CLONAZEPAM

Klonopin and others

***Benzodiazepine***

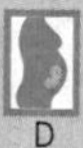

Yes Yes 3 D

**Tabs:** 0.5, 1, 2 mg

**Disintegrating oral tabs:** 0.125, 0.25, 0.5, 1, 2 mg; contains phenylalanine

**Oral suspension:** 100 mcg/mL

***Child < 10 yr or <30 kg:***

***Initial:*** 0.01–0.03 mg/kg/24 hr ÷ Q8 hr PO

***Increment:*** 0.25–0.5 mg/24 hr Q3 days, up to **max. maintenance dose** of 0.1–0.2 mg/kg/24 hr ÷ Q8 hr

***Child ≥ 10 yr or ≥ 30 kg and adult:***

***Initial:*** 1.5 mg/24 hr PO ÷ TID

***Increment:*** 0.5–1 mg/24 hr Q3 days; **max. dose:** 20 mg/24 hr

**Contraindicated** in severe liver disease and acute narrow-angle glaucoma. Drowsiness, behavior changes, increased bronchial secretions, GI, CV, GU, and hematopoietic toxicity (thrombocytopenia, leukopenia) may occur. **Use with**

*Continued*

CLONAZEPAM *continued*

caution in patients with renal impairment. **Do not** discontinue abruptly. $T_{1/2}$ = 24–36 hr.

Proposed therapeutic levels (not well established): 20–80 ng/mL. Recommended serum sampling time: Obtain trough level within 30 min prior to an oral dose. Steady-state is typically achieved after 5–8 days continuous therapy using the same dose.

Carbamazepine, phenytoin, and phenobarbital may decrease clonazepam levels and effect. Drugs that inhibit CYP 450 3A4 isoenzymes (e.g., erythromycin) may increase clonazepam levels and effects/toxicity.

## CLONIDINE

Catapres, Catapres TTS, Duraclon, and others

***Central alpha-adrenergic agonist, antihypertensive***

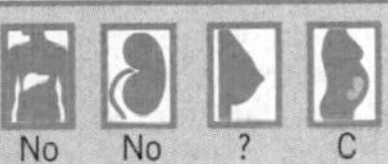


**Tabs:** 0.1, 0.2, 0.3 mg
**Oral suspension:** 0.1 mg/mL
**Transdermal patch (Catapres TTS):** 0.1, 0.2, 0.3 mg/24 hr (7 day patch)
**Injection, epidural (Duraclon):** 100, 500 mcg/mL (10 mL); preservative free

***Hypertension:***

***Child (PO):*** 5–10 mcg/kg/24 hr PO ÷ Q8–12 hr initially; if needed, increase at 5–7 day intervals to 5–25 mcg/kg/24 hr PO ÷ Q6 hr; **max. dose:** 25 mcg/kg/24 hr up to 0.9 mg/24 hr.

***Adult (PO):*** 0.1 mg BID initially; increase in 0.1 mg/24 hr increments at weekly intervals until desired response is achieved (usual range: 0.1–0.8 mg/24 hr ÷ BID); **max. dose:** 2.4 mg/24 hr

***Transdermal patch:***

***Child:*** Conversion to patch only after establishing an optimal oral dose first. Use a transdermal dosage closest to the established total oral daily dose.

***Adult:*** Initial 0.1 mg/24 hr patch for first wk. May increase dose by 0.1 mg/24 hr at 1–2 wk intervals PRN. Usual range: 0.1–0.3 mg/24 hr. Each patch lasts for 7 days. Doses > 0.6 mg/24 hr do not provide additional benefit.

***ADHD:***

***Child:*** Start with 0.05 mg QHS PO; if needed, increase by 0.05 mg every 3–7 days up to a **max. dose** of 0.4 mg/24 hr. Titrated doses may be divided TID-QID.

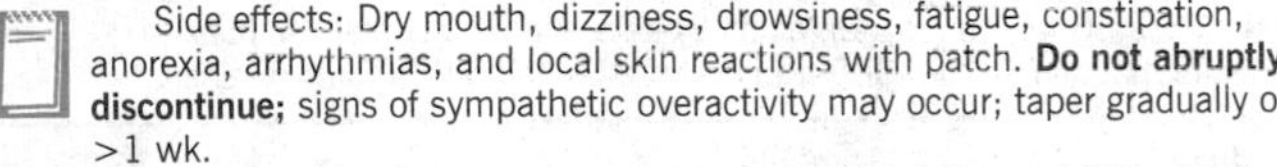

Side effects: Dry mouth, dizziness, drowsiness, fatigue, constipation, anorexia, arrhythmias, and local skin reactions with patch. **Do not abruptly discontinue;** signs of sympathetic overactivity may occur; taper gradually over >1 wk.

Beta-blockers may exacerbate rebound hypertension during and following the withdrawal of clonidine. If patient is receiving both clonidine and a beta-blocker and clonidine is to be discontinued, the beta-blocker should be withdrawn several days prior to tapering the clonidine. If converting from clonidine over to a beta-blocker, introduce the beta-blocker several days after discontinuing clonidine (following taper).

$T_{1/2}$: 44–72 hr (neonate), 6–20 hr (adult). Onset of action (antihypertensive): 0.5–1 hr for oral route, 2–3 days for transdermal route.

For explanation of icons, see p. 698.

## CLOTRIMAZOLE

Lotrimin AF, Cruex, Gyne-Lotrimin 3, Gyne-Lotrimin 7, Mycelex, Mycelex-7, and others
***Antifungal, imidazole***

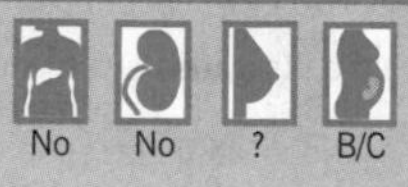


**Oral troche:** 10 mg
**Cream, topical (OTC):** 1% (12, 15, 24, 30, 45 g); contains benzyl alcohol
**Solution, topical (OTC):** 1% (10, 30 mL)
**Lotion, topical (OTC):** 1% (20 mL); contains benzyl alcohol
**Vaginal suppository (OTC):** 200 mg
**Vaginal cream (OTC):** 1% (15, 30, 45 g), 2% (21 g)
**Combination packs:**
Mycelex-7 Combination Pack (OTC): Vaginal suppository 100 mg (7) and vaginal cream 1% (7 g)
Gyne-Lotrimin 3 Combination Pack (OTC): Vaginal suppository 200 mg (3) and vaginal cream 1% (7 g)

***Topical:*** Apply to skin BID × 4–8 wk
***Vaginal candidiasis:*** (vaginal suppositories)
100 mg/dose QHS × 7 days, or
200 mg/dose QHS × 3 days, or
1 applicator dose (5 g) of 1% vaginal cream QHS × 7–14 days, or
1 applicator dose of 2% vaginal cream QHS × 3 days
***Thrush:***
***>3 yr–adult:*** Dissolve slowly (15–30 min) one troche in the mouth 5 times/24 hr × 14 days

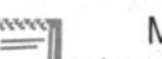

May cause erythema, blistering, or urticaria with topical use. Liver enzyme elevation, nausea and vomiting may occur with troches. **Avoid use** of condoms and diaphragms with vaginal cream or suppository as latex can be weakened. **Do not use** troches for systemic infections.
Pregnancy code is "B" for topical and vaginal dosage forms and "C" for troches.

## CODEINE

Various generics
***Narcotic, analgesic, antitussive***

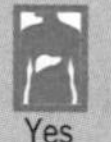

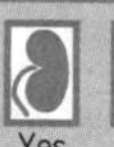

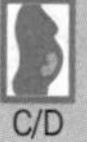


**Tabs:** 15, 30, 60 mg; as sulfate
**Injection:** 30, 60 mg/mL (2 mL); as phosphate and may contain sulfites
**Oral solution:** 15 mg/5 mL (500 mL); as phosphate and contains parabens

***Analgesic:***
***Child:*** 0.5–1 mg/kg/dose Q4–6 hr IM, SC, or PO; **max. dose:** 60 mg/dose
***Adult:*** 15–60 mg/dose Q4–6 hr IM, SC, or PO
***Antitussive (all doses PRN):*** 1–1.5 mg/kg/24 hr ÷ Q4–6 hr; alternatively dose by age:

*Continued*

CODEINE *continued*

*2–5 yr:* 2.5–5 mg/dose Q4–6 hr; **max. dose:** 30 mg/24 hr
*6–12 yr:* 5–10 mg/dose Q4–6 hr; **max. dose:** 60 mg/24 hr
*≥12 yr and adult:* 10–20 mg/dose Q4–6 hr; **max. dose:** 120 mg/24 hr

**Do not use** in children <2 yr old as antitussive. Not intended for IV use, due to large histamine release and cardiovascular effects. **Use with caution** in hypersensivity reactions to other opioids, respiratory disorders, and severe liver or renal insufficiency **(adjust dose in renal failure; see Chapter 31).** Side effects: CNS and respiratory depression, constipation, cramping, hypotension, and pruritis. May be habit forming.

Codeine's analgesic effect is due to its metabolism to morphine. For analgesia, use with acetaminophen orally. **See Chapter 6 for equianalgesic dosing.**

Pregnancy risk factor changes to "D" if used for prolonged periods or in high doses at term. Nursing infants whose mothers are taking codeine and are "ultra-rapid" metabolizers (CYP 450 2D6) of codeine may have a more rapid and complete conversion to morphine. This may increase the risk for morphine overdose to the nursing infant.

## CODEINE AND ACETAMINOPHEN

Tylenol #1, #2, #3, #4, and various generics
***Narcotic analgesic combination product***

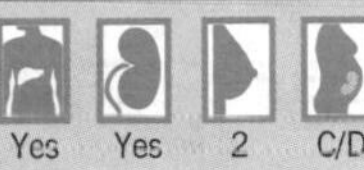


**Elixir (7% alcohol and saccharin), oral suspension, oral solution:** acetaminophen 120 mg and codeine phosphate 12 mg/5 mL (120, 473 mL)
**Tabs:** (all containing 300 mg acetaminophen per tab and may contain metabisulfite)
Tylenol #2: 15 mg codeine
Tylenol #3: 30 mg codeine
Tylenol #4: 60 mg codeine

See *Acetaminophen* and *Codeine* for additional dosing information.
***Analgesic:***
***Child:*** 0.5–1 mg codeine/kg/dose PO Q4–6 hr PRN
***Using elixir, oral suspension, or oral solution:***
*3–6 yr:* 5 mL (12 mg codeine and 120 mg acetaminophen) PO Q6–8 hr PRN
*7–12 yr:* 10 mL (24 mg codeine and 240 mg acetaminophen) PO Q6–8 hr PRN
*≥12 yr:* 15 mL (36 mg codeine and 360 mg acetaminophen) PO Q4 hr PRN
***Adult:*** 0.5–2 tablets (15–60 mg codeine; check tablet strength) PO Q4 hr PRN; **max. codeine dose:** 360 mg /24 hr, **max. acetaminophen dose:** 4 g/24 hr

See *Acetaminophen* and *Codeine*. Pregnancy category is "C" (changing to "D" if used for prolonged periods or in high doses at term) for codeine. **Do not use** combination product in renal impairment because codeine requires dosage adjustment; consider using each drug separately with proper dose adjustments.

For explanation of icons, see p. 698.

## CORTICOTROPIN

H.P. Acthar Gel

***Adrenocorticotropic hormone***

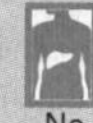 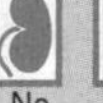 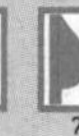 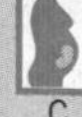

No No ? C

**Injection, repository gel:** 80 U/mL (5 mL)
1 unit = 1 mg

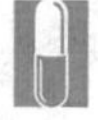

***Anti-inflammatory:***
0.8 U/kg/24 hr ÷ Q12–24 hr IM
***Infantile spasms:*** many regimens exist
20–40 U/24 hr IM QD × 6 wk or 150 U/$m^2$/24 hr ÷ BID for 2 wk; followed by a gradual taper.

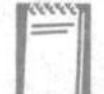

**Contraindicated** in acute psychoses, CHF, Cushing's disease, TB, peptic ulcer, ocular herpes, fungal infections, recent surgery, and sensitivity to porcine products. **Repository gel dosage form is only for IM route.**

Hypersensitivity reactions may occur. Similar adverse effects as corticosteroids.

## CORTISONE ACETATE

Various generics

***Corticosteroid***

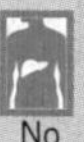 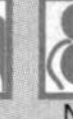 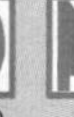 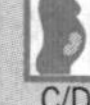 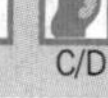

No No ? C/D

**Tabs:** 25 mg

***Anti-inflammatory/immunosuppressive:***
***PO:*** 2.5–10 mg/kg/24 hr ÷ Q6–8 hr

May produce glucose intolerance, Cushing's syndrome, edema, hypertension, adrenal suppression, cataracts, hypokalemia, skin atrophy, peptic ulcer, osteoporosis, and growth suppression.

Pregnancy category changes to "D" if used in the first trimester.

## CO-TRIMOXAZOLE

See *Sulfamethoxazole and Trimethoprim*

## CROMOLYN

Intal, Nasalcrom, Gastrocrom, Crolom, Opticrom, and various generics

***Anti-allergic agent, mast cell stabilizer***

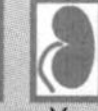 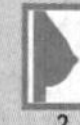 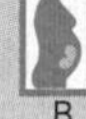

Yes Yes ? B

**Nebulized solution:** 10 mg/mL (2 mL)
**Aerosol inhaler:** 800 mcg/spray (112 inhalations, 8.1 g; 200 inhalations, 14.2 g)
**Oral concentrate (Gastrocrom):** 100 mg/5 mL
**Ophthalmic solution (Crolom, Opticrom):** 4% (2.5, 10, 15 mL)
**Nasal spray (Nasalcrom) [OTC]:** 4% (5.2 mg/spray) (100 sprays, 13 mL; 200 sprays, 26 mL); contains benzalkonium chloride and EDTA

*Continued*

CROMOLYN *continued*

***Nebulization:***

***Child ≥ 2 yr and adult:*** 20 mg Q6–8 hr

***Nasal:***

***Child ≥ 2 yr and adult:*** 1 spray each nostril TID-QID

***Aerosol inhaler:***

***Child 5–12 yr:*** 1–2 puffs TID-QID

***Child > 5 yr and adult:*** 2–4 puffs TID-QID

***Ophthalmic:***

***Child > 4 yr and adult:*** 1–2 gtts 4–6 times/24 hr

***Food allergy/inflammatory bowel disease:***

***2–12 yr:*** 100 mg PO QID; give 15–20 min AC and QHS; **max. dose:** 40 mg/kg/24 hr

***>12 yr and adult:*** 200–400 mg PO QID; give 15–20 min AC and QHS

***Systemic mastocytosis:***

***<2 yr:*** 20 mg/kg/24 hr ÷ QID PO; **max. dose:** 30 mg/kg/24 hr

***2–12 yr:*** 100 mg PO QID; give 30 min AC and QHS; **max. dose:** 40 mg/kg/24 hr

***>12 yr and adult:*** 200 mg PO QID; give 30 min AC and QHS; **max. dose:** 40 mg/kg/24 hr

May cause rash, cough, bronchospasm, and nasal congestion. May cause headache, diarrhea with oral use. **Use with caution** in patients with renal or hepatic dysfunction.

Therapeutic response often occurs within 2 wk, however, a 4- to 6-wk trial may be needed to determine max. benefit. For exercise-induced asthma, give no longer than 1 hr before activity. Oral concentrate can be diluted only in water. Nebulized solution can be mixed with albuterol nebs.

## CYANOCOBALAMIN/VITAMIN $B_{12}$

Cyanoject, Cyomin, Nascobal, Vitamin $B_{12}$ and others

***Vitamin (synthetic), water soluble***

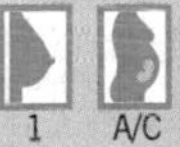


**Tabs (OTC):** 100, 500, 1000, 5000 mcg
**Sublingual tabs:** 1000 mcg
**Lozenges (OTC):** 50, 100, 250, 500 mcg
**Nasal spray (Nascobal):** 500 mcg/spray (2.3 mL delivers 8 doses); contains benzalkonium chloride
**Injection (Cyanoject, Cyomin):** 100, 1000 mcg/mL (10, 30 mL); some preparations may contain benzyl alcohol
Contains cobalt (4.35%)

***U.S. RDA:*** See Chapter 21.

***Vitamin $B_{12}$ deficiency, treatment:***

***Child (IM or deep SC):*** 100 mcg/24 hr × 10–15 days

***Maintenance:*** At least 60 mcg/mo

***Adult (IM or deep SC):*** 30–100 mcg/24 hr × 5–10 days

***Maintenance:*** 100–200 mcg/mo

***Pernicious anemia:***

***Child (IM or deep SC):*** 30–50 mcg/24 hr for at least 14 days to total dose of 1000 mcg

***Maintenance:*** 100 mcg/mo

*Continued*

For explanation of icons, see p. 698.

CYANOCOBALAMIN/VITAMIN $B_{12}$ *continued*

***Pernicious anemia (cont'd):***

***Adult (IM or deep SC):*** 100 mcg/24 hr × 7 days, followed by 100 mcg/dose QOD × 14 days, then 100 mcg/dose Q3–4 days until remission is complete.

***Maintenance:***

***IM/deep SC:*** 100–1000 mcg/mo
***Intranasal:*** 500 mcg in one nostril once weekly
***Sublingual:*** 1000–2000 mcg/24 hr

---

**Contraindicated** in optic nerve atrophy. May cause hypokalemia, hypersensitivity, pruritis, and vascular thrombosis. Pregnancy category changes to "C" if used in doses above the RDA.

Prolonged use of acid-suppressing medications may reduce cyanocobalamin oral absorption.

Protect product from light. Oral route of administration is generally **not recommended** for pernicious anemia and $B_{12}$ deficiency due to poor absorption. IV route of administration is **not recommended** because of a more rapid elimination. **See Chapter 21 for multivitamin preparations.**

## CYCLOPENTOLATE

Cyclogyl and others

***Anticholinergic, mydriatic agent***

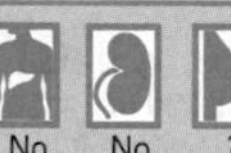
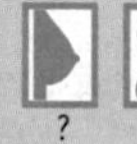
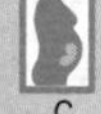

No No ? C

**Ophthalmic solution:** 0.5%, 1%, 2% (2, 5, 15 mL); may contain benzalkonium chloride

---

***Infant:*** Use cyclopentolate/phenylephrine (Cyclomydril) due to lower cyclopentolate concentration and reduced risk of systemic side effects.

***Child:*** 1 drop of 0.5%–1% OU, followed by repeat drop, if necessary, in 5 min.

***Adult:*** 1 drop of 1% OU followed by another drop OU in 5 min; use 2% solution for heavily pigmented iris.

---

**Do not use** in narrow-angle glaucoma. May cause a burning sensation, behavioral disturbance, tachycardia, and loss of visual accommodation. To minimize absorption, apply pressure over nasolacrimal sac for at least 2 min.

CNS and cardiovascular side effects are common with the 2% solution in children. **Avoid** feeding infants within 4 hr of dosing to prevent potential feeding intolerance.

Onset of action: 15–60 min. Duration of action: 6–24 hr; complete recovery of accommodation may take several days for some patients. Observe patient closely for at least 30 min after dose.

## CYCLOPENTOLATE WITH PHENYLEPHRINE

Cyclomydril

***Anticholinergic/sympathomimetic, mydriatic agent***

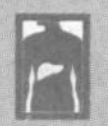
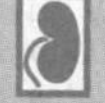
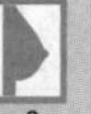
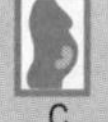

No No ? C

**Ophthalmic solution:** 0.2% cyclopentolate and 1% phenylephrine (2, 5 mL); contains 0.1% benzalkonium chloride, EDTA and boric acid

*Continued*

CYCLOPENTOLATE WITH PHENYLEPHRINE *continued*

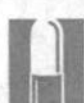

***Neonate–adult:*** 1 drop OU Q5–10 min; **max. dose:** 3 drops per eye

Used to induce mydriasis. See *Cyclopentolate* for additional remarks. Onset of action: 15–60 min. Duration of action: 4–12 hr.

## CYCLOSPORINE, CYCLOSPORINE MICROEMULSION, CYCLOSPORINE MODIFIED

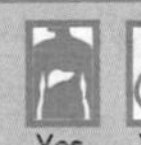
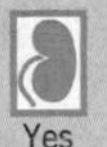
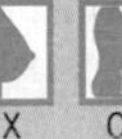

Yes Yes X C

Sandimmune, Gengraf, Neoral, and others

***Immunosuppressant***

**CYCLOSPORINE (Sandimmune and others):**

- **Injection:** 50 mg/mL; contains 32.9% alcohol and 650 mg/mL polyoxyethylated castor oil
- **Oral solution:** 100 mg/mL (50 mL); contains 12.5% alcohol
- **Caps:** 25, 50, 100 mg; contains 12.8% alcohol

**CYCLOSPORINE MICROEMULSION (Neoral):**

- **Caps:** 25, 100 mg
- **Oral solution:** 100 mg/mL (50 mL)
- Neoral products contain 11.9% alcohol

**CYCLOSPORINE MODIFIED (Gengraf):**

- **Caps:** 25, 100 mg; contains 12.8% alcohol
- **Oral solution:** 100 mg/mL (50 mL): contains castor oil

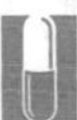

***Neoral manufacturer recommends a 1: 1 conversion ratio with Sandimmune. Due to its better absorption, however, lower doses of Neoral and Gengraf may be required. Exact dosing may vary depending on transplant type.***

***Oral:*** 15 mg/kg/24 hr as a single dose given 4–12 hr pretransplantation; give same daily dose for 1–2 wk posttransplantation, then reduce by 5% per wk to 3–10 mg/kg/24 hr ÷ Q12–24 hr

***IV:*** 5–6 mg/kg/24 hr as a single dose given 4–12 hr pretransplantation; administer over 2–6 hr; give same daily dose posttransplantation until patient is able to tolerate oral form.

May cause nephrotoxicity, hepatotoxicity, hypomagnesemia, hyperkalemia, hyperuricemia, hypertension, hirsutism, acne, GI symptoms, tremor, leukopenia, sinusitis, gingival hyperplasia, and headache. Encephalopathy, convulsions, vision and movement disturbances, and impaired consciousness have been reported, especially in liver transplant patients. Psoriasis patients previously treated with PUVA and, to a lesser extent, methotrexate or other immunosuppressive agents, UVB, coal tar, or radiation therapy, are at increased risk for skin malignancies when taking Neoral or Gengraf. **Use caution** with concomitant use of other nephrotoxic drugs (e.g., amphotericin B, aminoglycosides, nonsteroidal anti-inflammatory drugs, and tacrolimus).

Plasma concentrations increased with the use of fluconazole, ketoconazole, itraconazole, erythromycin, clarithromycin, diltiazem, verapamil, nicardipine, carvedilol, and corticosteroids. Plasma concentrations decreased with the use of carbamazepine, nafcillin, rifampin, phenobarbital, octreotide, and phenytoin. May increase methotrexate levels. Cyclosporine is a substrate for CYP 450 3A4.

Children may require dosages 2–3 times higher than adults. Plasma half-life 6–24 hr.

*Continued*

For explanation of icons, see p. 698.

CYCLOSPORINE, CYCLOSPORINE MICROEMULSION, CYCLOSPORINE MODIFIED *continued*

Monitor trough levels (just prior to a dose at steady-state). Steady-state is generally achieved after 3–5 days of continuous dosing. Interpretation will vary based on treatment protocol and assay methodology (RIA monoclonal vs. RIA polyclonal vs. HPLC) as well as whole blood vs. serum sample. Additional monitoring and dosage adjustments may be necessary in renal and hepatic impairment or when changing dosage forms.

## CYPROHEPTADINE

Various generics; previously available as Periactin

***Antihistamine***

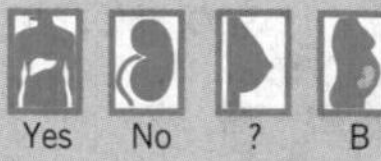

Yes No ? B

**Tabs:** 4 mg
**Syrup:** 2 mg/5 mL (473 mL); may contain alcohol

***Antihistaminic uses:***
***Child:*** 0.25 mg/kg/24 hr or 8 mg/m²/24 hr ÷ Q8–12 hr PO or by age:
***2–6 yr:*** 2 mg Q8–12 hr PO; **max. dose:** 12 mg/24 hr
***7–14 yr:*** 4 mg Q8–12 hr PO; **max. dose:** 16 mg/24 hr
***Adult:*** Start with 12 mg/24 hr ÷ TID PO; dosage range: 12–32 mg/24 hr ÷ TID PO; **max. dose:** 0.5 mg/kg/24 hr
***Migraine prophylaxis:*** 0.25–0.4 mg/kg/24 hr ÷ BID–TID PO up to following **max. doses:**
***2–6 yr:*** 12 mg/24 hr
***7–14 yr:*** 16 mg/24 hr
***Adult:*** 0.5 mg/kg/24 hr or 32 mg/24 hr
***Appetite stimulation:***
***4–8 yr (limited data):*** 2 mg Q8 hr PO
***>13 yr and adult:*** Start with 2 mg Q6 hr PO; dose may be gradually increased to 8 mg Q6 hr over a 3 wk period.

**Contraindicated** in neonates, patients currently on MAO inhibitors, and patients suffering from asthma, glaucoma, or GI/GU obstruction. May produce anti-cholinergic side effects including sedation and appetite stimulation. Consider reducing dosage with hepatic insufficiency.

Allow 4 to 8 wk of continuous therapy for assessing efficacy in migraine propylaxis.

## DANTROLENE

Dantrium

***Skeletal muscle relaxant***

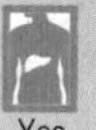
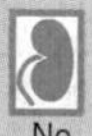
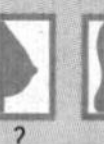
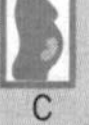

Yes No ? C

**Caps:** 25, 50, 100 mg
**Injection:** 20 mg; contains 3 g mannitol/20 mg drug
**Oral suspension:** 5 mg/mL

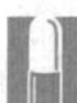

***Chronic spasticity:***
***Child (<5 yr):***
***Initial:*** 0.5 mg/kg/dose PO BID

*Continued*

DANTROLENE *continued*

***Increment:*** Increase frequency to TID–QID at 4- to 7-day intervals; then increase doses by 0.5 mg/kg/dose.

**Max. dose:** 3 mg/kg/dose PO BID–QID, up to 400 mg/24 hr

***Malignant hyperthermia:***

***Prevention:***

***PO:*** 4–8 mg/kg/24 hr ÷ Q6 hr × 1–2 days before surgery with last dose administered 3–4 hr prior to surgery.

***IV:*** 2.5 mg/kg over 1 hr beginning 1.25 hr before anesthesia, additional doses PRN

***Treatment:*** 1 mg/kg IV, repeat PRN to **max. cumulative dose** of 10 mg/kg, followed by a post-crisis regimen of 4–8 mg/kg/24 hr PO ÷ Q6 hr for 1–3 days

---

**Contraindicated** in active hepatic disease. Monitor transaminases for hepatotoxicity. **Use with caution** in children with cardiac or pulmonary impairment. May cause change in sensorium, weakness, diarrhea, constipation, incontinence, and enuresis.

**Avoid** unnecessary exposure of medication to sunlight. **Avoid** IV extravasation into tissues. A decrease in spasticity sufficient to allow daily function should be therapeutic goal. Discontinue if benefits are not evident in 45 days.

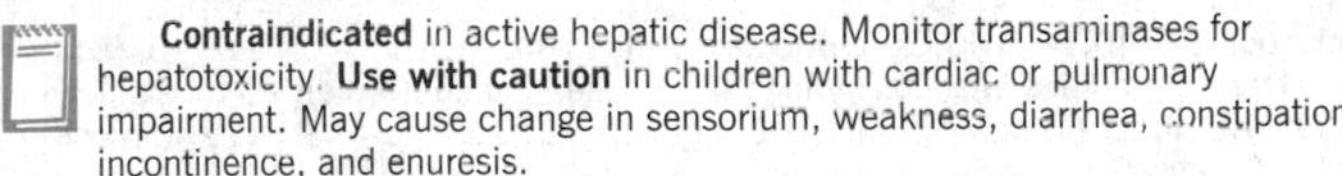

**DAPSONE**

Aczone, Diaminodiphenylsulfone, DDS

***Antibiotic, sulfone derivative***

No Yes 1 C

**Tabs:** 25, 100 mg

**Oral suspension:** 2 mg/mL

**Topical gel (Aczone):** 5% (30 g)

---

***Pneumocystis jiroveci (formerly carinii) prophylaxis:***

***Child > 1 mo:*** 2 mg/kg/24 hr PO QD; **max. dose:** 100 mg/24 hr. Alternative weekly dosing, 4 mg/kg/dose PO Q7 days; **max. dose:** 200 mg/dose

***Adult:*** 100 mg/24 hr PO ÷ QD–BID with pyrimethamine 50 mg PO Q7 days and leucovorin 25 mg PO Q monthly; other combination regimens with pyrimethamine and leucovorin can be used (see www.hivatis.org/trtgdlns.html#Opportunistic).

***Toxoplasma gondii prophylaxis:***

***Child ≥ 1 mo:*** 2 mg/kg/24 hr PO QD; **max. dose:** 25 mg/24 hr with pyrimethamine 1 mg/kg/24 PO QD and leucovorin 5 mg PO Q3 days.

***Adult:*** 50 mg PO QD with pyrimethamine 50 mg PO Q7 days and leucovorin 25 mg PO Q monthly; other combination regimens with pyrimethamine and leucovorin can be used (see www.hivatis.org/trtgdlns.html#Opportunistic).

***Leprosy (see www.who.int/lep/disease/disease.htm for latest recommendations including combination regimens such as rifampin ± clofazimine):***

***Child:*** 1–2 mg/kg/24 hr PO QD; **max. dose:** 100 mg/24 hr

***Adult:*** 50–100 mg PO QD

***Acne vulgaris:***

***≥12 yr:*** Apply small amount of topical gel onto clean, acne affected areas BID.

---

Patients with HIV, glutathione deficiency, or G6PD deficiency may be at increased risk for developing methemoglobinemia. Side effects include hemolytic anemia (dose related), agranulocytosis, methemoglobinemia, aplastic

*Continued*

For explanation of icons, see p. 698.

DAPSONE *continued*

anemia, nausea, vomiting, hyperbilirubinemia, headache, nephrotic syndrome, and hypersensitivity reaction (sulfone syndrome).

Didanosine, rifabutin and rifampin decreases dapsone levels. Trimethoprim increases dapsone levels. Pyrimethamine, nitrofurantoin, and primaquine increases risk for hematological side effects.

Oral suspension may not be absorbed as well as tablets.

## DARBEPOETIN ALFA

Aranesp

***Erythropoiesis stimulating protein***

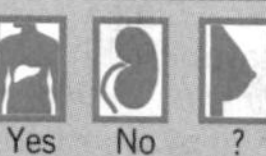
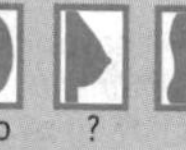


**Injection:** 25, 40, 60, 100, 200, 300 mcg/1 mL (1 mL), 150 mcg/0.75 mL (0.75 mL)
**Single-dose pre-filled injection syringe (27-gauge ½-inch needle):** 25 mcg/0.42 mL, 40 mcg/0.4 mL, 60 mcg/0.3 mL, 100 mcg/0.5 mL, 150 mcg/0.3 mL, 200 mcg/0.4 mL, 300 mcg/0.6 mL, 500 mcg/1 mL
Both dosage forms contain either albumin (2.5 mg/mL) or polysorbate (0.05 mg/mL).

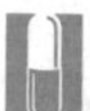

***Anemia in chronic renal failure:***

***Child and adult:*** Start with 0.45 mcg/kg/dose IV/SC once weekly and adjust dose according to the table that follows.

***Anemia associated with chemotherapy (patients with nonmyeloid malignancies):***

***Child (limited data) and adult:*** Start with 2.25 mcg/kg/dose SC once weekly and adjust dose according to the table that follows (discontinue use after completing chemotherapy course).

**DARBEPOETIN ALFA DOSE ADJUSTMENT**

| Response to Dose | Dose Adjustment |
|---|---|
| <1 g/dL increase in hemoglobin and below target range after 4 wk of therapy | Increase dose by 25% not more frequently than once monthly. Further increases, if needed, may be done at 4-wk intervals. |
| >1 g/dL increase in hemoglobin in any 2-wk period, or if hemoglobin is increasing and approaching 12 g/dL | Decrease dose by 25% |
| Hemoglobin continues to increase despite dosage reduction | Discontinue therapy; reinitiate therapy at a 25% lower dose of the previous dose after the hemoglobin starts to decrease |

Conversion from epoetin alfa to darbepoetin alfa. See table on next page.

**Contraindicated** in uncontrolled hypertension and patients hypersensitive to albumin/polysorbate 80 or epoetin alfa. Darbepoetin alfa is not intended for patients requiring acute correction of anemia. **Use with caution** in seizures and

*Continued*

DARBEPOETIN ALFA *continued*

**CONVERSION FROM EPOETIN ALFA TO DARBEPOEITIN ALFA**

| | Pediatric | Adult |
|---|---|---|
| **Previous Weekly Epoetin Alfa Dose (units/wk)*** | **Weekly Darbepoetin Alfa Dose (mcg/wk) Administered SC/IV Once Weekly†** | **Weekly Darbepoetin Alfa Dose (mcg/wk) Administered SC/IV Once Weekly†** |
| <1500 | Insufficient data | 6.25 |
| 1500–2499 | 6.25 | 6.25 |
| 2500–4999 | 10 | 12.5 |
| 5000–10,999 | 20 | 25 |
| 11,000–17,999 | 40 | 40 |
| 18,000–33,999 | 60 | 60 |
| 34,000–89,000 | 100 | 100 |
| ≥90,000 | 200 | 200 |

*200 units of epoetin alfa is equivalent to 1 mcg darbepoetin alfa.
†If patient was receiving epoetin alfa once weekly, darbepoetin alfa should be administered once every 2 wk.

liver disease. Evaluate serum iron, ferritin, and TIBC; concurrent iron supplementation may be necessary. Red cell aplasia and severe anemia associated with neutralizing antibodies to erythropoietin have been reported.

**USE IN CHRONIC RENAL FAILURE:** In pediatric patients, higher doses may be needed for individuals being switched from epoetin alfa compared to naïve patients. May cause edema, fatigue, GI disturbances, headache, blood pressure changes, fever, cardiac arrhythmia/arrest, infections and myalgia. Higher risk for mortality and serious cardiovascular events have been reported with higher targeted hemoglobin levels (13.5–14 g/dL). If hemoglobin levels do not increase or reach targeted levels despite appropriate dose titrations over a 12 wk period, (1) **do not** administer higher doses and use the lowest dose that will maintain hemoglobin levels to avoid the need for recurrent blood transfusions; (2) evaluate and treat other causes of anemia; (3) always follow the dose adjustment instructions; and (4) discontinue use if patient remains transfusion dependent.

**USE IN CANCER:** Use only for anemia due to myelosuppressive chemotherapy; not effective in reducing the need for transfusions in patients with anemia not due to chemotherapy. May cause fatigue, fever, edema, dizziness, headache, GI disturbances, arthralgia/myalgia, and rash. Use lowest dose to avoid transfusions and **do not exceed** hemoglobin levels > 12 g/dL; increased frequency of adverse events, including mortality and thrombotic vascular events have been reported. Shortened survival and time to tumor progression have also been reported in patients with various cancers.

Targeted hemoglobin in adults is 9–12 g/dL; **do not exceed** 12 g/dL. Monitor hemoglobin, BP, serum chemistries, and reticulocyte count. Increases in dose should **not** be made more frequently than once per mo. For IV administration, infuse over 1–3 min.

For explanation of icons, see p. 698.

## DEFEROXAMINE MESYLATE

Desferal

***Chelating agent***

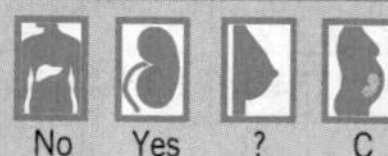

No Yes ? C

**Injection:** 500, 2000 mg

***Acute iron poisoning (if using IV route, convert to IM as soon as the patient's clinical condition permits):***

***Child:***

- ***IV:*** 15 mg/kg/hr or
- ***IM:*** 50 mg/kg/dose Q6 hr
- **Max. dose:** 6 g/24 hr

***Adult:***

- ***IV:*** 15 mg/kg/hr
- ***IM:*** 1 g × 1, then 0.5 g Q4 hr × 2; may repeat 0.5 g Q4–12 hr
- **Max. dose:** 6 g/24 hr

***Chronic iron overload (see remarks):***

***Child:***

- ***IV:*** 15 mg/kg/hr; **max. dose:** 6 g/24 hr
- ***SC:*** 20–40 mg/kg/dose QD as infusion over 8–12 hr; **max. dose:** 2 g/24 hr

***Adult:***

- ***IV:*** 15 mg/kg/hr; **max. dose:** 6 g/24 hr
- ***IM:*** 0.5–1 g/dose QD
- ***SC:*** 1–2 g/dose QD as infusion over 8–24 hr

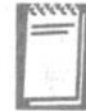

**Contraindicated** in severe renal disease or anuria. Not approved for use in primary hemochromatosis. May cause flushing, erythema, urticaria, hypotension, tachycardia, diarrhea, leg cramps, fever, cataracts, hearing loss, nausea, and vomiting. Iron mobilization may be poor in children < 3 yr.

High doses and concomitant low ferritin levels have also been associated with growth retardation. Growth velocity may resume to pretreatment levels by reducing the dosage. Acute respiratory distress syndrome has been reported following treatment with excessively high intravenous doses in patients with acute iron intoxication or thalassemia. Toxicity risk has been reported with infusions > 8 mg/kg/hr for > 4 days for thalassemia; and with infusions of 15 mg/kg/hr for > 1 day for acute iron toxicity. Pulmonary toxicity was not seen in 193 courses.

**Max. IV infusion rate:** 15 mg/kg/hr. SC route is via a portable controlled-infusion device and is **not recommended** in acute iron poisoning.

## DESLORATADINE

Clarinex, Clarinex RediTabs

***Antihistamine, less sedating***

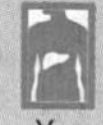
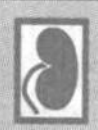
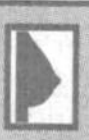
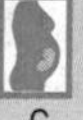

Yes Yes 1 C

**Tabs:** 5 mg

**Disintegrating tabs (RediTabs):** 2.5, 5 mg; contains phenylalanine

**Syrup:** 2.5 mg/5 mL (480 mL)

**Extended-release tabs of desloratadine and pseudoephedrine (PE):**

- Clarinex-D 12 Hour: 2.5 mg desloratadine + 120 mg pseudoephedrine
- Clarinex-D 24 Hour: 5 mg desloratadine + 240 mg pseudoephedrine

*Continued*

DESLORATADINE *continued*

***6–11 mo:*** 1 mg PO QD
***1–5 yr:*** 1.25 mg PO QD
***6–11 yr:*** 2.5 mg PO QD
***≥12 yr and adult:*** 5 mg PO QD
***Liver or renal impairment:*** administer age appropriate dose QOD.
***Extended-release tabs of desloratadine and pseudoephedrine:***
***≥12 yr and adult:***
***Clarinex-D 12 Hour:*** 1 tablet PO BID
***Clarinex-D 24 Hour:*** 1 tablet PO QD

**Contraindicated** in loratadine hypersensitivity. **Use with caution** in liver or renal disease (reduce dosage), glaucoma, prostatic hypertrophy, urinary retention and with other CNS depressants or anticholinergic drugs. Has **not** been implicated in causing cardiac arrhythmias when used with medications metabolized by hepatic microsomal enzymes (e.g., ketoconazole, erythromycin). May cause somnolence, fatigue, liver enzyme elevation, dizziness, tachycardia, palpitations, and other anticholinergic effects. Individuals with slow metabolism (reported as 7% of population and 20% of blacks from a clinical trial) may be susceptible to dose-related adverse effects.

All dosage forms may be administered regardless of food. For use of RediTabs, place tablet on tongue and allow it to disintegrate in the mouth with or without water. For Clarinex-D extended-release tabs, see *Pseudoephedrine* for additional remarks.

## DESMOPRESSIN ACETATE

DDAVP, Stimate, and others
***Vasopressin analog, synthetic; hemostatic agent***

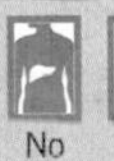
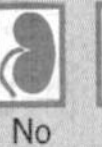
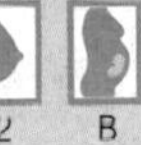

No No 2 B

**Tabs:** 0.1, 0.2 mg
**Nasal solution (with rhinal tube):** DDAVP, 100 mcg/mL (2.5 mL); contains 9 mg NaCl/mL
**Injection:** 4 mcg/mL (1, 10 mL); contains 9 mg NaCl/mL
**Nasal spray:**
100 mcg/mL, 10 mcg/spray (50 sprays, 5 mL); contains 7.5 mg NaCl/mL
Stimate: 1500 mcg/mL, 150 mcg/spray (25 sprays, 2.5 mL); contains 9 mg NaCl/mL
**Conversion:** 100 mcg = 400 IU arginine vasopressin

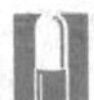

***Diabetes insipidus:***
***Oral:***
***Child ≤ 12 yr:*** Start with 0.05 mg/dose BID; titrate to effect; usual dose range: 0.1–0.8 mg/24 hr.
***Child > 12 yr and adult:*** Start with 0.05 mg/dose BID; titrate dose to effect; usual dose range: 0.1–1.2 mg/24 hr ÷ BID–TID.
***Intranasal:***
***3 mo–12 yr:*** 5–30 mcg/24 hr ÷ QD–BID
***>12 yr and adult:*** 10–40 mcg/24 hr ÷ QD–TID; titrate dose to achieve control of excessive thirst and urination. Morning and evening doses should be adjusted separately for diurnal rhythm of water turnover.
***IV/SC:***
***>12 yr and adult:*** 2–4 mcg/24 hr ÷ BID

*Continued*

For explanation of icons, see p. 698.

DESMOPRESSIN ACETATE *continued*

***Hemophilia A and von Willebrand's disease (see remarks):***
*Intranasal:* 2–4 mcg/kg/dose
*IV:* 0.2–0.4 mcg/kg/dose over 15–30 min
***Nocturnal enuresis (≥ 6 yr; see remarks):***
*Oral:* 0.2 mg at bedtime, titrated to a **max. dose** of 0.6 mg to achieve desired effect.
*Intranasal (see remarks):* 20 mcg at bedtime, range 10–40 mcg; divide dose by 2 and administer each one-half dose in each nostril.

---

**Use with caution** in hypertension and coronary artery disease. May cause headache, nausea, seizures, blood pressure changes, hyponatremia, nasal congestion, abdominal cramps, and hypertension.

**NOCTURNAL ENURESIS:** Intranasal formulations are no longer indicated by the FDA for primary nocturnal enuresis (children are susceptible to severe hyponatremia and seizures) or in patients with a history of hyponatremia. Patients using tablets should have their therapy interrupted during acute illnesses that may lead to fluid and/or electrolyte imbalance.

Injection may be used SC or IV at approximately 10% of intranasal dose. Adjust fluid intake to decrease risk of water intoxication and monitor serum sodium.

If switching stablized patient from intranasal route to IV/SC route, use 10% of intranasal dose. Peak effects: 1–5 hr with intranasal route; 1.5–3 hr with IV route; and 2–7 hr with PO route.

For hemophilia A and von Willebrand's disease, administer dose intranasally, 2 hr before procedure; IV, 30 min before procedure.

## DEXAMETHASONE

Decadron, Hexadrol, Maxidex, and many generics
***Corticosteroid***

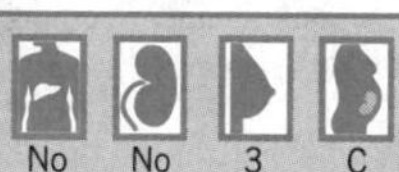


**Tabs (Decadron and other generics):** 0.25, 0.5, 0.75, 1, 1.5, 2, 4, 6 mg
**Injection (sodium phosphate salt):** 4, 10, 20 mg/mL (some preparations contain benzyl alcohol or methyl/propyl parabens)
**Elixir:** 0.5 mg/5 mL (some preparations contain 5% alcohol)
**Oral solution:** 0.1, 1 mg/mL (some preparations contain 30% alcohol)
**Ophthalmic solution:** 0.1% (5 mL)
**Ophthalmic suspension (Maxidex):** 0.1% (5 mL)

---

***Airway edema:*** 0.5–2 mg/kg/24 hr IV/IM ÷ Q6 hr (begin 24 hr before extubation and continue for 4–6 doses after extubation)
***Croup:*** 0.6 mg/kg/dose PO/IV/IM × 1
***Antiemetic (chemotherapy-induced):***
*Initial:* 10 mg/m²/dose IV; **max. dose:** 20 mg
*Subsequent:* 5 mg/m²/dose Q6 hr IV
***Anti-inflammatory:***
*Child:* 0.08–0.3 mg/kg/24 hr PO, IV, IM ÷ Q6–12 hr
*Adult:* 0.75–9 mg/24 hr PO, IV, IM ÷ Q6–12 hr
***Brain tumor associated cerebral edema:***
*Loading dose:* 1–2 mg/kg/dose IV/IM × 1
*Maintenance:* 1–1.5 mg/kg/24 hr ÷ Q4–6 hr; **max. dose:** 16 mg/24 hr
***Spinal cord compression with neurological abnormalities:***
*Child:* 2 mg/kg/24 hr IV ÷ Q6 hr

*Continued*

DEXAMETHASONE *continued*

***Ophthalmic use (child and adult):***

***Ointment:*** Apply a thin coating of ointment to the conjunctival sac of the affected eye(s) TID–QID. When a favorable response is achieved, reduce daily dosage to BID and later to QD as a maintenance dose sufficient to control symptoms.

***Solution:*** Instill 1 to 2 drops into the conjunctival sac of the affected eye(s) Q1 hr during the day and Q2 hr during the night as initial therapy. When a favorable response is achieved, reduce dosage to 1 drop Q4 hr. Further dose reduction to 1 drop TID–QID may be sufficient to control symptoms.

***Suspension:*** Shake well before using. Instill 1–2 drops in the conjunctival sac of the affected eye(s). For severe disease, drops may be Q1 hr, being tapered to discontinuation as inflammation subsides. For mild disease, drops may be used ≤ 4 to 6 times/24 hr.

---

**Not recommended** for systemic therapy in the prevention or treatment of chronic lung disease in infants with very low birth weight because of increase risk for adverse events (*Pediatrics* 2002;109(2):330–338). Dexamethasone is a substrate of CYP 450 3A3/4.

Toxicity: same as for prednisone without mineralcorticoid effects. **Contraindicated** in active untreated infections and fungal, viral, and mycobacterial ocular infections.

**OPHTHALMIC USE:** Use ophthalmic preparation only in consultation with an ophthalmologist. **Use with caution** in cornial/scleral thinning and glaucoma. Consider the possibility of persistent fungal infections of the cornea after prolonged use. Ophthalmic solution/suspension may be used in otitis externa.

Oral peak serum levels occur 1–2 hr and within 8 hr following IM administration. **For other uses, doses based on body surface area, and dose equvalence to other steroids, see Chapter 30, Table 30-1.**

## DEXTROAMPHETAMINE ± AMPHETAMINE

DextroStat, Dexedrine Spansules, and many other generics

In combination with amphetamine: Adderall, Adderall XR

***CNS stimulant***

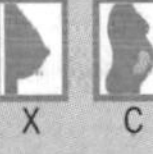


**Tabs:** 5, 10 mg

**Sustained-release caps (Dexedrine Spansules):** 5, 10, 15 mg

**In combination with amphetamine (Adderall):** Available as 1:1:1:1 mixture of dextroamphetamine sulfate, dextroamphetamine saccharate, amphetamine aspartate, and amphetamine sulfate salts; for example, the 5 mg tablet contains 1.25 mg dextroamphetamine sulfate, 1.25 mg dextroamphetamine saccharate, 1.25 mg amphetamine aspartate, and 1.25 mg amphetamine sulfate:

Tabs: 5, 7.5, 10, 12.5, 15, 20, 30 mg

Caps, extended-release (Adderal XR): 5, 10, 15, 20, 25, 30 mg

Oral suspension: 1 mg/mL

---

**Dosages are in terms of mgs of dextroamphetamine when using dextroamphetamine alone OR in terms of mgs of the total dextroamphetamine and amphetamine salts when using Adderall. Non-extended-release dosage forms are usually given BID–TID (first dose on awakening and subsequent doses at intervals of 4–6 hr later). Extended/sustained-release dosage forms are usually given QD, sometimes BID.**

*Continued*

For explanation of icons, see p. 698.

DEXTROAMPHETAMINE ± AMPHETAMINE *continued*

***Attention deficit hyperactivity disorder:***

***3–5 yr:*** 2.5 mg/24 hr QAM; increase by 2.5 mg/24 hr at weekly intervals to a **max. dose** of 40 mg/24 hr ÷ QD-TID.

***≥6 yr:*** 5 mg/24 hr QAM; increase by 5 mg/24 hr at weekly intervals to a **max. dose** of 40 mg/24 hr ÷ QD-TID.

***Narcolepsy:***

***6–12 yr:*** 5 mg/24 hr ÷ QD-TID; increase by 5 mg/24 hr at weekly intervals to a **max. dose** of 60 mg/24 hr

***>12 yr and adult:*** 10 mg/24 hr ÷ QD-TID; increase by 10 mg/24 hr at weekly intervals to a **max. dose** of 60 mg/24 hr

---

**Use with caution** in presence of hypertension or cardiovascular disease. **Avoid** use in known serious structural cardiac abnormalities, cardiomyopathy, serious heart rhythm abonormalities, coronary artery disease or other serious cardiac problems that may increase risk of sympathomimetic effects of amphetamines (sudden death, stroke, and MI have been reported). **Do not give** with MAO inhibitors or general anesthetics.

**Not recommended** for <3 yr. Medication should generally not be used in children <5 yr old as diagnosis of ADHD in this age group is extremely difficult (use in consultation with a specialist). Interrupt administration occasionally to determine need for continued therapy. Many side effects, including insomnia (**avoid** dose administration within 6 hr of bedtime), restlessness, anorexia, psychosis, visual disturbances, headache, vomiting, abdominal cramps, dry mouth, and growth failure. Tolerance develops. Same guidelines as for methylphenidate apply.

## DIAZEPAM

Valium, Diastat, Diastat AcuDial, and various generics

***Benzodiazepine; anxiolytic, anticonvulsant***

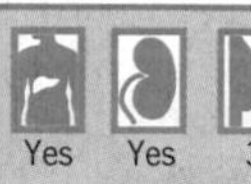
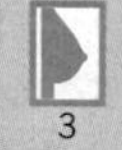
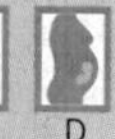

Yes Yes 3 D

**Tabs:** 2, 5, 10 mg

**Oral solution:** 1 mg/mL, 5 mg/mL (contains 19% alcohol)

**Injection:** 5 mg/mL (contains 40% propylene glycol, 10% alcohol, 5% sodium benzoate, and 1.5% benzyl alcohol)

**Pediatric rectal gel (Diastat):** 2.5, 5 mg (5 mg/mL concentration with 4.4 cm rectal tip delivery system; contains 10% alcohol, 1.5% benzyl alcohol, and propylene glycol); in twin packs.

**Pediatric/Adult rectal gel (Diastat AcuDial):**

**4.4 cm rectal tip delivery system (Pediatric/Adult):** 10 mg (5 mg/mL, delivers set doses of either 5, 7.5, or 10 mg); contains 10% alcohol, and 1.5% benzyl alcohol; in twin packs.

**6 cm rectal tip delivery system (Adult):** 20 mg (5 mg/mL, delivers set doses of either 10, 12.5, 15, 17.5, 20 mg); contains 10% alcohol, and 1.5% benzyl alcohol; in twin packs.

---

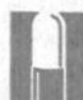

***Sedative/muscle relaxant:***

***Child:***

***IM or IV:*** 0.04–0.2 mg/kg/dose Q2–4 hr; **max. dose:** 0.6 mg/kg within an 8-hr period.

***PO:*** 0.12–0.8 mg/kg/24 hr ÷ Q6–8 hr

***Adult:***

***IM or IV:*** 2–10 mg/dose Q3–4 hr PRN

***PO:*** 2–10 mg/dose Q6–12 hr PRN

*Continued*

DIAZEPAM *continued*

***Status epilepticus:***

***Neonate:*** 0.3–0.75 mg/kg/dose IV Q15–30 min × 2–3 doses; **max. total dose:** 2 mg.

***Child >1 mo:*** 0.2–0.5 mg/kg/dose IV Q15–30 min; **max. total dose:** <5 yr: 5 mg; ≥ 5 yr: 10 mg. May repeat dosing in 2–4 hr as needed.

***Adult:*** 5–10 mg/dose IV Q10–15 min; **max. total dose:** 30 mg in an 8-hr period. May repeat dosing in 2–4 hr as needed.

***Rectal dose (using IV dosage form):*** 0.5 mg/kg/dose followed by 0.25 mg/kg/dose in 10 min PRN.

***Rectal gel:*** all doses rounded to the nearest available dosage strength; repeat dose in 4–12 hr PRN

***2–5 yr:*** 0.5 mg/kg/dose
***6–11 yr:*** 0.3 mg/kg/dose
***>12 yr and adult:*** 0.2 mg/kg/dose

Hypotension and respiratory depression may occur. **Use with caution** in hepatic and renal dysfunction, glaucoma, shock, and depression. **Do not use** in combination with protease inhibitors. Concurrent use with CNS depressants, cimetidine, erythromycin, itraconazole, and valproic acid may enhance the effects of diazepam. Diazepam is a substrate for CYP 450 2B6, 2C8, 2C9, and 3A5-7; and minor substrate and inhibitor for CYP 450 2C19 and 3A3/4. The active desmethyldiazepam metabolite is a CYP 450 2C19 substrate.

Administer the conventional IV product undiluted no faster than 2 mg/min. **Do not mix** with IV fluids.

In status epilepticus, diazepam must be followed by long-acting anticonvulsants. Onset of anticonvulsant effect: 1–3 min with IV route; 2–10 min with rectal route. **For management of status epilepticus, see Chapter 1, Table 1-5. For additional information, see Chapter 20, Table 20-7.**

## DIAZOXIDE

Proglycem

***Antihypertensive agent, antihypoglycemic agent***

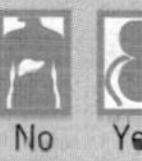
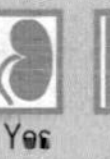
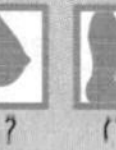

No Yes ? C

**Oral suspension:** 50 mg/mL (30 mL); contains 7.25% alcohol

***Hyperinsulinemic hypoglycemia (due to insulin-producing tumors; start at the lowest dose):***

***Newborn and infant:*** 8–15 mg/kg/24 hr ÷ Q8–12 hr PO
***Child and adult:*** 3–8 mg/kg/24 hr ÷ Q8–12 hr PO

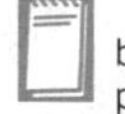

Hypoglycemia should be treated initially with IV glucose; diazoxide should be introduced only if refractory to glucose infusion. Should not be used in patients hypersensitive to thiazides unless benefit outweighs risk. **Use with caution** in renal impairment (clearance of drug is reduced); consider dosage reduction.

Sodium and fluid retention is common in young infants and adults and may precipitate CHF in patients with compromised cardiac reserve (usually responsive to diuretics). Hirsutism (reversible), GI disturbances, transient loss of taste, tachycardia, ketoacidosis, tachycardia, palpitations, rash, headache, weakness,and hyperuricemia may occur. Monitor BP closely for hypotension.

Hyperglycemic effect with PO administration occurs within 1 hr, with a duration of 8 hr.

For explanation of icons, see p. 698.

## DICLOXACILLIN SODIUM

Dycill, Pathocil, and others

***Antibiotic, penicillin (penicillinase-resistant)***

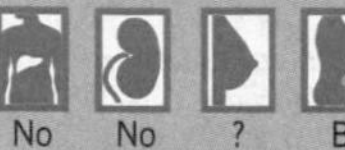


**Caps:** 250, 500 mg; contains 0.6 mEq Na/250 mg

***Child (<40 kg) (see remarks):***

***Mild/moderate infections:*** 12.5–25 mg/kg/24 hr PO ÷ Q6 hr

***Severe infections:*** 50–100 mg/kg/24 hr PO ÷ Q6 hr

***Adult (≥ 40 kg):*** 125–500 mg/dose PO Q6 hr; **max. dose:** 4 g/24 hr

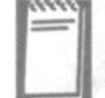

**Contraindicated** in patients with a history of penicillin allergy. **Use with caution** in cephalosporin hypersensitivity. May cause nausea, vomiting, and diarrhea.

Limited experience in neonates and very young infants. Higher doses (50–100 mg/kg/24 hr) are indicated following IV therapy for osteomyelitis.

Administer 1 hr before meals or 2 hr after meals.

## DIGOXIN

Lanoxin, Digitek, Lanoxicaps

***Antiarrhythmic agent, inotrope***

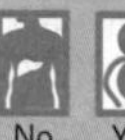
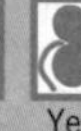
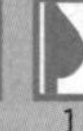
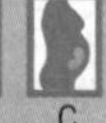


**Caps (Lanoxicaps):** 100, 200 mcg
**Tabs:** 125, 250 mcg
**Elixir:** 50 mcg/mL (60 mL); may contain 10% alcohol
**Injection:** 100, 250 mcg/mL; may contain propylene glycol and alcohol

***Digitalizing:*** Total digitalizing dose (TDD) and maintenance doses in mcg/kg/24 hr (see the table that follows):

**DIGOXIN DIGITALIZING AND MAINTENANCE DOSES**

| | TDD | | Daily Maintenance | |
|---|---|---|---|---|
| **Age** | **PO** | **IV/IM** | **PO** | **IV/IM** |
| Premature | 20 | 15 | 5 | 3–4 |
| Full term | 30 | 20 | 8–10 | 6–8 |
| <2 yr | 40–50 | 30–40 | 10–12 | 7.5–9 |
| 2–10 yr | 30–40 | 20–30 | 8–10 | 6–8 |
| >10 yr and <100 kg | 10–15 | 8–12 | 2.5–5 | 2–3 |

***Initial:*** ½ TDD, then ¼ TDD Q8–18 hr × 2 doses; obtain ECG 6 hr after dose to assess for toxicity

***Maintenance:***

***<10 yr:*** Give maintenance dose ÷ BID

***≥10 yr:*** Give maintenance dose QD

**Contraindicated** in patients with ventricular dysrhythmias. **Use with caution** in renal failure and with adenosine (enhanced depressant effects on SA and AV nodes). May cause AV block or dysrhythmias. In the patient treated

*Continued*

DIGOXIN *continued*

with digoxin, cardioversion, or calcium infusion may lead to ventricular fibrillation (pretreatment with lidocaine may prevent this). Decreased serum potassium and magnesium, or increased magnesium and calcium may increase risk for digoxin toxicity. For signs and symptoms of toxicity, see Chapter 2.

Excreted via the kidney; **adjust dose in renal failure (see Chapter 31).** Therapeutic concentration: 0.8–2 ng/mL. Higher doses may be required for supraventricular tachycardia. Neonates, pregnant women, and patients with renal, hepatic, or heart failure may have falsely elevated digoxin levels, due to the presence of digoxin-like substances.

$T_{1/2}$: Premature infants, 61–170 hr; full-term neonates, 35–45 hr; infants, 18–25 hr; and children, 35 hr.

Recommended serum sampling at steady-state: Obtain a single level from 6 hr postdose to just before the next scheduled dose following 5–8 days of continuous dosing. Levels obtained prior to steady-state may be useful in preventing toxicity.

## DIGOXIN IMMUNE FAB (OVINE)

Digibind, DigiFab

***Antidigoxin antibody***

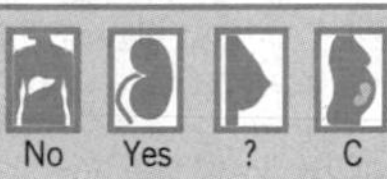


**Injection:**

Digibind: 38 mg
DigiFab: 40 mg

First, determine total body digoxin load (TBL):

TBL(mg) = serum digoxin level (ng/mL) × 5.6 × wt (kg) ÷ 1000, **OR** TBL (mg) = mg digoxin ingested × 0.8

Then, calculate digoxin immune Fab dose:

Dose in number of digoxin immune Fab vials (Digibind or DigiFab): # vials = TBL ÷ 0.5

Infuse IV over 15–30 min; administer through 0.22-micron filter only if using Digibind.

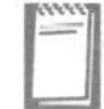

**Contraindicated** if hypersensitive to sheep products. **Use with caution** in renal or cardiac failure. May cause rapidly developing severe hypokalemia, decreased cardiac output, rash, and edema. Digoxin therapy may be reinstituted in 3–7 days, when toxicity has been corrected. Digoxin immune FAB will interfere with digitalis immunoassay measurements to result in misleading concentrations. See Chapter 2 for additional information.

## DILTIAZEM

Cardizem, Cardizem SR, Cardizem CD, Cardizem LA, Dilacor XR, Tiazac, and many others

***Calcium channel blocker, antihypertensive***

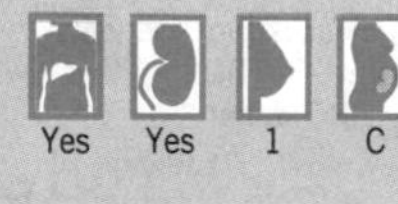


**Tabs:** 30, 60, 90, 120 mg

**Extended-release tabs:**

Cardizem LA: 120, 180, 240, 300, 360, 420 mg

**Extended-release caps:**

Various generics: 60, 90, 120, 180, 240, 300, 360, 420 mg
Cardizem CD: 120, 180, 240, 300, 360 mg
Dilacor XR: 120, 180, 240 mg
Tiazac: 120, 180, 240, 300, 360, 420 mg

*Continued*

For explanation of icons, see p. 698.

DILTIAZEM *continued*

**Oral liquid:** 12 mg/mL
**Injection:** 5 mg/mL (5, 10, 25 mL)

***Child:*** 1.5–2 mg/kg/24 hr PO ÷ TID–QID; **max. dose:** 3.5 mg/kg/24 hr, **alternative max. dose** of 6 mg/kg/24 hr up to 360 mg/24 hr has been recommended.

***Adolescent:***

***Immediate release:*** 30–120 mg/dose PO TID–QID; usual range 180–360 mg/24 hr.

***Extended release:*** 120–300 mg/24 hr PO ÷ QD–BID (BID dosing with Cardizem SR; QD dosing with Cardizem CD, Cardizem LA, Dilacor XR, Tiazac); **max. dose:** 540 mg/24 hr.

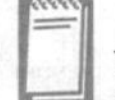

**Contraindicated** in acute MI with pulmonary congestion, second- or third-degree heart block, and sick sinus syndrome. **Use with caution** in CHF or renal and hepatic impairment. Dizziness, headache, edema, nausea, vomiting, heart block, and arrhythmias may occur.

Diltiazem is a substrate and inhibitor of the CYP 450 3A4 enzyme system. May increase levels and/or effect of buspirone, cyclosporine, carbamazepine, fentanyl, digoxin, quinidine, tacrolimus, benzodiazepines, and beta-blockers. Cimetidine may increase diltiazem serum levels. Rifampin may decrease diltiazem serum levels.

Maximal antihypertensive effect seen within 2 wk.

## DIMENHYDRINATE

Dramamine, Children's Dramamine, and other brand names

***Antiemetic, antihistamine***

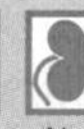

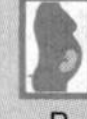

No No ? B

**Tabs (OTC):** 50 mg
**Chewable tabs (OTC):** 50 mg; contains 1.5 mg phenylalanine
**Oral liquid:** 12.5 mg/4 mL (OTC), 12.5 mg/5 mL (OTC), 15.62 mg/5 mL; some preparations may contain 5% alcohol
**Injection:** 50 mg/mL; contains benzyl alcohol and propylene glycol

***Child (<12 yr):*** 5 mg/kg/24 hr ÷ Q6 hr PO/IM/IV; alternative oral dosing by age:

***2–5 yr:*** 12.5–25 mg/dose Q6–8 hr PRN PO with the **max. dosage** in the subsequent list

***6–12 yr:*** 25–50 mg/dose Q6–8 hr PRN PO with the **max. dosage** in the subsequent list

***Adult:*** 50–100 mg/dose Q4–6 hr PRN PO/IM/IV

**Max. PO doses:**

***2–5 yr:*** 75 mg/24 hr
***6–12 yr:*** 150 mg/24 hr
***Adult:*** 400 mg/24 hr

**Max. IM dose:** 300 mg/24 hr

Causes drowsiness and anticholinergic side effects. May mask vestibular symptoms and cause CNS excitation in young children. **Caution** when taken with ototoxic agents or history of seizures. Use should be limited to management of prolonged vomiting of known etiology. **Not recommended** in children <2 yr. Toxicity resembles anti-cholinergic poisoning.

## DIMERCAPROL

BAL, British Anti-Lewisite

***Heavy metal chelator (arsenic, gold, mercury, lead)***

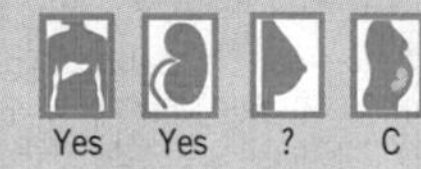


**Injection (in oil):** 100 mg/mL; contains 20% benzyl benzoate and peanut oil (3 mL)

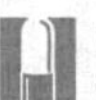

***Give all injections deep IM.***

***Lead poisoning:***

***Acute severe encephalopathy (lead level > 70 mcg/dL):*** 4 mg/kg/dose Q4 hr × 2–7 days with the addition of Ca-EDTA (given at separate site) at the time of the second dose.

***Less severe poisoning:*** 4 mg/kg × 1, then 3 mg/kg/dose Q4 hr × 2–7 days.

***Arsenic or gold poisoning:***

***Days 1 and 2:*** 2.5–3 mg/kg/dose Q6 hr

***Day 3:*** 2.5–3 mg/kg/dose Q12 hr

***Days 4–13:*** 2.5–3 mg/kg/dose Q24 hr

***Mercury poisoning:*** 5 mg/kg × 1, then 2.5 mg/kg/dose QD–BID × 10 days

**Contraindicated** in hepatic or renal insufficiency. May cause hypertension, tachycardia, GI disturbance, headache, fever (30% of children), nephrotoxicity, transient neutropenia. Symptoms are usually relieved by antihistamines. Urine should be kept alkaline to protect the kidneys. **Use with caution** with G6PD deficiency and peanut-sensitive patients. **Do not use** concomitantly with iron.

## DIPHENHYDRAMINE

Benadryl and many other brand names

***Antihistamine***

No Yes 3 B

**Elixir (OTC):** 12.5 mg/5 mL; may contain 5.6% alcohol
**Syrup:** 12.5 mg/5 mL; some may contain 5% alcohol
**Oral suspension:** 25 mg/5 mL; may contain phenylalanine
**Oral liquid/solution (OTC):** 12.5 mg/5 mL
**Caps/Tabs (OTC):** 25, 50 mg
**Tabs, orally disintegrating (OTC):** 12.5 mg; contains aspartame, phenylalanine
**Strips, orally disintegrating (OTC):** 12.5, 25 mg; may contain < 5% alcohol
**Chewable tabs:** 12.5 mg (OTC), 25 mg; contains aspartame, phenylalanine
**Injection:** 50 mg/mL
**Cream (OTC):** 1, 2% (14.2, 15, 28.35 g)
**Lotion (OTC):** 1% (180 mL)
**Topical gel (OTC):** 1% (37.5 g), 2% (15, 30, 118 g)
**Topical spray (OTC):** 1, 2% (60 mL)

***Child:*** 5 mg/kg/24 hr ÷ Q6 hr PO/IM/IV

**Max. dose:** 300 mg/24 hr

***Adult:*** 25–50 mg/dose Q4–8 hr PO/IM/IV

**Max. dose:** 400 mg/24 hr

***For anaphylaxis or phenothiazine overdose:*** 1–2 mg/kg IV slowly.

**Contraindicated** with concurrent MAO inhibitor use, acute attacks of asthma, GI or urinary obstruction. **Use with caution** in infants and young children, and **do not use** in neonates due to potential CNS effects. Side effects

*Continued*

For explanation of icons, see p. 698.

DIPHENHYDRAMINE *continued*

include sedation, nausea, vomiting, xerostoma, blurred vision and other reactions common to antihistamines. CNS side effects more common than GI disturbances. May cause paradoxical excitement in children. **Adjust dose in renal failure (see Chapter 31).**

## DIVALPROEX SODIUM

Depakote, Depakote ER

***Anticonvulsant***

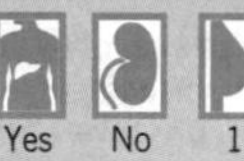

Yes No 1 D

**Delayed-release tabs:** 125, 250, 500 mg
**Extended-release tabs (Depakote ER):** 250, 500 mg
**Sprinkle caps:** 125 mg

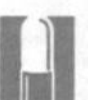

***Dose:*** See *Valproic Acid*

See *Valproic Acid*. Preferred over valproic acid for patients on ketogenic diet. Depakote ER is prescribed by a once daily interval; whereas Depakote is typically prescribed BID. Depakote and Depakote ER are not bioequivalent; see package insert for dose conversion.

## DOBUTAMINE

Various generics; previously available as Dobutrex

***Sympathomimetic agent***

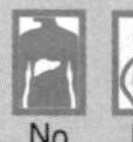
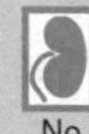
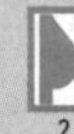
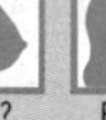
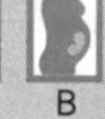

No No ? B

**Injection:** 12.5 mg/mL (20 mL); contains sulfites
**Prediluted in $D_5W$:** 1 mg/mL (250, 500 mL), 2 mg/mL (250 mL), 4 mg/mL (250 mL)

***Continuous IV infusion:*** 2.5–15 mcg/kg/min;
**Max. dose:** 40 mcg/kg/min.
***To prepare infusion:*** See the inside front cover.

**Contraindicated** in idiopathic hypertrophic subaortic stenosis (IHSS). Tachycardia, arrhythmias (PVCs), and hypertension may occasionally occur (especially at higher infusion rates). Correct hypovolemic states before use. Increases AV conduction, may precipitate ventricular ectopic activity.

Dobutamine has been shown to increase cardiac output and systemic pressure in pediatric patients of every age group. However, in premature neonates, dobutamine is less effective than dopamine in raising systemic blood pressure without causing undue tachycardia, and dobutamine has not been shown to provide any added benefit when given to such infants already receiving optimal infusions of dopamine.

Monitor BP and vital signs. $T_{1/2}$: 2 min. Peak effects in 10–20 min.

## DOCUSATE

Colace, Surfak, and many other brands

***Stool softener, laxative***

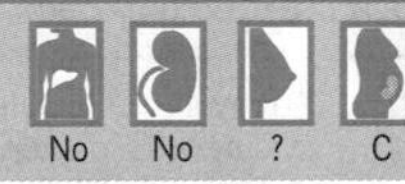


**Available as docusate sodium:**
**Caps (OTC):** 50, 100, 250 mg; sodium content (50 mg cap, 3 mg; 100 mg cap, ~5 mg)
**Tabs (OTC):** 100 mg
**Syrup (OTC):** 16.7 mg/5 mL, 20 mg/5 mL; may contain alcohol
**Oral liquid (OTC):** 10 mg/mL; contains 1 mg/mL sodium
**Rectal enema (Enemeez; OTC):** 283 mg/5 mL (5 mL)
**Available as docusate calcium:**
**Caps (Surfak; OTC):** 240 mg

---

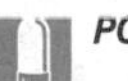

***PO:*** (take with liquids)
***<3 yr:*** 10–40 mg/24 hr ÷ QD–QID
***3–6 yr:*** 20–60 mg/24 hr ÷ QD–QID
***6–12 yr:*** 40–150 mg/24 hr ÷ QD–QID
***>12 yr and adult:*** 50–400 mg/24 hr ÷ QD–QID

***Rectal:***
***Older child and adult:*** add 50–100 mg of oral liquid (not syrup) to enema fluid.

---

Oral dosage effective only after 1–3 days of therapy. Incidence of side effects is exceedingly low. Oral liquid is bitter; give with milk, fruit juice, or formula to mask taste.

A few drops of the 10 mg/mL oral liquid may be used in the ear as a cerumenolyic. Effect is usually seen within 15 min.

## DOLASETRON

Anzemet

***Antiemetic agent, 5-HT$_3$ antagonist***

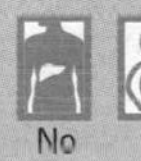
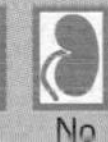
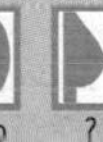
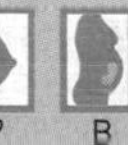


**Injection:** 20 mg/mL (0.625, 5, 25 mL)
**Tabs:** 50, 100 mg
**Oral suspension:** 10 mg/mL

---

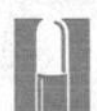

***Chemotherapy-induced nausea and vomiting prevention:***
***2 yr–adult:*** 1.8 mg/kg/dose IV/PO up to a **max. dose** of 100 mg. Administer IV doses 30 min prior to chemotherapy and administer PO doses 60 min prior to chemotherapy.

***Postoperative nausea and vomiting prevention:*** Administer IV doses 15 min prior to cessation of anesthesia or at onset of nausea and vomiting and PO doses 2 hr prior to surgery.

***2–16 yr:***
***IV:*** 0.35 mg/kg/dose (**max. dose:** 12.5 mg) × 1
***PO:*** 1.2 mg/kg/dose × 1 (**max. dose:** 100 mg) × 1

***Adult:***
***IV:*** 12.5 mg/dose × 1
***PO:*** 100 mg/dose × 1

*Continued*

For explanation of icons, see p. 698.

DOLASETRON *continued*

May cause hypotension and prolongation of cardiac conduction intervals; particularly QTc interval. Common side effects include dizziness, headache, sedation, blurred vision, fever, chills, and sleep disorders. Rare cases of sustained supraventricular and ventricular arrhythmias, fatal cardiac arrest and MI have been reported in children and adolescents.

**Avoid** concurrent use with other drugs that increase QTc interval (e.g., erythromycin, cisapride). Drug's active metabolite (hydrodolasetron) is a substrate for CYP 450 2D6 and 3A3/4 isoenzymes; concomitant use of enzyme inhibitors (e.g., cimetidine) may increase risk for side effects and use of enzyme inducers (e.g., rifampin) may decrease dolasetron's efficacy. Although no dosage adjustments are necessary, hydrodolasetron's clearance decreases 42% with severe hepatic impairment and 44% with severe renal impairment.

IV doses may be administered undiluted over 30 sec.

## DOPAMINE

Various generics; previously available as Intropin

***Sympathomimetic agent***

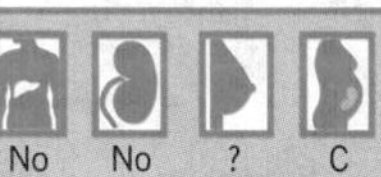


**Injection:** 40, 80, 160 mg/mL (5, 10, 20 mL)
**Prediluted in $D_5W$:** 0.8, 1.6, 3.2 mg/mL (250, 500 mL)

***Low dose:*** 2–5 mcg/kg/min IV; increases renal blood flow; minimal effect on heart rate and cardiac output
***Intermediate dose:*** 5–15 mcg/kg/min IV; increases heart rate, cardiac contractility, cardiac output, and to a lesser extent, renal blood flow.
***High dose:*** >20 mcg/kg/min IV; alpha-adrenergic effects are prominent; decreases renal perfusion.
**Max. dose recommended:** 20–50 mcg/kg/min IV
***To prepare infusion:*** See the inside front cover.

**Do not use** in pheochromocytoma, tachyarrhythmias, or hypovolemia. Monitor vital signs and blood pressure continuously. Correct hypovolemic states. Tachyarrhythmias, ectopic beats, hypertension, vasoconstriction, and vomiting may occur. **Use with caution** with phenytoin because hypotension and bradycardia may be exacerbated.

Newborn infants may be more sensitive to the vasoconstrictive effects of dopamine. Children < 2 yr of age clear dopamine faster and exhibit high variablity in neonates.

Should be administered through a central line or large vein. Extravasation may cause tissue necrosis; treat with phentolamine. **Do not administer** into an umbilical arterial catheter.

## DORNASE ALFA/DNASE

Pulmozyme

***Inhaled mucolytic***

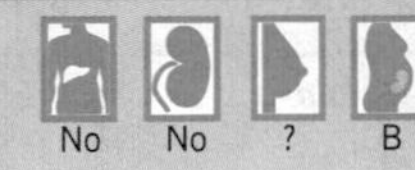

No No ? B

**Inhalation solution:** 1 mg/mL (2.5 mL)

***Child > 5 yr and adult:*** 2.5 mg via nebulizer QD. Some patients may benefit from 2.5 mg BID.

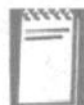

**Contraindicated** in patients with hypersensitivity to epoetin alfa. Voice alteration, pharyngitis, laryngitis may result. These are generally reversible without dose adjustment.

**Do not mix** with other nebulized drugs. A beta-agonist may be useful before administration to enhance drug distribution. Chest physiotherapy should be incorporated into treatment regimen. Use of the "Sidestream" nebulizer cup can significantly reduce the medication administration time.

## DOXAPRAM HCL

Dopram

***CNS stimulant***

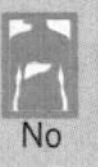 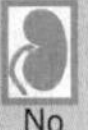 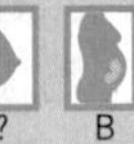

No No ? B

**Injection:** 20 mg/mL (20 mL); contains 0.9% benzyl alcohol

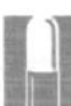

***Methylxanthine-refractory neonatal apnea:*** Load with 2.5–3 mg/kg over 15 min, followed by a continuous infusion of 1 mg/kg/hr titrated to the lowest effective dose; **max. dose:** 2.5 mg/kg/hr.

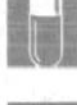

**Contraindicated** in seizures, proven or suspected pulmonary embolism, head injuries, cerebral vascular accident, cerebral edema, cardiovascular or coronary artery disease, severe hypertension, pheochromocytoma, hyperthyroidism, and in patients with mechanical disorders of ventilation. **Do not use** with general anesthetic agents that can sensitize the heart to catecholamines (e.g., halothane, cyclopropane, and enflurane) to reduce the risk of cardiac arrhythmias, including ventricular tachycardia and ventricular fibrillation. **Do not** initiate doxapram until the general anesthetic agent has been completely excreted.

Hypertension occurs with higher doses (> 1.5 mg/kg/hr). May also cause tachycardia, arrhythmias, seizure, hyperreflexia, hyperpyrexia, abdominal distension, bloody stools, and sweating. **Avoid** extravasation into tissues.

## DOXYCYCLINE

Vibramycin, Periostat, and others

***Antibiotic, tetracycline derivative***

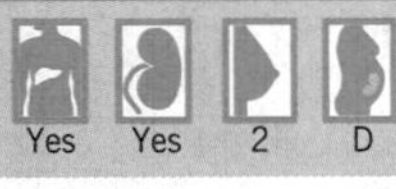

Yes Yes 2 D

**Caps:** 20 (Periostat), 50, 75, 100 mg
**Tabs:** 20 (Periostat), 50, 75, 100 mg
**Syrup:** 50 mg/5 mL (60 mL)
**Oral suspension:** 25 mg/5 mL (60 mL)
**Injection:** 100, 200 mg

*Continued*

For explanation of icons, see p. 698.

DOXYCYCLINE *continued*

***Initial:***

***≤45 kg:*** 2.2 mg/kg/dose BID PO/IV × 1 day to **max. dose** of 200 mg/ 24 hr

***>45 kg:*** 100 mg/dose BID PO/IV × 1 day

***Maintenance:***

***≤45 kg:*** 2.2–4.4 mg/kg/24 hr QD-BID PO/IV

***>45 kg:*** 100–200 mg/24 hr ÷ QD-BID PO/IV

**Max. adult dose:** 300 mg/24 hr

***PID:*** See Chapter 17.

***Anthrax (inhalation/systemic/cutaneous; see remarks):*** Initiate therapy with IV route and convert to PO route when clinically appropriate. Duration of therapy is 60 days (IV and PO combined):

***≤8 yr or ≤45 kg:*** 2.2 mg/kg/dose BID IV/PO; **max. dose:** 200 mg/24 hr

***>8 yr and >45 kg:*** 100 mg/dose BID IV/PO

***Malaria prophylaxis (start 1–2 days prior to exposure and continue for 4 wk after leaving endemic area):***

***>8 yr:*** 2 mg/kg/24 hr PO QD; **max. dose:** 100 mg/24 hr

***Adult:*** 100 mg PO QD

***Periodontitis:***

***Adult:*** 20 mg BID PO × ≤9 mo

**Use with caution** in hepatic and renal disease. May cause increased intracranial pressure. Generally **not recommended** for use in children <8 yr due to risk for tooth enamel hypoplasia and discoloration. However, the AAP *Red Book* recommends doxycycline as the drug of choice for rickettsial disease regardless of age. May cause GI symptoms, photosensitivity, hemolytic anemia, rash and hypersensitivity reactions.

Doxycycline is approved for the treatment of anthrax (*Bacillus anthracis*) in combination with one or two other antimicrobials. If meningitis is suspected, consider using an alternative agent because of poor CNS penetration. Consider changing to high-dose amoxicillin (25–35 mg/kg/dose TID PO) for penicillin-susceptible strains. See www.bt.cdc.gov for the latest information.

Rifampin, barbiturates, phenytoin, and carbamazepine may increase clearance of doxycycline. Doxycycline may enhance the hypoprothrombinemic effect of warfarin. See *Tetracycline* for additional drug/food interactions and remarks.

Infuse IV over 1–4 hr. **Avoid** prolonged exposure to direct sunlight.

For periodontitis, take capsules ≥ 1 hr prior to meals; and take tablets ≥ 1 hr prior or 2 hr after meals.

## DRONABINOL

Tetrahydrocannabinol, THC, Marinol

***Antiemetic***

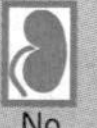
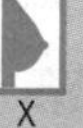
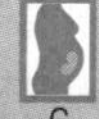

Yes No X C

**Caps:** 2.5, 5, 10 mg; contains sesame oil

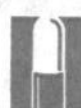

***Antiemetic:***

***Child and adult (PO):*** 5 mg/m$^2$/dose 1–3 hr prior to chemotherapy, then Q2–4 hr up to a **max. dose** of 6 doses/24 hr; doses may be gradually increased by 2.5 mg/m$^2$/dose increments up to a **max. dose** of 15 mg/m$^2$/dose if needed and tolerated

*Continued*

DRONABINOL *continued*

***Appetite stimulant:***

***Adult (PO):*** 2.5 mg BID 1 hr before lunch and dinner; if not tolerated, reduce dose to 2.5 mg QHS.

**Max. dose:** 20 mg/24 hr (**use caution** when increasing doses because of increased risk of dose-related adverse reactions at higher dosages)

**Contraindicated** in patients with history of substance abuse and mental illness, allergy to sesame oil. **Use with caution** in heart disease, seizures, hepatic disease (reduce dose if severe). Side effects: euphoria, dizziness, difficulty concentrating, anxiety, mood change, sedation, hallucinations, ataxia, paresthesia, hypotension, excessively increased appetite, and habit forming potential.

Onset of action: 0.5–1 hr. Duration of psychoactive effects 4–6 hr; appetite stimulation, 24 hr.

## DROPERIDOL

Inapsine and others

***Sedative, antiemetic***

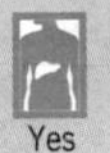
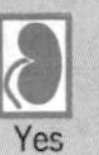
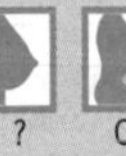
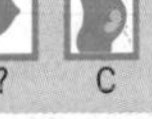

Yes Yes ? C

**Injection:** 2.5 mg/mL (1, 2 mL)

***Antiemetic/sedation:***

***Child:*** 0.03–0.07 mg/kg/dose IM or IV over 2–5 min; if needed, may give 0.1–0.15 mg/kg/dose; **initial max. dose:** 0.1 mg/kg/dose and **subsequent max. dose:** 2.5 mg/dose

***Dosage interval:***

***Antiemetic:*** PRN Q4–6 hr

***Sedation:*** Repeat dose in 15–30 min if necessary

***Adult:*** 2.5–5 mg IM or IV over 2–5 min; **initial max. dose** is 2.5 mg.

***Dosage interval:***

***Antiemetic:*** PRN Q3–4 hr

***Sedation:*** Repeat dose in 15–30 min if necessary.

**Use with caution** in renal and hepatic impairment; 75% of metabolites are excreted renally and drug is extensively metabolized in the liver. Side effects include hypotension, tachycardia, extrapyramidal side effects such as dystonia, feeling of motor restlessness, laryngospasm, bronchospasm. May lower seizure threshold. **Fatal arrhythmias and QT interval prolongation has been associated with use.**

Onset in 3–10 min. Peak effects within 10–30 min. Duration of 2–4 hr. Often given as adjunct to other agents.

## EDETATE (EDTA) CALCIUM DISODIUM

Calcium disodium versenate

***Chelating agent, antidote for lead toxicity***

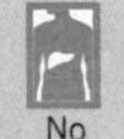
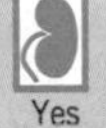
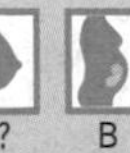

No Yes ? B

**Injection:** 200 mg/mL (5 mL)

*Continued*

For explanation of icons, see p. 698.

EDETATE (EDTA) CALCIUM DISODIUM *continued*

***Lead poisoning:***
***Lead level > 70 mcg/dL (use with dimercaprol):*** Initiate at the time of the second dimercaprol dose and treat for 3–5 days. May repeat a course as needed after 2–4 days of no EDTA.
***IM:*** 1000–1500 mg/m²/24 hr ÷ Q4 hr
***IV:*** 1000–1500 mg/m²/24 hr as an 8–24 hr infusion or divided Q12 hr. Use 1500 mg/m²/24 hr for 5 days in the presence of encephalopathy.
***Lead level 20–70 mcg/dL:*** 1000 mg/m²/24 hr IV as an 8–24 hr infusion OR intermittent dosing divided Q12 hr × 5 days. May repeat course as needed after 2–4 days of no EDTA.
**Max. daily dose:** 75 mg/kg/24 hr.

**Edetate (EDTA) calcium disodium is not interchangable with edetate disodium; erroneous substitutions have lead to fatalities.** Prescribe this product by its full name and **avoid** the EDTA abbreviation to prevent dispensing errors.

May cause renal tubular necrosis. **Do not use** if anuric. Dosage reduction is recommended with mild renal disease. Follow urinalysis and renal function. Monitor ECG continuously for arrhythmia when giving IV. Rapid IV infusion may cause sudden increase in intracranial pressure in patients with cerebral edema. May cause zinc and copper deficiency. Monitor $Ca^{2+}$ and $PO_4$.

IM route preferred. Give IM with 0.5% procaine.

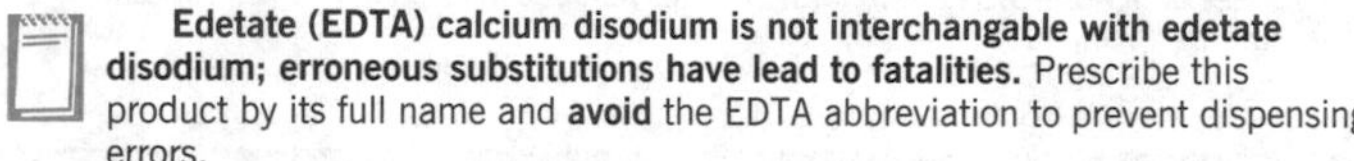

## EDROPHONIUM CHLORIDE

Tensilon, Enlon, Reversol

***Anticholinesterase agent, antidote for neuromuscular blockade***

No Yes ? C

**Injection:** 10 mg/mL (1, 10, 15 mL) (contains 0.45% phenol and 0.2% sulfite)

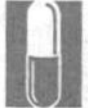

***Test for myasthenia gravis (IV):***
***Neonate:*** 0.1 mg single dose
***Infant and child:***
***Initial:*** 0.04 mg/kg/dose × 1
**Max. dose:** 1 mg for <34 kg; 2 mg for ≥34 kg
If no response after 1 min, may give 0.16 mg/kg/dose for a total of 0.2 mg/kg
**Total max. dose:** 5 mg for <34 kg; 10 mg for ≥34 kg
***Adult:*** 2 mg test dose IV; if no reaction, give 8 mg after 45 sec.

May precipitate cholinergic crisis, arrhythmias, and bronchospasm. Keep atropine available in syringe and have resuscitation equipment ready. Hypersensitivity to test dose (fasciculations or intestinal cramping) is indication to stop giving drug. **Contraindicated** in GI or GU obstruction, or arrhythmias. Dose may need to be reduced in chronic renal failure.

Reported doses for reversing neuromuscular blockade in children have ranged from 0.1–1.43 mg/kg/dose. Antagonism of nondepolarizing neuromuscular blocking drugs in children is more rapid than in adults.

Short duration of action with IV route (5–10 min). **Antidote:** atropine 0.01–0.04 mg/kg/dose.

## EMLA

See *Lidocaine* and *Prilocaine*

## ENALAPRIL MALEATE (PO), ENALAPRILAT (IV)

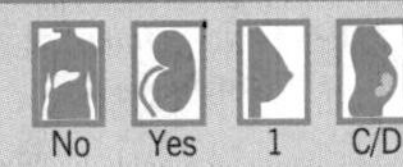


Enalapril: Vasotec and others
Enalaprilat: Vasotec IV and others
***Angiotensin converting enzyme inhibitor, antihypertensive***

**Enalapril:**
Tabs: 2.5, 5, 10, 20 mg
Oral suspension: 0.1, 1 mg/mL 
**Enalaprilat:**
Injection: 1.25 mg/mL (1, 2 mL); contains benzyl alcohol

***Infant and child:***
***PO:*** 0.1 mg/kg/24 hr up to 5 mg/24 hr ÷ QD–BID; increase PRN over 2 wk.
**Max. dose:** 0.6 mg/kg/24 hr up to 40 mg/24 hr
***IV:*** 0.005–0.01 mg/kg/dose Q8–24 hr
***Adolescent and adult:***
***PO:*** 2.5–5 mg/24 hr QD initially to **max. dose** of 40 mg/24 hr ÷ QD-BID
***IV:*** 0.625–1.25 mg/dose IV Q6 hr; doses as high as 5 mg Q6 hr is reported to be tolerated for up to 36 hr

**Use with caution** in bilateral renal artery stenosis. **Avoid** use with dialysis with high-flux membranes since anaphylactoid reactions have been reported. Side effects: nausea, diarrhea, headache, dizziness, hyperkalemia, hypoglycemia, hypotension, and hypersensitivity. Cough is a reported side effect of ACE inhibitors.

Enalapril (PO) is converted to its active form (Enalaprilat) by the liver. Administer IV over 5 min. **Adjust dose in renal impairment (see Chapter 31).**

Pregnancy category is "C" during the first trimester but changes to "D" during the second and third trimesters (fetal injury and death have been reported). Despite the pregnancy category, enalapril/enalaprilat should be discontinued as soon as possible when pregnancy is detected.

## ENOXAPARIN

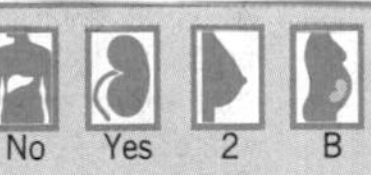


Lovenox
***Anticoagulant, low molecular weight heparin***

**Injection:** 100 mg/mL (3 mL); contains 15 mg/mL benzyl alcohol
**Injection (pre-filled syringes with 27-gauge × ½-inch needle):** 30 mg/0.3 mL, 40 mg/0.4 mL, 60 mg/0.6 mL, 80 mg/0.8 mL, 100 mg/1 mL, 120 mg/0.8 mL, 150 mg/1 mL
**Approximate anti-factor Xa activity:** 100 IU per 1 mg

*Continued*

For explanation of icons, see p. 698.

ENOXAPARIN *continued*

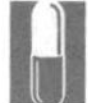

***DVT treatment:***

***Infant < 2 mo:*** 1.5 mg/kg/dose Q12 hr SC

***Infant ≥ 2 mo–adult:*** 1 mg/kg/dose Q12 hr SC; alternatively, 1.5 mg/kg/dose Q24 hr SC can be used in adults.

***Dosage adjustment to achieve target anti-factor Xa levels of 0.5–1 units/mL (see the following table):***

| Anti-factor Xa Level (units/mL) | Hold Next Dose? | Dose Change | Repeat Anti-factor Xa Level? |
|---|---|---|---|
| <0.35 | No | Increase by 25% | 4 hr post next new dose |
| 0.35–0.49 | No | Increase by 10% | 4 hr post next new dose |
| 0.5–1 | No | No | Next day, then 1 wk later at 4 hr post dose |
| 1.1–1.5 | No | Decrease by 20% | 4 hr post next new dose |
| 1.6–2 | 3 hr | Decrease by 30% | 4 hr post next new dose |
| >2 | Until anti-factor Xa reaches 0.5 units/mL (levels can be measured Q12 hr until it reaches ≤ 0.5 units/mL). | When anti-factor Xa reaches 0.5 units/mL, dose may be restarted at a dose 40% less than originally prescribed. | 4 hr post next new dose |

***DVT prophylaxis:***

***Infant < 2 mo:*** 0.75 mg/kg/dose Q12 hr SC

***Infant ≥ 2 mo–18 yr:*** 0.5 mg/kg/dose Q12 hr SC

***Adult:***

***Knee or hip replacement surgery:*** 30 mg BID SC × 7–14 days; initiate therapy 12–24 hr after surgery provided hemostasis is established. Alternatively for hip replacement surgery, 40 mg QD SC × 7–14 days initially up to 3 wk thereafter; initiate therapy 9–15 hr prior to surgery.

***Abdominal surgery:*** 40 mg QD SC × 7–12 days initiated 2 hr prior to surgery.

***Patients at risk due to severe restricted mobility during an acute illness:*** 40 mg QD SC × 6–14 days.

Inhibits thrombosis by inactivating factor Xa without significantly affecting bleeding time, platelet function, PT, or aPTT at recommended doses. Dosages of enoxaparin, heparin, or other low molecular weight heparins **cannot** be used interchangeably on a unit-for-unit (or mg-for-mg) basis because of differences in pharmacokinetics and activity. Peak anti-factor Xa activity is achieved 4 hr after a dose.

*Continued*

ENOXAPARIN *continued*

**Contraindicated** in major bleeding and drug-induced thrombocytopenia. **Use with caution** in uncontrolled arterial hypertension, bleeding diathesis, history of recurrent GI ulcers, diabetic retinopathy, and severe renal dysfunction (reduce dose by increasing the dosage interval from Q12 hr to Q24 hr if GFR < 30 mL/min). Prophylactic use is **not recommended** in patients with prosthetic heart valves (especially in pregnant women) because of reports of fatalities in patients and fetuses. **Concurrent use with spinal or epidural anesthesia or spinal puncture has resulted in long-term or permanent paralysis; potential benefits must be weighed against the risks.** May cause fever, confusion, edema, nausea, hemorrhage, thrombocytopenia, hypochromic anemia, and pain/erythema at injection site. **Protamine sulfate is the antidote;** 1 mg protamine sulfate neutralizes 1 mg enoxaparin.

Recommended anti-factor Xa levels obtained 4 hr after subcutaneous dose:

*DVT treatment:* 0.5–1 units/mL

*DVT prophylaxis:* 0.2–0.4 units/mL

Administer by deep SC injection by having the patient lie down. Alternate administration between the left and right anterolateral and left and right posterolateral abdominal wall. See package insert for detailed SC administration recommendations. To minimize bruising, **do not** rub the injection site. IV or IM route of administration is **not receommended.**

For additional information, see *Chest* 2004;126:645S-687S.

## EPINEPHRINE HCL

Adrenalin, Epi-pen, and others

***Sympathomimetic agent***

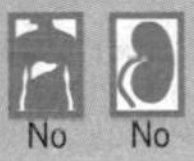
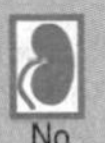
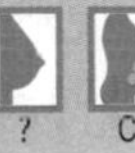
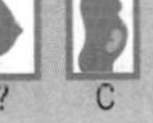

No No ? C

**Injection:**

1:1000 (aqueous): 1 mg/mL (1, 30 mL)

1:10,000 (aqueous): 0.1 mg/mL (10 mL pre-filled syringes with either 18-G 3.5 inch or 21-G 1.5 inch needles or 10 mL vials)

**Autoinjector:**

Epi-Pen: Delivers a single 0.3 mg (0.3 mL) dose (1 or 2 pack)

Epi-Pen Jr: Delivers a single 0.15 mg (0.3 mL) dose (1 or 2 pack)

**Aerosol:** 0.22 mg epinephrine base/spray (15, 22.5 mL); may contain alcohol

**Oral inhalation solution:** 1% (10 mg/mL or 1:100) (7.5 mL)

Some preparations may contain sulfites.

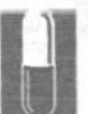

***Cardiac uses:***

***Neonate:***

***Asystole and bradycardia:*** 0.01–0.03 mg/kg of 1:10,000 solution (0.1–0.3 mL/kg) IV/ET Q3–5 min PRN.

***Infant and child:***

***Bradycardia/asystole and pulseless arrest:*** See inside front cover and algorithms.

***Bradycardia, asystole, and pulseless arrest (see remarks):***

***First dose:*** 0.01 mg/kg of 1:10,000 solution (0.1 mL/kg) IO/IV; **max. dose:** 1 mg (10 mL). Subsequent doses Q3–5 min PRN should be the same. High- dose epinephrine after failure of standard dose has not been shown to be effective (see remarks). Must circulate drug with CPR. See also ET route.

***All ET doses:*** 0.1 mg/kg of 1:1000 solution (0.1 mL/kg) ET Q3–5 min.

***Adult:***

***Asystole:*** 1–5 mg IV/ET Q3–5 min.

**IV drip (all ages):** 0.1–1 mcg/kg/min; titrate to effect; to prepare infusion, see inside front cover.

*Continued*

For explanation of icons, see p. 698.

EPINEPHRINE HCL *continued*

***Respiratory uses:***

***Bronchodilator:*** 1:1000 (aqueous):

***Infant and child:*** 0.01 mL/kg/dose SC (**max. single dose** 0.5 mL); repeat Q15 min × 3–4 doses or Q4 hr PRN

***Adult:*** 0.3–0.5 mg (0.3–0.5 mL)/dose SC Q20 min × 3 doses.

***Inhalation:*** 1–2 puffs Q4 hr PRN

***Nebulization:*** (alternative to racemic epinephrine): 0.5 mL/kg of 1:1000 solution diluted in 3 mL NS; **max. dose:** ≤4 yr: 2.5 mL/dose; >4 yr: 5 mL/dose

***Hypersensitivity reactions (see remarks for IV dosing):***

***Child:*** 0.01 mg/kg/dose IM/SC up to a **max. dose** of 0.5 mg/dose Q20 min–4 hr PRN. If using EpiPen or EpiPen Jr, administer only via the IM route using the following dosage:

***<30 kg:*** 0.15 mg

***≥30 kg:*** 0.3 mg

***Adult:*** Start with 0.1–0.5 mg IM/SC Q20 min–4 hr PRN; doses may be increased if necessary to a single **max. dose** of 1 mg.

High-dose rescue therapy for in-hospital cardiac arrest in children after failure of an initial standard dose has been reported to be of no benefit compared to standard dose (*N Engl J Med* 2004;350:1722–1730).

Hypersensitivity reactions: For bronchial asthma and certain allergic manifestations (e.g., angioedema, urticaria, serum sickness, anaphylactic shock) use epinephrine SC. Patients with anaphylaxis may benefit from IM administration. The adult IV dose for hypersensitivity reactions or to relieve bronchospasm usually ranges from 0.1 to 0.25 mg injected slowly over 5–10 min Q5–15 min as needed. Neonates may be given a dose of 0.01 mg/kg body weight; for infants, 0.05 mg is an adequate initial dose and this may be repeated at 20 to 30 min intervals in the management of asthma attacks.

May produce arrhythmias, tachycardia, hypertension, headaches, nervousness, nausea, vomiting. Necrosis may occur at site of repeated local injection.

Concomitant use of noncardiac selective beta-blockers or tricyclic antidepressants may enhance epinephrine's pressor response. Chlorpromazine may reverse the pressor response.

ETT doses should be diluted with NS to a volume of 3–5 mL before administration. Follow with several positive pressure ventilations.

EpiPen and EpiPen Jr should be administered IM into the anterolateral aspect of the thigh.

## EPINEPHRINE, RACEMIC

MicroNefrin, Nephron, S-2 Inhalant

***Sympathomimetic agent***

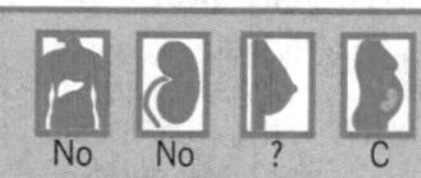


**Solution for inhalation:** 2.25% (1.25% epinephrine base) (15, 30 mL)
Contains sulfites

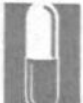

***<4 yr:***

***Croup (using 2.25% solution):*** 0.05 mL/kg/dose up to a **max. dose** of 0.5 mL/dose diluted to 3 mL with NS. Given via nebulizer over 15 min PRN but **not** more frequently than Q1–2 hr.

***≥4 yr:*** 0.5 mL/dose via nebulizer over 15 min Q3–4 hr PRN

*Tachyarrhythmias, headache, nausea, palpitations reported. Rebound symptoms may occur. Cardiorespiratory monitoring should be considered if administered more frequently than Q1–2 hr.*

## EPOETIN ALFA

Erythropoietin, Epogen, Procrit

***Recombinant human erythropoietin***

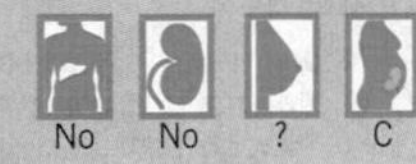


**Injection (single-dose, preservative-free vials):** 2000, 3000, 4000, 10,000, 40,000 U/mL (1 mL)
**Injection (multi-dose vials):** 10,000 U/mL (2 mL), 20,000 U/mL (1 mL); contains 1% benzyl alcohol
All dosage forms contains 2.5 mg albumin per 1 mL.

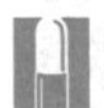

***Anemia in chronic renal failure (see remarks for dosage adjustment):*** SC/IV
***Initial dose:***
***Child:*** Start at 50 U/kg/dose 3 times per wk. Reported dosage range for children (3 mo–20 yr) not requiring dialysis, 50–250 U/kg/dose 3 times per wk. Reported dosage range for children receiving hemodialysis, 50–450 U/kg/dose 2–3 times per wk.
***Adult:*** Start at 50–100 U/kg/dose 3 times per wk
***Maintenance dose:*** Dose is individualized to achieve and maintain the lowest Hgb level sufficient to avoid transfusions and **not to exceed** 12 g/dL.

***Anemia in cancer (see remarks for dosage reduction and withholding therapy):***
***Initial dose:***
***Child:*** Start at 600 U/kg (**max. dose:** 40,000 U) IV once weekly.
***Adult:*** Start at 150 U/kg/dose SC 3 times per wk or 40,000 U SC once every wk.
***Increasing doses (if needed):***
***3 times a wk dosing:*** If no reduction in transfusion requirements or rise in Hgb after 8 wk, increase dosage to 300 U/kg/dose 3 times per wk.
***Weekly dosing:*** If no increase in Hgb > 1 g/dL after 8 wk of therapy, in the absence of a transfusion:
***Child:*** Increase dose to 900 U/kg/dose IV (**max. dose:** 60,000 U) once weekly.
***Adult:*** 60,000 U SC once weekly.

***AZT treated HIV patients (see remarks for dosage adjustment):*** SC/IV
***Child:*** Reported dosage range in children (8 mo–17 yr), 50–400 U/kg/dose 2–3 times per wk.
***Adult (with serum erythropoietin ≤ 500 milliunits/mL and receiving ≤ 4200 mg AZT per wk):*** Start at 100 U/kg/dose 3 times per wk × 8 wk.
***Dose increments, if needed:*** If response is not satisfactory in reducing transfusion requirements or increasing Hgb levels after 8 wk of therapy, dose may be increased by 50–100 U/kg/dose given 3 times per wk and reevaluate every 4-8 wk thereafter. Patients are unlikely to respond to doses > 300 U/kg/dose 3 times per wk.

***Anemia of prematurity (many regimens exist):***
25–100 U/kg/dose SC 3 times per wk; alternatively, 200–400 U/kg/dose IV/SC 3–5 times per wk for 2–6 wk (total dose per wk is 600–1400 U/kg).

Use the lowest dose to avoid transfusions and **do not exceed** hemoglobin levels > 12 g/dL. Increased risk for death, serious cardiovascular events, and thrombosis in cancer patients with Hgb levels > 12 g/dL have been reported with epoetin alfa and other erythropoiesis-stimulating agents. Shortened survival and time to tumor progression have also been reported in patients with various cancers.

Evaluate serum iron, ferritin, TIBC before therapy. Iron supplementation recommended during therapy unless iron stores are already in excess. Monitor Hct, BP, clotting times, platelets, BUN, serum creatinine. Peak effect in 2–3 wk.

*Continued*

For explanation of icons, see p. 698.

EPOETIN ALFA *continued*

Recommended Hgb treatment goals:

*Anemia in chronic renal failure:* 10–12 g/dL.

*Cancer:* Lowest Hgb level sufficient to avoid transfusion and ≤12 g/dL.

**DOSAGE ADJUSTMENTS:**

*Reduce dose by 25%:* when target Hgb is reached, OR when Hgb increases >1 g/dL in any 2-wk period.

*Increase dose:* when Hgb does not increase by 2 g/dL after 8 wk of therapy and Hgb remains at a level not sufficient to avoid the need for transfusion. Dosage increments should **not be** made more frequently than once per mo.

*Withholding therapy:* when Hgb > 12 g/dL; restart therapy at a 25% lower dose after Hgb decreases to target levels or < 11 g/dL.

May cause hypertension, seizure, hypersensitivity reactions, headache, edema, dizziness. SC route provides sustained serum levels compared to IV route.

## ERGOCALCIFEROL

Drisdol, Calciferol

***Vitamin $D_2$***

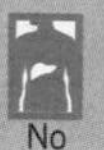
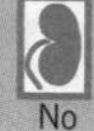
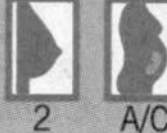

No No 2 A/C

**Caps:** 50,000 IU (1.25 mg)
**Drops (OTC):** 8000 IU/mL (200 mcg/mL) (60 mL); contains propylene glycol
1 mg = 40,000 IU vitamin D activity

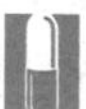

***Dietary supplementation:***

***Preterm:*** 400–800 IU/24 hr PO

***Infant and child:*** 400 IU/24 hr PO; please refer to Chapter 21 for details.

***Renal failure (CKD stages 3–4) and 25-OH vitamin D levels < 30 ng/mL:***

***25-OH vitamin D < 5 ng/mL:***

***Child:*** 8000 IU/24 hr PO × 4 wk or 50,000 IU every wk × 4 wk, followed by 4000 IU/24 hr or 50,000 IU twice monthly for a total of therapy of 3 mo.

***Adult:*** 50,000 IU every wk × 12 wk, followed by 50,000 IU every mo for a total therapy of 6 mo.

***25-OH vitamin D 5–15 ng/mL:***

***Child:*** 4000 IU/24 hr PO × 12 wk or 50,000 IU every other wk × 12 wk.

***Adult:*** 50,000 IU every wk × 4 wk followed by 50,000 IU every mo for a total therapy of 6 mo.

***25-OH vitamin D 16–30 ng/mL:***

***Child:*** 2000 IU/24 hr PO × 3 mo or 50,000 IU every mo × 3 mo.

***Adult:*** 50,000 IU every mo × 6 mo.

***Vitamin D dependent rickets:***

***Child:*** 3000–5000 IU/24 hr PO; **max. dose:** 60,000 IU/24 hr

***Adult:*** 10,000–60,000 IU/24 hr PO; some may require 500,000 IU/24 hr

***Nutritional rickets:***

***Child and adult with normal GI absorption:*** 2000–5000 IU/24 hr PO × 6–12 wk

***Malabsorption:***

***Child:*** 10,000–25,000 IU/24 hr PO

***Adult:*** 10,000–300,000 IU/24 hr PO

***Vitamin D resistant rickets (with phosphate supplementation):***

***Child:*** Initial dose 40,000–80,000 IU/24 hr PO; increase daily dose by 10,000–20,000 IU PO Q3–4 mo if needed.

***Adult:*** 10,000–60,000 IU/24 hr PO

*Continued*

ERGOCALCIFEROL *continued*

***Hypoparathyroidism (with calcium supplementation):***
***Child:*** 50,000–200,000 IU/24 hr PO
***Adult:*** 25,000–200,000 IU/24 hr PO

Monitor serum $Ca^{2+}$, $PO_4$, 25-OH vitamin D and alkaline phosphate. Serum $Ca^{2+}$, $PO_4$ product should be <70 mg/dL to avoid ectopic calcification. Titrate dosage to patient response. Watch for symptoms of hypercalcemia: weakness, diarrhea, polyuria, metastatic calcification, nephrocalcinosis. Vitamin $D_2$ is activated by 25-hydroxylation in liver and 1-hydroxylation in kidney.

Injectable dosage form is no longer available.

Pregnancy category changes to "C" if used in doses above the U.S. RDA.

## ERGOTAMINE TARTRATE ± CAFFEINE

Ergomar
In combination with caffeine: Cafergot and others
***Ergot alkaloid***

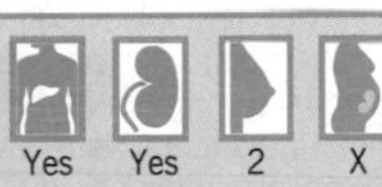


**Sublingual tabs (Ergomar):** 2 mg
**In combination with caffeine:**
**Tabs:** 1 mg and 100 mg caffeine
**Suppository:** 2 mg and 100 mg caffeine
Drug also available in combinations with belladonna alkaloids and/or phenobarbital.

***Older child and adolescent:***
***PO/SL:*** 1 mg at onset of migraine attack, then 1 mg Q30 min PRN up to **max. dose** of 3 mg per attack.
***Adult:***
***PO/SL:*** 2 mg at onset of migraine attack, then 1–2 mg Q30 min up to 6 mg per attack; **do not exceed** 10 mg per wk.
***Suppository:*** 2 mg at first sign of attack; follow with second 2 mg dose after 1 hr; **max. dose:** 4 mg per attack, **not to exceed** 10 mg/wk.

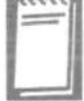

**Use with caution** in renal or hepatic disease. May cause paresthesias, GI disturbance, angina-like pain, rebound headache with abrupt withdrawal, or muscle cramps. **Contraindicated** in pregnancy and has **not been recommended** in breast-feeding. Concurrent administration with protease inhibitors, clarithromycin, erythromycin, or other CYP 450 3A4 inhibitors is **not recommended** owing to risk of ergotism (nausea, vomiting, vasospastic ischemia).

## ERTAPENEM

Invanz
***Antibiotic, carbapenem***

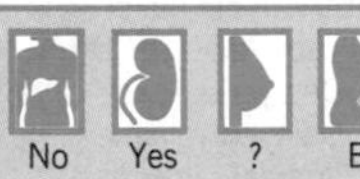


**Injection:** 1 g
Contains ~6 mEq Na/g drug

*Continued*

For explanation of icons, see p. 698.

ERTAPENEM *continued*

***3 mo–12 yr:*** 15 mg/kg/dose IV/IM Q12 hr; **max. dose:** 1 g/24 hr
***Adolescent and adult:*** 1 g IV/IM Q24 hr
***Recommended duration of therapy (all ages):***
***Complicated intra-abdominal infection:*** 5–14 days
***Complicated skin/subcutaneous tissue infections:*** 7–14 days
***Diabetic foot infection without osteomyelitis:*** Up to 28 days
***Community-acquired pneumonia, complicated UTI/pyelonephritis:*** 10–14 days
***Acute pelvic infection:*** 3–10 days

Ertapenem has poor activity against *P. aeruginosa, Acinetobacter,* MRSA, and *Enterococcus.* **Do not use** in meningitis due to poor CSF penetration. **Use with caution** with CNS disorders including seizures. Adjust dosage in renal impairment by decreasing dose by 50% when GFR < 30 mL/min.

Diarrhea, infusion complications, nausea, headache, vaginitis, phlebitis/thromobophlebitis, and vomiting are common. Seizures have been reported primarily in renal insufficiency and/or CNS disorders such as brain lesions or seizures. Decreases valproic acid levels. Probenecid may increase ertapenem levels. IM dosage form contains 1% lidocaine.

## ERYTHROMYCIN ETHYLSUCCINATE AND ACETYLSULFISOXAZOLE

Pediazole, Eryzole, and others
***Antibiotic, macrolide + sulfonamide derivative***

Yes Yes 1 C/D

**Oral suspension:** 200 mg erythromycin and 600 mg sulfa/5 mL (100, 150, 200, 250 mL)

***Otitis media:*** 50 mg/kg/24 hr (as erythromycin) and 150 mg/kg/24 hr (as sulfa) ÷ Q6 hr PO, or give 1.25 mL/kg/24 hr ÷ Q6 hr PO.
**Max. dose:** 2 g erythromycin, 6 g sulfisoxazole/24 hr

**Contraindicated** in liver dysfunction or porphyria. See adverse effects of *Erythromycin* and *Sulfisoxazole*. **Not recommended** in infants <2 mo. **Do not use** in renal impairment because dosage adjustments are inconsistent for sulfisoxazole and erythromycin.

Pregnancy category changes to "D" if administered near term.

## ERYTHROMYCIN PREPARATIONS

Erythrocin, Pediamycin, E-Mycin, Ery-Ped, and others
***Antibiotic, macrolide***

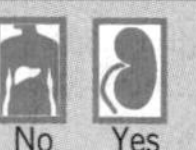
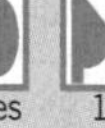
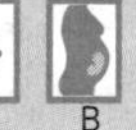

No Yes 1 B

**Erythromycin base:**
Tabs: 250, 500 mg
Delayed-release tabs: 250, 333, 500 mg
Delayed-release caps: 250 mg
Topical ointment: 2% (25 g)
Topical gel: 2% (30, 60 g); contains alcohol 92%
Topical solution: 1.5%, 2% (60 mL); may contain 44%–66% alcohol
Topical swab: 2% (60s)
Ophthalmic ointment: 0.5% (1, 3.5 g)
**Erythromycin ethyl succinate (EES):**
Suspension: 200, 400 mg/5 mL (100, 480 mL)

*Continued*

ERYTHROMYCIN PREPARATIONS *continued*

Oral drops: 100 mg/2.5 mL (50 mL)
Chewable tabs: 200 mg
Tabs: 400 mg

**Erythromycin estolate:**
Suspension: 125, 250 mg/5 mL (480 mL)

**Erythromycin stearate:**
Tabs: 250 mg

**Erythromycin lactobionate:**
Injection: 500, 1000 mg; may contain benzyl alcohol

---

***Oral:***
***Neonate:***
***<1.2 kg:*** 20 mg/kg/24 hr ÷ Q12 hr PO
***≥1.2 kg:***
***0–7 days:*** 20 mg/kg/24 hr ÷ Q12 hr PO
***>7 days:*** 30 mg/kg/24 hr ÷ Q8 hr PO
***Chlamydial conjunctivitis and pneumonia:*** 50 mg/kg/24 hr ÷ Q6 hr PO × 14 days.
***Child:*** 30–50 mg/kg/24 hr ÷ Q6–8 hr; **max. dose:** 2 g/24 hr
***Adult:*** 1–4 g/24 hr ÷ Q6 hr; **max. dose:** 4 g/24 hr

***Parenteral:***
***Child:*** 20–50 mg/kg/24 hr ÷ Q6 hr IV
***Adult:*** 15–20 mg/kg/24 hr ÷ Q6 hr IV
**Max. dose:** 4 g/24 hr

***Rheumatic fever prophylaxis:*** 500 mg/24 hr ÷ Q12 hr PO
***Ophthalmic:*** Apply 0.5 inch ribbon to affected eye BID-QID
***Pertussis:*** Estolate salt: 50 mg/kg/24 hr ÷ Q6 hr PO × 14 days
***Preoperative bowel prep:*** 20 mg/kg/dose PO erythromycin base × 3 doses, with neomycin, 1 day before surgery
***Prokinetic agent:*** 10–20 mg/kg/24 hr PO ÷ TID-QID (QAC or QAC and QHS)

---

**Avoid** IM route (pain, necrosis). GI side effects common (nausea, vomiting, abdominal cramps). **Use with caution** in liver disease. Estolate may cause cholestatic jaundice, although hepatotoxicity is uncommon (2% of reported cases). Inhibits CYP 450 1A2, 3A3/4 isoenzymes. May produce elevated digoxin, theophylline, carbamazapine, clozapine, cyclosporine, and methylprednisolone levels. **Avoid** use with astemizole, cisapride, pimozide or terfenadine. Hypertrophic pyloric stenosis in neonates receiving prophylactic therapy for pertussis; and life-threatening episodes of ventricular tachycardia associated with prolonged QTc interval have been reported.

Oral therapy should replace IV as soon as possible. Give oral doses after meals. Because of different absorption characteristics, higher oral doses of EES are needed to achieve therapeutic effects. May produce false positive urinary catecholamines.

**Adjust dose in renal failure (see Chapter 31).**

## ERYTHROPOIETIN

See *Epoetin Alfa*

For explanation of icons, see p. 698.

## ESMOLOL HCL

Brevibloc

***Beta-1-selective adrenergic blocking agent, antihypertensive agent, class II antiarrhythmic***

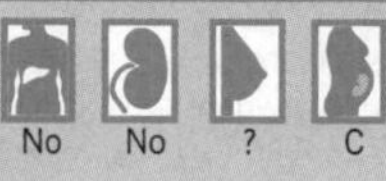


**Injection:** 10 mg/mL (10 mL), 20 mg/mL (5 mL)
**Injection, premixed infusion in iso-osmotic sodium chloride:** 10 mg/mL (250 mL), 20 mg/mL (100 mL)

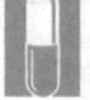

**Titrate to individual response (limited information).**
***Loading dose:*** 100–500 mcg/kg IV over 1 min.
***Maintenance dose:*** 25–100 mcg/kg/min as infusion.
If inadequate response, may readminister loading dose and/or increase maintenance dose by 25–50 mcg/kg/min in increments of Q5–10 min.
***Usual maintenance dose range:*** 50–500 mcg/kg/min; dosages as high as 1000 mcg/kg/min have been administered.

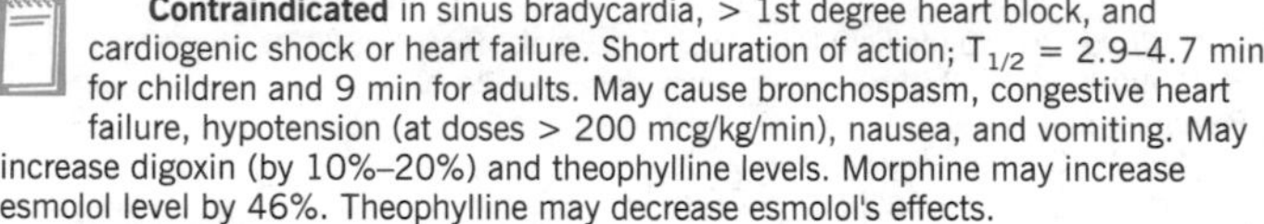

**Contraindicated** in sinus bradycardia, > 1st degree heart block, and cardiogenic shock or heart failure. Short duration of action; $T_{1/2}$ = 2.9–4.7 min for children and 9 min for adults. May cause bronchospasm, congestive heart failure, hypotension (at doses > 200 mcg/kg/min), nausea, and vomiting. May increase digoxin (by 10%–20%) and theophylline levels. Morphine may increase esmolol level by 46%. Theophylline may decrease esmolol's effects.

**Administer only in a monitored setting.** Concentration for administration is typically ≤ 10 mg/mL; however, 20 mg/mL has been administered in pediatric patients.

## ESOMEPRAZOLE

Nexium

***Gastric acid proton pump inhibitor***

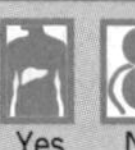

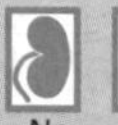

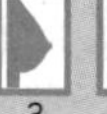

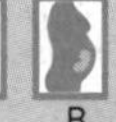


**Caps, delayed-release:** 20, 40 mg; contains magnesium
**Powder for oral suspension:** 20, 40 mg packets (30s); contains magnesium
**Injection:** 20, 40 mg; contains EDTA

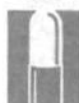

***Child (PO/IV):***
***GERD:***
***<12 yr:*** Limited data from 12 patients treated for cystinosis related gastric acid hypersecretion over 16 wk; mean age 5.8 yr, range: 2.4–9.8 yr. A final dosage range of 0.7–2.75 mg/kg/24 hr (mean: 1.7 mg/kg/24 hr) was observed from the following recomendations:
***<10 yr:*** 10 mg PO BID; if needed, increase dose by 50% at 4-wk intervals up to a **max. dose** of 20 mg BID.
***10–12 yr:*** 20 mg PO BID; if needed, increase dose by 50% at 4-wk intervals up to a **max. dose** of 40 mg BID.
***12–17 yr:*** 20–40 mg QD for up to 8 wk (short-term therapy).

***Adult (PO/IV):***
***GERD:*** 20–40 mg QD × 4–8 wk.
***Prevention of NSAID-induced gastric ulcers:*** 20–40 mg QD for up to 6 mo.
***Pathological hypersecretory conditions (e.g., Zollinger-Ellison syndrome):*** 40 mg BID; doses up to 240 mg/24 hr have been used.
***Hepatic impairment:*** Patients with severe hepatic function impairment (Child-Pugh class C) **should not exceed** 20 mg/24 hr.

*Continued*

ESOMEPRAZOLE *continued*

Cross-allergic reactions with other proton pump inhibitors (e.g., lansoprazole, pantoprazole, rabeprazole). **Use with caution** in liver impairment (see dosage adjustment recommendation in dosing section). GI disturbances and headache are common. Erythema multiforme, Stevens-Johnson syndrome, TEN, and pancreatitis have been reported. Drug is a substrate and inhibitor of CYP 450 2C19 and substrate of CYP 450 3A4. May decrease the absorption of atazanavir, ketoconazole, itraconazole, and iron salts. May increase the effect/toxicity of diazepam, midazolam, digoxin, carbamazepine, and warfarin. Voriconazole may increase the effects of esomeprazole. May be used in combination with clarithromycin and amoxicillin for *H. pylori* infections.

Administer all doses before meals. Administer 30 min before sucralfate. **Do not** crush or chew capsules. IV doses may be given as fast as 3 min or infused over 10–30 min.

## ETANERCEPT

Enbrel

***Antirheumatic, immunomodulatory agent, tumor necrosis factor receptor p75 Fc fusion protein***

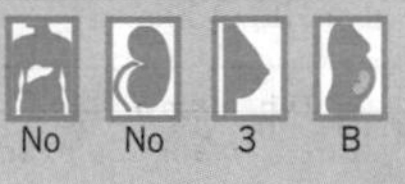


**Pre-filled injection:** 25 mg (0.51 mL of 50 mg/mL solution), 50 mg (0.98 mL of 50 mg/mL solution); contains sucose, L-arginine
**Injection (powder):** 25 mg with diluent (1 mL bacteriostatic water containing 0.9% benzyl alcohol); contains mannitol, sucrose, tromethamine

***JRA:***

***Child 4–17 yr:*** 0.4 mg/kg/dose SC twice weekly administered 72–96 hr apart; **max. dose:** 25 mg. Alternative once weekly dose of 0.8 mg/kg/dose SC (**max. dose:** 50 mg/wk and **max. single injection site dose** of 25 mg) may be used.

***Rheumatoid arthritis, psoriatic arthritis, ankylosing spondylitis:***

***Adult:*** 25 mg SC twice weekly administered 72–96 hr apart. Alternative once weekly dose of 50 mg SC (**max. single injection site dose** of 25 mg) may be used.

***Plaque psoriasis:***

***Adult:*** Start with 50 mg SC twice weekly administered 72–96 hr apart × 3 mo, followed by a reduced maintenance dose of 50 mg SC per wk. Starting doses of 25 mg or 50 mg per wk have also been shown to be effective.

**Max. single injection site dose:** 25 mg.

**Contraindicated** in serious infections, sepsis, or hypersensitivity to any of medication components. **Use with caution** in patients with history of recurrent infections or underlying conditions that may predispose them to infections (including concomitant immunosuppressive therapy), CNS demyelinating disorders, malignancies, immune-related diseases, and latex allergy. Common adverse effects in children include headache, abdominal pain, vomiting, and nausea. Injection site reactions (e.g., discomfort, itching, swelling), rhinitis, dizziness, rash, depression, infections (varicella, aseptic meningitis, rare cases of TB, and fatal/serious infections and sepsis), bone marrow suppression (e.g., aplastic anemia), vertigo, and CNS demyelinating disorder have also been reported.

**Do not** administer live vaccines concurrently with this drug. In JRA, it is recommended that the patient be brought up to date with all immunizations in agreement with current immunization guidelines prior to initiating therapy.

Onset of action is 1–4 wk, with peak effects usually within 3 mo.

*Continued*

For explanation of icons, see p. 698.

ETANERCEPT *continued*

Patients must be properly instructed on preparing and administering the medication. Drug requires reconstitution by gently swirling its contents with the supplied diluent (**do not** shake or vigorously agitate) as some foaming will occur. Reconstituted solutions should be clear and colorless and used within 6 hr. Drug is administered subcutaneously by rotating injection sites (thigh, abdomen, or upper arm) with a **max. single injection site dose** of 25 mg. Administer new injections ≥ 1 inch from an old site and **never** where the skin is tender, bruised, red, or hard.

## ETHAMBUTOL HCL

Myambutol

***Antituberculosis drug***

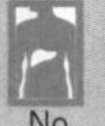
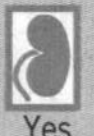
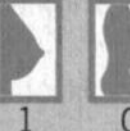

No Yes 1 C

**Tabs:** 100, 400 mg

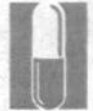

***Tuberculosis:***

***Infant, child, adolescent, and adult:*** 15–25 mg/kg/dose PO QD or 50 mg/kg/dose PO twice weekly

**Max. dose:** 2.5 g/24 hr

***Nontuberculous mycobacterial infection:***

***Child, adolescent, and adult:*** 15–25 mg/kg/24 hr PO; **max. dose:** 1 g/24 hr

***M. avium complex prophylaxis in AIDS (use in combination with other medications):***

***Infant, child, adolescent, and adult:*** 15 mg/kg/dose PO QD; **max. dose:** 900 mg/dose

May cause reversible optic neuritis, especially with larger doses. Obtain baseline ophthalmologic studies before beginning therapy and then monthly. Follow visual acuity, visual fields, and (red-green) color vision. **Do not use** in optic neuritis and in children whose visual acuity cannot be assessed. **Discontinue** if any visual deterioration occurs. Monitor uric acid, liver function, heme status, and renal function. Hyperuricemia, GI disturbances and mania are common. Coadministration with aluminum hydroxide can reduce ethambutol's absorption; space administration by 4 hr. Give with food. **Adjust dose with renal failure (see Chapter 31).**

## ETHOSUXIMIDE

Zarontin

***Anticonvulsant***

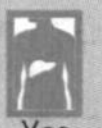
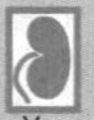
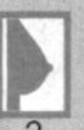
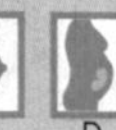

Yes Yes 2 D

**Caps:** 250 mg

**Syrup:** 250 mg/5 mL

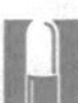

***Oral:***

***≤6 yr:*** Initial: 15 mg/kg/24 hr ÷ BID; **max. dose:** 500 mg/24 hr; increase as needed Q4–7 days. Usual maintenance dose: 15–40 mg/kg/24 hr ÷ BID

***>6 yr and adult:*** 250 mg BID; increase by 250 mg/24 hr as needed Q4–7 days; usual maintenance dose: 20–40 mg/kg/24 hr ÷ BID

**Max. dose:** 1500 mg/24 hr

*Continued*

ETHOSUXIMIDE *continued*

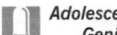

**Use with caution** in hepatic and renal disease. Ataxia, anorexia, drowsiness, sleep disturbances, rashes, and blood dyscrasias are rare idiosyncratic reactions. May cause lupus-like syndrome; may increase frequency of grand mal seizures in patients with mixed type seizures. Cases of birth defects have been reported; ethosuximide crosses the placenta. Drug of choice for absence seizures. Carbamazepine, phenytoin, primidone, phenobarbital, valproic acid, nevirapine, and ritonavir may decrease ethosuximide levels.

Therapeutic levels: 40–100 mg/L. $T_{1/2}$ = 24–42 hr. Recommended serum sampling time at steady-state: obtain trough level within 30 min prior to the next scheduled dose after 5–10 days of continuous dosing.

To minimize GI distress, may administer with food or milk. Abrupt withdrawal of drug may precipitate absence status.

## FAMCICLOVIR

Famvir

***Antiviral***

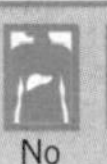
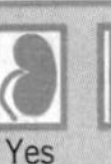
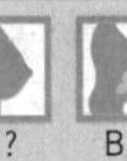

No Yes ? B

**Tabs:** 125, 250, 500 mg

***Adolescent:***

***Genital herpes, first episode:*** 250 mg Q8 hr PO × 7–10 days
***Episodic recurrent genital herpes:*** 125 mg Q12 hr PO × 3–5 days
***Daily suppressive therapy:*** 250 mg Q12 hr PO up to 1 yr; then reassess HSV recurrence

***Adult:***

***Herpes zoster:*** 500 mg Q8 hr PO × 7 days; initiate therapy promptly as soon as diagnosis is made (initiation within 48 hr after rash onset is ideal; currently no data for starting treatment > 72 hr after rash onset).
***Recurrent genital herpes:*** 1000 mg Q12 hr PO × 1 day; initiate therapy at first sign or symptom. Efficacy has not been established when treatment is initiated > 6 hr after onset of symptoms or lesions.
***Suppression of recurrent genital herpes:*** 250 mg Q12 hr PO up to 1 yr
***Recurrent mucocutaneous herpes in HIV:*** 500 mg Q12 hr PO × 7 days

Drug is converted to its active form (penciclovir). Better absorption than PO acyclovir. May cause headache, diarrhea, nausea, and abdominal pain. Concomitant use with probenecid and other drugs eliminated by active tubular secretion may result in decreased penciclovir clearance. **Reduce dose in renal impairment (see Chapter 31).**

Safety and efficacy in suppression of recurrent genital herpes have not been established beyond 1 yr. May be administered with or without food.

## FAMOTIDINE

Pepcid, Pepcid AC [OTC], Pepcid Complete [OTC], Pepcid RPD, and others

***Histamine-2-receptor antagonist***

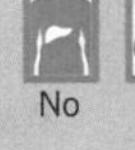
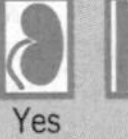
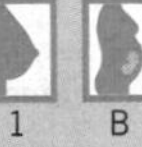

No Yes 1 B

**Injection:** 10 mg/mL (2, 4, 20 mL); multidose vials contain 0.9% benzyl alcohol
**Premixed injection:** 20 mg/50 mL in iso-osmotic sodium chloride
**Oral suspension:** 40 mg/5 mL (contains parabens)

*Continued*

For explanation of icons, see p. 698.

FAMOTIDINE *continued*

**Tabs:** 10 (OTC), 20 (OTC), 40 mg
**Gel caps:** 10 mg (OTC)
**Disintegrating oral tabs** (Pepcid RPD): 20, 40 mg; contains aspartame
**Chewable tabs:** 10 mg (OTC); contains aspartame
Pepcid Complete (OTC): 10 mg famotidine with 800 mg calcium carbonate and 165 mg magnesium hydroxide

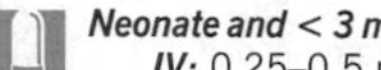

***Neonate and < 3 mo:***
*IV:* 0.25–0.5 mg/kg/dose Q24 hr
*PO:* 0.5–1 mg/kg/dose Q24 hr
***≥3 mo–1 yr (GERD):*** 0.5 mg/kg/dose PO Q12 hr

***Child:***
*IV:* Initial: 0.6–0.8 mg/kg/24 hr ÷ Q8–12 hr up to a **max. dose** of 40 mg/24 hr
*PO:* Initial: 1–1.2 mg/kg/24 hr ÷ Q8–12 hr up to a **max. dose** of 40 mg/24 hr
*Peptic ulcer:* 0.5 mg/kg/24 hr PO QHS or ÷ Q12 hr up to a **max. dose** of 40 mg/24 hr
*GERD:* 1–2 mg/kg/24 hr PO ÷ Q12 hr up to a **max. dose** of 80 mg/24 hr

***Adolescent and adult:***
*Duodenal ulcer:*
*PO:* 20 mg BID or 40 mg QHS × 4–8 wk, then maintenance therapy at 20 mg QHS
*IV:* 20 mg BID
*GERD:* 20 mg BID PO × 6 wk
*Esophagitis:* 20–40 mg BID PO × 12 wk

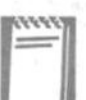

A Q12-hr dosage interval is generally recommended; however, infants and young children may require a Q8-hr interval because of enhanced elimination. Headaches, dizziness, constipation, diarrhea, and drowsiness have occurred.

**Dosage adjustment is required in severe renal failure (see Chapter 31).**

Shake oral suspension well prior to each use. Disintegrating oral tablets should be placed on the tongue to be disintegrated and subsequently swallowed. Doses may be administered with or without food.

## FELBAMATE

Felbatol
***Anticonvulsant***

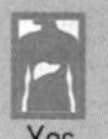
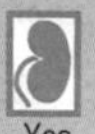
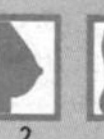
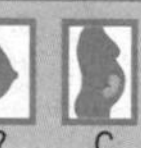

Yes Yes ? C

**Tabs:** 400, 600 mg
**Oral suspension:** 600 mg/5 mL

***Lennox-Gastaut for child 2–14 yr (adjunctive therapy):***
Start at 15 mg/kg/24 hr PO ÷ TID-QID; increase dosage by 15 mg/kg/24 hr increments at weekly intervals up to a **max. dose** of 45 mg/kg/24 hr or 3600 mg/24 hr (whichever is less). See remarks.

***Child ≥ 14 yr–adult:***
*Adjunctive therapy:* start at 1200 mg/24 hr PO ÷ TID-QID; increase dosage by 1200 mg/24 hr at weekly intervals up to a **max. dose** of 3600 mg/day. See remarks.
*Monotherapy (as initial therapy):* Start at 1200 mg/24 hr PO ÷ TID-QID. Increase dose under close clinical supervision at 600 mg increments Q2 wk to 2400 mg/24 hr. **Max. dose:** 3600 mg/24 hr.

*Continued*

FELBAMATE *continued*

**_Conversion to monotherapy:_** Start at 1200 mg/24 hr ÷ PO TID-QID for 2 wk; then increase to 2400 mg/24 hr for 1 wk. At wk 3, increase to 3600 mg/24 hr. See remarks for dose reduction instructions of other antiepileptic drugs.

Drug should be prescribed under strict supervision by a specialist. **Contraindicated** in blood dyscrasias or hepatic dysfunction (prior or current); and hypersensitivity to meprobamate. Aplastic anemia and hepatic failure leading to death have been associated with drug. May cause headache, fatigue, anxiety, GI disturbances, gingival hyperplasia, increased liver enzymes, and bone marrow suppression. Suicidal behavior or ideation have been reported. **Obtain serum levels of concurrent anticonvulsants.** Monitor liver enzymes, bilirubin, CBC with differential, platelets at baseline and every 1–2 wk. **Doses should be decreased by 50% in renally impaired patients.**

When initiating adjunctive therapy (all ages), doses of other antiepileptic drugs (AEDs) are reduced by 20% to control plasma levels of concurrent phenytoin, valproic acid, phenobarbital and carbamazepine. Further reductions of concomitant AED dosages may be necessary to minimize side effects caused by drug interactions.

When converting to monotherapy, reduce other AEDs by one third at start of felbamate therapy. Then after 2 wk and at the start of increasing the felbamate dosage, reduce other AEDs by an additional one third. At wk 3, continue to reduce other AEDs as clinically indicated.

Carbamazepine levels may be decreased; whereas phenytoin and valproic acid levels may be increased. Phenytoin and carbamazepine may increase felbamate clearance; valproic acid may decrease its clearance.

Doses can be administered with or without food.

## FENTANYL

Sublimaze, Duragesic, Fentora, Actiq, and many generics

***Narcotic; analgesic, sedative***

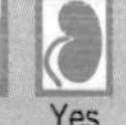
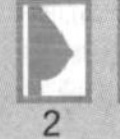
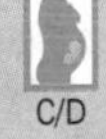

No Yes 2 C/D

**Injection:** 50 mcg/mL
**SR patch (Duragesic and others):** 12.5, 25, 50, 75, 100 mcg/hr (5s)
**Tabs for buccal administration:**
Fentora: 100, 200, 300, 400, 600, 800 mcg (28s)
**Lozenge on a stick:**
Actiq and others: 200, 400, 600, 800, 1200, 1600 mcg (30s)

**_Titrate dose to effect._**

**_Neonate and younger infant:_**

**_Sedation/analgesia:_** 1–4 mcg/kg/dose IV Q2–4 hr PRN.

**_Continuous IV infusion:_** 1–5 mcg/kg/hr; tolerance may develop.

**_Older infant and child:_**

**_Sedation/analgesia:_** 1–2 mcg/kg/dose IV/IM Q30–60 min PRN.

**_Continuous IV infusion:_** 1 mcg/kg/hr; titrate to effect; usual infusion range 1–3 mcg/kg/hr.

**_To prepare infusion:_** Use the following formula:

$$50 \times \frac{\text{Desired dose (mcg/kg/hr)}}{\text{Desired infusion rate (mL/hr)}} \times \text{Wt (kg)} = \frac{\text{mcg Fentanyl}}{\text{50 mL fluid}}$$

*Continued*

For explanation of icons, see p. 698.

FENTANYL *continued*

***Oral, breakthrough cancer pain for opioid-intolerant patients (see remarks):***

***Buccal tabs (≥18 yr):*** Start with 100 mcg by placing tablet in the buccal cavity (above a rear molar, between the upper cheek and gum) and letting the tablet dissolve for 15–25 min. A second 100 mcg dose, if needed, may be administered 30 min after the start of the first dose. If needed, increase dose initially in multiples of 100 mcg tablet when patients require > 1 dose per breakthrough pain episode for several consecutive episodes. If titration requires > 400 mcg/dose, use 200 mcg tabs.

***Lozenges (≥16 yr):*** Start with 200 mcg by placing lozenge in the mouth between the cheek and lower gum. If needed, may repeat dose 15 min after the completion of the first dose (30 min after start of prior dose). If therapy requires > 1 lozenge per episode, consider increasing the dose to the next higher strength. **Do not** give more than 2 doses for each episode of breakthrough pain and re-evaluate long-acting opioid therapy if patient requires > 4 doses/ 24 hr.

***Transdermal (see remarks):*** Safety has not been established in children < 2 yr and should be administered in children ≥ 2 yr who are opioid tolerant. Use is **contraindicated** in acute or post-operative pain in opiate-naïve patients.

***Opioid-tolerant child receiving at least 60 mg morphine equivalents/24 hr:*** Use 25 mcg/hr patch Q72 hr. Patch titration should not occur before 3 days of administration of the initial dose or more frequently than every 6 days thereafter.

See Chapter 6 for equianalgesic dosing and PCA dosing.

---

**Use with caution** in bradycardia, respiratory depression, and increased intracranial pressure. **Adjust dose in renal failure (see Chapter 31).** Fatalities and life-threatening respiratory depression have been reported with inappropriate use (overdoses, use in opioid-naïve patients, changing the patch too frequently and exposing the patch to a heat source) of the transdermal route.

Highly lipophilic and may deposit into fat tissue. IV onset of action 1–2 min with peak effects in 10 min. IV duration of action 30–60 min. Give IV dose over 3–5 min. Rapid infusion may cause respiratory depression and chest wall rigidity. Respiratory depression may persist beyond the period of analgesia. Transdermal onset of action 6–8 hr with a 72-hr duration of action. See Chapter 6 for pharmacodynamic information with transmucosal and transdermal routes.

Buccal tabs and oral lozenges are indicated only for the management of breakthrough cancer pain in patients who are already receiving and who are tolerant to opioid therapy. Buccal tabs (Fentora) and lozenge dosage forms are **NOT** bioequivalent; see package insert for conversion.

Fentanyl is a substrate for the CYP 450 3A4 enzyme. Be aware of medications that inhibit or induce this enzyme, for it may increase or decrease the effects of fentanyl, respectively.

Pregnancy category changes to "D" if drug is used for prolonged periods or in high doses at term.

## FERRIC GLUCONATE

See *Iron—Injectable Preparations*

## FERROUS SULFATE

See *Iron—Oral Preparations*

F

FORMULARY

## FEXOFENADINE ± PSEUDOEPHEDRINE

Allegra, Allegra ODT, Allegra-D 12 Hour, Allegra-D 24 Hour, and other generics

***Antihistamine, less-sedating ± decongestant***

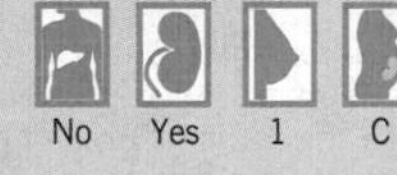

No Yes 1 C

**Tabs:** 30, 60, 180 mg
**Tabs, orally disintegrating** (Allegra ODT): 30 mg; contains phenylalanine
**Oral suspension:** 6 mg/mL (30, 300 mL)
**Extended-release tab in combination with pseudoephedrine (PE):**
Allegra-D 12 Hour: 60 mg fexofenadine + 120 mg pseudoephedrine
Allegra-D 24 Hour: 180 mg fexofenadine + 240 mg pseudoephedrine

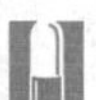

***Fexofenadine:***
***6 mo–<2 yr:*** 15 mg PO BID
***2–11 yr:*** 30 mg PO BID
***≥12 yr–adult:*** 60 mg PO BID; 180 mg PO QD may be used in seasonal rhinitis.

***Extended-release tabs of fexofenadine and pseudoephedrine:***
***≥12 yr–adult:***
***Allegra-D 12 Hour:*** 1 tablet PO BID
***Allegra-D 24 Hour:*** 1 tablet PO QD

May cause drowsiness, fatigue, headache, dyspepsia, nausea, and dysmenorrhea. Has **not** been implicated in causing cardiac arrhythmias when used with other drugs that are metabolized by hepatic microsomal enzymes (e.g., ketoconazole, erythromycin). **Reduce dose to 30 mg PO QD for child 6–11 yr old and 60 mg PO QD for ≥12 yr old if CrCl <40 mL/min.** For use of Allegra-D 12 Hour and decreased renal function, an initial dose of 1 tablet PO QD is recommended. See *Pseudoephedrine* for additional remarks if using the combination product.

Medication as the single agent may be administered with or without food. **Do not** administer antacids with or within 2 hr of fexofenadine dose. The extended-release combination product should be swallowed whole without food.

## FILGRASTIM

Neupogen, G-CSF

***Colony stimulating factor***

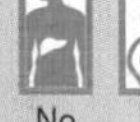
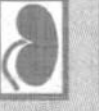
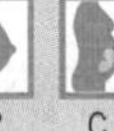

No No ? C

**Injection:** 300 mcg/mL (1, 1.6 mL)
**Injection, prefilled syringes with 27-gauge ½-inch needles:** 600 mcg/mL (0.5, 0.8 mL)
All dosage forms are preservative free.

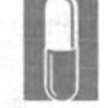

**Individual protocols may direct dosing.**
***IV/SC:*** 5–10 mcg/kg/dose QD × 14 days or until ANC > 10,000/mm$^3$. Dosage may be increased by 5 mcg/kg/24 hr if desired effect is not achieved within 7 days.
Discontinue therapy when ANC > 10,000/mm$^3$.

May cause bone pain, fever, and rash. Monitor CBC, uric acid, and LFTs. **Use with caution** in patients with malignancies with myeloid characteristics. **Contraindicated** for patients sensitive to *E. coli*-derived proteins. **Do not** administer 24 hr before or after administration of chemotherapy. *Continued*

For explanation of icons, see p. 698.

FILGRASTIM *continued*

SC routes of administration are preferred because of prolonged serum levels over IV route. If used via IV route and G-CSF final concentration < 15 mcg/mL, add 2 mg albumin/1 mL of IV fluid to prevent drug adsorption to the IV administration set.

## FLECAINIDE ACETATE

Tambocor and others

***Antiarrhythmic, class Ic***

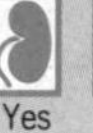
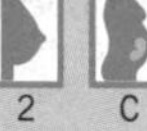

No Yes 2 C

**Tabs:** 50, 100, 150 mg
**Oral suspension:** 5, 20 mg/mL

***Child:*** Initial: 1–3 mg/kg/24 hr ÷ Q8 hr PO; usual range: 3–6 mg/kg/24 hr ÷ Q8 hr PO, monitor serum levels to adjust dose if needed.

***Adult:***

***Sustained V tach:*** 100 mg PO Q12 hr; may increase by 50 mg Q12 hr every 4 days to **max. dose** of 600 mg/24 hr.

***Paroxysmal SVT/paroxysmal AF:*** 50 mg PO Q12 hr; may increase dose by 50 mg Q12 hr every 4 days to **max. dose** of 300 mg/24 hr.

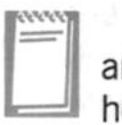

May aggravate LV failure, sinus bradycardia, preexisting ventricular arrhythmias. May cause AV block, dizziness, blurred vision, dyspnea, nausea, headache, and increased PR or QRS intervals. **Reserve for life-threatening cases.**

Flecainide is a substrate for the CYP 450 2D6 enzyme. Be aware of medications that inhibit or induce this enzyme for it may increase or decrease the effects of flecainide, respectively.

Therapeutic trough level: 0.2–1 mg/L. Recommended serum sampling time at steady-state: Obtain trough level within 30 min prior to the next scheduled dose after 2–3 days of continuous dosing for children; after 3–5 days for adults. **Adjust dose in renal failure (see Chapter 31).**

## FLUCONAZOLE

Diflucan and others

***Antifungal agent***

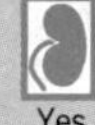
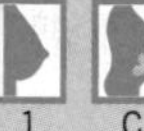
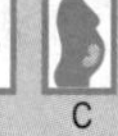

No Yes 1 C

**Tabs:** 50, 100, 150, 200 mg
**Injection:** 2 mg/mL (100, 200 mL); contains 9 mEq Na/2 mg drug
**Oral suspension:** 10 mg/mL (35 mL), 40 mg/mL (35 mL)

***Neonate:***

***Loading dose:*** 12 mg/kg IV/PO,

***Maintenance dose:*** 6 mg/kg IV/PO with the following dosing intervals (see following table)

*Continued*

FLUCONAZOLE *continued*

| Post-Conceptional Age (wk) | Postnatal Age (days) | Dosing Interval (hr) and Time (hr) to Start 1st Maintenance Dose after Load |
|---|---|---|
| ≤29 | 0–14 | 72 |
| | >14 | 48 |
| 30–36 | 0–14 | 48 |
| | >14 | 24 |
| 37–44 | 0–7 | 48 |
| | >7 | 24 |
| ≥45 | >0 | 24 |

***Child (IV/PO):***

| Indication | Loading Dose | Maintenance Dose to Begin 24 Hr after Loading Dose |
|---|---|---|
| Oropharyngeal Candidiasis | 6 mg/kg | 3 mg/kg |
| Esophageal Candidiasis | 12 mg/kg | 6 mg/kg |
| Invasive Systemic Candidiasis and Cryptococcal meningitis | 12 mg/kg | 6-12 mg/kg |
| Suppressive Therapy for HIV Infected with Cryptococcal Meningitis | 6 mg/kg | 6 mg/kg |

**Max. dose:** 12 mg/kg/24 hr

***Adult:***

***Oropharyngeal and esophageal candidiasis:*** Loading dose of 200 mg PO/IV followed by 100 mg QD 24 hr after; doses up to **max. dose** of 400 mg/24 hr should be used for esophageal candidiasis

***Systemic candidiasis and cryptococcal meningitis:*** Loading dose of 400 mg PO/IV, followed by 200–800 mg QD 24 hr later

***Bone marrow transplant prophylaxis:*** 400 mg PO/IV Q24 hr

***Suppressive therapy in for HIV infected with cryptococcal meningitis:*** 200 mg QD PO/IV Q24 hr

***Vaginal candidiasis:*** 150 mg PO × 1

Cardiac arrhythmias may occur when used with cisapride; concomitant use is **contraindicated**. May cause nausea, headache, rash, vomiting, abdominal pain, hepatitis, cholestasis, and diarrhea. Neutropenia, agranulocytosis, and thrombocytopenia have been reported.

Inhibits CYP 450 2C9/10 and CYP 450 3A3/4 (weak inhibitor). May increase effects, toxicity, or levels of cyclosporine, midazolam, phenytoin, rifabutin, tacrolimus, theophylline, warfarin, oral hypoglycemics, and AZT. Rifampin increases fluconazole metabolism.

Pediatric to adult dose equivalency: every 3 mg/kg pediatric dosage is equal to 100 mg adult dosage. **Adjust dose in renal failure (see Chapter 31).**

For explanation of icons, see p. 698.

## FLUCYTOSINE

Ancobon, 5-FC, 5-Fluorocytosine

***Antifungal agent***

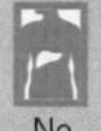 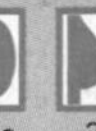 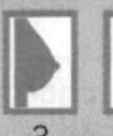 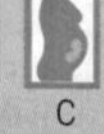

No Yes 3 C

**Caps:** 250, 500 mg
**Oral liquid:** 10 mg/mL

***Neonate:*** 80–160 mg/kg/24 hr ÷ Q6 hr PO
***Child and adult:*** 50–150 mg/kg/24 hr ÷ Q6 hr PO

Monitor CBC, BUN, serum creatinine, alkaline phosphatase, AST, and ALT. Common side effects: nausea, vomiting, diarrhea, rash, CNS disturbance, anemia, leukopenia, and thrombocytopenia. Use is **contraindicated** in the first trimester of pregnancy.

Therapeutic levels: 25–100 mg/L. Recommended serum sampling time at steady-state: Obtain peak level 2–4 hr after oral dose following 4 days of continuous dosing. Peak levels of 40–60 mg/L have been recommended for systemic candidiasis. Maintain trough levels above 25 mg/L. Prolonged levels above 100 mg/L can increase risk for bone marrow suppression. Bone marrow suppression in immunosuppressed patients can be irreversible and fatal.

Flucytosine interferes with creatinine assay tests using the dry-slide enzymatic method (Kodak Ektachem analyzer). **Adjust dose in renal failure (see Chapter 31).**

## FLUDROCORTISONE ACETATE

Florinef acetate, 9-Fluorohydrocortisone, Fluohydrisone, and various generics

***Corticosteroid***

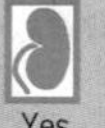 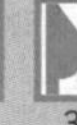 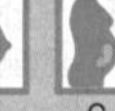

No Yes 3 C

**Tabs:** 0.1 mg

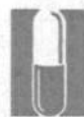

***Infant and child:*** 0.05–0.1 mg/24 hr QD PO
***Congenital adrenal hyperplasia:*** 0.05–0.3 mg/24 hr QD PO
***Adult:*** 0.05–0.2 mg/24 hr QD PO

**Contraindicated** in CHF and systemic fungal infections. Has primarily mineralocorticoid activity. **Use with caution** in hypertension, edema or renal dysfunction. May cause hypertension, hypokalemia, acne, rash, bruising, headaches, GI ulcers, and growth suppression.

Monitor BP and serum electrolytes. See Chapter 30 for steroid potency comparison.

Drug interactions: Drug's hypokalemic effects may induce digoxin toxicity; phenytoin and rifampin may increase fludrocortisone metabolism.

Doses 0.2–2 mg/24 hr have been used in the management of severe orthostatic hypotension in adults. Use a gradual dosage taper when discontinuing therapy.

## FLUMAZENIL

Romazicon and other generics
***Benzodiazepine antidote***

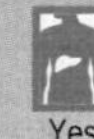 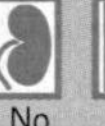 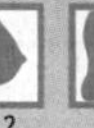 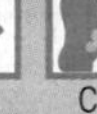
Yes No ? C

**Injection:** 0.1 mg/mL (5, 10 mL); contains parabens

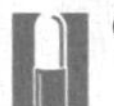

***Child, IV; Reversal of benzodiazepine sedation:***
***Initial dose:*** 0.01 mg/kg (**max. dose:** 0.2 mg) given over 15 sec, then 0.01 mg/kg (**max. dose:** 0.2 mg) given Q1 min to a **max. total cumulative dose** of 0.05 mg/kg or 1 mg, whichever is lower. Usual total dose: 0.08–1 mg (average 0.65 mg). Doses may be repeated in 20 min up to a **max. dose** of 3 mg in 1 hr.

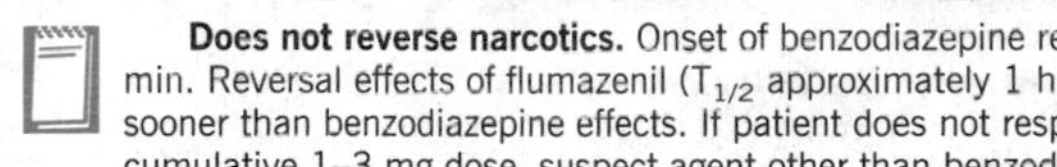

**Does not reverse narcotics.** Onset of benzodiazepine reversal occurs in 1–3 min. Reversal effects of flumazenil ($T_{1/2}$ approximately 1 hr) may wear off sooner than benzodiazepine effects. If patient does not respond after cumulative 1–3 mg dose, suspect agent other than benzodiazepines.

May precipitate seizures, especially in patients taking benzodiazepines for seizure control or in patients with tricyclic antidepressant overdose. Fear, panic attacks in patients with history of panic disorders have been reported. **Use with caution** in liver dysfunction; flumazenil's clearance is significantly reduced.

See Chapter 2 for complete management of suspected ingestions.

## FLUNISOLIDE

Nasarel, Aerospan, Aerobid, Aerobid-M
***Corticosteroid***

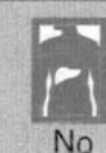 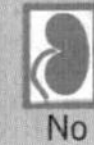 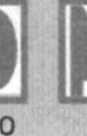 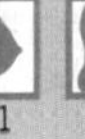 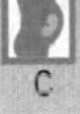
No No 1 C

**Nasal solution:**
Nasarel and others: 25 mcg/spray (200 sprays/bottle) (25 mL)
**Oral aerosol inhaler:**
Aerospan: 80 mcg/dose (60 doses/5.1 g, 120 doses/8.9 g); CFC-free (HFA)
Aerobid, Aerobid-M: 250 mcg/dose (100 doses/inhaler) (7 g), contains CFCs
Aerobid-M: Contains menthol flavoring

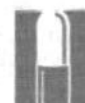

**For all dosage forms, after symptoms are controlled, reduce to lowest effective maintenance dose to control symptoms.**
***Nasal solution:***
***Child (6–14 yr):***
***Initial:*** 1 spray per nostril TID or 2 sprays per nostril BID; **max. dose:** 4 sprays per nostril/24 hr.
***Adult:***
***Initial:*** 2 sprays per nostril BID; **max. dose:** 8 sprays per nostril/24 hr.
***Inhaler (see remarks):***
***Aerobid or Aerobid-M:***
***Child (6–15 yr):*** 2 puffs BID; **max. dose:** 4 puffs/24 hr
***≥16 yr and adult:*** 2 puffs BID; **max. dose:** 8 puffs/24 hr
***Aerospan:***
***Child (6–11 yr):*** 1 puff BID; **max. dose:** 4 puffs/24 hr
***Adult:*** 2 puffs BID; **max. dose:** 8 puffs/24 hr

*Continued*

For explanation of icons, see p. 698.

FLUNISOLIDE *continued*

May cause a reduction in growth velocity. Shake inhaler or nasal solution well before use. Patients using nasal solution should clear nasal passages before use.

**Aerobid and Aerospan are not interchangable on a mcg per mcg basis.** Spacer devices may enhance drug delivery of Aerobid/Aerobid-M. **Do not use** a spacer with Aerospan because the product has a self-contained spacer. Rinse mouth after administering drug by inhaler to prevent thrush.

## FLUORIDE

Luride, Fluoritab, Pediaflor, and others

***Mineral***

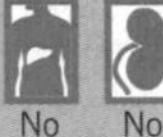
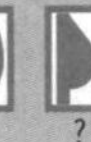
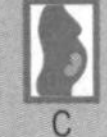

No No ? C

**Concentrations and strengths based on fluoride ion.**
**Drops:** 0.125 mg/drop, 0.25 mg/drop, 0.5 mg/mL
**Oral solution:** 0.2 mg/mL
**Chewable tabs:** 0.25, 0.5, 1 mg
**Tabs:** 1 mg
**Lozenges:** 1 mg
See Chapter 21 for fluoride-containing multivitamins.

***All doses/24 hr (see following table):***
Recommendations from American Academy of Pediatrics and American Dental Association.

| | **Concentration of Fluoride in Drinking Water (ppm)** | | |
|---|---|---|---|
| **Age** | **<0.3** | **0.3–0.6** | **>0.6** |
| Birth–6 mo | 0 | 0 | 0 |
| 6 mo–3 yr | 0.25 mg | 0 | 0 |
| 3–6 yr | 0.5 mg | 0.25 mg | 0 |
| 6–16 yr | 1 mg | 0.5 mg | 0 |

**Contraindicated** in areas where drinking water fluoridation is > 0.7 ppm. **Acute overdose:** GI distress, salivation, CNS irritability, tetany, seizures, hypocalcemia, hypoglycemia, cardiorespiratory failure. Chronic excess use may result in mottled teeth or bone changes.

Take with food, but **not** milk, to minimize GI upset. The doses have been decreased owing to concerns over dental fluorosis.

**FLUOXETINE HYDROCHLORIDE**

Prozac, Sarafem, Prozac Weekly, and various generics

***Antidepressant, selective serotonin reuptake inhibitor***

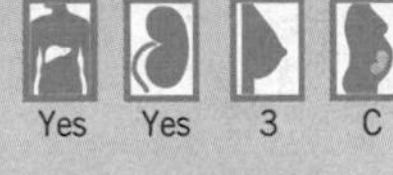


**Oral solution:** 20 mg/5 mL; may contain alcohol
**Caps:** 10, 20, 40 mg
**Delayed-release caps (Prozac Weekly):** 90 mg
**Tabs:** 10, 20 mg

***Depression:***

***Child, 8–18 yr:*** Start at 10–20 mg QD PO. If started on 10 mg/24 hr, may increase dose to 20 mg/24 hr after 1 wk. Use lower 10 mg/24 hr initial dose for lower weight children; if needed, increase to 20 mg/24 hr after several wk.

***Adult:*** Start at 20 mg QD PO. May increase after several wk by 20 mg/24 hr increments to **max. dose** of 80 mg/24 hr. Doses > 20 mg/24 hr should be divided BID.

***Obsessive-compulsive disorder:***

***Child, 7–18 yr:***

***Lower weight child:*** Start at 10 mg QD PO. May increase after several wk. Usual dose range: 20–30 mg/24 hr. There is very minimal experience with doses > 20 mg/24 hr and no expereince with doses > 60 mg/24 hr.

***Higher weight child and adolescent:*** Start at 10 mg QD PO and increase dose to 20 mg/24 hr after 2 wk. May further increase dose after several wk. Usual dose range: 20–60 mg/24 hr.

***Bulimia:***

***Adult:*** 60 mg QAM PO; it is recommended to titrate up to this dose over several days.

***Premenstrual dysphoric disorder:***

***Adult:*** Start at 20 mg QD PO using the Sarafem product. **Max. dose:** 80 mg/24 hr. Systematic evaluation has shown that efficacy is maintained for periods of 6 mo at a dose of 20 mg/day. Reassess patients periodically to determine the need for continued treatment.

**Contraindicated** in patients taking MAO inhibitors due to possibility of seizures, hyperpyrexia, and coma. **Use with caution** in patients receiving diuretics, or with liver (reduce dose with cirrhosis) or renal impairment. May increase the effects of tricyclic antidepressants. May cause headache, insomnia, nervousness, drowsiness, GI disturbance, and weight loss. Increased bleeding diathesis with unaltered prothrombin time may occur with warfarin. Hyponatremia has been reported. Monitor for clinical worsening of depression and suicidal ideation/behavior following the initiation of therapy or after dose changes.

May displace other highly protein-bound drugs. Inhibits CYP 450 2C19, 2D6, and 3A3/4 drug metabolism isoenzymes, which may increase the effects or toxicity of drugs metabolized by these enzymes.

Delayed-release capsule is currently indicated for depression and is dosed at 90 mg Q7 days. It is unknown if weekly dosing provides the same protection from relapse as does daily dosing.



For explanation of icons, see p. 698.

## FLUTICASONE PROPIONATE

Flonase HFA, Cutivate, Flovent Diskus, and others

***Corticosteroid***

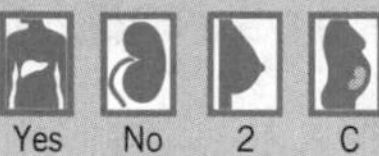


**Nasal spray (Flonase and other generics):** 50 mcg/actuation (16 g = 120 doses)
**Topical cream (Cutivate and others):** 0.05% (15, 30, 60 g)
**Topical ointment (Cutivate and others):** 0.005% (15, 30, 60 g)
**Topical lotion (Cutivate):** 0.05% (60 mL)
**Aerosol inhaler (MDI) (Flovent HFA) :** 44 mcg/actuation, 110 mcg/actuation, 220 mcg/actuation (7.9 g = 60 doses/inhaler, 13 g = 120 doses/inhaler)
**Dry-powder inhalation (DPI) (Flovent Diskus):** 50 mcg/dose, 100 mcg/dose, 250 mcg/dose; all strengths come in a package of 15 Rotadisks; each Rotadisk provides 4 doses for a total of 60 doses per package.

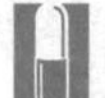

***Intranasal (allergic rhinitis):***

***≥4 yr and adolescent:*** 1 spray (50 mcg) per nostril QD. Dose can be increased to 2 sprays (100 mcg) per nostril QD if inadequate response or severe symptoms. Reduce to 1 spray per nostril QD once symptoms are controlled.

**Max. dose:** 2 sprays (100 mcg) per nostril/24 hr

***Adult:*** Initial 200 mcg/24 hr [2 sprays (100 mcg) per nostril QD; OR 1 spray (50 mcg) per nostril BID]. Reduce to 1 spray per nostril QD once symptoms are controlled.

**Max dose:** 2 sprays (100 mcg) per nostril/24 hr

***Oral inhalation (asthma):*** **Divide all 24 hr doses BID.** If desired response is not seen after 2 wk of starting therapy, increase dosage. Then reduce to the lowest effective dose when asthma symptoms are controlled. Administration of MDI with aerochamber enhances drug delivery.

**Recommended dosages for asthma (see following table):**

**RECOMMENDED DOSAGES FOR ASTHMA**

| Age | Previous Use of Bronchodilators Only (max. dose) | Previous Use of Inhaled Corticosteroid (max. dose) | Previous Use of Oral Corticosteroid (max. dose) |
|---|---|---|---|
| Child (4–11 yr) | MDI: 88 mcg/24 hr (176 mcg/24 hr)<br>DPI: 100 mcg/24 hr (200 mcg/24 hr) | MDI: 88 mcg/24 hr (176 mcg/24 hr)<br>DPI: 100 mcg/24 hr (200 mcg/24 hr) | Dose not available. |
| ≥12 yr and adult | MDI: 176 mcg/24 hr (880 mcg/24 hr)<br>DPI: 200 mcg/24 hr (1000 mcg/24 hr) | MDI: 176–440 mcg/24 hr (880 mcg/24 hr)<br>DPI: 200–500 mcg/24 hr (1000 mcg/24 hr) | MDI: 880 mcg/24 hr (1760 mcg/24 hr)<br>DPI: 1000–2000 mcg/24 hr (2000 mcg/24 hr) |

MDI, metered dose inhaler; DPI, dry powder inhaler.

*Continued*

FLUTICASONE PROPIONATE *continued*

***Topical:***

***Cream (see Chapter 30 for topical steroid comparisons):***

***≥3 mo and adult:*** Apply thin film to affected areas BID; then reduce to a less potent topical agent when symptoms are controlled.

***Lotion:***

***≥1 yr and adult:*** Apply thin film to affected areas QD.

***Ointment:***

***Adult:*** Apply thin film to affected areas BID.

---

Concurrent administration with ritonavir and other CYP 450 3A4 inhibitors may increase fluticasone levels resulting in Cushing syndrome and adrenal suppression. **Use with caution** and monitor closely in hepatic impairment.

Intranasal: Clear nasal passages prior to use. May cause epistaxis and nasal irritation, which are usually transient. Taste and smell alterations, rare hypersensitivity reactions (angioedema, pruritis, urticaria, wheezing, dyspnea), and nasal septal perforation have been reported in post-marketing studies.

Oral inhalation: Rinse mouth after each use. May cause dysphonia, oral thrush, and dermatitis. Compared to beclomethasone, has been shown to have less of an effect on suppressing linear growth in asthmatic children. Eosinophilic conditions may occur with the withdrawal or decrease of oral corticosteroids after the initiation of inhaled fluticasone.

Topical use: **Avoid** application/contact to face, eyes, and open skin. Occlusive dressings are **not recommended**.

## FLUTICASONE PROPIONATE AND SALMETEROL

Advair Diskus, Advair HFA

***Corticosteroid and long-acting beta-2 adrenergic agonist***

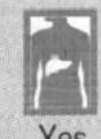
Yes
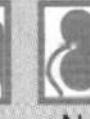
No
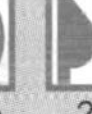
2
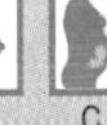
C

**Dry powder inhalation (DPI) (Advair Diskus):**

100 mcg fluticasone propionate + 50 mcg salmeterol per inhalation (28, 60 inhalations)

250 mcg fluticasone propionate + 50 mcg salmeterol per inhalation (28, 60 inhalations)

500 mcg fluticasone propionate + 50 mcg salmeterol per inhalation (28, 60 inhalations)

**Aerosol inhaler (MDI) (Advair HFA):**

45 mcg fluticasone propionate + 21 mcg salmeterol per inhalation (12 g delivers 120 doses)

115 mcg fluticasone propionate + 21 mcg salmeterol per inhalation (12 g delivers 120 doses)

230 mcg fluticasone propionate + 21 mcg salmeterol per inhalation (12 g delivers 120 doses)

---

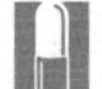

***Asthma:***

***Without prior inhaled steroid use:***

***Dry powder inhalation (DPI):***

***4 yr–adult:*** Start with 1 inhalation BID of 100 mcg fluticasone propionate + 50 mcg salmeterol.

*Continued*

For explanation of icons, see p. 698.

FLUTICASONE PROPIONATE AND SALMETEROL *continued*

***Asthma (cont'd):***

***Aerosol inhaler (MDI):***

***≥12 yr and adult:*** 2 inhalations BID of 45 mcg fluticasone + 21 mcg salmeterol, OR 115 mcg fluticasone + 21 mcg salmeterol; **max. dose:** 2 inhalations BID of 230 mcg fluticasone + 21 mcg salmeterol.

***With prior inhaled steroid use (conversion from other inhaled steroids; see following table):***

| Inhaled Corticosteroid | Current Daily Dose | Recommended Strength of Fluticasone Propionate + Salmeterol Diskus (DPI) (Advair Diskus) Administered at 1 Inhalation BID | Recommended Strength of Fluticasone Propionate + Salmeterol Aerosol Inhaler (MDI) (Advair HFA) Administered at 2 Inhalations BID |
|---|---|---|---|
| Beclomethasone dipropionate (Qvar; CFC-free, HFA) | 160 mcg | 100 mcg + 50 mcg | 45 mcg + 21 mcg |
| | 320 mcg | 250 mcg + 50 mcg | 115 mcg + 21 mcg |
| | 640 mcg | 500 mcg + 50 mcg | 230 mcg + 21 mcg |
| Budesonide | ≤400 mcg | 100 mcg + 50 mcg | 45 mcg + 21 mcg |
| | 800–1200 mcg | 250 mcg + 50 mcg | 115 mcg + 21 mcg |
| | 1600 mcg | 500 mcg + 50 mcg | 230 mcg + 21 mcg |
| Flunisolide (Aerobid, Aerobid-M; containing CFCs) | ≤1000 mcg | 100 mcg + 50 mcg | 45 mcg + 21 mcg |
| | 1250–2000 mcg | 250 mcg + 50 mcg | 115 mcg + 21 mcg |
| Flunisolide (Aerospan; CFC-free, HFA) | ≤320 mcg | 100 mcg + 50 mcg | 45 mcg + 21 mcg |
| | 640 mcg | 250 mcg + 50 mcg | 115 mcg + 21 mcg |

*Continued*

FLUTICASONE PROPIONATE AND SALMETEROL *continued*

| Inhaled Corticosteroid | Current Daily Dose | Recommended Strength of Fluticasone Propionate + Salmeterol Diskus (DPI) (Advair Diskus) Administered at 1 Inhalation BID | Recommended Strength of Fluticasone Propionate + Salmeterol Aerosol Inhaler (MDI) (Advair HFA) Administered at 2 Inhalations BID |
|---|---|---|---|
| Fluticasone propionate aerosol (MDI) | ≤176 mcg | 100 mcg + 50 mcg | 45 mcg + 21 mcg |
| | 440 mcg | 250 mcg + 50 mcg | 115 mcg + 21 mcg |
| | 660–880 mcg | 500 mcg + 50 mcg | 230 mcg + 21 mcg |
| Fluticasone propionate dry powder (DPI) | ≤200 mcg | 100 mcg + 50 mcg | 45 mcg + 21 mcg |
| | 500 mcg | 250 mcg + 50 mcg | 115 mcg + 21 mcg |
| | 1000 mcg | 500 mcg + 50 mcg | 230 mcg + 21 mcg |
| Mometasone furoate | 220 mcg | 100 mcg + 50 mcg | 45 mcg + 21 mcg |
| | 440 mcg | 250 mcg + 50 mcg | 115 mcg + 21 mcg |
| | 880 mcg | 500 mcg + 50 mcg | 230 mcg + 21 mcg |
| Triamcinolone | ≤1000 mcg | 100 mcg + 50 mcg | 45 mcg + 21 mcg |
| | 1100–1600 mcg | 250 mcg + 50 mcg | 115 mcg + 21 mcg |

**Max. dose:**

***Dry powder inhalation (DPI):*** 1 inhalation BID of 500 mcg fluticasone propionate + 50 mcg salmeterol.

***Aerosol inhaler (MDI):*** 2 inhalations BID of 230 mcg fluticasone propionate + 21 mcg salmeterol.

See *Fluticasone Propionate* and *Salmeterol* for remarks. Titrate to the lowest effective strength after asthma is adequately controlled. Proper patient education including dosage administration technique is essential; see patient package insert for detailed instructions. Rinse mouth after each use.

For explanation of icons, see p. 698.

## FLUVOXAMINE

Many generics; previously available as Luvox
***Antidepressant, selective serotonin reuptake inhibitor***

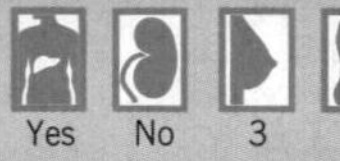
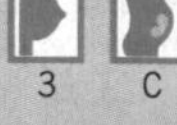
Yes No 3 C

**Tabs:** 25, 50, 100 mg

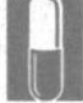

***Obsessive compulsive disorder:***
***>8–17 yr:*** Start at 25 mg PO QHS. Dose may be increased by 25 mg/24 hr Q4–7 days. Total daily doses > 50 mg/24 hr should be divided BID. Female patients may require lower dosages compared to males.
**Max. dose:** Child: 8–11 yr: 200 mg/24 hr; and child ≥12–17 yr: 300 mg/24 hr
***Adult:*** Start at 50 mg PO QHS. Dose may be increased by 50 mg/24 hr Q4–7 days up to a **max. dose** of 300 mg/24 hr. Total daily doses > 100 mg/24 hr should be divided BID.

Contraindicated with coadministration of cisapride, pimozide, thioridazine, tizanidine, or MAO inhibitors. **Use with caution** in hepatic disease (dosage reduction may be necessary); drug is extensively metabolized by the liver.

Monitor for clinical worsening of depression and suicidal ideation/behavior following the initiation of therapy or after dose changes.

Inhibits CYP 450 1A2, 2C19, 2D6, and 3A3/4, which may increase the effects or toxicity of drugs metabolized by these enzymes. Dose-related use of thioridazine with fluvoxamine may cause prolongation of QT interval and serious arrhythmias. May increase warfarin plasma levels by 98% and prolong PT. May increase toxicity and/or levels of theophylline, caffeine, and tricyclic antidepressants. Side effects include: headache, insomnia, somnolence, nausea, diarrhea, dyspepsia, and dry mouth.

Titrate to lowest effective dose.

## FOLIC ACID

Folvite and many others
***Water-soluble vitamin***

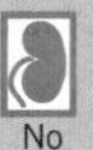
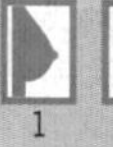
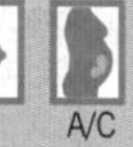
No No 1 A/C

**Tabs (OTC):** 0.4, 0.8, 1 mg
**Oral solution:** 50 mcg/mL
**Injection:** 5 mg/mL; contains 1.5% benzyl alcohol

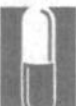

**For U.S. RDA, see Chapter 21.**
***Folic acid deficiency PO, IM, IV, SC (see following table)***

| Infant | Child 1–10 yr | Child ≥ 11 yr and adult |
|---|---|---|
| **INITIAL DOSE** | | |
| 15 mcg/kg/ dose; **max. dose:** 50 mcg/24 hr | 1 mg/dose | 1 mg/dose |
| **MAINTENANCE** | | |
| 30–45 mcg/24 hr QD | 0.1–0.4 mg/24 hr QD | 0.5 mg/24 hr QD; pregnant/lactating women: 0.8mg/24 hr QD |

*Continued*

FOLIC ACID *continued*

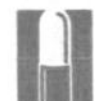

Normal levels: see Chapter 21. May mask hematologic effects of vitamin $B_{12}$ deficiency, but will not prevent progression of neurologic abnormalities. High-dose folic acid may decrease the absorption of phenytoin.

Women of child-bearing age considering pregnancy should take at least 0.4 mg QD before and during pregnancy to reduce risk of neural tube defects in the fetus. Pregnancy category changes to "C" if used in doses above the RDA.

## FOMEPIZOLE

Antizol and others

***Antidote for ethylene glycol or methanol toxicity***

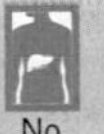
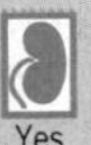
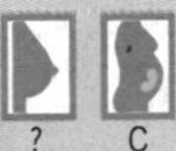

No Yes ? C

**Injection:** 1 g/mL (1.5 mL)

***Adults not requiring hemodialysis (IV, all doses administered over 30 min):***

*Load:* 15 mg/kg/dose × 1

*Maintenance:* 10 mg/kg/dose Q12 hr × 4 doses, then 15 mg/kg/dose Q12 hr until ethylene glycol level decreases to < 20 mg/dL and the patient is asymptomatic with normal pH

***Adults requiring hemodialysis (IV following the recommended doses at the intervals indicated here. Fomepizole is removed by dialysis. All doses administered over 30 min):***

***Dosing at the beginning of hemodialysis:***

If <6 hr since last fomepizole dose: **DO NOT** administer dose.

If ≥6 hr since last fomepizole dose: Administer next scheduled dose.

***Dosing during hemodialysis:*** Administer Q4 hr or as continuous infusion of 1–1.5 mg/kg/hr.

***Dosing at the time hemodialysis is completed (based on the time between last dose and end of hemodialysis):***

<1 hr: **DO NOT** administer dose at end of hemodialysis.

1–3 hr: Administer ½ of next scheduled dose.

>3 hr: Administer next scheduled dose.

***Maintenance dose off hemodialysis:*** Give next scheduled dose 12 hr from last dose administered.

Works by competitively inhibiting alcohol dehydrogenase. Safety and efficacy in pediatrics have not been established. **Contraindicated** in hypersensitivity to any components or other pyrazole compounds. Most frequent side effects include headache, nausea, and dizziness. Fomepizole is extensively eliminated by the kidneys (**use with caution in renal failure**) and removed by hemodialysis.

Drug product may solidify at temperatures < 25° C (77° F); vial can be liquefied by running it under warm water (efficacy, safety, and stability are not affected). All doses must be diluted with at least 100 mL of $D_5W$ or NS to prevent vein irritation.



For explanation of icons, see p. 698.

## FORMOTEROL

Foradil Aerolizer, Perforomist

***Beta-2 adrenergic agonist (long acting)***

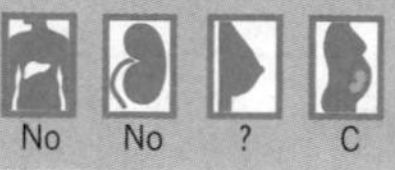


**Inhalation powder in capsules** (Foradil Aerolizer): 12 mcg (12s and 60s); contains lactose. Use with Aerolizer inhaler.
**Inhalation solution** (Perforomist): 20 mcg/2 mL (60s)

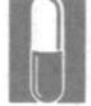

***≥5 yr and adult:***
***Asthma/Bronchodilation:***
***Foradil Aerolizer:*** 12 mcg Q12 hr; **max. dose:** 24 mcg/24 hr (12 mcg spaced 12 hr apart)
***Perforomist:*** 20 mcg Q12 hr; **max. dose:** 40 mcg/24 hr (20 mcg spaced 12 hr apart)
***Prevention of exercise-induced asthma for patients NOT receiving maintenance long-acting beta-2 agonists (e.g., formoterol or salmeterol):***
***Foradil Aerolizer:*** 12 mcg 15 min prior to exercise. If needed, an additional dose may be given AFTER 12 hr. **Max. dose:** 24 mcg/24 hr (12 mcg spaced 12 hr apart). Consider alternative therapy if max. dosage is not effective.

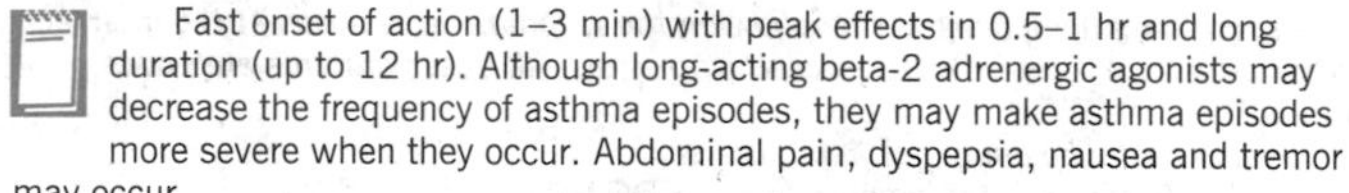

Fast onset of action (1–3 min) with peak effects in 0.5–1 hr and long duration (up to 12 hr). Although long-acting beta-2 adrenergic agonists may decrease the frequency of asthma episodes, they may make asthma episodes more severe when they occur. Abdominal pain, dyspepsia, nausea and tremor may occur.

**WARNING: Long-acting beta-2 agonists may increase the risk of asthma-related death.** Use formoterol only as additional therapy for patients not adequately controlled on other asthma-controller medications (e.g., low- to medium-dose inhaled corticosteroids) or whose disease severity clearly requires initiation of treatment with 2 maintenance therapies. Should **not** be used in conjunction with an inhaled, long-acting beta-2 agonist and is **not** a substitute for inhaled or systemic corticosteroids. See Chapter 24 for recommendations for asthma controller therapy.

## FOSCARNET

Foscavir

***Antiviral agent***

No Yes 3 C

**Injection:** 24 mg/mL (250, 500 mL)

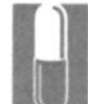

***Adolescent and adult, IV:***
***CMV retinitis:***
***Induction:*** 180 mg/kg/24 hr ÷ Q8 hr × 14–21 days
***Maintenance:*** 90–120 mg/kg/24 hr QD
***Acyclovir-resistant herpes simplex:*** 40 mg/kg/dose Q8 hr or 40–60 mg/kg/dose Q12 hr for up to 3 wk or until lesions heal

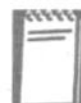

**Use with caution** in patients with renal insufficiency. **Discontinue** use in adults if serum Cr ≥ 2.9 mg/dL. **Adjust dose in renal failure (see Chapter 31).**

May cause peripheral neuropathy, seizures, hallucinations, GI disturbance, increased LFTs, hypertension, chest pain, ECG abnormalities, coughing,

*Continued*

FOSCARNET *continued*

dyspnea, bronchospasm, and renal failure (adequate hydration and avoiding nephrotoxic medications may reduce risk). Hypocalcemia (increased risk if given with pentamidine), hypokalemia, and hypomagnesemia may also occur. Use with ciprofloxacin may increase risk for seizures.

## FOSPHENYTOIN

Cerebyx and others

***Anticonvulsant***

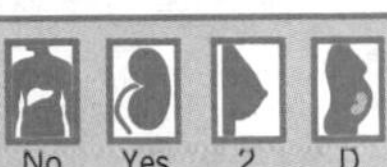


**Injection:** 50 mg phenytoin equivalent (75 mg fosphenytoin)/1 mL (2, 10 mL).
1 mg phenytoin equivalent provides 0.0037 mmol phosphate.

**All doses are expressed as phenytoin sodium equivalents (PE) (see remarks for dose administration information).**

***Child:*** **See Phenytoin and use the conversion of 1 mg phenytoin = 1 mg PE**

***Adult:***

***Loading dose:***

***Status epilepticus:*** 15–20 mg PE/kg IV

***Nonemergent loading:*** 10–20 mg PE/kg IV/IM

***Initial maintenance dose:*** 4–6 mg PE/kg/24 hr IV/IM

**All doses should be prescribed and dispensed in terms of mg phenytoin sodium equivalents (PE) to avoid medication errors. Safety in pediatrics has not been fully established.**

**Use with caution** in patients with porphyria, consider amount of phosphate delivered by fosphenytoin in patients with phosphate restrictions. Drug is also metabolized to liberate small amounts of formaldehyde, which is considered clinically insignificant with short-term use (e.g., 1 wk). Side effects: hypokalemia (with rapid IV administration), slurred speech, dizziness, ataxia, rash, exfoliative dermatitis, nystagmus, diplopia, and tinnitus. Increased unbound phenytoin concentrations may occur in patients with renal disease or hypoalbuminemia; measure "free" or "unbound" phenytoin levels in these patients.

Abrupt withdrawal may cause status epilepticus. BP and ECG monitoring should be present during IV loading dose administration. **Max. IV infusion rate:** 3 mg PE/kg/min up to a **max.** of 150 mg PE/min. Administer IM via 1 or 2 injection sites and IM route is **not recommended** in status epilepticus.

Therapeutic levels: 10–20 mg/L (free and bound phenytoin) **OR** 1–2 mg/L (free only). Recommended peak serum sampling times: 4 hr following an IM dose or 2 hr following an IV dose.

See *Phenytoin* remarks for drug interactions. Drug is more safely administered via peripheral IV than phenytoin.

## FUROSEMIDE

Lasix and many other generics

***Loop diuretic***

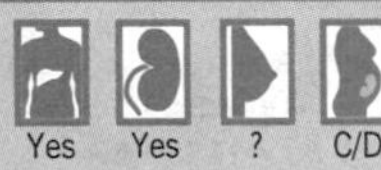


**Tabs:** 20, 40, 80 mg
**Injection:** 10 mg/mL (2, 4, 10 mL)
**Oral solution:** 10 mg/mL (60, 120 mL), 40 mg/5 mL (5, 10, 500 mL)

*Continued*

For explanation of icons, see p. 698.

FUROSEMIDE *continued*

***IM, IV:***
***Neonate:*** 0.5–1 mg/kg/dose Q8–24 hr; **max. dose:** 2 mg/kg/dose
***Infant and child:*** 0.5–2 mg/kg/dose Q6–12 hr
***Adult:*** 20–40 mg/24 hr ÷ Q6–12 hr; **max. dose:** 600 mg/24 hr or 80 mg/dose

***PO:***
***Neonate:*** Bioavailability by this route is poor; doses of 1–4 mg/kg/dose QD to BID have been used.
***Infant and child:*** Start at 2 mg/kg/dose; may increase by 1–2 mg/kg/dose no sooner than 6–8 hr following the previous dose. **Max. dose:** 6 mg/kg/dose. Dosages have ranged from 1–6 mg/kg/dose Q12–24 hr.
***Adult:*** 20–80 mg/dose Q6–12 hr; **max. dose:** 600 mg/24 hr.

***Continuous IV infusion:***
***Infant and child:*** 0.05 mg/kg/hr, titrate to effect.
***Adult:*** 0.1 mg/kg/hr; titrate to effect; **max. dose:** 0.4 mg/kg/hr.

**Contraindicated** in anuria and hepatic coma. **Use with caution** in hepatic disease; cirrhotic patients may require higher than usual doses. Ototoxicity may occur in presence of renal disease, especially when used with aminoglycosides.

May cause hypokalemia, alkalosis, dehydration, hyperuricemia, and increased calcium excretion. Prolonged use in premature infants may result in nephrocalcinosis.

Furosemide-resistant edema in pediatric patients may benefit with the addition of metolazone. Some of these patients may have an exaggerated response leading to hypovolemia, tachycardia, and orthostatic hypotension requiring fluid replacement. Severe hypokalemia has been reported with a tendency for diuresis persisting for up to 24 hr after discontinuing metolazone.

**Max. rate of intermittent IV dose:** 0.5 mg/kg/min.

Pregnancy category changes to "D" if used in pregnancy-induced hypertension.

## GABAPENTIN
Neurontin, Gabarone
***Anticonvulsant***

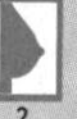
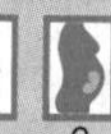
No Yes ? C

**Caps:** 100, 300, 400 mg
**Tabs:** 100, 300, 400, 600, 800 mg
**Oral solution:** 250 mg/5 mL (480 mL)

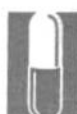

***Seizures (max. time between doses should not exceed 12 hr):***
***3–12 yr (PO, see remarks):***
***Day 1:*** 10–15 mg/kg/24 hr ÷ TID, then gradually titrate dose upward to the following dosages over a 3-day period:
***3–4 yr:*** 40 mg/kg/24 hr ÷ TID
***≥5–12 yr:*** 25–35 mg/kg/24 hr ÷ TID
**Dosages up to 50 mg/kg/24 hr have been well tolerated.**
***>12 yr and adult (PO, see remarks):*** Start with 300 mg TID; if needed, increase dose up to 1800 mg/24 hr ÷ TID. Usual effective doses: 900–1800 mg/24 hr ÷ TID. Doses as high as 3.6 g/24 hr have been tolerated.

***Neuropathic pain:***
***Child (PO; limited data):***
***Day 1:*** 5 mg/kg/dose at bedtime
***Day 2:*** 5 mg/kg/dose BID

*Continued*

GABAPENTIN *continued*

*Day 3:* 5 mg/kg/dose TID; then titrate dose to effect. Usual dosage range: 8–35 mg/kg/24 hr. **Max. daily dose has not been evaluated.**

*Adult (PO):*

*Day 1:* 300 mg at bedtime

*Day 2:* 300 mg BID

*Day 3:* 300 mg TID; then titrate dose to effect. Usual dosage range: 1800–2400 mg/24 hr; **max. dose:** 3600 mg/24 hr. For post-herpetic neuralgia, dose may be titrated up PRN for pain relief to a daily dose of 1800 mg/24 hr ÷ TID (efficacy has been shown from 1800–3600 mg/24 hr, however no additional benefit has been shown for doses > 1800 mg/24 hr).

Generally used as adjunctive therapy for partial and secondary generalized seizures, and neuropathic pain.

Somnolence, dizziness, ataxia, fatigue, and nystagmus were common in use for seizures (≥ 12 yr). Viral infections, fever, nausea and/or vomiting, somnolence, and hostility have been reported in patients 3–12 yr receiving other antiepileptics. Dizziness, somnolence, and peripheral edema are common side effects in adults with post-herpetic neuralgia.

**Do not withdraw medication abruptly** (gradually over a minimum of 1 wk). Drug is not metabolized by the liver and is primarily excreted in the urine unchanged.

May be taken with or without food. In TID dosing schedule, interval between doses **should not exceed** 12 hr. **Adjust dose in renal impairment (see Chapter 31).**

## GANCICLOVIR

Cytovene

***Antiviral agent***

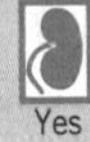
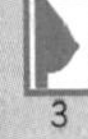
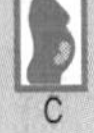

No Yes 3 C

**Injection:** 500 mg; contains 4 mEq Na per 1 g drug
**Caps:** 250, 500 mg
**Oral solution:** 25, 100 mg/mL

***Cytomegalovirus (CMV) infections:***

*Neonate (congenital CMV):* 12 mg/kg/24 hr ÷ Q12 hr IV × 6 wk

*Child > 3 mo and adult:*

*Induction therapy (duration 14–21 days):* 10 mg/kg/24 hr ÷ Q12 hr IV

*IV maintenance therapy:* 5 mg/kg/dose QD IV or 6 mg/kg/dose QD IV for 5 days/wk

*Oral maintenance therapy following induction:*

*6 mo–16 yr:* 30 mg/kg/dose PO Q8 hr with food

*Adult:* 1000 mg PO TID with food

***Prevention of CMV in transplant recipients:***

*Child and adult:*

*Induction therapy (duration 7–14 days):* 10 mg/kg/24 hr ÷ Q12 hr IV

*IV maintenance therapy:* 5 mg/kg/dose QD IV or 6 mg/kg/dose QD IV for 5 days/wk for 100–120 days post-transplant

*Oral maintenance therapy:* See oral doses for CMV treatment.

***Prevention of CMV in HIV-infected individuals (see www.hivatis.org for latest recommendations) :***

*Infant and child:*

*First episode prophylaxis:* 30 mg/kg/dose PO Q8 hr with food; consider valganciclovir

*Recurrence prophylaxis:* 5 mg/kg/dose IV QD

*Continued*

For explanation of icons, see p. 698.

GANCICLOVIR *continued*

***Prevention of CMV in HIV-infected individuals (cont'd):***
***Adolescent and adult:***
***First episode prophylaxis:*** 1000 mg PO TID with food
***Recurrence prophylaxis:*** 5–6 mg/kg/dose IV QD for 5–7 days/wk; or 1000 mg PO TID

Limited experience with use in children <12 yr old. **Contraindicated** in severe neutropenia (ANC < 500/microliter) or severe thrombocytopenia (platelets < 25,000/microliter). **Use with extreme caution. Reduce dose in renal failure (see Chapter 31).** Oral absorption is poor; consider the more bioavailable pro-drug, valganciclovir.

Common side effects: Neutropenia, thrombocytopenia, retinal detachment, confusion. Drug reactions alleviated with dose reduction or temporary interruption. Ganciclovir may increase didanosine and zidovudine levels, whereas didanosine and zidovudine may decrease ganciclovir levels. Immunosuppressive agents may increase hematologic toxicities. Amphotericin B, cyclosporine, and tacrolimus increase risk for nephrotoxicity. Imipenem/cilastatin may increase risk for seizures.

Minimum dilution is 10 mg/mL and should be infused IV over ≥ 1 hr. IM and SC administration are **contraindicated** because of high pH (pH = 11).

## GCSF

See *Filgrastim*

## GENTAMICIN

Garamycin and many others
***Antibiotic, aminoglycoside***

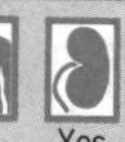
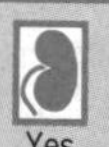
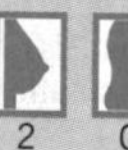
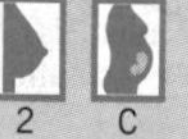
No Yes 2 C

**Injection:** 10 mg/mL (2 mL), 40 mg/mL (2, 20 mL); some products may contain sodium metabisulfite
**Pre-mixed injection in NS:** 40 mg (50 mL), 60 mg (50, 100 mL), 70 mg (50 mL), 80 mg (50, 100 mL), 90 mg (100 mL), 100 mg (50, 100 mL), 120 mg (50, 100 mL)
**Ophthalmic ointment:** 0.3% (3.5 g)
**Ophthalmic drops:** 0.3% (1, 5, 15 mL)
**Topical ointment:** 0.1% (15, 30 g)
**Topical cream:** 0.1% (15, 30 g)

***Parenteral (IM or IV):***
***Neonate and Infant (see table next page):***
***Child:*** 7.5 mg/kg/24 hr ÷ Q8 hr
***Adult:*** 3–6 mg/kg/24 hr ÷ Q8 hr
***Cystic fibrosis:*** 7.5–10.5 mg/kg/24 hr ÷ Q8 hr
***Intrathecal/intraventricular (use preservative-free product only):***
***Newborn:*** 1 mg QD
***>3 mo:*** 1–2 mg QD
***Adult:*** 4–8 mg QD
***Ophthalmic ointment:*** Apply Q8–12 hr
***Ophthalmic drops:*** 1–2 drops Q2–4 hr

*Continued*

GENTAMICIN *continued*

**NEONATE/INFANT**

| Post-conceptual Age (wk) | Postnatal Age (days) | Dose (mg/kg/dose) | Interval (hr) |
|---|---|---|---|
| ≤29* | 0–7 | 5 | 48 |
| | 8–28 | 4 | 36 |
| | >28 | 4 | 24 |
| 30–33 | 0–7 | 4.5 | 36 |
| | >7 | 4 | 24 |
| 34–37 | 0–7 | 4 | 24 |
| | >7 | 4 | 18–24 |
| ≥38 | 0–7 | 4 | 24 |
| | >7 | 4 | 12–18 |

*Or significant asphyxia, PDA, indomethicin use, poor cardiac output, reduced renal function.

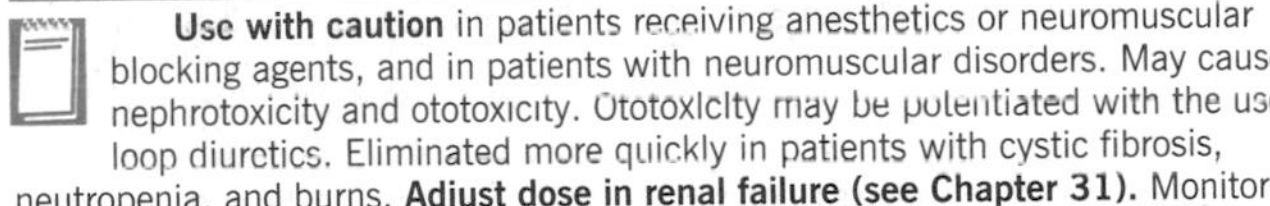

**Use with caution** in patients receiving anesthetics or neuromuscular blocking agents, and in patients with neuromuscular disorders. May cause nephrotoxicity and ototoxicity. Ototoxicity may be potentiated with the use of loop diuretics. Eliminated more quickly in patients with cystic fibrosis, neutropenia, and burns. **Adjust dose in renal failure (see Chapter 31).** Monitor peak and trough levels.

Therapeutic peak levels:

*6–10 mg/L general*

*8–10 mg/L in pulmonary infections, cystic fibrosis, neutropenia, osteomyelitis, and severe sepsis*

Therapeutic trough levels: <2 mg/L. Recommended serum sampling time at steady state: trough within 30 min prior to the 3rd consecutive dose and peak 30–60 min after the administration of the 3rd consecutive dose.

## GLUCAGON HCL

GlucaGen, Glucagon Emergency Kit

***Antihypoglycemic agent***

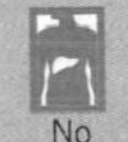 No 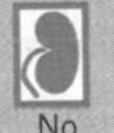 No 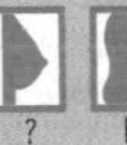 ? 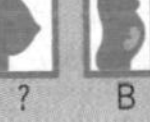 B

**Injection:** 1 mg vial (requires reconstitution)
1 unit = 1 mg

***Hypoglycemia, IM, IV, SC:***

***Neonate, infant, and child < 20 kg:*** 0.5 mg/dose (or 0.02–0.03 mg/kg/dose) Q20 min PRN

***Child ≥ 20 kg and adult:*** 1 mg/dose Q20 min PRN

For beta-blocker and calcium channel blocker overdose, see Chapter 2.

**Use with caution** in insulinoma and/or pheochromocytoma. Drug product is genetically engineered and identical to human glucagon. High doses have cardiac stimulatory effect and have had some success in beta-blocker and calcium channel blocker overdose. May cause nausea, vomiting, urticaria, and respiratory distress. **Do not delay** glucose infusion; dose for hypoglycemia is 2–4 mL/kg of dextrose 25%.

Onset of action: IM: 8–10 min; IV: 1 min. Duration of action: IM: 12–27 min; IV: 9–17 min.

For explanation of icons, see p. 698.

## GLYCERIN

Fleet Babylax, Sani-Supp, and others

***Osmotic Laxative***

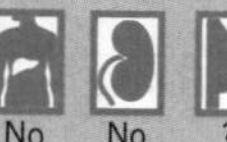  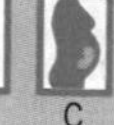

No No ? C

**Rectal solution (OTC):** 4 mL per application (6 doses), 7.5 mL per application (4 doses)

**Suppository (OTC):**

Infant/pediatric (10s, 12s, 24s, 25s, 50s)
Adult (10s, 12s, 18s, 24s, 25s, 48s, 50s)

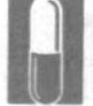

***Constipation:***

***Neonate:*** 0.5 mL/kg/dose rectal solution PR as an enema QD–BID PRN or half of infant suppository PR QD PRN

***Child < 6 yr:*** 2–5 mL rectal solution PR as an enema or 1 infant suppository PR QD–BID PRN

***>6 yr–adult:*** 5–15 mL rectal solution PR as an enema or 1 adult suppository PR QD–BID PRN

Onset of action: 15-30 min. May cause rectal irritation, abdominal pain, bloating, and dizziness. Insert suppository high into rectum and retain for 15 min.

## GLYCOPYRROLATE

Robinul

***Anticholinergic agent***

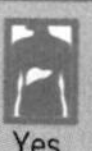 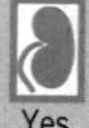 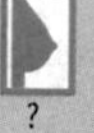 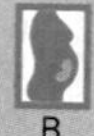

Yes Yes ? B

**Tabs:** 1, 2 mg

**Injection:** 0.2 mg/mL (1, 2, 5, 20 mL); some multidose vials contain 0.9% benzyl alcohol

***Respiratory antisecretory:***

***IM/IV:***

***Child:*** 0.004–0.01 mg/kg/dose Q4–8 hr
***Adult:*** 0.1–0.2 mg/dose Q4–8 hr
**Max. dose:** 0.2 mg/dose or 0.8 mg/24 hr

***Oral:***

***Child:*** 0.04–0.1 mg/kg/dose Q4–8 hr
***Adult:*** 1–2 mg/dose BID-TID

***Reverse neuromuscular blockade:***

***Child and adult:*** 0.2 mg IV for every 1 mg neostigmine or 5 mg pyridostigmine

**Use with caution** in hepatic and renal disease, ulcerative colitis, asthma, glaucoma, ileus, or urinary retention. Atropine-like side effects: tachycardia, nausea, constipation, confusion, blurred vision, and dry mouth. These may be potentiated if given with other drugs with anticholinergic properties. IV dosage form may be used orally.

Onset of action: PO: within 1 hr; IM/SC: 15–30 min; IV: 1 min. Duration of antisialogogue effect: PO: 8–12 hr; IM/SC/IV: 7 hr.

## GRANISETRON

Kytril and others

***Antiemetic agent, 5-HT$_3$ antagonist***

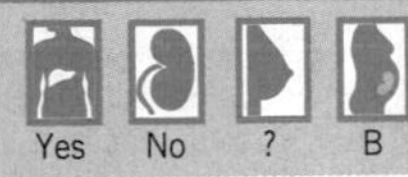


**Injection:** 1 mg/mL (1, 4 mL); 4 mL vials contain benzyl alcohol
**Tabs:** 1 mg
**Oral liquid:** 0.2 mg/mL (30 mL); contains sodium benzoate

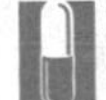

***Chemotherapy-induced nausea and vomiting:***

*IV:*

***Child ≥ 2 yr and adult:*** 10–20 mcg/kg/dose 15–60 min before chemotherapy; the same dose may be repeated 2–3 times at ≥ 10-min intervals following chemotherapy (within 24 hr after chemotherapy) as a treatment regimen. **Max. dose:** 3 mg/dose or 9 mg/24 hr. Alternatively, a single 40 mcg/kg/dose 15–60 min before chemotherapy has been used.

*PO:*

***Adult:*** 2 mg/24 hr ÷ QD-BID; initiate first dose 1 hr prior to chemotherapy.

***Post-operative nausea and vomiting prevention (dosed prior to anesthesia or immediately before anesthesia reversal) and treatment (IV):***

***≥4 yr:*** 20–40 mcg/kg/dose (**max. dose:** 1 mg) × 1
***Adult:*** 1 mg ×1

***Radiation-induced nausea and vomiting prevention:***

***Adult:*** 2 mg QD PO administered 1 hr before radiation.

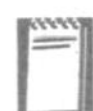

**Use with caution** in liver disease. May cause hypertension, hypotension, arrythmias, agitation, and insomnia. Inducers or inhibitors of the CYP 450 3A3/4 drug metabolizing enzymes may increase or decrease, respectively, the drug's clearance.

Onset of action: IV: 4–10 min. Duration of action: IV: ≤ 24 hr.

## GRISEOFULVIN

Grifulvin V, Grisactin, Fulvicin U/F, Fulvicin P/G, Gris-PEG, and others

***Antifungal agent***

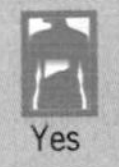
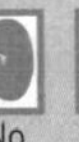
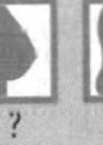


**Microsize:**

**Tabs (Grifulvin V):** 500 mg
**Oral suspension (Grifulvin V, Griseofulvin Microsize):** 125 mg/5 mL (120 mL); contains 0.2% alcohol, parabens and propylene glycol

**Ultramicrosize (250 mg ultramicrosize is approximately 500 mg microsize):**

**Tabs (Gris-PEG):** 125, 250 mg

***Microsize:***

***Child >2 yr:*** 10–20 mg/kg/24 hr PO ÷ QD-BID; give with milk, eggs, fatty foods. Some have recommended a higher dose of 20–25 mg/kg/24 hr PO for tinea capitis to improve efficacy due to relative resistance of the organism.
***Adult:*** 500–1000 mg/24 hr PO ÷ QD-BID
**Max. dose:** 1 g/24 hr

***Ultramicrosize:***

***Child >2 yr:*** 10–15 mg/kg/24 hr PO ÷ QD-BID
***Adult:*** 330–750 mg/24 hr PO ÷ QD-BID
**Max. dose:** 750 mg/24 hr

*Continued*

For explanation of icons, see p. 698.

GRISEOFULVIN *continued*

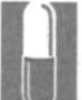

**Contraindicated** in porphyria, pregnancy and hepatic disease. Monitor hematologic, renal, and hepatic function. May cause leukopenia, rash, headache, paresthesias, and GI symptoms. Possible cross-reactivity in penicillin-allergic patients. Usual treatment period is 8 wk for tinea capitis and 4–6 mo for tinea unguium. Photosensitivity reactions may occur. May reduce effectiveness or decrease level of oral contraceptives, warfarin, and cyclosporine. Induces CYP 450 1A2 isoenzyme. Phenobarbital may enhance clearance of griseofulvin. Coadministration with fatty meals will increase the drug's absorption.

## HALOPERIDOL

Haldol, Haldol Decanoate 50, Haldol Decanoate 100, and other generics
***Antipsychotic agent***

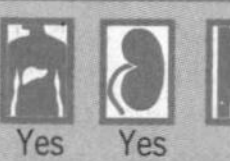

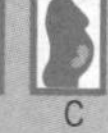

Yes Yes 3 C

**Injection (IM use only):**
Lactate: 5 mg/mL (1, 10 mL); may contain parabens
Decanoate (long acting): 50, 100 mg/mL (1, 5 mL); in sesame oil with 1.2% benzyl alcohol
**Tabs:** 0.5, 1, 2, 5, 10, 20 mg
**Oral solution:** 2 mg/mL (15, 120 mL)

***Child 3–12 yr:***
***PO:*** Initial dose at 0.025–0.05 mg/kg/24 hr ÷ BID–TID. If necessary, increase daily dosage by 0.25–0.5 mg/24 hr Q5–7 days PRN up to a **max. dose** of 0.15 mg/kg/24 hr. Usual maintenance doses for specific indications include the following:
***Agitation:*** 0.01–0.03 mg/kg/24 hr QD PO
***Psychosis:*** 0.05–0.15 mg/kg/24 hr ÷ BID-TID PO
***Tourette's syndrome:*** 0.05–0.075 mg/kg/24 hr ÷ BID-TID PO; may increase daily dose by 0.5 mg Q5–7 days.
***IM, as lactate, for 6–12 yr:*** 1–3 mg/dose Q4–8 hr; **max. dose:** 0.15 mg/kg/24 hr

***>12 yr:***
***Acute agitation:*** 2–5 mg/dose IM as lactate or 1–15 mg/dose PO; repeat in 1 hr PRN
***Psychosis:*** 2–5 mg/dose Q4–8 hr IM PRN or 1–15 mg/24 hr ÷ BID-TID PO
***Tourette's:*** 0.5–2 mg/dose BID-TID PO

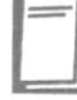

**Use with caution** in patients with cardiac disease (risk of hypotension), renal or hepatic dysfunction, thyrotoxicosis, and in patients with epilepsy since the drug lowers the seizure threshold. Extrapyramidal symptoms, drowsiness, headache, tachycardia, ECG changes, nausea, and vomiting can occur. Higher than recommended doses are associated with a higher risk of QT-prolongation and torsades de pointes.

Drug is metabolized by CYP 450 1A2, 2D6, and 3A3/4 isoenzymes. May also inhibit CYP 450 2D6 and 3A3/4 isoenzymes. Serotonin specific reuptake inhibitors (e.g., fluoxetine) may increase levels and effects of haloperidol. Carbamazepine and phenobarbital may decrease levels and effects of haloperidol.

Acutely agitated patients may require doses as often as Q60 min. **Decanoate salt is given every 3–4 wk in doses that are 10–15 times the individual patient's stablized oral dose.**

## HEPARIN SODIUM

Various trade names

***Anticoagulant***

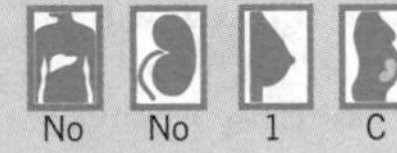


**Injection:**

Porcine intestinal mucosa: 1000, 2000, 2500, 5000, 7500, 10,000, 20,000, 40,000 U/mL (some products may be preservative-free; multi-dosed vials contain benzyl alcohol)

**Lock flush solution (porcine based):** 1, 10, 100 U/mL (some products may be preservative-free or contain benzyl alcohol)

**Injection for IV infusion (porcine based):**

$D_5W$: 40 U/mL (500 mL), 50 U/mL (500 mL), 100 U/mL (100, 250 mL); contains bisulfite

NS (0.9% NaCl): 2 U/mL (500, 1000 mL)

0.45% NaCl: 50 U/mL (250, 500 mL), 100 U/mL (250 mL); contains EDTA

120 U = approximately 1 mg

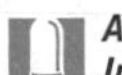

***Anticoagulation (see Chapter 14, Table 14-7 for dosage adjustments):***

***Infant and child:***

***Initial:*** 75 U/kg IV bolus over 10 min.

***Maintenance IV infusion (preferred):***

***<1 yr:*** 28 U/kg/hr

***≥1 yr:*** 20 U/kg/hr; use 18 U/kg/hr for older children

***Maintenance intermittent:*** 75–100 U/kg/dose Q4 hr IV

***Adult:***

***Initial:*** 50–100 U/kg IV bolus

***Maintenance:*** 15–25 U/kg/hr as IV infusion or 75–125 U/kg/dose Q4 hr IV

See remarks.

***DVT prophylaxis:***

***Adult:*** 5000 U/dose SC Q8–12 hr until ambulatory

***Heparin flush (dose should be less than heparinizing dose):***

***Younger child:*** lower doses should be used to **avoid** systemic heparinization.

***Older child and adult:***

***Peripheral IV:*** 1–2 mL of 10 U/mL solution Q4 hr

***Central lines:*** 2–3 mL of 100 U/mL solution Q24 hr

***TPN (central line) and arterial line:*** Add heparin to make final concentration of 0.5–1 U/mL

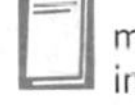

Adjust dose to give aPTT 1.5–2.5 times control value. aPTT is best measured 6–8 hr after initiation or changes in infusion rate. For intermittent injection, aPTT is measured 3.5–4 hr after injection. Toxicities: bleeding, allergy, alopecia, thrombocytopenia.

Use preservative-free heparin in neonates. **Note:** Heparin flush doses may alter aPTT in small patients; consider using more dilute heparin in these cases.

**Antidote: Protamine sulfate** (1 mg per 100 U heparin in previous 4 hr). For low molecular weight heparin, see *Enoxaparin.*



For explanation of icons, see p. 698.

## HYALURONIDASE

Amphadase, Hydase, Hylenex, Vitrase

***Antidote, extravasation***

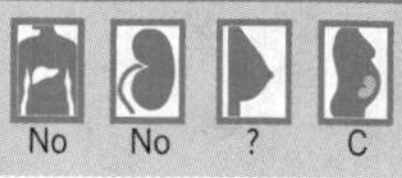

No No ? C

**Injection:**

Amphadase, Hydase: 150 U/mL (1 mL); bovine source and may contain thimerosal
Hylenex: 150 U/mL (1 mL); recombinant human source
Vitrase: 200 U/mL (2 mL); ovine source, preservative-free

**Powder for injection (Vitrase):** 6200 U; ovine source

Pharmacy can make a 15 U/mL dilution.

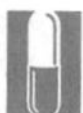

***Infant and child:*** Dilute to 15 U/mL; give 1 mL (15 U) by injecting 5 separate injections of 0.2 mL (3 U) at borders of extravasation site SC or intradermal using a 25- or 26-gauge needle. Alternatively, a 150 U/mL concentration has been used with the same dosing instructions.

**Contraindicated** in dopamine and alpha-agonist extravasation and hypersensitivity to the respective product sources (bovine or ovine). May cause urticaria. Patients receiving large amounts of salicylates, cortisone, ACTH, estrogens, or antihistamines may decrease the effects of hyaluronidase (larger doses may be necessary). Administer as early as possible (minutes to 1 hr) after IV extravasation.

## HYDRALAZINE HYDROCHLORIDE

Apresoline and others

***Antihypertensive, vasodilator***

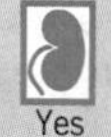
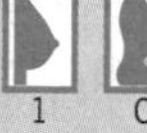
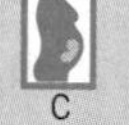

No Yes 1 C

**Tabs:** 10, 25, 50, 100 mg
**Injection:** 20 mg/mL (1 mL)
**Oral liquid:** 1.25, 4 mg/mL
Some dosage forms may contain tartrazines or sulfites.

**Hypertensive crisis (may result in severe and prolonged hypotension, see Chapter 4, Table 4-7 for alternatives):**

***Child:*** 0.1–0.2 mg/kg/dose IM or IV Q4–6 hr PRN; **max. dose:** 20 mg/dose. Usual IV/IM dosage range is 1.7–3.5 mg/kg/24 hr.

***Adult:*** 10–40 mg IM or IV Q4–6 hr PRN

***Chronic hypertension:***

***Infant and child:*** Start at 0.75–1 mg/kg/24 hr PO ÷ Q6–12 hr (**max. dose:** 25 mg/dose). If necessary, increase dose over 3–4 wk up to a **max. dose** of 5 mg/kg/24 hr for infants and 7.5 mg/kg/24 hr for children; or 200 mg/24 hr

***Adult:*** 10–50 mg/dose PO QID; **max. dose:** 300 mg/24 hr

**Use with caution** in severe renal and cardiac disease. Slow acetylators, patients receiving high-dose chronic therapy, and those with renal insufficiency are at highest risk of lupus-like syndrome (generally reversible). May cause reflex tachycardia, palpitations, dizziness, headaches, and GI discomfort. MAO inhibitors and beta-blockers may increase hypotensive effects. Indomethacin may decrease hypotensive effects.

Drug undergoes first pass metabolism. Onset of action: PO: 20–30 min; IV: 5–20 min. Duration of action: PO: 2–4 hr; IV: 2–6 hr. **Adjust dose in renal failure (see Chapter 31).**

## HYDROCHLOROTHIAZIDE

Hydrodiuril and many generics

***Diuretic, thiazide***

No Yes 1 B/D

**Tabs:** 12.5, 25, 50, 100 mg
**Caps:** 12.5 mg

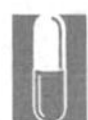

***Edema:***

***Neonate and infant < 6 mo:*** 2–4 mg/kg/24 hr ÷ BID PO; **max. dose:** 37.5 mg/24 hr

***≥6 mo and child:*** 2 mg/kg/24 hr ÷ BID PO; **max. dose:** 100 mg/24 hr

***Adult:*** 25–100 mg/24 hr ÷ QD–BID PO; **max. dose:** 200 mg/24 hr

***Hypertension:***

***Infant and child:*** Start at 0.5–1 mg/kg/24 hr QD PO; dose may be increased to a **max. dose** of 3 mg/kg/24 hr up to 50 mg/24 hr.

***Adult:*** 12.5–25 mg/dose QD–BID PO; doses > 50 mg/24 hr often result in hypokalemia.

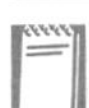

See Chlorothiazide. May cause fluid and electrolyte imbalances, and hyperuricemia. Drug may not be effective when creatinine clearance is less than 25–50 mL/min.

Hydrochlorothiazide is also available in combination with potassium-sparing diuretics (e.g., spironolactone), ACE inhibitors, angiotensin II receptor antagonists, hydralazine, methyldopa, reserpine, and beta-blockers.

Pregnancy category is "D" if used in pregnancy-induced hypertension.

## HYDROCORTISONE

Solu-Cortef, Cortef, Cortifoam, and many others

***Corticosteroid***

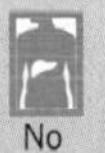 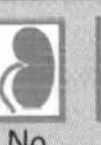 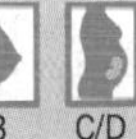

No No 3 C/D

**Hydrocortisone base:**

Tabs: 5, 10, 20 mg
Oral suspension: 2.5 mg/mL
Rectal cream: 1%
Rectal suspension: 100 mg/60 mL (7s)
Topical ointment: 0.5% (OTC), 1% (OTC), 2.5%
Topical cream: 0.5% (OTC), 1% (OTC), 2.5%
Topical lotion: 1% (OTC), 2.5%

**Na Succinate (Solu-Cortef):**

Injection: 100, 250, 500, 1000 mg/vial; contains benzyl alcohol

**Acetate:**

Topical ointment (OTC): 0.5%, 1%
Topical cream (OTC): 0.5%, 1%
Rectal cream: 1%
Suppository: 25, 30 mg
Rectal foam aerosol (Cortifoam): 10% (90 mg/dose) (15 g)

*Continued*

For explanation of icons, see p. 698.

HYDROCORTISONE *continued*

***Status asthmaticus:***
***Child:***
***Load (optional):*** 4–8 mg/kg/dose IV; **max. dose:** 250 mg
***Maintenance:*** 8 mg/kg/24 hr ÷ Q6 hr IV
***Adult:*** 100–500 mg/dose Q6 hr IV
***Physiologic replacement:*** See Chapter 30 for dosing.
***Anti-inflammatory/immunosuppressive:***
***Child:***
***PO:*** 2.5–10 mg/kg/24 hr ÷ Q6–8 hr
***IM/IV:*** 1–5 mg/kg/24 hr ÷ Q12–24 hr
***Adolescent and adult:***
***PO/IM/IV:*** 15–240 mg/dose Q12 hr
***Acute adrenal insufficiency:*** See Chapters 10 and 30 for dosing.
***Topical Use:***
***Child and adult:*** Apply to affected areas BID–QID, depending on severity

For doses based on body surface area and topical preparations (with comparisons), see Chapter 30. Pregnancy category changes to "D" if used in first trimester.

## HYDROMORPHONE HCL

Dilaudid, Dilaudid-HP, and other generics
***Narcotic, analgesic***

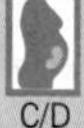


**Tabs:** 2, 4, 8 mg
**Injection:** 1, 2, 4, 10 mg/mL (may contain methyl- and propylparabens)
**Powder for injection (Dilaudid-HP):** 250 mg
**Suppository:** 3 mg
**Oral solution:** 1 mg/mL

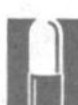

***Analgesia, titrate to effect:***
***Child:***
***IV:*** 0.015 mg/kg/dose Q4–6 hr PRN
***PO:*** 0.03–0.08 mg/kg/dose Q4–6 hr PRN; **max. dose:** 5 mg/dose
***Adolescent and adult:***
***IM, IV, SC:*** 1–2 mg/dose Q4–6 hr PRN
***PO:*** 1–4 mg/dose Q4–6 hr PRN

Refer to Chapter 6 for equianalgesic doses and for patient-controlled analgesia dosing. Less pruritus than morphine. Similar profile of side effects to other narcotics. **Use with caution** in infants and young children, and **do not use** in neonates due to potential CNS effects. Dose reduction recommended in renal insufficiency or severe hepatic impairment. Pregnancy category changes to "D" if used for prolonged periods or in high doses at term.

## HYDROXYCHLOROQUINE

Plaquenil, Quineprox

***Antimalarial, antirheumatic agent***

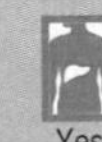 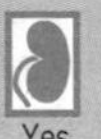 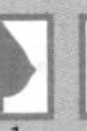 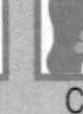

Yes Yes 1 C

**Tabs:** 200 mg (155 mg base)
**Oral suspension:** 25 mg/mL (19.375 mg/mL base)

**Doses expressed in mg of hydroxychloroquine base.**

***Malaria prophylaxis (start 1 wk prior to exposure and continue for 4 wk after leaving endemic area):***

*Child:* 5 mg/kg/dose PO once weekly; **max. dose:** 310 mg
*Adult:* 310 mg PO once weekly

***Malaria treatment (acute uncomplicated cases):***

For treatment of malaria, consult with ID specialist or see the latest edition of the AAP *Red Book.*

*Child:* 10 mg/kg/dose (**max. dose:** 620 mg) PO × 1 followed by 5 mg/kg/dose (**max. dose:** 310 mg) 6 hr later. Then 5 mg/kg/dose (**max. dose:** 310 mg) Q24 hr × 2 doses starting 24 hr after the first dose.

*Adult:* 620 mg PO × 1 followed by 310 mg 6 hr later. Then 310 mg Q24 hr × 2 doses starting 24 hr after the first dose.

***Juvenile rheumatoid arthritis or systemic lupis erythematosus:***

*Child:* 2.325–3.875 mg/kg/24 hr PO ÷ QD–BID; **max. dose:** 310 mg/24 hr **not to exceed** 5.425 mg/kg/24 hr

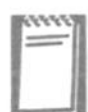

**Contraindicated** in psoriasis, porphyria, retinal or visual field changes, and 4-aminoquinoline hypersensitivity. **Use with caution** in liver disease, G6PD deficiency, concomitant hepatic toxic drugs, renal impairment, metabolic acidosis or hematologic disorders.

Long-term use in children is **not recommended**. May cause headaches, myopathy, GI disturbances, skin and mucosal pigmentation, agranulocytosis, visual disturbances, and increased digoxin serum levels.

For SLE and JRA, lower doses can be utilized when used in combination with other immunosuppressive agents.

## HYDROXYZINE

Vistaril and various generics

***Antihistamine, anxiolytic, antiemetic***

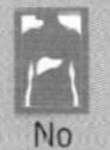 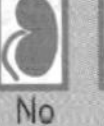 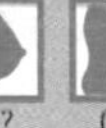 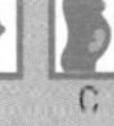

No No ? C

**Tabs (HCl salt):** 10, 25, 50 mg
**Caps (pamoate salt):** 25, 50, 100 mg
**Syrup (HCl salt):** 10 mg/5 mL (118, 473 mL); may contain alcohol
**Oral suspension (pamoate salt):** 25 mg/5 mL (120, 473 mL)
**Injection (HCl salt):** 25, 50 mg/mL; may contain benzyl alcohol
**NOTE:** Pamoate and HCl salts are equivalent in regards to mg of hydroxyzine.

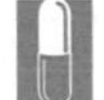

***Pruritus and anxiety:***

***Oral:***

*Child:* 2 mg/kg/24 hr ÷ Q6–8 hr PRN, OR alternative dosing by age:
*<6 yr:* 50 mg/24 hr ÷ Q6–8 hr PRN
*≥6 yr:* 50–100 mg/24 hr ÷ Q6–8 hr PRN

*Adult:* 25 mg/dose TID–QID PRN; **max. dose:** 600 mg/24 hr

*Continued*

For explanation of icons, see p. 698.

HYDROXYZINE *continued*

***Pruritis and anxiety (cont'd):***

***IM:***

***Child:*** 0.5–1 mg/kg/dose Q4–6 hr PRN

***Adult:*** 25–100 mg/dose Q4–6 hr PRN; **max. dose:** 600 mg/24 hr

May potentiate barbiturates, meperidine, and other CNS depressants. May cause dry mouth, drowsiness, tremor, convulsions, blurred vision, and hypotension. May cause pain at injection site.

Onset of action within 15–30 min. Duration of action: 4–6 hr.

**IV administration is not recommended**.

## IBUPROFEN

PO: Motrin, Advil, Children's Advil, Children's Motrin, and others

IV: NeoProfen

***Nonsteroidal anti-inflammatory agent***

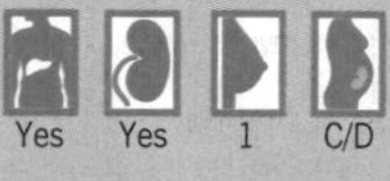


**Oral suspension [OTC]:** 100 mg/5 mL (60, 120, 480 mL)
**Oral drops [OTC]:** 40 mg/mL (7.5, 15 mL)
**Chewable tabs [OTC]:** 50, 100 mg
**Caplets [OTC]:** 100, 200 mg
**Tabs:** 100 [OTC], 200 [OTC], 400, 600, 800 mg
**Capsules [OTC]:** 200 mg
**Injection (NeoProfen, as lysine salt):** 10 mg ibuprofen base/1 mL (2 mL)

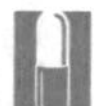

***PO:***

***Child:***

***Analgesic/antipyretic:*** 5–10 mg/kg/dose Q6–8 hr PO; **max. dose:** 40 mg/kg/24 hr PO.

***JRA:*** 30–50 mg/kg/24 hr ÷ Q6 hr PO; **max. dose:** 2400 mg/24 hr.

***Adult:***

***Inflammatory disease:*** 400–800 mg/dose Q6–8 hr PO; **max. dose:** 800 mg/dose or 3.2 g/24 hr.

***Pain/fever/dysmenorrhea:*** 200–400 mg/dose Q4–6 hr PRN PO; **max. dose:** 1.2 g/24 hr.

***IV:***

***Closure of ductus arteriosus:***

***<32 wk of gestation and 0.5–1.5 kg (use birth weight to calculate all doses and infuse all doses over 15 min; see remarks):*** 10 mg/kg/dose IV × 1 followed by two doses of 5 mg/kg/dose each, after 24 and 48 hr. Hold second or third dose if urinary output is < 0.6 mL/kg/hr; dosing should resume when laboratory studies indicate the return of normal renal function. If the ductus arteriosus fails to close or reopens, a second course of ibuprofen, the use of IV indomethacin, or surgery may be necessary.

**Contraindicated** with active GI bleeding and ulcer disease. **Use caution** with aspirin hypersensitivity, or hepatic/renal insufficiency, heart disease (risk for MI and stroke with prolonged use), dehydration, and in patients receiving anticoagulants. GI distress (lessened with milk), rashes, ocular problems, granulocytopenia, and anemia may occur. Inhibits platelet aggregation. Consumption of more than three alcoholic beverages per day, use with corticosteroids or anticoagulants may increase risk for GI bleeding.

*Continued*

IBUPROFEN *continued*

May increase serum levels and effects of digoxin, methotrexate, and lithium. May decrease the effects of antihypertensives, aspirin (anti-platelet effects), furosemide, and thiazide diuretics.

Pregnancy category changes to "D" if used in third trimester or near delivery.

**IV USE for PDA: Contraindicated** in untreated infections, congenital heart diseases requiring a patent ductus arteriosus to facilitate satisfactory pulmonary and systemic blood flow, active intracranial or gastrointestinal bleeds, thrombocytopenia, coagulation defects, suspected/active NEC, and significant renal impairment. **Use with caution** in hyperbilirubinemia. Not indicated for IVH prophylaxis. When compared to IV indomethacin, renal side effects are generally less frequent and severe.

## IMIPENEM AND CILASTATIN

Primaxin IV, Primaxin IM

***Antibiotic, carbapenem***

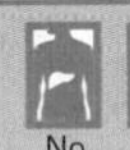 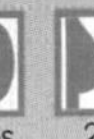 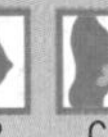 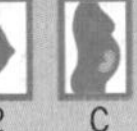

No Yes 2 C

**Injection:**

Primaxin IV: 250, 500 mg; contains 3.2 mEq Na/g drug

Primaxin IM: 500, 750 mg; contains 2.8 mEq Na/g drug

Each 1 mg drug contains 1 mg imipenem and 1 mg cilastatin.

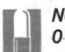

***Neonate:***

***0–4 wk old and < 1.2 kg:*** 50 mg/kg/24 hr ÷ Q12 hr IV

***<1 wk old and ≥ 1.2 kg:*** 50 mg/kg/24 hr ÷ Q12 hr IV

***≥1 wk old and ≥ 1.2 kg:*** 75 mg/kg/24 hr ÷ Q8 hr IV

***Child (4 wk–3 mo):*** 100 mg/kg/24hr ÷ Q6 hr IV

***Child (> 3 mo):*** 60–100 mg/kg/24 hr ÷ Q6 hr IV; **max. dose:** 4 g/24 hr

***Cystic fibrosis:*** 90 mg/kg/24 hr ÷ Q6 hr IV; **max. dose:** 4 g/24 hr

***Adult:***

***IV:*** 250–1000 mg/dose Q6–8 hr; **max. dose:** 4 g/24 hr or 50 mg/kg/24 hr, whichever is less.

***IM:*** 500–750 mg/dose Q12 hr

For IV use, give slowly over 30–60 min. Use IM preparation with **caution** since it contains lidocaine. Adverse effects: pruritus, urticaria, GI symptoms, seizures, dizziness, hypotension, elevated LFTs, blood dyscrasias, and penicillin allergy. CSF penetration is variable but best with inflamed meninges.

**Do not administer with** probenecid (increases imipenem/cilastatin levels) and ganciclovir (increase risk for seizures).

**Adjust dose in renal failure (see Chapter 31).**

## IMIPRAMINE

Tofranil, Tofranil-PM, and many generics

***Antidepressant, tricyclic***

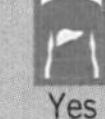 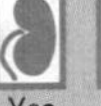 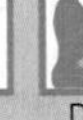 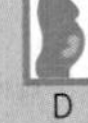

Yes Yes 3 D

**Tabs (HCl):** 10, 25, 50 mg

**Caps (Tofranil-PM, pamoate):** 75, 100, 125, 150 mg; strengths are expressed as imipramine HCl equivalent

*Continued*

For explanation of icons, see p. 698.

IMIPRAMINE *continued*

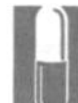

***Antidepressant:***

***Child:***

***Initial:*** 1.5 mg/kg/24 hr ÷ TID PO; increase 1–1.5 mg/kg/24 hr Q3–4 days to a **max. dose** of 5 mg/kg/24 hr

***Adolescent:***

***Initial:*** 25–50 mg/24 hr ÷ QD-TID PO; **max. dose:** 200 mg/24 hr. Dosages exceeding 100 mg/24 hr are generally not necessary.

***Adult:***

***Initial:*** 75–100 mg/24 hr ÷ TID PO

***Maintenance:*** 50–300 mg/24 hr QHS PO; **max. dose:** 300 mg/24 hr

***Enuresis (≥6 yr):***

***Initial:*** 10–25 mg QHS PO

***Increment:*** 10–25 mg/dose at 1- to 2-wk intervals until **max. dose** for age or desired effect achieved. Continue × 2–3 mo, then taper slowly

**Max. dose:**

***6–12 yr:*** 50 mg/24 hr

***12–14 yr:*** 75 mg/24 hr

***Augment analgesia for chronic pain:***

***Initial:*** 0.2–0.4 mg/kg/dose QHS PO; increase 50% every 2–3 days to a **max. dose** of 1–3 mg/kg/dose QHS PO

**Contraindicated** in narrow-angle glaucoma and patients who used MAO inhibitors within 14 days. See Chapter 2 for management of toxic ingestion. Monitor for clinical worsening of depression and suicidal ideation/behavior following the initiation of therapy or after dose changes. **Use with caution** in renal or hepatic impairment. Side effects include sedation, urinary retention, constipation, dry mouth, dizziness, drowsiness, and arrhythmia. QHS dosing during first weeks of therapy will reduce sedation. Monitor ECG, BP, CBC at start of therapy and with dose changes. Tricyclics may cause mania.

Therapeutic reference range (sum of imipramine and desipramine) = 150–250 ng/mL. Levels > 1000 ng/mL are toxic, however, toxicity may occur at > 300 ng/mL.

Recommended serum sampling times at steady-state: Obtain trough level within 30 min prior to the next scheduled dose after 5–7 days of continuous therapy. Carbamazepine may reduce imipramine levels; and cimetidine, fluoxetine, fluvoxamine, labetolol, quinidine may increase imipramine levels.

Onset of antidepressant effects: 1–3 wk. **Do not discontinue abruptly** in patients receiving long-term high-dose therapy.

## IMMUNE GLOBULIN

***Immune globulins***

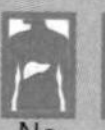
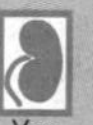
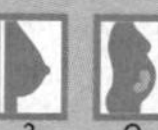

No Yes ? C

**IM preparations:**

GamaSTAN S/D: 150–180 mg/mL (2, 10 mL); contains 0.21-0.32 M glycine

**IV preparations in solution:**

Flebogamma 5% (50 mg/mL): contains 50 mg/mL sorbitol and ≤ 6 mg/mL polyethylene glycol

Gamunex: 10% (100 mg/mL); contains 0.16–0.24 M glycine

Gammagard liquid: 10% (100 mg/mL)

Octagam: 5% (50 mg/mL); contains 100 mg/mL maltose

*Continued*

IMMUNE GLOBULIN *continued*

**IV preparations in powder for reconstitution:**

Carimune NF: 1, 3, 6, 12 g (contains 1.67 g sucrose and < 20 mg NaCl per 1 g Ig); dilute to 3, 6, 9 or 12%

Polygam S/D: 2.5, 5, 10 g (contains 3 mg/mL albumin, 22.5 mg/mL glycine, 20 mg/mL glucose, 2 mg/mL polyethylene glycol, 1 mcg/mL tri-n-butyl phosphate, 1 mcg/mL octoxynol 9, and 100 mcg/mL polysorbate 80); dilute to 5% or 10%

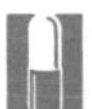

See indications and doses in Chapter 15.

General guidelines for administration (see package insert of specific products): Begin infusion at 0.01 mL/kg/min, double rate every 15–30 min, up to **max.** of 0.08 mL/kg/min. If adverse reactions occur, stop infusion until side effects subside and may restart at rate that was previously tolerated.

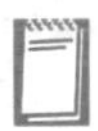

May cause flushing, chills, fever, headache, and hypotension. Hypersensitivity reaction may occur when IV form is administered rapidly. Gamimune-N contains maltose and may cause an osmotic diuresis. May cause **anaphylaxis** in IgA-deficient patients due to varied amounts of IgA. Some products are IgA depleted; consult a pharmacist.

Intravenous preparations containing sucrose **should not be infused** at a rate such that the amount of sucrose exceeds 3 mg/kg/min to decrease risk of renal dysfunction including acute renal failure.

Delay immunizations after IVIG administration (see 2007 *Red Book* for details).

## INDOMETHACIN

Indocin, Indocin SR, Indocin I.V., and various generics

***Nonsteroidal anti-inflammatory agent***

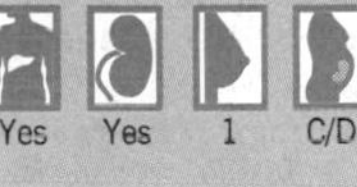


**Caps:** 25, 50 mg
**Sustained-release caps (Indocin SR and others):** 75 mg
**Oral suspension:** 25 mg/5 mL (237 mL); contains 1% alcohol
**Suppositories:** 50 mg (30s)
**Injection (Indocin I.V.):** 1 mg

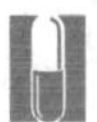

***Anti-inflammatory/rheumatoid arthritis:***

***≥2 yr old:*** Start at 1–2 mg/kg/24 hr ÷ BID-QID PO; **max. dose:** the lesser of 4 mg/kg/24 hr or 200 mg/24 hr

***Adult:*** 50–150 mg/24 hr ÷ BID-QID PO; **max. dose:** 200 mg/24 hr

***Closure of ductus arteriosus:***

Infuse intravenously over 20–30 min:

| | Dose (mg/kg/dose Q12–24 hr) | | |
|---|---|---|---|
| **Postnatal Age** | **#1** | **#2** | **#3** |
| <48 hr | 0.2 | 0.1 | 0.1 |
| 2–7 days | 0.2 | 0.2 | 0.2 |
| >7 days | 0.2 | 0.25 | 0.25 |

In infants <1500 g, 0.1–0.2 mg/kg/dose IV Q24 hr may be given for an additional 3–5 days.

*Continued*

For explanation of icons, see p. 698.

INDOMETHACIN *continued*

***Intraventricular hemorrhage prophylaxis:*** 0.1 mg/kg/dose IV Q24 hr × 3 doses, initiated at 6–12 hr of age (give in consultation with a neonatologist).

**Contraindicated** in active bleeding, coagulation defects, necrotizing enterocolitis, and renal insufficiency. **Use with caution** in cardiac dysfunction, hypertension, heart disease (risk for MI and stroke with prolonged use), and renal or hepatic impairment. May cause (especially in neonates) decreased urine output, platelet dysfunction, decreased GI blood flow, and reduce the antihypertensive effects of beta-blockers, hydralazine, and ACE inhibitors. **Fatal hepatitis reported in treatment of JRA**. Monitor renal and hepatic function before and during use.

**Reduction in cerebral blood flow associated with rapid IV infusion**; infuse all IV doses over 20–30 min.

Sustained-release capsules are dosed QD-BID. Pregnancy category changes to "D" if used for > 48 hr or after 34 wk gestation or close to delivery.

## INSULIN PREPARATIONS
***Pancreatic hormone***

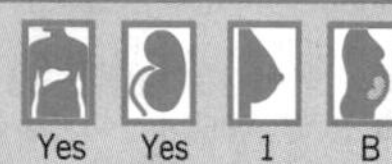


**Many preparations, at concentrations of 40, 100, 500 U/mL**

: Diluted concentrations of 1 U/mL or 10 U/mL may be necessary for neonates and infants.

***Insulin preparations:*** See Chapter 30, Table 30-4.
***Hyperkalemia:*** See Chapter 11, Figure 11-2.
***DKA:*** See Chapter 10, Figure 10-1.

When using insulin drip with new IV tubing, fill the tubing with the insulin infusion solution and wait for 30 min (before connecting tubing to the patient). Then flush the line and connect the IV line to the patient to start the infusion. This will ensure proper drug delivery. **Adjust dose in renal failure (see Chapter 31). Use with caution** and monitor closely in hepatic impairment.

## IODIDE

See *Potassium Iodide*

## IOHEXOL
Omnipaque 140, Omnipaque 240, Omnipaque 300, and Omnipaque 350
***Radiopaque agent, contrast media***

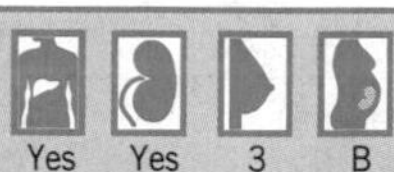


**Injection:**
Omnipaque 140: 302 mg iohexol equivalent to 140 mg iodine/mL (50 mL)

*Continued*

IOHEXOL *continued*

Omnipaque 240: 518 mg iohexol equivalent to 240 mg iodine/mL (10, 20, 50, 100, 150, 200 mL)
Omnipaque 300: 647 mg iohexol equivalent to 300 mg iodine/mL (10, 30, 50, 75, 100, 125, 150 mL)
Omnipaque 350: 755 mg iohexol equivalent to 350 mg iodine/mL (50, 75, 100, 125, 150, 200, 250 mL)

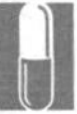

***Contrast enhanced CT scan of the abdomen:***
***Oral (administered prior to IV dose):***

***Child:*** Mix 20 mL of Omnipaque 350 with 500 mL of noncarbonated beverage of patient's choice (apple juice works well for younger patients). Administer diluted contrast media PO 30–60 min prior to the IV dose and image acquisition using the following dosage:

***<6 mo:*** 40–60 mL
***6–18 mo:*** 120–160 mL
***18 mo–3 yr:*** 165–240 mL
***3 yr–12 yr:*** 250–360 mL
***>12 yr:*** 480–520 mL

***Adult:*** Mix 50 mL of Omnipaque 350 with ½ gallon of noncarbonated beverage of patient's choice. Give 2–4 cups containing 480 mL (16 oz) of the diluted contrast media PO 20–40 min prior to the IV dose and image acquisition.

***IV (administered after PO dose):***

***Child:*** 1–2 mL/kg IV of Omnipaque 240 or Omnipaque 300 given 30–60 min after the oral dose. **Max. dose:** 3 mL/kg.
***Adult:*** 100–150 mL IV of Omnipaque 300 given 20–40 min after the oral dose.

**Use with caution** in dehydration, previous allergic reaction to a contrast medium, iodine senistivity, asthma, hay fever, food allergy, congestive heart failure, severe liver or renal impairment, diabetic nephropathy, multiple myeloma, pheochromocytoma, hyperthyroidism, and sickle cell disease. Allergic reactions, arrhythmias, and nephrotoxicity have been rarely reported. Children at higher risk for adverse events with contrast medium administration may include those having asthma, sensitivity to medication and/or allergens, congestive heart failure, serum creatinine > 1.5 mg/dL, or < 12 mo.

Use **NOT** recommended with drugs that lower seizure threshold (e.g., phenothiazines), amiodarone (increase risk of cardiotoxicity), and metformin (lactic acidosis and acute renal failure).

Many other uses exist, see package insert for additional information. Iohexol is particularly useful when barium sulfate is **contraindicated** in patients with suspected bowel perforation or those where aspiration of contrast medium is of concern. Oral dose is poorly absorbed from the normal GI tract (0.1%–0.5%); absorption increases with bowel perforation or bowel obstruction. Concentrations ≥ 518 mg iohexol/mL are hyperosmolar (1.8–3 times that of plasma).

## IPECAC

Various generic brands
***Emetic agent***

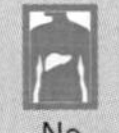
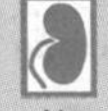
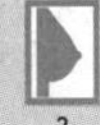
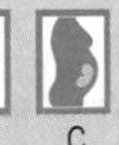

No No ? C

**Syrup (OTC):** 70 mg/mL (15, 30 mL); contains 1.5%–2% alcohol

*Continued*

FORMULARY

For explanation of icons, see p. 698.

IPECAC *continued*

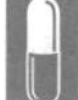

See Chapter 2 for indications.
All doses are administered × 1 and may be repeated once if vomiting does not occur within 20–30 min. If vomiting does not occur within 30–45 min after the second dose, perform gastric lavage.
***6–12 mo:*** 5–10 mL ipecac followed by 10–20 mL/kg or 120–240 mL water.
***1–12 yr:*** 15 mL ipecac followed by 10–20 mL/kg or 120–240 mL water.
***≥12 yr and adult:*** 15–30 mL ipecac followed by 200–300 mL of water.

Routine use of ipecac in poisoned patient **has not been recommended** by the American Academy of Clinical Toxicology. Use may delay and decrease the efficacy of activated charcoal, oral antidotes and whole bowel irrigation. The AAP now recommends ipecac should no longer be routinely used as a home treatment strategy.

**Do not** administer if patient is unconscious or has potential for decline in mental status, lacks a gag reflex, has seizures, or has ingested corrosives, strong acids or bases, volatile oils. May cause GI irritation, cardiotoxicity, myopathy. **Do not use** ipecac fluid extract as it is 14 times more potent. **Do not** administer with milk or carbonated beverages.

Onset of action: 15–30 min. Duration of action: 20 min to 1 hr.

## IPRATROPIUM BROMIDE

Atrovent and other generics

***Anticholinergic agent***

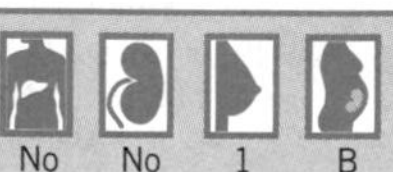


**Aerosol (HFA):** 17 mcg/dose (200 actuations per canister, 12.9 g)
**Nebulized solution:** 0.02% (500 mcg/2.5 mL, 25s, 60s)
**Nasal spray:** 0.03% (21 mcg per actuation, 30 mL); 0.06% (42 mcg per actuation, 15 mL)
**In combination with albuterol (DuoNeb and others):**
Nebulized solution: 0.5 mg ipratropium bromide and 2.5 mg albuterol in 3 mL (30s, 60s)

***Acute use in the ED or ICU:***
***Nebulizer treatments:***
***<12 yr:*** 250 mcg/dose Q20 min × 3, then Q2–4 hr PRN
***≥12 yr:*** 500 mcg/dose Q30 min × 3, then Q2–4 hr PRN
***Inhaler:***
***Child and adult:*** 4–8 puffs PRN
***Nonacute use:***
***Inhaler:***
***<12 yr:*** 1–2 puffs Q6 hr; **max. dose:** 12 puffs/24 hr
***≥12 yr:*** 2–3 puffs Q6 hr; **max. dose:** 12 puffs/24 hr
***Nebulized treatments:***
***Infant:*** 125–250 mcg/dose Q8 hr
***Child ≤ 12 yr:*** 250 mcg/dose Q6–8 hr
***>12 yr and adult:*** 250–500 mcg/dose Q6–8 hr
***Nasal spray:***
***Allergic and nonallergic rhinitis:***
***≥6 yr and adult:*** 2 sprays of 0.03% strength (42 mcg) per nostril BID–TID
***Rhinitis associated with common cold:***
***5–11 yr:*** 2 sprays of 0.06% strength (84 mcg) per nostril TID × 4 days.

*Continued*

IPRATROPIUM BROMIDE *continued*

**≥12 yr and adult:** 2 sprays of 0.06% strength (84 mcg) per nostril TID–QID × 4 days.

**Contraindicated** in soy or peanut allergy (for aerosol inhaler) and atropine hypersensitivity. **Use with caution** in narrow-angle glaucoma or bladder neck obstruction, though ipratropium has fewer anticholinergic systemic effects than atropine. May cause anxiety, dizziness, headache, GI discomfort, and cough with inhaler or nebulized use. Epistaxis, nasal congestion, and dry mouth/throat have been reported with the nasal spray. Reversible anisocoria may occur with unintentional aerosolization of drug to the eyes; particularly with mask nebulizers. Proven efficacy of nebulized solution in pediatrics is currently limited to reactive airway disease management in the emergency room and intensive care unit areas.

Bronchodilation onset of action is 1–3 min with peak effects within 1.5–2 hr and duration of action of 4–6 hr.

Shake inhaler well prior to use with spacer. Nebulized solution may be mixed with albuterol (or use DuoNeb).

Breast-feeding safety **extrapolated** from safety of atropine.

## IRON DEXTRAN

See *Iron—Injectable Preparations*

## IRON SUCROSE

See *Iron—Injectable Preparations*

## IRON—INJECTABLE PREPARATIONS

Ferric gluconate: Ferrlecit
Iron dextran: INFeD, DexFerrum
Iron sucrose: Venofer
***Parenteral iron***

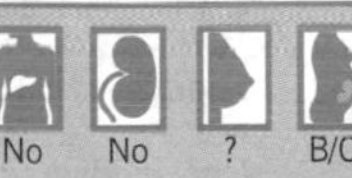


**Injection:**

Ferric gluconate (Ferrlecit): 62.5 mg/mL (12.5 mg elemental Fe/mL) (5 mL); contains 9 mg/mL benzyl alcohol and 20% sucrose
Iron dextran (INFeD, DexFerrum): 50 mg/mL (50 mg elemental Fe/mL) (1, 2 mL); products containing phenol 0.5% are only for IM administration; products containing sodium chloride 0.9% can be administered via the IM or IV route.
Iron sucrose (Venofer): 20 mg/mL (20 mg elemental Fe/mL) (5 mL); contains 300 mg/mL sucrose

***FERRIC GLUCONATE (IV):***

**Iron deficiency anemia in patents undergoing chronic hemodialysis who are receiving supplemental erythropoietin therapy (most require 8 doses at 8 sequential dialysis treatments to achieve a favorable response):**

***Child ≥ 6 yr:*** 1.5 mg/kg elemental Fe (0.12 mL/kg) IV; **max. dose:** 125 mg elemental Fe/dose. Dilute dose in 25 mL NS and infuse over 1 hr.
***Adult:*** 125 mg elemental Fe in 100 mL NS IV; infuse over 1 hr. Most require a minimum cumulative dose of 1 g elemental Fe administered over 8 sessions.

*Continued*

FORMULARY
For explanation of icons, see p. 698.

IRON—INJECTABLE PREPARATIONS *continued*

***IRON DEXTRAN (IV or IM):***

***Iron deficiency anemia:***

***Test dose:*** 25 mg (12.5 mg for infants) IV (over 5 min) or IM. May initiate treatment dose 1 hr after test dose.

Total replacement dose of iron dextran (mL) = 0.0476 × lean body wt (kg) × (desired Hgb [g/dL] – measured Hgb [g/dL]) + 1 mL per 5 kg lean body weight (up to **max.** of 14 mL).

***Acute blood loss:*** Total replacement dose of iron dextran (mL) = 0.02 × blood loss (mL) × hematocrit expressed as decimal fraction. Assumes 1 mL of RBC = 1 mg elemental iron.

If no reaction to test dose, give remainder of replacement dose ÷ over 2–3 daily doses.

**Max. daily (IM) dose:**

***<5 kg:*** 0.5 mL (25 mg)

***5–10 kg:*** 1 mL (50 mg)

***>10 kg:*** 2 mL (100 mg)

***IM administration:*** Use "Z-track" technique.

***IV administration:*** Dilute in NS at a **max.** concentration of 50 mg/mL and infuse over 1–6 hr at a **max.** rate of 50 mg/min.

***IRON SUCROSE (IV):***

***Iron deficiency anemia in patients with chronic kidney disease:***

***Child (limited data from 14 children with ESRD on hemodialysis):*** 1 mg/kg/dialysis was adequate for correcting ferritin levels and 0.3 mg/kg/dialysis was successful in maintaining ferritin levels between 193 and 250 mcg/L. Doses were administered during the last hr of each dialysis and are recommended at a frequency of 3 times a wk. A 10 mg test dose was administered.

***Adult:***

***Hemodialysis-dependent:*** 100 mg elemental Fe 1–3 times a wk during dialysis up to a total cumulative dose of 1000 mg. May continue to administer at lowest dose to maintain target Hb, Hct, and iron levels.

***Nonhemodialysis-dependent:*** 200 mg elemental Fe on 5 different days over a 2 wk period (total cumulative dose: 1000 mg).

***IV administration:*** May administer undiluted over 2–5 min. For an infusion, dilute each 100 mg with a **max.** of 100 mL NS and infuse over at least 15 min.

---

Oral therapy with iron salts is preferred, injectable routes are painful. Gluconate and sucrose salts may be better tolerated than iron dextran. Adverse effects include hypotension, GI disturbances, fever, rash, myalgia, arthralgias, cramps and headaches. Hypersensitivity reactions have been reported.

**IM administration is possible only with iron dextran salt.** Follow infusion recommendations for specific product. Monitor vital signs during IV infusion. TIBC levels may not be meaningful within 3 wk after dosing.

Pregnancy category is "B" for ferric gluconate and iron sucrose and "C" for iron dextran.

## IRON—ORAL PREPARATIONS

Fergon, Fer-In-Sol, Feosol, Niferex, Slow FE, and many others

***Oral iron supplements***

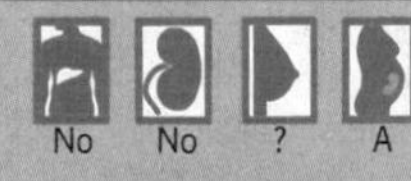


**Ferrous sulfate (20% elemental Fe):**

Drops (Fer-In-Sol, OTC): 75 mg (15 mg Fe)/0.6 mL (50 mL); contains 0.2% alcohol and sodium bisulfite
Elixir (OTC): 220 mg (44 mg Fe)/5 mL; contains 5% alcohol
Oral liquid (OTC): 300 mg (60 mg Fe)/5 mL
Tabs (OTC): 300 mg (60 mg Fe), 324 mg (65 mg Fe), 325 mg (65 mg Fe)

**Ferrous gluconate (12% elemental Fe):**

Tabs (OTC): 240 mg (27 mg Fe, as Fergon), 246 mg (28 mg Fe), 300 mg (34 mg Fe), 325 mg (36 mg Fe)

**Ferrous sulfate, exsiccated/dried (30% elemental Fe):**

Tabs (OTC): 200 mg (65 mg Fe)
Extended-release tabs (Slow FE, OTC): 160 mg (50 mg Fe)

**Ferrous fumarate (33% elemental Fe):**

Tabs (OTC): 90 mg (29.5 mg Fe), 200 mg (66 mg Fe), 324 mg (106 mg Fe), 325 mg (106 mg Fe), 350 mg (115 mg Fe)
Chewable tabs: 100 mg (33 mg Fe)
Timed-release tabs (OTC): 150 mg (50 mg Fe)

**Polysaccharide-iron complex and ferrous bis-glycinate chelate (Niferex) (expressed in mg elemental Fe):**

Caps (OTC): 60, 150 mg; 150 mg strength contains 50 mg vitamin C
Elixir (OTC): 100 mg/5 mL (237 mL); contains 10% alcohol

---

***Iron deficiency anemia:***

***Premature infant:*** 2–4 mg elemental Fe/kg/24 hr ÷ QD–BID PO; **max. dose:** 15 mg elemental Fe/24 hr
***Child:*** 3–6 mg elemental Fe/kg/24 hr ÷ QD–TID PO
***Adult:*** 60–100 mg elemental Fe BID PO up to 60 mg elemental Fe QID

***Prophylaxis:***

***Child:*** Give dose below PO ÷ QD–TID
***Premature:*** 2 mg elemental Fe/kg/24 hr; **max. dose:** 15 mg elemental Fe/24 hr
***Full-term:*** 1–2 mg elemental Fe/kg/24 hr; **max. dose:** 15 mg elemental Fe/24 hr
***Adult:*** 60–100 mg elemental Fe/24 hr PO ÷ QD–BID

---

**Contraindicated** in hemolytic anemia and hemochromatosis. **Avoid** use in GI tract inflammation.

Iron preparations are variably absorbed. Less GI irritation when given with or after meals. Vitamin C, 200 mg per 30 mg iron, may enhance absorption. Liquid iron preparations may stain teeth. Give with dropper or drink through straw. May produce constipation, dark stools (false positive guaiac is controversial), nausea, and epigastric pain. Iron and tetracycline inhibit each other's absorption. Antacids may decrease iron absorption.

FORMULARY

For explanation of icons, see p. 698.

## ISONIAZID

INH, Nydrazid, Laniazid, and others

***Antituberculous agent***

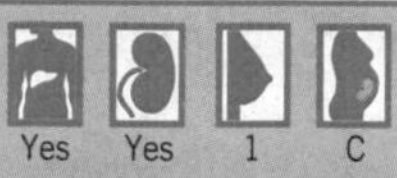


**Tabs:** 100, 300 mg
**Syrup:** 50 mg/5 mL (473 mL)
**Injection:** 100 mg/mL (10 mL); contains 0.25% chlorobutanol

See most recent edition of the AAP *Red Book* for details and length of therapy.

***Prophylaxis:***

***Infant and child:*** 10 mg/kg (**max. dose:** 300 mg) PO QD. After 1 mo of daily therapy and in cases where daily compliance cannot be assured, may change to 20–40 mg/kg (**max. dose:** 900 mg) per dose PO, given twice weekly.

***Adult:*** 300 mg PO QD

***Treatment:***

***Infant and child:*** 10–15 mg/kg (**max. dose:** 300 mg) PO QD or 20–30 mg/kg (**max. dose:** 900 mg) per dose twice weekly with rifampin for uncomplicated pulmonary tuberculosis in compliant patients. Additional drugs are necessary in complicated disease.

***Adult:*** 5 mg/kg (**max. dose:** 300 mg) PO QD or 15 mg/kg (**max. dose:** 900 mg) per dose twice weekly with rifampin. Additional drugs are necessary in complicated disease.

***For INH-resistant TB:*** Discuss with Health Dept., or consult ID specialist.

**Should not be used alone for treatment. Contraindicated** in acute liver disease and previous isoniazid-associated hepatitis. Peripheral neuropathy, optic neuritis, seizures, encephalopathy, psychosis, hepatic side effects may occur with higher doses, especially in combination with rifampin. Follow LFTs monthly. Supplemental pyridoxine (1–2 mg/kg/24 hr) is recommended. May cause false-positive urine glucose test.

Inhibits CYP 450 1A2, 2C9, 2C19, and 3A3/4 microsomal enzymes; decrease dose of carbamazepine, diazepam, phenytoin, and prednisone. Prednisone may decrease isoniazid's effects. Also a substrate and inducer of CYP 450 2E1 and may potentiate acetaminophen hepatotoxicity.

May be given IM (same as oral doses) when oral therapy is not possible. Administer oral doses 1 hr prior to and 2 hr after meals. Aluminum salts may decrease absorption. **Adjust dose in renal failure (see Chapter 31).**

## ISOPROTERENOL

Isuprel and other generics

***Adrenergic agonist***

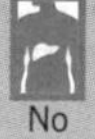
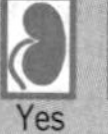
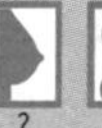
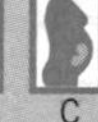

No Yes ? C

**Isoproterenol HCl:**

Injection, prefilled syringes: 0.02 mg/mL (10 mL); contains sulfites
Injection: 0.2 mg/mL (1, 5, 10 mL); contains sulfites

*Continued*

ISOPROTERENOL *continued*

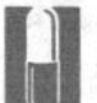

**NOTE: The dosage units for adults are in mcg/min, compared to mcg/kg/min for children.**
***IV infusion:***
***Neonate–child:*** 0.05–2 mcg/kg/min; start at minimum dose and increase every 5–10 min by 0.1 mcg/kg/min until desired effect or onset of toxicity; **max. dose:** 2 mcg/kg/min.
***Adult:*** 2–20 mcg/min.

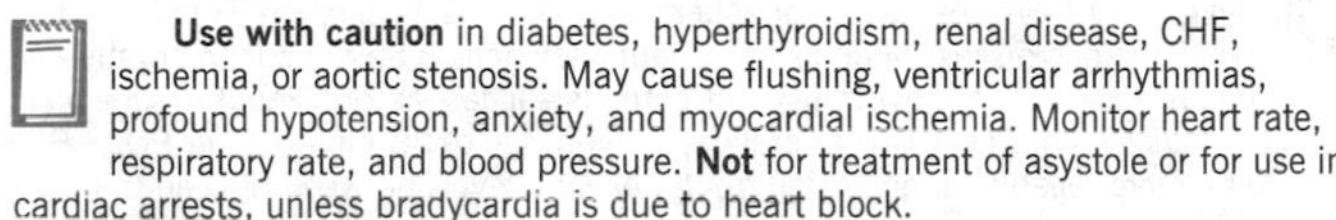

**Use with caution** in diabetes, hyperthyroidism, renal disease, CHF, ischemia, or aortic stenosis. May cause flushing, ventricular arrhythmias, profound hypotension, anxiety, and myocardial ischemia. Monitor heart rate, respiratory rate, and blood pressure. **Not** for treatment of asystole or for use in cardiac arrests, unless bradycardia is due to heart block.

Continuous infusion for bronchodilatation must be gradually tapered over a 24–48 hr period to prevent rebound bronchospasm. Tolerance may occur with prolonged use. Clinical deterioration, myocardial necrosis, congestive heart failure and **death** have been reported with continuous infusion use in refractory asthmatic children.

## ISOTRETINOIN

Accutane, Amnesteem, Claravis, Sotret
***Retinoic acid, vitamin A derivative***

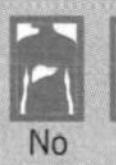 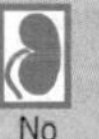 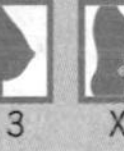

No No 3 X

**Caps:** 10, 20, 30, 40 mg, may contain soybean oil, EDTA, and parabens

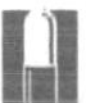

***Cystic acne:***
***Child and adult:*** 0.5–2 mg/kg/24 hr ÷ BID PO × 15–20 wk
Dosages as low as 0.05 mg/kg/24 hr have been reported to be beneficial.

**Contraindicated during pregnancy; known teratogen. Use with caution** in females during childbearing years. May cause conjunctivitis, xerosis, pruritus, photosensitivity reactions (**avoid** expose to sunlight and use sunscreen), epistaxis, anemia, hyperlipidemia, pseudotumor cerebri (especially in combination with tetracyclines, **avoid** this combination), cheilitis, bone pain, muscle aches, skeletal changes, lethargy, nausea, vomiting, elevated ESR, mental depression, aggressive/violent behavior, and psychosis.

To **avoid** additive toxic effects, **do not** take vitamin A concomitantly. Increases clearance of carbamazepine. Hormonal birth control (oral, injectable, and implantable) failures have been reported with concurrent use. Monitor CBC, ESR, triglycerides, and LFTs.

Prescribers, site pharmacists, patients, and wholesalers must register with the iPLEDGE system (a risk minimization program) at www.ipledgeprogram.com or 1-866-495-0654 before doses are dispensed. Prescriptions may not be written for more than a 1 mo supply.



For explanation of icons, see p. 698.

## ITRACONAZOLE

Sporanox

***Antifungal agent***

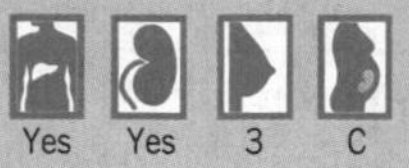


**Caps:** 100 mg
**Oral solution:** 10 mg/mL (150 mL); contains sacharin and sorbitol

***Child (limited data):*** 3–5 mg/kg/24 hr PO ÷ QD-BID; dosages as high as 5–10 mg/kg/24 hr have been used for aspergillus prophylaxis in chronic granulomatous disease. Population pharmacokinetic data in pediatric cystic fibrosis and bone marrow transplant patients suggest an oral liquid dosage of 10 mg/kg/24 hr PO ÷ BID or oral capsule dosage of 20 mg/kg/24 hr PO ÷ BID to be more reliable for achieving trough plasma levels between 500 and 2000 ng/mL.

***Prophylaxis for recurrence of opportunistic disease in HIV:***

***Cryptococcus neoformans:*** 2–5 mg/kg/dose PO Q12–24 hr

***Histoplasma capsulatum or Coccidioides immitis:*** 2–5 mg/kg/dose PO Q12–48 hr

***Adult:***

***Blastomycosis and nonmeningeal histoplasmosis:***

***PO:*** 200 mg QD up to a **max. dose** of 400 mg/24 hr ÷ BID (**max. dose:** 200 mg/dose)

***IV:*** 400 mg/24 hr ÷ BID × 2 days, followed by 200 mg QD; switch to oral therapy as soon as possible.

***Aspergillosis and severe infections:***

***PO:*** 600 mg/24 hr ÷ TID × 3–4 days, followed by 200–400 mg/24 hr ÷ BID; **max. dose:** 600 mg/24 hr ÷ TID.

***IV:*** 400 mg/24 hr ÷ BID × 2 days, followed by 200 mg QD; switch to oral therapy as soon as possible

***Empiric therapy in febrile, neutropenic patients:*** 400 mg/24 hr IV ÷ BID × 2 days, followed by 200 mg QD for up to 14 days; continue with the oral solution at 200 mg PO BID until resolution.

Oral solution and capsule dosage form should **NOT** be used interchangeably; oral solution is more bioavailable. Only the oral solution has been demonstrated effective for oral and/or esophageal candidasis. **Use with caution** in hepatic impairment. May cause GI symptoms, headaches, rash, liver enzyme elevation, hepatitis, and hypokalemia.

Like ketoconazole, it inhibits the activity of the CYP 450 3A4 drug metabolizing isoenzyme. Thus the coadministration of cisapride, dofetilide, pimozide, quinidine, triazolam, lovastatin, simvastatin, ergot derivatives, and oral midazolam is **contraindicated**. See remarks in *Ketoconazole* for additional drug interaction information.

Steady-state trough serum concentrations of > 250 ng/mL itraconazole and > 1000 ng/mL hydroxyitraconazole (metabolite) have been recommended. Recommended serum sampling time at steady-state: Trough level after 2 wk of continuous dosing.

IV dosage form should **not** be used in patients with GFR < 30 mL/min because the hydoxypropyl-beta-cyclodextrin excipient has reduced clearance in patients with renal failure. IV form should be diluted with NS (**not** compatible with $D_5W$ or LR) and infused over 1 hr.

Administer oral solution on an empty stomach, but administer capsules with food. Achlorhydria reduces absorption of the drug.

## KANAMYCIN

Kantrex and others

***Antibiotic, aminoglycoside***

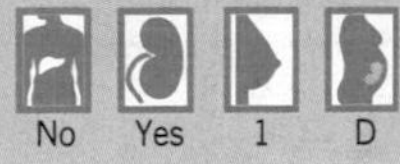


**Caps:** 500 mg
**Injection:** 37.5, 250, 333, 500 mg/mL; may contain sulfites

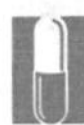

***Neonate IV/IM administration (see following table):***

| Birth Weight (kg) | <7 Days | ≥7 Days |
|---|---|---|
| <2 | 15 mg/kg/ 24 hr ÷ Q12 hr | 22.5 mg/kg/ 24 hr ÷ Q8 hr |
| ≥2 | 20 mg/kg/ 24 hr ÷ Q12 hr | 30 mg/kg/ 24 hr ÷ Q8 hr |

***Infant and child:*** IM/IV: 15–30 mg/kg/24 hr ÷ Q8–12 hr
***Adult:*** IV/IM: 15 mg/kg/24 hr ÷ Q8–12 hr
***PO administration for GI bacterial overgrowth:*** 150–250 mg/kg/24 hr ÷ Q6 hr; **max. dose:** 4 g/24 hr

Renal toxicity and ototoxicity may occur. Give over 30 min if IV route is used. **Use with caution** in neuromuscular disorders, anesthesia and muscle-relaxant medications and hypermagnesemia. **Adjust dose in renal failure (see Chapter 31).** Poorly absorbed orally, PO used to treat GI bacterial overgrowth. Oral route is **contraindicated** in intestinal obstructions.

Therapeutic levels: peak: 15–30 mg/L; trough: <5–10 mg/L. Recommended serum sampling time at steady-state: trough within 30 min prior to the 3rd consecutive dose and peak 30–60 min after the administration of the 3rd consecutive dose.

## KETAMINE

Ketalar and various generics

***General anesthetic***

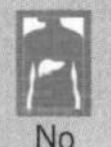

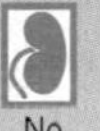

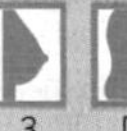


**Injection:** 10 mg/mL (20 mL), 50 mg/mL (10 mL), 100 mg/mL (5 mL); contains benzethonium chloride

***Child:***
***Sedation:***
- ***PO:*** 5 mg/kg × 1
- ***IV (see remarks):*** 0.25–0.5 mg/kg
- ***IM:*** 1.5–2 mg/kg × 1

***Adult:***
***Analgesia with sedation:***
- ***IV (see remarks):*** 0.2–1 mg/kg
- ***IM:*** 0.5–4 mg/kg

*Continued*

For explanation of icons, see p. 698.

KETAMINE *continued*

**Contraindicated** in elevated ICP, hypertension, aneurysms, thyrotoxicosis, CHF, angina, and psychotic disorders. May cause hypertension, hypotension, emergence reactions, tachycardia, laryngospasm, respiratory depression, and stimulation of salivary secretions. Intravenous use may induce general anesthesia. Benzodiazepine may be added to prevent emergence phenomenon. Anticholinergic agent may be added to decrease hypersalivation. Rate of IV infusion **should not exceed** 0.5 mg/kg/min and should **not be administered** in less than 60 sec. For additional information including onset and duration of action, see Chapter 6, Table 6-10.

## KETOCONAZOLE

Nizoral, Nizoral A-D and others

***Antifungal agent, imidazole***

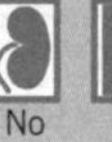
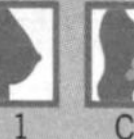

No No 1 C

**Tabs:** 200 mg
**Oral suspension:** 100 mg/5 mL
**Cream:** 2% (15, 30, 60 g); contains sulfites
**Shampoo:** 1% [Nizoral A-D, OTC] (120, 210 mL), 2% (120 mL)

***Oral:***
***Child ≥ 2 yr:*** 3.3–6.6 mg/kg/24 hr QD
***Adult:*** 200–400 mg/24 hr QD
**Max. dose:** 800 mg/24 hr ÷ BID
***Topical:*** 1–2 applications/24 hr
***Shampoo:*** Twice weekly for 4 wk with at least 3 days between applications; intermittently as needed to maintain control.
***Suppressive therapy against mucocutaneous candidiasis in HIV:***
***Child:*** 5–10 mg/kg/24 hr ÷ QD-BID PO; **max. dose:** 800 mg/24 hr ÷ BID
***Adolescent and adult:*** 200 mg/dose QD PO

Monitor LFTs in long-term use. Drugs that decrease gastric acidity will decrease absorption. May cause nausea, vomiting, rash, headache, pruritus, and fever. Inhibits CYP 450 3A4. **Contraindicated** when used with cisapride, quinidine, terfinadine, and pimozide because of risk for cardiac arrhythmias. May increase levels/effects of phenytoin, digoxin, cyclosporine, corticosteroids, nevirapine, protease inhibitors, and warfarin. Achlorhydria, phenobarbital, rifampin, isoniazid, $H_2$ blockers, antacids, and omeprazole can decrease levels of ketoconazole.

Administering oral doses with food or acidic beverages and 2 hr prior to antacids will increase absorption.

To use shampoo, wet hair and scalp with water, apply sufficient amount to scalp and gently massage for about 1 min. Rinse hair thoroughly, reapply shampoo and leave on the scalp for an additional 3 min; then rinse.

## KETOROLAC

Many generics (previously available as Toradol), Acular, Acular LS, Acular PF

***Nonsteroidal anti-inflammatory agent***

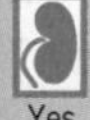
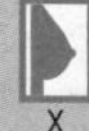
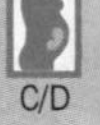

Yes Yes X C/D

**Injection:** 15 mg/mL (1 mL), 30 mg/mL (1, 2 mL); contains 10% alcohol
**Tabs:** 10 mg

*Continued*

KETOROLAC *continued*

**Ophthalmic:**
Acular: 0.5% (3, 5, 10 mL); contains benzalkonium chloride
Acular PF: 0.5% (0.4 mL); preservative-free
Acular LS: 0.4% (5 mL); contains benzalkonium chloride

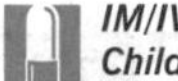

***IM/IV:***
***Child:*** 0.5 mg/kg/dose IM/IV Q6 hr. **Max. dose:** 30 mg Q6 hr or 120 mg/24 hr
***Adult:*** 30 mg IM/IV Q6 hr. **Max. dose:** 120 mg/24 hr

***PO:***
***Child >50 kg and adult:*** 10 mg PRN Q6 hr; **max. dose:** 40 mg/24 hr

***Ophthalmic (see remarks):***
***≥3 yr–adult:*** 1 drop in each affected eye QID

**Ketorolac therapy is not to exceed 5 days (IM, IV, PO).** May cause GI bleeding, nausea, dyspepsia, drowsiness, decreased platelet function, and interstitial nephritis. **Not recommended** in patients at increased risk of bleeding. **Do not use** in hepatic or renal failure. **Use with caution** in heart disease (risk for MI and stroke with prolonged use).

Use Acular PF for incisional refractive surgery and Acular LS for corneal refractive surgery. Duration of therapy for ophthalmic use: 14 days after cataracts surgery; up to 4 days after corneal refractive surgery; and up to 3 days after incisional refractive surgery.

Pregnancy category changes to "D" if used in the third trimester.

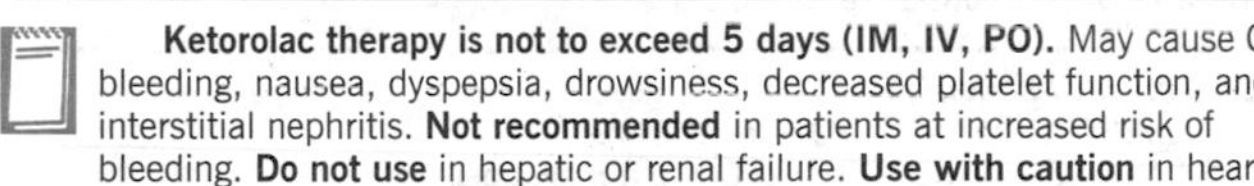

## LABETALOL
Normodyne, Trandate, and various generics
***Adrenergic antagonist (alpha and beta), antihypertensive***

Yes | No | 1 | C/D

**Tabs:** 100, 200, 300 mg
**Injection:** 5 mg/mL (20, 40 mL); contains parabens
**Oral suspension:** 10, 40 mg/mL

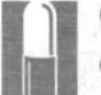

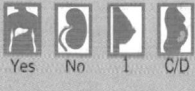

***Child:***
***PO:*** Initial: 4 mg/kg/24 hr ÷ BID. May increase up to 40 mg/kg/24 hr
***IV:*** Hypertensive emergency (start at lowest dose and titrate to effect; see Chapter 4):
***Intermittent dose:*** 0.2–1 mg/kg/dose Q10 min PRN; **max. dose:** 20 mg/dose
***Infusion (hypertensive emergencies):*** 0.4–1 mg/kg/hr, to a **max. dose** of 3 mg/kg/hr; may initiate with a 0.2–1 mg/kg bolus; **max. bolus:** 20 mg.

***Adult:***
***PO:*** 100 mg BID, increase by 100 mg/dose Q2–3 days PRN to a **max. dose** of 2.4 g/24 hr. Usual range: 200–800 mg/24hr ÷ BID
***IV:*** Hypertensive emergency (start at lowest dose and titrate to effect):
***Intermittent dose:*** 20–80 mg/dose (begin with 20 mg) Q10 min PRN; **max. dose:** 300 mg total dose
***Infusion:*** 2 mg/min, increase to titrate to response.

**Contraindicated** in asthma, pulmonary edema, cardiogenic shock, and heart block. May cause orthostatic hypotension, edema, CHF, bradycardia, AV conduction disturbances, bronchospasm, urinary retention, and skin tingling. **Use with caution** in hepatic disease (dose reduction may be necessary);

*Continued*



For explanation of icons, see p. 698.

LABETALOL *continued*

diabetes, liver function test elevation, hepatic necrosis, hepatitis, and cholestatic jaundice have been reported.

Patient should remain supine for up to 3 hr after IV administration. Pregnancy category changes to "D" if used in second or third trimesters.

Onset of action: PO: 1–4 hr; IV: 5–15 min.

## LACTULOSE

Cephulac, Chronulac, Enuloase, and other generics

***Ammonium detoxicant, hyperosmotic laxative***

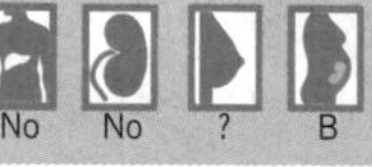


**Syrup:** 10 g/15 mL (30, 237, 473, 960, 1893 mL); contains galactose, lactose, and other sugars

**Crystals for reconstitution:** 10 g (30s), 20 g (30s)

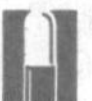

***Chronic constipation:***

- ***Child:*** 7.5 mL/24 hr PO after breakfast
- ***Adult:*** 15–30 mL/24 hr PO QD to a **max. dose** of 60 mL/24 hr.

***Portal systemic encephalopathy (adjust dose to produce 2–3 soft stools/day):***

- ***Infant:*** 2.5–10 mL/24 hr PO ÷ TID–QID
- ***Child:*** 40–90 mL/24 hr PO ÷ TID–QID
- ***Adult:*** 30–45 mL/dose PO TID–QID; acute episodes 30–45 mL Q1–2 hr until 2–3 soft stools/day
- ***Rectal (adult):*** 300 mL diluted in 700 mL water or NS in 30–60 min retention enema; may give Q4–6 hr

**Contraindicated** in galactosemia. **Use with caution** in diabetes mellitus. GI discomfort and diarrhea may occur. For portal systemic encephalopathy, monitor serum ammonia, serum potassium, and fluid status.

Adjust dose to achieve 2–3 soft stools per day. **Do not use** with antacids. Dissolve crystal dosage form with 4 ounces of water or juice. All doses may be administered with juice, milk, or water.

## LAMIVUDINE

Epivir, Epivir-HBV, 3TC

***Antiviral agent, nucleoside analogue reverse transcriptase inhibitor***

Yes Yes 3 C

**Tabs:** 100 mg (Epivir-HBV), 150, 300 mg

**Oral solution:** 5 mg/mL (Epivir-HBV), 10 mg/mL; contains parabens

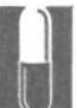

***HIV:*** See www.aidsinfo.nih.gov/guidelines.

***Chronic hepatitis B (see remarks):***

- ***2–17 yr:*** 3 mg/kg/dose PO QD up to a **max. dose** of 100 mg/dose
- ***Adult:*** 100 mg/dose PO QD

See aidsinfo.nih.gov/guidelines for remarks for use in HIV.

May cause headache, fatigue, GI disturbances, rash, and myalgia/arthralgia. Lactic acidosis, severe hepatomegaly with steatosis, post-treatment exacerbations of hepatitis B and ALT elevations, pancreatitis, and emergence of resistant viral strains have been reported. Concomitant use with cotrimoxazole (TMP/SMX) may result in increase lamivudine levels.

*Continued*

LAMIVUDINE *continued*

**Use Epivir-HBV product for chronic hepatitis B indication.** Safety and effectiveness beyond 1 yr have not been determined. Patients with both HIV and hepatitis B should use the higher HIV doses along with an appropriate combination regimen.

May be administered with food. **Adjust dose in renal impairment (see Chapter 31).**

## LAMOTRIGINE

Lamictal

***Anticonvulsant***

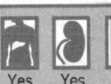

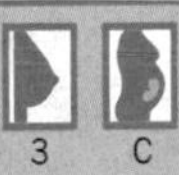


**Chewable tabs:** 2, 5, 25 mg
**Tabs:** 25, 100, 150, 200 mg
**Oral suspension:** 1 mg/mL

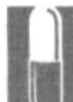

***Child 2–12 yr adjunctive therapy (see remarks):***
***WITH anti-epileptic drugs (AEDs) other than carbamazepine, phenytoin, phenobarbital, primidone, or valproic acid:***

***Wk 1 and 2:*** 0.3 mg/kg/24 hr PO ÷ BID; rounded down to the nearest whole tablet.

***Wk 3 and 4:*** 0.6 mg/kg/24 hr PO ÷ BID; rounded down to the nearest whole tablet.

***Usual maintenance dose:*** 4.5–7.5 mg/kg/24 hr PO ÷ BID titrate to effect; to achieve the usual maintenance dose, increase doses Q1–2 wk by 0.6 mg/kg/24 hr (rounded down to the nearest whole tablet) as needed.

**Max. dose:** 300 mg/24 hr ÷ BID.

***WITH enzyme-inducing AEDs WITHOUT valproic acid:***

***Wk 1 and 2:*** 0.6 mg/kg/24 hr PO ÷ BID; rounded down to the nearest whole tablet.

***Wk 3 and 4:*** 1.2 mg/kg/24 hr PO ÷ BID; rounded down to the nearest whole tablet.

***Usual maintenance dose:*** 5–15 mg/kg/24 hr PO ÷ BID titrate to effect; to achieve the usual maintenance dose, increase doses Q1–2 wk by 1.2 mg/kg/24 hr (rounded down to the nearest whole tablet) as needed.

**Max. dose:** 400 mg/24 hr ÷ BID.

***WITH AEDs WITH valproic acid:***

***Wk 1 and 2:*** 0.15 mg/kg/24 hr PO ÷ QD–BID; rounded down to the nearest whole tablet (see following table)

***Wk 3 and 4:*** 0.3 mg/kg/24 hr PO ÷ QD–BID; rounded down to the nearest whole tablet (see following table)

| Weight (kg) | Weeks 1 and 2 | Weeks 3 and 4 |
|---|---|---|
| 6.7–14 | 2 mg QOD | 2 mg QD |
| 14.1–27 | 2 mg QD | 4 mg/24 hr ÷ QD–BID |
| 27.1–34 | 4 mg/24 hr ÷ QD–BID | 8 mg/24 hr ÷ QD–BID |
| 34.1–40 | 5 mg QD | 10 mg/24 hr ÷ QD–BID |

*Continued*

For explanation of icons, see p. 698.

LAMOTRIGINE *continued*

***Child 2–12 yr adjunctive therapy (cont'd):***

***WITH AEDs WITH valproic acid (cont'd):***

***Usual maintenance dose:*** 1–5 mg/kg/24 hr PO ÷ QD-BID titrate to effect; to achieve the usual maintenance dose, increase doses Q1–2 wk by 0.3 mg/kg/24 hr (rounded down to the nearest whole tablet) as needed. If adding lamotrigine with valproic acid alone, usual maintenance dose is 1–3 mg/kg/24 hr.

**Max. dose:** 200 mg/24 hr.

***>12 yr and adult adjunctive therapy:***

***WITH AEDs other than carbamazepine, phenytoin, phenobarbital, primidone, or valproic acid:***

***Wk 1 and 2:*** 25 mg QD PO

***Wk 3 and 4:*** 50 mg QD PO

***Usual maintenance dose:*** 225–375 mg/24 hr ÷ BID PO titrate to effect; to achieve the usual maintenance dose, increase doses Q1–2 wk by 50 mg/24 hr as needed.

***WITH enzyme-inducing AEDs WITHOUT valproic acid:***

***Wk 1 and 2:*** 50 mg QD PO

***Wk 3 and 4:*** 50 mg BID PO

***Usual maintenance dose:*** 300–500 mg/24 hr ÷ BID PO titrate to effect; to achieve the usual maintenance dose, increase doses Q1–2 wk by 100 mg/24 hr as needed. Doses as high as 700 mg/24 hr ÷ BID have been used.

***WITH AEDs WITH valproic acid:***

***Wk 1 and 2:*** 25 mg QOD PO

***Wk 3 and 4:*** 25 mg QD PO

***Usual maintenance dose:*** 100–400 mg/24 hr ÷ QD-BID PO titrate to effect; to achieve the usual maintenance dose, increase doses Q1–2 wk by 25–50 mg/24 hr as needed. If adding lamotrigine to valproic acid alone, usual maintenance dose is 100–200 mg/kg/24 hr.

***Converting from a single enzyme-inducing AED to lamotrigine monotherapy for child ≥ 16 yr and adult (titrate lamotrigine to maintenance dose; then gradually withdraw enzyme-inducing AED by 20% decrements over a 4-wk period):***

***Wk 1 and 2:*** 50 mg QD PO

***Wk 3 and 4:*** 50 mg BID PO

***Usual maintenance dose:*** 500 mg/24 hr ÷ BID PO titrate to effect; to achieve the usual maintenance dose, increase doses Q1–2 wk by 100 mg/24 hr as needed.

***Bipolar disease:***

***≥18 yr and adult (see table on next page):***

---

Enzyme-inducing anti-epileptic drugs (AEDs) include carbamazepine, phenytoin, and phenobarbital. Stevens-Johnson syndrome, toxic epidermal necrolysis, and other potentially life-threatening rashes have been reported in children (0.8%) and adults (0.3%) for adjunctive therapy in seizures. Reported rates for adults treated for bipolar/mood disorders as monotherapy and adjunctive therapy are 0.08% and 0.13%, respectively. May cause fatigue, drowsiness, ataxia, rash (especially with valproic acid), headache, nausea, vomiting, and abdominal pain. Diplopia, nystagmus, and alopecia have also been reported. Use during the first 3 mo of pregnancy may result in a higher chance for cleft lip or cleft palate in the newborn. Suicidal behavior or ideation has been reported.

*Continued*

LAMOTRIGINE *continued*

| | Weeks 1 and 2 | Weeks 3 and 4 | Week 5 | Week 6 and thereafter |
|---|---|---|---|---|
| Patient NOT receiving enzyme-inducing drugs (e.g., carbamazepine) OR valproic acid | 25 mg/24 hr PO | 50 mg/24 hr PO | 100 mg/24 hr PO | 200 mg/24 hr PO (target dose) |
| Patents receiving enzyme-inducing drugs (e.g., carbamazepine) WITHOUT valproic acid | 50 mg/24 hr PO | 100 mg/24 hr PO ÷ QD–BID | 200 mg/24 hr PO ÷ QD–BID | Wk 6: 300 mg/24 hr PO ÷ QD–BID<br>Wk 7 and thereafter: may increase to 400 mg/24 hr PO ÷ QD–BID (target dose)* |
| Patients receiving valproic acid | 25 mg QOD PO | 25 mg/24 hr PO | 50 mg/24 hr PO | 100 mg/24 hr PO (target dose)† |

*If carbamazepine or other enzyme-inducing drug is discontinued, maintain current lamotrigine dose for 1 wk, then decrease daily lamotrigine dose in 100 mg increments at weekly intervals until 200 mg/24 hr.

†If valproic acid is discontinued, increase lamotrigine by 50 mg weekly intervals up to 200 mg/24 hr.

Reduce maintenance dose in renal failure. Reduce all doses (initial, escalation, and maintenance) in liver dysfunction defined by the Child-Pugh grading system as follows:

*Grade B:* moderate dysfunction, decrease dose by ~50%
*Grade C:* severe dysfunction, decrease dose by ~75%

Withdrawal symptoms may occur if discontinued suddenly. A stepwise dose reduction over ≥ 2 wk (~50% per wk) is recommended unless safety concerns require a more rapid withdrawal.

Acetaminophen, carbamazepine, oral contraceptives (ethinylestradiol), phenobarbital, primidone, phenytoin, and rifampin may decrease levels of lamotrigine. Valproic acid may increase levels.

## LANSOPRAZOLE

Prevacid

***Gastric acid pump inhibitor***

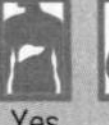
Yes
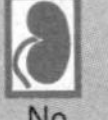
No

?
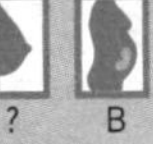
B

**Caps, delayed-release:** 15, 30 mg
**Tabs, disintegrating delayed-release:** 15, 30 mg; contains aspartame
**Granules for delayed-release oral suspension:** 15, 30 mg packets (30s)
**Oral suspension:** 3 mg/mL ; contains ~0.3 mEq sodium bicarbonate per 1 mg drug
**Injection:** 30 mg; contains 60 mg mannitol

*Continued*

For explanation of icons, see p. 698.

LANSOPRAZOLE *continued*

***1–11 yr (short-term treatment of GERD and erosive esophagitis, for up to 8 wk):***
***<10 kg:*** 7.5 mg PO QD
***11–30 kg:*** 15 mg PO QD–BID; dosage may be increased to 30 mg PO BID after ≥ 2 wk of therapy without response at a lower dose
***>30 kg:*** 30 mg PO QD–BID

***12 yr–adult:***
***GERD:*** 15 mg PO QD for up to 8 wk
***Erosive esophagitis:***
***PO:*** 30 mg QD × 8–16 wk; maintenance dose: 15 mg PO QD
***IV:*** 30 mg QD for up to 7 days and convert to PO as soon as possible.
***Duodenal ulcer:*** 15 mg PO QD × 4 wk
***Gastric ulcer:*** 30 mg PO QD for up to 8 wk
***Hypersecretory conditions:*** 60 mg PO QD; dosage may be increased up to 90 mg PO BID.

Common side effects include GI discomfort, headache, fatigue, rash, and taste perversion. Microscopic colitis resulting in watery diarrhea has been reported and switching to an alternative proton-pump inhibitor may be beneficial in resolving diarrhea.

Drug is a substrate for CYP 450 2C19 and 3A3/4. May decrease absorption of itraconazole, ketoconazole, iron salts and ampicillin esters; and increase the effects of warfarin. Theophylline clearance may be enhanced. Reduce dose in severe hepatic impairment. May be used in combination with clarithromycin and amoxicillin for *H. pylori* infections.

Administer all oral doses before meals and 30 min prior to sucralfate. **Do not** crush or chew the granules (all dosage forms). Capsule may be opened and intact granules may be administered in an acidic beverage (e.g., apple or cranberry juice) or apple sauce. The extemporaneously compounded oral suspension may be less bioavailable owing to the loss of the enteric coating. For IV use, use a 1.2 micron in-line filter.

## LEVALBUTEROL

Xopenex, Xopenex HFA
***Beta-2 adrenergic agonist***

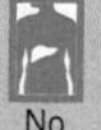
No
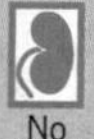
No
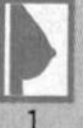
1
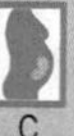
C

**Prediluted nebulized solution:** 0.31 mg in 3 mL, 0.63 mg in 3 mL, 1.25 mg in 3 mL (24s)
**Concentrated nebulized solution:** 1.25 mg/0.5 mL (0.5 mL)
**Aerosol inhaler (MDI; Xopenex HFA):** 45 mcg/actuation (15 g delivers 200 doses)

***Nebulizer:***
***<6 yr:*** See remarks.
***6–11 yr:*** Start at 0.31 mg inhaled TID (Q6–8 hr) PRN; dose may be increased to 0.63 mg TID PRN
***≥12 yr and adult:*** Start at 0.63 mg inhaled TID (Q6–8 hr) PRN; dose may be increased to 1.25 mg inhaled TID PRN

***Aerosol inhaler (MDI):***
***≥4 yr and adult:*** 1–2 puffs Q4–6 hr PRN.

For use in acute exacerbations, more aggressive dosing may be employed.

*Continued*

LEVALBUTEROL *continued*

R-isomer of racemic albuterol. Side effects include tachycardia, palpitations, tremor, insomnia, nervousness, nausea, and headache.

Current clinical data in children indicate levalbuterol is as effective as albuterol with fewer cardiac side effects at equi-potent doses (0.31–0.63 mg levalbuterol ~ 2.5 mg albuterol). Limited data from a single dose, randomized, double blind crossover study in children 2–11 yr indicate that 0.16–1.25-mg inhalations were used safely with clinical improvement.

More frequent dosing may be necessary in asthma exacerbation.

## LEVETIRACETAM

Keppra

***Anticonvulsant***

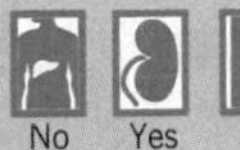
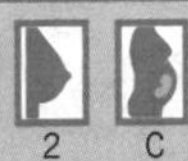

No Yes 2 C

**Tabs:** 250, 500, 750, 1000 mg
**Oral solution:** 100 mg/mL (480 mL); dye free and contains parabens
**Injection:** 100 mg/mL (5 mL); contains 45 mg sodium chloride and 8.2 mg sodium acetate trihydrate per 100 mg drug

***Partial seizures (adjunctive therapy):***
***Child 4–15 yr:*** Start at 10 mg/kg/dose PO BID; may increase by 10 mg/kg/dose BID every 2 wk as tolerated up to a **max. dose** of 30 mg/kg/dose BID.
***16 yr–adult:*** Start at 500 mg PO BID; may increase by 500 mg/dose BID every 2 wk as tolerated up to a **max. dose** of 1500 mg BID.
***Myoclonic seizure (adjunctive therapy):***
***≥12 yr and adult:*** Start at 500 mg PO BID; then increase dosage by 500 mg/dose BID every 2 wk to the reach the target dosage of 1500 mg BID.
***Tonic-clonic seizure (primary generalized, adjunctive therapy):***
***Child 6–15 yr:*** Start at 10 mg/kg/dose PO BID; may increase by 10 mg/kg/dose BID every 2 wk to reach the target dosage of 30 mg/kg/dose BID.
***16 yr–adult:*** Start at 500 mg PO BID; then increase dosage by 500 mg/dose BID every 2 wk to reach the target dosage of 1500 mg BID.
***Refractory seizures (add-on therapy; data limited to):*** See remarks.

**Do not** abruptly withdraw therapy to reduce risk for seizures. **Use with caution** in renal impairment **(reduce dose; see Chapter 31)**, hemodialysis, and neuropsychiatric conditions.

May cause loss of appetite, vomiting, dizziness, headaches, somnolence, agitation, depression and mood swings. Drowsiness, fatigue, nervousness and aggressive behavior have been reported in children. Suicidal behavior or ideation, and hematologic abnormalities have been reported. Levetiracetam may decrease carbamazepine's effects. Ginkgo may decrease levetiracetam's effects.

Use in children 6 mo–4 yr has been reported in refractory seizures of various types and as an add-on therapy. The following dosage has been used: Start at 5–10 mg/kg/24 hr PO ÷ BID-TID; if needed and tolerated, increase dose by 10 mg/kg/24 hr at weekly intervals up to a **max. dose** of 60 mg/kg/24 hr.

Drug has excellent PO absorption. For IV use, use similar PO dosages only when the oral route of administration is not feasible.

For explanation of icons, see p. 698.

## LEVOFLOXACIN

Levaquin, Quixin, Iquix

***Antibiotic, quinolone***

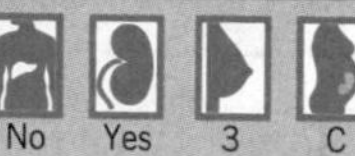


**Tabs:** 250, 500, 750 mg
**Oral solution:** 25 mg/mL (480 mL)
**Injection:** 25 mg/mL (20, 30 mL)
**Prediluted injection in $D_5W$:** 250 mg/50 mL, 500 mg/100 mL, 750 mg/150 mL
**Ophthalmic drops:**
Quixin: 0.5% (2.5, 5 mL)
Iquix: 1.5% (5 mL)

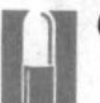

***Child:***

***Recurrent or persistent acute otitis media (6 mo–<5 yr):*** 10 mg/kg/dose PO Q12 hr × 10 days; **max. dose:** 500 mg/24 hr

***Community-acquired pneumonia (see remarks) and data from a single-dose pharmacokinetic study to provide similar drug exposures associated with clinical efficacy and safety as seen in adults:***

***6 mo–<5 yr:*** 10 mg/kg/dose PO/IV Q12 hr

***5–12 yr:*** 10 mg/kg/dose PO/IV Q24 hr; **max. dose:** 500 mg/24 hr

***Adult:***

***Community-acquired pneumonia:*** 500 mg PO/IV Q24 hr × 7–14 days; OR 750 mg PO/IV Q24 hr × 5 days

***Complicated UTI/acute pyelonephritis:*** 250 PO/IV Q24 hr × 10 days; OR 750 mg PO/IV Q24 hr × 5 days

***Uncomplicated UTI:*** 250 mg PO/IV Q24 hr × 3 days

***Uncomplicated skin/skin structure infection:*** 500 mg PO/IV Q24 hr × 7–10 days

***Acute bacterial sinusitis:*** 500 mg PO/IV Q24 hr × 10–14 days; OR 750 mg PO/IV Q24 hr × 5 days

***Inhalational anthrax (post-exposure):*** 500 mg PO/IV Q24 hr × 60 days.

***Conjunctivitis:***

***≥1 yr and adult:*** Instill 1–2 drops of the 0.5% solution to affected eye(s) Q2 hr up to 8 times/24 hr while awake for the first 2 days, then Q4 hr up to 4 times/24 hr while awake for the next 5 days.

***Corneal ulcer:***

***≥6 yr and adult:*** Instill 1–2 drops of the 1.5% solution to affected eye(s) Q30 min–2 hr while awake and 4 and 6 hr after retiring for the first 3 days, then Q1–4 hr while awake.

**Contraindicated** in hypersensitivity to other quinolones. **Avoid** in patients with history of QTc prolongation or taking QTc prolonging drugs, and excessive sunlight exposure. **Use with caution** in diabetes, seizures, children < 18 yr, and renal impairment **(adjust dose, see Chapter 31)**. May cause GI disturbances, headache, and blurred vision with the ophthalmic solution. Like other quinolones, tendon rupture can occur during or after therapy (risk increases with concurrent corticosteroids). Use with NSAIDs may increase risk of CNS stimulation and seizures.

Levofloxacin was well tolerated with equal efficacy in a comparative study to standard-of-care antibiotics in children 0.5 to 16 yr with community-acquired pneumonia. Long-term safety trials are underway in children treated for pneumonia and otitis media.

Infuse IV over 1–1.5 hr; **avoid** IV push or rapid infusion because of risk of hypotension. **Do not** administer antacids or other divalent salts with or within 2 hr of oral levofloxacin dose; otherwise may be administered with or without food.

L



## LEVOTHYROXINE ($T_4$)

Synthroid, Levothroid, Levoxyl, and others

***Thyroid product***

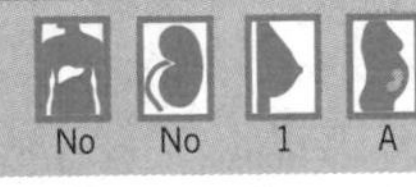


**Tabs:** 25, 50, 75, 88, 100, 112, 125, 137, 150, 175, 200, 300 mcg
**Injection:** 200, 500 mcg
**Oral suspension:** 25 mcg/mL

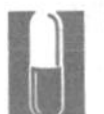

***Child PO dosing:***
***0–6 mo:*** 8–10 mcg/kg/dose QD
***6–12 mo:*** 6–8 mcg/kg/dose QD
***1–5 yr:*** 5–6 mcg/kg/dose QD
***6–12 yr:*** 4–5 mcg/kg/dose QD
***>12 yr:*** 2–3 mcg/kg/dose QD

***IM/IV dose:*** 50%–75% of oral dose QD

***Adult:***

***PO:*** Start with 12.5–50 mcg/dose QD. Increase by 25–50 mcg/24 hr at intervals of Q2–4 wk until euthyroid. Usual adult dose: 100–200 mcg/24 hr.

***IM/IV dose:*** 50% of oral dose QD

***Myxedema coma or stupor:*** 200–500 mcg IV × 1, then 75–100 mcg IV QD; convert to oral therapy once patient is stabilized.

**Contraindications** include acute MI, thyrotoxicosis, and uncorrected adrenal insufficiency. May cause hyperthyroidism, rash, growth disturbances, hypertension, arrhythmias, diarrhea, and weight loss. Pseudotumor cerebri has been reported in children. Overtreatment may cause craniosynostosis in infants and premature closure of the epiphyses in children.

Total replacement dose may be used in children unless there is evidence of cardiac disease; in that case, begin with one fourth of maintenance and increase weekly. Titrate dosage with clinical status and serum $T_4$ and TSH. Increases the effects of warfarin. Phenytoin, rifampin, and carbamazepine may decrease levothyroxine levels. Tricyclic antidepressants and SSRIs may enhance toxic effects.

**100 mcg levothyroxine = 65 mg thyroid USP.** Administer oral doses on an empty stomach and tablets with a full glass of water. Iron and calcium supplements and antacids may decrease absorption; **do not** administer within 4 hr of these agents. Excreted in low levels in breast milk; preponderance of evidence suggest no clinically significant effect in infants.

## LIDOCAINE

Xylocaine, L-M-X, Lidoderm, and various generics

***Anti-arrhythmic class Ib, local anesthetic***

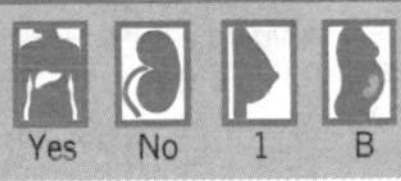


**Injection:** 0.5%, 1%, 1.5%, 2%, 4%, 10%, 20% (1% sol = 10 mg/mL)
**IV infusion (in $D_5W$):** 0.4% (4 mg/mL) (250, 500 mL); 0.8% (8 mg/mL) (250, 500 mL)
**Injection with 1:50,000 epi:** 2%
**Injection with 1:100,000 epi:** 1%, 2%
**Injection with 1:200,000 epi:** 0.5%, 1%, 1.5%, 2%
**Ointment:** 5% (50 g)
**Cream, topical:** 3% (30 g), 4% (L-M-X-4) [OTC] (5, 15, 30 g); may contain benzyl alcohol
**Cream, rectal:** 5% (L-M-X-5; 15, 30 g); contains benzyl alcohol
**Jelly:** 2% (5, 15, 30 mL); may contain benzalkonium chloride

*Continued*

For explanation of icons, see p. 698.

LIDOCAINE *continued*

**Liquid (topical):** 2.5% (7.5 mL)
**Liquid (viscous):** 2% (20, 100 mL)
**Solution (topical):** 2% (180 mL), 4% (50 mL)
**Topical spray:** 0.5% (60 mL), 9.6% (13 mL)
**Topical 2.5% (with 2.5% prilocaine):** See *Lidocaine* and *Prilocaine*
**Transdermal patch (Lidoderm):** 5% (30s)

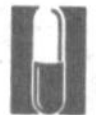

***Anesthetic:***
***Injection:***
***Without epinephrine:*** **max. dose** of 4.5 mg/kg/dose (up to 300 mg); **do not** repeat within 2 hr.
***With epinephrine:*** **max. dose** of 7 mg/kg/dose (up to 500 mg); **do not** repeat within 2 hr.

***Topical:*** 3 mg/kg/dose no more frequently than Q2 hr
***Antiarrhythmic:*** Bolus with 1 mg/kg/dose (**max. dose:** 100 mg) slowly IV; may repeat in 10–15 min × 2; **max. total dose** 3–5 mg/kg within the first hr. ETT dose = 2–3 × IV dose.
***Continuous infusion:*** 20–50 mcg/kg/min IV/IO (**do not exceed** 20 mcg/kg/min for patients with shock or CHF); see inside front cover for infusion preparation. Administer a 1 mg/kg bolus when infusion is initiated if bolus has not been given within previous 15 min.
***Oral use:***
***Adult:*** 15 mL swish and spit Q3 hr PRN up to a **max. dose** of 8 doses/24 hr

**Contraindicated** in Stokes-Adams attacks, SA, AV, or intraventricular heart block without a pacemaker. Side effects include hypotension, asystole, seizures, and respiratory arrest.

CYP 450 2D6 and 3A3/4 substrate. Decrease dose in hepatic failure or decreased cardiac output. **Do not use** topically for teething. Prolonged infusion may result in toxic accumulation of lidocaine, especially in infants. **Do not use** epinephrine-containing solutions for treatment of arrhythmias.

Therapeutic levels 1.5–5 mg/L. Toxicity occurs at >7 mg/L. Toxicity in neonates may occur at >5 mg/L. Elimination $T_{1/2}$: premature infant: 3.2 hr; adult: 1.5–2 hr.

## LIDOCAINE AND PRILOCAINE

EMLA, Eutectic mixture of lidocaine and prilocaine
***Topical analgesic***

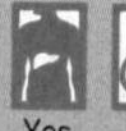
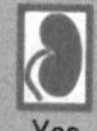
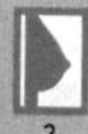
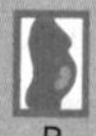

Yes Yes ? B

**Cream:** Lidocaine 2.5% + prilocaine 2.5%; 5 g kit (with dressings); 30 g tube
**Topical anesthetic disc:** Lidocaine 2.5% + prilocaine 2.5%; 1 g (contact surface ~ 10 cm²) (box of 2s or 10s)

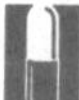

See Chapter 6, Table 6-5, for general use information.
***Newborn ≥ 37 wk of gestation, child, and adult:***
***Minor procedures:*** 2.5 g/site for at least 60 min.
***Painful procedures:*** 2 g/10 $cm^2$ of skin for at least 2 hr
See following table for **max. dose** and application information.

*Continued*

LIDOCAINE AND PRILOCAINE *continued*

| Age and Weight | Max. Total EMLA Dose (g) | Max. Application Area ($cm^2$) | Max. Application Time |
|---|---|---|---|
| Birth–3 mo or < 5 kg | 1 | 10 | 1 hr |
| 3–12 mo and > 5 kg* | 2 | 20 | 4 hr |
| 1–6 yr and > 10 kg | 10 | 100 | 4 hr |
| 7–12 yr and > 20 kg | 20 | 200 | 4 hr |

*If patient is > 3 mo and is not > 5 kg, use the **max. total dose** that corresponds to the patient's weight.

**Should not be** used in neonates < 37 wk of gestation nor in infants < 12 mo old receiving treatment with methoglobin-inducing agents (e.g., sulfa drugs, acetaminophen, nitrofurantoin, nitroglycerin, nitroprusside, phenobarbital, phenytoin). **Use with caution** in patients with G6PD deficiency, patients treated with class I or III anti-arrhythmic drugs (additive or toxic cardiac effects), and in patients with renal and hepatic impairment. Prilocaine has been associated with methemoglobinemia. Long duration of application, large treatment area, small patients, or impaired elimination may result in high blood levels.

Apply topically to intact skin and cover with occlusive dressing; **avoid** mucous membranes or the eyes. Wipe cream off before procedure.

## LINDANE

Various brands, Gamma benzene hexachloride

***Scabicidal agent, pediculocide***

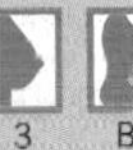


**Shampoo:** 1% (30, 60, 473 mL)
**Lotion:** 1% (30, 60, 473 mL)

***Scabies:*** Apply thin layer of lotion to skin. Bathe and rinse off medication in adults after 8–12 hr; children 6–8 hr. May repeat × 1 in 7 days PRN.

***Pediculosis capitis:*** Apply 15–30 mL of shampoo, lather for 4–5 min, rinse hair and comb with fine comb to remove nits. May repeat × 1 in 7 days PRN.

***Pediculosis pubis:*** May use lotion or shampoo (applied locally) as for scabies and pediculosis capitis.

**Contraindicated** in premature infants and seizure disorders. **Use with caution** with drugs that lower seizure threshold. Systemically absorbed. Risk of toxic effects is greater in young children; use other agents (permethrin) in infants, young children, and during pregnancy. Lindane is considered second-line therapy owing to side-effect risk. May cause a rash; rarely may cause seizures or aplastic anemia. For scabies, change clothing and bedsheets after starting treatment and treat family members. For pediculosis pubis, treat sexual contacts.

**Avoid** contact with face, urethral meatus, damaged skin, or mucous membranes. **Do not use** any covering that does not breathe (e.g., plastic lining or clothing) over the applied lindane.

For explanation of icons, see p. 698.

## LINEZOLID

Zyvox

***Antibiotic, oxazolidinone***

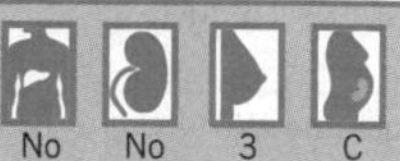


**Tabs:** 400, 600 mg; contains ~0.45 mEq Na per 200 mg drug
**Oral suspension:** 100 mg/5 mL (150 mL); contains phenylalanine and sodium benzoate and 0.8 mEq Na per 200 mg drug
**Injection, premixed:** 200 mg in 100 mL, 400 mg in 200 mL, 600 mg in 300 mL; contains 1.7 mEq Na per 200 mg drug

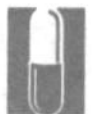

***Neonate < 7 days old:*** 10 mg/kg/dose IV/PO Q12 hr; if response is suboptimal, increase dose to 10 mg/kg/dose Q8 hr.
***Neonate ≥ 7 days old–11 yr:***
***Pneumonia, bacteremia, complicated skin/skin structure infections, Vancomycin-resistant E. faecium (VRE):*** 10 mg/kg/dose IV/PO Q8 hr. Duration of therapy: 10–14 days, except for VRE (14–28 days).
***Uncomplicated skin/skin structure infections:***
***<5 yr:*** 10 mg/kg/dose PO Q8 hr × 10–14 days
***5–11 yr:*** 10 mg/kg/dose PO Q12 hr × 10–14 days
***≥12 yr and adult:***
***MRSA Infections:*** 600 mg Q12 hr IV/PO
***Vancomycin-resistant E. faecium:*** 600 mg Q12 hr IV/PO × 14–28 days.
***Community-acquired and nosocomial pneumonia; and bacteremia:*** 600 mg Q12 hr IV/PO × 10–14 days
***Uncomplicated skin infections:***
***≥12 yr and adolescent:*** 600 mg Q12 hr PO × 10–14 days.
***Adult:*** 400 mg Q12 hr PO × 10–14 days.

Most common side effects include diarrhea, headache, and nausea. Anemia, leukopenia, pancytopenia, thrombocytopenia may occur in patients who are at risk for myelosuppression and who receive regimens > 2 wk. Complete blood count monitoring is recommended in these individuals. Pseudomembranous colitis and neuropathy (peripheral and optic) have also been reported.

**Avoid** use with SSRIs (e.g., fluoxetine, paroxetine), tricyclic antidepressants, venlafaxine, and trazodone; may cause serotonin syndrome. **Use caution** when using adrenergic (epinephrine, pseudoephedrine) agents or consuming large amounts of foods and beverages containing tyramine; may increase blood pressure. Dosing information in severe hepatic failure and renal impairment with multi-doses have not been completed.

Protect all dosage forms from light and moisture. Oral suspension product must be gently mixed by inverting the bottle 3–5 times prior to each use (**do not shake**). All oral doses may be administered with or without food.

## LISINOPRIL

Prinivil, Zestril, and others

***Angiotensin converting enzyme inhibitor, antihypertensive***

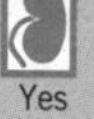
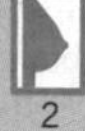
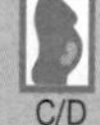


**Tabs:** 2.5, 5, 10, 20, 30, 40 mg
**Oral suspension:** 1, 2 mg/mL

*Continued*

LISINOPRIL *continued*

***Hypertension:***

***6–16 yr:*** Start with 0.07 mg/kg/dose PO QD; **max. initial dose:** 5 mg/dose. If needed, titrate dose upward to doses up to 0.61 mg/kg/24 hr or 40 mg/24 hr (higher doses have not been evaluated).

***Adult:*** Start with 10 mg PO QD. Usual dosage range: 20–40 mg/24 hr.
**Max. dose:** 80 mg/24 hr.

**Contraindicated** in hypersensitivity and history of angioedema with other ACE inhibitors. **Avoid** use with dialysis with high-flux membranes because of anaphylactoid reactions have been reported. **Use with caution** in aortic or bilateral renal artery stenosis. Side effects include cough, dizziness, headache, hyperkalemia, hypotension (especially with concurrent diuretic or antihypertensive agent use), rash and GI disturbances. Use with diabetic patients treated with oral antidiabetic agents should be monitored for hypoglycemia, especially during the first mo of use. NSAIDs (e.g., indomethacin) may decrease lisinopril's effects. **Adjust dose in renal impairment (see Chapter 31).**

Use lower initial dose if using with a diuretic. Onset of action: 1 hr with maximal effect in 6–8 hr. Pregnancy category is "C" during the first trimester but changes to "D" for the second and third trimesters. Despite the pregnancy category, an increased risk for major congenital malformations has been reported with use of ACE inhibitors during the first trimester. Lisinopril should be discontinued as soon as possible when pregnancy is detected.

## LITHIUM

Lithobid and many other generics (previously available as Eskalith)

***Antimanic agent***

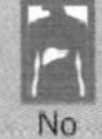
No
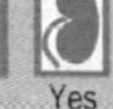
Yes
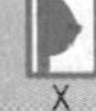
X
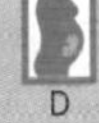
D

**Carbonate:**

300 mg carbonate = 8.12 mEq lithium
**Caps:** 150, 300, 600 mg
**Tabs:** 300 mg
**Extended-release tabs:** 300 mg (Lithobid), 450 mg

**Citrate:**

**Syrup:** 8 mEq/5 mL (5, 10, 480 mL); 5 mL is equivalent to 300 mg lithium carbonate

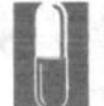

***Child:***

***Initial:*** 15–60 mg/kg/24 hr ÷ TID–QID PO. Adjust as needed (weekly) to achieve therapeutic levels.

***Adolescent:*** 600–1800 mg/24 hr ÷ TID–QID PO (divided BID using controlled/slow-release tablets)

***Adult:***

***Initial:*** 300 mg TID PO. Adjust as needed to achieve therapeutic levels. Usual dose is about 300 mg TID–QID. **Max. dose:** 2.4 g/24 hr or 900–1800 mg/24 hr with controlled/slow-release tablets.

*Continued*

For explanation of icons, see p. 698.

LITHIUM *continued*

**Contraindicated** in severe cardiovascular or renal disease. Decreased sodium intake or increased sodium wasting will increase lithium levels. May cause goiter, nephrogenic diabetes insipidus, hypothyroidism, arrhythmias, or sedation at therapeutic doses.

Co-administration with thiazide diuretics, metronidazole, ACE inhibitors, or nonsteroidal anti-inflammatory drugs may increase risk for lithium toxicity. Iodine may increase risk for hypothyroidism. If used in combination with haloperidol, closely monitor neurologic toxicities because an encephalopathic syndrome followed by irreversible brain damage has been reported.

**Therapeutic levels:** 0.6–1.5 mEq/L. In either acute or chronic toxicity, confusion, and somnolence may be seen at levels of 2–2.5 mEq/L. **Seizures or death** may occur at levels >2.5 mEq/L. Recommended serum sampling: trough level within 30 min prior to the next scheduled dose. Steady-state is achieved within 4–6 days of continuous dosing. **Adjust dose in renal failure (see Chapter 31).**

## LOPERAMIDE

Imodium, Imodium AD, and others

***Antidiarrheal***

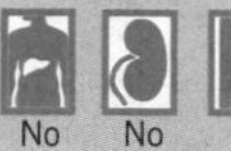
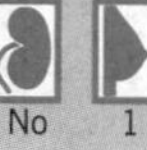
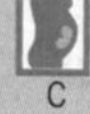

No No 1 C

**Caps (OTC):** 2 mg
**Tabs (OTC):** 2 mg
**Caplets (OTC):** 2 mg
**Liquid (OTC):** 1 mg/5 mL, 1 mg/7.5 mL; may contain alcohol (60, 120 mL)

***Active diarrhea:***

***Child (initial doses within the first 24 hr):***

***2–5 yr (13–20 kg):*** 1 mg PO TID
***6–8 yr (20–30 kg):*** 2 mg PO BID
***9–12 yr (>30 kg):*** 2 mg PO TID
**Max. single dose:** 2 mg
Follow initial day's dose with 0.1 mg/kg/dose after each loose stool (**not to exceed** the aforementioned initial doses).

***Adult:*** 4 mg/dose × 1, followed by 2 mg/dose after each stool up to **max. dose** of 16 mg/24 hr.

***Chronic diarrhea:***

***Child:*** 0.08–0.24 mg/kg/24 hr ÷ BID-TID; **max. dose:** 2 mg/dose

**Contraindicated** in acute dysentery; acute ulcerative colitis; bacterial enterocolitis caused by *Salmonella, Shigella, Campylobacter,* and *C. difficile*; and abdominal pain in the absence of diarrhea. **Avoid** use in children <2 yr due to reports of paralytic ileus associated with abdominal distention. Rare hypersensitivity reactions including anaphylactic shock have been reported. May cause nausea, rash, vomiting, constipation, cramps, dry mouth, and CNS depression. **Discontinue use if no clinical improvement is observed within 48 hr.** Naloxone may be administered for CNS depression.

## LORATADINE ± PSEUDOEPHEDRINE

Claritin, Claritin Children's Allergy, Claritin RediTabs, Claritin-D 12 Hour, Claritin-D 24 Hour, and others

***Antihistamine, less sedating ± decongestant***

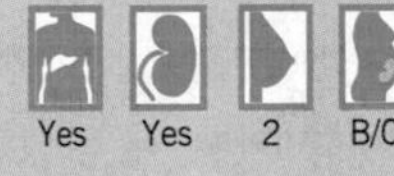


**Tabs (OTC):** 10 mg
**Chewable tabs (Claritin Children's Allergy) (OTC):** 5 mg; contains aspartame
**Disintegrating tabs (RediTabs) (OTC):** 5, 10 mg; contains aspartame
**Syrup (OTC):** 1 mg/mL (480 mL)
**Time-release tabs in combination with pseudoephedrine (PE):**
Claritin-D 12 Hour (OTC): 5 mg loratadine + 120 mg PE
Claritin-D 24 Hour (OTC): 10 mg loratadine + 240 mg PE

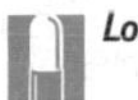

***Loratadine:***
***2–5 yr:*** 5 mg PO QD
***≥6 yr and adult:*** 10 mg PO QD
***Time-release tabs of loratadine and pseudoephedrine:***
***≥12 yr and adult:***
***Claritin-D 12 Hour:*** 1 tablet PO BID
***Claritin-D 24 Hour:*** 1 tablet PO QD

May cause drowsiness, fatigue, dry mouth, headache, bronchospasms, palpitations, dermatitis, and dizziness. Has **not** been implicated in causing cardiac arrhythmias when used with other drugs that are metabolized by hepatic microsomal enzymes (e.g., ketoconazole, erythromycin). May be administered safely in patients who have allergic rhinitis and asthma.

In hepatic and renal function impairment (GFR < 30 mL/min), prolong loratadine (single agent) dosage interval to QOD. **Adjust dose in renal failure (see Chapter 31).**

For time-release tablets of the combination product (loratadine and pseudoephedrine), prolong dosage interval in renal impairment (GFR < 30 mL/min) as follows: Claritin-D 12 Hour: 1 tablet PO QD; Claritin-D 24 Hour: 1 tablet PO QOD. **Do not use** the combination product in hepatic impairment because drugs cannot be individually titrated.

Administer doses on an empty stomach. For use of RediTabs, place tablet on tongue and allow it to disintegrate in the mouth with or without water. For Claritin-D, also see remarks in Pseudoephedrine.

Pregnancy category is "B" for loratadine and "C" for the combination product.

## LORAZEPAM

Ativan and many generics

***Benzodiazepine anticonvulsant***

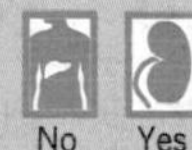
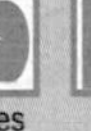
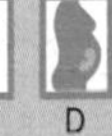
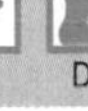


**Tabs:** 0.5, 1, 2, mg
**Injection:** 2, 4 mg/mL (each contains 2% benzyl alcohol and propylene glycol)
**Oral solution:** 2 mg/mL (10, 30 mL); alcohol and dye free

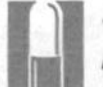

***Status epilepticus:***
***Neonate, infant, child, and adolescent:*** 0.05–0.1 mg/kg/dose IV over 2–5 min. May repeat 0.05 mg/kg × 1 in 10–15 min.
**Max. dose:** 2 mg/dose.
***Adult:*** 4 mg/dose given slowly over 2–5 min. May repeat in 10–15 min. **Usual total max. dose** in 12-hr period is 8 mg.

*Continued*

For explanation of icons, see p. 698.

LORAZEPAM *continued*

***Antiemetic adjunct therapy:***

***Child:*** 0.02–0.05 mg/kg/dose IV Q6 hr PRN; **max. single dose:** 2 mg.

***Anxiolytic/sedation:***

***Child:*** 0.05 mg/kg/dose Q4–8 hr PO/IV; **max. dose:** 2 mg/dose. May also give IM for preprocedure sedation.

***Adult:*** 1–10 mg/24 hr PO ÷ BID-TID

**Contraindicated** in narrow-angle glaucoma and severe hypotension. **Use with caution** in renal insufficiency (glucoronide metabolite clearance is reduced), compromised pulmonary function, and use of CNS depressant medications. May cause respiratory depression, especially in combination with other sedatives. May also cause sedation, dizziness, mild ataxia, mood changes, rash, and GI symptoms. Paradoxical excitation has been reported in chlidren (10%–30% of patients < 8 yr old).

Significant respiratory depression and/or hypotension has been reported when used in combination with loxapine. Probenecid and valproic acid may increase the effects/toxicity of lorazepam and oral contraceptive steroids may decrease lorazepam's effects.

Injectable product may be given rectally. Benzyl alcohol and propylene glycol may be toxic to newborns at high doses.

Onset of action for sedation: PO, 20–30 min; IM, 30–60 min; IV, 1–5 min. Duration of action: 6–8 hr. **Flumazenil is the antidote.**

## LOSARTAN

Cozaar

***Angiotensin II receptor antagonist***

Yes Yes ? C/D

**Tabs:** 25, 50, 100 mg

**Oral suspension:** 2.5 mg/mL

Contains 2.12 mg potassium per 25 mg drug

***Hypertension (see remarks):***

***≥6 yr:*** Start with 0.75 mg/kg/dose PO QD up to 50 mg/24 hr. Adjust dose to desired blood pressure response. **Max. dose:** 1.4 mg/kg/24 hr or 100 mg/24 hr.

***Adult:*** Start with 50 mg PO QD. Usual maintenance dose is 25–100 mg/24 hr PO ÷ QD–BID

**Use with caution** in angioedema (current or past), excessive hypotension (volume depletion), hepatic (use lower starting dose) or renal (contains potassium) impairment, hyperkalemia, renal artery stenosis and severe CHF.

**Not recommended** in patients < 6 yr or in children with GFR < 30 mL/min/1.73 m$^2$ due to the lack of data.

**Discontinue use** as soon as possible when pregnancy is detected because injury and death to developing fetus may occur. Pregnancy category is "C" during the first trimester but changes to "D" for the second and third trimesters.

Diarrhea, asthenia, dizziness, fatigue and hypotension are common. Thrombocytopenia, rhabdomyolysis and angioedema have been rarely reported. Losartan is a substrate for CYP 450 2C9 (major) and 3A4. Fluconazole and cimetidine may increase losartan effects/toxicity. Rifampin, phenobarbital and indomethacin may decrease its effects. Losartan may increase the risk of lithium toxicity.

## LOW MOLECULAR WEIGHT HEPARIN

See *Enoxaparin*

## MAGNESIUM CITRATE

Various, 16.17% Elemental Magnesium

***Laxative/cathartic***

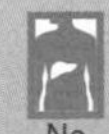
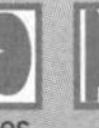
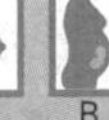

No Yes 1 B

**Oral solution (OTC):** 1.75 g/30 mL (300 mL); 5 mL = 3.9–4.7 mEq Mg

***Cathartic:***

***<6 yr:*** 2–4 mL/kg/24 hr PO ÷ QD-BID
***6–12 yr:*** 100–150 mL/24 hr PO ÷ QD-BID
***>12 yr and adult:*** 150–300 mL/24 hr PO ÷ QD-BID

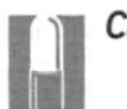

**Use with caution** in renal insufficiency and patients receiving digoxin. May cause hypermagnesemia, diarrhea, muscle weakness, hypotension, and respiratory depression. Up to about 30% of dose is absorbed. May decrease absorption of $H_2$ antagonists, phenytoin, iron salts, tetracycline, steroids, benzodiazepines, and quinolone antibiotics.

## MAGNESIUM HYDROXIDE

Milk of Magnesia and various generics, 41.69% Elemental Magnesium

***Antacid, laxative***

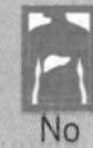
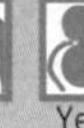
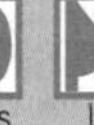
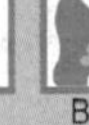
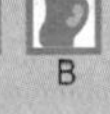

No Yes 1 B

**Oral liquid (OTC):** 400 mg/5 mL (Milk of Magnesia and others)
**Concentrated oral liquid (OTC):** 800 mg/5 mL (Milk of Magnesia concentrate)
**Chewable tabs (OTC):** 311 mg
400 mg magnesium hydroxide is equivalent to 166.76 mg elemental magnesium
Combination product with aluminum hydroxide: *See Aluminum Hydroxide.*

***Laxative (all liquid mL doses based on 400 mg/5 mL magnesium hydroxide, unless noted otherwise):***
Dose/24 hr ÷ QD-QID PO

***<2 yr:*** 0.5 mL/kg
***2–5 yr:*** 5–15 mL OR 311–622 mg (1–2 chewable tabs)
***6–11 yr:*** 15–30 mL OR 933–1244 mg (3–4 chewable tabs)
***≥12 yr and adult:*** 30–60 mL OR 1866–2488 mg (6–8 chewable tabs)

***Antacid:***

***Child:***

***Liquid:*** 2.5–5 mL/dose QD-QID PO
***Tabs:*** 311 mg QD-QID PO

***Adult:***

***Liquid:*** 5–15 mL/dose QD-QID PO
***Concentrated liquid:*** 2.5–7.5 mL/dose QD-QID PO
***Tabs:*** 622–1244 mg/dose QD-QID PO

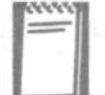

See *Magnesium Citrate*

For explanation of icons, see p. 698.

## MAGNESIUM OXIDE

Mag-200, Mag-Ox 400, Uro-Mag, and others

60.32% Elemental Magnesium

***Oral magnesium salt***

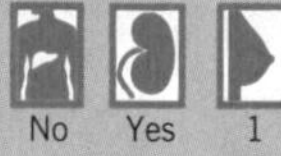

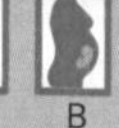


**Tabs (OTC):** 200, 400, 420, 500 mg
**Caps (Uro-Mag and others; OTC):** 140 mg
400 mg magnesium oxide is equivalent to 241.3 mg elemental Mg or 20 mEq Mg

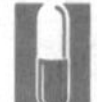

**Doses expressed in magnesium oxide salt.**

***Magnesium supplementation:***

***Child:*** 5–10 mg/kg/24 hr ÷ TID-QID PO
***Adult:*** 400–800 mg/24 hr ÷ BID-QID PO

***Hypomagnesemia:***

***Child:*** 65–130 mg/kg/24 hr ÷ QID PO
***Adult:*** 2000 mg/24 hr ÷ QID PO

See *Magnesium Citrate*. For dietary recommended intake (U.S. RDA) for magnesium, see Chapter 21.

## MAGNESIUM SULFATE

Epsom salts and others

9.9% Elemental Magnesium

***Magnesium salt***

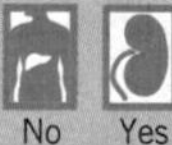
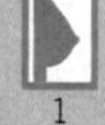
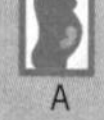


**Injection:** 100 mg/mL (0.8 mEq/mL), 125 mg/mL (1 mEq/mL), 500 mg/mL (4 mEq/mL)
**Injection, pre-diluted in sterile water for injection; ready to use:** 40 mg/mL (0.325 mEq/mL) (100, 500, 1000 mL); 80 mg/mL (0.65 mEq/mL) (50 mL)
**Injection, pre-diluted in $D_5W$; ready to use:** 10 mg/mL (0.081 mEq/mL) (100 mL); 20 mg/mL (0.163 mEq/mL) (500, 1000 mL)
**Granules:** Approx. 40 mEq Mg per 5 g (120, 454, 1810 g)
500 mg magnesium sulfate is equivalent to 49.3 mg elemental Mg or 4.1 mEq Mg

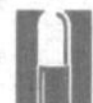

**All doses expressed in magnesium sulfate salt.**

***Cathartic:***

***Child:*** 0.25 g/kg/dose PO Q4–6 hr
***Adult:*** 10–30 g/dose PO Q4–6 hr

***Hypomagnesemia or hypocalcemia:***

***IV/IM:*** 25–50 mg/kg/dose Q4–6 hr × 3–4 doses; repeat PRN.
**Max. single dose:** 2 g
***PO:*** 100–200 mg/kg/dose QID PO

***Daily maintenance:***

30–60 mg/kg/24 hr or 0.25–0.5 mEq/kg/24 hr IV
**Max. dose:** 1 g/24 hr

***Adjunctive therapy for moderate to severe reactive airway disease exacerbation (bronchodilation):***

***Child:*** 25–75 mg/kg/dose (**max. dose:** 2 g) × 1 IV over 20 min.
***Adult:*** 2 g/dose × 1 IV over 20 min.

When given IV, **beware** of hypotension, respiratory depression, complete heart block, and/or hypermagnesemia. Calcium gluconate (IV) should be available as **antidote. Use with caution** in patients with renal insufficiency and with patients on digoxin. **Serum level dependent toxicity** includes the

*Continued*

MAGNESIUM SULFATE *continued*

following: >3 mg/dL: CNS depression; >5 mg/dL: decreased deep tendon reflexes, flushing, somnolence; and >12 mg/dL: respiratory paralysis, heart block.

**Max. IV intermittent infusion rate:** 1 mEq/kg/hr or 125 mg $MgSO_4$ salt/kg/hr.

## MANNITOL

Osmitrol, Resectisol, and various generics

***Osmotic diuretic***

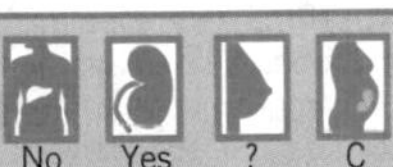


**Injection:** 50, 100, 150, 200, 250 mg/mL (5%, 10%, 15%, 20%, 25%)

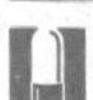

***Anuria/oliguria:***

***Test dose to assess renal function:*** 0.2 g/kg/dose IV; **max. dose:** 12.5 g over 3–5 min. If there is no diuresis within 2 hr, discontinue mannitol.

***Initial:*** 0.5–1 g/kg/dose

***Maintenance:*** 0.25–0.5 g/kg/dose Q4–6 hr IV

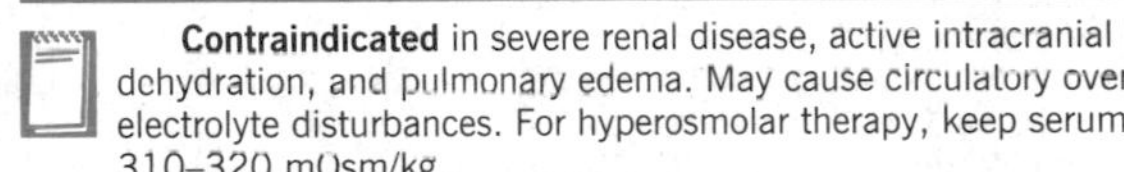

**Contraindicated** in severe renal disease, active intracranial bleed, dehydration, and pulmonary edema. May cause circulatory overload and electrolyte disturbances. For hyperosmolar therapy, keep serum osmolality at 310–320 mOsm/kg.

**Caution:** May crystallize at low temperatures with concentrations ≥ 15%; redissolve crystals by warming solution up to 70° C with agitation. Use an in-line filter. May cause hypovolemia, headache, and polydipsia. Reduction in ICP occurs in 15 min and lasts 3–6 hr.

## MEBENDAZOLE

Vermox and others

***Anthelmintic***

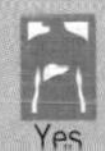
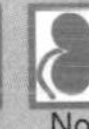
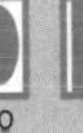
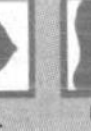
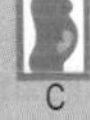


**Chewable tabs:** 100 mg (may be swallowed whole or chewed) (boxes of 12s, 60s)

***Child (> 2 yr) and adult:***

***Pinworms (Enterobius):*** 100 mg PO × 1; repeat in 2 wk if not cured.

***Hookworms, roundworms (Ascaris), and whipworm (Trichuris):*** 100 mg PO BID × 3 days. Repeat in 3–4 wk if not cured. Alternatively, may administer 500 mg PO ×1.

***Capillariasis:*** 200 mg PO BID × 20 days

***Visceral larva migrans (Toxocariasis):*** 100–200 mg PO BID × 5 days

***Trichinellosis (Trichinella spiralis):*** 200–400 mg PO TID × 3 days, then 400–500 mg PO TID × 10 days; use with steroids for severe symptoms

***Ancylostoma caninum (Eosinophilic enterocolitis):*** 100 mg PO BID × 3 days.

See latest edition of the AAP *Red Book* for additional information.

Experience in children <2 yr is limited. May cause rash, headache, diarrhea and abdominal cramping in cases of massive infection. Liver function test elevations and hepatitis have been reported with prolonged courses; monitor hepatic function with prolonged therapy. Family may need to be treated as a group. Therapeutic effect may be decreased if administered to patients receiving carbamazepine or phenytoin. Administer with food.

For explanation of icons, see p. 698.

## MEDROXYPROGESTERONE

Depo-Provera, Provera, and various generics;
Depo-Sub Q Provera 104.
***Contraceptive, progestin***

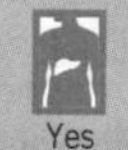 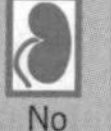 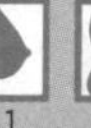 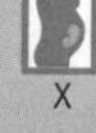

Yes No 1 X

**Tabs (Provera and others):** 2.5, 5, 10 mg
**Injection, suspension as acetate:**
Depo-Provera and others, for IM use only: 150 mg/mL (1 mL), 400 mg/mL (2.5, 10 mL); may contain parabens
**Injection, pre-filled syringe:**
Depo-Sub Q Provera 104, for SC use only: 104 mg (0.65 mL of 160 mg/mL); contains parabens

***Adolescent and adult:***
***Contraception:*** Initiate therapy during the first 5 days after onset of a normal menstrual period, within 5 days postpartum if not breast-feeding, or if breast-feeding, at 6 wk postpartum. When converting contraceptive method to Depo-Sub Q Provera, dose should be administered within 7 days after the last day of using the previous method (pill, ring, patch).
***IM (Depo-Provera):*** 150 mg Q3 mo
***SC (Depo-Sub Q Provera 104):*** 104 mg Q3 mo (every 12–14 wk)
***Amenorrhea:*** 5–10 mg PO QD × 5–10 days
***Abnormal uterine bleeding:*** 5–10 mg PO QD × 5–10 days initiated on the 16th or 21st day of the menstrual cycle.
***Endometriosis-associated pain:*** Depo-Sub Q Provera 104: 104 mg SC Q3 mo. **Do not use** longer than 2 yr due to impact on bone mineral density.

Consider patient's risk for osteoporosis because of the potential for decrease in bone mineral density with long-term use. **Contraindicated** in pregnancy, breast or genital cancer, liver disease, missed abortion, thrombophlebitis, thromboembolic disorders, cerebral vascular disease and undiagnosed vaginal bleeding. **Use with caution** in patients with family history of breast cancer, depression, diabetes, and fluid retention. May cause dizziness, headache, insomnia, fatigue, nausea, weight increase, appetite changes, amenorrhea, and breakthrough bleeding. Cholestatic jaundice and increased intracranial pressure have been reported.

Aminoglutethimide may decrease medroxyprogesterone levels. May alter thyroid and liver function tests, prothrombin time, factors VII, VIII, IX and X, and metyrapone test.

**Do not** inject IM or SC product intravenously. Shake IM injection vial well before use and administer in the upper arm or buttock. Administer SC injection product into the anterior thigh or abdomen. Administer oral doses with food.

## MEFLOQUINE HCL

Lariam and others
***Antimalarial***

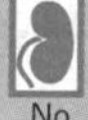 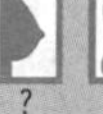 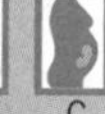

Yes No ? C

**Tabs:** 250 mg (228 mg base)

*Continued*

MEFLOQUINE HCL *continued*

**Doses expressed in mg mefloquine HCl salt**
***Malaria prophylaxis (start 1 wk prior to exposure and continue for 4 wk after leaving endemic area):***
***Child (PO, administered Q weekly):***
***<10 kg:*** 5 mg/kg
***10–19 kg:*** 62.5 mg (¼ tablet)
***20–30 kg:*** 125 mg (½ tablet)
***31–45 kg:*** 187.5 mg (¾ tablet)
***>45 kg:*** 250 mg (1 tablet)
***Adult:*** 250 mg PO Q weekly
***Malaria treatment:***
***<45 kg:*** 15 mg/kg ×1 PO followed by 10 mg/kg × 1 PO 8–12 hr later
***Adult:*** 750 mg × 1 PO followed by 500 mg × 1 PO 12 hr later
See latest edition of the *Red Book* for additional information.

**Contraindicated** in active or recent history of depression, anxiety disorders, psychosis or schizophrenia, seizures, or hypersensitivity to quinine or quinidine. **Use with caution** in cardiac dysrhythmias and neurologic disease. May cause dizziness, headache, syncope, seizures, ocular abnormalities, GI symptoms, leukopenia, and thrombocytopenia. Monitor liver enzymes and ocular exams for therapies greater than 1 yr. Mefloquine may reduce valproic acid levels. ECG abnormalities may occur when used in combination with quinine, quinidine, chloroquine, halofantrine, and beta-blockers. If any of the aforementioned antimalarial drugs is used in the initial treatment of severe malaria, initiate mefloquine at least 12 hours after the last dose of any of these drugs.

**Do not take** on an empty stomach. Administer with at least 240 mL (8 oz) water. Treatment failures in children may be related to vomiting of administered dose. If vomiting occurs less than 30 min after the dose, administer a second full dose. If vomiting occurs 30–60 min after the dose, administer an additional half-dose. If vomiting continues, monitor patient closely and consider alternative therapy.

## MEPERIDINE HCL

Demerol and many generics
***Narcotic, analgesic***

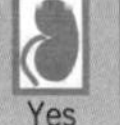
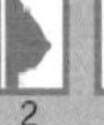
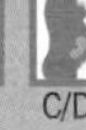
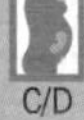
Yes Yes 2 C/D

**Tabs:** 50, 100 mg
**Syrup and oral solution:** 50 mg/5 mL
**Injection:** 10, 25, 50, 75, and 100 mg/mL

***PO, IM, IV, and SC:***
***Child:***
1–1.5 mg/kg/dose Q3–4 hr PRN
**Max. dose:** 100 mg
***Adult:***
50–150 mg/dose Q3–4 hr PRN

See Chapter 6 for details of use and equianalgesic dosing. **Contraindicated** in cardiac arrhythmias, asthma, and increased ICP. Potentiated by MAO inhibitors (use **contraindicated**), acyclovir, tricyclic antidepressants, cimetidine, ritonavir, phenothiazines, and other CNS-acting agents. Phenytoin may increase the clearance of meperidine. Meperidine may increase the adverse effects of isoniazid. May cause nausea, vomiting, respiratory depression, smooth muscle spasm, pruritis, palpitations, hypotension, constipation, and lethargy. *Continued*

For explanation of icons, see p. 698.

MEPERIDINE HCL *continued*

Drug is metabolized by the liver and its metabolite (normeperidine) is renally eliminated. **Caution:** In renal and hepatic failure, sickle cell disease, and seizure disorders, accumulation of normeperidine metabolite may precipitate seizures.

**Adjust dose in renal failure (see Chapter 31).** Pregnancy category changes to "D" if used for prolonged periods or in high doses at term. Onset of action: PO/IM/SC, 10–15 min; IV, 5 min.

## MEROPENEM

Merrem

***Carbapenem antibiotic***

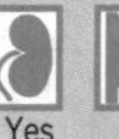
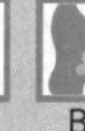
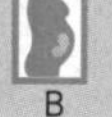

No Yes ? B

**Injection:** 0.5, 1 g
Contains 3.92 mEq Na/g drug

***Neonate:*** 20 mg/kg/dose IV using the following dosage intervals:
***<7 days old:*** Q12 hr
***≥7 days old:***
***1.2–2 kg:*** Q12 hr
***>2 kg:*** Q8 hr

***Infant > 3 mo and child:***
***Skin and subcutaneous tissue infections:*** 30 mg/kg/24 IV ÷ Q8 hr; **max. dose:** 1.5 g/24 hr
***Intra-abdominal and mild/moderate infections:*** 60 mg/kg/24 hr IV ÷ Q8 hr; **max. dose:** 3 g/24 hr
***Meningitis and severe infections:*** 120 mg/kg/24 hr IV ÷ Q8 hr; **max. dose:** 6 g/24 hr

***Adult:***
***Skin and subcutaneous tissue infections:*** 1.5 g/24 hr IV ÷ Q8 hr
***Intra-abdominal and mild/moderate infections:*** 3 g/24 hr IV ÷ Q8 hr
***Meningitis and severe infections:*** 6 g/24 hr IV ÷ Q8 hr

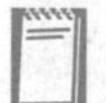

**Contraindicated** in patients sensitive to carbapenems, or with a history of anaphylaxis to beta-lactam antibiotics. **Use with caution** in meningitis and CNS disorders (may cause seizures) and renal impairment (**adjust dose; see Chapter 31**). Drug penetrates well into the CSF.

May cause diarrhea, rash, nausea, vomiting, oral moniliasis, glossitis, pain and irritation at the IV injection site, and headache. Hepatic enzyme and bilirubin elevation, leukopenia, thrombocytopenia (in renal dysfunction) and neutropenia have been reported. Probenecid may increase serum meropenem levels. May reduce valproic acid levels.

## MESALAMINE

Asacol, Canasa, Lialda, Pentasa, Rowasa, FIV-ASA, and others; 5-aminosalicylic acid, 5-ASA

***Salicylate, GI anti-inflammatory agent***

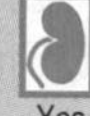
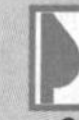
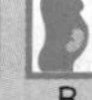

Yes Yes 2 B

**Caps, controlled-release (Pentasa):** 250, 500 mg
**Tabs, delayed-release:** 400 mg (Asacol), 1200 mg (Lialda)
**Suppository (Canasa, FIV-ASA):** 500, 1000 mg (30s)
**Rectal suspension (Rowasa and others):** 4 g/60 mL (7s, 28s); contains sulfites and sodium benzoate

*Continued*

MESALAMINE *continued*

***Child:***
***Caps, controlled-release:*** 50 mg/kg/24 hr ÷ Q6–12 hr PO
***Tabs, delayed-release:*** 50 mg/kg/24 hr ÷ Q8–12 hr PO

***Adult:***
***Caps, controlled-release:*** 1 g QID PO up to 8 wk
***Tabs, delayed-release:***
***Asacol:*** 800 mg TID PO for 6 wk; for ulcerative colitis remission, use 1.6 g/24 hr ÷ BID-QID. PO up to 6 mo.
***Lialda:*** 2.4–4.8 g QD PO up to 8 wk.
***Suppository:*** 500 mg BID PR × 3–6 wk; may increase dose to TID if inadequate response for 2 wk. Alternately, 1000 mg QHS PR may be used. Retain each dose in the rectum for 1–3 hr or longer.
***Rectal suspension:*** 60 mL (4 g) QHS × 3–6 wk, retaining each dose for about 8 hr; lie on left side during administration to improve delivery to the sigmoid colon.

Generally **not recommended** in children < 16 yr with chicken pox or flu-like symptoms (risk of Reye's syndrome). **Contraindicated** in active peptic ulcer disease, severe renal failure, and salicylate hypersensitivity. Rectal suspension **should not** be used in patients with history of sulfite allergy. **Use with caution** in sulfasalazine hypersensitivity, impaired hepatic or renal function, pyloric stenosis, and concurrent thrombolytics. May cause headache, GI discomfort, pancreatitis, pericarditis, rash, and Stevens-Johnson syndrome.

**Do not administer** with lactulose or other medications that can lower intestinal pH. Oral capsules are designed to release medication throughout the GI tract and oral tablets release medication at the terminal ileus and beyond. 400 mg PO mesalamine is equivalent to 1 g sulfasalazine PO. Tablets should be swallowed whole.

## METFORMIN

Glucophage, Glucophage XR, Fortamet, Riomet, and others
***Antidiabetic, biguanide***

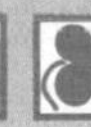 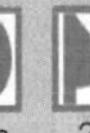 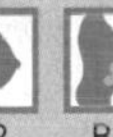 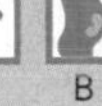

Yes Yes 2 B

**Tabs:** 500, 850, 1000 mg
**Tabs, extended-release (Glucophage XR, Fortamet, and others):** 500, 750, 1000 mg
**Oral suspension (Riomet):** 100 mg/mL (120, 480 mL), contains saccharin

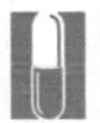

**Administer all doses with meals (e.g., BID: morning and evening meals).**
***Child (10–16 yr) (see remarks):*** Start with 500 mg BID; may increase dose weekly by 500 mg/24 hr in 2 divided doses up to a **max. dose** of 2000 mg/24 hr.

***Child ≥ 17 yr and adult (see remarks):***
***500 mg tabs:*** Start with 500 mg PO BID; may increase dose weekly by 500 mg/24 hr in 2 divided doses up to a **max. dose** of 2500 mg/24 hr. Administer 2500 mg/24 hr doses by dividing daily dose TID with meals.
***850 mg tabs:*** Start with 850 mg PO QD with morning meal; may increase by 850 mg every 2 wk up to a **max. dose** of 2550 mg/24 hr (first dosage increment: 850 mg PO BID; second dosage increment: 850 mg PO TID).
***Extended-release tabs:*** Start with 500 mg PO QD with evening meal; may increase by 500 mg every wk up to a **max. dose** of 2000 mg/24 hr (if glycemic control is not achieved at **max. dose**, divide dose to 1000 mg PO BID). If a dose > 2000 mg is needed, switch to nonextended-release tablets in divided doses and increase dose to a **max. dose** of 2550 mg/24 hr.

*Continued*



For explanation of icons, see p. 698.

METFORMIN *continued*

**Contraindicated** in renal impairment, CHF, metabolic acidosis and during radiology studies using iodinated contrast media. **Use with caution** when transferring patients from chlorpropamide therapy (potential hypoglycemia risk), excessive alcohol intake, hypoxemia, dehydration, surgical procedures, hepatic disease, anemia and thyroid disease.

**Fatal lactic acidosis** (diarrhea; severe muscle pain, cramping; shallow and fast breathing; unusual weakness and sleepiness) and decrease in vitamin $B_{12}$ levels have been reported. May cause GI discomfort (~50% incidence), anorexia and vomiting. Transient abdominal discomfort or diarrhea has been reported in 40% of pediatric patients. Cimetidine, furosemide, and nifedipine may increase the effects/toxicity of metformin. In addition to monitoring serum glucose and glycosylated hemoglobin, monitor renal function and hematologic parameters (baseline and annual).

Adult patients initiated on 500 mg PO BID may also have their dose increased to 850 mg PO BID after 2 wk.

**COMBINATION THERAPY WITH SULFONYLUREAS:** If patient has not responded to 4 wk of maximum doses of metformin monotherapy, consider gradual addition of an oral sulfonylurea with continued maximum metformin dosing (even if failure with sulfonylurea has occurred). Attempt to identify the minimum effective dosage for each drug (metformin and sulfonylurea), since the combination can increase risk for sulfonylurea-induced hypoglycemia. If patient does not respond to 1–3 mo of combination therapy with maximum metformin doses, consider discontinuing combination therapy and initiating insulin therapy.

Administer all doses with food.

## METHADONE HCL

Dolophine, Methadose, and others

***Narcotic, analgesic***

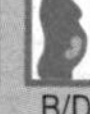

No Yes 2 B/D

**Tabs:** 5, 10 mg
**Tabs (dispersible):** 40 mg
**Oral solution:** 5 mg/5 mL, 10 mg/5 mL; contains 8% alcohol
**Concentrated solution:** 10 mg/mL
**Injection:** 10 mg/mL (20 mL), contains 0.5% chlorobutanol

***Analgesia:***

***Child:*** 0.7 mg/kg/24 hr ÷ Q4–6 hr PRN pain PO, SC, IM, or IV. **Max. dose:** 10 mg/dose.

***Adult:*** 2.5–10 mg/dose Q3–4 hr PRN pain PO, SC, IM, or IV.

***Detoxification or maintenance:*** See package insert.

Unintential overdoses have resulted in fatalities and severe adverse events such as respiratory depression and cardiac arrhythmias. May cause respiratory depression, sedation, increased intracranial pressure, hypotension, and bradycardia. Average $T_{1/2}$: children, 19 hr; adults, 35 hr. Oral duration of action is 6–8 hr initially and 22–48 hr after repeated doses. Respiratory effects last longer than analgesia. Accumulation may occur with continuous use, making it necessary to adjust dose. Nevirapine may decrease serum levels of methadone. Methadone is a substrate for CYP 450 3A3/4, 2D6, 1A2; and inhibitor of 2D6.

See Chapter 6 for equianalgesic dosing and onset of action. **Adjust dose in renal failure (see Chapter 31).** Pregnancy category changes to "D" if used for prolonged period or in high doses at term.

## METHIMAZOLE

Tapazole and others

***Antithyroid agent***

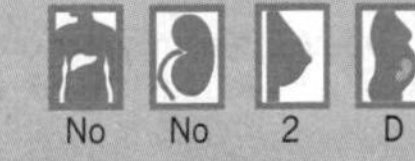


**Tabs:** 5, 10 mg

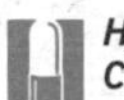

***Hyperthyroidism:***

***Child:***

***Initial:*** 0.4–0.7 mg/kg/24 hr or 15–20 mg/m²/24 hr PO ÷ Q8 hr

***Maintenance:*** ⅓–⅔ of initial dose PO ÷ Q8 hr

**Max. dose:** 30 mg/24 hr

***Adult:***

***Initial:*** 15–60 mg/24 hr PO ÷ TID

***Maintenance:*** 5–15 mg/24 hr PO ÷ TID

Readily crosses placental membranes and distributes into breast milk (maternal doses ≤ 20 mg/24 hr is considered safe but there is insufficient data to support safe use with maternal doses > 20 mg/24 hr). Blood dyscrasias, dermatitis, hepatitis, arthralgia, CNS reactions, pruritis, nephritis, hypoprothrombinemia, agranulocytosis, headache, fever, and hypothyroidism may occur.

May increase the effects of oral anticoagulants. When correcting hyperthyroidism, existing beta-blocker, digoxin, and theophylline doses may need to be reduced to avoid potential toxicities.

Switch to maintenance dose when patient is euthyroid. Administer all doses with food.

## METHYLDOPA

Various brand names

***Central alpha-adrenergic blocker, antihypertensive***

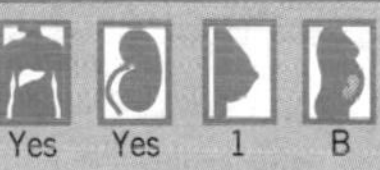


**Tabs:** 250, 500 mg

**Injection:** 50 mg/mL; may contain sulfites

**Oral suspension:** 50 mg/ mL

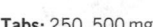

***Hypertension:***

***Child:*** 10 mg/kg/24 hr ÷ Q6–12 hr PO; increase PRN Q2 days.

**Max. dose:** 65 mg/kg/24 hr or 3 g/24 hr, whichever is less.

***Adult:*** 250 mg/dose BID-TID PO. Increase PRN Q2 days to **max. dose** of 3 g/24 hr.

***Hypertensive crisis:***

***Child:*** 2–4 mg/kg/dose IV to a **max. dose** of 5–10 mg/kg/dose IV Q6–8 hr. **Max. dose** (whichever is less): 65 mg/kg/24 hr or 3 g/24 hr.

***Adult:*** 250–1000 mg IV Q6–8 hr. **Max. dose:** 4 g/24 hr.

**Contraindicated** in pheochromocytoma and active liver disease. **Use with caution** if patient is receiving haloperidol, propranolol, lithium, sympathomimetics. Positive Coombs' test rarely associated with hemolytic anemia. Fever, leukopenia, sedation, memory impairment, hepatitis, GI disturbances, orthostatic hypotension, black tongue, and gynecomastia may occur. May interfere with lab tests for creatinine, urinary catecholamines, uric acid, and AST.

*Continued*

For explanation of icons, see p. 698.

METHYLDOPA *continued*

**Do not co-administer** oral doses with iron; decreases methyldopa absorption. **Adjust dose in renal failure (see Chapter 31).**

## METHYLENE BLUE

Urolene Blue and many generics

***Antidote, drug-induced methemoglobinemia, and cyanide toxicity***

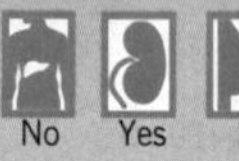
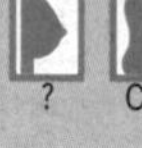
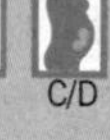


**Tabs (Urolene Blue):** 65 mg
**Injection:** 10 mg/mL (1%) (1, 10 mL)

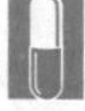

***Methemoglobinemia:***
***Child and adult:*** 1–2 mg/kg/dose or 25–50 mg/$m^2$/dose IV over 5 min. May repeat in 1 hr if needed.

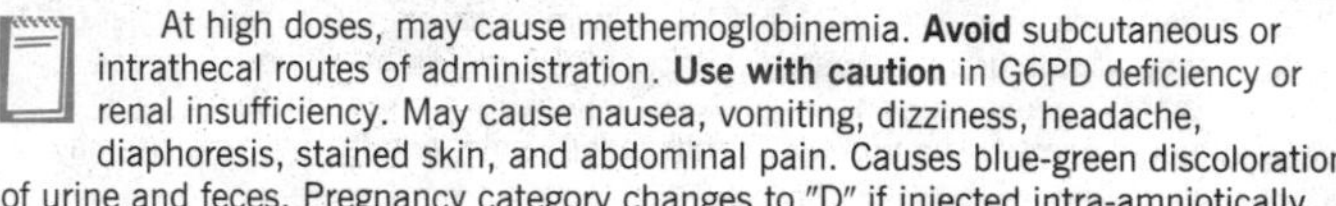

At high doses, may cause methemoglobinemia. **Avoid** subcutaneous or intrathecal routes of administration. **Use with caution** in G6PD deficiency or renal insufficiency. May cause nausea, vomiting, dizziness, headache, diaphoresis, stained skin, and abdominal pain. Causes blue-green discoloration of urine and feces. Pregnancy category changes to "D" if injected intra-amniotically.

## METHYLPHENIDATE HCL

Ritalin, Methylin, Metadate ER, Methylin ER, Concerta, Ritalin SR, Metadate CD, Ritalin LA, Daytrana, and others

***CNS stimulant***

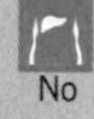
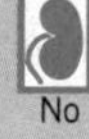
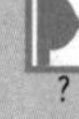
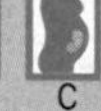


**Tabs:** 5, 10, 20 mg
**Chewable tabs:** 2.5, 5, 10 mg; contains phenylalanine
**Oral solution (Methylin):** 1 mg/mL, 2 mg/mL
**Extended-release tabs:**
- 8-hr duration (Metadate ER, Methylin ER): 10, 20 mg
- 24-hr duration (Concerta): 18, 27, 36, 54 mg

**Sustained-release tabs:**
- 8-hr duration (Ritalin SR): 20 mg

**Extended-release caps:**
- 24-hr duration (Metadate CD, Ritalin LA): 10, 20, 30, 40, 50, 60 mg

**Transdermal patch (Daytrana):** 10 mg/9 hr (each 12.5 $cm^2$ patch contains 27.5 mg), 15 mg/9 hr (each 18.75 $cm^2$ patch contains 41.3 mg), 20 mg/9 hr (each 25 $cm^2$ patch contains 55 mg), 30 mg/9 hr (each 37.5 $cm^2$ patch contains 82.5 mg) (10s and 30s)

***Attention deficit hyperactivity disorder:***
***≥6 yr:***
- ***Initial:*** 0.3 mg/kg/dose (or 2.5–5 mg/dose) given before breakfast and lunch. May increase by 0.1 mg/kg/dose PO (or 5–10 mg/24 hr) weekly until maintenance dose achieved. May give extra afternoon dose if needed.
- ***Maintenance dose range:*** 0.3–1 mg/kg/24 hr
- **Max. dose:** 2 mg/kg/24 hr or 60 mg/24 hr

*Continued*

METHYLPHENIDATE HCL *continued*

***Once daily dosing (Concerta), ≥6 yr:***

***Patients new to methylphenidate:*** Start with 18 mg PO QAM, dosage may be increased at weekly intervals at 18 mg increments up to the following **max. dose:**

***6–12 yr:*** 54 mg/24 hr

***13–17 yr:*** 72 mg/24 hr **not to exceed** 2 mg/kg/24 hr

***Patients currently receiving methylphenidate:*** See following table.

RECOMMENDED DOSE CONVERSION FROM METHYLPHENIDATE REGIMENS TO CONCERTA

| Previous Methylphenidate Daily Dose | Recommended Concerta Dose |
|---|---|
| 5 mg PO BID–TID or 20 mg SR PO QD | 18 mg PO QAM |
| 10 mg PO BID–TID or 40 mg SR PO QD | 36 mg PO QAM |
| 15 mg PO BID–TID or 60 mg SR PO QD | 54 mg PO QAM |

After 1 wk of receiving the recommended Concerta dose, dose may be increased in 18 mg increments at weekly intervals up to a **max.** of 54 mg/24 hr for 6–12 yr old and 72 mg/24 hr (**not to exceed** 2 mg/kg/24 hr) for 13–17 yr old.

***Transdermal patch (Daytrana):*** Apply to the hip 2 hr before the effect is needed and remove 9 hr later. Patch may be removed before 9 hours if shorter duration of effect is desired or if late day adverse effects appear.

***6–12 yr:*** Start with 10 mg/9 hr patch QD. Increase dose PRN Q7 days by increasing to the next dosage strength.

**Contraindicated** in glaucoma, anxiety disorders, motor tics and Tourette's syndrome. Medication should generally **not** be used in children < 5 yr old as diagnosis of ADHD in this age group is extremely difficult and should be only done in consultation with a specialist. **Sudden death** (children, adolescents, and adults), stroke (adults), and MI (adults) have been reported in patients with pre-existing structural cardiac abnormalities or other serious heart problems. **Use with caution** in patients with hypertension, psychiatric conditions, and epilepsy. Insomnia, weight loss, anorexia, rash, nausea, emesis, abdominal pain, hyper- or hypotension, tachycardia, arrhythmias, palpitations, restlessness, headaches, fever, tremor, visual disturbances, and thrombocytopenia may occur. Abnormal liver function, cerebral arteritis and/or occlusion, leukopenia and/or anemia, transient depressed mood, and scalp hair loss have been reported. Skin irritation may occur with transdermal route. High doses may slow growth by appetite suppression. GI obstruction has been reported with Concerta.

May increase serum concentrations of tricyclic antidepressants, phenytoin, phenobarbital, and warfarin. Effect of methylphenidate may be potentiated by MAO inhibitors; hypertensive crisis may also occur if used within 14 days of discontinuance of the MAO inhibitor.

**Extended/sustained-release dosage forms have either an 8- or 24-hour dosage interval (as stipulated previously).** Concerta dosage form delivers 22.2% of its dose as an immediate-release product with the remaining amounts as an extended-release product (e.g., 18 mg strength: 4 mg as immediate release and 14 mg as extended release). **Do not expose transdermal application site to external heat sources** (e.g., electric blankets, heating pads); this may increase drug release.

For explanation of icons, see p. 698.

## METHYLPREDNISOLONE

Medrol, Medrol Dosepack, Solu-Medrol, Depo-Medrol, and others
***Corticosteroid***

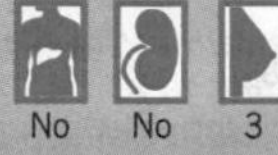
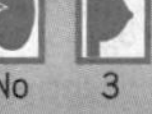

No No 3 C

**Tabs:** 2, 4, 8, 16, 24, 32 mg
**Tabs, dose pack (Medrol Dosepack and others):** 4 mg (21s)
**Injection, Na succinate (Solu-Medrol and others):** 40, 125, 500, 1000, 2000 mg (IV or IM use); may contain benzyl alcohol
**Injection, Acetate (Depo-Medrol and others):** 20, 40, 80 mg/mL (IM repository)

***Anti-inflammatory/immunosuppressive:***
***PO/IM/IV:*** 0.5–1.7 mg/kg/24 hr ÷ Q6–12 hr.
***Asthma exacerbations (2007 National Heart, Lung, and Blood Institute Guideline Recommendations; dose until peak expiratory flow reaches 70% of predicted or personal best):***
***Child ≤ 12 yr (IM/IV/PO):*** 1 mg/kg/24 hr ÷ Q12 hr (**max. dose:** 60 mg/24 hr). Higher alternative regimen of 1 mg/kg/dose Q6 hr × 48 hr followed by 1–2 mg/kg/24 hr (**max. dose:** 60 mg/24 hr) ÷ Q12 hr has been suggested.
***>12 yr and adult (IV/IM/PO):*** 40–80 mg/24 hr ÷ Q12–24 hr. Higher alternative regimen of 120–180 mg/24 hr ÷ Q6–8 hr × 48 hr followed by 60–80 mg/24 hr ÷ Q12 hr has been suggested.
***Outpatient asthma exacerbation burst therapy (longer durations may be necessary):***
***PO:***
***Child ≤ 12 yr:*** 1–2 mg/kg/24 hr ÷ Q12–24 hr (**max. dose:** 60 mg/24 hr) × 3–10 days.
***Child > 12 yr and adult:*** 40–60 mg/24 hr ÷ Q12–24 hr × 5–10 days.
***IM (use methylprednisolone acetate product) for patients vomiting or with adherence issues:***
***Child ≤ 12 yr:*** 7.5 mg/kg (**max. dose:** 240 mg) IM × 1
***Child > 12 yr and adult:*** 240 mg IM × 1.
***Acute spinal cord injury:***
30 mg/kg IV over 15 min followed in 45 min by a continuous infusion of 5.4 mg/kg/hr × 23 hr.

See Chapter 30 for relative, steroid potencies and doses based on body surface area. Acetate form may also be used for intra-articular and intralesional injection and has longer times to max. effect and duration of action; it should **NOT** be given IV. Like all steroids, may cause hypertension, pseudotumor cerebri, acne, Cushing syndrome, adrenal axis suppression, GI bleeding, hyperglycemia, and osteoporosis.

Barbiturates, phenytoin, and rifampin may enhance methylprednisolone clearance. Erythromycin, itraconazole, and ketoconazole may increase methylprednisone levels. Methylprednisolone may increase cyclosporine and tacrolimus levels.

## METOCLOPRAMIDE

Reglan, Maxolon, and many other generics
***Antiemetic, prokinetic agent***

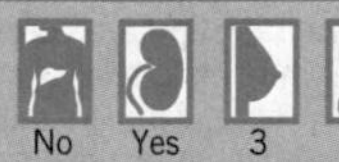

No Yes 3 B

**Tabs:** 5, 10 mg
**Injection:** 5 mg/mL (2, 10, 20, 30 mL)
**Syrup:** 5 mg/5 mL

*Continued*

METOCLOPRAMIDE *continued*

***Gastroesophageal reflux (GER) or GI dysmotility:***
- ***Infant and child:*** 0.1–0.2 mg/kg/dose up to QID IV/IM/PO; **max. dose:** 0.8 mg/kg/24 hr
- ***Adult:*** 10–15 mg/dose QAC and QHS IV/IM/PO

***Antiemetic (all ages):***
1–2 mg/kg/dose Q2–6 hr IV/IM/PO. Premedicate with diphenydramine to reduce EPS.

***Postoperative nausea and vomiting:***
- ***Child:*** 0.1–0.2 mg/kg/dose Q6–8 hr PRN IV
- ***>14 yr and adult:*** 10 mg Q6–8 hr PRN IV

**Contraindicated** in GI obstruction, seizure disorder, pheochromocytoma, or in patients receiving drugs likely to cause extrapyramidal symptoms (EPS). May cause EPS, especially at higher doses. Sedation, headache, anxiety, depression, leukopenia, and diarrhea may occur. Rare occurrences of neuroleptic malignant syndrome have been reported.

For GER, give 30 min before meals and at bedtime. **Reduce dose in renal impairment (see Chapter 31).**

## METOLAZONE

Zaroxolyn and many other generics

***Diuretic, thiazide-like***

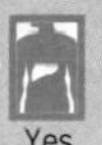
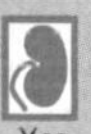
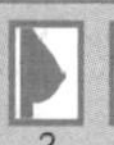
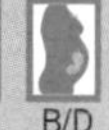

Yes Yes 2 B/D

**Tabs:** 2.5, 5, 10 mg
**Oral suspension:** 1 mg/mL

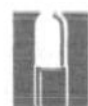

***Dosage based on Zaroxolyn (for oral suspension, see remarks):***
- ***Child:*** 0.2–0.4 mg/kg/24 hr ÷ QD-BID PO
- ***Adult:***
  - ***Hypertension:*** 2.5–5 mg QD PO
  - ***Edema:*** 2.5–20 mg QD PO

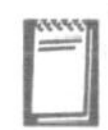

**Contraindicated** in patients with anuria, hepatic coma, or hypersensitivity to sulfonamides or thiazides. **Use with caution** in severe renal disease, impaired hepatic funciton, gout, lupus erythematosus, diabetes mellitus, and elevated cholesterol and triglycerides. Electrolyte imbalance, GI disturbance, hyperglycemia, marrow suppression, chills, hyperuricemia, chest pain, hepatitis and rash may occur.

Oral suspension has increased bioavailability; therefore, lower doses may be necessary when using these dosage forms. More effective than thiazide diuretics in impaired renal function; may be effective in GFRs as low as 20 mL/min. Furosemide-resistant edema in pediatric patients may benefit with the addition of metolazone.

Pregnancy category changes to "D" if used for pregnancy-induced hypertension.

For explanation of icons, see p. 698.

## METOPROLOL

Lopressor, Toprol-XL, and others

***Adrenergic blocking agent (beta-1 selective), class II antiarrhythmic***

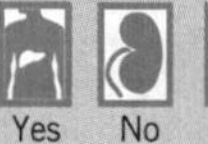 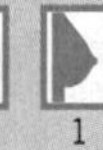 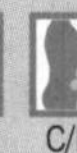 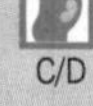

Yes No 1 C/D

**Tabs:** 25, 50, 100 mg
**Extended-release tabs (Toprol-XL and others):** 25, 50, 100, 200 mg
**Oral liquid:** 10 mg/mL
**Injection:** 1 mg/mL (5 mL)

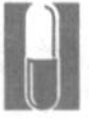

***Hypertension:***
***Child ≥ 1 yr and adolescent (nonextended-release oral dosage forms):*** Start at 1–2 mg/kg/24 hr PO ÷ BID; **max. dose:** 6 mg/kg/24 hr **up to** 200 mg/24 hr.
***Adult:***
***Nonextended-release tabs:*** Start at 50–100 mg/24 hr PO ÷ QD-BID; if needed, increase dosage at weekly intervals to desired blood pressure. Effective dosage range is 100–450 mg/24 hr. Doses > 450 mg/24 hr have not been studied. Patients with bronchospastic diseases should receive the lowest possible daily dose divided TID.
***Extended-release tabs:*** Start at 25–100 mg/24 hr PO QD; if needed, increase dosage at weekly intervals to desired blood pressure. Usual dosage range is 50–100 mg/24 hr. Doses > 400 mg/24 hr have not been studied.

**Contraindicated** in sinus bradycardia, heart block > 1st degree, sick sinus syndrome (except with functioning pacemaker), cardiogenic shock and uncompensated CHF. **Use with caution** in hepatic dysfunction, peripheral vascular disease, history of severe anaphylactic hypersensitivity drug reactions, pheochromocytoma, and concurrent use with verapamil, diltiazem or anesthetic agents that may decrease myocardial function. Reserpine and other drugs that deplete catecholamines (e.g., MAO inhibitors) may increase the effects of metoprolol. Metoprolol is a CYP 450 2D6 substrate.

**Avoid** abrupt cessation of therapy in ischemic heart disease; angina and MI have occurred. Common side effects include bradyarrhythmia, heart block, heart failure, pruritus, rash, GI disturbances, dizziness, fatigue, and depression. Bronchospasm, dyspnea and elevations in transaminase, alkaline phosphatase and LDH have all been reported.

Pregnancy category changes to "D" if used in second or third trimester.

## METRONIDAZOLE

Flagyl, Flagyl ER, Protostat, MetroGel, MetroLotion, MetroCream, Noritate, MetroGel-Vaginal, and others

***Antibiotic, antiprotozoal***

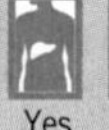 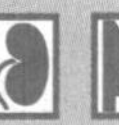  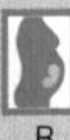

Yes Yes 3 B

**Tabs:** 250, 500 mg
**Tabs, extended-release (Flagyl ER):** 750 mg
**Caps:** 375 mg
**Oral suspension:** 20 mg/mL or 50 mg/mL
**Injection:** 500 mg; contains 830 mg mannitol/g drug
**Ready to use injection:** 5 mg/mL (100 mL); contains 28 mEq Na/g drug
**Gel, topical (MetroGel):** 0.75% (28, 45 g)
**Lotion (MetroLotion):** 0.75% (60 mL); contains benzyl alcohol

*Continued*

METRONIDAZOLE *continued*

**Cream, topical:**
MetroCream: 0.75% (45 g); contains benzyl alcohol
Noritate: 1% (30 g)
**Gel, vaginal (MetroGel-Vaginal):** 0.75% (70 g with 5 applicators)

---

***Amebiasis:***
***Child:*** 35–50 mg/kg/24 hr PO ÷ TID × 10 days
***Adult:*** 500–750 mg/dose PO TID × 10 days
***Anaerobic infection:***
***Neonate:*** **PO/IV:**
*<7 days:*
***<1.2 kg:*** 7.5 mg/kg/dose Q48 hr
***1.2–2 kg:*** 7.5 mg/kg/dose Q24 hr
***≥2 kg:*** 15 mg/kg/24 hr ÷ Q12 hr
***≥7 days:***
***<1.2 kg:*** 7.5 mg/kg/dose Q24 hr
***1.2–2 kg:*** 15 mg/kg/24 hr ÷ Q12 hr
***≥2 kg:*** 30 mg/kg/24 hr ÷ Q12 hr
***Infant/child/adult:***
***IV/PO:*** 30 mg/kg/24 hr ÷ Q6 hr
**Max. dose:** 4 g/24 hr
***Other parasitic infections:***
***Infant/child:*** 15–30 mg/kg/24 hr PO ÷ Q8 hr
***Adult:*** 250 mg PO Q8 hr or 2 g PO × 1
***Bacterial vaginosis:***
***Adolescent and adult:***
***PO:*** 500 mg BID × 7 days or 2 g × 1 dose
***Vaginal:*** 5 g (1 applicator full) BID × 5 days
***Giardiasis:***
***Child:*** 15 mg/kg/24 hr PO ÷ TID × 5 days; **max. dose:** 750 mg/24 hr
***Adult:*** 250 mg PO TID × 5 days
***Trichomoniasis:*** Treat sexual contacts.
***Child:*** 15 mg/kg/24 hr PO ÷ TID × 7 days
***Adolescent/adult:*** 2 g PO × 1 or 250 mg PO TID or 375 mg PO BID × 7 days
***C. difficile infection (IV may be less efficacious):***
***Child:*** 30 mg/kg/24 hr ÷ Q6 hr PO/IV x 10 days
***Adult:*** 250–500 mg TID-QID PO × 10–14 days, or 500 mg Q8 hr IV × 10–14 days
***H. pylori infection (use in combination with amoxicillin and bismuth subsalicylate):***
***Child:*** 15–20 mg/kg/24 hr ÷ BID PO × 4 wk
***Adult:*** 250–500 mg TID PO × 14 days
***Inflammatory bowel disease (as alternative to sulfasalazine):***
***Adult:*** 400 mg BID PO
***Topical use:*** Apply and rub a thin film to affected areas at the following frequencies specific to product concentration.
***0.75% cream:*** BID
***1% cream:*** QD

---

**Avoid** use in first trimester of pregnancy. **Use with caution** in patients with CNS disease, blood dyscrasias, severe liver or **renal disease (GFR <10 mL/min), see Chapter 31**. Nausea, diarrhea, urticaria, dry mouth, leukopenia, vertigo, metallic taste and peripheral neuropathy may occur. Candidiasis may worsen. May discolor urine. Patients **should not** ingest alcohol for 24–48 hr after dose (disulfuram-type reaction).

*Continued*

For explanation of icons, see p. 698.

METRONIDAZOLE *continued*

May increase levels or toxicity of phenytoin, lithium, and warfarin. Phenobarbital and rifampin may increase metronidazole metabolism.

IV infusion must be given slowly over 1 hr. For intravenous use in all ages, some references recommend a 15 mg/kg loading dose.

## MICAFUNGIN SODIUM

Mycamine

***Antifungal, echinocandin***

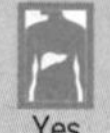 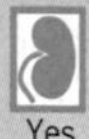 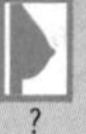 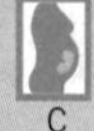

Yes Yes ? C

**Injection:** 50, 100 mg; contains lactose

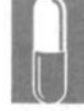

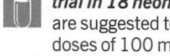

***Premature infant > 1000 g (based on single dose pharmacokinetic and safety trial in 18 neonates, 26 ± 2.4 wk of gestation):*** 5 mg/kg and 7 mg/kg doses are suggested to provide similar AUC drug exposure of adults receiving daily doses of 100 mg and 150 mg. Dosages ranging from 0.75–3 mg/kg were well tolerated in this study.

***Esophageal candidiasis:***

***<50 kg:*** 3 mg/kg/dose IV QD; **max. dose:** 150 mg/dose

***≥50 kg:*** 150 mg IV QD; mean duration for successful therapy was 15 days (range: 10–30 days).

***Invasive candidiasis:***

***<40 kg:*** 2–3 mg/kg/dose IV QD; **max. dose:** 150 mg/24 hr

***≥40 kg:*** 100–150 mg IV QD

***Candida prophylaxis in hematopoietic stem cell transplant:***

***<50 kg:*** 1–2 mg/kg/dose IV QD; **max. dose:** 50 mg/dose

***≥50 kg:*** 50 mg IV QD; mean duration 19 days (range: 6–51 days)

***Invasive aspergillosis (doses under investigation):***

***<50 kg:*** 3–4 mg/kg/dose IV QD

***≥50 kg:*** 150 mg IV QD

Prior hypersensitivity to other echinocandins (anidulafungin, caspofungin) increases risk; anaphylaxis with shock has been reported. **Use with caution** in hepatic and renal impairment. No dosing adjustments are required based on race or gender, or in patients with severe renal dysfunction or mild to moderate hepatic function impairment. Effect of severe hepatic function impairment on micafungin pharmacokinetics has not been evaluated.

May cause GI disturbances, phlebitis, rash, hyperbilirubinemia, liver function test elevation, headache, fever, and rigor. Anemia, leukopenia, neutropenia, thrombocytopenia, and hemolysis have been reported. Micafungin is a CYP 450 3A isoenzyme substrate and weak inhibitor. May increase the effects/toxicity of nifedipine and sirolimus.

## MICONAZOLE

Monistat and others

Topical products: Micatin, Lotrimin AF, and others

***Antifungal agent***

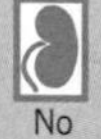  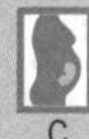

No No ? C

**Cream (OTC):** 2% (15, 30, 90 g)
**Lotion (OTC):** 2% (30, 60 mL)
**Ointment (OTC):** 2% (28.4 g)
**Solution (OTC):** 2% with alcohol (7.39, 29.57 mL)
**Gel (OTC):** 2% with alcohol (24 g)

*Continued*

MICONAZOLE *continued*

**Topical solution (OTC):** 2% with alcohol (7.4, 29.6 mL)
**Powder (OTC):** 2% (70, 90 g)
**Spray, liquid (OTC):** 2% (105 mL); contains alcohol
**Spray, powder (OTC):** 2% (85, 90, 100 g); contains alcohol
**Vaginal cream (OTC):** 2% (15, 25, 45 g)
**Vaginal suppository (OTC):** 100 mg (7s), 200 mg (3s)
**Vaginal combination packs:**
Monistat 1 (Rx): 1200 mg suppository (1) and 2% cream (9 g)
M-Zole 3, Monistat 3, Vagistat-3 (OTC): 200 mg suppository (3s) and 2% cream (9 g)
Monistat 7, M-Zole 7 (OTC): 100 mg suppository (7s) and 2% cream (9 g)

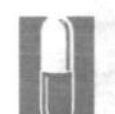

***Topical:*** Apply BID × 2–4 wk
***Vaginal:*** 1 applicator full of cream or 100 mg suppository QHS × 7 days or 200 mg suppository QHS × 3 days
***Monistat 1:*** 1200 mg suppository ×1 at bedtime or during the day.

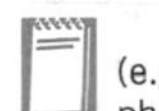

**Use with caution** in hypersensitivity to other imidazole antifungal agents (e.g., clotrimazole, ketoconazole). Side effects include pruritis, rash, burning, phlebitis, headaches, and pelvic cramps.

Drug is a substrate and inhibitor of the CYP 450 3A3/4 isoenzymes. Vaginal use with concomitant warfarin use has also been reported to increase warfarin's effect. Vegetable oil base in vaginal suppositories may interact with latex products (e.g., condoms and diaphragms); consider switching to the vaginal cream.

## MIDAZOLAM

Various generics; previously available as Versed
***Benzodiazepine***

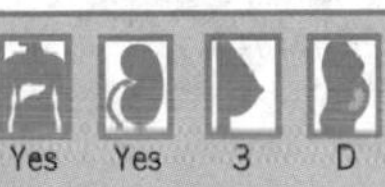


**Injection:** 1, 5 mg/mL; some preparations may contain 1% benzyl alcohol
**Oral syrup:** 2 mg/mL, contains sodium benzoate

**Titrate to effect under controlled conditions.**
See Chapter 6 for additional routes of administration.
***Sedation for procedures:***
***Child:***
*IV:*
***6 mo–5 yr:*** 0.05–0.1 mg/kg/dose over 2–3 min. May repeat dose PRN in 2–3 min intervals up to a **max. total dose** of 6 mg. A total dose up to 0.6 mg/kg may be necessary for desired effect.
***6–12 yr:*** 0.025–0.05 mg/kg/dose over 2–3 min. May repeat dose PRN in 2–3 min intervals up to a **max. total dose** of 10 mg. A total dose up to 0.4 mg/kg may be necessary for desired effect.
***>12–16 yr:*** Use adult dose; up to **max. total dose** of 10 mg.
*PO:*
***≥6 mo:*** 0.25–0.5 mg/kg/dose × 1; **max. dose:** 20 mg. Younger patients (6 mo–5 yr) may require higher doses of 1 mg/kg/dose, whereas older patients (6–15 yr) may require only 0.25 mg/kg/dose. Use 0.25 mg/kg/dose for patients with cardiac or respiratory compromise, concurrent CNS depressive drug, or high-risk surgery.
***Adult:***
***IV:*** 0.5–2 mg/dose over 2 min. May repeat PRN in 2–3 min intervals until desired effect. Usual total dose: 2.5–5 mg. **Max. total dose:** 10 mg.

*Continued*

For explanation of icons, see p. 698.

MIDAZOLAM *continued*

***Sedation with mechanical ventilation:***

***Intermittent:***

***Infant and child:*** 0.05–0.15 mg/kg/dose Q1–2 hr PRN

***Continuous IV infusion (initial doses, titrate to effect):***

***Neonate:***

***<32 wk of gestation:*** 0.5 mcg/kg/min

***≥32 wk of gestation:*** 1 mcg/kg/min

***Infant and child:*** 1–2 mcg/kg/min

***Refractory status epilepticus:***

***≥2 mo and child:*** Load with 0.15 mg/kg IV × 1 followed by a continuous infusion of 1 mcg/kg/min and titrate dose upward Q5 min to effect (mean dose of 2.3 mcg/kg/min with a range of 1–18 mcg/kg/min has been reported).

---

**Contraindicated** in patients with narrow-angle glaucoma and shock. **Use with caution** in CHF, **renal impairment (adjust dose; see Chapter 31)**, pulmonary disease, hepatic dysfunction, and in neonates. Causes respiratory depression, hypotension and bradycardia. Cardiovascular monitoring is recommended. Use lower doses or reduce dose when given in combination with narcotics or in patients with respiratory compromise.

Drug is a substrate for CYP 450 3A4. Serum concentrations may be increased by cimetidine, clarithromycin, diltiazem, erythromycin, itraconazole, ketoconazole, and protease inhibitors. Sedative effects may be antagonized by theophylline. **Effects can be reversed by flumazenil.** For pharmacodynamic information, see Chapter 6.

## MILRINONE

Primacor

***Inotrope***

No Yes ? C

**Injection:** 1 mg/mL (10, 20, 50 mL)

**Pre-mixed injection in $D_5W$:** 200 mcg/mL (100, 200 mL)

---

***Child (limited data):*** 50 mcg/kg IV bolus over 15 min, followed by a continuous infusion of 0.5–0.75 mcg/kg/min and titrate to effect.

***Adult:*** 50 mcg/kg IV bolus over 10 min, followed by a continuous infusion of 0.375–0.75 mcg/kg/min and titrate to effect. **Max. dose:** 1.13 mg/kg/24 hr.

---

**Contraindicated** in severe aortic stenosis, severe pulmonic stenosis, and acute MI. May cause headache, dysrhythmias, hypotension, hypokalemia, nausea, vomiting, anorexia, abdominal pain, hepatotoxicity, and thrombocytopenia. Pediatric patients may require higher mcg/kg/min doses because of a faster elimination $T_{1/2}$ and larger volume of distribution, when compared to adults. Hemodynamic effects can last up to 3–5 hr after discontinuation of infusion in children. **Reduce dose in renal impairment.**

## MINERAL OIL

Kondremul, Fleet Mineral Oil, and others

***Laxative, lubricant***

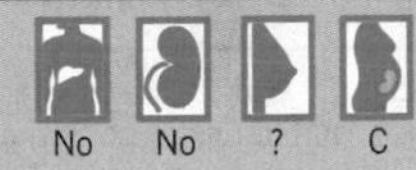


**Liquid, oral (OTC):** 180, 480 mL
**Emulsion, oral (Kondremul; OTC):** 480 mL
**Rectal liquid (Fleet Mineral Oil, OTC):** 133 mL

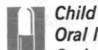

***Child 5–11 yr:***
***Oral liquid:*** 5–15 mL/24 hr ÷ QD-TID PO
***Oral emulsion (Kondremul):*** 10–25 mL/24 hr ÷ QD-TID PO
***Rectal:*** 30–60 mL as single dose
***Child ≥ 12 yr and adult:***
***Oral liquid:*** 15–45 mL/24 hr ÷ QD-TID PO
***Oral emulsion (Kondremul):*** 30–75 mL/24 hr ÷ QD-TID PO
***Rectal:*** 60–150 mL as single dose

May cause diarrhea, cramps, and lipid pneumonitis via aspiration. Use as a laxative **should not exceed** > 1 wk. Onset of action is approximately 6–8 hr. Higher doses may be necessary to achieve desired effect. Do **not** give QHS dose and **use with caution** in children <5 yr to minimize risk of aspiration. May impair the absorption of fat-soluble vitamins, calcium, phosphorus, oral contraceptives, and warfarin. Emulsified preparations are more palatable and are dosed differently than the oral liquid preparation.

For disimpaction, doses up to 1 ounce (30 mL) per yr of age (**max. dose** of 240 mL) BID can be given.

## MINOCYCLINE

Minocin, Dynacin, Arestin, and others

***Antibiotic, tetracycline derivative***

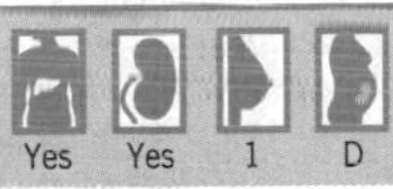


**Tabs:** 50, 75, 100 mg
**Caps:** 50, 75, 100 mg
**Extended-release tabs:** 45, 90, 135 mg
**Caps (pellet filled):** 50, 100 mg
**Sustained-release microspheres (Arestin):** 1 mg (12s)
**Oral suspension:** 50 mg/5 mL (60 mL); contains 5% alcohol

***General infections:***
***Child (8–12 yr):*** 4 mg/kg/dose × 1 PO, then 2 mg/kg/dose Q12 hr PO; **max. dose:** 200 mg/24 hr
***Adolescent and adult:*** 200 mg/dose × 1 PO, then 100 mg Q12 hr PO
***Chlamydia trachomatis/Ureaplasma urealyticum:***
***Adolescent and adult:*** 100 mg PO Q12 hr × 7 days
***Acne (≥12 yr–adult):***
***Immediate-release dosage forms:*** 50-100 mg PO QD-BID
***Extended-release tabs:***
***45–59 kg:*** 45 mg PO QD
***60–90 kg:*** 90 mg PO QD
***91–136 kg:*** 135 mg PO QD

*Continued*



For explanation of icons, see p. 698.

MINOCYCLINE *continued*

**Not recommended** for children < 8 yr and during the last half of pregnancy due to risk of permanent tooth discoloration. **Use with caution** in renal failure; lower dosage may be necessary. High incidence of vestibular dysfunction (30%–90%). Nausea, vomiting, allergy, increased intracranial pressure, photophobia and injury to developing teeth may occur. Hepatitis, including autoimmune hepatitis, and liver failure have been reported.

May increase effects/toxicity of warfarin and decrease the efficacy of live attenuated oral typhoid vaccine. May be administered with food but **NOT** with milk or dairy products. See *Tetracycline* for additional drug/food interactions and remarks.

## MINOXIDIL

Various generics (previously available as Loniten), Rogaine, Men's Rogaine Extra Strength

***Antihypertensive agent, hair growth stimulant***

No Yes 2 C

**Tabs:** 2.5, 10 mg

**Topical solution:**

Rogaine (OTC): 2% (60 mL)

Men's Rogaine Extra Strength (OTC): 5% (60 mL); contains 30% alcohol

**Topical aerosol foam:**

Men's Rogaine Extra Strength (OTC): 5% (60 g); contains alcohol

***Child < 12 yr:***

Start with 0.1–0.2 mg/kg/24 hr PO QD; **max. dose:** 5 mg/24 hr. Dose may be increased in increments of 0.1–0.2 mg/kg/24 hr at 3-day intervals. Usual effective range: 0.25–1 mg/kg/24 hr PO ÷ QD-BID; **max. dose:** 50 mg/24 hr.

***≥12 yr and adult:***

***Oral:*** Start with 5 mg QD. Dose may be gradually increased at 3-day intervals. Usual effective range: 10–40 mg/24 hr ÷ QD-BID; **max. dose:** 100 mg/24 hr.

***Topical (alopecia):*** Apply 1 mL to the total affected areas of the scalp BID (QAM and QHS). **Max. dose:** 2 mL/24 hr.

**Contraindicated** in acute MI, dissecting aortic aneurysm, and pheochromocytoma. Concurrent use with a beta-blocker and diuretic is recommended to prevent reflex tachycardia and reduce water retention, respectively. May cause drowsiness, dizziness, CHF, pulmonary edema, pericardial effusion, pericarditis, thrombocytopenia, leukopenia, Stevens-Johnson syndrome, and hypertrichosis (reversible) with systemic use. Concurrent use of guanethidine may cause profound orthostatic hypotension; use with other antihypertensive agents may cause additive hypotension. Patients with renal failure or receiving dialysis may require a dosage reduction. Antihypertensive onset of action within 30 min and peak effects within 2–8 hr.

**TOPICAL USE:** Local irritation, contact dermatitis may occur. **Do not use** in conjunction with other topical agents including topical corticosteroids, retinoids or petrolatum, or agents that are known to enhance cutaneous drug absorption. Onset of hair growth (topical use) is 4 mo. The 5% solution is flammable.

M

**MOMETASONE FUROATE**
Asmanex Twisthaler, Nasonex, Elocon, and other generic topical products
***Corticosteroid***

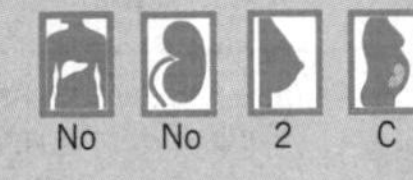


**Nasal spray (Nasonex):** 0.05%, 50 mcg per actuation (17 g = 120 doses)
**Powder for inhalation (Asmanex Twisthaler):** 220 mcg per actuation (14, 30, 60, 120 units); contains lactose
**Topical cream and ointment (Elocon and others):** 0.1% (15, 45 g)
**Topical lotion and solution (Elocon and others):** 0.1% (30, 60 mL); contains isopropyl alcohol

***Intranasal (allergic rhinitis):*** Patients with known seasonal allergic rhinitis should initiate therapy 2–4 wk prior to anticipated pollen season.
***2–11 yr:*** 50 mcg (1 spray) each nostril QD
***≥12 yr:*** 100 mcg (2 sprays) each nostril QD

***Oral inhalation:***
***≥12 yr:*** Max. effects may not be achieved until 1–2 wk or longer. Titrate doses to the lowest effective dose once asthma is stabilized.
***Previously treated with bronchodilators alone or with inhaled corticosteroids:*** Start with 220 mcg (1 inhalation) QD in the evening. Dose may be increased up to a **max. dose** of 440 mcg/24 hr ÷ QD in the evening or BID.
***Previously treated with oral corticosteroids:*** Start with 440 mcg BID; **max. dose:** 880 mcg/24 hr.

***Topical:***
***Cream and ointment:***
***≥2 yr:*** Apply a thin film to affected area QD. Safety and efficacy for > 3 wk has not been established for pediatric patients.
***Lotion:***
***≥12 yr:*** Apply a few drops to affected area and massage lightly into skin until it disappears QD.

Concurrent administration with ketoconazole and other CYP 450 3A4 inhibitors may increase mometasone levels, resulting in Cushing syndrome and adrenal suppression.

**INTRANASAL:** Clear nasal passages and shake nasal spray well before each use. Onset of action for nasal symptoms of allergic rhinitis has been shown to occur within 11 hr after the first dose. Nasal burning and irritation may occur. Nasal septal perforation, taste and smell disturbances have been rarely reported.

**ORAL INHALATION:** Rinse mouth after each use. Musculoskeletal pain, oral candidiasis, arthralgia, and fatigue may occur.

**TOPICAL USE: Avoid** application/contact to face, eyes, underarms, groin, and open skin. Occlusive dressings and use in diaper dermatitis are **not recommended.**

**MONTELUKAST**
Singulair
***Anti-asthmatic, anti-allergy, leukotriene receptor antagonist***

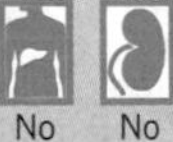

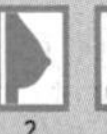


**Chewable tabs:** 4, 5 mg; contains phenylalanine
**Tabs:** 10 mg
**Oral granules:** 4 mg per packet (30s)

*Continued*

FORMULARY

For explanation of icons, see p. 698.

MONTELUKAST *continued*

***Asthma and seasonal allergic rhinitis:***
***Child (6 mo–5 yr):*** 4 mg (oral granules or chewable tablet) PO QHS
***Child (6–14 yr):*** 5 mg (chewable tablet) PO QHS
***>14 yr and adult:*** 10 mg PO QHS
***Prevention of exercise-induced bronchospasm:***
***≥15 yr and adult:*** 10 mg PO at least 2 hr prior to exercise; additional doses **should not** be administered within 24 hr.

Chewable tablet dosage form is **contraindicated** in phenylketonuric patients. Side effects include: headache, abdominal pain, dyspepsia, fatigue, dizziness, cough, and elevated liver enzymes. Diarrhea, eosinophilia, hypersensitivity reactions, pharyngitis, nausea, otitis, sinusitis, and viral infections have been reported in children. Drug is a substrate for CYP 450 3A4 and 2C9. Phenobarbital and rifampin may induce hepatic metabolism to increase the clearance of montelukast.

Doses may administered with or without food.

## MORPHINE SULFATE
Roxanol, MS Contin, Oramorph SR, and many others
***Narcotic, analgesic***

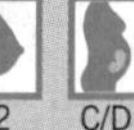

No Yes 2 C/D

**Oral solution:** 10 mg/5 mL, 20 mg/5 mL
**Concentrated oral solution:** 100 mg/5 mL
**Caps/tabs:** 15, 30 mg
**Controlled-release tabs (MS Contin, Oramorph SR):** 15, 30, 60, 100*, 200* mg
**Extended-release tabs:** 15, 30, 60, 100*, 200* mg
**Soluble tabs:** 10, 15, 30 mg
**Extended-release caps:** 30, 60*, 90*, 120* mg
**Sustained-release pellets in caps:** 10, 20, 30, 50, 60, 100*, 200* mg
**Rectal suppository:** 5, 10, 20, 30 mg
**Injection:** 0.5, 1, 2, 4, 5, 8, 10, 15, 25, 50 mg/mL
*Use only for opioid-tolerant patients

**Titrate to effect.**
***Analgesia/tetralogy (cyanotic) spells:***
***Neonate:*** 0.05–0.2 mg/kg/dose IM, slow IV, SC Q4 hr
***Neonatal opiate withdrawal:*** 0.08–0.2 mg/dose Q3–4 hr PRN
***Infant and child:***
***PO:*** 0.2–0.5 mg/kg/dose Q4–6 hr PRN (immediate release) or 0.3–0.6 mg/kg/dose Q12 hr PRN (controlled release)
***IM/IV/SC:*** 0.1–0.2 mg/kg/dose Q2–4 hr PRN; **max. dose:** 15 mg/dose.
***Adult:***
***PO:*** 10–30 mg Q4 hr PRN (immediate release) or 15–30 mg Q8–12 hr PRN (controlled release)
***IM/IV/SC:*** 2–15 mg/dose Q2–6 hr PRN
***Continuous IV infusion:*** (dosing ranges, titrate to effect)
***Neonate:*** 0.01–0.02 mg/kg/hr
***Infant and child:***
***Postoperative pain:*** 0.01–0.04 mg/kg/hr
***Sickle cell and cancer:*** 0.04–0.07 mg/kg/hr
***Adult:*** 0.8–10 mg/hr

*Continued*

MORPHINE SULFATE *continued*

**To prepare infusion for neonates, infants, and children:** Use the following formula:

$$50 \times \frac{\text{Desired dose (mg/kg/hr)}}{\text{Desired infusion rate (mL/hr)}} \times \text{Wt (kg)} = \frac{\text{mg morphine}}{\text{50 mL fluid}}$$

Dependence, CNS and respiratory depression, nausea, vomiting, urinary retention, constipation, hypotension, bradycardia, increased ICP, miosis, biliary spasm, and allergy may occur. **Naloxone may be used to reverse effects, especially respiratory depression**. Causes histamine release resulting in itching and possible bronchospasm. Low-dose naloxone infusion may be used for itching. Inflammatory masses (e.g. granulomas) have been reported with continuous infusions via indwelling intrathecal catheters.

See Chapter 6 for equianalgesic dosing. Pregnancy category changes to "D" if used for prolonged periods or in higher doses at term. Rectal dosing is same as oral dosing but is **not recommended** due to poor absorption.

Controlled/sustained-release oral tablets must be administered whole. Controlled-release oral capsules may be opened and the entire contents sprinkled on applesauce immediately prior to ingestion. **Adjust dose in renal failure (see Chapter 31).**

## MUPIROCIN

Bactroban, Bactroban Nasal, and others

***Topical antibiotic***

No No ? B

**Ointment:** 2% (15, 22, 30 g); contains polyethylene glycol
**Cream:** 2% (15, 30 g); contains benzyl alcohol
**Nasal ointment:** 2% (1 g), as calcium salt

***Topical:***
***≥3 mo–adult:*** Apply small amount TID to affected area × 5–14 days. Ointment may be used in infants > 2 mo.
***Intranasal:*** Apply small amount intranasally 2–4 times/24 hr for 5–14 days.

**Avoid** contact with the eyes. Topical cream is **not** intended for use in lesions > 10 cm in length or 100 $cm^2$ in surface area. **Do not use** topical ointment preparation on open wounds because of concerns about systemic absorption of polyethylene glycol. May cause minor local irritation and dry skin. Intranasal route may cause nasal stinging, taste disorder, headache, rhinitis, and pharyngitis.

If clinical response is not apparent in 3–5 days with topical use, reevaluate infection. Intranasal administration may be used to eliminate carriage of *S. aureus*, including MRSA.

## MYCOPHENOLATE

Mycophenolate mofetil: CellCept
Mycophenolate sodium: Myfortic

***Immunosuppressant agent***

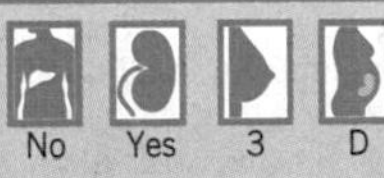


**Mycophenolate mofetil:**
**Caps:** 250 mg

*Continued*

For explanation of icons, see p. 698.

MYCOPHENOLATE *continued*

***Mycophenolate mofetil (cont'd):***
**Tabs:** 500 mg
**Oral suspension:** 200 mg/mL (225 mL); contains phenylalanine (0.56 mg/mL) and methylparabens
**Injection:** 500 mg
**Mycophenolate sodium:**
**Delayed-release tabs (Myfortic):** 180, 360 mg

---

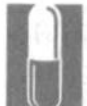

***Child (see remarks):***
***Caps, tabs, or suspension:*** 600 mg/m$^2$/dose PO BID up to a **max. dose** of 2000 mg/24 hr; alternatively, patients with body surface areas (BSAs) $\geq$ 1.25 m$^2$ may be dosed as follows:
***1.25–1.5 m$^2$:*** 750 mg PO BID
***$>$1.5 m$^2$:*** 1000 mg PO BID
***Delayed-release tabs (Myfortic):*** 400 mg/m$^2$/dose PO BID; **max. dose:** 720 mg BID; **not recommended** in patients with BSAs $<$ 1.19 m$^2$. Alternatively, patients with body surface areas $\geq$ 1.19 m$^2$ may be dosed as follows:
***1.19–1.58 m$^2$:*** 540 mg PO BID
***$>$1.58 m$^2$:*** 720 mg PO BID

***Adult (in combination with corticosteroids and cyclosporine):***
***IV:*** 2000–3000 mg/24 hr ÷ BID
***Oral:***
***Caps, tabs, or suspension:*** 2000–3000 mg/24 hr PO ÷ BID
***Delayed-release tabs (Myfortic):*** 720 mg PO BID

---

Check specific transplantation protocol for specific dosage. Mycophenolate mofetil is a pro-drug for mycophenolic acid. Due to differences in absorption, the delayed-release tablets **should not** be interchanged with the other oral dosage forms on an equivalent mg-to-mg basis. Increases risk of first trimester pregnancy loss and increased risk of congenital malformations (especialy external ear and facial abnormalities including cleft lip and palate, and anomalies of the distal limbs, heart, and esophagus).

Common side effects may include headache, hypertension, diarrhea, vomiting, bone marrow suppression, anemia, fever, opportunistic infections, and sepsis. May also increase the risk for lymphomas or other malignancies. GI bleeds and increased risk for rejection in heart transplant patients switched from calicineurin inhibitors (e.g., cyclosporine and tacrolimus) and CellCept to sirolimus and CellCept have been reported.

**Use with caution** in patients with active GI disease or renal impairment (GFR $<$ 25 mL/min/1.73 m$^2$) outside of the immediate post-transplant period. In adults with renal impairment, **avoid** doses $>$ 2 g/24 hr and observe carefully. No dose adjustment is needed for patients experiencing delayed graft function postoperatively.

**Drug interactions:** (1) Displacement of phenytoin or theophylline from protein binding sites will decrease total serum levels and increase free serum levels of these drugs. Salicylates displace mycophenolate to increase free levels of mycophenolate. (2) Competition for renal tubular secretion results in increased serum levels of acyclovir, ganciclovir, probenecid, and mycophenolate (when any of these are used together). (3) **Avoid** live and live attenuated vaccines (including influenza); decreases vaccine effectiveness.

Administer oral doses on an empty stomach. Cholestyramine and antacid use may decrease mycophenolic acid levels. Infuse intravenous doses over 2 hr. Oral suspension may be administered via NG tube with a minimum size of 8 French.

## NAFCILLIN

Unipen, Nallpen, and others

***Antibiotic, penicillin (penicillinase resistant)***

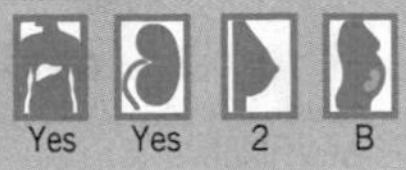


**Caps:** 250 mg
**Injection:** 1, 2, 10 g; contains 2.9 mEq Na/g drug
**Injection, premixed in iso-osmotic dextrose:** 1 g in 50 mL, 2 g in 100 mL

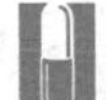

***Neonate:*** **IM/IV**
***≤7 days:***
***<2 kg:*** 50 mg/kg/24 hr ÷ Q12 hr
***≥2 kg:*** 75 mg/kg/24 hr ÷ Q8 hr
***>7 days:***
***<1.2 kg:*** 50 mg/kg/24 hr ÷ Q12 hr
***1.2–2 kg:*** 75 mg/kg/24 hr ÷ Q8 hr
***≥2 kg:*** 100 mg/kg/24 hr ÷ Q6 hr
***Infant and child:***
***PO:*** 50–100 mg/kg/24 hr ÷ Q6 hr
***IM/IV:***
***Mild to moderate infections:*** 50–100 mg/kg/24 hr ÷ Q6 hr
***Severe infections:*** 100–200 mg/kg/24 hr ÷ Q4–6 hr
**Max. dose:** 12 g/24 hr
***Adult:***
***PO:*** 250–1000 mg Q4–6 hr
***IV:*** 500–2000 mg Q4–6 hr
***IM:*** 500 mg Q4–6 hr
**Max. dose:** 12 g/24 hr

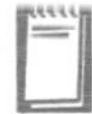

Allergic cross-sensitivity with penicillin. **Oral route not recommended because of unpredictable absorption.** Solutions containing dextrose may be **contraindicated** in patients with known allergy to corn or corn products. High incidence of phlebitis with IV dosing. CSF penetration is poor unless meninges are inflamed. **Use with caution** in patients with combined renal and hepatic impairment (reduce dose by 33%–50%). Nafcillin may increase elimination of cyclosporine and warfarin. Acute interstitial nephritis is rare. May cause rash and bone marrow suppression.

## NALOXONE

Narcan and many generics

***Narcotic antagonist***

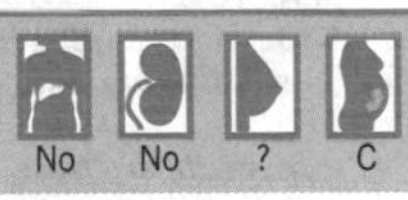


**Injection:** 0.4 mg/mL (1, 10 mL); some preparations may contain parabens
**Injection, in syringe:** 1 mg/mL (2 mL)

***Opiate intoxication (see remarks):***
***Neonate, infant, child <20 kg:*** IM/IV/SC/ETT: 0.1 mg/kg/dose. May repeat PRN Q2–3 min.
***Child ≥ 20 kg or >5 yr:*** 2 mg/dose. May repeat PRN Q2–3 min.
***Continuous infusion (child and adult):*** 0.005 mg/kg loading dose followed by infusion of 0.0025 mg/kg/hr has been recommended. A range of 0.0025–0.16 mg/kg/hr has been reported. Taper gradually to avoid relapse.

*Continued*

For explanation of icons, see p. 698.

NALOXONE *continued*

***Opioate intoxication (cont'd):***

***Adult:*** 0.4–2 mg/dose. May repeat PRN Q2–3 min. Use 0.1- to 0.2-mg increments in opiate-dependent patients.

---

Short duration of action may necessitate multiple doses. For severe intoxication, doses of 0.2 mg/kg may be required. If no response is achieved after a cumulative dose of 10 mg, reevaluate diagnosis. **In the nonarrest situation, use the lowest dose effective (may start at 0.001 mg/kg/dose). See Chapter 6 for additional information.**

Will produce narcotic withdrawal syndrome in patients with chronic dependence. **Use with caution** in patients with chronic cardiac disease. Abrupt reversal of narcotic depression may result in nausea, vomiting, diaphoresis, tachycardia, hypertension, and tremulousness.

May be used simultaneously with opiates at lower dosages (~0.25–2 mcg/kg/hr) to abate opiate-related side effects.

## NAPROXEN/NAPROXEN SODIUM

Naprosyn, Anaprox, EC-Naprosyn, Naprelan, Aleve [OTC], and many others

***Nonsteroidal anti-inflammatory agent***

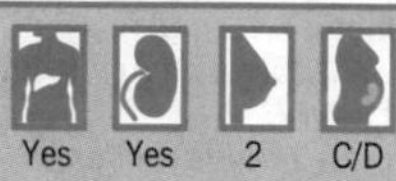


**Naproxen:**

Tabs: 250, 375, 500 mg

Delayed-release tabs (EC-Naprosyn): 375, 500 mg

Oral suspension: 125 mg/5 mL; contains 0.34 mEq Na/1 mL and parabens

**Naproxen Sodium:**

Tabs:

Aleve and others (OTC): 220 mg (200 mg base); contains 0.87 mEq Na

Anaprox: 275 mg (250 mg base), 550 mg (500 mg base); contains 1 mEq, 2 mEq Na, respectively

Controlled-release tabs (Naprelan): 412.5 mg (375 mg base), 550 mg (500 mg base)

---

***All doses based on naproxen base.***

***Child >2 yr:***

***Analgesia:*** 5–7 mg/kg/dose Q8–12 hr PO

***JRA:*** 10–20 mg/kg/24 hr ÷ Q12 hr PO

**Usual max. dose:** 1250 mg/24 hr

***Rheumatoid arthritis, ankylosing spondylitis:***

***Adult:***

***Immediate-release forms:*** 250–500 mg BID PO

***Delayed-release tabs (EC-Naprosyn):*** 375–500 mg BID PO

***Controlled-release tabs (Naprelan):*** 750–1000 mg QD PO; **max. dose:** 1500 mg/24 hr

***Dysmenorrhea:***

500 mg × 1, then 250 mg Q6–8 hr PO; **max. dose:** 1250 mg/24 hr.

---

**Contraindicated** in treating perioperative pain for coronary artery bypass graft surgery. May cause GI bleeding, thrombocytopenia, heartburn, headache, drowsiness, vertigo, and tinnitus. **Use with caution** in patients with GI disease, cardiac disease (risk for thrombotic events, MI, stroke), renal or hepatic impairment, and those receiving anticoagulants. See *Ibuprofen* for other side effects.

Pregnancy category changes to "D" if used in the third trimester or near delivery. Administer doses with food or milk to reduce GI discomfort.

## NEOMYCIN SULFATE

Mycifradin, Neo-fradin, Neo-Tabs, and others

***Antibiotic, aminoglycoside; ammonium detoxicant***

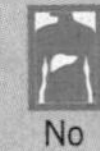 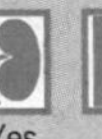 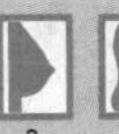 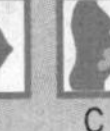

No Yes ? C

**Tabs (Neo-Tabs):** 500 mg
**Oral solution (Mycifradin, Neo-Fradin):** 125 mg/5 mL; contains parabens

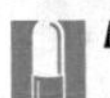

***Diarrhea:***

***Preterm and newborn:*** 50 mg/kg/24 hr ÷ Q6 hr PO

***Hepatic encephalopathy:***

***Infant and child:*** 50–100 mg/kg/24 hr ÷ Q6–8 hr PO × 5–6 days.
**Max. dose:** 12 g/24 hr
***Adult:*** 4–12 g/24 hr ÷ Q4–6 hr PO × 5–6 days

***Bowel prep:***

***Child:*** 90 mg/kg/24 hr PO ÷ Q4 hr × 2–3 days
***Adult:*** 1 g Q1 hr PO × 4 doses, then 1 g Q4 hr PO × 5 doses. (Many other regimens exist.)

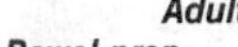

**Contraindicated** in ulcerative bowel disease, intestinal obstruction, or aminoglycoside hypersensitivity. Monitor for nephrotoxicity and ototoxicity. Oral absorption is limited, but levels may accumulate. Consider dosage reduction in the presence of renal failure. May cause itching, redness, edema, colitis, candidiasis, or poor wound healing if applied topically. Prevalence of neomycin hypersensitivity has increased. May decrease absorption of penicillin V, potassium, vitamin $B_{12}$, digoxin, and methotrexate. May potentiate oral anticoagulants and the adverse effects of other neurotoxic, ototoxic, or nephrotoxic drugs.

## NEOMYCIN/POLYMYXIN B/ ± BACITRACIN

Neosporin GU Irrigant, Neosporin, Neosporin Ophthalmic, and others

***Topical antibiotic***

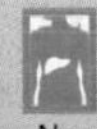 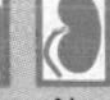 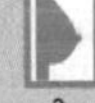 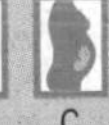

No No ? C

**Solution, genitourinary irrigant:** 40 mg neomycin sulfate, 200,000 U polymyxin B/mL (1, 20 mL); multidose vial contains methylparabens
**In combination with bacitracin:**
**Ointment, topical (Neosporin) (OTC):** 3.5 mg neomycin sulfate, 400 U bacitracin, 5000 U polymyxin B/g (0.9, 14, 28 g)
**Ointment, ophthalmic (Neosporin Ophthalmic):** 3.5 mg neomycin sulfate, 400 U bacitracin, 10,000 U polymyxin B/g (3.5 g)

***Topical:*** Apply to minor wounds and burns QD-TID
***Ophthalmic:*** Apply small amount to conjunctiva Q3–4 hr × 7–10 days, depending on the severity of infection.
***Bladder irrigation:***

***Adult:*** Mix 1 mL in 1000 ml NS and administer via a 3-way catheter at a rate adjusted to the patient's urine output. **Do not exceed** 10 days of continuous use.

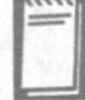

**Do not use** for extended periods. May cause superinfection, delayed healing. See *Neomycin* for additional remarks. Ophthalmic preparation may cause stinging and sensitivity to bright light. **Avoid** use of bladder irrigant in patients with defects in the bladder mucosa or wall.

For explanation of icons, see p. 698.

## NEOSTIGMINE

Prostigmin and others

***Anticholinesterase (cholinergic) agent***

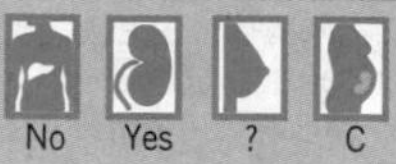


**Tabs:** 15 mg (bromide)
**Injection:** 0.25, 0.5, 1 mg/mL (methylsulfate); may contain parabens or phenol

***Myasthenia gravis diagnosis:*** Use with atropine (see remarks).
- ***Child:*** 0.025–0.04 mg/kg IM × 1
- ***Adult:*** 0.02 mg/kg IM × 1

***Treatment:***
- ***Child:***
  - ***IM/IV/SC:*** 0.01–0.04 mg/kg/dose Q2–4 hr PRN
  - ***PO:*** 2 mg/kg/24 hr ÷ Q3–4 hr; **max. dose:** 375 mg/24 hr.
- ***Adult:***
  - ***IM/IV/SC:*** 0.5–2.5 mg/dose Q1–3 hr PRN up to **max. dose** of 10 mg/24 hr.
  - ***PO:*** Start with 15 mg/dose TID. May increase every 1–2 days. Dosage requirements may vary from 15–375 mg/24 hr with an average of 150 mg/24 hr. Some patients may require as much as 30–40 mg Q2–4 hr.

***Reversal of nondepolarizing neuromuscular blocking agents:*** Administer with atropine or glycopyrrolate.
- ***Infant:*** 0.025–0.1 mg/kg/dose IV
- ***Child:*** 0.025–0.08 mg/kg/dose IV
- ***Adult:*** 0.5–2.5 mg/dose IV
- **Max. dose:** 5 mg/dose

**Contraindicated** in GI and urinary obstruction. **Caution** in asthmatics. May cause cholinergic crisis, bronchospasm, salivation, nausea, vomiting, diarrhea, miosis, diaphoresis, lacrimation, bradycardia, hypotension, fatigue, confusion, respiratory depression, and seizures. Titrate for each patient, but **avoid** excessive cholinergic effects.

For diagnosis of myasthenia gravis (MG), administer atropine 0.011 mg/kg/dose IV immediately before or IM (0.011 mg/kg/dose) 30 min before neostigmine. For treatment of MG, patients may need higher doses of neostigmine at times of greatest fatigue.

**Antidote:** Atropine 0.01–0.04 mg/kg/dose. Atropine and epinephrine should be available in the event of a hypersensitivity reaction.

**Adjust dose in renal failure (see Chapter 31).**

## NEVIRAPINE

Viramune, NVP

***Antiviral, non-nucleoside reverse transcriptase inhibitor***

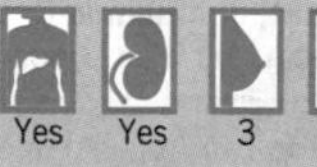
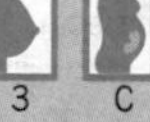


**Tabs:** 200 mg
**Oral suspension:** 10 mg/mL (240 mL); contains parabens

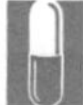

***HIV:*** See www.aidsinfo.nih.gov/guidelines
***Prevention of vertical transmission:*** See Chapter 17.

*Continued*

NEVIRAPINE *continued*

See www.aidsinfo.nih.gov/guidelines for additional remarks.

**Use with caution** in patients with hepatic or renal dysfunction. Most frequent side effects include: skin rash (may be life-threatening, including Stevens-Johnson syndrome; **permanently discontinue and never restart**), fever, abnormal liver function tests, headache, and nausea. **Discontinue therapy** if a severe rash or a rash with fever, blistering, oral lesions, conjunctivitis or muscle aches occur. **Life-threatening** hepatotoxicity has been reported primarily during the first 12 wk of therapy. Patients with increased serum transaminase or a history of hepatitis B or C infection prior to nevirapine are at greater risk for hepatotoxicity. Women, including pregnant women, with $CD_4$ counts > 250 cells/mm$^3$ or men with $CD_4$ counts > 400 cells/mm$^3$ are at risk for hepatotoxicity. Monitor liver function tests and CBCs.

Nevirapine induces the CYP 450 3A4 drug metabolizing isoenzyme to cause an autoinduction of its own metabolism within the first 2–4 wk of therapy and has the potential to interact with many drugs. **Carefully review the patient's drug profile for other drug interactions each time nevirapine is initiated or when a new drug is added to a regimen containing nevirapine.**

Doses can be administered with food and concurrently with didanosine.

## NIACIN/VITAMIN $B_3$

Niacor, Niaspan, Slo-Niacin, Nicotinic acid, Vitamin $B_3$, and many other generics

***Vitamin, water soluble***

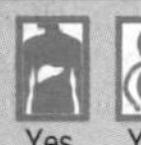
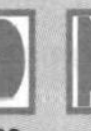
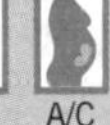

Yes Yes ? A/C

**Tabs (OTC):** 50, 100, 250, 500 mg
**Timed or extended-release tabs (all OTC except 1000 mg):** 250, 500, 750, 1000 mg
**Timed or extended-release caps (OTC):** 125, 250, 400, 500 mg

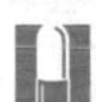

***U.S. RDA:*** **See Chapter 21.**
***Pellagra (PO):***
***Child:*** 50–100 mg/dose TID
***Adult:*** 50–100 mg/dose TID-QID
**Max. dose:** 500 mg/24 hr

**Contraindicated** in hepatic dysfunction, active peptic ulcer, and severe hypotension. **Use with caution** in unstable angina, acute MI (especially if receiving vasoactive drugs), renal dysfunction, and in patients with history of jaundice, hepatobiliary disease, or peptic ulcer. Adverse reactions of flushing, pruritis or GI distress may occur with PO administration. May cause hyperglycemia, hyperuricemia, blurred vision, abnormal liver function tests, dizziness, and headaches. May cause false-positive urine catecholamines (fluorometric methods) and urine glucose (Benedict's reagent).

Pregnancy category changes to "C" if used in doses above the RDA or for typical doses used for lipid disorders. See Chapter 21 for multivitamin preparations.



For explanation of icons, see p. 698.

## NICARDIPINE

Cardene, Cardene SR, and others

***Calcium channel blocker, antihypertensive***

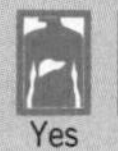 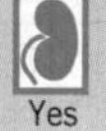  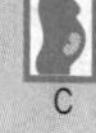

Yes Yes 2 C

**Caps (immediate release):** 20, 30 mg
**Sustained-release caps:** 30, 45, 60 mg
**Injection:** 2.5 mg/mL (10 mL)

***Child (see remarks):***
***Hypertension:***
***Continuous IV infusion:*** 0.5–5 mcg/kg/min

***Adult:***
***Hypertension:***
***Oral:***
***Immediate release:*** 20 mg PO TID, dose may be increased after 3 days to 40 mg PO TID if needed.
***Sustained release:*** 30 mg PO BID, dose may be increased after 3 days to 60 mg PO BID if needed.
***Continuous IV infusion:*** Start at 5 mg/hr, increase dose as needed by 2.5 mg/hr Q5–15 min up to a **max. dose** of 15 mg/hr. Following attainment of desired BP, decrease infusion to 3 mg/hr and adjust rate as needed to maintain desired response.

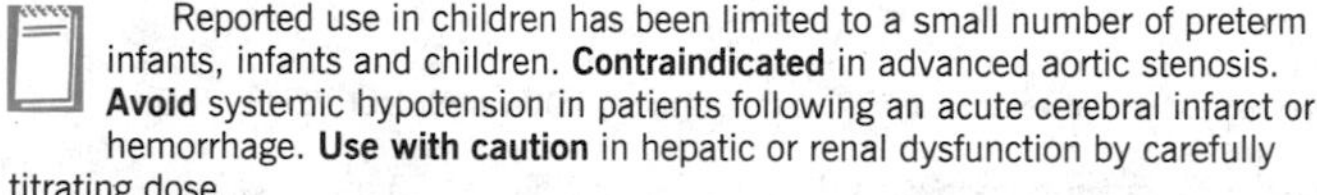

Reported use in children has been limited to a small number of preterm infants, infants and children. **Contraindicated** in advanced aortic stenosis. **Avoid** systemic hypotension in patients following an acute cerebral infarct or hemorrhage. **Use with caution** in hepatic or renal dysfunction by carefully titrating dose.

The drug undergoes significant first pass metabolism through the liver and is excreted in the urine (60%). May cause headache, dizziness, asthenia, peripheral edema, and GI symptoms. **See *Nifedipine* for drug and food interactions.** Onset of action for PO administration is 20 min with peak effects in 0.5–2 hr. IV onset of action is 1 min. Duration of action following a single IV or PO dose is 3 hr. For additional information, see Chapter 4.

## NIFEDIPINE

Adalat CC, Nifediac CC, Procardia, Procardia XL, and many others

***Calcium channel blocker, antihypertensive***

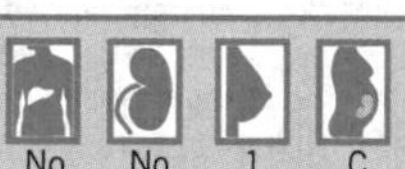

No No 1 C

**Caps (Procardia and others):** 10 mg (0.34 mL), 20 mg (0.45 mL)
**Sustained-release tabs: (Adalat CC, Nifediac CC, Procardia XL, and others):** 30, 60, 90 mg.

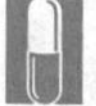

***Child (see remarks for precautions):***
***Hypertensive urgency:*** 0.25–0.5 mg/kg/dose Q4–6 hr PRN PO/SL. **Max. dose:** 10 mg/dose or 1–2 mg/kg/24 hr.
***Hypertension:***
***Sustained release:*** Start with 0.25–0.5 mg/kg/24 hr ÷ Q12–24 hr. May increase to **max. dose:** 3 mg/kg/24 hr up to 120 mg/24 hr.
***Hypertrophic cardiomyopathy:*** 0.6–0.9 mg/kg/24 hr ÷ Q6–8 hr PO/SL.

*Continued*

NIFEDIPINE *continued*

***Adult:***

***Hypertension:***

***Caps:*** Start with 10 mg/dose PO TID. May increase to 30 mg/dose PO TID-QID.

**Max. dose:** 180 mg/24 hr

***Sustained release:*** Start with 30–60 mg PO QD. May increase to **max. dose:** 120 mg/24 hr.

---

Use of immediate-release dosage form in children is controversial and has been abandoned by some. **Use with caution** in children with acute CNS injury due to increased risk for stroke, seizure, and altered level of consciousness. To prevent rapid decrease in blood pressure in children, an initial dose of ≤ 0.25 mg/kg is recommended.

**Use with caution** in patients with CHF and aortic stenosis. May cause severe hypotension, peripheral edema, flushing, tachycardia, headaches, dizziness, nausea, palpitations, and syncope. Although overall use in adults has been abandoned, the immediate-release dosage form is **contraindicated** in adults with severe obstructive coronary artery disease or recent MI, and hypertensive emergencies.

Nifedipine is a substrate for CYP 450 3A3/4 and 3A5-7. **Do not administer** with grapefruit juice; may increase bioavailability and effects. Itraconazole and ketoconazole may increase nifedipine levels/effects. Nifedipine may increase phenytoin, cyclosporine, and digoxin levels. For hypertensive emergencies, see Chapter 4.

For sublingual administration, capsule must be punctured and liquid expressed into mouth. A small amount is absorbed via the SL route. Most effects are due to swallowing and oral absorption. **Do not** crush or chew sustained-release tablet dosage form.

## NITROFURANTOIN

Furadantin, Macrodantin, Macrobid, and others

***Antibiotic***

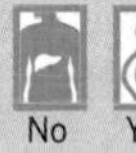
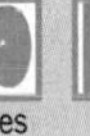
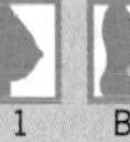
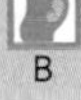

No Yes 1 B

**Caps (macrocrystals; Macrodantin):** 25, 50, 100 mg
**Caps (dual release; Macrobid):** 100 mg (25 mg macrocrystal/75 mg monohydrate)
**Oral suspension (Furadantin):** 25 mg/5 mL (470 mL); contains parabens and saccharin

---

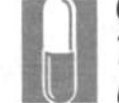

***Child (> 1 mo):***
***Treatment:*** 5–7 mg/kg/24 hr ÷ Q6 hr PO; **max. dose:** 400 mg/24 hr
***UTI prophylaxis:*** 1–2 mg/kg/dose QHS PO; **max. dose:** 100 mg/24 hr
***≥12 yr and adult:***
***Macrocrystals:*** 50–100 mg/dose Q6 hr PO
***Dual release:*** 100 mg/dose Q12 hr PO
***UTI prophylaxis (macrocrystals):*** 50–100 mg/dose PO QHS

---

**Contraindicated** in severe renal disease, infants <1 mo of age, GFR < 60 mL/min (reduced drug distribution in the urine), and pregnant women at term. **Use with caution** in G6PD deficiency, anemia, lung disease, and peripheral neuropathy. May cause nausea, hypersensitivity reactions, vomiting, cholestatic jaundice, headache, hepatotoxicity, polyneuropathy, and hemolytic anemia.

Anticholinergic drugs and high-dose probenecid may increase nitrofurantoin toxicity. Magnesium salts may decrease nitrofurantoin absorption. Causes false-positive urine glucose with Clinitest. Administer doses with food or milk.

For explanation of icons, see p. 698.

## NITROGLYCERIN

Nitro-Bid, Nitrostat, Nitro-Time, Nitro-Dur, NitroMist, and many others

***Vasodilator, antihypertensive***

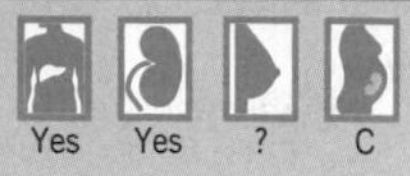


**Injection:** 5 mg/mL (5, 10 mL); may contain alcohol or propylene glycol
**Prediluted injection in $D_5W$:** 100 mcg/mL, 200 mcg/mL, 400 mcg/mL (250, 500 mL)
**Sublingual tabs (Nitrostat and others):** 0.3, 0.4, 0.6 mg
**Sustained-release caps (Nitro-Time and others):** 2.5, 6.5, 9 mg
**Ointment, topical (Nitro-Bid and others):** 2% (1, 30, 60 g)
**Patch (Nitro-Dur and others):** 2.5 mg/24 hr (0.1 mg/hr), 5 mg/24 hr (0.2 mg/hr), 7.5 mg/24 hr (0.3 mg/hr), 10 mg/24 hr (0.4 mg/hr), 15 mg/24 hr (0.6 mg/hr), 20 mg/24 hr (0.8 mg/hr)
**Spray, translingual:** 0.4 mg per metered spray (4.9, 12 g; delivers 60 and 200 doses, respectively); may contain 20% alcohol
NitroMist: 0.4 mg per metered spray (8.5 g; delivers 230 doses)

---

***Child:***
***Continuous IV infusion:*** Begin with 0.25–0.5 mcg/kg/min; may increase by 0.5–1 mcg/kg/min Q3–5 min PRN. Usual dose: 1–5 mcg/kg/min. **Max. dose:** 20 mcg/kg/min.

***Adult:***
***Continuous IV infusion:*** 5 mcg/min IV, then increase Q3–5 min PRN by 5 mcg/min up to 20 mcg/min. If no response, increase by 10 mcg/min Q3–5 min PRN up to a **max.** of 200 mcg/min.

**Note: The dosage units for adults are in mcg/min; compared to mcg/kg/min for children.**

***Sublingual:*** 0.2–0.6 mg Q5 min. **Max.** of three doses in 15 min.
***Oral:*** 2.5–9 mg BID-TID; up to 26 mg QID
***Ointment:*** Apply 1–2 inches Q8 hr, up to 4–5 inches Q4 hr
***Patch:*** 0.2–0.4 mg/hr initially, then titrate to 0.4–0.8 mg/hr; apply new patch daily (tolerance is minimized by removing patch for 10–12 hr/24 hr)

---

**Contraindicated** in glaucoma and severe anemia. In small doses (1–2 mcg/kg/min) acts mainly on systemic veins and decreases preload. At 3–5 mcg/kg/min acts on systemic arterioles to decrease resistance. May cause headache, flushing, GI upset, blurred vision, and methemoglobinemia. **Use with caution** in severe renal impairment, increased ICP, and hepatic failure. IV nitroglycerin may antagonize anticoagulant effect of heparin.

Decrease dose gradually in patients receiving drug for prolonged periods to **avoid** withdrawal reaction. Must use polypropylene infusion sets to **avoid** adsorption of drug to plastic tubing.

Onset (duration) of action: IV: 1–2 min. (3–5 min.); sublingual: 1–3 min. (30–60 min); PO sustained release: 40 min (4–8 hr); topical ointment: 20–60 min (2–12 hr); and transdermal patch: 40–60 min (18–24 hr).

## NITROPRUSSIDE

Nitropress and others (previously available as Nipride)

***Vasodilator, antihypertensive***

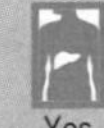 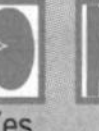 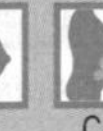 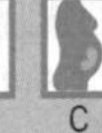

Yes Yes ? C

**Injection:** 25 mg/mL (2 mL)

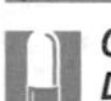

***Child and adult:*** IV, continuous infusion
***Dose:*** Start at 0.3–0.5 mcg/kg/min, titrate to effect. Usual dose is 3–4 mcg/kg/min. **Max. dose:** 10 mcg/kg/min.

**Contraindicated** in patients with decreased cerebral perfusion and in situations of compensatory hypertension (increased ICP). Monitor for hypotension and acidosis. Dilute with $D_5W$ and protect from light.

Nitroprusside is nonenzymatically converted to cyanide, which is converted to thiocyanate. Cyanide may produce metabolic acidosis and methemoglobinemia; thiocyanate may produce psychosis and seizures. Monitor thiocyanate levels if used for > 48 hr or if dose ≥ 4 mcg/kg/min. **Thiocyanate levels should be < 50 mg/L.** Monitor **cyanide levels (toxic levels > 2 mcg/mL)** in patients with hepatic dysfunction and thiocyanate levels in patients with renal dysfunction.

Onset of action is 2 min with a 1- to 10-min duration of effect.

## NOREPINEPHRINE BITARTRATE

Levophed and others

***Adrenergic agonist***

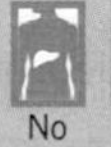 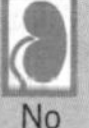 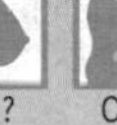 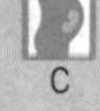

No No ? C

**Injection:** 1 mg/mL as norepinephrine base (4 mL); contains sulfites

***Child:*** Continuous IV infusion **doses as norepinephrine base**. Start at 0.05–0.1 mcg/kg/min. Titrate to effect. **Max. dose:** 2 mcg/kg/min.
***Adult:*** Continuous IV infusion **doses as norepinephrine base**. Start at 4 mcg/min and titrate to effect. Usual dosage range: 8–12 mcg/min.

**NOTE: The dosage units for adults are in mcg/min; compared to mcg/kg/min for children.**

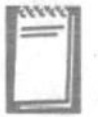

May cause cardiac arrhythmias, hypertension, hypersensitivity, headaches, vomiting, uterine contractions, and organ ischemia. May cause decreased renal blood flow and urine output. **Avoid** extravasation into tissues; may cause severe tissue necrosis. If this occurs, treat locally with phentolamine.

## NORFLOXACIN

Noroxin, Chibroxin

***Antibiotic, quinolone***

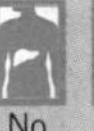 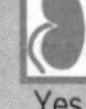 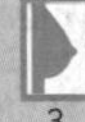 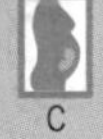

No Yes 3 C

**Tabs:** 400 mg
**Ophthalmic drops (Chibroxin):** 3 mg/mL (5 mL)

*Continued*

For explanation of icons, see p. 698.

NORFLOXACIN *continued*

***Child:***
***UTI (limited data in children 5 mo–19 yr):*** 9–14 mg/kg/24 hr PO ÷ Q12 hr; **max. dose:** 800 mg/24 hr. For UTI prophylaxis, give 2–6 mg/kg/24 hr.
***Adult:***
**UTI:** 400 mg PO Q12 hr (× 7–10 days for uncomplicated cases and × 10–21 days for complicated cases)
**Prostatitis:** 400 mg PO Q12 hr × 28 days
**N. gonorrheae (uncomplicated):** 800 mg PO × 1
***Ophthalmic:***
***≥1 yr–adult:*** 1–2 drops QID × ≤ 7 days. May give up to Q2 hr for severe infections during the first day of therapy.

Like other quinolones, there is concern regarding development of arthropathy. Norfloxacin does **not** adequately treat chlamydia co-infections. UTI dosing can be used for BK virus nephropathy in immunocompromised patients. **Use with caution** in children <18 yr, seizures, proarrythmic conditions, diabetes, patients receiving Class Ia or Class III antiarrhythmics and impaired renal function **(adjust dose in renal failure; see Chapter 31).**

Inhibits CYP 450 1A2. May increase serum theophylline levels. May prolong PT in patients on warfarin. See *Ciprofoxacin* for common side effects and drug interactions. QTc prolongation, peripheral neuropathy and tendon rupture (especially with corticosteroid use) have been reported.

Ophthalmic dosage form may cause local burning or discomfort, photophobia and bitter taste. Administer oral doses on an empty stomach.

## NORTRIPTYLINE HYDROCHLORIDE

Pamelor, Aventyl, and various generics
***Antidepressant, tricyclic***

Yes No 3 D

**Caps:** 10, 25, 50, 75 mg; may contain benzyl alcohol, EDTA
**Oral solution:** 10 mg/5 mL; contains up to 4% alcohol

***Depression:***
***Child 6–12 yr:*** 1–3 mg/kg/24 hr ÷ TID-QID PO or 10–20 mg/24 hr ÷ TID-QID PO
***Adolescent:*** 1–3 mg/kg/24 hr ÷ TID-QID PO or 30–50 mg/24 hr ÷ TID-QID PO
***Adult:*** 75–100 mg/24 hr ÷ TID-QID PO
**Max. dose:** 150 mg/24 hr
***Nocturnal enuresis:***
***6–7 yr (20–25 kg):*** 10 mg PO QHS
***8–11 yr (26–35 kg):*** 10–20 mg PO QHS
***>11 yr (36–54 kg):*** 25–35 mg PO QHS

See *Imipramine* for **contraindications** and common side effects. Fewer CNS and anticholinergic side effects than amitriptyline. Lower doses and slower dose titration is recommended in hepatic impairment. Therapeutic antidepressant effects occur in 7–21 days. Monitor for clinical worsening of depression and suicidal ideation/behavior following the initiation of therapy or after dose changes. **Do not** discontinue abruptly. Nortriptyline is a substrate for the CYP 450 1A2 and 2D6 drug metabolizing enzymes.

*Continued*

NORTRIPTYLINE HYDROCHLORIDE *continued*

Therapeutic nortriptyline levels for depression: 50–150 ng/mL. Recommended serum sampling time: obtain a single level 8 or more hr after an oral dose (following 4 days of continuous dosing for children and after 9–10 days for adults).

Administer with food to decrease GI upset.

## NYSTATIN

Mycostatin, Nilstat, and others

***Antifungal agent***

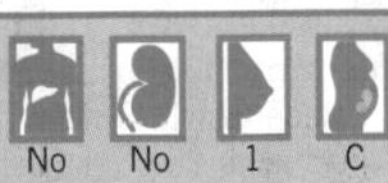


**Tabs:** 500,000 U
**Troches/pastilles:** 200,000 U
**Oral suspension:** 100,000 U/mL (5, 60, 480 mL)
**Cream/ointment:** 100,000 U/g (15, 30 g)
**Topical powder:** 100,000 U/g (15, 30 g)
**Vaginal tabs:** 100,000 U (15s)

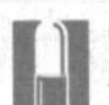

***Oral:***
***Preterm infant:*** 0.5 mL (50,000 U) to each side of mouth QID
***Term infant:*** 1 mL (100,000 U) to each side of mouth QID
***Child/adult:***
***Suspension:*** 4–6 mL (400,000–600,000 U) swish and swallow QID
***Troche:*** 200,000–400,000 U 4–5 ×/24 hr
***Vaginal:***
***Adolescent and adult:*** 1 tab QHS × 14 days
***Topical:*** Apply to affected areas BID-QID

May produce diarrhea and GI side effects. Local irritation, contact dermatitis and Stevens-Johnson syndrome have been reported. Treat until 48–72 hr after resolution of symptoms. Drug is poorly absorbed through the GI tract. **Do not** swallow troches whole (allow to dissolve slowly). Oral suspension should be swished about the mouth and retained in the mouth as long as possible before swallowing.

## OCTREOTIDE ACETATE

Sandostatin, Sandostatin LAR Depot

***Somatostatin analog, antisecretory agent***

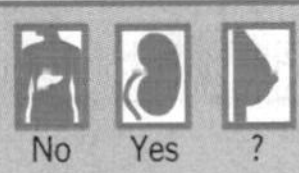


**Injection (amps):** 0.05, 0.1, 0.5 mg/mL (1 mL)
**Injection (multi-dose vials):** 0.2, 1 mg/mL (5 mL)
**Injection, microspheres for suspension (Sandostatin LAR Depot):** 10, 20, 30 mg (in kits with 2 mL diluent and 1.5 inch 20-gauge needles)

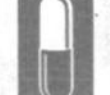

***Infant and child (limited data):***
***Intractable diarrhea:***
***IV/SC:*** 1–10 mcg/kg/24 hr ÷ Q12–24 hr. Dose may be increased within the recommended range by 0.3 mcg/kg/dose every 3 days as needed. **Max. dose:** 1500 mcg/24 hr.
***IV continuous infusion:*** 1 mcg/kg/dose bolus followed by 1 mcg/kg/hr has been used in diarrhea associated with graft versus host disease.

*Continued*

For explanation of icons, see p. 698.

OCTREOTIDE ACETATE *continued*

Cholelithiasis, hyperglycemia, hypoglycemia, hypothyroidism, nausea, diarrhea, abdominal discomfort, headache, dizziness, and pain at injection site may occur. Growth hormone suppression may occur with long-term use.

Bradycardia in patients with acromegaly, and pancreatitis have been reported. Cyclosporine levels may be reduced in patients receiving this drug. May increase the effects/toxicity of bromocriptine.

Patients with severe renal failure requiring dialysis may require dosage adjustments due to an increase in half-life. The effects of hepatic dysfunction on octreotide have not been evaluated.

Sandostatin LAR Depot is administered once every 4 wk **only** by the IM route and is currently indicated for use in adults who have been stabilized on IV/SC therapy. See package insert for details.

## OFLOXACIN

Floxin, Floxin Otic, Ocuflox, and others

***Antibiotic, quinolone***

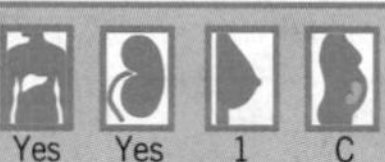


**Otic solution (Floxin Otic):** 0.3% (5, 10 mL)
**Ophthalmic solution (Ocuflox):** 0.3% (1, 5, 10 mL)
**Tabs:** 200, 300, 400 mg
**Prediluted injection in $D_5W$:** 200 mg/50 mL, 400 mg/100 mL

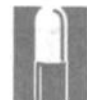

***Otitic use:***

***Otitis externa:***

***1–12 yr:*** 5 drops to affected ear(s) BID × 10 days

***≥12 yr:*** 10 drops to affected ear(s) BID × 10 days

***Chronic suppurative otitis media:***

***≥12 yr:*** 10 drops to affected ear(s) BID × 14 days

***Acute otitis media with tympanostomy tubes:***

***1–12 yr:*** 5 drops to affected ear(s) BID × 10 days

***Ophthalmic use:***

***>1 yr:*** 1–2 drops to affected eye(s) Q2–4 hr × 2 days, then QID for an additional 5 days.

Pruritus, local irritation, taste perversion, dizziness, earache have been reported with otic use. Ocular burning/discomfort is frequent with ophthalmic use. Consult with ophthalmology in corneal ulcers.

When using otic solution, warm solution by holding the bottle in the hand for 1–2 min. Cold solutions may result in dizziness. For otitis externa, patient should lie with affected ear upward before instillation and remain in the same position after dose administration for 5 min to enhance drug delivery. For acute otitis media with tympanostomy tubes, patient should lie in the same position prior to instillation and the tragus should be pumped 4 times after the dose to assist in drug delivery to the middle ear.

**Adjust dose in severe renal or hepatic impairment (max. dose: 400 mg/24 hr) with systemic use.** Systemic use of ofloxacin is typically replaced by its S-isomer, levofloxacin, which has a more favorable side effect profile than ofloxacin. See *Levofloxacin.*

## OLOPATADINE
Patanol
***Antihistamine***

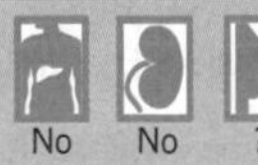
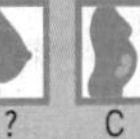

No No ? C

**Ophthalmic solution:** 0.1% (5 mL), 0.2% (2.5 mL)

***Allergic conjunctivitis:***
***≥3 yr and adult:***
***0.1% solution:*** 1–2 drops in affected eye(s) BID (spaced 6–8 hr apart).
***0.2% solution:*** 1 drop in affected eye(s) QD.

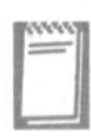

**DO NOT** use while wearing contact lenses; wait at least 10 min after instilling drops before inserting lenses. Ocular side effects include burning or stinging, dry eye, foreign body sensation, hyperemia, keratitis, lid edema and pruritis. May also cause headaches, asthenia, pharyngitis, rhinitis, and taste perversion.

## OLSALAZINE
Dipentum, Di-mesalazine, Di-5-ASA
***Salicylate, GI anti-inflammatory agent***

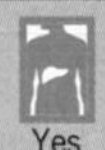
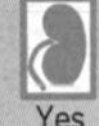

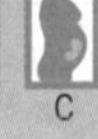

Yes Yes 2 C

**Caps:** 250 mg

***Ulcerative colitis:***
***Child:*** See remarks.
***Adult:*** 500 mg PO BID

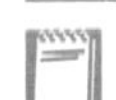

Drug is converted to 5-aminosalicylic acid (mesalamine) by colonic bacteria. 1 g olsalazine generally delivers 0.9 g of mesalamine to the colon. Only 1%–3% of olsalazine is systemically absorbed.

**Contraindicated** in salicylate hypersensitivity. **Use with caution** in severe liver disease, renal dysfunction, sulfasalazine hypersensitivity and bronchial asthma. Diarrhea is the most common dose related side effect. May also cause GI discomfort, headaches, rash, dizziness, and increase risk of bleeding with low molecular weight heparins or heparinoids and warfarin. Use with 6-mercaptopurine or thioguanine may increase risk of myelosuppression. Pancreatitis in children and hepatotoxicity have been reported. Monitor urinalysis and renal function.

Administer all doses with food to enhance efficacy.

Use in children (2–18 yr) has been limited to a trial where olsalazine 30 mg/kg/24 hr (**max. dose:** 2 g/24 hr) was found to be less efficacious than sulfasalazine 60 mg/kg/24 hr (**max. dose:** 4 g/24 hr) in treating mild/moderate ulcerative colitis. This may suggest inadequate dosing in this trial; additional studies are needed.

## OMEPRAZOLE
Prilosec, Prilosec OTC, and others
In combination with sodium bicarbonate: Zegerid
***Gastric acid pump inhibitor***

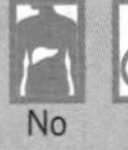
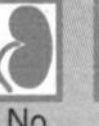
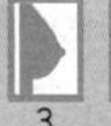
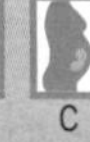

No No 3 C

**Caps, sustained-release:** 10, 20, 40 mg
**Tabs, delayed-release (OTC):** 20 mg

*Continued*

For explanation of icons, see p. 698.

OMEPRAZOLE *continued*

**Oral suspension:** 2 mg/mL ; contains ~ 0.5 mEq sodium bicarbonate per 1 mg drug

**In combination with sodium bicarbonate:**

**Powder for oral suspension (Zegerid):** 20, 40 mg packets (30s); each packet (regardless of strength) contains 1680 mg (20 mEq) sodium bicarbonate

**Caps, immediate-release (Zegerid):** 20, 40 mg; each capsule (regardless of strength) contains 1100 mg (13.1 mEq) sodium bicarbonate

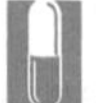

***Child:***

***Esophagitis, GERD, or ulcers:*** 1 mg/kg/24 hr PO ÷ QD-BID. Reported effective range: 0.2–3.5 mg/kg/24 hr. Children 1–6 yr may require higher doses due to enchanced drug clearance. Alternative dosing for patients ≥ 2 yr:

***<20 kg:*** 10 mg PO QD

***≥20 kg:*** 20 mg PO QD

***Adult:***

***Duodenal ulcer or GERD:*** 20 mg/dose PO QD × 4–8 wk; may give up to 12 wk for errosive esophagitis

***Gastric ulcer:*** 40 mg/24 hr PO ÷ QD-BID × 4–8 wk

***Pathological hypersecretory conditions:*** Start with 60 mg/24 hr PO QD. If needed, dose may be increased up to 120 mg/24 hr PO ÷ TID. Daily doses > 80 mg should be administered in divided doses.

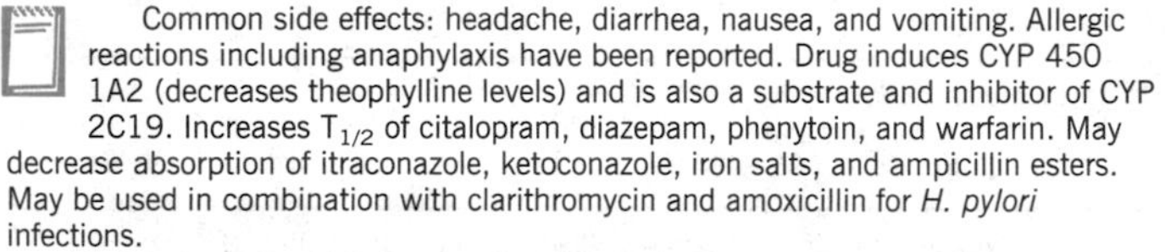

Common side effects: headache, diarrhea, nausea, and vomiting. Allergic reactions including anaphylaxis have been reported. Drug induces CYP 450 1A2 (decreases theophylline levels) and is also a substrate and inhibitor of CYP 2C19. Increases $T_{1/2}$ of citalopram, diazepam, phenytoin, and warfarin. May decrease absorption of itraconazole, ketoconazole, iron salts, and ampicillin esters. May be used in combination with clarithromycin and amoxicillin for *H. pylori* infections.

Administer all doses before meals. Administer 30 min prior to sulcralfate. Capsules contain enteric-coated granules to ensure bioavailability. **Do not** chew or crush capsule. For doses unable to be divided by 10 mg, capsule may be opened and intact pellets may be administered in an acidic beverage (e.g., apple juice, cranberry juice) or apple sauce. The extemporaneously compounded oral suspension product may be less bioavailable due to the loss of the enteric coating.

## OMNIPAQUE

See *Iohexol*

## ONDANSETRON

Zofran

***Antiemetic agent, 5-HT$_3$ antagonist***

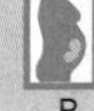

Yes No ? B

**Injection:** 2 mg/mL (2, 20 mL); may contain parabens

**Premixed injection in $D_5W$:** 32 mg/50 mL

**Tabs:** 4, 8, 16, 24 mg

**Tabs, orally disintegrating (ODT):** 4, 8 mg; contains aspartame

**Oral solution:** 4 mg/5 mL (50 mL); contains sodium benzoate

*Continued*

ONDANSETRON *continued*

***Preventing nausea and vomiting associated with chemotherapy:***
***Oral (give initial dose 30 min before chemotherapy):***
***Child, dose based on body surface area:***
- ***<0.3 m²:*** 1 mg TID PRN nausea
- ***0.3–0.6 m²:*** 2 mg TID PRN nausea
- ***0.6–1 m²:*** 3 mg TID PRN nausea
- ***>1 m²:*** 4–8 mg TID PRN nausea

***Dose based on age:***
- ***<4 yr:*** Use dose based on body surface area from preceding dosages.
- ***4–11 yr:*** 4 mg TID PRN nausea
- ***>11 yr and adult:*** 8 mg TID PRN nausea

***IV (child and adult):***
- ***Moderately emetogenic drugs:*** 0.15 mg/kg/dose at 30 min before, 4 and 8 hr after emetogenic drugs. Then same dose Q4 hr PRN.
- ***Highly emetogenic drugs:*** 0.45 mg/kg/dose (**max. dose:** 32 mg/dose) 30 min before emetogenic drugs. Then 0.15 mg/kg/dose Q4 hr PRN.

***Preventing nausea and vomiting associated with surgery (see remarks):***
***IV/IM (administered prior to anesthesia over 2–5 min):***
***Child (2–12 yr):***
- ***≤40 kg:*** 0.1 mg/kg/dose ×1
- ***>40 kg:*** 4 mg × 1

***Adult:*** 4 mg × 1
***PO:***
- ***Adult:*** 16 mg × 1, 1 hr prior to induction of anesthesia

***Preventing nausea and vomiting associated with radiation therapy (adult):***
- ***Total body irradiation:*** 8 mg PO 1–2 hr prior to radiation QD
- ***Single high-dose fraction radiation to abdomen:*** 8 mg PO 1–2 hr prior to radiation with subsequent doses Q8 hr after first dose × 1–2 days after completion of radiation.
- ***Daily fractionated radiation to abdomen:*** 8 mg PO 1–2 hr prior to radiation with subsequent doses Q8 hr after first dose for each day radiation is given.

***Vomiting in acute gastroenteritis (PO route is preferred, use IV when PO is not possible):***
***PO (use oral disintegrating tablet):***
- ***8–15 kg:*** 2 mg × 1
- ***>15 and ≤ 30 kg:*** 4 mg × 1
- ***>30 kg:*** 8 mg × 1

***IV:*** 0.1–0.5 mg/kg/dose × 1; **max. dose:** 4 mg/dose

Bronchospasm, tachycardia, hypokalemia, seizures, headaches, lightheadedness, constipation, diarrhea and transient increases in AST, ALT, and bilirubin may occur. Transient blindness (resolution within a few min up to 48 hr) and rare/transient ECG changes (including QT interval prolongation) have been reported with IV route of administration. Data limited for use in children < 3 yr.

Ondansetron is a substrate for CYP 450 1A2, 2D6, 2E1, and 3A3/4 drug metabolizing enzymes. It is likely that the inhibition/loss of one of the previously listed enzymes will be compensated by others and may result in insignificant changes to ondansetron's elimination. Ondansetron's elimination may be affected by CYP 450 enzyme inducers. Follow theophylline, phenytoin, or warfarin levels closely, if used in combination.

Additional post-operative doses for controlling nausea and vomiting may not provide any benefits.

*Continued*



For explanation of icons, see p. 698.

ONDANSETRON *continued*

In severe hepatic impairment (Child-Pugh score ≥ 10), extend dosage interval up to QD and limit **max. dose** to 8 mg/dose.

Administer orally disintegrating tablet by placing it on the tongue and swallowing it without taking liquids (higher incidence of headache has been reported when taken with water).

## OPIUM TINCTURE

Deodorized tincture of opium

***Narcotic, analgesic***

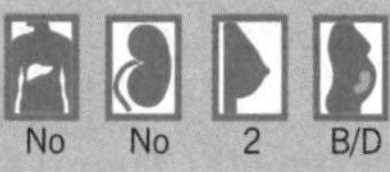


**Oral liquid:** 10% opium. Contains 17%–21% alcohol (1 mL equivalent to 10 mg morphine)

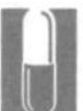

**Dilute 25-fold with water to make a final concentration of 0.4 mg/mL morphine equivalent.**

***Neonatal opiate withdrawal:***

Start with 0.08–0.12 mg (or 0.2–0.3 mL)/dose Q3–4 hr, increase dose by 0.02 mg (or 0.05 mL)/dose Q3–4 hr until symptoms abate; **max. dose:** 0.28 mg (or 0.7 mL)/dose

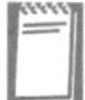

**Use 25-fold dilution** to treat neonatal abstinence syndrome (NAS). Follow neonatal abstinence scores. **Doses for the dilution are equivalent to paregoric doses.** Morphine may also be used to treat NAS. May cause respiratory depression, hypotension, bradycardia, and CNS depression. Pregnancy category changes to "D" if used for prolonged periods or in high doses at term.

## OSELTAMIVIR PHOSPHATE

Tamiflu

***Antiviral***

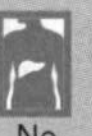
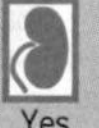
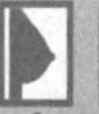
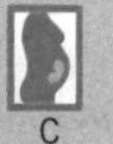

No Yes ? C

**Caps:** 75 mg

**Oral suspension:** 12 mg/mL (25 mL); contains saccharin and sodium benzoate

***Treatment of influenza (initiate therapy within 2 days of onset of symptoms):***

***Child ≥ 1 yr:*** See following table.

***≥12 yr and adult:*** 75 mg PO BID × 5 days.

| Weight (kg) | Dosage for 5 Days | Volume of Oral Suspension |
|---|---|---|
| ≤15 | 30 mg PO BID | 2.5 mL |
| >15–23 | 45 mg PO BID | 3.75 mL |
| >23–40 | 60 mg PO BID | 5 mL |
| >40 | 75 mg PO BID | 6.25 mL |

***Prophylaxis of influenza (see remarks):***

***≥13 yr and adult:*** 75 mg PO QD for a minimum of 7 days and up to 6 wk; initiate therapy within 2 days of exposure.

*Continued*

OSELTAMIVIR PHOSPHATE *continued*

Currently indicated for the treatment of influenza A and B strains. **Do not use** in children < 1 yr due to concerns of fatalities related to excessive CNS penetration in 7-day-old rats. Nausea and vomiting generally occuring within the first 2 days are the most common adverse effects. Insomnia, vertigo, seizures, neuropsychiatric events (may result in fatal outcomes), arrhythmias, rash, and toxic epidermal necrolysis have also been reported. Reduce treatment dose if GFR is 10–30 mL/min to 75 mg PO QD × 5 days. **(See Chapter 31.)**

**PROPHYLAXIS USE:** Oseltamivir is **not** a substitute for annual flu vaccination. Safety and efficacy have been demonstrated for ≤ 6 wk; duration of protection lasts for as long as dosing is continued. Adjust prophylaxis dose if GFR is 10–30 mL/min to 75 mg PO QOD.

Probenecid increases oseltamivir levels. Oseltamivir decreases the efficacy of the nasal influenza vaccine (FluMist); discontinue oseltamivir 48 hr before and **do not** restart for at least 1–2 wk after FluMist administration.

Dosage adjustments in hepatic impairment, severe renal disease and dialysis have not been established for either treatment or prophylaxis use. The safety and efficacy of repeated treatment or prophylaxis courses have not been evaluated. Doses may be administered with or without food.

## OXACILLIN

Various generic brands

***Antibiotic, penicillin (penicillinase resistant)***

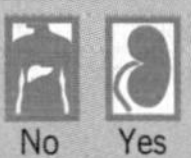
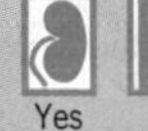
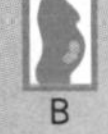

No Yes 2 B

**Oral solution:** 250 mg/5 mL (100 mL); contains 0.8 mEq Na per 250 mg drug and may contain saccharin
**Injection:** 0.5, 1, 2, 10 g
**Injection, premixed in iso-osmotic dextrose:** 1 g/50 mL, 2 g/50 mL
Injectable products contain 2.8–3.1 mEq Na per 1 g drug

**Neonate, *IM/IV:***
***≤7 days:***
- ***<1.2 kg:*** 50 mg/kg/24 hr ÷ Q12 hr
- ***1.2–2 kg:*** 50–100 mg/kg/24 hr ÷ Q12 hr
- ***≥2 kg:*** 75–150 mg/kg/24 hr ÷ Q8 hr

***>7 days:***
- ***<1.2 kg:*** 50 mg/kg/24 hr ÷ Q12 hr
- ***1.2–2 kg:*** 75–150 mg/kg/24 hr ÷ Q8 hr
- ***≥2 kg:*** 100–200 mg/kg/24 hr ÷ Q6 hr

***Infant and child:***
- ***Oral:*** 50–100 mg/kg/24 hr ÷ Q6 hr
- ***IM/IV:*** 100–200 mg/kg/24 hr ÷ Q4–6 hr
- **Max. dose:** 12 g/24 hr

***Adult:***
- ***Oral:*** 500–1000 mg/dose Q4–6 hr
- ***IM/IV:*** 250–2000 mg/dose Q4–6 hr

Rash and GI disturbances are common. Leukopenia, reversible hepatotoxicity, and acute interstitial nephritis have been reported. Hematuria and azotemia have occurred in neonates and infants with high doses. May cause false-positive urinary and serum proteins.

CSF penetration is poor unless meninges are inflamed. Use the lower end of the usual dosage range for patients with creatinine clearances < 10 mL/min. Oral form should be administered on an empty stomach. **Adjust dose in renal failure (see Chapter 31).**

For explanation of icons, see p. 698.

## OXCARBAZEPINE

Trileptal

***Anticonvulsant***

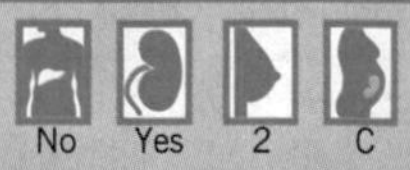


**Tabs:** 150, 300, 600 mg
**Oral suspension:** 300 mg/5 mL (250 mL); contains saccharin and ethanol

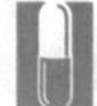

***Child (2–<4 yr):***

***Adjunctive therapy:*** Start with 8–10 mg/kg/24 hr PO ÷ BID up to a **max. dose** of 600 mg/24 hr. For children < 20 kg, may consider using a starting dose of 16–20 mg/kg/24 hr PO ÷ BID; gradually increase the dose over a 2–4 wk period and **do not exceed** 60 mg/kg/24 hr ÷ BID.

***Child (4–16 yr, see remarks):***

***Adjunctive therapy:*** Start with 8–10 mg/kg/24 hr PO ÷ BID up to a **max. dose** of 600 mg/24 hr. Then gradually increase the dose over a 2-wk period to the following maintenance doses:

***20–29 kg:*** 900 mg/24 hr PO ÷ BID
***29.1–39 kg:*** 1200 mg/24 hr PO ÷ BID
***>39 kg:*** 1800 mg/24 hr PO ÷ BID

***Conversion to monotherapy:*** Start with 8–10 mg/kg/24 hr PO ÷ BID and simultaneously initiate dosage reduction of concomitant AEDs and withdrawal completely over 3–6 wk. Dose may be increased at weekly intervals, as clinically indicated, by a **max.** of 10 mg/kg/24 hr to achieve the recommended monotherapy maintenance dose as described in the following table.

***Initiation of monotherapy:*** Start with 8–10 mg/kg/24 hr PO ÷ BID. Then increase by 5 mg/kg/24 hr every 3 days up to the recommended monotherapy maintenance dose as described in the following table.

**RECOMMENDED MONOTHERAPY MAINTENANCE DOSES FOR CHILDREN BY WEIGHT**

| Weight (kg) | Daily Oral Maintenance Dose (mg/24 hr) Divided BID |
|---|---|
| 20 | 600–900 |
| 25–30 | 900–1200 |
| 35–40 | 900–1500 |
| 45 | 1200–1500 |
| 50–55 | 1200–1800 |
| 60–65 | 1200–2100 |
| 70 | 1500–2100 |

***Adult:***

***Adjunctive therapy:*** Start with 600 mg/24 hr PO ÷ BID. Dose may be increased at weekly intervals, as clinically indicated, by a **max.** of 600 mg/24 hr. Usual maintenance dose is 1200 mg/24 hr PO ÷ BID. Doses ≥ 2400 mg/24 hr are generally **not** well tolerated due to CNS side effects.

***Conversion to monotherapy:*** Start with 600 mg/24 hr PO ÷ BID and simultaneously initiate dosage reduction of concomitant AEDs. Dose may be increased at weekly intervals, as clinically indicated, by a **max.** of 600 mg/24 hr to achieve a dose of 2400 mg/24 hr PO ÷ BID. Concomitant AEDs should be terminated gradually over approximately 3–6 wk.

***Initiation of monotherapy:*** Start with 600 mg/24 hr PO ÷ BID. Then increase by 300 mg/24 hr every 3 days up to 1200 mg/24 hr PO ÷ BID.

*Continued*

OXCARBAZEPINE *continued*

**Clinically significant hyponatremia may occur; generally seen within the first 3 mo of therapy.** May also cause headache, dizziness, drowsiness, ataxia, fatigue, nystagmus, urticaria, diplopia, abnormal gait and GI discomfort. About 25% to 30% of patients with cabamazepine hypersensitivity will experience a cross reaction with oxcarbazepine. Serious dermatological reactions (Stevens-Johnson and TEN), multi-organ hypersensitivity reactions, rare cases of anaphylaxis and angioedema, and suicidal behavior or ideation have been reported.

Inhibits CYP 450 2C19 and induces CYP 450 3A4/5 drug metabolizing enzymes. Carbamazepine, phenobarbital, phenytoin, valproic acid and verapamil may decrease oxcarbazepine levels. Oxcarbazepine may increase phenobarbital and phenytoin levels. Oxcarbazepine can decrease the effects of oral contraceptives, felodipine and lamotrigine.

A median pediatric maintenance dose of 31 mg/kg/24 hr (range: 6–51 mg/kg/24 hr) was achieved in a clinical trial. Adjust dosage if GFR < 30 mL/min by administering 50% of the normal starting dose (**max. dose:** 300 mg/24 hr) followed by a slower than normal increase in dose if necessary. **(See Chapter 31.)** No dosage adjustment is required in mild/moderate hepatic impairment.

Doses may be administered with or without food.

## OXYBUTYNIN CHLORIDE

Ditropan, Ditropan XL, Oxytrol, and others

***Anticholinergic agent, antispasmodic***

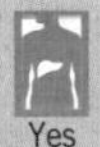
Yes

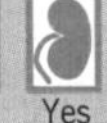
Yes

?

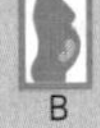
B

**Tabs:** 5 mg
**Tabs, extended-release (Ditropan XL and others):** 5, 10, 15 mg
**Syrup:** 1 mg/mL (473 mL); contains parabens
**Transdermal system (Oxytrol):** delivers 3.9 mg/24 hr (8s); contains 36 mg per system

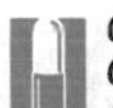

***Child ≤ 5 yr:*** 0.2 mg/kg/dose BID-QID PO; **max. dose:** 15 mg/24 hr
***Child >5 yr:*** 5 mg/dose BID-TID PO; **max. dose:** 15 mg/24 hr
***Adult:***
- ***Immediate release:*** 5 mg/dose BID QID PO
- ***Extended release (Ditropan XL):*** 5–10 mg/dose QD PO up to a **max. dose** of 30 mg/dose QD PO.
- ***Transdermal system:*** 1 patch (3.9 mg/24 hr) every 3–4 days (twice weekly)

**Use with caution** in hepatic or renal disease, hyperthyroidism, IBD, or cardiovascular disease. Anticholinergic side effects may occur, including drowsiness and hallucinations. **Contraindicated** in glaucoma, GI obstruction, megacolon, myasthenia gravis, severe colitis, hypovolemia, and GU obstruction. Oxybutynin is a CYP 450 3A4 substrate; inhibitors and inducers of CYP 450 3A4 may increase and decrease the effects of oxybutynin, respectively.

Dosage adjustments for the extended-release dosage form are at weekly intervals. **Do not** crush, chew, or divide the extended-release tablets. Apply transdermal system on dry intact skin on the abdomen, hip, or buttock by rotating the site and avoiding same site application within 7 days.

For explanation of icons, see p. 698.

## OXYCODONE

Roxicodone, OxyContin, and many others

***Narcotic, analgesic***

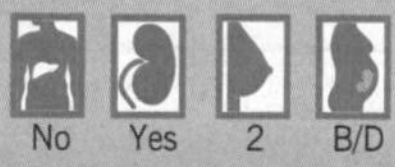


**Solution:** 1 mg/mL (5, 500 mL); contains alcohol
**Concentrated solution:** 20 mg/mL (30 mL); may contain saccharin
**Tabs:** 5, 15, 30 mg
**Controlled-release tabs (OxyContin and others):** 10, 20, 40, 80 mg (80 mg strength for opioid-tolerant patients only)
**Caps:** 5 mg

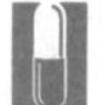

**Dose based upon oxycodone salt:**
***Child:*** 0.05–0.15 mg/kg/dose Q4–6 hr PRN up to 5 mg/dose PO
***Adult:*** 5–10 mg Q4–6 hr PRN PO; see remarks for use of controlled-release tablets.

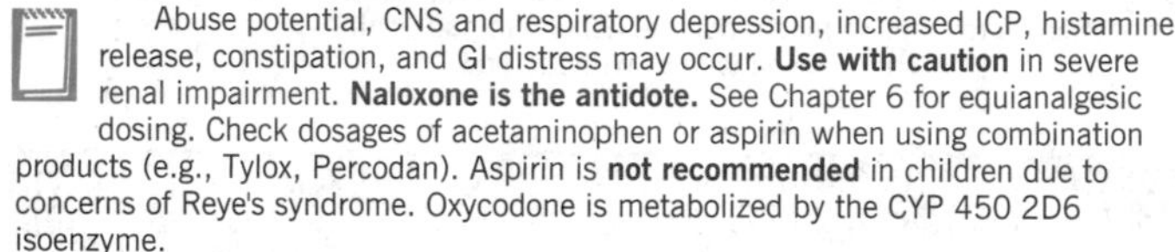

Abuse potential, CNS and respiratory depression, increased ICP, histamine release, constipation, and GI distress may occur. **Use with caution** in severe renal impairment. **Naloxone is the antidote.** See Chapter 6 for equianalgesic dosing. Check dosages of acetaminophen or aspirin when using combination products (e.g., Tylox, Percodan). Aspirin is **not recommended** in children due to concerns of Reye's syndrome. Oxycodone is metabolized by the CYP 450 2D6 isoenzyme.

When using controlled-release tablets (Oxycontin), determine patient's total 24-hr requirements and divide by 2 to administer on a Q12 hr dosing interval. Oxycontin 80 mg tablet is **USED ONLY** for opioid-tolerant patients; this strength can cause fatal respiratory depression in opioid-naïve patients. Controlled-release dosage form **should not be used** as a PRN analgesic and must be swallowed whole.

Pregnancy category changes to "D" if used for prolonged periods or in high doses at term.

## OXYCODONE AND ACETAMINOPHEN

Tylox, Roxilox, Percocet, Endocet, Roxicet, and many others

***Combination analgesic with a narcotic***

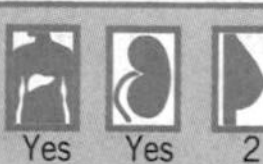


**Capsule (Tylox, Roxilox)/caplet:** Oxycodone HCl 5 mg + acetaminophen 500 mg
**Tabs (Percocet, Endocet, and others):**
Most common strength: Oxycodone HCl 5 mg + acetaminophen 325 mg
Other strengths:
Oxycodone HCl 2.5 mg + acetaminophen 325 mg
Oxycodone HCl 7.5 mg + acetaminophen 325 mg or 500 mg
Oxycodone HCl 10 mg + acetaminophen 325 mg or 650 mg
**Oral solution (Roxicet):** Oxycodone HCl 5 mg + acetaminophen 325 mg/5 mL (5, 500 mL); contains 0.4% alcohol and saccharin

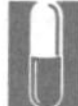

Dose based on amount of oxycodone and acetaminophen.

*Continued*

OXYCODONE AND ACETAMINOPHEN *continued*

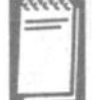

See *Oxycodone* and *Acetaminophen*.

## OXYCODONE AND ASPIRIN

Percodan, Roxiprin, and many others

***Combination analgesic (narcotic and salicylate)***

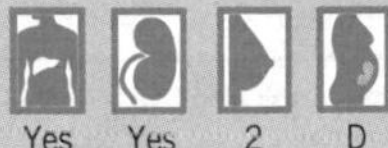

Yes Yes 2 D

**Tabs:**

Percodan, Roxiprin, and others: Oxycodone HCl 4.5 mg, oxycodone tereph 0.38 mg, and aspirin 325 mg

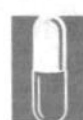

Dose based on amount of oxycodone (combined salts) and aspirin.

See *Oxycodone* and *Aspirin*. **Do not use** in children <16 yr because of risk for Reye's syndrome.

## OXYMETAZOLINE

Nasal: Afrin, Duramist 12-Hr Nasal, Neo-Synephrine 12-Hour Nasal, Nostrilla, and many others

Ophthalmic: Visine LR

***Nasal decongestant, vasoconstrictor***

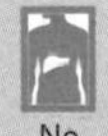

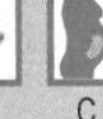

No No ? C

**Nasal spray [OTC]:** 0.05% (15, 30 mL)
**Ophthalmic drops [OTC]:** 0.025% (15, 30 mL); contains benzalkonium chloride and EDTA

***Nasal decongestant* (not to exceed 3 days in duration):**
***≥6 yr–adult:*** 2–3 sprays or 2–3 drops or 1–2 metered sprays (Nostrilla) in each nostril BID. **Do not exceed** 2 doses/24 hr period.
***Ophthalmic:***
***≥6 yr–adult:*** Instill 1–2 drops in the affected eye(s) Q6 hr.

**Contraindicated** in patients on MAO inhibitor therapy. Rebound nasal congestion may occur with excessive use (> 3 days) via the nasal route. Systemic absorption may occur with either route of administration. Headache, dizziness, hypertension, transient burning, stinging, dryness, nasal mucosa ulceration, sneezing, blurred vision and mydriasis have occurred. **Do not use** ophthalmic solution if it changes color or becomes cloudy.

For explanation of icons, see p. 698.

## PALIVIZUMAB

Synagis

***Monoclonal antibody***

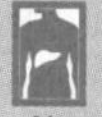 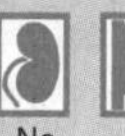 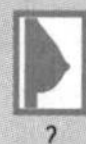 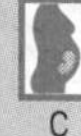

No No ? C

**Injection, solution:** 100 mg/mL (0.5, 1 mL; single use); contains glycine and histidine.

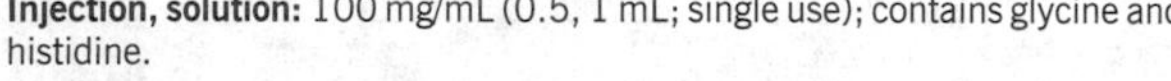

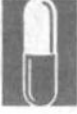

**RSV prophylaxis (see latest edition of *Red Book* for most recent indications):** ***Chronic lung disease ≤ 2 yr, premature infants (≤28 wk of gestation) < 12 mo of age, premature infants (29–32 wk of gestation) < 6 mo of age, or hemodynamically significant cyanotic and acyanotic congenital heart disease ≤ 2 yr:*** 15 mg/kg/dose IM Q monthly just prior to and during the RSV season.

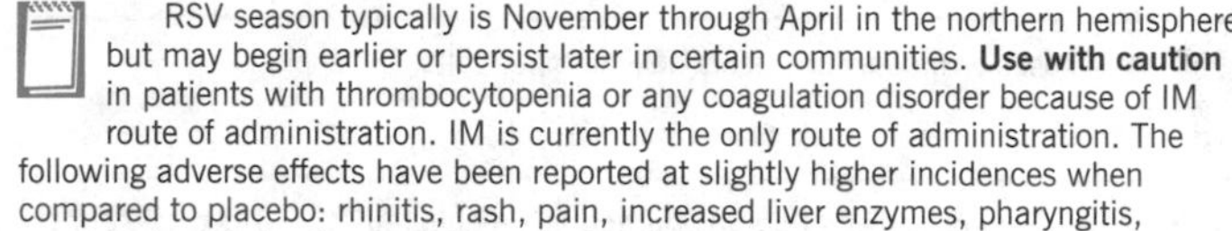

RSV season typically is November through April in the northern hemisphere but may begin earlier or persist later in certain communities. **Use with caution** in patients with thrombocytopenia or any coagulation disorder because of IM route of administration. IM is currently the only route of administration. The following adverse effects have been reported at slightly higher incidences when compared to placebo: rhinitis, rash, pain, increased liver enzymes, pharyngitis, cough, wheeze, diarrhea, vomiting, conjunctivitis and anemia.

Does not interfere with the response to routine childhood vaccines. Palivizumab is currently indicated for RSV prophylaxis in high-risk infants only. Efficacy and safety have not been demonstrated for treatment of RSV.

Each dose should be administered IM in the anterolateral aspect of the thigh. It is recommended to divide doses with total injection volumes > 1 mL. **Avoid** injection in the gluteal muscle because of risk for damage to the sciatic nerve.

## PANCREATIC ENZYMES

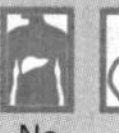 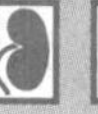 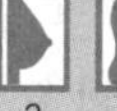 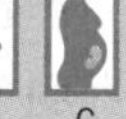

No No 2 C

**See Chapter 30 for description and contents of lipase, protease, and amylase.**

***Initial doses:*** (actual requirements are patient specific)

***Enteric-coated microspheres and microtabs:***

***Infant:*** 2000–4000 U lipase per 120 mL formula or per breast-feeding.

***Child <4 yr:*** 1000 U lipase/kg/meal

***Child ≥ 4 yr and adult:*** 500 U lipase/kg/meal

**Max. dose:** 2500 U lipase/kg/meal

The total daily dose should include approximately three meals and two to three snacks per day. Snack doses are approximately half of meal doses.

May cause occult GI bleeding, allergic reactions to porcine proteins, hyperuricemia and hyperuricosuria with high doses. Dose should be titrated to eliminate diarrhea and to minimize steatorrhea. **Do not** chew microspheres or microtabs. Concurrent administration with $H_2$ antagonists or gastric acid pump inhibitors may enhance enzyme efficacy. Doses higher than 6000 U lipase/kg/meal have been associated with colonic strictures in children <12 yr. Powder dosage form is **not** preferred due to potential GI mucosal ulceration. **Avoid use** of generic pancreatic enzyme products, since they have been associated with treatment failures.

## PANCURONIUM BROMIDE

Various generic brands

***Nondepolarizing neuromuscular blocking agent***

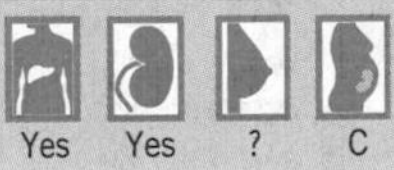


**Injection:** 1 mg/mL (10 mL), 2 mg/mL (2, 5 mL); contains benzyl alcohol

***Neonate:***

***Initial:*** 0.02 mg/kg/dose IV

***Maintenance:*** 0.05–0.1 mg/kg/dose Q0.5–4 hr PRN

***1 mo–adult:***

***Initial:*** 0.04–0.1 mg/kg/dose IV

***Maintenance:*** 0.015–0.1 mg/kg/dose IV Q30–60 min

***Continuous IV infusion:*** 0.1 mg/kg/hr

Onset of action is 1–2 min. May cause tachycardia, salivation, and wheezing.

Drug effects may be accentuated by hypothermia, acidosis, neonatal age, decreased renal function, halothane, succinylcholine, hypokalemia, hyponatremia, hypocalcemia, clindamycin, tetracycline, and aminoglycoside antibiotics. Drug effects may be antagonized by alkalosis, hypercalcemia, peripheral neuropathies, diabetes mellitus, demyelinating lesions, carbamazepine, phenytoin, theophylline, anticholinesterases (e.g., neostigmine, pyridostigmine) and azathioprine.

**Antidote is neostigmine** (with atropine or glycopyrrolate). **Avoid** use in severe renal impairment (<10 mL/min). Patients with cirrhosis may require a high initial dose to achieve adequate relaxation but muscle paralysis will be prolonged.

## PANTOPRAZOLE

Protonix and others

***Gastric acid pump inhibitor***

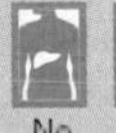
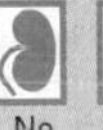
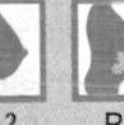


**Tab, enteric coated:** 20, 40 mg

**Injection:** 40 mg; contains edetate sodium

**Oral suspension:** 2 mg/mL ; contains 0.25 mEq sodium bicarbonate per 1 mg drug

**Powder for delayed-release oral suspension:** 20 mg (90s), 40 mg (30s)

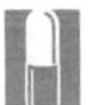

***Child:***

***GERD with erosive esophagitis (limited data):*** 0.5–1 mg/kg/dose PO QD × 28 days; dosed as 20 mg PO QD in 15 children 6–13 yr weighing 20–40 kg.

***IV (data limited to pharmacokinetic trials):*** Some doses ranging from 0.32–1.88 mg/kg/dose have been reported from three separate trials (total N = 31; 0.01–16.4 yr). Patients with Systemic Inflammatory Response Syndrome (SIRS) cleared the drug more slowly, resulting in higher $T_{1/2}$ and AUC, than patients without. Despite limited data, 1–2 mg/kg/24 hr ÷ Q12–24 hr have been used. Additional studies are needed.

***Adult:***

***GERD:*** 40 mg PO QD × 8–16 wk or 40 mg IV QD × 7–10 days.

***Peptic ulcer:*** 40–80 mg PO QD × 4–8 wk

*Continued*

For explanation of icons, see p. 698.

PANTOPRAZOLE *continued*

***Adult (cont'd):***

***Hypersecretory conditions:***

***PO:*** 40 mg BID; dose may be increased as needed up to a **max. dose** of 240 mg/24 hr.

***IV:*** 80 mg Q12 hr; dose may be increased as needed to Q8 hr (**max. dose:** 240 mg/24 hr). Therapy > 6 days at 240 mg/24 hr has not been evaluated.

---

Convert from IV to PO therapy as soon as patient is able to tolerate PO. Common side effects include diarrhea and headache. May cause transient elevation in LFTs. Drug is a substrate for CYP 450 2C19 and 3A3/4 isoenzymes. May decrease the absorption of itraconazole, ketoconazole, iron salts and ampicillin esters.

All oral doses may be taken with or without food. **Do not** crush or chew tablets. The extemporaneously compounded oral suspension may be less bioavailable owing to the loss of the enteric coating. Powder for delayed-release oral suspension product may be mixed with 5 mL apple juice (administer immediately followed by rinsing container with more apple juice), or sprinkled on 1 teaspoonful of apple sauce (administer within 10 min); see package insert for NG administration.

For IV infusion, doses may be administered over 15 min at a concentration of 0.4–0.8 mg/mL or over 2 min at a concentration of 4 mg/mL. Midazolam and zinc are **not compatible** with the IV dosage form. Parenteral routes other than IV are **not recommended**.

## PAREGORIC

Camphorated opium tincture

***Narcotic, analgesic***

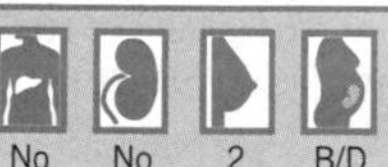


**Camphorated tincture:** 2 mg (morphine equivalent)/5 mL (contains 45% alcohol and may contain benzoic acid or camphor) (473 mL)

---

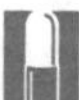

***Analgesia:***

***Child:*** 0.1–0.2 mg/kg (or 0.25–0.5 mL/kg)/dose PO QD-QID

***Adult:*** 2–4 mg (or 5–10 mL)/dose PO QD-QID

***Neonatal opiate withdrawal:***

Start with 0.08–0.12 mg (or 0.2–0.3 mL)/dose Q3–4 hr, increase dose by 0.02 mg (or 0.05 mL)/dose Q3–4 hr until symptoms abate; **max. dose:** 0.28 mg (or 0.7 mL)/dose. Maintain withdrawal dose for 3–5 days and then gradually taper dosage by maintaining same dosage amount and widen dosing interval over a 2- to 4-wk period.

---

Morphine or DTO is preferred over paregoric because of excipients found in paregoric. Each 5 mL paregoric contains 2 mg morphine equivalent, 0.02 mL anise oil, 20 mg benzoic acid, 20 mg camphor, 0.2 mL glycerin and alcohol. The final concentration of morphine equivalent is 0.4 mg/mL. This is 25-fold less potent than undiluted deodorized tincture of opium (DTO: 10 mg morphine equivalent/mL). **If using DTO to treat neonatal abstinence, must dilute 25-fold prior to use.** Similar side effects to morphine. After symptoms are controlled for several days, dose for opiate withdrawal should be decreased gradually over a 2- to 4-wk period (e.g., by 10% Q2–3 days). Monitor neonatal abstinence scores for NAS. Pregnancy category changes to "D" if used for prolonged periods or in high doses.

P

## PAROMOMYCIN SULFATE

Humatin

***Amebicide, antibiotic (aminoglycoside)***

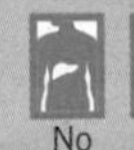
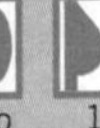
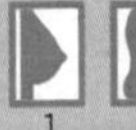
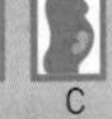

No No 1 C

**Caps:** 250 mg

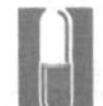

***Intestinal amebiasis (Entamoeba histolytica), Dientamoeba fragilis, and Giardia lamblia infection:***

***Child and adult:*** 25–35 mg/kg/24 hr PO ÷ Q8 hr × 7 days

***Tapeworm (T. saginata, T. solium, D. latum, and D. caninum):***

***Child:*** 11 mg/kg/dose PO Q15 min × 4 doses

***Adult:*** 1 g PO Q15 min × 4 doses

***Tapeworm (Hymenolepis nana):***

***Child and adult:*** 45 mg/kg/dose PO QD × 5–7 days

***Cryptosporidial diarrhea:***

***Adult:*** 1.5–2.25 g/24 hr PO ÷ 3–6 × daily. Duration varies from 10–14 days to 4–8 wk. Maintenance therapy has also been used. Alternatively, 1 g PO BID × 12 wk in conjunction with azithromycin 600 mg PO QD × 4 wk has been used in patients with AIDS.

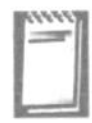

**Contraindicated** in intestinal obstruction. **Use with caution** in ulcerative bowel lesions to avoid renal toxicity via systemic absorption. Drug is generally poorly absorbed and therefore **not** indicated for sole treatment of extraintestinal amebiasis. Side effects include GI disturbance, hematuria, rash, ototoxicity and hypocholesterolemia. May decrease the effects of digoxin.

## PAROXETINE

Paxil, Pexeva, Paxil CR, and others

***Antidepressant, selective serotonin reuptake inhibitor***

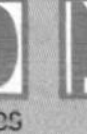

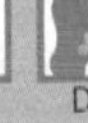

Yes Yes 3 D

**Tabs:** 10, 20, 30, 40 mg

**Controlled-release tabs (Paxil CR):** 12.5, 25, 37.5 mg

**Oral suspension:** 10 mg/5 mL (250 mL); contains saccharin and parabens

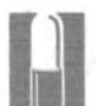

***Child:***

***Depression:*** Well-controlled clinical trials have failed to demonstrate efficacy in children. The FDA recommends that paroxetine **not** be used for this indication.

***Obsessive compulsive disorder (limited data, based on a 10-wk randomized controlled trial in 207 children 7–17 yr; mean age 11.1 ± 3.03 yr):*** Start with 10 mg PO QD. If needed, adjust upward by increasing dose no more than 10 mg/24 hr no more frequently than Q7 days up to a **max. dose** of 50 mg/24 hr. Mean doses of 20.3 mg/24 hr (children) and 26.8 mg/24 hr (adolescents) were used.

***Social anxiety disorder (8–17 yr):*** Start with 10 mg PO QD. If needed, increase dose by 10 mg/24 hr no more frequently than Q7 days up to a **max. dose** of 50 mg/24 hr.

***Adult:***

***Depression:*** Start with 20 mg PO QAM × 4 wk. If no clinical improvement, increase dose by 10 mg/24 hr Q7 days PRN up to a **max. dose** of 50 mg/24 hr.

***Paxil CR:*** Start with 25 mg PO QAM × 4 wk. If no improvement, increase dose by 12.5 mg/24 hr Q7 days PRN up to a **max. dose** of 62.5 mg/24 hr.

*Continued*

FORMULARY

For explanation of icons, see p. 698.

PAROXETINE *continued*

***Adult (cont'd):***

***Obsessive compulsive disorder:*** Start with 20 mg PO QD; increase dose by 10 mg/24 hr Q 7 days PRN up to a **max. dose** of 60 mg/24 hr. Usual dose is 40 mg PO QD.

***Panic disorder:*** Start with 10 mg PO QAM; increase dose by 10 mg/24 hr Q7 days PRN up to a **max. dose** of 60 mg/24 hr.

***Paxil CR:*** Start with 12.5 mg PO QAM; increase dose by 12.5 mg/24 hr Q7 days PRN up to a **max. dose** of 75 mg/24 hr.

---

**Contraindicated** in patients taking MAO inhibitors, within 14 days of discontinuing MAO inhibitors, or thioridazine. **Use with caution** in patients with history of seizures, renal or hepatic impairment, cardiac disease, suicidal concerns, mania/hypomania, and diuretic use. Patients with severe renal or hepatic impairment should initiate therapy at 10 mg/24 hr and increase dose as needed up to a **max.** of 40 mg/24 hr.

Common side effects include anxiety, nausea, anorexia, and decreased appetite. Monitor for clinical worsening of depression and suicidal ideation/behavior following the initiation of therapy or after dose changes.

Paroxetine is an inhibitor and substrate for CYP 450 2D6. May increase the effects/toxicity of tricyclic antidepressants, theophylline, and warfarin. Cimetidine, ritonavir, MAO inhibitors (fatal serotonin syndrome), dextromethorphan, phenothiazines and type 1C antiarrhythmics may increase the effect/toxicity of paroxetine. Weakness, hyperreflexia and poor coordination have been reported when taken with sumatriptan.

**Do not discontinue therapy abruptly**; may cause sweating, dizziness, confusion, and tremor. May be taken with or without food.

## PENICILLAMINE

Cuprimine, Depen

***Heavy metal chelator***

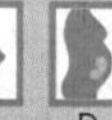
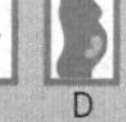


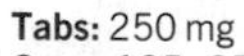

**Tabs:** 250 mg
**Caps:** 125, 250 mg
**Oral suspension:** 50 mg/mL

---

***Lead chelation therapy (third-line therapy):***

***Child:*** 30–40 mg/kg/24 hr or 600–750 mg/m$^2$/24 hr PO ÷ TID–QID; **max. dose:** 1.5 g/24 hr. Administer doses 2 hr before or 3 hr after meals.

***Adult:*** 1–1.5 g/24 hr PO ÷ BID–TID

Durations of treatment vary from 1 to 6 mo.

***Wilson's disease (see remarks for titration information):***

***Infant and child:*** 20 mg/kg/24 hr PO ÷ BID–QID; **max. dose:** 1 g/24 hr.

***Adult:*** 250 mg/dose PO QID; **max. dose:** 2 g/24 hr.

***Arsenic poisoning:***

***Child:*** 100 mg/kg/24 hr PO ÷ Q6 hr × 5 days; **max. dose:** 1 g/24 hr.

***Cystinuria (see remarks for titration information):***

***Infant and young child:*** 30 mg/kg/24 hr ÷ QID PO; **max. dose:** 4 g/24 hr.

***Older child and adult:*** 1–4 g/24 hr ÷ QID PO.

***Primary biliary cirrhosis (adult):***

***Initial:*** 250 mg/24 hr PO; increase by 250 mg Q2 wk to a total of 1 g/24 hr (given as 250 mg QID).

***Juvenile rheumatoid arthritis:***

5 mg/kg/24 hr ÷ QD–BID PO × 2 mo, then 10 mg/kg/24 hr ÷ QD–BID PO × 4 mo.

*Continued*

PENICILLAMINE *continued*

Dose should be given 1 hr before or 2 hr after meals. **AAP relegates this drug as a third-line agent for lead chelation indicated only after unacceptable reaction with oral succimer and calcium EDTA.** If used, must be in lead-free environment, since it can increase absorption of lead if present in GI tract. **Avoid use** if patient's creatinine clearance is < 50 mL/min. Follow CBC, LFTs, and urinalysis; and monitor the patient's skin, lymph nodes, and body temperature. Can cause optic neuritis, fever, rash, GI disturbances, altered taste, vomiting, lupus-like syndrome, nephrotic syndrome, peripheral neuropathy, leukopenia, eosinophilia, and thrombocytopenia. May reduce serum digoxin levels. **Avoid** concomitant administration with iron, antacids, and food.

Patients treated for Wilson's disease, rheumatoid arthritis, or cystinuria should be treated with pyridoxine 25–50 mg/24 hr. Titrate urinary copper excretion to >1 mg/24 hr for patients with Wilson's disease. Patients with cystinuria should have doses titrated to maintain urinary cystine excretion at <100–200 mg/24 hr.

## PENICILLIN G PREPARATIONS—AQUEOUS POTASSIUM AND SODIUM

Pfizerpen and others

***Antibiotic, aqueous penicillin***

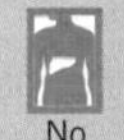
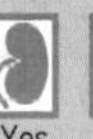
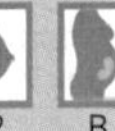
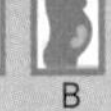

No Yes 2 B

**Injection ($K^+$):** 5, 20 million units (contains 1.7 mEq K and 0.3 mEq Na/1 million units penicillin G)
**Premixed frozen injection ($K^+$):** 1 million units in 50 mL dextrose 4%; 2 million units in 50 mL dextrose 2.3%; 3 million units in 50 mL dextrose 0.7% (contains 1.7 mEq K and 0.3 mEq Na/1 million units penicillin G)
**Injection ($Na^+$):** 5 million units (contains 2 mEq Na/1 million units penicillin G)
Conversion: 250 mg = 400,000 U

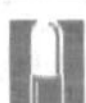

***Neonate (IM/IV):***
***≤7 days:***
***≤2 kg:*** 50,000–100,000 U/kg/24 hr ÷ Q12 hr
***>2 kg:*** 75,000–150,000 U/kg/24 hr ÷ Q8 hr
***>7 days:***
***<1.2 kg:*** 50,000–100,000 U/kg/24 hr ÷ Q12 hr
***1.2–2 kg:*** 75,000–150,000 U/kg/24 hr ÷ Q8 hr
***≥2 kg:*** 100,000–200,000 U/kg/24 hr ÷ Q6 hr
***Group B streptococcal meningitis:***
***≤7 days:*** 250,000–450,000 U/kg/24 hr ÷ Q8 hr
***>7 days:*** 450,000–500,000 U/kg/24 hr ÷ Q4–6 hr
***Congenital syphilis, neurosyphilis:*** See Chapter 17.
***Infant and child:***
***IM/IV:*** 100,000–400,000 U/kg/24 hr ÷ Q4–6 hr; **max. dose:** 24 million U/24 hr
***Adult (IM/IV):*** 4–24 million U/24 hr ÷ Q4–6 hr

Use penicillin V potassium for oral use. Side effects: anaphylaxis, urticaria, hemolytic anemia, interstitial nephritis, Jarisch-Herxheimer reaction (syphilis). $T_{1/2}$ = 30 min; may be prolonged by concurrent use of probenecid. For meningitis, use higher daily dose at shorter dosing intervals. For the treatment of anthrax (*Bacillus anthracis*), see www.bt.cdc.gov for additional information. **Adjust dose in renal impairment (see Chapter 31).**

*Continued*

For explanation of icons, see p. 698.

PENICILLIN G PREPARATIONS—AQUEOUS POTASSIUM AND SODIUM *continued*

Tetracyclines, chloramphenicol and erythromycin may antagonize penicillin's activity. Probenecid increases penicillin levels. May cause false-positive or negative urinary glucose (Clinitest method), false-positive direct Coombs' test, and false-positive urinary and/or serum proteins.

## PENICILLIN G PREPARATIONS—BENZATHINE

Bicillin L-A

***Antibiotic, penicillin (very long-acting IM)***

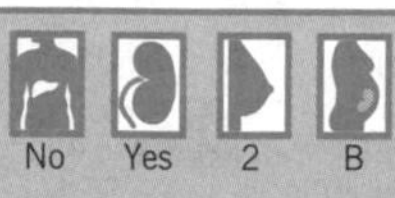


**Injection:** 600,000 U/mL (1, 2, 4 mL); contains parabens and povidone
**Injection should be IM only.**

***Group A streptococci:***
***Infant and child:*** 25,000–50,000 U/kg/dose IM × 1. **Max. dose:** 1.2 million U/dose **OR**
***>1 mo and <27 kg:*** 600,000 U/dose IM × 1
***≥27 kg and adult:*** 1.2 million U/dose IM × 1

***Rheumatic fever prophylaxis:***
***Infant and child:*** 25,000–50,000 U/kg/dose IM Q3–4 wk. **Max. dose:** 1.2 million U/dose
***Adult:*** 1.2 million U/dose IM Q3–4 wk or 600,000 U/dose IM Q2 wk

***Syphilis:*** Early acquired and >1 yr duration; see Chapter 17.

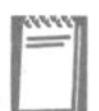

Provides sustained levels for 2–4 wk. **Use with caution** in renal failure, asthma, and cephalosporin hypersensitivity. Side effects and drug interactions same as for penicillin G preparations—aqueous potassium and sodium.

Injection site reactions are common. **Do not administer intravenously (cardiac arrest and death may occur)** and **do not inject** into or near an artery or nerve (may result in permanent neurological damage).

## PENICILLIN G PREPARATIONS—PENICILLIN G BENZATHINE AND PENICILLIN G PROCAINE

Bicillin C-R, Bicillin C-R 900/300

***Antibiotic, penicillin (very long-acting IM)***

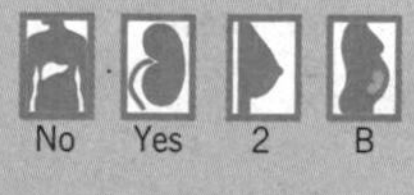


**Bicillin CR:** 300,000 U penicillin G procaine + 300,000 U penicillin G benzathine/mL to provide 600,000 U penicillin per 1 mL (1, 2 mL tubex, 4 mL syringe)
**Bicillin CR (900/300):** 150,000 U penicillin G procaine + 450,000 U penicillin G benzathine/mL (2 mL tubex)
All preparations contain parabens and povidone.
**Injection should be for IM use only.**

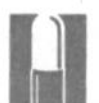

***Dosage based on total amount of penicillin.***
***Group A streptococci:***
***Child < 14 kg:*** 600,000 U/dose IM × 1
***Child 14–27 kg:*** 900,000–1,200,000 U/dose IM × 1
***Child >27 kg and adult:*** 2,400,000 U/dose IM × 1

*Continued*

PENICILLIN G PREPARATIONS—PENICILLIN G BENZATHINE AND PENICILLIN G PROCAINE *continued*

This preparation provides early peak levels in addition to prolonged levels of penicillin in the blood. **Do not use this product to treat syphilis because of treatment failure. Use with caution** in renal failure, asthma, significant allergies, and cephalosporin hypersensitivity. The addition of procaine penicillin has not been shown to be more efficacious than benzathine alone. However, it may reduce injection discomfort. **Do not administer intravenously** (cardiac arrest and death may occur) and **do not inject** into or near an artery or nerve (may result in permanent neurological damage).

Side effects and drug interactions same as for penicillin G preparations—aqueous potassium and sodium. Immune hypersensitivity reaction has been reported.

## PENICILLIN G PREPARATIONS—PROCAINE

Wycillin and others

***Antibiotic, penicillin (long-acting IM)***

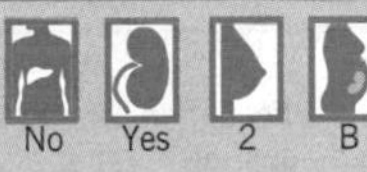


**Injection:** 600,000 U/mL (1, 2 mL); may contain parabens, phenol, povidone, and formaldehyde)
Contains 120 mg procaine per 300,000 U penicillin.
**Injection should be for IM use only.**

***Newborn (see remarks):*** 50,000 U/kg/24 hr IM QD
***Infant and child:*** 25,000–50,000 U/kg/24 hr ÷ Q12–24 hr IM. **Max. dose:** 4.8 million U/24 hr
***Adult:*** 0.6–4.0 million U/24 hr ÷ Q12–24 hr IM
***Congenital syphilis, syphilis, neurosyphilis:*** See Chapter 17.

Provides sustained levels for 2–4 days. **Use with caution** in renal failure, asthma, significant allergies, cephalosporin hypersensitivity, and in neonates (higher incidence of sterile abscess at injection site and risk of procaine toxicity). Side effects and drug interactions similar to penicillin G preparations—aqueous potassium and sodium. In addition, may cause CNS stimulation and seizures. Immune hypersensitivity reaction has been reported.

**Do not administer intravenously (cardiac arrest and death may occur)** and **do not inject** into or near an artery or nerve (may result in permanent neurological damage). Large doses may be administered in two injection sites. No longer recommended for empiric treatment of gonorrhea due to resistant strains.

## PENICILLIN V POTASSIUM

Veetids and others

***Antibiotic, penicillin***

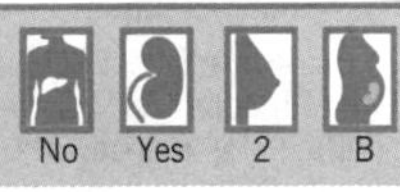


**Tabs:** 250, 500 mg
**Oral solution:** 125 mg/5 mL, 250 mg/5 mL (100, 200 mL); may contain saccharin
Contains 0.7 mEq potassium/ 250 mg drug
250 mg = 400,000 U

*Continued*

For explanation of icons, see p. 698.

PENICILLIN V POTASSIUM *continued*

***Child:*** 25–50 mg/kg/24 hr ÷ Q6–8 hr PO. **Max. dose:** 3 g/24 hr
***Adolescent and adult:*** 250–500 mg/dose PO Q6–8 hr
***Acute group A streptococcal pharyngitis (see remarks):***
***Child < 27 kg:*** 250 mg PO BID–TID × 10 days
***≥27 kg, adolescent and adult:*** 500 mg PO BID–TID × 10 days
***Rheumatic fever prophylaxis, and pneumococcal prophylaxis for sickle cell disease and functional or anatomical asplenia (regardless of immunization status):***
***2 mo–<3 yr:*** 125 mg PO BID
***3–5 yr:*** 250 mg PO BID; for sickle cell and asplenia, use may be discontinued after 5 yr of age if child received recommended pneumococcal immunizations and did not experience invasive pneumococcal infection.
***Recurrent rheumatic fever prophylaxis:***
***Child and adult:*** 250 mg PO BID

See *Penicillin G Preparations—Aqueous Potassium and Sodium* for side effects and drug interactions. GI absorption is better than penicillin G. **NOTE:** Must be taken 1 hr before or 2 hr after meals. Penicillin will prevent rheumatic fever if started within 9 days of the acute illness. The BID regimen for streptococcal pharyngitis should be used only if good compliance is expected. **Adjust dose in renal failure (see Chapter 31).**

## PENTAMIDINE ISETHIONATE

Pentam 300, NebuPent
***Antibiotic, antiprotozoal***

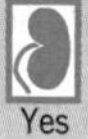
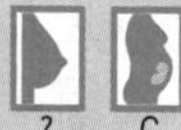

No Yes ? C

**Injection (Pentam 300 and others):** 300 mg
**Inhalation (NebuPent):** 300 mg

***Treatment:***
***Pneumocystis jiroveci (formerly carinii):*** 4 mg/kg/24 hr IM/IV QD × 14–21 days (IV is the preferred route)
***Trypanosomiasis (T. gambiense, T. rhodesiense):*** 4 mg/kg/24 hr IM QD × 10 days
***Visceral leishmaniasis (L. donovani, L. infantum, L. chagasi):*** 4 mg/kg/dose IM QD or QOD × 15–30 doses
***Cutaneous leishmaniasis (L. [V.] panamensis):*** 2–3 mg/kg/dose IM QD or QOD × 4–7 doses
***Prophylaxis:***
***Pneumocystis jiroveci (formerly carinii):***
***IM/IV:*** 4 mg/kg/dose Q2–4 wk
***Inhalation:***
***≥5 yr:*** 300 mg in 6 mL $H_2O$ via inhalation Q mo. Use with a Respigard II nebulizer.
**Max. single dose:** 300 mg

**Use with caution** in ventricular tachycardia, Stevens-Johnson syndrome, and daily doses > 21 days. May cause hypoglycemia, hyperglycemia, hypotension (both IV and IM administration), nausea, vomiting, fever, mild hepatotoxicity, pancreatitis, megaloblastic anemia, nephrotoxicity, hypocalcemia and granulocytopenia. Additive nephrotoxicity with aminoglycosides, amphotericin B, cisplatin and vancomycin may occur. Aerosol administration may also cause bronchospasm, cough, oxygen desaturation, dyspnea and loss of appetite.

*Continued*

PENTAMIDINE ISETHIONATE *continued*

Infuse IV over 1–2 hr to reduce the risk of hypotension. Sterile abscess may occur at IM injection site.

**Adjust dose in renal impairment (see Chapter 31) with systemic use.**

## PENTOBARBITAL

Nembutal and others

***Barbiturate***

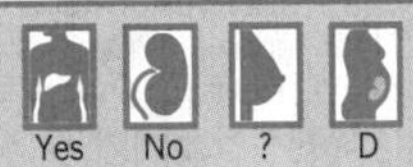

Yes No ? D

**Injection:** 50 mg/mL (2 mL); contains prophylene glycol and 10% alcohol

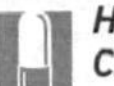

***Hypnotic:***

***Child:***

***IM:*** 2–6 mg/kg/dose. **Max. dose:** 100 mg

***Adult:***

***IM:*** 150–200 mg

***Pre-procedure sedation:***

***Child:***

***IM:*** 2–6 mg/kg/dose. **Max. dose:** 150 mg

***IV:*** 1–3 mg/kg/dose. **Max. dose:** 150 mg

***Barbiturate coma:***

***Child and adult:***

***IV: Load:*** 10–15 mg/kg given slowly over 1–2 hr

***Maintenance:*** Begin at 1 mg/kg/hr. Dose range: 1–3 mg/kg/hr as needed.

**Contraindicated** in liver failure and history of porphyria. **Use with caution** in hypovolemic shock, CHF, hypotension, and hepatic impairment. No advantage over phenobarbital for control of seizures. Adjunct in treatment of ICP. May cause drug-related isoelectric EEG. **Do not administer** for >2 wk in treatment of insomnia. May cause hypotension, arrhythmias, hypothermia, respiratory depression, and dependence.

Onset of action: IM: 10–15 min, IV: 1 min. Duration of action: IV: 15 min. Administer IV at a rate of <50 mg/min.

Therapeutic serum levels: Sedation: 1–5 mg/L; Hypnosis: 5–15 mg/L; Coma: 20–40 mg/L (steady-state is achieved after 4–5 days of continuous IV dosing).

## PERMETHRIN

Elimite, Acticin, Nix, and others

***Scabicidal agent***

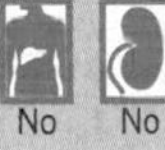
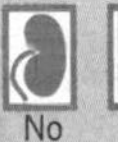
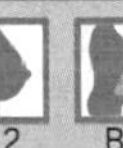

No No 2 B

**Cream (Elimite, Acticin):** 5% (60 g); contains 0.1% formaldehyde

**Liquid cream rinse (Nix-OTC):** 1% (60 mL with comb); contains 20% isopropyl alcohol

**Lotion (OTC):** 1% (60 mL with comb)

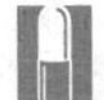

***Pediculus capitis, Phthirus pubis:***

***Head lice:*** Saturate hair and scalp with 1% cream rinse after shampooing, rinsing, and towel drying hair. Leave on for 10 min, then rinse. May repeat in 7–10 days. May be used for lice in other areas of the body (e.g., pubic lice) in same fashion.

***Scabies (see remarks):*** Apply 5% cream from neck to toe (head to toe for infants and toddlers); wash off with water in 8–14 hr. May repeat in 7 days.

*Continued*

For explanation of icons, see p. 698.

PERMETHRIN *continued*

Ovicidal activity generally makes single-dose regimen adequate. However, resistance to permethrin has been reported. **Avoid** contact with eyes during application. Shake well before using. May cause pruritus, hypersensitivity, burning, stinging, erythema, and rash. For either lice or scabies, instruct patient to launder bedding and clothing. For lice, treat symptomatic contacts only. For scabies, treat all contacts even if asymptomatic. The 5% cream has been used safely in children < 1 mo with neonatal scabies (a 6-hr application time was utilized). Topical cream dosage form contains formaldehyde. Dispense 60 g per adult or 2 small children.

## PHENAZOPYRIDINE HCL

Pyridium, Azo-Standard [OTC], and others

***Urinary analgesic***

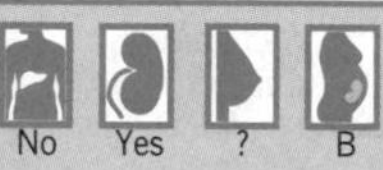

No Yes ? B

**Tabs:** 95 mg [OTC], 97.2 mg, 100 mg [OTC and Rx], 150 mg, 200 mg
**Oral suspension:** 10 mg/mL

***UTI (use with an appropriate antibacterial agent):***

***Child 6–12 yr:*** 12 mg/kg/24 hr ÷ TID PO until symptoms of lower urinary tract irritation are controlled or 2 days.

***Adult:*** 100–200 mg TID PO until symptoms are controlled or 2 days.

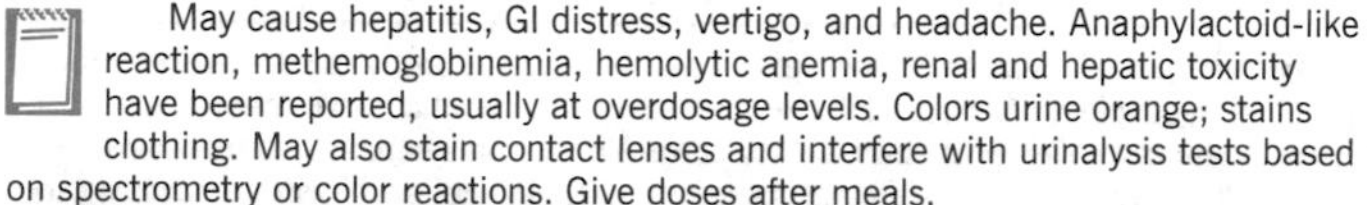

May cause hepatitis, GI distress, vertigo, and headache. Anaphylactoid-like reaction, methemoglobinemia, hemolytic anemia, renal and hepatic toxicity have been reported, usually at overdosage levels. Colors urine orange; stains clothing. May also stain contact lenses and interfere with urinalysis tests based on spectrometry or color reactions. Give doses after meals.

**Avoid use in moderate/severe renal impairment; adjust dose in mild renal impairment (see Chapter 31).**

## PHENOBARBITAL

Luminal and many others

***Barbiturate***

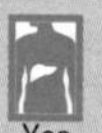 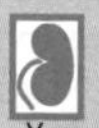 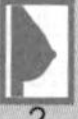 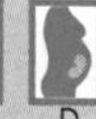

Yes Yes 2 D

**Tabs:** 15, 16, 30, 60, 90, 100 mg
**Caps:** 16 mg
**Elixir:** 20 mg/5 mL; contains alcohol
**Injection:** 60, 65, 130 mg/mL; may contain 10% alcohol and propylene glycol

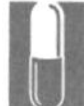

***Status epilepticus:***

***Loading dose, IV:***

***Neonate, infant, and child:*** 15–20 mg/kg/dose in a single or divided dose. May give additional 5 mg/kg doses Q15–30 min to a **max. total** of 30 mg/kg.

***Maintenance dose, PO/IV:*** Monitor levels.

***Neonate:*** 3–5 mg/kg/24 hr ÷ QD-BID
***Infant:*** 5–6 mg/kg/24 hr ÷ QD-BID
***Child 1–5 yr:*** 6–8 mg/kg/24 hr ÷ QD-BID
***Child 6–12 yr:*** 4–6 mg/kg/24 hr ÷ QD-BID
***>12 yr:*** 1–3 mg/kg/24 hr ÷ QD-BID

*Continued*

PHENOBARBITAL *continued*

***Hyperbilirubinemia (<12 yr):*** 3–8 mg/kg/24 hr PO ÷ BID-TID. Doses up to 12 mg/kg/24 hr have been used.
***Preoperative sedation (child):*** 1–3 mg/kg/dose IM/IV/PO × 1. Give 60–90 min prior to procedure.

**Contraindicated** in porphyria, severe respiratory disease with dyspnea or obstruction. **Use with caution** in hepatic or renal disease (reduce dose). IV administration may cause respiratory arrest or hypotension. Side effects include drowsiness, cognitive impairment, ataxia, hypotension, hepatitis, skin rash, respiratory depression, apnea, megaloblastic anemia and anti-convulsant hypersensitivity syndrome. Paradoxical reaction in children (not dose related) may cause hyperactivity, irritability, insomnia. Induces several liver enzymes (CYP 450 1A2, 2B6, 2C8, 3A3/4, 3A5-7), thus decreases blood levels of many drugs (e.g., anticonvulsants). IV push **not to exceed** 1 mg/kg/min.

$T_{1/2}$ is variable with age: neonates, 45–100 hr; infants, 20–133 hr; children, 37–73 hr. Due to long half-life, consider other agents for sedation for procedures.

Therapeutic levels: 15–40 mg/L. Recommended serum sampling time at steady-state: trough level obtained within 30 min prior to the next scheduled dose after 10–14 days of continuous dosing.

**Adjust dose in renal failure (see Chapter 31).**

## PHENTOLAMINE MESYLATE

Regitine and others

***Adrenergic blocking agent (alpha); antidote, extravasation***

No No ? C

**Injection:** 5 mg vial; may contain mannitol

***Treatment of alpha adrenergic drug extravasation (most effective within 12 hr of extravasation)***

***Neonate:*** Make a solution of 0.25–0.5 mg/mL with preservative-free normal saline. Inject 1 mL (in 5 divided doses of 0.2 mL) SC around site of extravasation within 12 hr of extravasation; **max. total dose:** 0.1 mg/kg or 2.5 mg total.

***Infant, child, and adult:*** Make a solution of 0.5–1 mg/mL with preservative-free normal saline. Inject 1–5 mL (in 5 divided doses) SC around site of extravasation within 12 hr of extravasation; **max. total dose:** 0.1–0.2 mg/kg or 5 mg total.

***Diagnosis of pheochromocytoma, IM/IV:***

***Child:*** 0.05–0.1 mg/kg/dose up to a **max. dose** of 5 mg.
***Adult:*** 5 mg/dose

***Hypertension, prior to surgery for pheochromocytoma, IM/IV:***

***Child:*** 0.05–0.1 mg/kg/dose up to a **max. dose** of 5 mg 1–2 hr prior to surgery, repeat Q2–4 hr PRN.
***Adult:*** 5 mg/dose 1–2 hr prior to surgery; repeat Q2–4 hr PRN.

**Contraindicated** in MI, coronary insufficiency and angina. **Use with caution** in hypotension, arrhythmias and cerebral vascular spasm/occlusion.

For diagnosis of pheochromocytoma, patient should be resting in a supine position. A blood pressure reduction of more than 35 mm Hg systolic and 24 mm Hg diastolic is considered a positive test for pheochromocytoma. For treatment of extravasation, use 27- to 30-gauge needle with multiple small injections and monitor site closely as repeat doses may be necessary.

For explanation of icons, see p. 698.

## PHENYLEPHRINE HCL

Neo-Synephrine and many others

***Adrenergic agonist***

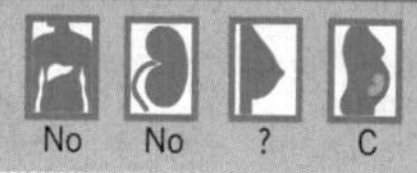


**Nasal drops [OTC]:** 0.125, 0.25, 0.5, 1% (15, 30 mL)
**Nasal spray [OTC]:** 0.25, 0.5, 1% (15, 30 mL)
**Note:** For Neo-Synephrine 12-hr Nasal, see *Oxymetazoline*
**Ophthalmic drops:** 0.12% [OTC] (0.3, 20 mL), 2.5% (2, 3, 5, 15 mL), 10% (2, 5 mL)
**Injection:** 10 mg/mL (1%) (1, 5 mL); may contain bisulfites
**Tabs (Sudafed PE) (OTC):** 10 mg
**Chewable tabs (AH-chew):** 10 mg
**Orally disintegrating tabs (Nasop):** 10 mg; contains phenylalanine
**Oral liquid:** 7.5 mg/5 mL (472); contains phenylalanine
**Oral solution (OTC):** 2.5 mg/5 mL
**Oral drops (OTC):** 2.5 mg/1 mL
**Orally disintegrating filmstrip (OTC):** 1.25, 2.5, 10 mg
**Oral suspension (Phenylephrine Tannate):**
- **AH-chewD:** 10 mg/5 mL (118 mL)
- **NaSop:** 7.5 mg/5 mL (120 mL)

---

***Hypotension:***
***Child:***
- ***IV bolus:*** 5–20 mcg/kg/dose Q10–15 min PRN
- ***IV drip:*** 0.1–0.5 mcg/kg/min; titrate to effect
- ***IM/SC:*** 0.1 mg/kg/dose Q1–2 hr PRN; **max. dose:** 5 mg

***Adult:***
- ***IV bolus:*** 0.1–0.5 mg/dose Q10–15 min PRN
- ***IV drip:*** Initial rate at 100–180 mcg/min; titrate to effect. Usual maintenance dose: 40–60 mcg/min.
- ***IM/SC:*** 2–5 mg/dose Q1–2 hr PRN; **max. dose:** 5 mg

***To prepare infusion:*** See inside front cover.

**Note: The dosage units for adults are in mcg/min; compared to mcg/kg/min for children.**

***Pupillary dilation:*** 2.5% solution; 1 drop in each eye 15 min before exam.

***Nasal decongestant (in each nostril; give up to 3 days):***
- ***Infant (> 6 mo):*** 1–2 drops of 0.16% solution (see remarks) Q3 hr PRN
- ***Child 1–6 yr:*** 2–3 drops of 0.125% solution Q4 hr PRN
- ***Child 6–12 yr:*** 2–3 drops or 1–2 sprays of 0.25% solution Q4 hr PRN
- ***>12 yr–adult:*** 2–3 drops or 1–2 sprays of 0.25% or 0.5% solution Q4 hr PRN

***Oral decongestant (see remarks):***

***2–<6 yr:***
- ***Oral drops (2.5 mg/mL):*** 1 mL (2.5 mg) PO Q4 hr; **not to exceed** 6 doses in 24 hr.
- ***Oral liquid (7.5 mg/5 mL):*** 2.5 mL (3.75 mg) PO Q6 hr up to 10 mL (15 mg) per 24 hr.
- ***Oral solution (2.5 mg/5 mL):*** 5 mL (2.5 mg) PO Q4 hr, up to 30 mL (15 mg) per 24 hr.
- ***Oral suspension (Phenylephrine Tannate):***
  - ***NaSop (7.5 mg/5 mL):*** 1.25–2.5 mL (1.88-3.75 mg) PO Q12 hr.

***≥6–<12 yr:***
- ***Oral liquid (7.5 mg/5 mL):*** 5 mL (7.5 mg) PO Q6 hr up to 20 mL (30 mg) per 24 hr.
- ***Oral solution (2.5 mg/5 mL):*** 10 mL (5 mg) PO Q4 hr up to 60 mL (30 mg) per 24 hr.

*Continued*

PHENYLEPHRINE HCL *continued*

***Oral suspension (Phenylephrine Tannate):***
***AH-chewD (10 mg/5 mL):*** 2.5–5 mL (5–10 mg) PO Q12 hr
***NaSop (7.5 mg/5 mL):*** 2.5–5 mL (3.75–7.5 mg) PO Q12 hr
***Tabs or chewable tabs:*** 10 mg PO Q4 hr
***≥12 yr and adult:***
***Tabs or chewable tabs:*** 10-20 mg PO Q4 hr
***Oral liquid (7.5 mg/5 mL):*** 10 mL (15 mg) PO Q6 hr up to 40 mL (60 mg) per 24 hr.
***Oral suspension (Phenylephrine Tannate):***
***AH-chewD (10 mg/5 mL):*** 5–10 mL (10–20 mg) PO Q12 hr
***NaSop (7.5 mg/5 mL):*** 5–10 mL (7.5–15 mg) PO Q12 hr

**Use with caution** in presence of arrhythmias, hyperthyroidism, or hyperglycemia. May cause tremor, insomnia, palpitations. Metabolized by MAO. **Contraindicated** in pheochromocytoma and severe hypertension. Injectable product may contain sulfites.

Nasal decongestants may cause rebound congestion with excessive use (>3 days). The 0.16% nasal drops are no longer available; may use the 0.125% solution or dilute the 0.25% or 0.5% concentrations with normal saline.The 1% nasal spray can be used in adults with extreme congestion.

Oral phenylephrine is found in a variety of combination cough and cold products and has replaced pseudoephedrine and phenylpropanolamine. Over the counter (OTC or nonprescription) use of this product is **not recommended** for children < 6 yr old due to reports of serious adverse effects (cardiac and respiratory distress, convulsions, and hallucinations) and fatalities (from unintentional overdosages, including combined use of other OTC products containing the same active ingredients).

## PHENYTOIN

Dilantin, Dilantin Infatab, Phenytek, and others
***Anticonvulsant, class Ib antiarrhythmic***

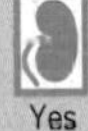
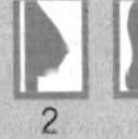
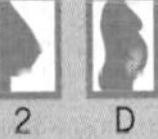
Yes Yes 2 D

**Chewable tabs (Infatab):** 50 mg
**Prompt-release caps:** 100 mg
**Extended-release caps:** 30, 100, 200, 300 mg
**Oral suspension:** 125 mg/5 mL (240 mL); contains ≤ 0.6% alcohol
**Injection:** 50 mg/mL; contains alcohol and propylene glycol

***Status epilepticus:*** **See Chapter 1.**
***Loading dose (all ages):*** 15–20 mg/kg IV
**Max. dose:** 1500 mg/24 hr
***Maintenance for seizure disorders:***
***Neonate:*** Start with 5 mg/kg/24 hr PO/IV ÷ Q12 hr; usual range 5–8 mg/kg/24 hr PO/IV ÷ Q8–12 hr.
***Infant/child:*** Start with 5 mg/kg/24 hr ÷ BID-TID PO/IV; usual dose range (doses divided BID-TID):
***6 mo–3 yr:*** 8–10 mg/kg/24 hr
***4–6 yr:*** 7.5–9 mg/kg/24 hr
***7–9 yr:*** 7–8 mg/kg/24 hr
***10–16 yr:*** 6–7 mg/kg/24 hr
**Note:** Use QD–BID dosing with extended-release caps.

*Continued*

For explanation of icons, see p. 698.

PHENYTOIN *continued*

***Status epilepticus (cont'd):***

***Adult:*** Start with 100 mg/dose Q8 hr IV/PO and carefully titrate (if needed) by 100 mg increments Q2–4 wk to 300–600 mg/24 hr (or 6–7 mg/kg/24 hr) ÷ Q8–24 hr IV/PO.

***Anti-arrhythmic (secondary to digitalis intoxication):***

***Load (all ages):*** 1.25 mg/kg IV Q5 min up to a total of 15 mg/kg

***Maintenance:***

***Child (IV/PO):*** 5–10 mg/kg/24 hr ÷ Q8–12 hr

***Adult:*** 250 mg PO QID × 1 day, then 250 mg PO Q12 hr × 2 days, then 300–400 mg/24 hr ÷ Q6–24 hr.

---

**Contraindicated** in patients with heart block or sinus bradycardia. IM administration is **not recommended** because of erratic absorption and pain at injection site; consider fosphenytoin. Side effects include gingival hyperplasia, hirsutism, dermatitis, blood dyscrasia, ataxia, lupus-like and Stevens-Johnson syndromes, lymphadenopathy, liver damage and nystagmus. Many drug interactions: levels may be increased by cimetidine, chloramphenicol, INH, sulfonamides, trimethoprim, etc. Levels may be decreased by some antineoplastic agents. Phenytoin induces hepatic microsomal enzymes (CYP 450 1A2, 2C8/9/19, and 3A3/4) leading to decreased effectiveness of oral contraceptives, quinidine, valproic acid, theophylline, and other substrates to the previously listed CYP 450 hepatic enzymes.

Suggested dosing intervals for specific oral dosage forms: extended-release caps (QD–BID); chewable and immediate-release tablets, and oral suspension (TID). Oral absorption reduced in neonates. $T_{1/2}$ is variable (7–42 hr) and dose-dependent. Drug is highly protein-bound; free fraction of drug will be increased in patients with hypoalbuminemia.

For seizure disorders, therapeutic levels: 10–20 mg/L (free and bound phenytoin) **OR** 1–2 mg/L (free only). Monitor free phenytoin levels in hypoalbuminemia or renal insufficiency. Recommended serum sampling times: trough level (PO/IV) within 30 min prior to the next scheduled dose; peak or post-load level (IV) 1 hr after the end of IV infusion. Steady-state is usually achieved after 5–10 days of continuous dosing. For routine monitoring, measure trough.

IV push/infusion rate: **Not to exceed** 0.5 mg/kg/min in neonates, or 1 mg/kg/min infants, children, and adults with **max.** of 50 mg/min; may cause cardiovascular collapse. Consider fosphenytoin in situations of tenuous IV access and risk for extravasation.

## PHOSPHORUS SUPPLEMENTS

NeutraPhos, NeutraPhos-K, K-PHOS Neutral, K-PHOS M.F., K-PHOS No. 2, Uro-KP-Neutral, Sodium Phosphate, Potassium Phosphate, and many generics for injections

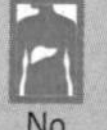
No
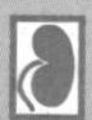
Yes
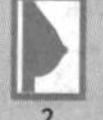
?
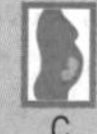
C

**Oral:** (reconstitute in 75 mL $H_2O$ per capsule or packet)

**Na and K phosphate:**

NeutraPhos; caps, powder (OTC): 250 mg (8 mM) P, 7.125 mEq Na, 7.125 mEq K per capsule or packet of powder

Uro-KP-Neutral; tabs: 250 mg (8 mM) P, 10.9 mEq Na, 1.27 mEq K

*Continued*

PHOSPHORUS SUPPLEMENTS *continued*

***Na and K phosphate (cont'd):***

K-PHOS Neutral; tabs: 250 mg P (8 mM), 13 mEq Na, 1.1 mEq K
K-PHOS M.F.; tabs: 125.6 mg (4 mM) P, 2.9 mEq Na, 1.1 mEq K
K-PHOS No. 2; tabs: 250 mg (8 mM) P, 5.8 mEq Na, 2.3 mEq K

**K Phosphate:**

NeutraPhos-K; caps, powder (OTC): 250 mg (8 mM) P, 14.25 mEq K per capsule or packet of powder

**Injection:**

Na phosphate: 3 mM (94 mg) P, 4 mEq Na/mL
K phosphate: 3mM (94 mg) P, 4.4 mEq K/mL

**Conversion: 31 mg P = 1 mM P**

---

***Acute hypophosphatemia:*** 0.16–0.32 mM/kg/dose (or 5–10 mg/kg/dose) IV over 6 hr

***Maintenance/replacement:***

***Child:***

***IV:*** 0.5–1.5 mM/kg (or 15–45 mg/kg) over 24 hr
***PO:*** 30–90 mg/kg/24 hr (or 1–3 mM/kg/24 hr) ÷ TID–QID

***Adult:***

***IV:*** 50–65 mM (or 1.5–2 g) over 24 hr
***PO:*** 3–4.5 g/24 hr (or 100–150 mM/24 hr) ÷ TID–QID

***Recommended infusion rate:*** ≤ 0.1 mM/kg/hr (or 3.1 mg/kg/hr) of phosphate. When potassium salt is used, the rate will be limited by the **max.** potassium infusion rate. **Do not** co-infuse with calcium-containing products.

---

May cause tetany, hyperphosphatemia, hyperkalemia, hypocalcemia. **Use with caution** in patients with renal impairment. Be aware of sodium and/or potassium load when supplementing phosphate. IV administration may cause hypotension and renal failure, or arrhythmias, heart block, cardiac arrest with potassium salt. PO dosing may cause nausea, vomiting, abdominal pain, or diarrhea. See Chapter 21 for daily requirements and Chapter 11 for additional information on hypophosphatemia and hyperphosphatemia.

## PHYSOSTIGMINE SALICYLATE

Antilirium

***Cholinergic agent***

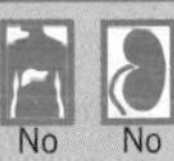
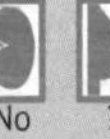
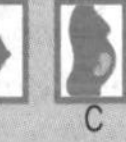

No No ? C

**Injection:** 1 mg/mL (2 mL); contains 2% benzyl alcohol and 0.1% sodium bisulfite

---

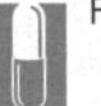

For antihistamine overdose or anticholinergic poisoning, see Chapter 2.

---

**Physostigmine antidote:** Atropine always should be available. **Contraindicated** in asthma, gangrene, diabetes, cardiovascular disease, GI or GU tract obstruction, any vagotonic state, and patients receiving choline esters or depolarizing neuromuscular blocking agents (e.g., decamethonium, succinylcholine). May cause seizures, arrythmias, bradycardia, GI symptoms, and other cholingeric effects.

For explanation of icons, see p. 698.

## PHYTONADIONE/VITAMIN $K_1$

Mephyton and others

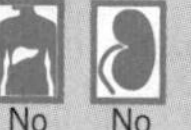
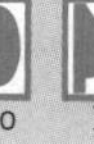
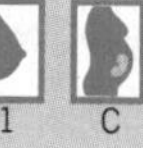
No No 1 C

**Tabs (Mephyton):** 5 mg
**Oral suspension:** 1 mg/mL
**Injection, emulsion:** 2 mg/mL (0.5 mL), 10 mg/mL (1 mL); contains 0.9% benzyl alcohol

***Neonatal hemorrhagic disease:***
***Prophylaxis:*** 0.5–1 mg IM × 1 within 1 hr after birth
***Treatment:*** 1–2 mg/24 hr IM/SC/IV
***Oral anticoagulant overdose:***
***Infant and child:*** 0.5–5 mg/dose PO/IM/SC/IV
***INR >8 (no bleeding or minor bleeding):*** 0.5–2.5 mg
***Major bleeding:*** 5 mg
***Adult:*** 2.5–10 mg/dose PO/IM/SC/IV
Dose may be repeated 12–48 hr after PO dose or 6–8 hr after parenteral dose
***Vitamin K deficiency:***
***Infant and child:***
***PO:*** 2.5–5 mg/24 hr
***IM/SC/IV:*** 1–2 mg/dose × 1
***Adult:***
***PO:*** 2.5–25 mg/24 hr
***IM/SC/IV:*** 10 mg/dose × 1

Monitor PT/PTT. Large doses (10–20 mg) in newborns may cause hyperbilirubinemia and severe hemolytic anemia. Blood coagulation factors increase within 6–12 hr after oral doses and within 1–2 hr following parenteral administration.

IV injection rate **not to exceed** 3 mg/m$^2$/min or 1 mg/min. IV or IM doses may cause flushing, dizziness, cardiac/respiratory arrest, hypotension and anaphylaxis. IV or IM administration is indicated only when other routes of administration are not feasible (or in emergency situations).

Mineral oil may decrease GI absorption of vitamin K with concurrent oral administration. Protect product from light. See Chapter 21 for multivitamin preparations.

## PILOCARPINE HCL

Akarpine, Isopto Carpine, Pilocar, Salagen, and others
***Cholinergic agent***

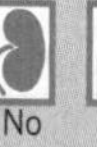
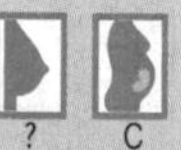
Yes No ? C

**Ophthalmic solution:** 0.25% (15 mL), 0.5% (15, 30 mL), 1% (1, 2, 15, 30 mL), 2% (1, 2, 15, 30 mL), 3% (15, 30 mL), 4% (1, 2, 15, 30 mL), 5% (15 mL), 6% (15, 30 mL), 8% (2, 15 mL), 10% (15 mL); may contain benzalkonium chloride
**Ophthalmic gel:** 4% (3.5 g); contains benzalkonium chloride
**Tab (Salagen and others):** 5, 7.5 mg

*Continued*

PILOCARPINE HCL *continued*

***For elevated intraocular pressure:***
***Drops:*** 1–2 drops in each eye 4–6 times a day; adjust concentration and frequency as needed.
***Gel:*** 0.5-inch ribbon applied to lower conjunctival sac QHS. Adjust dose as needed.

***Xerostomia:***
***Adult:*** 5 mg/dose PO TID; dose may be titrated to 10 mg/dose PO TID in patients who do not respond to lower dose and who are able to tolerate the drug.

**Contraindicated** in acute iritis or anterior chamber inflammation and uncontrolled asthma. May cause stinging, burning, lacrimation, headache and retinal detachment with ophthalmic use. **Use with caution** in patients with corneal abrasion or significant cardiovascular disease. Use with topical NSAIDs (e.g., ketorolac) may decrease topical pilocarpine effects. Sweating, nausea, rhinitis, chills, flushing, urinary frequency, dizziness, asthenia and headaches have also been reported with oral dosing. Reduce oral dosing in the presence of mild hepatic insufficiency (Child-Pugh score of 5–6); use in severe hepatic insufficiency is **not recommended**.

## PIMECROLIMUS

Elidel
***Topical immunosuppressant***

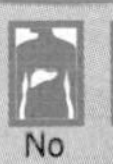
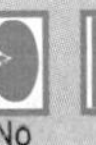
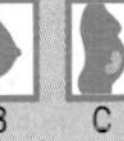
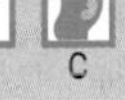

No No 3 C

**Cream:** 1% (30, 60, 100 g); contains benzyl alcohol and propylene glycol

***≥2 yr and adult:*** Apply a thin layer to affected area BID and rub in gently and completely. Reevaluate patient in 6 wk if lesions are not healed.

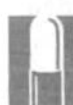

**Do not use** in children < 2 yr (higher rate of upper respiratory infections), immunocompromised patients, or with occlusive dressings (promotes systemic absorption). Approved as a second-line therapy for atopic dermatitis for patients who fail to respond, or do not tolerate, other approved therapies. Use medication for short periods of time by using the minimum amounts to control symptoms; long-term safety is unknown. **Avoid** contact with eyes, nose, mouth, and cut, infected, or scrapped skin. Minimize and **avoid** exposure to natural and artificial sunlight, respectively.

Most common side effects include burning at the application site, headache, viral infections, and pyrexia. Skin discoloration, skin flushing associated with alcohol use, anaphylactic reactions, occular irritation after application to the eyelids or near the eyes, angioneurotic edema, and facial edema have been reported. Although the risk is uncertain, the FDA has issued an alert about the potential cancer risk with the use of this product. See www.fda.gov/medwatch for the latest information. Drug is a CYP 450 3A3/4 substrate.



For explanation of icons, see p. 698.

## PIPERACILLIN

Pipracil and others

***Antibiotic, penicillin (extended spectrum)***

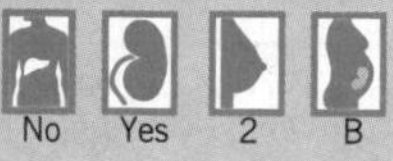


**Injection:** 2, 3, 4, 40 g
Contains 1.85 mEq Na/g drug

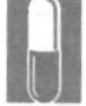

***Neonate, IV:***
***≤7 days:***
***≤36 wk of gestation:*** 150 mg/kg/24 hr ÷ Q12 hr
***>36 wk of gestation:*** 225 mg/kg/24 hr ÷ Q8 hr
***>7 days:***
***≤36 wk of gestation:*** 225 mg/kg/24 hr ÷ Q8 hr
***>36 wk of gestation:*** 300 mg/kg/24 hr ÷ Q6 hr
***Infant and child:*** 200–300 mg/kg/24 hr IM/IV ÷ Q4–6 hr; **max. dose:** 24 g/24 hr
***Cystic fibrosis:*** 350–600 mg/kg/24 hr IM/IV ÷ Q4–6 hr; **max. dose:** 24 g/24 hr
***Adult:*** 2–4 g/dose IV Q4–6 hr or 1–2 g/dose IM Q6 hr; **max. dose:** 24 g/24 hr

Similar to penicillin. Like other penicillins, CSF penetration occurs only with inflammed meninges. Thrombophlebitis, injection site pain, rash, diarrhea, headache and fever are common. Seizures (higher doses), prolonged bleeding time, bone marrow suppression, LFT elevations and acute interstitial nephritis have been reported. Cystic fibrosis patients have an increased risk for fever and rash.

Coagulation parameters should be tested more frequently and monitored regularly with high doses of heparin, warfarin, or other drugs affecting blood coagulation or thrombocyte function. May falsely lower aminoglycoside serum levels if the drugs are infused close to one another; allow a minimum of 2 hr between infusions to prevent this interaction.

For IM use, drug may be diluted to 400 mg/mL with 0.5 or 1% lidocaine without epinephrine. **Adjust dose in renal impairment (see Chapter 31).**

## PIPERACILLIN WITH TAZOBACTAM

Zosyn

***Antibiotic, penicillin (extended spectrum with beta-lactamase inhibitor)***

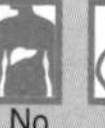
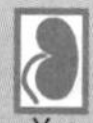
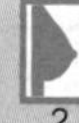
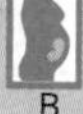


**8:1 ratio of piperacillin to tazobactam:**
**Injection, powder:** 2 g piperacillin and 0.25 g tazobactam; 3 g piperacillin and 0.375 g tazobactam; 4 g piperacillin and 0.5 g tazobactam; 36 g piperacillin and 4.5 g tazobactam
**Injection, premixed in iso-osmotic dextrose:** 2 g piperacillin and 0.25 g tazobactam in 50 mL; 3 g piperacillin and 0.375 g tazobactam in 50 mL; 4 g piperacillin and 0.5 g tazobactam in 100 mL
Contains 2.35 mEq Na/g piperacillin

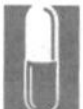

**All doses based on piperacillin component.**
***Infant <6 mo:*** 150–300 mg/kg/24 hr IV ÷ Q6–8 hr
***Infant >6 mo and child:*** 300–400 mg/kg/24 hr IV ÷ Q6–8 hr
***Adult:***
***Intra-abdomininal or soft tissue infections:*** 3 g IV Q6 hr
***Nosocomial pneumonia:*** 4 g IV Q6 hr

*Continued*

PIPERACILLIN WITH TAZOBACTAM *continued*

***Cystic fibrosis:*** See *Piperacillin*

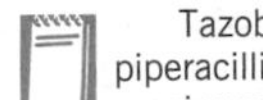

Tazobactam is a beta-lactamase inhibitor, thus extending the spectrum of piperacillin. Like other penicillins, CSF penetration occurs only with inflammed meninges. See *Piperacillin* and *Penicillin G Preparations—Aqueous Potassium and Sodium* for additional remarks.

**Adjust dose in renal impairment (see Chapter 31).**

## POLYCITRA

See *Citrate Mixtures*

## POLYETHYLENE GLYCOL—ELECTROLYTE SOLUTION

GoLYTELY, CoLyte, NuLYTELY, OCL, TriLyte, MiraLax, and others

***Bowel evacuant, osmotic laxative***

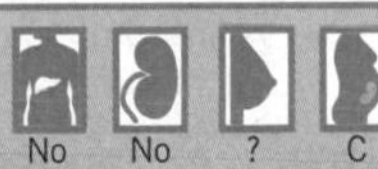


**Powder for oral solution:**

GoLYTELY: Polyethylene glycol 3350 236 g, Na sulfate 22.74 g, Na bicarbonate 6.74 g, NaCl 5.86 g, KCl 2.97 g. Contents vary somewhat. See package insert for specific contents of other products.

MiraLax and others: Polyethylene glycol 3350 (255, 527 g)

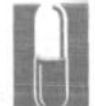

**Bowel cleansing (use products containing supplemental electrolytes for bowel cleansing such as GoLYTELY, CoLyte, NuLYTELY, OCL, TriLyte; and patients should be NPO 3–4 hr prior to dosing).**

***Child:***

***Oral/nasogastric:*** 25–40 mL/kg/hr until rectal effluent is clear (usually in 4–10 hr)

***Adult:***

***Oral:*** 240 ml PO Q10 min up to 4 L or until rectal effluent is clear

***Nasogastric:*** 20–30 ml/min (1.2–1.8 L/hr) up to 4 L

***Constipation (MiraLax; see remarks):***

***Child (limited data in 20 children with chronic constipation, 18 mo–11 yr; see remarks):*** A mean effective dose of 0.84 g/kg/24 hr PO ÷ BID for 8 wk (range: 0.25–1.42 g/kg/24 hr) was used to yield 2 soft stools per day. **Do not exceed** 17 g/24 hr. If patient > 20 kg, use adult dose.

***Adult:*** 17 g (1 heaping tablespoonful) mixed in 240 mL of water, juice, soda, coffee, or tea PO QD

**Contraindicated** in polyethylene glycol hypersensitivity. Monitor electrolytes, BUN, serum glucose, and urine osmolality with prolonged administration.

**BOWEL CLEANSING: Contraindicated** in toxic megacolon, gastric retention, colitis and bowel perforation. **Use with caution** in patients prone to aspiration or with impaired gag reflex. Effect should occur within 1–2 hr. Solution generally more palatable if chilled. MiraLax at higher dosages of 1–1.5 g/kg/24 hr (**max. dose:** 100 g/24 hr) PO × 3 days has been shown to be safe and effective in treating childhood fecal impaction.

*Continued*

FORMULARY
For explanation of icons, see p. 698.

POLYETHYLENE GLYCOL—ELECTROLYTE SOLUTION *continued*

**CONSTIPATION (MiraLax): Contraindicated** in bowel obstruction.

**Child:** Dilute powder using the ratio of 17 g powder to 240 mL of water, juice or milk. An onset of action within 1 wk in 12 of 20 patients, with the remaining 8 patients reporting improvement during the second wk of therapy. Side effects reported in this trial included diarrhea, flatulence, and mild abdominal pain. (See *J Pediatr* 2001;139[3]:428-432 for additional information.)

**Adult:** 2 to 4 days may be required to produce a bowel movement. Most common side effects include nausea, abdominal bloating, cramping and flatulence. Use beyond 2 wk has not been studied.

## POLYMYXIN B SULFATE AND BACITRACIN

See *Bacitracin* ± *Polymyxin B*

## POLYMYXIN B SULFATE AND TRIMETHOPRIM SULFATE

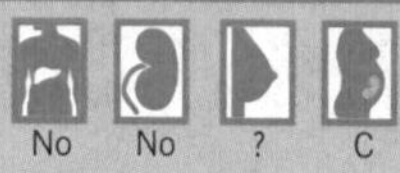


Polytrim Ophthalmic Solution and various others

***Topical antibiotic (ophthalmic preparations listed)***

**Ophthalmic solution:** Polymyxin B sulfate 10,000 U, trimethoprim sulfate 1 mg/mL (10 mL); some preparations may contain 0.04 mg/mL benzalkonium chloride

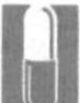

***≥2 mo and adult:*** Instill 1 drop in the affected eye(s) Q3 hr (**max.** of 6 doses/24 hr) × 7–10 days.

**Not indicated** for the prophylaxis or treatment of ophthalmia neonatorum. Local irritation consisting of redness, burning, stinging, and/or itching is common. Hypersensitivity reactions consisting of lid edema, itching, increased redness, tearing, and/or circumocular rash has been reported.

Apply finger pressure to lacrimal sac during and for 1–2 min after dose application.

## POLYMYXIN B SULFATE, NEOMYCIN SULFATE, HYDROCORTISONE

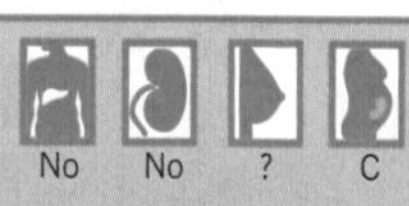


Cortisporin Otic, AK-Spore H.C. Otic, PediOtic, and many others

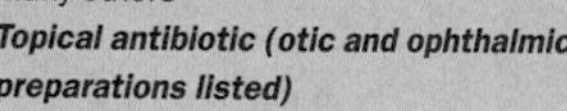

***Topical antibiotic (otic and ophthalmic preparations listed)***

**Otic solution or suspension:** Polymyxin B sulfate 10,000 U, neomycin sulfate 5 mg (3.5 mg neomycin base), hydrocortisone 10 mg/mL (10 mL); some preparations may contain thimerosol and metabisulfite.

**Ophthalmic suspension:** Polymyxin B sulfate 10,000 U, neomycin sulfate 5 mg (3.5 mg neomycin base), hydrocortisone 10 mg/mL (7.5 mL); may contain thimerosol and propylene glycol

*Continued*

POLYMYXIN B SULFATE, NEOMYCIN SULFATE, HYDROCORTISONE *continued*

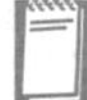

***Otitis externa:***

***≥2 yr–adult:*** 3–4 drops TID-QID × 7–10 days. If preferred, a cotton wick may be saturated and inserted into ear canal. Moisten wick with antibiotic every 4 hr. Change wick Q24 hr.

***Ophthalmic:***

***Adolescent and adult:*** Instill 1–2 drops into the affected eye(s) Q3–4 hr.

Neomycin may cause sensitization. Prolonged treatment may result in overgrowth of nonsusceptible organisms and fungi. May cause cutaneous sensitization.

**OTIC USE:** Shake suspension well before use. **Contraindicated** in patients with active varicella and herpes simplex and in cases with perforated eardrum (possible ototoxicity). **Use with caution** in chronic otitis media and when the integrity of the tympanic membrane is in question. Metabisulfite-containing products may cause allergic reactions in susceptible individuals. Hypersensitivity (itching, skin rash, redness, swelling, or other signs of irritation in or around the ear) may occur. Warm the medication to body temperature prior to use.

**OPHTHALMIC USE: Use with caution** in glaucoma. Blurred vision, burning, and stinging may occur. Increased intraocular pressure and mycosis may occur with prolonged use. Apply finger pressure to lacrimal sac during and for 1–2 min after dose application.

## POLYTRIM OPHTHALMIC SOLUTION

See *Polymixin B Sulfate and Trimethoprim Sulfate*

## PORACTANT ALFA

See *Surfactant, Pulmonary/Poractant Alfa*

## POTASSIUM IODIDE

Iosat, Pima, SSKI, ThyroShield, ThyroSafe, and others

***Antithyroid agent***

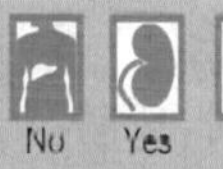

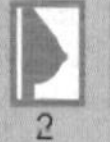

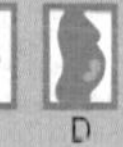

No Yes 2 D

**Tabs:**

ThyroSafe (OTC): 65 mg (50 mg iodine)

Iosat: 130 mg

**Syrup (Pima):** 325 mg/5 mL (249 mg iodide/5 mL) (473 mL, 4000 mL)

**Oral solution:**

ThyroShield: 65 mg/mL (30 mL); contains parabens and saccharin

Saturated solution (SSKI): 1000 mg/mL (30, 240 mL); 10 drops = 500 mg potassium iodide

Lugol's (strong iodine) solution: Iodine 50 mg and potassium iodide 100 mg per mL (15, 473 mL)

Potassium content is 6 mEq (234 mg) $K^+$/g potassium iodide.

*Continued*



For explanation of icons, see p. 698.

POTASSIUM IODIDE *continued*

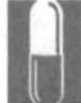

***Neonatal Grave's disease:*** 1 drop strong iodine (Lugol's solution) PO Q8 hr
***Thyrotoxicosis:***
***Child:*** 50–250 mg PO TID (about 1–5 drops of SSKI TID)
***Adult:*** 50–500 mg PO TID (1–10 drops SSKI PO TID)
***Cutaneous or lymphocutaneous sporotrichosis (see remarks):***
***Child and adult:*** Start with 250 mg PO TID. Doses may be gradually increased as tolerated to the following **max. doses:**
***Child max.:*** 1250–2000 mg PO TID
***Adult max.:*** 2000–2500 mg PO TID

**Contraindicated** in pregnancy, hyperkalemia, iodine-induced goiter, and hypothyroidism. **Use with caution** in cardiac disease and renal failure. GI disturbance, metallic taste, rash, salivary gland inflammation, headache, lacrimation and rhinitis are symptoms of iodism. Give with milk or water after meals. Monitor thyroid function tests. Onset of antithyroid effects: 1–2 days.

Lithium carbonate and iodide-containing medications may have synergistic hypothyroid activity. Potassium-containing medications, potassium-sparing diuretics, and ACE inhibitors may increase serum potassium levels.

For sporotrichosis, continue treatment for 4–6 wk after lesions have completely healed. Increase dose until either **max. dose** is achieved or signs of intolerance appear.

For use as a thyroid blocking agent in radiation emergencies, see www.fda.gov/cder/guidance/4825fnl.pdf.

## POTASSIUM SUPPLEMENTS

Many brand names
***Electrolyte***

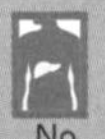
No
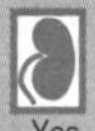
Yes
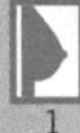
1
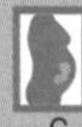
C

**Potassium chloride (40 mEq K = 3 g KCl):**
Sustained-release caps: 8, 10 mEq
Sustained-release tabs: 8, 10, 15, 20 mEq
Powder: 15, 20, 25 mEq/packet
Oral solution: 10% (6.7 mEq/5 mL), 20% (13.3 mEq/5 mL)
Concentrated injection: 2 mEq/mL
**Potassium gluconate: (40 mEq K = 9.4 g K gluconate):**
Tabs (OTC): 500 mg (2.15 mEq) , 595 mg (2.56 mEq)
Oral liquid: 20 mEq/15 mL; may contain alcohol
**Potassium acetate (40 mEq K = 3.9 g K acetate):**
Concentrated injection: 2 mEq/mL
**Potassium bicarbonate (10 mEq K = 1 g K bicarbonate):**
Effervescent tab for oral solution: 10, 20 mEq
**Potassium phosphate:**
See *Phosphorus Supplements*

***Normal daily requirements:*** **See Chapter 21.**
***Replacement:*** Determine based on maintenance requirements, deficit and ongoing losses. **See Chapter 11.**

*Continued*

POTASSIUM SUPPLEMENTS *continued*

***Hypokalemia:***

***Oral:***

***Child:*** 1–4 mEq/kg/24 hr ÷ BID-QID. Monitor serum potassium.
***Adult:*** 40–100 mEq/24 hr ÷ BID-QID

***IV:*** **MONITOR SERUM K CLOSELY.**

***Child:*** 0.5–1 mEq/kg/dose given as an infusion of 0.5 mEq/kg/hr × 1–2 hr.
**Max. IV infusion rate:** 1 mEq/kg/hr. This may be used in critical situations (i.e., hypokalemia with arrhythmia).

***Adult:***

***Serum K ≥ 2.5 mEq/L:*** Replete at rates up to 10 mEq/hr. **Total dosage not to exceed** 200 mEq/24 hr.
***Serum K < 2 mEq/L:*** Replete at rates up to 40 mEq/hr. **Total dosage not to exceed** 400 mEq/24 hr.

**Max. peripheral IV solution concentration:** 40 mEq/L
**Max. concentration for central line administration:** 150–200 mEq/L

---

PO administration may cause GI disturbance and ulceration. Oral liquid supplements should be diluted in water or fruit juice prior to administration. Sustained-release tablets must be swallowed whole, and **NOT** dissolved in the mouth or chewed.

**Do not administer** IV potassium undiluted. IV administration may cause irritation, pain, and phlebitis at the infusion site. **Rapid or central IV infusion may cause cardiac arrhythmias.** Patients receiving infusion >0.5 mEq/kg/hr (>20 mEq/hr for adults) should be placed on an ECG monitor.

## PRALIDOXIME CHLORIDE

Protopam, 2-PAM
***Antidote, organophosphate poisoning***

No Yes ? C

**Injection:** 1000 mg

---

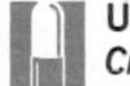

**Use with atropine.**
***Child:*** 20–50 mg/kg/dose × 1 IM/IV/SC. May repeat in 1–2 hr if muscle weakness is not relieved, and then at Q10–12 hr if cholinergic signs reappear.
***Adult:*** 1–2 g/dose × 1 IM/IV/SC. May repeat in 1–2 hr if muscle weakness is not relieved, then at Q10–12 hr if cholinergic signs reappear.
Continuous infusions have also been recommended; see package insert.

---

**Contraindicated** in poisonings due to phosphorus, inorganic phosphates, or organic phosphates without anticholinesterase activity. **Do not use** as an antidote for carbamate classes of pesticides. Removal of secretions and maintaining a patent airway is critical. May cause muscle rigidity, laryngospasm, and tachycardia after rapid IV infusion. Drug is generally ineffective if administered 36–48 hr after exposure. Additional doses may be necessary.

For IV administration, dilute to 50 mg/mL or less and infuse over 15–30 min (**not to exceed** 200 mg/min). Reduce dosage in renal impairment since 80%–90% of the drug is excreted unchanged in the urine 12 hr after administration.

For explanation of icons, see p. 698.

## PREDNISOLONE

Orapred, Orapred ODT, Prelone, Pediapred, and others

***Corticosteroid***

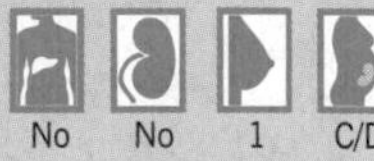


**Tabs:** 5 mg
**Syrup (Prelone and others):** 5 mg/5 mL (120 mL), 15 mg/5 mL (240 mL); may contain alcohol and saccharin
**Tablets, orally disintegrating (as Na phosphate) (Orapred ODT):** 10, 15, 30 mg
**Oral solution (as Na phosphate):**
Pediapred: 5 mg/5 mL (120 mL); may contain alcohol and is dye free
Orapred and others: 15 mg /5 mL (237 mL); may contain 2% alcohol and is dye free
**Ophthalmic suspension (as acetate):** 0.12% (5, 10 mL), 1% (1, 5, 10, 15 mL); contains benzalkonium chloride and may contain bisulfites
**Ophthalmic solution (as Na phosphate):** 1% (5, 10, 15 mL); contains benzalkonium chloride

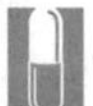

**See *Prednisone* for oral dosing (equivalent dosing).**
***Ophthalmic (consult ophthalmologist before use):***
***Child and adult:*** Start with 1–2 drops Q1 hr during the day and Q2 hr during the night until favorable response, then reduce dose to 1 drop Q4 hr. Dose may be further reduced to 1 drop TID-QID.

See *Prednisone* for remarks. See Chapter 30 for relative steroid potencies. Pregnancy category changes to "D" if used in the first trimester. Orapred oral solution product should be stored in the refrigerator.

**OPHTHALMIC USE: Contraindicated** in viral (e.g., herpes simplex, vaccinia, and varicella), fungal, and mycobacterial infections of the cornea and conjunctiva. Increase in intraoccular pressure, cataract formation, and delayed wound healing may occur.

## PREDNISONE

Orasone, Deltasone, Liquid Pred, and others

***Corticosteroid***

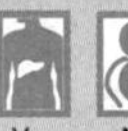
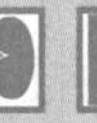
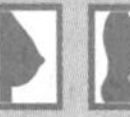
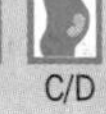


**Tabs:** 1, 2.5, 5, 10, 20, 50 mg
**Oral syrup/solution:** 1 mg/mL (120, 240, 500 mL); contains 5% alcohol and saccharin
**Concentrated solution:** 5 mg/mL (30 mL); contains 30% alcohol

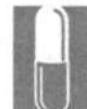

***Anti-inflammatory/immunosuppressive:***
***Child:*** 0.5–2 mg/kg/24 hr PO ÷ QD–BID
***Acute asthma:***
***Child:*** 2 mg/kg/24 hr PO ÷ QD-BID × 5–7 days; **max. dose:** 80 mg/24 hr. Patients may benefit from tapering if therapy exceeds 5–7 days.

***Asthma exacerbations (2007 National Heart, Lung, and Blood Institute Guideline Recommendations; dose until peak expiratory flow reaches 70% of predicted or personal best):***
***Child ≤ 12 yr:*** 1 mg/kg/24 hr PO ÷ Q12 hr (**max. dose:** 60 mg/24 hr).
***>12 yr and adult:*** 40–80 mg/24 hr PO ÷ Q12–24 hr.

*Continued*

PREDNISONE *continued*

***Outpatient asthma exacerbation burst therapy (longer durations may be necessary):***
***Child ≤ 12 yr:*** 1–2 mg/kg/24 hr PO ÷ Q12–24 hr (**max. dose:** 60 mg/24 hr) × 3–10 days.
***Child > 12 yr and adult:*** 40–60 mg/24 PO hr ÷ Q12–24 hr × 5–10 days.
***Nephrotic syndrome:***
***Child:*** Starting doses of 2 mg/kg/24 hr PO (**max. dose:** 80 mg/24 hr) are recommended. Further treatment plans are individualized. Consult a nephrologist.

See Chapter 30 for physiologic replacement, relative steroid potencies, and doses based on body surface area. Methylprednisolone is preferable in hepatic disease because prednisone must be converted to methylprednisolone in the liver.

Side effects may include: mood changes, seizures, hyperglycemia, diarrhea, nausea, abdominal distension, GI bleeding, HPA axis suppression, osteopenia, cushingoid effects and cataracts with prolonged use. Prednisone is a CYP 450 3A3/4 substrate and inducer. Barbiturates, carbamazepine, phenytoin, rifampin, isoniazid may reduce the effects of prednisone, whereas estrogens may enhance the effects. Pregnancy category changes to "D" if used in the first trimester.

## PRIMAQUINE PHOSPHATE

Various generic brands
***Antimalarial***

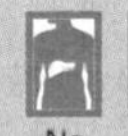
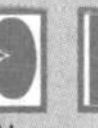
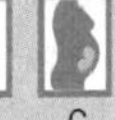

No No ? C

**Tabs:** 26.3 mg (15 mg base)

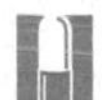

**Doses expressed in mg of primaquine base.**
***Malaria:***
***Prevention of relapses for P. vivax or P. ovale only (initiate therapy during the last 2 wk of, or following a course of, suppression with chloroquine or comparable drug):***
***Child:*** 0.5 mg/kg/dose (**max. dose:** 30 mg/dose) PO QD × 14 days
***Adult:*** 30 mg PO QD × 14 days
***Prevention of chloroquine-resistant strains (initiate 1 day prior to departure and continue until 3–7 days after leaving endemic area):***
***Child:*** 0.5 mg/kg/dose PO QD; **max. dose:** 30 mg/24 hr.
***Adult:*** 30 mg PO QD
***Pneumocystis jiroveci (formerly carinii) pneumonia (in combination with clindamycin):***
***Adult:*** 30 mg PO QD × 21 days

**Contraindicated** in granulocytopenia (e.g., rheumatoid arthritis, lupus erythematosus) and bone marrow suppression. **Avoid use** with quinacrine and with other drugs that have a potential for causing hemolysis or bone marrow suppression. **Use with caution** in G6PD and NADH methemoglobin-reductase deficient patients due to increased risk for hemolytic anemia and leukopenia, respectively. Use in pregnancy is **not recommended** by the AAP *Red Book*. Cross sensitivity with iodoquinol.

May cause headache, visual disturbances, nausea, vomiting and abdominal cramps. Hemolytic anemia, leukopenia and methemoglobinemia have been reported. Administer all doses with food to mask bitter taste.

For explanation of icons, see p. 698.

## PRIMIDONE

Mysoline and others

***Anticonvulsant, barbiturate***

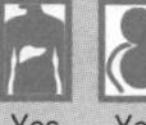 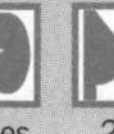 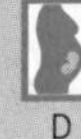

Yes Yes 2 D

**Tabs:** 50, 250 mg

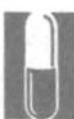

| Day of Therapy | <8 Yr | ≥8 Yr and Adult |
|---|---|---|
| Days 1–3 | 50 mg PO QHS | 100–125 mg PO QHS |
| Days 4–6 | 50 mg PO BID | 100–125 mg PO BID |
| Days 7–9 | 100 mg PO BID | 100–125 mg PO TID |
| Day 10 and thereafter | 125–250 mg PO TID or 10–25 mg/kg/ 24 hr ÷ TID-QID | 250 mg PO TID-QID; **max. dose:** 2 g/24 hr |

**Use with caution** in renal or hepatic disease and pulmonary insufficiency. Primidone is metabolized to phenobarbital and has the same drug interactions and toxicities (see *Phenobarbital*). Additionally, primidone may cause vertigo, nausea, leukopenia, malignant lymphoma-like syndrome, diplopia, nystagmus, systemic lupus-like syndrome. Acetazolamide may decrease primidone absorption. **Adjust dose in renal failure (see Chapter 31).**

Follow both primidone and phenobarbital levels. Therapeutic levels: 5–12 mg/L of primidone and 15–40 mg/L of phenobarbital. Recommended serum sampling time at steady-state: trough level obtained within 30 min prior to the next scheduled dose after 1–4 days of continuous dosing.

## PROBENECID

Various generic brands

***Penicillin therapy adjuvant, uric acid lowering agent***

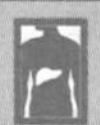 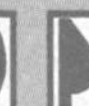 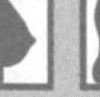 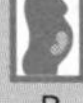

No Yes ? B

**Tabs:** 500 mg

***To prolong penicillin levels:***

***Child (2–14 yr):*** 25 mg/kg PO × 1, then 40 mg/kg/24 hr ÷ QID; **max. dose:** 500 mg/dose. Use adult dose if > 50 kg.

***Adult:*** 500 mg PO QID

***Hyperuricemia:***

***Adult:*** 250 mg PO BID × 1 wk, then 500 mg PO BID; may increase by 500 mg increments Q4 wk PRN up to a **max. dose** of 2–3 g/24 hr ÷ BID.

***Gonorrhea (just prior to antibiotic):***

***≤45 kg:*** 23 mg/kg/dose PO × 1 just prior to antibiotic

***>45 kg:*** 1 g PO × 1

**Use with caution** in patients with peptic ulcer disease. **Contraindicated** in children < 2 yr and patients with renal insufficiency. **Do not use** if GFR < 30 mL/min.

*Continued*

PROBENECID *continued*

Increases uric acid excretion. Inhibits renal tubular secretion of acyclovir, ganciclovir, ciprofloxacin, levofloxacin, nalidixic acid, moxifloxacin, organic acids, penicillins, cephalosporins, AZT, dapsone, methotrexate, nonsteroidal anti-inflammatory agents, and benzodiazepines. Salicylates may decrease probenecid's activity. Alkalinize urine in patients with gout. May cause headache, GI symptoms, rash, anemia, and hypersensitivity. False-positive glucosuria with Clinitest may occur.

## PROCAINAMIDE

Pronestyl, Procanbid, and various generic brands

***Antiarrhythmic, class Ia***

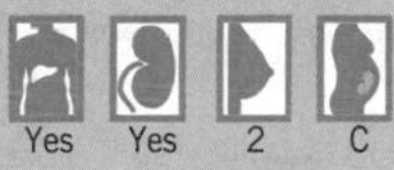


**Tabs (Pronestyl):** 375, 500 mg
**Sustained-release tabs (Procanbid):** 250, 500, 750, 1000 mg
**Caps:** 250, 375, 500 mg
**Injection:** 500 mg/mL; contains methylparabens and bisulfites
**Oral suspension:** 5, 50, 100 mg/mL

***Child:***

***V. tach with poor perfusion:*** Consider 15 mg/kg/dose IV × 1 over 30–60 min if cardioversion ineffective; follow with continuous infusion if effective (see information that follows).

***IM:*** 20–30 mg/kg/24 hr ÷ Q4–6 hr; **max. dose:** 4 g/24 hr (peak effect in 1 hr).

***IV: Load:*** 2–6 mg/kg/dose over 5 min (**max. dose:** 100 mg/dose); repeat dose Q5–10 min PRN up to a total **max. dose** of 15 mg/kg. **Do not exceed** 500 mg in 30 min.

***Maintenance:*** 20–80 mcg/kg/min by continuous infusion; **max. dose:** 2 g/24 hr.

***PO:*** 15–50 mg/kg/24 hr ÷ Q3–6 hr; **max. dose:** 4 g/24 hr

***Adult:***

***IM:*** 50 mg/kg/24 hr ÷ Q3–6 hr

***IV: Load:*** 50–100 mg/dose; repeat dose Q5 min PRN to a **max. dose** of 1000–1500 mg.

***Maintenance:*** 1–6 mg/min by continuous infusion

**NOTE: The IV infusion dosage units for adults are in mg/min; compared to mcg/kg/min for children.**

***PO:*** Usual dose: 50 mg/kg/24 hr

***Immediate release:*** 250–500 mg/dose Q3–6 hr

***Sustained release:*** 500–1000 mg/dose Q6 hr

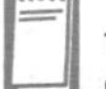

**Contraindicated** in myasthenia gravis, complete heart block, SLE, and torsade de pointes. **Use with caution** in asymptomatic premature ventricular contractions, digitalis intoxication, CHF, renal or hepatic dysfunction. **Adjust dose in renal failure (see Chapter 31).**

May cause lupus-like syndrome, positive Coombs' test, thrombocytopenia, arrhythmias, GI complaints, and confusion. Increased LFTs and liver failure have been reported. Monitor BP and ECG when using IV. QRS widening by >0.02 sec suggests toxicity.

Cimetidine, ranitidine, amiodarone, beta-blockers, and trimethoprim may increase procainamide levels. Procainamide may enhance the effects of skeletal muscle relaxants and anticholinergic agents. Therapeutic levels: 4–10 mg/L of procainamide or 10–30 mg/L of procainamide and NAPA levels combined.

*Continued*

For explanation of icons, see p. 698.

PROCAINAMIDE *continued*

Recommended serum sampling times:
*IM/PO intermittent dosing:* Trough level within 30 min prior to the next scheduled dose after 2 days of continuous dosing (steady-state).
*IV continuous infusion:* 2 and 12 hr after start of infusion and at 24-hr intervals thereafter.

## PROCHLORPERAZINE

Compazine and others

***Antiemetic, phenothiazine derivative***

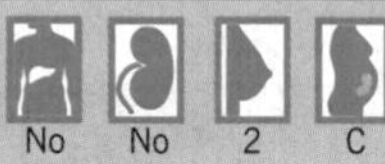


**Tabs (as maleate):** 5, 10 mg
**Slow-release caps (as maleate):** 10, 15 mg
**Syrup (as edisylate):** 5 mg/5 mL (120 mL)
**Suppository:** 2.5, 5, 25 mg (12s)
**Injection (as edisylate):** 5 mg/mL (2, 10 mL); may contain bisulfites and benzyl alcohol

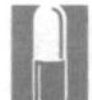

***Antiemetic doses:***
***Child (>10 kg or >2 yr):***
*PO or PR:* 0.4 mg/kg/24 hr ÷ TID–QID or alternative dosing by weight:
***10–14 kg:*** 2.5 mg QD–BID; **max. dose:** 7.5 mg/24 hr
***15–18 kg:*** 2.5 mg BID–TID; **max. dose:** 10 mg/24 hr
***19–39 kg:*** 2.5 mg TID or 5 mg BID; **max. dose:** 15 mg/24 hr
*IM:* 0.1–0.15 mg/kg/dose TID–QID; **max. dose:** 40 mg/24 hr
***Adult:***
*PO:*
*Immediate release:* 5–10 mg/dose TID–QID
*Extended release:* 10 mg/dose BID or 15 mg/dose QD
*PR:* 25 mg/dose BID
*IM:* 5–10 mg/dose Q3–4 hr
*IV:* 2.5–10 mg/dose; may repeat Q3–4 hr
*Max. IM/IV dose:* 40 mg/24 hr
***Psychoses:***
***Child 2–12 yr:***
*PO or PR:* Start with 2.5 mg BID–TID with a **max. first day dose** of 10 mg/24 hr. Dose may be increased as needed to 20 mg/24 hr for children 2–5 yr and 25 mg/24 hr for 6–12 yr.
*IM:* 0.13 mg/kg/dose × 1 and convert to PO immediately.
***Adult:***
*PO:* 5–10 mg TID–QID; may be increased as needed to a **max. dose** of 150 mg/24 hr
*IM:* 10–20 mg Q2–4 hr PRN convert to PO immediately.

Toxicity as for other phenothiazines (see *Chlorpromazine*). Extrapyramidal reactions (reversed by diphenhydramine) or orthostatic hypotension may occur. May mask signs and symptoms of overdosage of other drugs and may obscure the diagnosis and treatment of conditions such as intestinal obstruction, brain tumor and Reye's syndrome. May cause false-positive test for phenylketonuria, urinary amylase, uroporphyrins and urobilinogen. **Do not use** IV route in children. Use only in management of prolonged vomiting of known etiology.

A 0.15 mg/kg/dose IV over 10 min was effective in migraine headaches presenting in emergency departments for children 5–18 yr (see *Ann Emerg Med* 2004;43:256–262).

## PROMETHAZINE

Phenergan and others

***Antihistamine, antiemetic, phenothiazine derivative***

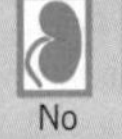
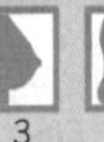
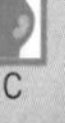

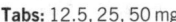

No No 3 C

**Tabs:** 12.5, 25, 50 mg
**Syrup:** 6.25 mg/5 mL (473 mL); contains alcohol
**Suppository:** 12.5, 25, 50 mg (12s)
**Injection:** 25, 50 mg/mL (1 mL); may contain sulfites

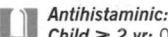

***Antihistaminic:***
***Child ≥ 2 yr:*** 0.1 mg/kg/dose (**max. dose:** 12.5 mg/dose) Q6 hr PO during the day hours and 0.5 mg/kg/dose (**max. dose:** 25 mg/dose) QHS PO PRN
***Adult:*** 12.5 mg PO TID and 25 mg QHS

***Nausea and vomiting PO/IM/IV/PR (see remarks):***
***Child ≥ 2 yr:*** 0.25–1 mg/kg/dose Q4–6 hr PRN; **max. dose:** 25 mg/dose
***Adult:*** 12.5–25 mg Q4–6 hr PRN

***Motion sickness: (first dose 0.5–1 hr before departure):***
***Child ≥ 2 yr:*** 0.5 mg/kg/dose Q12 hr PO/PR PRN; **max. dose:** 25 mg/dose
***Adult:*** 25 mg PO Q8–12 hr PRN

**Avoid** use in children < 2 yr because of risk for fatal respiratory depression. Toxicity similar to other phenothiazines (see *Chlorpromazine*). **Do not** administer SQ or intra-arterially because of severe local reactions. IV route of administration is **not recommended** (IM preferred) due to severe tissue injury (tissue necrosis and gangrene). If using IV route, dilute 25 mg/mL strength product with 10–20 mL NS and administer over 10–15 min, consider lower initial doses, administer through a large-bore vein and check patency of line before administering, administer through an IV line at the port farthest from the patient's vein, and monitor for burning or pain during or after injection. Administer oral doses with meals to decrease GI irritation.

May cause profound sedation, blurred vision, respiratory depression (use lowest effective dose in children and **avoid** concomitant use of respiratory depressants), and dystonic reactions (reversed by diphenhydramine). Cholestatic jaundice and neuroleptic malignant syndrome has been reported. May intefere with pregnancy tests (immunologic reactions between hCG and anti-hCG). For nausea and vomiting, use only in management of prolonged vomiting of known etiology.

## PROPRANOLOL

Inderal and many other generics

***Adrenergic blocking agent (beta), class II antiarrhythmic***

Yes Yes 1 C/D

**Tabs:** 10, 20, 40, 60, 80, 90 mg
**Extended-release caps:** 60, 80, 120, 160 mg
**Oral solution:** 20, 40 mg/5 mL; contains parabens and saccharin
**Concentrated solution:** 80 mg/mL; alcohol and dye free
**Injection:** 1 mg/mL (1 mL)

*Continued*

For explanation of icons, see p. 698.

PROPRANOLOL *continued*

***Arrhythmias:***

***Child:***

***IV:*** 0.01–0.1 mg/kg/dose IV push over 10 min, repeat Q6–8 hr PRN
**Max. dose:** 1 mg/dose for infants; 3 mg/dose for children
***PO:*** Start at 0.5–1 mg/kg/24 hr ÷ Q6–8 hr; increase dosage Q3–5 days PRN. Usual dosage range: 2–4 mg/kg/24 hr ÷ Q6–8 hr
**Max. dose:** 60 mg/24 hr or 16 mg/kg/24 hr

***Adult:***

***IV:*** 1 mg/dose Q5 min up to total 5 mg
***PO:*** 10–20 mg/dose TID-QID; increase PRN. Usual dosage range 40–320 mg/24 hr ÷ TID-QID

***Hypertension:***

***Child:***

***PO:*** Initial: 0.5–1 mg/kg/24 hr ÷ Q6–12 hr. May increase dose Q3–5 days PRN; **max. dose:** 8 mg/kg/24 hr

***Adult:***

***PO:*** 40 mg/dose PO BID or 60–80 mg/dose (sustained-release capsule) PO QD. May increase 10–20 mg/dose Q3–5 days; **max. dose:** 640 mg/24 hr.

***Migraine prophylaxis:***

***Child:***

***<35 kg:*** 10–20 mg PO TID
***≥35 kg:*** 20–40 mg PO TID

***Adult:*** 80 mg/24 hr ÷ Q6–8 hr PO; increase dose by 20–40 mg/dose Q3–4 wk PRN. Usual effective dose range: 160–240 mg/24 hr.

***Tetralogy spells:***

***IV:*** 0.15–0.25 mg/kg/dose slow IV push. May repeat in 15 min × 1. See also Chapter 7.
***PO:*** Start at 2–4 mg/kg/24 hr ÷ Q6 hr PRN. Usual dose range: 4–8 mg/kg/24 hr ÷ Q6 hr PRN. Doses as high as 15 mg/kg/24 hr have been used with careful monitoring.

***Thyrotoxicosis:***

***Neonate:*** 2 mg/kg/24 hr PO ÷ Q6–12 hr

***Adolescent and adult:***

***IV:*** 1–3 mg/dose over 10 min. May repeat in 4–6 hr.
***PO:*** 10–40 mg/dose PO Q6 hr

---

**Contraindicated** in asthma, Raynaud's syndrome, heart failure, and heart block. **Not indicated** for the treatment of hypertensive emergencies. **Use with caution** in presence of obstructive lung disease, diabetes mellitus, renal or hepatic disease. May cause hypoglycemia, hypotension, nausea, vomiting, depression, weakness, impotence, bronchospasm, and heart block. Cutaneous reactions, including Stevens-Johnson syndrome, TEN, exfoliative dermatitis, erythema multiforme, and utricaria have been reported. Acute hypertension have occurred after insulin-induced hypoglycemia in patients on propranolol.

Therapeutic levels: 30–100 ng/mL. Drug is metabolized by CYP 450 1A2, 2C18, 2C19 and 2D6 isoenzymes. Concurrent administration with barbiturates, indomethacin, or rifampin may cause decreased activity of propranolol. Concurrent administration with cimetidine, hydralazine, flecainide, quinidine, chlorpromazine, or verapamil may lead to increased activity of propranolol. **Avoid** IV use of propranolol with calcium channel blockers; may increase effect of calcium channel blocker.

Pregnancy category changes to "D" if used in second or third trimesters.

## PROPYLTHIOURACIL

PTU

***Antithyroid agent***

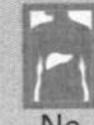 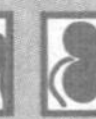 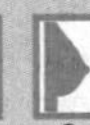 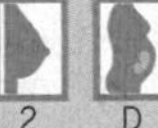
No Yes 2 D

**Tabs:** 50 mg
**Oral suspension:** 5 mg/mL
100 mg PTU = 10 mg methimazole

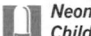

***Neonate:*** 5–10 mg/kg/24 hr ÷ Q8 hr PO
***Child:***
***Initial:*** 5–7 mg/kg/24 hr ÷ Q8 hr PO, OR by age:
***6–10 yr:*** 50–150 mg/24 hr ÷ Q8 hr PO
***>10 yr:*** 150–300 mg/24 hr ÷ Q8 hr PO
***Maintenance:*** Generally begins after 2 mo. Usually ⅓–⅔ the initial dose in divided doses (Q8–12 hr) when the patient is euthyroid.
***Adult:***
***Initial:*** 300–450 mg/24 hr ÷ Q8 hr PO; some may require larger doses of 600–1200 mg/24 hr
***Maintenance:*** 100–150 mg/24 hr ÷ Q8–12 hr PO

May cause blood dyscrasias, fever, liver disease, dermatitis, urticaria, malaise, CNS stimulation or depression, and arthralgias. Glomerulonephritis, interstitial pneumonitis, exfoliative dermatitis, and erythema nodosum have also been reported. May decrease the effectiveness of warfarin. Monitor thyroid function. Dosages should be adjusted as required to achieve and maintain $T_4$, TSH levels in normal ranges. A dose reduction of beta-blocker may be necessary when the hyperthyroid patient becomes euthyroid.

For neonates, crush tablets, weigh appropriate dose, and mix in formula/breast milk. **Adjust dose in renal failure (see Chapter 31).**

## PROSTAGLANDIN $E_1$

See *Alprostadil*

## PROTAMINE SULFATE

Various generic brands

***Antidote, heparin***

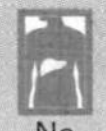 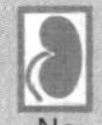 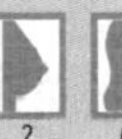
No No ? C

**Injection:** 10 mg/mL (5, 25 mL); preservative free

***Heparin antidote, IV:***
1 mg protamine will neutralize 115 U porcine intestinal heparin or 90 U beef lung heparin.
*Consider time since last heparin dose:*
***If < 0.5 hr:*** Give 100% of specified dose
***If within 0.5–1 hr:*** Give 50%–75% of aforementioned dose
***If within 1–2 hr:*** Give 37.5%–50% of aforementioned dose
***If ≥ 2 hr:*** Give 25%–37.5% of aforementioned dose
**Max. dose:** 50 mg IV
**Max. infusion rate:** 5 mg/min
**Max. IV concentration:** 10 mg/mL

*Continued*

For explanation of icons, see p. 698.

PROTAMINE SULFATE *continued*

*If heparin was administered by deep SC injection, give 1–1.5 mg protamine per 100 U heparin as follows:*
Load with 25–50 mg via slow IV infusion followed by the rest of the calculated dose via continuous infusion over 8–16 hr or the expected duration of heparin absorption.

*Enoxaparin overdosage, IV (see remarks):* Approximately 1 mg protamine will neutralize 1 mg enoxaparin.

***Consider time since last enoxaparin dose:***
***If < 8 hr:*** Give 100% of aforementioned dose.
***If within 8–12 hr:*** Give 50% of aforementioned dose.
***If > 12 hr:*** Protamine not required
If aPTT remains prolonged 2–4 hr after the first protamine dose, a second infusion of 0.5 mg protamine per 1 mg enoxaparin may be given.
**Max. dose:** 50 mg. See Heparin antidote IV dosage for **max.** administration concentration and rate.

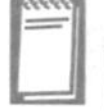

Risk factors for protamine hypersensitivity include known hypersensitivity to fish, and exposure to protamine-containing insulin or prior protamine therapy. May cause hypotension, bradycardia, dyspnea, and anaphylaxis. Monitor aPTT or ACT. Heparin rebound with bleeding has been reported to occur 8–18 hr later.

Use in enoxaparin overdose may not be complete despite using multiple doses of protamine.

## PSEUDOEPHEDRINE

Sudafed, Efidac/24-Pseudoephedrine, and others

***Sympathomimetic, nasal decongestant***

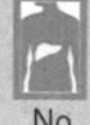
No
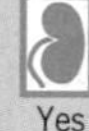
Yes
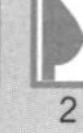
2
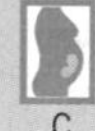
C

**Tabs (OTC):** 30, 60 mg
**Chewable tabs (OTC):** 15 mg; contains phenylalanine
**Extended-release tabs (OTC):** 120 mg, 240 mg (Efidac/24)
**Caps (OTC):** 30, 60 mg
**Sustained-release caps (OTC):** 120 mg
**Liquid (OTC):** 15, 30 mg/5 mL (120, 473 mL)
**Syrup (OTC):** 15 mg/5 mL (118 mL); contains parabens
**Drops (OTC):** 7.5 mg/0.8 mL (15, 30 mL)
**Purchases of OTC products are limited to behind the pharmacy counter sales with monthly sale limits due to the methamphetamine epidemic.**

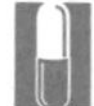

***Child <12 yr:*** 4 mg/kg/24 hr ÷ Q6 hr PO or by age:
***<2 yr:*** 4 mg/kg/24 hr ÷ Q6 hr PO
***2–5 yr:*** 15 mg/dose Q6 hr PO; **max. dose:** 60 mg/24 hr
***6–12 yr:*** 30 mg/dose Q6 hr PO; **max. dose:** 120 mg/24 hr

***Child ≥ 12 yr and adult:***
***Immediate release:*** 30–60 mg/dose Q6 hr PO; **max. dose:** 240 mg/24 hr
***Sustained release:*** 120 mg PO Q12 hr
***Efidac/24:*** 240 mg PO Q24 hr

**Contraindicated** with MAO inhibitor drugs and in severe hypertension and severe coronary artery disease. **Use with caution** in mild/moderate hypertension, hyperglycemia, hyperthyroidism, and cardiac disease. May cause dizziness, nervousness, restlessness, insomnia, and arrhythmias.

Pseudoephedrine is a common component of OTC cough and cold preparations and is

*Continued*

PSEUDOEPHEDRINE *continued*

combined with several antihistamines. Since drug and active metabolite are primarily excreted renally, **doses should be adjusted in renal impairment**. May cause false-positive test for amphetamines (EMIT assay).

## PSYLLIUM

Metamucil, Fiberall, Serutan, Konsyl, Perdiem Fiber Therapy, and many others

***Bulk-forming laxative***

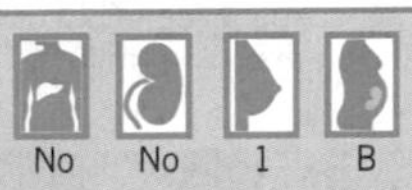


**Granules [OTC]:** Serutan: 2.5 g/rounded teaspoon (170, 540 g), Perdiem: 4.03 g/rounded teaspoon (100, 250 g)
**Powder [OTC]:** 50% psyllium, 50% dextrose (sugar-free version available) (Metamucil: 3.4 g/rounded teaspoon); 100% psyllium (Konsyl: 6 g/rounded teaspoon); for other products check label for the amount of psyllium per unit of measurement
**Wafers [OTC]:** 3.4 g
**Caps:** 0.52 g

***Child*** (granules or powder must be mixed with a full glass of water or juice):
***<6 yr:*** 1.25–2.5 g/dose PO QD-TID; **max. dose:** 7.5 g/24 hr
***6–11 yr:*** 2.5–3.75 g/dose PO QD-TID; **max. dose:** 15 g/24 hr
***≥12 yr:*** 2.5–7.5 g/dose PO QD-TID; **max. dose:** 30 g/24 hr

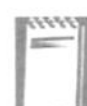

**Contraindicated** in cases of fecal impaction or GI obstruction. **Use with caution** in patients with esophageal strictures and rectal bleeding. Phenylketonurics should be aware that certain preparations may contain aspartame. Should be taken with a full glass (240 mL) of liquid. Onset of action: 12–72 hr.

## PYRANTEL PAMOATE

Antiminth, Reese's Pinworm, Pamix, Pin-Rid, and Pin-X

***Anthelmintic***

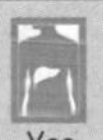
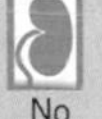
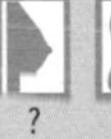
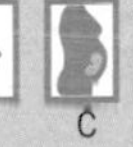


**Oral suspension (OTC):** 50 mg/mL pyrantel base (144 mg/mL pyrantel pamoate) (30, 60 mL)
**Liquid (OTC):** 50 mg/mL pyrantel base (144 mg/mL pyrantel pamoate) (30 mL); may contain parabens
**Caps (OTC) and tabs (OTC):** 62.5 mg pyrantel base (180 mg pyrantel pamoate)

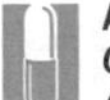

**All doses expressed in terms of pyrantel base.**
***Child and adult:***
***Ascaris (roundworm) and Trichostrongylus:*** 11 mg/kg/dose PO × 1
***Enterobius (pinworm):*** 11 mg/kg/dose PO × 1. Repeat same dose 2 wk later.
***Hookworm or eosinophilic enterocolitis:*** 11 mg/kg/dose PO QD × 3 days
**Max. dose (all indications):** 1 g/dose

*Continued*

For explanation of icons, see p. 698.

PYRANTEL PAMOATE *continued*

**Use with caution** in liver dysfunction. **Do not use** in combination with piperazine because of antagonism. May cause nausea, vomiting, anorexia, transient AST elevations, headaches, rash, and muscle weakness. Limited experience in children < 2 yr. May increase theophylline levels. Drug may be mixed with milk or fruit juice and may be taken with food.

## PYRAZINAMIDE

Pyrazinoic acid amide

***Antituberculous agent***

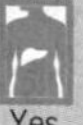 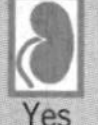 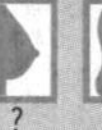 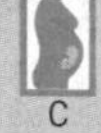

Yes Yes ? C

**Tab:** 500 mg

**Oral suspension:** 10, 100 mg/mL

**In combination with isoniazid and rifampin (Rifater):**

**Tab:** 300 mg with 50 mg isoniazid and 120 mg rifampin; contains povidone and propylene glycol

***Tuberculosis:*** Use as part of a multidrug regimen for tuberculosis. See latest edition of the AAP *Red Book* for recommended treatment for tuberculosis.

***Child:***

***Daily dose:*** 20–40 mg/kg/24 hr PO ÷ QD-BID; **max. dose:** 2 g/24 hr

***Twice-weekly dose:*** 50 mg/kg/dose PO 2 × per wk; **max. dose:** 2 g/dose

***Adult:***

***Daily dose:*** 15–30 mg/kg/24 hr PO ÷ QD-QID; **max. dose:** 2 g/24 hr

***Twice-weekly dose:*** 50–70 mg/kg/dose PO 2 × per wk; **max. dose:** 4 g/dose

***Mycobacterium tuberculosis in HIV, prophylaxis to prevent first episode:***

***Adolescent and adult:*** 15–20 mg/kg/24 hr PO QD × 2 mo in combination with either rifampin 600 mg PO QD × 2 mo or rifampin 300 mg PO QD × 2 mo

See latest edition of the AAP *Red Book* for recommended treatment for tuberculosis. **Contraindicated** in severe hepatic damage and acute gout. The CDC and ATS **do not recommend** the combination of pyrazinamide and rifampin for latent TB infections. **Use with caution** in patients with renal failure (dosage reduction has been recommended), gout or diabetes mellitus. Monitor liver function tests (baseline and periodic) and serum uric acid.

Hepatoxicity is most common dose-related side effect; doses ≤ 30 mg/kg/24 hr minimize effect. Hyperuricemia, maculopapular rash, arthralgia, fever, acne, porphyria, dysuria and photosensitivity may occur. Severe hepatic toxicity may occur with rifampin use. May decrease isoniazid levels.

## PYRETHRINS

Tisit, A-200, Pyrinyl, Pronto, RID, and others

***Pediculicide***

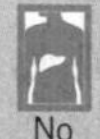 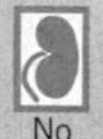 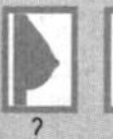 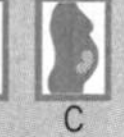

No No ? C

**All products are available without a prescription.**

**Lotion (Tisit):** 0.3% pyrethrins and 2% piperonyl butoxide (59, 118 mL); contains petroleum distillate and equivalent to 1.6% ether

*Continued*

PYRETHRINS *continued*

**Gel (Tisit):** 0.3% pyrethrins and 3% piperonyl butoxide (30 mL)
**Shampoo (Tisit, RID, Pronto, A-200):** 0.33% pyrethrins and 4% piperonyl butoxide (60, 120, 240 mL); may contain alcohol
**Mousse (RID):** 0.33% pyrethrins and 4% piperonyl butoxide (165 mL); contains alcohol

***Pediculosis:*** Apply to hair or affected body area for 10 min; then wash thoroughly and comb with fine-tooth comb or nit-removing comb; repeat in 7–10 days.

**Contraindicated** in ragweed hypersensitivity; drug is derived from the chrysanthemum flower. For topical use only. **Avoid** use in and around the eyes, mouth, nose, or vagina. **Avoid** repeat applications in < 24 hr. Low ovicidal activity requires repeat treatment. Dead nits require mechanical removal. Wash bedding and clothing to eraticate infestation.

Local irritation including erythema, pruritis, urticaria, edema, and eczema may occur.

## PYRIDOSTIGMINE BROMIDE

Mestinon and others
***Cholinergic agent***

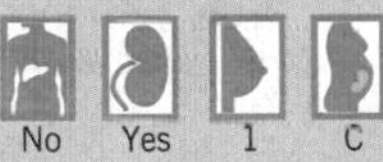

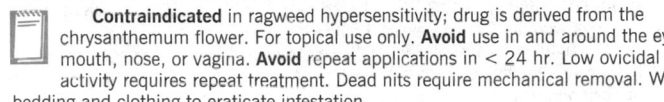

**Syrup:** 60 mg/5 mL (480 mL); contains 5% alcohol
**Tabs:** 60 mg
**Sustained-release tab:** 180 mg
**Injection:** 5 mg/mL; may contain 0.2% parabens

***Myasthenia gravis:***
***Neonate:***
- ***PO:*** 5 mg/dose Q4–6 hr
- ***IM/IV:*** 0.05–0.15 mg/kg/dose Q4–6 hr; **max. single IM/IV dose:** 10 mg

***Child:***
- ***PO:*** 7 mg/kg/24 hr in 5–6 divided doses
- ***IM/IV:*** 0.05–0.15 mg/kg/dose Q4–6 hr; **max. single IM/IV dose:** 10 mg

***Adult:***
- ***PO (immediate release):*** 60 mg TID; increase Q48 hr PRN. Usual effective dose: 60–1500 mg/24 hr.
- ***PO (sustained release):*** 180–540 mg QD-BID
- ***IM/IV:*** 2–5 mg/dose Q2–3 hr

**Contraindicated** in mechanical intestinal or urinary obstruction. **Use with caution** in patients with epilepsy, asthma, bradycardia, hyperthyroidism, arrhythmias, or peptic ulcer. May cause nausea, vomiting, diarrhea, rash, headache, and muscle cramps. Pyridostigmine is mainly excreted unchanged by the kidney. Therefore, lower doses titrated to effect in renal disease may be necessary.

Changes in oral dosages may take several days to show results. **Atropine is the antidote.**

For explanation of icons, see p. 698.

## PYRIDOXINE

Aminoxin, Vitamin $B_6$, and various others

***Vitamin, water soluble***

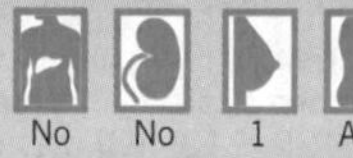

No No 1 A/C

**Tabs (HCl) [OTC]:** 25, 50, 100, 250, 500 mg
**Tabs, enteric-coated (pyridoxal-5'-phosphate) (Aminoxin) [OTC]:** 20 mg
**Oral solution (HCl):** 1 mg/mL
**Injection (HCl):** 100 mg/mL (1 mL); contains chlorobutanol

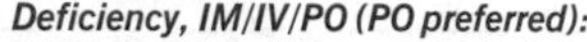

***Deficiency, IM/IV/PO (PO preferred):***
***Child:*** 5–25 mg/24 hr × 3 wk, followed by 1.5–-2.5 mg/24 hr as maintenance therapy (via multivitamin preparation)
***Adult:*** 10–20 mg/24 hr × 3 wk, followed by 2–5 mg/24 hr as maintenance therapy (via multivitamin preparation)

***Drug-induced neuritis, PO:***
- ***Prophylaxis:***
  - ***Child:*** 1–2 mg/kg/24 hr
  - ***Adult:*** 25–100 mg/24 hr
- ***Treatment:***
  - ***Child:*** 10–50 mg/24 hr
  - ***Adult:*** 100–300 mg/24 hr

***Sideroblastic anemia:***
***Adult:*** 200–600 mg/24 hr PO × 1–2 mo. If adequate response, dose may be reduced to 30–50 mg/24 hr.

***Pyridoxine dependent seizures:***
- ***Neonate and infant:***
  - ***Initial:*** 50–100 mg/dose IM or rapid IV × 1
  - ***Maintenance:*** 50–100 mg/24 hr PO

***Recommended daily allowance: See Chapter 21.***

**Use caution** with concurrent levodopa therapy. Chronic administration has been associated with sensory neuropathy. Nausea, headache, increased AST, decreased serum folic acid level and allergic reaction may occur. May lower phenobarbital and phenytoin levels. **See Chapter 20 for management of neonatal seizures.** Pregnancy category changes to "C" if dosage exceeds U.S. RDA recommendation.

## PYRIMETHAMINE ± SULFADOXINE

Daraprim

In combination with sulfadoxine: Fansidar

***Antiparasitic agent ± sulfonamide antibiotic***

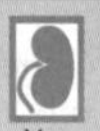 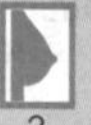 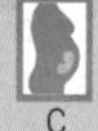

Yes Yes 2 C

**Tabs:** 25 mg
**Suspension:** 2 mg/mL
**In combination with sulfadoxine:**
**Tabs (Fansidar):** Pyrimethamine 25 mg and sulfadoxine 500 mg

***PYRIMETHAMINE:***
***Congenital toxoplasmosis (administer with sulfadiazine; see remarks):***
***Load:*** 2 mg/kg/24 hr PO ÷ Q12 hr × 2 days

*Continued*

PYRIMETHAMINE ± SULFADOXINE *continued*

***Maintenance:*** 1 mg/kg/24 hr PO QD × 2–6 mo, then 1 mg/kg/24 hr 3 × per wk to complete total 12 mo of therapy

***Toxoplasmosis (administer with sulfadiazine or trisulfapyrimidines):***

***Child:***

***Load:*** 2 mg/kg/24 hr PO ÷ BID × 3 days; **max. dose:** 100 mg/24 hr

***Maintenance:*** 1 mg/kg/24 hr PO ÷ QD-BID × 4 wk; **max. dose:** 25 mg/24 hr

***Adult:*** 50–75 mg/24 hr × 3–4 wk depending on response. After response, decrease dose by 50% and continue for an additional 4–5 wk.

***PYRIMETHAMINE AND SULFADOXINE:***

***Malaria treatment (acute uncomplicated P. falciparum with suspected chloroquine resistance) > 2 mo of age as a single dose PO:***

***Child:***

***5–10 kg:*** ½ tab
***11–20 kg:*** 1 tab
***21–30 kg:*** 1.5 tabs
***31–45 kg:*** 2 tabs
***>45 kg:*** 3 tabs

***Adult:*** 2–3 tabs

***Malaria prophylaxis (for areas of chloroquine-resistant P. falciparum used as a single dose for self-treatment of febrile illness when medical care is not immediately available):***

***Child:***

***2–11 mo:*** ¼ tab
***1–3 yr:*** ½ tab
***4–8 yr:*** 1 tab
***9–14 yr:*** 2 tabs
***>14 yr:*** 3 tabs

***Adult:*** 3 tabs

---

Pyrimethamine is a folate antagonist. Supplementation with folinic acid leucovorin at 5–15 mg/24 hr is recommended. **Contraindicated** in megaloblastic anemia secondary to folate deficiency. **Use with caution** in G6PD deficiency, malabsorption syndromes, alcoholism, pregnancy, and renal or hepatic impairment. Pyrimethamine can cause glossitis, bone marrow suppression, seizures, rash, and photosensitivity. For congenital toxoplasmosis, see *Clin Infect Dis* 1994;18:38–72. Zidovudine and methotrexate may increase risk for bone marrow suppression. Aurothioglucose, trimethoprim, and sulfamethoxazole may increase risk for blood dyscrasias. Administer doses with meals. Most cases of acquired toxoplasmosis **do not** require specific antimicrobial therapy.

**PYRIMETHAMINE AND SULFADOXINE:** Effective against certain strains of *P. falciparum* that are resistant to chloroquine. Resistance has been reported in Southeast Asia, the Amazon basin, sub-Saharan Africa, Bangladesh, and Oceania. **Contraindicated** (in addition to previously listed contraindications) in sulfa hypersensitivity, porphyria, severe renal or hepatic impairment, infants < 2 mo, and pregnancy at term. May cause (in addition to previously listed causes) erythema multiforme, Stevens-Johnson syndrome, toxic epidermal necrolysis, elevated ALT and AST, and renal impairment. Aminobenzoic acid (PABA), benzocaine, and tetracaine may decrease effects of sulfadoxine. Administer doses with meals.

For explanation of icons, see p. 698.

## QUINIDINE

Quinidex and various generic brands

***Class Ia antiarrhythmic***

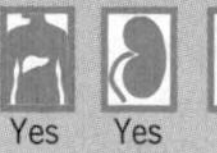
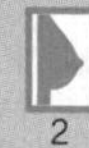
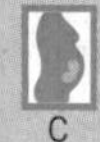

Yes Yes 2 C

**As gluconate (62% quinidine):**

**Slow-release tabs:** 324 mg

**Injection:** 80 mg/mL (50 mg/mL quinidine) (10 mL); contains phenol

**As sulfate (83% quinidine):**

**Tabs:** 200, 300 mg

**Slow-release tab (Quinidex):** 300 mg

**Oral suspension:** 10 mg/mL

Equivalents: 200 mg sulfate = 267 mg gluconate

**All doses expressed as salt forms.**

***Antiarrhythmic:***

***Child (give PO as sulfate; give IM/IV as gluconate):***

***Test dose:*** 2 mg/kg × 1 IM/PO; **max. dose:** 200 mg

***Therapeutic dose:***

***IV (as gluconate):*** 2–10 mg/kg/dose Q3–6 hr PRN

***PO (as sulfate):*** 15–60 mg/kg/24 hr ÷ Q6 hr

***Adult (give PO as sulfate; give IM/IV as gluconate):***

***Test dose:*** 200 mg × 1 IM/PO.

***Therapeutic dose:***

***As sulfate:***

***PO, immediate-release:*** 100–600 mg/dose Q4–6 hr. Begin at 200 mg/dose and titrate to desired effect.

***PO, sustained-release:*** 300–600 mg/dose Q8–12 hr.

***As gluconate:***

***IM:*** 400 mg/dose Q4–6 hr

***IV:*** 200–400 mg/dose, infused at a rate of ≤ 10 mg/min

***PO:*** 324–972 mg Q8–12 hr

***Malaria:***

***Child and adult (give IV as gluconate; see remarks):***

***Loading dose:*** 10 mg/kg/dose (**max. dose:** 600 mg) IV over 1–2 hr followed by maintenance dose. Omit or decrease load if patient has received quinine or mefloquine.

***Maintenance dose:*** 0.02 mg/kg/min IV as continuous infusion until oral therapy can be initiated. If more than 48 hr of IV therapy is required, reduce dose by 30%–50%.

Test dose is given to assess for idiosyncratic reaction to quinidine. Toxicity indicated by increase of QRS interval by ≥ 0.02 sec (skip dose or stop drug). May cause GI symptoms, hypotension, tinnitus, TTP, rash, heart block and blood dyscrasias. When used alone, may cause 1:1 conduction in atrial flutter leading to ventricular fibrillation. May get idiosyncratic ventricular tachycardia with low levels, especially when initiating therapy.

Quinidine is a substrate of CYP 450 3A3/4 and 3A5–7 enzymes, and an inhibitor of CYP 450 2D6 and 3A3/4 enzymes. Can cause increase in digoxin levels. Quinidine potentiates the effect of neuromuscular blocking agents, beta-blockers, anticholinergics, and warfarin. Amiodarone, antacids, delavirdine, diltiazem, grapefruit juice, saquinavir, ritonavir, verapamil, or cimetidine may enhance the drug's effect. Barbiturates, phenytoin, cholinergic drugs, nifedipine, sucralfate, or rifampin may reduce quinidine's effect. **Use with caution** in renal insufficiency (15%–25% of drug is eliminated unchanged in the urine), myocardial depression, sick sinus syndrome, G6PD deficiency, and hepatic dysfunction.

*Continued*

R

FORMULARY

QUINIDINE *continued*

Therapeutic levels: 3–7 mg/L. Recommended serum sampling times at steady-state: trough level obtained within 30 min prior to the next scheduled dose after 1–2 days of continuous dosing (steady-state).

**MALARIA USE:** Continuous monitoring of ECG, blood pressure and serum glucose are recommended; especially in pregnant women and young children.

## QUINUPRISTIN AND DALFOPRISTIN

Synercid

***Antibiotic, streptogramin***

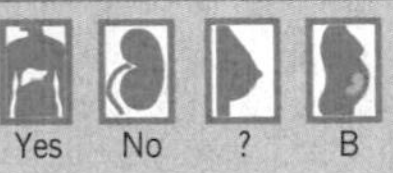


**Injection:** 500 mg (150 mg quinupristin and 350 mg dalfopristin)

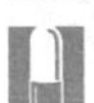

**Doses expressed in mg of combined quinupristin and dalfopristin.**

***Child < 16 yr (limited data), ≥ 16 yr and adult:***

***Vancomycin-resistant Enterococcus faecium (VREF):*** 7.5 mg/kg/dose IV Q8 hr

***Complicated skin infections:*** 7.5 mg/kg/dose IV Q12 hr for at least 7 days

***Peritonitis associated with CAPD (≥ 16 yr and adult):*** 5–10 mg/kg/dose IV Q12 hr × 14 days

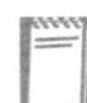

**Not active** against *Enterococcus faecalis.* **Use with caution** in hepatic impairment; dosage reduction may be necessary. Most common side effects include pain, burning, inflammation and edema at the IV infusion site, thrombophlebitis, thrombosis, GI disturbances, rash, arthralgia, myalgia, increased liver enzymes, hyperbilirubinemia, and headache. Dose frequency reductions (Q8 hr to Q12 hr) or discontinuation can improve severe cases of arthralgia and myalgia.

Drug is an inhibitor to the CYP 450 3A4 isoenzyme. **Avoid use** with CYP 450 3A4 substrates, which can prolong QTc interval (e.g., cisapride). May increase the effects/toxicity of cyclosporine, tacrolimus, sirolimus, delavirdine, nevirapine, indinavir, ritonavir, diazepam, midazolam, carbamazepine, methylprednisolone, vinca alkaloids, docetaxel, paclitaxel, quinidine, and some calcium channel blockers.

**Pediatric pharmacokinetic studies have not been completed.** Reduce dose for patients with hepatic cirrhosis (Child-Pugh A or B).

Drug is compatible with $D_5W$ and incompatible with saline and heparin. Infuse each dose over 1 hr using the following **max.** IV concentrations: peripheral line: 2 mg/mL; central line: 5 mg/mL. If injection site reaction occurs, dilute infusion to < 1 mg/mL.

## RANITIDINE HCL

Zantac, Zantac 75 [OTC], Zantac 150 Maximum Strength [OTC], and many generics

***Histamine-2-antagonist***

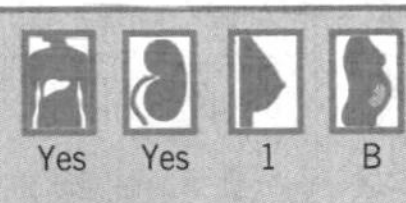


**Tabs:** 75 [OTC], 150 [OTC and Rx], 300 mg
**Effervescent tabs:** 25, 150 mg
**Syrup:** 15 mg/mL (480 mL); contains 7.5% alcohol and parabens
**Oral liquid:** 15 mg/mL (473 mL); contains parabens and may contain alcohol

*Continued*

For explanation of icons, see p. 698.

RANITIDINE HCL *continued*

**Carbohydrate-free oral solution:** 5, 10 mg/mL [dissolve 150 mg effervescent granules with 30 mL (5 mg/mL) or 15 mL (10 mg/mL) water; solution good for 24 hr] 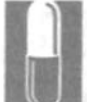
**Injection:** 25 mg/mL (2, 6 mL); contains 0.5% phenol
**Injection (pre-mixed):** 1 mg/mL (preservative-free in ½ normal saline, 50 mL)

***Neonate:***
*PO:* 2–4 mg/kg/24 hr ÷ Q8–12 hr
*IV:* 2 mg/kg/24 hr ÷ Q6–8 hr
***≥1 mo–16 yr:***
***Duodenal/gastric ulcer (see remarks):***
*PO:*
*Treatment:* 2–4 mg/kg/24 hr ÷ Q12 hr; **max. dose:** 300 mg/24 hr
*Maintenance:* 2–4 mg/kg/24 hr ÷ Q12 hr; **max. dose:** 150 mg/24 hr
*IV/IM:* 2–4 mg/kg/24 hr ÷ Q6–8 hr; **max. dose:** 200 mg/24 hr
***GERD/erosive esophagitis:***
*PO:* 5–10 mg/kg/24 hr ÷ Q8–12 hr; GERD **max. dose:** 300 mg/24 hr, erosive esophagitis **max. dose:** 600 mg/24 hr
*IV/IM:* 2–4 mg/kg/24 hr ÷ Q6–8 hr; **max. dose:** 200 mg/24 hr
***Adult:***
*PO:* 150 mg/dose BID or 300 mg/dose QHS
*IM/IV:* 50 mg/dose Q6–8 hr; **max. dose:** 400 mg/24 hr
***Continuous infusion, all ages:*** Administer daily IV dosage over 24 hr (may be added to parenteral nutrition solutions).

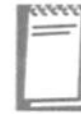

May cause headache and GI disturbance, malaise, insomnia, sedation, arthralgia and hepatotoxicity. May increase levels of nifedipine. May decrease levels of ketoconazole, itraconazole and delavirdine. May cause false-positive urine protein test (Multistix).

Duodenal/gastric ulcer doses for ≥ 1 mo–16 yr are extrapolated from clinical adult trials and pharmacokinetic data in children. Extemporaneously compounded carbohydrate-free oral solution dosage form is useful for patients receiving the ketogenic diet. The syrup dosage form has a peppermint flavor and may not be tolerated. **Adjust dose in renal failure (see Chapter 31).**

## RASBURICASE

Elitek

***Antihyperuricemic agent***

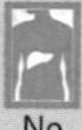 No 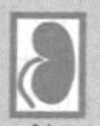 No 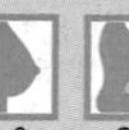 ? 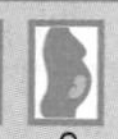 C

**Injection:** 1.5, 7.5 mg; contains mannitol

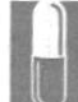

***Hyperuricemia:*** 0.1–0.2 mg/kg/dose (rounded down to the nearest whole 1.5 mg multiple) IV over 30 min × 1. Patients generally respond to 1 dose but, if needed, dose may be repeated Q24 hr for up to 4 additional doses.

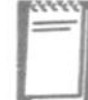

**Contraindicated** in G6PD deficiency or history of hypersensitivity, hemolytic reactions, or methemoglobinemia with rasburicase. **Use with caution** in asthma, allergies, hypersensitivity with other medications, and children < 2 yr (decreased efficacy and increased risk for rash, vomiting, diarrhea, and fever).

Common side effects include nausea, vomiting, abdominal pain, discomfort, diarrhea, constipation, mucositis, fever, and rash.

During therapy, uric acid blood samples must be sent to the laboratory immediately. Blood should be collected in prechilled tubes containing heparin, and placed in an ice-water bath to avoid potential falsely low uric acid levels

*Continued*

RASBURICASE *continued*

(degradation of plasma uric acid occurs in the presence of rasburicase at room temperature). Centrifugation in a precooled centrifuge (4°C) is indicated. Plasma samples must be assayed within 4 hr of sample collection.

## $Rh_o$ (D) IMMUNE GLOBULIN INTRAVENOUS (HUMAN)

WinRho SDF

***Immune Globulin***

No No ? C

**Injection:** 600, 1500, 2500, 5000, 15,000 IU
Conversion: 1 mcg = 5 IU

***Immune thrombocytopenic purpura*** (nonsplenectomized $Rh_o$(D)-positive patients):

***Initial dose (may given in two divided doses on separate days or as a single dose):***

- ***Hemoglobin ≥ 10 mg/dL:*** 250 IU/kg/dose IV × 1
- ***Hemoglobin < 10 mg/dL:*** 125–200 IU/kg/dose IV × 1. See remarks for hemoglobin < 8 mg/dL.

***Additional doses:*** 125–300 IU/kg/dose IV; actual dose and frequency of adminstration is determined by the patient's response and subsequent hemoglobin level.

WinRho SDF is currently the only $Rh_o$ (D) immune globulin product indicated for ITP. **Contraindicated** in IgA deficiency. **Use with extreme caution** in patients with a hemoglobin < 8 mg/dL and thrombocytopenia or bleeding disorders. Adverse events associated with ITP include headache, chills, fever and reduction in hemoglobin (due to the destruction of $Rh_o$ (D) antigen-positive red cells). Intravascular hemolysis resulting in anemia and renal insufficiency has been reported. May interfere with immune response to live virus vaccines (e.g., MMR, varicella). $Rh_o$(D) positive patients should be monitored for signs and symptoms of intravascular hemolysis, anemia, and renal insufficiency. Administer IV doses over 3–5 min.

## RIBAVIRIN

Oral: Rebetol, Copegus, Ribaspheres, and others

Inhalation: Virazole

***Antiviral agent***

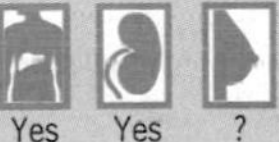


**Oral solution (Rebetol):** 200 mg/5 mL (100 mL); contains sodium benzoate
**Oral caps (Rebetol, Ribaspheres):** 200 mg
**Tabs (Copegus, Ribaspheres):** 200, 400, 600 mg
**Aerosol (Virazole):** 6 g

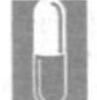

***Hepatitis C (PO, see remarks):***

***Child ≥3 yr*** *(in combination with interferon alfa-2b at 3 million units 3 × per wk SC using oral solution or capsule):*

- ***25–36 kg:*** 200 mg BID
- ***37–49 kg:*** 200 mg QAM and 400 mg QPM
- ***50–61 kg:*** 400 mg BID
- ***>61 kg:*** Use adult dose

***Dosage modification for toxicity:*** See remarks.

*Continued*

For explanation of icons, see p. 698.

RIBAVIRIN *continued*

***Hepatitis C (cont'd):***

***Adult:***

***Oral capsules in combination with interferon alfa-2b at 3 million units 3 × per wk SC:***

***≤75 kg:*** 400 mg QAM and 600 mg QPM

***>75 kg:*** 600 mg BID

***Oral capsules in combination with Peginterferon alfa-2b:*** 400 mg BID

***Oral tablets in combination with Peginterferon alfa-2a for hepatitis C genotype 1, 4:***

***≤75 kg:*** 500 mg BID × 48 wk

***>75 kg:*** 600 mg BID × 48 wk

***Oral tablets in combination with Peginterferon alfa-2a for genotype 2, 3:*** 400 mg BID × 24 wk

***Dosage modification for toxicity:*** See remarks.

***Inhalation:***

***Continuous:*** Administer 6 g by aerosol over 12–18 hr QD for 3–7 days. The 6 g ribavirin vial is diluted in 300 mL preservative-free sterile water to a final concentration of 20 mg/mL. **Must be administered** with Viratek Small Particle Aerosol Generator (SPAG-2).

***Intermittent (for nonventilated patients):*** Administer 2 g by aerosol over 2 hr TID for 3–7 days. The 6 g ribavirin vial is diluted in 100 mL preservative-free sterile water to a final concentration of 60 mg/mL. The intermittent use is **not recommended** in patients with endotracheal tubes.

---

**ORAL RIBAVIRIN: Contraindicated** in pregnancy, significant or unstable cardiac disease, autoimmune hepatitis, hepatic decompensation (Child-Pugh score > 6; class B or C), hemoglobinopathies, and creatinine clearance < 50 mL/min. **Use with caution** in pre-exisiting cardiac disease, pulmonary disease and sarcoidosis. Anemia (most common), insomnia, depression, irritability and suicidal behavior (higher in adolescent and pediatric patients) have been reported with the oral route. Tinnitus, hearing loss, vertigo and severe hypertriglyceridemia have been reported in combination with interferon. May decrease the effects of zidovudine, stavudine; and increase risk for lactic acidosis with nucleoside analogues.

**Reduce or discontinue dosage for toxicity as follows:**

Patient with no cardiac disease:

*Hgb < 10 g/dL and ≥ 8.5 g/dL:*

*Child:* 7.5 mg/kg/dose PO QD

*Adult:* 600 mg PO QD (capsules or solution) or 200 mg PO QAM and 400 mg PO QPM (tablets)

*Hgb < 8.5 g/dL:* Discontinue therapy permanently.

Patient with cardiac disease:

*≥2 mg/dL decrease in Hgb during any 4-wk period during therapy:*

*Child:* 7.5 mg/kg/dose PO QD

*Adult:* 600 mg PO QD (capsules or solution) or 200 mg PO QAM and 400 mg PO QPM (tablets)

*Hgb < 12 g/dL after 4 wk of reduced dose:* Discontinue therapy permanently.

**INHALED RIBAVIRIN:** Use of ribavirin for RSV is controversial and **not** routinely indicated. Aerosol therapy may be considered for selected infants and young children at high risk for serious RSV disease (see recommendations in *Pediatrics* 1996; 97:137–140 and most recent edition of the AAP *Red Book*). Most effective if begun early in course of RSV infection; generally in the first 3 days. May cause worsening respiratory distress, rash, conjunctivitis, mild bronchospasm, hypotension, anemia and cardiac arrest. **Avoid** unnecessary occupational exposure to ribavirin due to its teratogenic effects. Drug can precipitate in the respiratory equipment.

R

## RIBOFLAVIN

Vitamin $B_2$ and various brands

***Water-soluble vitamin***

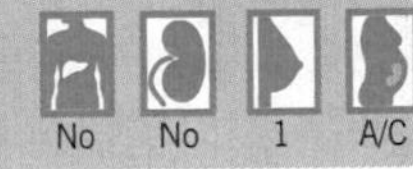


**Tabs [OTC]:** 50, 100 mg

***Riboflavin deficiency:***
- ***Child:*** 2.5–10 mg/24 hr ÷ QD-BID PO
- ***Adult:*** 5–30 mg/24 hr ÷ QD-BID PO

***U.S. RDA requirements: See Chapter 21.***

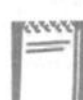

Hypersensitivity may occur. Administer with food. Causes yellow to orange discoloration of urine. For multivitamin information, see Chapter 21.

Pregnancy category changes to "C" if used in doses above the RDA.

## RIFABUTIN

Mycobutin

***Antituberculous agent***

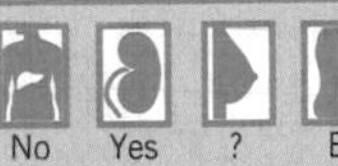


**Caps:** 150 mg
**Oral suspension:** 10, 20 mg/mL

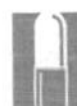

***MAC prophylaxis for first episode and recurrence of opportunistic disease in HIV (may be used in combination with a macrolide antibiotic; see www.aidsinfo.nih.gov/guideline):***
- ***<6 yr:*** 5 mg/kg/24 hr PO QD; **max. dose:** 300 mg/24 hr
- ***≥6 yr and adult:*** 300 mg PO QD; doses may be administered as 150 mg PO BID if GI upset occurs.

***MAC prophylaxis for recurrence of opportunistic disease in HIV (in combination with ethambutol and a macrolide antibiotic):***
- ***Infant and child:*** 5 mg/kg/24 hr PO QD; **max. dose:** 300 mg/24 hr
- ***Adolescent and adult:*** 300 mg PO QD

***MAC treatment:***
- ***Child:*** 5–10 mg/kg/24 hr PO QD; **max. dose:** 300 mg/24 hr as part of a multi-drug regimen.
- ***Adult:*** 300 mg PO QD; may be used in combination with azithromycin and ethambutol.
  - ***In combination with non-nucleoside reverse transcriptase inhibitors:***
    - ***With efavirenz:*** 450 mg PO QD or 600 mg PO 3 × per wk
    - ***With nevirapine:*** 300 mg PO 3 × per wk
  - ***In combination with protease inhibitors:***
    - ***With amprenavir, indinavir, or nelfinavir:*** 150 mg PO QD or 300 mg PO 3 × per wk
    - ***With ritonavir boosted regimens (e.g., saquinavir/ritonavir, or lopinavir/ritonavir):*** 150 mg PO QOD or 150 mg PO 3 × per wk

**Should not be used** for MAC prophylaxis with active TB. May cause GI distress, discoloration of skin and body fluids (brown-orange color) and marrow suppression. **Use with caution** in renal failure. **Adjust dose in renal impairment (see Chapter 31).** May permanently stain contact lenses. Uveitis can occur when using high doses (>300 mg/24 hr in adults) in combination with macrolide antibiotics.

*Continued*



For explanation of icons, see p. 698.

RIFABUTIN *continued*

Rifabutin is an inducer of CYP 450 3A enzyme and is structurally similar to rifampin (similar drug interactions, see *Rifampin*). Clarithromycin, fluconazole, itraconazole, nevirapine, and protease inhibitors increase rifabutin levels. Efavirenz may decrease rifabutin levels. May decrease effectiveness of dapsone, delavirdine, nevirapine, amprenavir, indinavir, nelfinavir, saquinavir, itraconazole, warfarin, oral contraceptives, digoxin, cyclosporine, ketoconazole, and narcotics.

Doses may be administered with food if patient experiences GI intolerance.

## RIFAMPIN

Rimactane, Rifadin, and others

***Antibiotic, antituberculous agent, rifamycin***

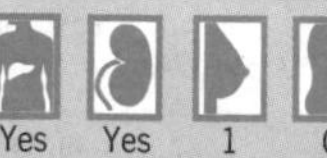


**Caps:** 150, 300 mg
**Oral suspension:** 10, 15, 25 mg/mL 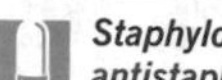
**Injection:** 600 mg

***Staphylococcus aureus infections (as part of synergistic therapy with other antistaphylococcal agents):***

***0–1 mo:***

*IV:* 10–20 mg/kg/24 hr ÷ Q12 hr

*PO:* 10–20 mg/kg/dose Q24 hr

***>1 mo:*** 10–20 mg/kg/24 hr ÷ Q12 hr IV/PO; **max. dose:** 600 mg/24 hr

***Adult:*** 300–600 mg Q12 hr IV/PO

***Prosthetic valve endocarditis:*** 300–400 mg Q8 hr IV/PO in combination with antistaphylococcal penicillin with or without gentamicin

***Tuberculosis:*** (see latest edition of the AAP *Red Book*, for duration of therapy and combination therapy). Twice weekly therapy may be used after 1–2 mo of daily therapy.

***Child:***

***Daily therapy:*** 10–20 mg/kg/24 hr ÷ Q12–24 hr IV/PO

***Twice weekly therapy:*** 10–20 mg/kg/24 hr PO twice weekly

**Max. daily dose:** 600 mg/24 hr

***Adult:***

***Daily therapy:*** 10 mg/kg/24 hr QD PO

***Twice weekly therapy:*** 10 mg/kg/24 hr QD twice weekly

**Max. daily dose:** 600 mg/24 hr

***Prophylaxis for N. meningitidis (see latest edition of the AAP* Red Book *additional information):***

***0–1 mo:*** 10 mg/kg/24 hr ÷ Q12 hr PO × 2 days

***>1 mo:*** 20 mg/kg/24 hr ÷ Q12 hr PO × 2 days

***Adult:*** 600 mg PO Q12 hr × 2 days

**Max. dose** (all ages): 1200 mg/24 hr

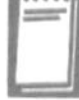

**Never** use as monotherapy except when used for prophylaxis. Patients with latent tuberculosis infection should **not** be treated with rifampin and pyrazinamide because of the risk of severe liver injury. Use is **not recommended** in porphyria.

May cause GI irritation, allergy, headache, fatigue, ataxia, confusion, fever, hepatitis, blood dyscrasias, interstitial nephritis, and elevated BUN and uric acid. Causes red discoloration of body secretions such as urine, saliva and tears (which can permanently stain contact lenses). Induces hepatic enzymes (CYP 450 2C9, 2C19, and 3A4), which may decrease plasma concentration of digoxin, corticosteroids, buspirone, benzodiazepines, fentanyl, calcium channel blockers, beta-blockers,

*Continued*

RIFAMPIN *continued*

cyclosporine, tacrolimus, itraconazole, ketoconazole, oral anticoagulants, barbiturates, and theophylline. May reduce the effectiveness of oral contraceptives and anti-retroviral agents (protease inhibitors and non-nucleoside reverse transcriptase inhibitors). Hepatotoxicity is a concern when used in combination with pyrazinamide.

**Adjust dose in renal failure (see Chapter 31).** Reduce dose in hepatic impairment. Give 1 hr before or 2 hr after meals.

For *H. influenza* prophylaxis, see latest edition of the *Red Book*.

## RIMANTADINE

Flumadine

***Antiviral agent***

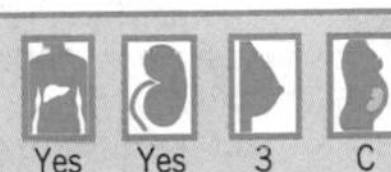


**Syrup:** 50 mg/ 5 mL (240 mL); contains saccharin and parabens
**Tabs:** 100 mg

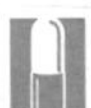

***Influenza A prophylaxis (for at least 10 days after known exposure; usually for 6–8 wk during influenza A season or local outbreak):***
***Child:***
***1–9 yr:*** 5 mg/kg/24 hr PO QD; **max. dose:** 150 mg/24 hr
***≥10 yr:***
***<40 kg:*** 5 mg/kg/24 hr PO ÷ QD-BID; **max. dose:** 150 mg/24 hr
***≥40 kg:*** 100 mg/dose PO BID
***Adult:*** 100 mg PO BID
***Influenza A treatment (within 48 hr of illness onset):***
Use the aforementioned prophylaxis dosage × 5–7 days.

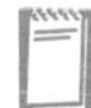

Individuals immunized with live attenuated influenza vaccine (e.g., FluMist) should **not** receive rimantadine prophylaxis for 14 days after the vaccine. Chemoprophylaxis does not interfere with immune response to inactivated influenza vaccine.

May cause GI disturbance, xerostomia, dizziness, headache and urinary retention. CNS disturbances are less than with amantadine. **Contraindicated** in amantadine hypersensitivity. **Use with caution** in renal or hepatic insufficiency; dosage reduction may be necessary. A dosage reduction of 50% has been recommended in severe hepatic or renal impairment.

## RISPERIDONE

Risperdal, Risperdal M-Tab, and Risperdal Consta

***Atypical antipsychotic, serotonin (5-$HT_2$) and dopamine ($D_2$) antagonist***

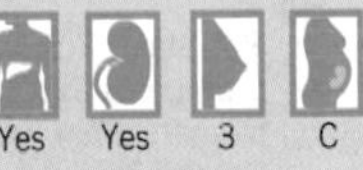


**Tabs:** 0.25, 0.5, 1, 2, 3, 4 mg
**Oral solution:** 1 mg/mL (30 mL)
**Orally disintegrating tabs (Risperdal M-Tab):** 0.5, 1, 2, 3, 4 mg; contains phenylalanine
**Injection (Risperdal Consta):** 25, 37.5, 50 mg (pre-filled syringe with 2 mL diluent); for IM administration only

*Continued*

For explanation of icons, see p. 698.

RISPERIDONE *continued*

***Irritability associated with autistic disorder:***
***5–16 yr (PO daily doses may be administered QD-BID; patients experiencing somnolence may benefit from QHS or BID dosing or dose reduction):***
***Initial dose:***

***<20 kg:*** 0.25 mg/24 hr PO for a minimum of 4 days; **use with caution** if < 15 kg as dosing recommendation is not established.
***≥20 kg:*** 0.5 mg/24 hr PO for a minimum of 4 days

***Dose increment (if needed) after 4 days of initial dose:***

***<20 kg:*** 0.5 mg/24 hr PO for a minimum of 14 days; if additional increments needed, increase dose by 0.25 mg/24 hr at intervals of at least 14 days.
***≥20 kg:*** 1 mg/24 hr PO for a minimum of 14 days; if additional increments needed, increase dose by 0.5 mg/24 hr at intervals of at least 14 days.

***Max. daily dose for plateau of therapeutic effect (from one pivotal clinical trial):***

***<20 kg:*** 1 mg/24 hr
***≥20–45 kg:*** 2.5 mg/24 hr
***>45 kg:*** 3 mg/24 hr

***Bipolar mania:*** Oral doses may be administered QD-BID and patients experiencing somnolence may benefit from QHS or BID dosing or dose reduction. Long-term use beyond 3 wk and doses (all ages) > 6 mg/24 hr have not been evaluated.

***Child (10–17 yr):*** Start with 0.5 mg/24 hr PO QD (QAM or QHS). If needed, increase dose at intervals not < 24 hr in increments of 0.5 or 1 mg/24 hr, as tolerated, up to a recommended dose of 2.5 mg/24 hr. Although efficacy has been demonstrated between 0.5–6 mg/24 hr, no additional benefit was seen above 2.5 mg/24 hr. Higher doses were associated with more adverse effects.
***Adult:*** Start with 2–3 mg PO QD. Dosage increases or decreases of 1 mg/24 hr can be made at 24-hr intervals. Dosage range: 1–6 mg/24 hr.

***Schizophrenia:*** Oral doses may be administered QD-BID and patients experiencing somnolence may benefit from BID dosing (see remarks).

***Adolescent (13–17 yr):*** No data are available to support long-term use of > 8 wk.

***PO:*** Start with 0.5 mg QD (QAM or QHS). If needed, increase dose at intervals not < 24 hr in increments of 0.5 to 1 mg/24 hr, as tolerated, to a recommended dose of 3 mg/24 hr. Although efficacy has been demonstrated between 1–6 mg/24 hr, no additional benefit was seen above 3 mg/24 hr. Doses > 6 mg/24 hr have not been studied.

***Adult:***

***PO:*** Start with 1 mg BID on day 1; if tolerated, increase to 2 mg BID on day 2 and to 3 mg BID thereafter. Dosage increases or decreases of 1–2 mg can be made on a weekly basis if needed. Usual effective dose: 4–8 mg/24 hr. Doses above 16 mg/24 hr have not been evaluated.
***IM:*** Start with 25 mg Q2 wk; if no response, dose may be increased to 37.5 mg or 50 mg at 4-wk intervals. **Max. IM dose:** 50 mg Q2 wk.

**Use with caution** in cardiovascular disorders, diabetes, renal or hepatic impairment (dose reduction necessary), hypothermia or hyperthermia, seizures, breast cancer or other prolactin-dependent tumors, and dysphagia. Common side effects include abdominal pain and other GI disturbances, arthralgia, anxiety, dizziness, headache, insomnia, somnolence (use QHS dosing), EPS, cough, fever, pharyngitis, rash, rhinitis, sexual dysfunction, tachycardia, and weight gain. Weight gain, somnolence, and fatigue were common side effects reported in the autism studies.

*Continued*

RISPERIDONE *continued*

In the presence of severe renal or hepatic impairment or risk for hypotension, the following adult dosing has been recommended: Start with 0.5 mg PO BID. Increase dose, if needed and tolerated, in increments no more than 0.5 mg BID. Increases to doses > 1.5 mg BID should occur at intervals of at least 1 wk; slower titration may be required in some patients.

Limited studies in pediatric related Tourette's syndrome, schizophrenia, and aggressive behavior in psychiatric disorders are reported. Autistic disorder safety and efficacy in children < 5 yr have not been established. If therapy has been discontinued for a period of time, therapy should be reinitiated with the same initial titration regimen.

Drug is a CYP 450 2D6 and 3A4 isoenzyme substrate. Concurrent use of isoenzyme inhibitors (e.g., fluoxetine, paroxetine, sertraline, cimetidine) and inducers (e.g., carbamazepine, rifampin, phenobarbital, phenytoin) may increase and decrease the effects of risperidone, respectively. Alcohol, CNS depressants, and St. John's wort may potentiate the drug's side effect. Risperidone may enhance the hypotensive effects of levodopa and dopamine agonists.

Oral dosage forms may be administered with or without food. Oral solution can be mixed in water, coffee, orange juice, or low-fat milk but is incompatible with cola or tea. **Do not** split or chew the orally disintegrating tablet. Use IM suspension preparation within 6 hr after reconstitution.

## ROCURONIUM

Zemuron

***Nondepolarizing neuromuscular blocking agent***

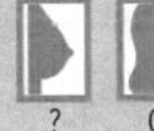
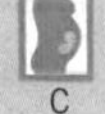

Yes No ? C

**Injection:** 10 mg/mL (5, 10 mL)

***Infant:***

*IV:* 0.5 mg/kg/dose; may repeat Q20–30 min PRN

***Child:***

*IV:* 0.6 mg/kg/dose × 1; if needed, give maintenance doses of 0.075–0.125 mg/kg/dose Q20–30 min.

***Adolescent and adult:***

*IV:* Start with 0.6–1.2 mg/kg/dose × 1; if needed, maintenance doses at 0.1–0.2 mg/kg/dose Q20–30 min.

***Continuous IV infusion:***

***Child and adult:*** Start at 10–12 mcg/kg/min and titrate to effect. Maintenance infusion rates have ranged from 4–16 mcg/kg/min in adults.

**Use with caution** in hepatic impairment and history of anaphylaxis with other neuromuscular blocking agents. Hypertension, hypotension, arrhythmia, tachycardia, nausea, vomiting, bronchospasm, wheezing, hiccups, rash, and edema at the injection site may occur. Increased neuromuscular blockade may occur with concomitant use of aminoglycosides, clindamycin, tetracycline, magnesium sulfate, quinine, quinidine, succinylcholine and inhalation anesthetics (for continuous infusion, reduce infusion by 30%–50% at 45–60 min after intubating dose). Caffeine, calcium, carbamazepine, phenytoin, phenylephrine, azathioprine and theophylline may reduce neuromuscular blocking effects.

Use must be accompanied by adequate anesthesia or sedation. Peak effects occur in 0.5–1 min for children and in 1–3.7 min for adults. Duration of action: 30–40 min in children and 20–94 min in adults (longer in geriatrics). Recovery time in children 3 mo to 1 yr is similar to adults. In obese patients, use actual body weight for dosage calculation.

For explanation of icons, see p. 698.

## SALMETEROL

Serevent Diskus

***Beta-2-adrenergic agonist (long acting)***

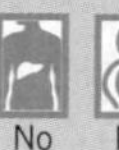 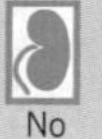  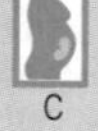

No No 2 C

**Dry powder inhalation (DPI; Diskus):** 50 mcg/inhalation (28, 60 inhalations)
In combination with fluticasone: See *Fluticasone Propionate and Salmeterol*

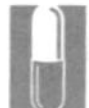

***Persistent asthma (see remarks):***

***≥4 yr and adult:*** 1 inhalation (50 mcg) Q12 hr

***Exercise-induced bronchospasm:***

***≥4 yr and adult:*** 1 inhalation 30–60 min before exercise. Additional dose should **not** be used for another 12 hr.

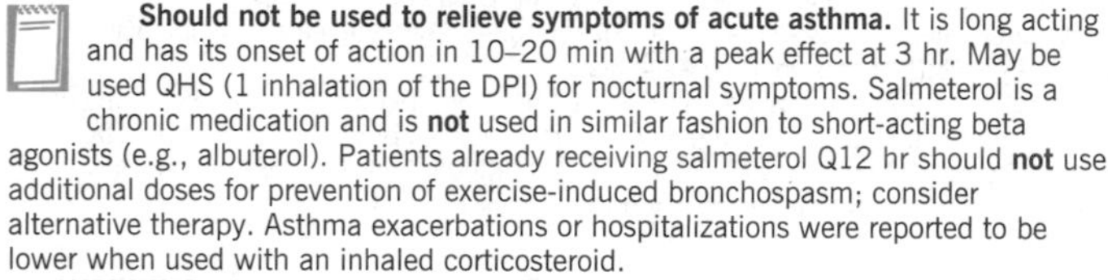

**Should not be used to relieve symptoms of acute asthma.** It is long acting and has its onset of action in 10–20 min with a peak effect at 3 hr. May be used QHS (1 inhalation of the DPI) for nocturnal symptoms. Salmeterol is a chronic medication and is **not** used in similar fashion to short-acting beta agonists (e.g., albuterol). Patients already receiving salmeterol Q12 hr should **not** use additional doses for prevention of exercise-induced bronchospasm; consider alternative therapy. Asthma exacerbations or hospitalizations were reported to be lower when used with an inhaled corticosteroid.

**WARNING: Long-acting beta-2-agonists may increase the risk of asthma-related death.** A subgroup analysis suggested higher risk in African-American patients compared to caucasions. Use salmeterol only as additional therapy for patients not adequately controlled on other asthma-controller medications (e.g., low- to medium-dose inhaled corticosteroids) or whose disease severity clearly requires initiation of treatment with 2 maintenance therapies. **Should not be used** in conjunction with an inhaled, long-acting beta-2 agonist and is **not** a substitute for inhaled or systemic corticosteroid.

Proper patient education is essential. Side effects are similar to albuterol. Hypertension and arrhythmias have been reported. See Chapter 24 for recommendations for asthma controller therapy.

## SCOPOLAMINE HYDROBROMIDE

Transderm Scop, Isopto Hyoscine, Scopace, and others

***Anticholinergic agent***

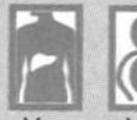 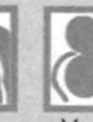 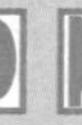 

Yes Yes 2 C

**Injection:** 0.3, 0.4, 0.86, 1 mg/mL; may contain alcohol
**Transdermal:** 1.5 mg/patch (10s and 24s); delivers ~1 mg over 3 days
**Ophthalmic solution (Isopto Hyoscine):** 0.25% (5, 15 mL); contains benzalkonium chloride
**Tabs, soluble (Scopace):** 0.4 mg

***Antiemetic (SC/IM/IV):***
***Child:*** 6 mcg/kg/dose Q6–8 hr PRN; **max. dose:** 300 mcg/dose
***Adult:*** 0.32–0.65 mg/dose Q6–8 hr PRN
***Transdermal (≥ 12 yr) (see remarks):***
***Motion sickness:*** Apply patch behind the ear at least 4 hr prior to exposure to motion; remove after 72 hr.
***Antiemetic prior to surgery:*** Apply patch behind the ear on the evening before surgery.

*Continued*

SCOPOLAMINE HYDROBROMIDE *continued*

***Antiemetic prior to cesarean section:*** Apply patch behind the ear 1 hr prior to minimize infant exposure.

***Ophthalmic:***

***Child refraction:*** 1 drop BID for 2 days before procedure

***Child iridocyclitis:*** 1 drop up to TID

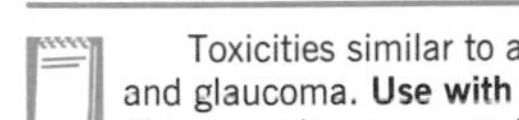

Toxicities similar to atropine. **Contraindicated** in urinary or GI obstruction and glaucoma. **Use with caution** in hepatic or renal dysfunction, cardiac disease, seizures or psychoses. May cause dry mouth, drowsiness, and blurred vision.

Transdermal route should **NOT** be used in children <12 yr. Drug withdrawal symptoms (nausea, vomiting, headache and vertigo) have been reported following removal of transdermal patch in patients using the patch for > 3 days. For perioperative use, the patch should be kept in place for 24 hr following surgery. Systemic effects have been reported with both transdermal and ophthalmic preparations. Compress nasolacrimal ducts to minimize systemic effects when using ophthalmic preparations.

## SELENIUM SULFIDE

Selsun and others

***Topical antiseborrheic agent***

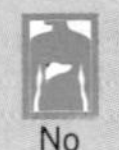 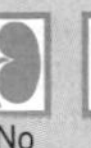 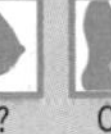 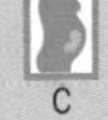

No No ? C

**Lotion/Shampoo:** 1% [OTC] (210, 325, 400 mL)

**Lotion:** 2.5% (120 mL)

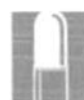

***Seborrhea/Dandruff:*** Massage 5–10 mL of 1% or 2.5% into wet scalp and leave on scalp × 2–3 min. Rinse thoroughly and repeat. Shampoo twice weekly × 2 wk. Maintenance applications once every 1–4 wk.

***Tinea versicolor:*** Apply 2.5% lotion to affected areas of skin. Allow to remain on skin × 30 min. Rinse thoroughly. Repeat QD × 7 days. Follow with monthly applications for 3 mo to prevent recurrences.

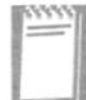

Rinse hands and body well after treatment. May cause local irritation, hair loss, and hair discoloration. **Avoid** eyes, genital areas and skin folds. Shampoo may be used for tinea capitis to reduce risk of transmission to others (does **not** eradicate tinea infection).

For tinea versicolor, 15%–25% sodium hyposulfite or thiosulfate (Tinver lotion) applied to affected areas BID × 2–4 wk is an alternative. Topical antifungals (e.g., clotrimazole, miconazole) may be used for small, focal infections. **Do not use** for tinea versicolor during pregnancy.

## SENNA/SENNOSIDES

Senokot, Senna-Gen, Lax-Pills, Fletcher's Castoria, and many others

***Laxative, stimulant***

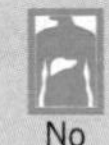 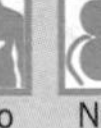 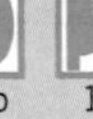 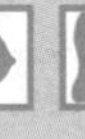

No No 1 C

**Based on mg of senna (all products are OTC):**

Granules: 326 mg/tsp

Syrup: 176 mg/5 mL, 218 mg/5 mL (60 mL, 240 mL)

Tabs: 187, 217, 374 mg

*Continued*

For explanation of icons, see p. 698.

SENNA/SENNOSIDES *continued*

**Based on mg of senna (cont'd):**
Liquid concentrate (Fletcher's Castoria): 33.3 mg/mL (75 mL); contains sodium benzoate
187 mg senna extract is approximately 8.6 mg sennosides.
**Based on mg of sennosides (all products are OTC):**
Granules: 15 mg/tsp, 20 mg /tsp
Syrup: 8.8 mg/5 mL (60 mL, 240 mL)
Tabs: 6, 8.6, 15, 17, 25 mg
Chewable tabs: 10, 15 mg
8.6 mg sennosides is approximately 187 mg senna extract.

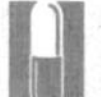

***Dosing based on mg senna:***
***Child:***
***Oral:*** 10–20 mg/kg/dose PO QHS (**max. dose:** as shown here) or dosage by age:
***1 mo–1 yr:*** 55–109 mg PO QHS to **max. dose:** 218 mg/24 hr
***1–5 yr:*** 109–218 mg PO QHS to **max. dose:** 436 mg/24 hr
***5–15 yr:*** 218–436 mg PO QHS to **max. dose:** 872 mg/24 hr
***Adult:***
***Granules:*** 326 mg (1 tsp) PO at bedtime; **max. dose:** 652 mg (2 tsp) BID
***Syrup:*** 436–654 mg PO at bedtime; **max. dose:** 654 mg (15 mL) BID
***Tabs:*** 374 mg PO at bedtime; **max. dose:** 748 mg BID
***Dosing based on mg sennosides:***
***Child:***
***Syrup:***
***1 mo–2 yr:*** 2.2–4.4 mg PO QHS to **max. dose:** 8.8 mg/24 hr
***2–5 yr:*** 4.4–6.6 mg PO QHS to **max. dose:** 6.6 mg BID
***6–12 yr:*** 8.8–13.2 mg PO QHS to **max. dose:** 13.2 mg BID
***Tabs:***
***2–5 yr:*** 4.3 mg PO QHS to **max. dose:** 8.6 mg BID
***6–12 yr:*** 8.6 mg PO QHS to **max. dose:** 17.2 mg BID
***>12 yr and adult:***
***Granules:*** 15 mg PO QHS to **max. dose:** 30 mg BID
***Syrup:*** 17.6–26.4 mg PO QHS to **max. dose:** 26.4 mg BID
***Tabs:*** 17.2 mg PO QHS to **max. dose:** 34.4 mg BID

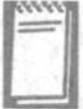

Effects occur within 6–24 hr after oral administration. May cause nausea, vomiting, diarrhea, abdominal cramps. Active metabolite stimulates Auerbach's plexus. Syrup may be administered with juice, milk, or mixed with ice cream. Granules may be sprinkled onto food or mixed with drinks.

## SERTRALINE HCL

Zoloft and many generics
***Antidepressant (selective serotonin reuptake inhibitor)***

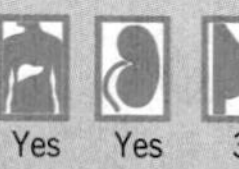
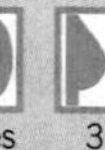
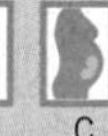

Yes Yes 3 C

**Tabs:** 25, 50, 100 mg
**Oral concentrate solution:** 20 mg/mL (60 mL); contains alcohol and menthol

*Continued*

SERTRALINE HCL *continued*

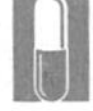

***Depression:***
***Child ≥ 6–12 yr (data limited in this age group):*** Start at 12.5–25 mg PO QD. May increase dosage by 25 mg at 1-wk intervals up to a **max. dose** of 200 mg/24 hr.
***Child ≥ 13 yr and adult:*** Start at 50 mg PO QD. May increase dosage by 50 mg at 1-wk intervals up to a **max. dose** of 200 mg/24 hr.
***Obsessive compulsive disorder:***
***Child ≥ 6–12 yr:*** Start at 25 mg PO QD. May increase dosage by 25 mg at 3–4 day intervals or by 50 mg at 7-day intervals up to a **max. dose** of 200 mg/24 hr.
***Child ≥ 13 yr and adult:*** Start at 50 mg PO QD. May increase dosage by 50 mg at 1-wk intervals up to **max. dose** of 200 mg/24 hr.

This drug should **NOT** be used in combination with an MAO inhibitor (or within 14 days of discontinuing an MAO inhibitor) or pimozide. **Use with caution** in patients with hepatic or renal impairment. Adverse effects include nausea, diarrhea, tremor and increased sweating. Hyponatremia and platelet dysfunction have been reported. Monitor for clinical worsening of depression and suicidal ideation/behavior following the initiation of therapy or after dose changes.

Use with drugs that interfere with hemostasis (e.g., NSAIDs, aspirin, and warfarin) may increase risk for GI bleeds. Use with warfarin may increase PT. Inhibits the CYP 450 2D6 drug metabolizing enzyme. Serotonin syndrome may occur when taken with selective serotonin reuptake inhibitors (e.g., amitriptyline, amphetamines, buspirone, dihydroergotamine, sumatriptan, sympathomimetics).

Mix oral concentrate solution with 4 oz. of water, ginger ale, lemon/lime soda, lemonade or orange juice. After mixing, a slight haze may appear; this is normal. This dosage form should be **used cautiously** in patients with latex allergy because the dropper contains dry natural rubber.

## SILDENAFIL

Revatio, Viagra
***Phosphodiesterase type 5 (PDE5) inhibitor***

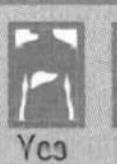
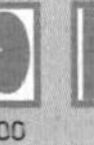
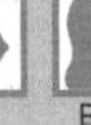
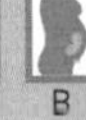

Yes Yes ? B

**Tabs:**
**Revatio:** 20 mg
**Viagra:** 25, 50, 100 mg
**Oral suspension:** 2.5 mg/mL

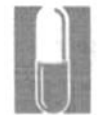

***Pulmonary hypertension (limited data from case reports and small clinical trials):***
***Neonate:*** Several dosages have been reported and have ranged from 0.3–1 mg/kg/dose Q6–12 hr PO. A single 3 mg/kg/dose PO has been used in select patients to facilitate weaning from inhaled nitric oxide.
***Infant and child:*** Several dosages have been reported. Start at 0.25–0.5 mg/kg/dose Q4–8 hr PO; if needed and tolerated, increase to 1 mg/kg/dose Q4–8 hr PO. Doses as high as 2 mg/kg/dose Q4 hr PO have been given in case reports.

**Contraindicated** with concurrent use of nitrates (e.g., nitroglycerin) and other nitric oxide donors; potentiates hypotensive effects. **Use with caution** in sepsis (high levels of cGMP may potentiate hypotension), and with concurrent CYP 450 3A4 inhibiting medications (see discussion that follows) and anti-hypertensive medications. Hepatic insufficiency or severe renal impairment (GFR < 30 mL/min) significantly reduces sildenafil clearance.

*Continued*

For explanation of icons, see p. 698.

SILDENAFIL *continued*

In adults, a transient impairment of color discrimination may occur; this effect could increase risk of severe retinopathy of prematurity in neonates. Common side effects reported in adults have included flushing, rash, diarrhea, indigestion, headache, abnormal vision and nasal congestion.

Sildenafil is substrate for CYP 450 3A4 (major) and 2C8/9 (minor). Azole antifungals, cimetidine, ciprofloxacin, clarithromycin, erythromycin, nicardipine, propofol, protease inhibitors, quinidine, verapamil, and grapefruit juice may increase the effects/toxicity of sildenafil. Bosentin, efavirenz, carbamazepine, phenobarbital, phenytoin, rifampin, St. John's wort, and high-fat meals decrease sildenafil effects.

## SILVER SULFADIAZINE

Silvadene, Thermazene, SSD Cream, SSD AF Cream

***Topical antibiotic***

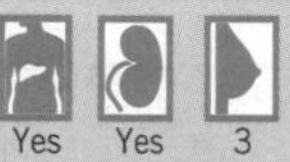


**Cream:** 1% (20, 25, 50, 85, 400, 1000 g); contains methylparabens

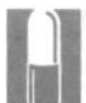

Cover affected areas completely QD–BID. Apply cream to a thickness of 1⁄16 inch using sterile technique.

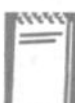

**Contraindicated** in premature infants and infants ≤2 mo of age due to concerns of kernicterus and in pregnancy (approaching term). **Use with caution** in G6PD and renal and hepatic impairment. Discard product if cream has darkened. Significant systemic absorption may occur in severe burns. Adverse effects include pruritus, rash, bone marrow suppression, hemolytic anemia, and interstitial nephritis. **NOT** for ophthalmic use. See Chapter 4 for more information.

## SIMETHICONE

Mylicon, Phazyme, Mylanta Gas, Gas-X, and others

***Antiflatulent***

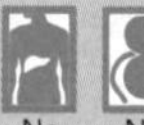
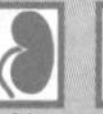
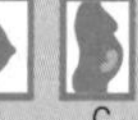
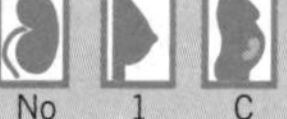


All dosage forms available OTC.
**Oral drops:** 40 mg/0.6 mL (30 mL)
**Caps:** 125, 180 mg
**Tabs:** 60, 95 mg
**Chewable tabs:** 80, 125 mg
**Strip, orally disintegrating:** 62.5 mg (18s)

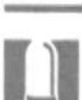

***Infant and child < 2 yr:*** 20 mg PO QID PRN; **max. dose:** 240 mg/24 hr
***2–12 yr:*** 40 mg PO QID PRN
***>12 yr and adult:*** 40–125 mg PO QPC and QHS PRN; **max. dose:** 500 mg/24 hr

Efficacy has not been demonstrated for treating infant colic. **Avoid** carbonated beverages and gas-forming foods. Oral liquid may be mixed with water, infant formula, or other suitable liquids for ease of oral administration.

## SIROLIMUS

Rapamune

***Immunosuppressant agent***

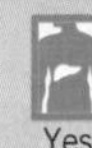
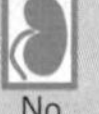
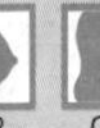
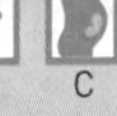

Yes No 3 C

**Tabs:** 1, 2 mg
**Oral solution:** 1 mg/mL (60 mL); contains 1.5%–2.5% ethanol

***Child ≥ 13 yr and < 40 kg:*** 3 mg/m²/dose PO × 1 immediately after transplantation, followed by 1 mg/m²/24 hr PO ÷ Q12–24 hr on the next day. Adjust dose to achieve desired trough blood levels.

***Adult:***

***Patients at low/moderate immunologic risk:***

***In combination with cyclosporine:*** 6 mg PO × 1 immediately after transplantation, followed by 2 mg PO QD on the next day. Adjust dose to achieve desired trough blood levels.

***Patients at high immunologic risk:***

***In combination with cyclosporine:*** 15 mg PO × 1 immediately after transplantation, followed by 5 mg PO QD on the next day. Adjust dose to achieve desired trough blood levels.

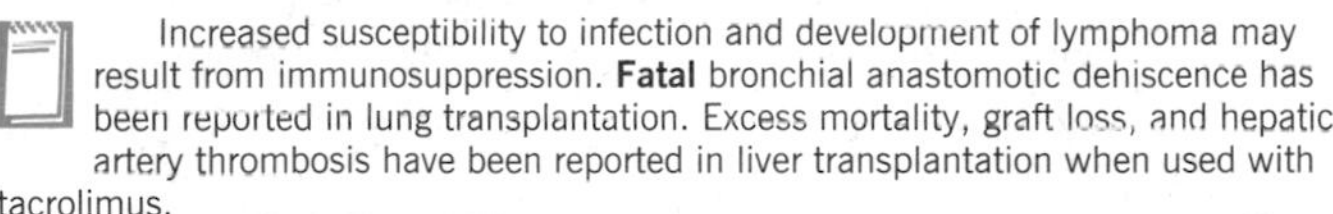

Increased susceptibility to infection and development of lymphoma may result from immunosuppression. **Fatal** bronchial anastomotic dehiscence has been reported in lung transplantation. Excess mortality, graft loss, and hepatic artery thrombosis have been reported in liver transplantation when used with tacrolimus.

Monitor whole blood trough levels (just prior to a dose at steady-state); especially with pediatric patients; hepatic impairment; concurrent use of CYP 450 3A4 and/or P-gp inducers and inhibitors; and/or if cyclosporine dosage is markedly changed or discontinued. Steady state is generally achieved after 5–7 days of continuous dosing. Interpretation will vary based on treatment protocol and assay methodology (HPLC vs. immunoassay vs. LC/MS/MS). Younger children may exhibit faster sirolimus clearance compared to adolescents.

Sirolimus is a substrate for CYP 450 3A4 and P-gp. Cyclosporine, diltiazem, protease inhibitors, erythromycin, grapefruit juice and other inhibitors of CYP 3A4 may increase the toxicity of sirolimus. Phenobarbital, carbamazepine, phenytoin, and St. John's wort may decrease the effects of sirolimus. Strong inhibitors (e.g., azole antifungals and clarithromycin) and strong inducers (e.g., rifamycins) are **not recommended**.

Hypertension, peripheral edema, increased serum creatinine, dyspnea, epistaxis, headache, anemia, thrombocytopenia, hyperlipidemia, hypercholesterolemia, and arthralgia may occur. Urinary tract infections have been reported in pediatric renal transplant patients with high immunologic risk.

2 mg of the oral solution has been demonstrated to be clinically equivalent to the 2 mg tablets. However, it is not known whether they are still therapeutically equivalent at higher doses. Reduce maintenance dosage by ⅓ in the presence of hepatic function impairment. Administer doses consistently with or without food. When administered with cyclosporine, give dose 4 hr after cyclosporine. **Do not** crush or split tablets. Measure the oral liquid dosage form with an amber oral syringe and dilute in a cup with 60 mL of water or orange juice only. Take dose immediately after mixing, add/mix additional 120 mL diluent into the cup, and drink immediately after mixing.

For explanation of icons, see p. 698.

## SODIUM BICARBONATE

Neut and many other generics

***Alkalinizing agent, electrolyte***

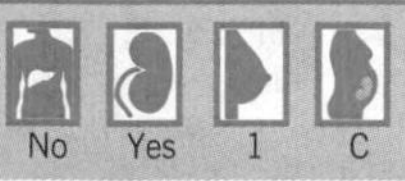


**Injection:** 4% (Neut) (0.48 mEq/mL) (5 mL), 4.2% (0.5 mEq/mL) (10 mL), 7.5% (0.89 mEq/mL) (50 mL), 8.4% (1 mEq/mL) (10, 50 mL)
**Injection, pre-mixed:** 5% (0.6 mEq/mL) (500 mL)
**Tabs:** 325 mg (3.8 mEq), 650 mg (7.6 mEq)
**Powder:** 120, 480 g; contains 30 mEq $Na^+$ per 1/2 teaspoon
Each 1 mEq bicarbonate provides 1 mEq $Na^+$.

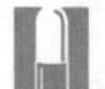

***Cardiac arrest:*** See inside front cover.
***Correction of metabolic acidosis:*** Calculate patient's dose with the following formulas.

***Neonate, infant and child:***

$HCO_3^-$ (mEq) = 0.3 × weight (kg) × base deficit (mEq/L), **OR**
$HCO_3^-$ (mEq) = 0.5 × weight (kg) × [24 – serum $HCO_3^-$ (mEq/L)]

***Adult:***

$HCO_3^-$ (mEq) = 0.2 × weight (kg) × base deficit (mEq/L), **OR**
$HCO_3^-$ (mEq) = 0.5 × weight (kg) × [24 – serum $HCO_3^-$ (mEq/L)]

***Urinary alkalinization (titrate dose accordingly to urine pH):***

***Child:*** 84–840 mg (1–10 mEq)/kg/24 hr PO ÷ QID
***Adult:*** 4 g (48 mEq) × 1 followed by 1–2 g (12–24 mEq) PO Q4 hr. Doses up to 16 g (192 mEq)/24 hr have been used.

**Contraindicated** in respiratory alkalosis, hypochloremia and inadequate ventilation during cardiac arrest. **Use with caution** in CHF, renal impairment, cirrhosis, hypocalcemia, hypertension and concurrent corticosteroids. Maintain high urine output. Monitor acid-base balance and serum electrolytes. May cause hypernatremia (contains sodium), hypokalemia, hypomagnesemia, hypocalcemia, hyperreflexia, edema and tissue necrosis (extravasation). Oral route of administration may cause GI discomfort and gastric rupture from gas production.

For direct IV administration (cardiac arrest) in neonates and infants, use the 0.5 mEq/mL (4.2%) concentration or dilute the 1 mEq/mL (8.4%) concentration 1:1 with sterile water for injection and infuse at a rate **no greater than** 10 mEq/min. The 1 mEq/mL (8.4%) concentration may be used in children and adults for direct IV administration.

For IV infusions (for all ages), dilute to a **max. concentration** of 0.5 mEq/mL in dextrose or sterile water for injection and infuse over 2 hr using a **max. rate** of 1 mEq/kg/hr.

Sodium bicarbonate should **not** be mixed with or be in contact with calcium, norepinephrine, or dobutamine.

## SODIUM PHOSPHATE

Fleet, Fleet Phospho-Soda, Visicol, OsmoPrep, and others

***Laxative, enema/oral***

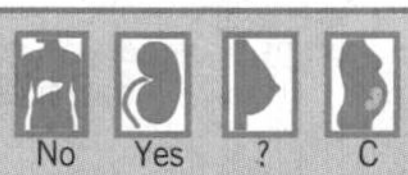


**Enema (Fleet) [OTC]:** 7 g dibasic sodium phosphate and 19 g monobasic sodium phosphate/118 mL; contains 4.4 g sodium per 118 mL

**Pediatric size:** 66 mL
**Adult size:** 133 mL

*Continued*

SODIUM PHOSPHATE *continued*

**Oral solution (Fleet Phospho-Soda) [OTC]:** 2.4 g monobasic sodium phosphate and 0.9 g dibasic sodium phosphate/5 mL (45, 90, 240 mL); contains 96.4 mEq Na per 20 mL and 62.25 mEq phospate/5 mL
**Oral tablets (Visicol, OsmoPrep):** 1.5 g

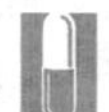

**Not to be used for phosphorus supplementation.** See *Phosphorus Supplements.*
***Enema:***
***2–12 yr:*** 66 mL enema × 1. May repeat × 1.
***>12 yr and adult:*** 133 mL enema × 1. May repeat × 1.
***Oral laxative (Fleet Phospho-Soda); mix with equal volume of water:***
***5–9 yr:*** 5 mL PO × 1
***10–12 yr:*** 10 mL PO × 1
***≥12 yr:*** 20–30 mL PO × 1

**Contraindicated** in patients with severe renal failure, megacolon, bowel obstruction and congestive heart failure. May cause hyperphosphatemia, hypernatremia, hypocalcemia, hypotension, dehydration, and acidosis. **Avoid** retention of enema solution and **do not exceed** recommended doses, as this may lead to severe electrolyte disturbances due to enhanced systemic absorption. Rare but serious form of kidney failure has been reported with the use of Fleet Phospho-Soda and Visicol.

Onset of action: PO, 3–6 hr; PR, 2–5 min.

## SODIUM POLYSTYRENE SULFONATE

Kayexalate, SPS, Kionex, and others
***Potassium-removing resin***

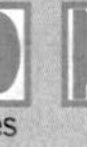
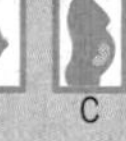
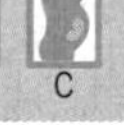

No Yes 2 C

**Powder:** 454, 480 g
**Suspension:** 15 g/60 mL (60, 120, 200, 500 mL); contains 21.5 mL sorbitol per 60 mL and 0.1%–0.3% alcohol
Contains 4.1 mEq $Na^+$/g drug

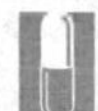

***Child:***
***Usual dose:*** 1 g/kg/dose Q6 hr PO or Q2–6 hr PR
***Adult:***
***PO:*** 15 g QD–QID
***PR:*** 30–50 g Q6 hr

**Note:** Suspension may be given PO or PR. Practical exchange ratio is 1 mEq K per 1 g resin. May calculate dose according to desired exchange.

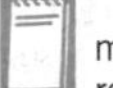

**Contraindicated** in obstructive bowel disease, neonates with reduced gut motility, and oral administration in neonates. **Use cautiously** in presence of renal failure, CHF, hypertension or severe edema. May cause hypokalemia, hypernatremia, hypomagnesemia and hypocalcemia.

1 mEq Na delivered for each mEq K removed. **Do not administer** with antacids or laxatives containing $Mg^{2+}$ or $Al^{3+}$. Systemic alkalosis may result. Retain enema in colon for at least 30–60 min.

For explanation of icons, see p. 698.

## SPIRONOLACTONE

Aldactone and others

***Diuretic, potassium sparing***

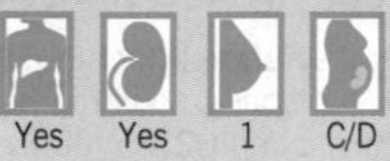


**Tabs:** 25, 50, 100 mg
**Oral suspension:** 1, 2, 2.5, 5, 25 mg/mL

***Diuretic:***
***Neonate:*** 1–3 mg/kg/24 hr ÷ QD–BID PO
***Child:*** 1–3.3 mg/kg/24 hr ÷ QD–QID PO
***Adult:*** 25–200 mg/24 hr ÷ QD–QID PO (see remarks)
**Max. dose:** 200 mg/24 hr

***Diagnosis of primary aldosteronism:***
***Child:*** 125–375 mg/m²/24 hr ÷ BID–QID PO
***Adult:*** 400 mg QD PO × 4 days (short test) or 3–4 wk (long test), then 100–400 mg QD maintenance.

***Hirsutism in women:***
***Adult:*** 50–200 mg/24 hr ÷ QD–BID PO

**Contraindicated in severe renal failure (see Chapter 31). Use with caution** in dehydration, hyponatremia, and renal or hepatic dysfunction. May cause hyperkalemia, GI distress, rash and gynecomastia. May potentiate ganglionic blocking agents and other antihypertensives. Monitor potassium levels and be aware of other $K^+$ sources, $K^+$ sparing diuretics and angiotensin-converting enzyme inhibitors (all can increase $K^+$). May cause false elevation in serum digoxin levels measured by radioimmunoassay.

Although TID–QID regimens have been recommended, data suggests QD–BID dosing to be adequate. Pregnancy category changes to "D" if used in pregnancy-induced hypertension.

## STREPTOKINASE

Streptase

***Thrombolytic enzyme***

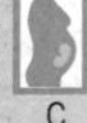
No No ? C

**Injection:** 250,000; 750,000; 1,500,000 IU; contains gelatin polypeptides, sodium L-glutamate, and albumin

***Thrombolytic:*** **Should be used in consultation with a hematologist.** Duration of therapy will depend on clinical response and generally does not exceed 3 days.
***Child:*** 2000 U/kg load IV over 30 min followed by 2000 U/kg/hr for 6–12 hr. Alternatively, 3500–4000 U/kg over 30 min, followed by 1000–1500 U/kg/hr has been used. Duration of infusion is individualized based on response.

Pediatric safety and efficacy information is limited. **Contraindicated** with intracranial or intraspinal surgery, history of internal bleeding, recent streptococcal infection or CVA within previous 2 mo. May cause hemorrhage, urticaria, itching, flushing, musculoskeletal pain, bronchospasm and anaphylaxis. Monitor fibrinogen, thrombin clotting time, PT, and aPTT when used as a thrombolytic.

Newborns have reduced plasminogen levels (~50% of adult values) which decrease the thrombolytic effects of streptokinase. Plasminogen supplementation may be necessary.

*Continued*

STREPTOKINASE *continued*

**Not recommended** in restoring patency of intravenous catheters. Hypotension, hypersensitivity reactions, apnea, and bleeding, some of which were life threatening, have been reported when used in this manner.

## STREPTOMYCIN SULFATE

Various

***Antibiotic, aminoglycoside; antituberculous agent***

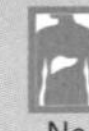 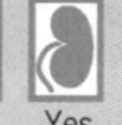 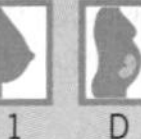 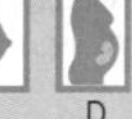

No Yes 1 D

**Injection:** 400 mg/mL (2.5 mL)
**Powder for injection:** 1 g

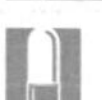

***Tuberculosis:*** Use as part of multidrug regimen; see latest edition of AAP *Red Book*

***Infant, child, and adolescent:***

***Daily therapy:*** 20–40 mg/kg/24 hr IM QD

**Max. daily dose:** 1 g/24 hr

***Twice weekly therapy:*** 20–40 mg/kg/dose IM twice weekly

**Max. daily dose:** 1.5 g/24 hr

***Adult:***

***Daily therapy:*** 15 mg/kg/24 hr IM QD

**Max. daily dose:** 1 g/24 hr

***Twice weekly therapy:*** 25–30 mg/kg/dose IM twice weekly

**Max. daily dose:** 1.5 g/24 hr

***Brucellosis, tularemia, plague, and rat bite fever:*** See latest edition of the *Red Book*.

**Contraindicated** with aminoglycoside and sulfite hypersensitivity. **Use with caution** in pre-existing vertigo, tinnitus, hearing loss and neuromuscular disorders. Drug is administered via deep IM injection only. Follow auditory status. May cause CNS depression, other neurologic problems, myocarditis, serum sickness, nephrotoxicity, and ototoxicity. Concomitant neurotoxic, ototoxic, or nephrotoxic drugs and dehydration may increase risk for toxicity.

Therapeutic levels: peak 15–40 mg/L; trough: <5 mg/L. Recommended serum sampling time at steady-state: trough within 30 min prior to the third consecutive dose and peak 30–60 min after the administration of the third consecutive dose. Therapeutic levels are **not** achieved in CSF.

**Adjust dose in renal failure (see Chapter 31).**

## SUCCIMER

Chemet, DMSA [dimercaptosuccinic acid]

***Chelating agent***

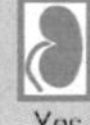 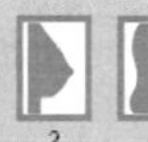 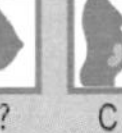

Yes Yes ? C

**Caps:** 100 mg

***Lead chelation, child:***

10 mg/kg/dose (or 350 mg/m$^2$/dose) PO Q8 hr × 5 days, then 10 mg/kg/dose (or 350 mg/m$^2$/dose) PO Q12 hr × 14 days.

*Manufacturer recommends (see following table):*

*Continued*



For explanation of icons, see p. 698.

SUCCIMER *continued*

| Weight (kg) | Dose (mg) |
|---|---|
| 8–15 | 100 |
| 16–23 | 200 |
| 24–34 | 300 |
| 35–44 | 400 |
| ≥45 | 500 |

Give aforementioned dose every 8 hr for 5 days. Then give the same dose Q12 hr for an additional 14 days.

**Use caution** in patients with compromised renal or hepatic function. Repeated courses may be necessary. Follow serum lead levels. Allow minimum of 2 wk between courses, unless blood levels require more aggressive management. Side effects: GI symptoms, increased LFTs (10%), rash, headaches, and dizziness. **Coadministration with other chelating agents is not recommended**. Treatment of iron deficiency is recommended as well as environmental remediation. Contents of capsule may be sprinkled on food for those who are unable to swallow capsule.

## SUCCINYLCHOLINE

Anectine and Quelicin

***Neuromuscular blocking agent***

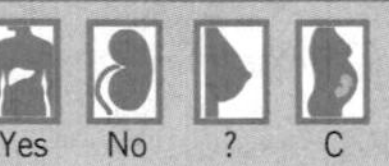


**Injection:** 20 mg/mL (5, 10 mL), 50 mg/mL (10 mL), 100 mg/mL (5, 10 mL); may contain parabens and/or benzyl alcohol
**Powder for infusion:** 500, 1000 mg

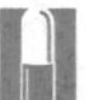

***Paralysis for intubation (see remarks):***
***Infant and Child:***
***Initial:***
***IV:*** 1–2 mg/kg/dose × 1
***IM:*** 2.5–4 mg/kg/dose × 1
**Max dose:** 150 mg/dose
***Maintenance:*** 0.3–0.6 mg/kg/dose IV Q5–10 min PRN. **Continuous infusion not recommended** due to risk of malignant hyperthermia.
***Adult:***
***Initial:***
***IV:*** 0.3–1.1 mg/kg/dose × 1
***IM:*** 2.5–4 mg/kg/dose × 1
**Max dose:** 150 mg/dose
***Maintenance:*** 0.04–0.07 mg/kg/dose IV Q5–10 min PRN. **Continuous infusion not recommended**.

Pretreatment with atropine is recommended to reduce incidence of bradycardia. For rapid sequence intubation, see Chapter 1.

**Contraindicated** after the acute phase of an injury following major burns, multiple trauma, extensive denervation of skeletal muscle, or upper motor neuron injury because severe hyperkalemia and subsequent **cardiac arrest** may occur.

**Cardiac arrest** has been reported in children and adolescents primarily with skeletal muscle myopathies (e.g., Duchenne's muscular dystrophy). Identify developmental delays suggestive of a myopathy prior to use. Pre-dose creatine kinase

*Continued*

SUCCINYLCHOLINE *continued*

may be useful for identifying patients at risk. Monitoring of ECG for peaked T-waves may be useful in detecting early signs of this adverse effect.

May cause malignant hyperthermia (use dantrolene to treat), bradycardia, hypotension, arrhythmia, and hyperkalemia. **Use with caution** in patients with severe burns, paraplegia or crush injuries and in patients with preexisting hyperkalemia. Beware of prolonged depression in patients with liver disease, malnutrition, pseudocholinesterase deficiency, hypothermia and those receiving aminoglycosides, phenothiazines, quinidine, beta-blockers, amphotericin B, cyclophosphamide, diuretics, lithium, acetylcholine, and anticholinesterases. Diazepam may decrease neuromuscular blocking effects. Prior use of succinylcholine may enhance the neuromuscular blocking effect of vecuronium and its duration of action. Duration of action 4–6 min IV, 10–30 min IM. Must be prepared to intubate within 1 min.

## SUCRALFATE

Carafate and many other generics

***Oral anti-ulcer agent***

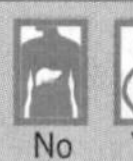
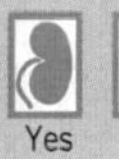
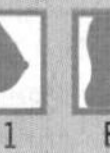
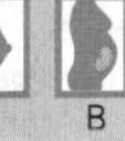

No Yes 1 B

**Tabs:** 1 g
**Suspension:** 100 mg/mL (420 mL); contains sorbitol and parabens

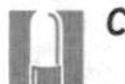

***Child:***

***Duodenal or gastric ulcer:*** 40–80 mg/kg/24 hr ÷ Q6 hr PO
***Stomatitis:*** 5–10 mL (500–1000 mg of suspension) swish and spit or swish and swallow QID

***Adult:***

***Duodenal ulcer:***
***Treatment:*** 1 g PO QID 1 hr before meals and QHS or 2 g PO BID × 4–8 wk
***Maintenance/prophylaxis:*** 1 g PO BID

***Stress ulcer:***
***Treatment:*** 1 g PO Q4 hr
***Prophylaxis:*** 1 g PO QID

***Stomatitis:*** 10 mL (1000 mg of suspension) swish and spit or swish and swallow QID

***Proctitis (use oral suspension as rectal enema):*** 20 mL (2 g) PR QD–BID

May cause vertigo, constipation and dry mouth. Aluminum may accumulate in patients with renal failure. This may be augmented by the use of aluminum-containing antacids. Decreases absorption of phenytoin, digoxin, theophylline, cimetidine, fat-soluble vitamins, ketoconazole, omeprazole, quinolones and oral anticoagulants. Administer these drugs at least 2 hr before or after sucralfate doses.

Drug requires an acidic environment to form a protective polymer coating for damaged GI tract mucosa. Administer oral doses on an empty stomach (1 hr before meals and QHS).

For explanation of icons, see p. 698.

## SULFACETAMIDE SODIUM OPHTHALMIC

AK-Sulf, Bleph 10, Ocusulf-10, and various generic products

***Ophthalmic antibiotic, sulfonamide derivative***

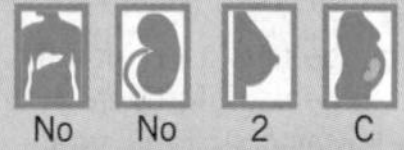


**Ophthalmic solution:** 10% (2, 2.5, 5, 15 mL); may contain methylparaben and propylparaben
**Ophthalmic ointment:** 10% (3.5 g); may contain phenylmecuric acetate

***Ophthalmic (usual duration of therapy for ophthalmic use is 7–10 days):***
***>2 mo and adult:***
***Ointment:*** Apply ribbon QID and QHS (5× per 24 hr).
***Drops:*** 1–2 drops Q2–3 hr to affected eye(s)

See *Sulfisoxazole*. 10% solution is used most frequently. Hypersensitivity reactions between different sulfonamides can occur regardless of route of administration. May cause local irritation, stinging, burning, conjunctival hyperemia, excessive tear production and eye pain. Rare toxic epidermal necrolysis and Stevens-Johnson syndrome have been reported. Sulfacetamide preparations are incompatible with silver preparations.

## SULFADIAZINE

Various trade names

***Antibiotic, sulfonamide derivative***

Yes Yes 2 C/D

**Tabs:** 500 mg
**Oral suspension:** 100 mg/mL 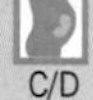

***Congenital toxoplasmosis*** (administer with pyrimethamine and folinic acid; see *Pyrimethamine* for dosage information) (from *Clin Infect Dis* 1994; 18:38):
***Infant:*** 100 mg/kg/24 hr PO ÷ BID × 12 mo
***Toxoplasmosis (administer with pyrimethamine and folinic acid):*** See *Pyrimethamine* for dosage information.
***Child:*** 100–200 mg/kg/24 hr ÷ Q6 hr PO × 3–4 wk
***Adult:*** 4–6 g/24 hr PO ÷ Q6 hr × 3–4 wk
***Rheumatic fever prophylaxis:***
***≤27 kg:*** 500 mg PO QD
***>27 kg:*** 1000 mg PO QD

Most cases of acquired toxoplasmosis do not require specific antimicrobial therapy. **Contraindicated** in porphyria and hypersensitivity to sulfonamides. **Use with caution** in premature infants and infants <2 mo because of risk of hyperbilirubinemia, and in hepatic or renal dysfunction (30%–44% eliminated in urine). Maintain hydration. May cause fever, rash, hepatitis, SLE-like syndrome, vasculitis, bone marrow suppression, and hemolysis in patients with G6PD deficiency, and Stevens-Johnson syndrome.

May cause increased effects of warfarin, methotrexate, thiazide diuretics, uricosuric agents, and sulfonylureas due to drug displacement from protein binding sites. Large quantities of vitamin C or acidifying agents (e.g., cranberry juice) may cause crystalluria. Pregnancy category changes from "C" to "D" if administered near term. Administer on an empty stomach with plenty of water.

## SULFAMETHOXAZOLE AND TRIMETHOPRIM

Trimethoprim-sulfamethoxazole, Co-Trimoxazole, TMP-SMX; Bactrim, Septra, Sulfatrim, and others

***Antibiotic, sulfonamide derivative***

Yes Yes 1 C/D

**Tabs (regular strength):** 80 mg TMP/400 mg SMX
**Tabs (double strength):** 160 mg TMP/800 mg SMX
**Suspension:** 40 mg TMP/200 mg SMX per 5 mL (20, 100, 150, 200, 480 mL)
**Injection:** 16 mg TMP/mL and 80 mg SMX/mL (5, 10, 20, 30 mL); some preparations may contain propylene glycol and benzyl alcohol

***Doses based on TMP component.***
***Minor/moderate infections (PO or IV):***
***Child:*** 8–12 mg/kg/24 hr ÷ BID
***Adult (>40 kg):*** 160 mg/dose BID
***Severe infections (PO or IV):***
***Child and adult:*** 20 mg/kg/24 hr ÷ Q6–8 hr
***UTI prophylaxis:***
***Child:*** 2–4 mg/kg/24 hr PO QD
***Pneumocystic jiroveci (formerly carinii) pneumonia (PCP):***
***Treatment (PO/IV):*** 20 mg/kg/24 hr ÷ Q6–8 hr
***Prophylaxis (PO or IV):***
***≥1 mo and child:*** 5–10 mg/kg/24 hr ÷ BID or 150 mg/m$^2$/24 hr ÷ BID for 3 consecutive days/wk; **max. dose:** 320 mg/24 hr
***Adult:*** 80–160 mg QD or 160 mg 3 days/wk

**Not recommended** for use with infants <2 mo (excluding PCP prophylaxis). **Contraindicated** in patients with sulfonamide or trimethoprim hypersensitivity, and megaloblastic anemia due to folate deficiency. May cause kernicterus in newborns; may cause blood dyscrasias, crystalluria, glossitis, renal or hepatic injury, GI irritation, rash, Stevens-Johnson syndrome, hemolysis in patients with G6PD deficiency. Hyperkalemia may appear in HIV/AIDS patients. **Do not use drug at term during pregnancy.** Pregnancy risk factor changes to "D" if administered near term. **Use with caution** in renal and hepatic impairment, and G6PD deficiency.

**Reduce dose in renal impairment (see Chapter 31).** See Chapter 17 for PCP prophylaxis guidelines.

## SULFASALAZINE

Salicylazosulfapyridine, SAS, Azulfidine, Azulfidine EN-tabs, and others

***Anti-inflammatory agent***

No Yes 2 B/D

**Tabs:** 500 mg
**Enteric-coated tabs (Azulfidine EN-tabs):** 500 mg

***Ulcerative colitis:***
***Child ≥ 6 yr:***
***Initial dosing:***
***Mild:*** 40–50 mg/kg/24 hr ÷ Q6 hr PO
***Moderate/severe:*** 50–75 mg/kg/24 hr ÷ Q4–6 hr PO; **max. dose:** 6 g/24 hr
***Maintenance:*** 30–50 mg/kg/24 hr ÷ Q4–8 hr PO; **max. dose:** 2 g/24 hr

*Continued*



For explanation of icons, see p. 698.

SULFASALAZINE *continued*

***Ulcerative colitis (cont'd):***

***Adult:***

***Initial:*** 3–4 g/24 hr ÷ Q4–6 hr PO
***Maintenance:*** 2 g/24 hr ÷ Q6–12 hr PO
**Max. dose:** 6 g/24 hr

***Juvenile rheumatoid arthritis:***

***Child > 6 yr:*** Start with 10 mg/kg/24 hr ÷ BID PO and increase by 10 mg/kg/24 hr Q7 days until planned maintenance dose is achieved. Usual maintenance dose is 30–50 mg/kg/24 hr ÷ BID PO up to a **max.** of 2 g/24 hr.

---

**Contraindicated** in sulfa or salicylate hypersensitivity, porphyria and GI or GU obstruction. **Use with caution** in renal impairment, blood dyscrasias, or asthma. Maintain hydration. May cause orange-yellow discoloration of urine and skin. May permanently stain contact lenses. May cause photosensitivity, hypersensitivity, blood dyscrasias, CNS changes, nausea, vomiting, anorexia, diarrhea and renal damage. Hepatotoxicity has been reported. May cause hemolysis in patients with G6PD deficiency. Decreases folic acid absorption; and reduces serum digoxin and cyclosporine levels. Slow acetylators may require lower dosage due to accumulation of active sulfapyridine metabolite. Pregnancy category changes to "D" if administered near term.

## SULFISOXAZOLE

Gantrisin and others
***Antibiotic, sulfonamide derivative***

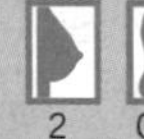
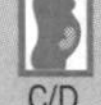

Yes Yes 2 C/D

**Tabs:** 500 mg
**Suspension:** 500 mg/5 mL (480 mL); contains 0.3% alcohol and parabens
**Ophthalmic solution:** 4% (40 mg/mL) (15 mL)
For combination product with erythromycin, see *Erythromycin Ethylsuccinate and Acetylsulfisoxazole.*

---

***Child ≥ 2 mo:*** 75 mg/kg/dose PO × 1 followed by 120–150 mg/kg/24 hr OR 4 g/m$^2$/24 hr ÷ Q4–6 hr PO; **max. dose:** 6 g/24 hr

***Otitis media prophylaxis:*** 50 mg/kg/dose QHS PO
***UTI prophylaxis:*** 10–20 mg/kg/24 hr ÷ Q12 hr

***Adult:*** 2–4 g PO × 1 followed by 4–8 g/24 hr ÷ Q4–6 hr PO

***Rheumatic fever prophylaxis:***

***<27 kg:*** 500 mg PO QD
***≥27 kg:*** 1000 mg PO QD

***Ophthalmic solution (usual duration of therapy is 7–10 days):***

***Conjunctivitis or other superficial ocular infections:*** 1–2 drops Q1–4 hr; increase the time interval between doses as the condition improves.
***Trachoma (with systemic sulfonamide therapy):*** 2 drops Q2 hr.

---

**Contraindicated** in urinary obstruction, porphyria, or near term pregnancy. **Use with caution** in infants <2 mo, in the presence of renal or liver disease, or in G6PD deficiency. Maintain adequate fluid intake. See *Sulfadiazine* for toxicities and drug interactions. Interferes with folate absorption. Usual duration of therapy for ophthalmic use is 7–10 days.

**Adjust dose in renal impairment with systemic use (see Chapter 31).** Pregnancy category changes to "D" if administered near term pregnancy. **For combination with erythromycin, see *Erythromycin Ethylsuccinate and Acetylsulfisoxazole.*** Administer oral doses on an empty stomach with plenty of water.

## SUMATRIPTAN SUCCINATE

Imitrex

***Antimigraine agent, selective serotonin agonist***

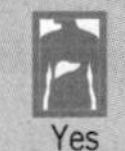 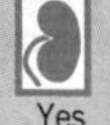 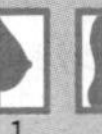

Yes Yes 1 C

**Injection:** 8, 12 mg/mL (0.5 mL)
**Tabs:** 25, 50, 100 mg
**Oral suspension:** 5 mg/mL
**Nasal spray (as a unit-dose spray device):** 5 mg dose in 100 microliters (6 units per pack); 20 mg dose in 100 microliters (6 units per pack)

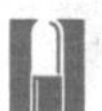

***Adolescent and adult (see remarks):***
***PO:*** 25 mg as soon as possible after onset of headache. If no relief in 2 hr, give 25–100 mg Q2 hr up to a **daily max.** of 200 mg.
**Max. single dose:** 100 mg/dose.
**Max. daily dose:** 200 mg/24 hr (with exclusive PO dosing or with an initial SC dose and subsequent PO dosing).
***SC:*** 6 mg × 1 as soon as possible after onset of headache. If no response, may give an additional dose of ≤ 6 mg 1 hr later.
**Max. daily dose:** 12 mg/24 hr.
***Nasal:*** 5–20 mg/dose into one nostril or divided into each nostril after onset of headache. Dose may be repeated in 2 hr up to a **max.** of 40 mg/24 hr.

**Contraindicated** with concomitant administration of ergotamine derivatives, MAO inhibitors (and use within the past 2 wk) or other vasoconstrictive drugs. **Not** for migraine prophylaxis. **Use with caution** in renal or hepatic impairment. A **max. single dose** of 50 mg has been recommended in adults with hepatic dysfunction. Acts as selective agonist for serotonin receptor. Induration and swelling at the injection site, flushing, dizziness, chest, jaw and neck tightness may occur with SC administration. Weakness, hyper-reflexia, incoordination, and serotonin syndrome have been reported with use in combination with selective serotonin reuptake inhibitors (e.g., fluoxetine, fluvoxamine, paroxetine, sertraline).

May cause coronary vasospasm if administered IV. **Use injectable form SC only!** Onset of action is 10–120 min SC, and 60–90 min PO. For nasal use, the safety of treating more than 4 headaches in a 30-day period has not been established.

Oral and nasal efficacy were not established in placebo-controlled trial in adolescents. Some **do not recommend** use in patients < 18 yr due to poor efficacy and reports of serious adverse events (e.g., stroke, visual loss and death) in both children and adults.

## SURFACTANT, PULMONARY/BERACTANT

Survanta

***Bovine lung surfactant***

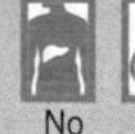 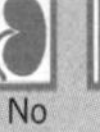 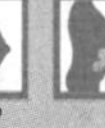 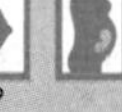

No No ?

**Suspension for inhalation:** 25 mg/mL (4, 8 mL); contains 0.5–1.75 mg triglycerides, 1.4–3.5 mg free fatty acids and < 1 mg protein/1 mL drug

***Prophylactic therapy:*** 4 mL/kg/dose intratracheally as soon as possible; up to 4 doses may be given at intervals no shorter than Q6 hr during the first 48 hr of life.
***Rescue therapy:*** 4 mL/kg/dose intratracheally, immediately following the diagnosis of respiratory distress syndrome (RDS). May repeat dose as needed Q6 hr to **max.** of 4 doses total.

*Continued*

For explanation of icons, see p. 698.

SURFACTANT, PULMONARY/BERACTANT *continued*

***Method of administration for previously listed therapies (see remarks):*** Suction infant prior to administration. Each dose is divided into four 1 mL/kg aliquots; administer 1 mL/kg in each of four different positions (slight downward inclination with head turned to the right, head turned to the left; slight upward inclination with the head turned to the right, head turned to the left).

Transient bradycardia, $O_2$ desaturation, pallor, vasoconstriction, hypotension, endotracheal tube blockage, hypercarbia, hypercapnea, apnea and hypertension may occur during the administration process. Other side effects may include pulmonary interstitial emphysema, pulmonary air leak, and post-treatment nosocomial sepsis. Monitor heart rate and transcutaneous $O_2$ saturation during dose administration; and arterial blood gases for post-dose hyperoxia and hypocarbia after administration.

All doses are administered intratracheally via a 5 french feeding catheter. If the suspension settles during storage, gently swirl the contents—**do not shake.** Drug is stored in the refrigerator, protected from light, and needs to be warmed by standing at room temperature for at least 20 min or warm in the hand for at least 8 min. Artificial warming methods should **NOT** be used.

## SURFACTANT, PULMONARY/CALFACTANT

Infasurf

***Bovine lung surfactant***

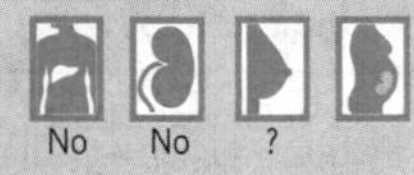


**Intratracheal suspension:** 35 mg/mL (3, 6 mL); contains 26 mg phosphatidylcholine and 0.26 mg surfactant protein B per 1 mL

***Prophylactic therapy:*** 3 mL/kg/dose intratracheally as soon as possible; up to a total of 3 doses may be given Q12 hr.

***Rescue therapy (see remarks):*** 3 mL/kg/dose intratracheally immediately after the diagnosis of respiratory distress syndrome (RDS). May repeat dose as needed Q12 hr to **max.** of 3 doses total.

***Method of administration for previously listed therapies (see remarks):*** Suction infant prior to administration. Manufacturer recommends administration through a side-port adapter into the endotracheal tube with two attendants (one to instill drug and another to monitor and position patient). Each dose is divided into two 1.5-mL/kg aliquots; administer 1.5 mL/kg in each of two different positions (infant positioned to the right or left side dependent). Drug is administered while ventilation is continued over 20–30 breaths for each aliquot, with small bursts timed only during the inspiratory cycles. A pause followed by evaluation of respiratory status and repositioning should separate the two aliquots. The drug has also been administered by divided dose into four equal aliquots and administered with repositioning in the prone, supine, right and left lateral positions.

Common adverse effects include cyanosis, airway obstruction, bradycardia, reflux of surfactant into the ET tube, requirement for manual ventilation, and reintubation. Monitor $O_2$ saturation and lung compliance after each dose such that oxygen therapy and ventilator pressure are adjusted as necessary.

All doses administered intratracheally via a 5 french feeding catheter. If suspension settles during storage, gently swirl the contents—**do not shake**. Drug is

*Continued*

SURFACTANT, PULMONARY/CALFACTANT *continued*

stored in the refrigerator, protected from light, and does not need to be warmed before administration. Unopened vials that have been warmed to room temperature (once only) may be refrigerated within 24 hr and stored for future use.

For rescue therapy, repeat doses may be administered as early as 6 hr after the previous dose for a total of up to 4 doses if the infant is still intubated and requires at least 30% inspired oxygen to maintain a $PaO_2 \geq 80$ torr.

## SURFACTANT, PULMONARY/PORACTANT ALFA

Curosurf

***Porcine lung surfactant***

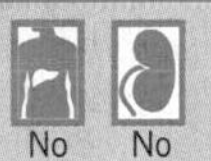
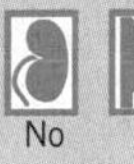
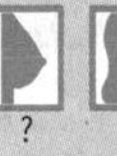
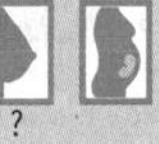

No No ?

**Intratracheal suspension:** 80 mg/mL (1.5, 3 mL): contains 0.3 mg sufactant protein B per 1 mL drug

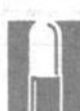

***Prophylaxis therapy:*** 2.5 mL/kg/dose× 1 intratracheally as soon as possible; up to 2 subsequent 1.25 mL/kg/doses may be given at 12-hr intervals for a **max. total dose** of 5 mL/kg.

***Rescue therapy:*** 2.5 mL/kg/dose × 1 intratracheally, immediately following the diagnosis of respiratory distress syndrome (RDS). May administer 1.25 mL/kg/dose Q12 hr × 2 doses as needed up to a **max. total dose** of 5 mL/kg.

***Method of administration for previously listed therapies (see remarks):*** Suction infant prior to administration. Each dose is divided into two aliquots, with each aliquot administered into one of the two main bronchi by positioning the infant with either the right or left side dependent. After the first aliquot is administered, remove the catheter from the ET tube and manually ventilate the infant with 100% oxygen at a rate of 40–60 breaths/min for 1 min. When the infant is stable, reposition the infant and administer the second dose. Then remove the catheter without flushing.

Transient episodes of bradycardia, decreased oxygen saturation, reflux of surfactant into the ET tube, and airway obstruction have occurred during dose administration. Monitor $O_2$ saturation and lung compliance after each dose, and adjust oxygen therapy and ventilator pressure as necessary.

All doses administered intratracheally via a 5 french feeding catheter. Suction infant prior to administration and 1 hr after surfactant instillation (unless signs of significant airway obstruction).

Drug is stored in the refrigerator and protected from light. Each vial of drug should be slowly warmed to room temperature and gently turned upside-down for uniform suspension **(do not shake)** before administration. Unopened vials that have been warmed to room temperature (once only) may be refrigerated within 24 hr and stored for future use.

## TACROLIMUS

Prograf, FK506, Protopic

***Immunosuppressant***

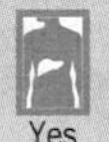
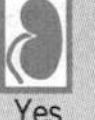
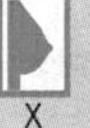
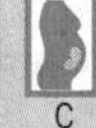

Yes Yes X C

**Caps:** 0.5, 1, 5 mg
**Oral suspension:** 0.5 mg/mL
**Injection:** 5 mg/mL (1 mL); contains alcohol and polyoxyl 60 hydrogenated castor oil
**Topical ointment (Protopic):** 0.03%, 0.1% (30, 60, 100 g)

*Continued*

For explanation of icons, see p. 698.

TACROLIMUS *continued*

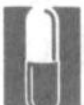

***Child:***
***Liver transplantation without pre-existing renal or hepatic dysfunction (initial doses; titrate to therapeutic levels):***
***IV:*** 0.03–0.15 mg/kg/24 hr by continuous infusion
***PO:*** 0.15–0.2 mg/kg/24 hr ÷ Q12 hr
***Adult (initial doses; titrate to therapeutic levels):***
***IV:*** 0.03–0.1 mg/kg/24 hr by continuous infusion
***PO:*** 0.15–0.3 mg/kg/24 hr ÷ Q12 hr
***Liver transplantation:*** 0.1–0.15 mg/kg/24 hr ÷ Q12 hr
***Kidney transplantation:*** 0.2 mg/kg/24 hr ÷ Q12 hr.
***Atopic dermatitis (continue treatment for 1 wk after clearing of signs and symptoms; see remarks*):**
***Child ≥ 2 yr old:*** Apply a thin layer of the 0.03% ointment to the affected skin areas BID and rub in gently and completely.
***Adult:*** Apply a thin layer of the 0.03% or 0.1% ointment to the affected skin areas BID and rub in gently and completely.

IV dosage form **contraindicated** in patients allergic to polyoxyl 60 hydrogenated castor oil. Experience in pediatric kidney transplantation is limited. Pediatric patients have required higher mg/kg doses than adults. For BMT use (beginning 1 day before BMT), dose and therapeutic levels similar to those in liver transplantation have been used.

Major adverse events include tremor, headache, insomnia, diarrhea, constipation, hypertension, nausea and renal dysfunction. Hypokalemia, hypomagnesemia, hyperglycemia, confusion, depression, infections, lymphoma, liver enzyme elevation and coagulation disorders may also occur. Tacrolimus is a substrate of the CYP 450 3A4 drug metabolizing enzyme. Calcium channel blockers, imidazole antifungals (ketoconazole, itraconazole, fluconazole, clotrimazole, posaconazole), macrolide antibiotics (erythromycin, clarithromycin, troleandomycin), cisapride, cimetidine, cyclosporine, danazol, methylprednisolone and grapefruit juice can increase tacrolimus serum levels. In contrast, carbamazepine, caspofungin, phenobarbital, phenytoin, rifampin, rifabutin, and sirolimus may decrease levels. Reduce dose in renal or hepatic insufficiency.

Monitor trough levels (just prior to a dose at steady-state). Steady-state is generally achieved after 2–5 days of continuous dosing. Interpretation will vary based on treatment protocol and assay methodology (whole blood ELISA vs. MEIA vs. HPLC). Whole blood trough concentrations of 5–20 ng/mL have been recommended in liver transplantation at 1–12 mo. Trough levels of 7–20 ng/mL (whole blood) for the first 3 mo and 5–15 ng/mL after 3 mo have been recommended in renal transplantation.

Tacrolimus therapy generally should be initiated 6 hr or more after transplantation. PO is the preferred route of administration and should be administered on an empty stomach. IV infusions should be administered at concentrations between 0.004 and 0.02 mg/mL diluted NS or $D_5W$.

**TOPICAL USE: Do not use** in children < 2 yr, immunocompromised patients, or with occlusive dressings (promotes systemic absorption). Approved as a second-line therapy for short-term and intermittent treatment of atopic dermatitis for patients who fail to respond, or do not tolerate, other approved therapies. Long-term safety is unknown. Skin burn sensation, pruritus, flu-like symptoms, allergic reaction, skin erythema, headache and skin infection are the most common side effects. Although the risk is uncertain, the FDA has issued an alert about the potential cancer risk with the use of this product. See www.fda.gov/medwatch for the latest information.

## TERBUTALINE

Brethine and others

***Beta-2-adrenergic agonist***

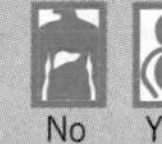
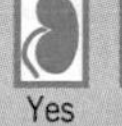

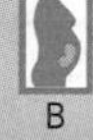
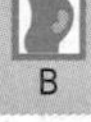

No Yes 1 B

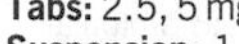

**Tabs:** 2.5, 5 mg
**Suspension:** 1 mg/mL
**Injection:** 1 mg/mL (1 mL)

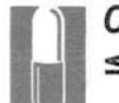

***Oral:***
***≤12 yr:*** Initial: 0.05 mg/kg/dose Q8 hr, increase as required.
**Max. dose:** 0.15 mg/kg/dose Q8 hr or total of 5 mg/24 hr.
***>12 yr and adult:*** 2.5–5 mg/dose PO Q6–8 hr
**Max. dose:**
***12–15 yr:*** 7.5 mg/24 hr
***>15 yr:*** 15 mg/24 hr

***Nebulization:***
***<2 yr:*** 0.5 mg in 2.5 mL NS Q4–6 hr PRN
***2–9 yr:*** 1 mg in 2.5 mL NS Q4–6 hr PRN
***>9 yr:*** 1.5–2.5 mg in 2.5 mL NS Q4–6 hr PRN

***SC injection:***
***≤12 yr:*** 0.005–0.01 mg/kg/dose (**max. dose:** 0.4 mg/dose) Q15–20 min × 3; if needed, Q2–6 hr PRN.
***>12 yr and adult:*** 0.25 mg/dose Q15–30 min PRN × 3.

***Continuous infusion, IV:*** 2–10 mcg/kg loading dose followed by infusion of 0.1–0.4 mcg/kg/min. May titrate in increments of 0.1–0.2 mcg/kg/min Q30 min depending on clinical response. Doses as high as 10 mcg/kg/min have been used.

***To prepare infusion:*** See inside front cover.

Nervousness, tremor, headache, nausea, tachycardia, arrhythmias and palpitations may occur. Paradoxical bronchoconstriction may occur with excessive use; if it occurs, discontinue drug immediately. Injectable product may be used for nebulization. For acute asthma, nebulizations may be given more frequently than Q4–6 hr. Use spacer device with inhaler to optimize drug delivery.

Monitor heart rate, blood pressure, respiratory rate and serum potassium when using the continuous IV infusion route of administration. **Adjust dose in renal failure (see Chapter 31).**

## TETRACYCLINE HCL

Sumycin and various generics

***Antibiotic***

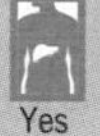
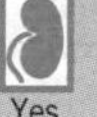
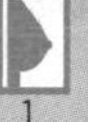
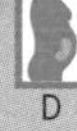

Yes Yes 1 D

**Caps:** 250, 500 mg
**Oral suspension:** 125 mg/5 mL (480 mL); contains saccharin and sodium metabisulfite

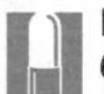

**Do not use in children <8 yr.**
***Child ≥ 8 yr:*** 25–50 mg/kg/24 hr PO ÷ Q6 hr; **max. dose:** 3 g/24 hr
***Adult:*** 1–2 g/24 hr PO ÷ Q6–12 hr

*Continued*

For explanation of icons, see p. 698.

TETRACYCLINE HCL *continued*

**Not recommended** in patients <8 yr due to tooth staining and decreased bone growth. Also **not recommended** for use in pregnancy because these side effects may occur in the fetus. The risk for these adverse effects are highest with long-term use. May cause nausea, GI upset, hepatotoxicity, stomatitis, rash, fever and superinfection. Photosensitivity reaction may occur. **Avoid** prolonged exposure to sunlight.

**Never use outdated tetracyclines** because they may cause Fanconi-like syndrome. **Do not** give with dairy products or with any divalent cations (i.e., $Fe^{2+}$, $Ca^{2+}$, $Mg^{2+}$). Give 1 hr before or 2 hr after meals.

May decrease the effectiveness of oral contraceptives, increase serum digoxin levels, and increase effects of warfarin. Use with methoxyflurane increases risk for nephrotoxicity and use with isotretinoin is associated with pseudotumor cerebri. **Adjust dose in renal failure (see Chapter 31).**

## THEOPHYLLINE

Theo-24, Theochron, Uniphyl, TheoCap, Elixophyllin, and many others

***Bronchodilator, methylxanthine***

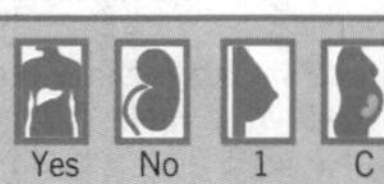


**Other dosage forms may exist.**

**Immediate release:**

Elixir (Elixophyllin): 80 mg/15 mL. Contains up to 20% alcohol.
Injection: 0.8, 1.6, 2, 3.2, 4 mg/mL

**Sustained/extended release (see remarks):**

Tabs: 100, 200, 300, 450, 600 mg
Caps: 100, 125, 200, 300, 400 mg
Sustained-release forms should **not** be chewed or crushed. Capsules may be opened and contents may be sprinkled on food.

***Dosing intervals are for immediate-release preparations.***

For sustained-release preparations, divide daily dose > Q8–24 hr based on product.

***Neonatal apnea:***

***Load:*** 5 mg/kg/dose PO × 1
***Maintenance:*** 3–6 mg/kg/24 hr PO ÷ Q6–8 hr

***Bronchospasm; PO:***

***Loading dose:*** 1 mg/kg/dose for each 2 mg/L desired increase in serum theophylline level.

***Maintenance, infant (< 1 yr):***

***Preterm:***

***<24 days old (postnatal):*** 1 mg/kg/dose PO Q12 hr
***≥24 days old (postnatal):*** 1.5 mg/kg/dose PO Q12 hr

***Full-term up to 1 yr old:*** Total daily dose (mg) = [(0.2 × age in weeks) + 5] × (kg body weight)

*Continued*

THEOPHYLLINE *continued*

***≤6 mo:*** Divide daily dose Q8 hr
***>6 mo:*** Divide daily dose Q6 hr

***Maintenance, child > 1 yr and adult without risk factors for altered clearance (see remarks)*:**

***<45 kg:*** Begin therapy at 12–14 mg/kg/24 hr ÷ Q4–6 hr up to **max. dose** of 300 mg/24 hr. If needed based on serum levels, gradually increase to 16–20 mg/kg/24 hr ÷ Q4–6 hr.
**Max. dose:** 600 mg/24 hr.
***≥45 kg:*** Begin therapy with 300 mg/24 hr ÷ Q6–8 hr. If needed based on serum levels, gradually increase to 400–600 mg/24 hr ÷ Q6–8 hr.

Drug metabolism varies widely with age, drug formulation, and route of administration. Most common side effects and toxicities are nausea, vomiting, anorexia, abdominal pain, gastroesophageal reflux, nervousness, tachycardia, seizures and arrhythmias.

Serum levels should be monitored. Therapeutic levels: bronchospasm: 10–20 mg/L; apnea: 7–13 mg/L. Half-life is age-dependent: 30 hr (newborns); 6.9 hr (infants); 3.4 hr (children); 8.1 hr (adults). See *Aminophylline* for guidelines for serum level determinations. Liver impairment, cardiac failure and sustained high fever may increase theophylline levels. Theophylline is a substrate for CYP 450 1A2. Levels are increased with allopurinol, alcohol, ciprofloxacin, cimetidine, clarithromycin, disulfiram, erythromycin, estrogen, isoniazid, propranolol, thiabendazole, and verapamil. Levels are decreased with carbamazepine, isoproterenol, phenobarbital, phenytoin, and rifampin. May cause increased skeletal muscle activity, agitation, and hyperactivity when used with doxapram.

Use ideal body weight in obese patients when calculating dosage because of poor distribution into body fat. Risk factors for increased clearance include: smoking, cystic fibrosis, hyperthyroidism, and high-protein carbohydrate diet. Factors for decreased clearance include CHF, correction of hyperthyroidism, fever, viral illness, and sepsis.

Suggested dosage intervals for sustained-release products (see following table):

**THEOPHYLLINE SUSTAINED-RELEASE PRODUCTS**

| Trade Name | Available Strengths | Dosage Interval |
|---|---|---|
| **CAPSULES** | | |
| Theo-24 | 100, 200, 300, 400 mg | Q24 hr |
| TheoCap | 125, 200, 300 mg | Q12–24 hr |
| Various generics | 125, 200 mg | Q12–24 hr |
| **TABLETS** | | |
| Theocron | 100, 200, 300, 450 mg | Q12–24 hr |
| Uniphyl | 400, 600 mg | Q24 hr |
| Various generics | 100, 200, 300, 450 mg | Q12–24 hr |

For explanation of icons, see p. 698.

## THIABENDAZOLE
Mintezol
***Anthelmintic***

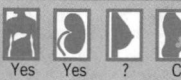

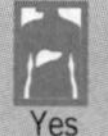 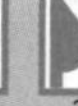 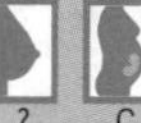
Yes Yes ? C

**Oral suspension:** 500 mg/5 mL
**Chew tabs:** 500 mg; contains saccharin
**Topical suspension:** 10%–15%
**Topical ointment:** 10% in white petrolatum

***Child and adult:*** 50 mg/kg/24 hr PO ÷ BID; **max. dose:** 3 g/24 hr
***Duration of therapy (consecutive days):***
***Strongyloides:*** × 2 days (5 days for disseminated disease)
***Cutaneous larva migrans:*** × 2–5 days
***Visceral larva migrans:*** × 5–7 days
***Trichinosis:*** × 2–4 days
***Angiostrongylosis:*** 75 mg/kg/24 hr PO ÷ BID-TID × 3 days; **max. dose:** 3 g/24 hr
***Dracunculosis:*** 50–75 mg/kg/24 hr PO ÷ BID × 3 days; **max. dose:** 3 g/24 hr

***Topical therapy for cutaneous larva migrans:*** Apply sparingly to all lesions 4–6 × per 24 hr until lesions are inactivated. See *Arch Dermatol* 1993;129:588 for additional information.

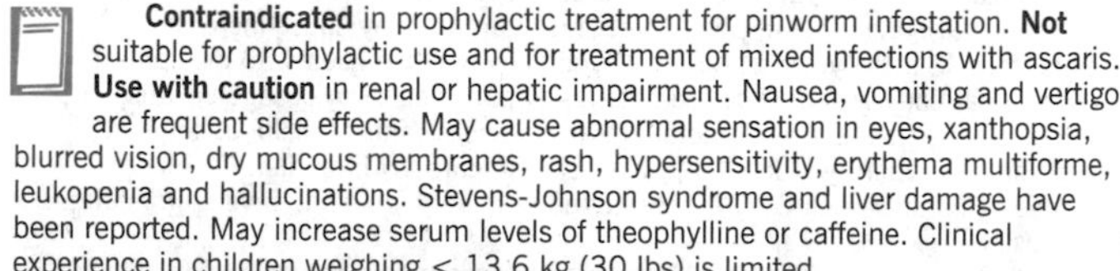

**Contraindicated** in prophylactic treatment for pinworm infestation. **Not** suitable for prophylactic use and for treatment of mixed infections with ascaris. **Use with caution** in renal or hepatic impairment. Nausea, vomiting and vertigo are frequent side effects. May cause abnormal sensation in eyes, xanthopsia, blurred vision, dry mucous membranes, rash, hypersensitivity, erythema multiforme, leukopenia and hallucinations. Stevens-Johnson syndrome and liver damage have been reported. May increase serum levels of theophylline or caffeine. Clinical experience in children weighing < 13.6 kg (30 lbs) is limited.

## THIAMINE
Vitamin $B_1$, Thiamilate, and others
***Water-soluble vitamin***

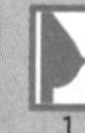 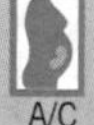
No No 1 A/C

**Tabs (OTC):** 50, 100, 250, 500 mg
**Enteric-coated tabs (OTC; Thiamilate):** 20 mg
**Injection:** 100 mg/mL (1, 2 mL); contains benzyl alcohol

For U.S. RDA, see Chapter 21.
***Beriberi (thiamine deficiency):***
***Child:*** 10–25 mg/dose IM/IV QD (if critically ill) or 10–50 mg/dose PO QD × 2 wk, followed by 5–10 mg/dose QD × 1 mo.
***Adult:*** 5–30 mg/dose IM/IV TID (if critically ill) × 2 wk, followed by 5–30 mg/24 hr PO ÷ QD or TID × 1 mo.

***Wernicke's encephalopathy syndrome (adult):*** 100 mg IV × 1, then 50–100 mg IM/IV QD until patient resumes a normal diet. (Administer thiamine before starting glucose infusion.)

Multivitamin preparations contain amounts meeting RDA requirements. Allergic reactions and anaphylaxis may occur, primarily with IV administration. Therapeutic range: 1.6–4 mg/dL. High carbohydrate diets or IV dextrose solutions may increase thiamine requirements. Large doses may interfere with

*Continued*

THIAMINE *continued*

serum theophylline assay. Pregnancy category changes to "C" if used in doses above the RDA.

## THIOPENTAL SODIUM

Pentothal and others

***Barbiturate***

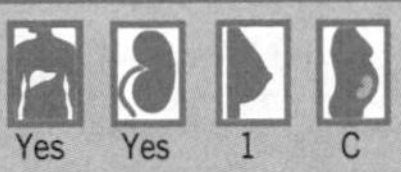


**Injection:** 250, 400, 500 mg, 1, 2.5, 5 g (reconstituted to 20 mg/mL or 25 mg/mL)
**Rectal solution:** 100 mg/mL (3.6 mL sterile water for injection in 400 mg of the injectable powder)

***Cerebral edema (child):*** 1.5–5 mg/kg/dose IV. Repeat PRN for increased ICP.
***Anesthesia induction (child and adult):***
*IV:* 2–6 mg/kg. Use lower doses in patients with hemodynamic instability. See Chapter 1 for rapid sequence intubation.
***Deep sedation:***
***Child:*** 30 mg/kg PR × 1; **max. dose:** 1 g/dose

**Contraindicated** in acute intermittent porphyria. **Use with caution** with severe cardiovascular disease, and hepatic or renal dysfunction **(adjust dose in renal failure; see Chapter 31)**. May cause respiratory depression, hypotension, anaphylaxis and decreased cardiac output. The injectable dosage form is alkaline and **cannot** be mixed with acidic drugs (e.g., vecuronium). **Avoid** IV extravasations or intra-arterial injections.

Onset of action: 30–60 sec for IV; 7–10 min for PR. Duration of action: 5–30 min for IV; 90 min for PR.

## THIORIDAZINE

Various generics; previously available as Mellaril

***Antipsychotic, phenothiazine derivative***

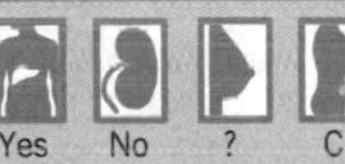


**Tabs:** 10, 15, 25, 50, 100, 150, 200 mg

***Child 2–12 yr:*** Start with 0.5 mg/kg/24 hr PO ÷ BID–TID; dosage range: 0.5–3 mg/kg/24 hr PO ÷ BID–TID. **Max. dose:** 3 mg/kg/24 hr.
***>12 yr and adult:*** Start with 75–300 mg/24 hr PO ÷ TID. Then gradually increase PRN to **max. dose** of 800 mg/24 hr ÷ BID–QID.

Indicated for schizophrenia unresponsive to standard therapy. **Contraindicated** in severe CNS depression, brain damage, narrow-angle glaucoma, blood dyscrasias, and severe liver or cardiovascular disease. **DO NOT** co-administer with drugs which may inhibit the CYP 450 2D6 isoenzymes (e.g., SSRIs such as fluoxetine, fluvoxamine, paroxetine; and beta-blockers such as propranolol and pindolol); drugs which may widen the QTc interval (e.g., disopyramide, procainamide, quinidine); and in patients with known reduced activity of CYP 450 2D6.

May cause drowsiness, extrapyramidal reactions, autonomic symptoms, ECG changes (QTc prolongation in a dose-dependent manner), arrhythmias, paradoxical reactions, and endocrine disturbances. Long-term use may cause tardive dyskinesia. Pigmentary retinopathy may occur with higher doses; a periodic eye exam is recommended. More autonomic symptoms and fewer extrapyramidal effects than

*Continued*

For explanation of icons, see p. 698.

THIORIDAZINE *continued*

chlorpromazine. Concurrent use with epinephrine can cause hypotension. Increased cardiac arrhythmias may occur with tricyclic antidepressants.

In an overdose situation, monitor ECG and avoid drugs that can widen QTc interval.

## TIAGABINE

Gabitril

***Anticonvulsant***

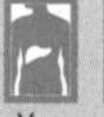
Yes
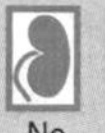
No
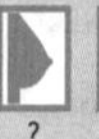
?
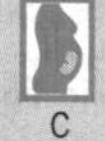
C

**Tabs:** 2, 4, 12, 16 mg
**Oral suspension:** 1 mg/mL

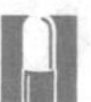

***Adjunctive therapy for refractory seizures (see remarks):***
***Child ≥ 2 yr (limited data from a safety and tolerability study in 52 children 2–17 yr, mean 9.3 ± 4.1):*** Initial dose of 0.25 mg/kg/24 hr PO ÷ TID × 4 wk. Dosage was increased at 4-wk intervals to 0.5, 1, and 1.5 mg/kg/24 hr until an effective and well-tolerated dose was established. Criteria for dose increase required tolerance of the current dosage level and <50% reduction in seizures. Patients receiving enzyme-inducing antiepileptic drugs (AEDs) received a **max. daily dose** of 0.73 ± 0.44 mg/kg/24 hr and patients receiving non-enzyme inducing AEDs received a **max.** of 0.61 ± 0.32 mg/kg/24 hr.
***Adjunctive therapy for partial seizures (dosage based on use with enzyme-inducing AEDs; see remarks).*** **Note:** Patients receiving non-enzyme-inducing AEDs result in tiagabine blood levels about two times higher than patients receiving enzyme-inducing AEDs.
***≥12 yr and adult:*** Start at 4 mg PO QD × 7 days. If needed, increase dose to 8 mg/24 hr PO ÷ BID. Dosage may be increased further by 4–8 mg/24 hr at weekly intervals (daily doses may be divided BID-QID) until a clinical response is achieved or up to specified **max. dose**.

**Max. dose:**
***12–18 yr:*** 32 mg/24 hr
***Adult:*** 56 mg/24 hr

**Use with caution** in hepatic insufficiency (may need to reduce dose and/or increase dosing interval). Most common side effects include dizziness, somnolence, depression, confusion, and asthenia. Nervousness, tremor, nausea, abdominal pain, confusion, and difficulty in concentrating may also occur. Cognitive/neuropsychiatric symptoms resulting in nonconvulsive status epilepticus requiring subsequent dose reduction or drug discontinuation have been reported. Suicidal behavior or ideation has been reported. **Off-label use in patients WITHOUT epilepsy is discouraged** due to reports of seizures in these patients.

Tiagabine's clearance is increased by concurrent hepatic enzyme-inducing antiepileptic drugs (e.g., phenytoin, carbamazepine and barbiturates). Lower doses or a slower titration for clinical response may be necessary for patients receiving non-enzyme-inducing drugs (e.g., valproate, gabapentin, and lamotrigine). **Avoid** abrupt discontinuation of drug.

TID dosing schedule may be preferred since BID schedule may not be well tolerated. Doses should be administered with food.

## TICARCILLIN

Ticar

***Antibiotic, penicillin (extended spectrum)***

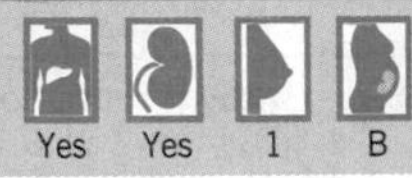


**Injection:** 3 g
Each gram contains 5.2–6.5 mEq Na.

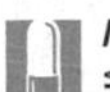

***Neonate, IM/IV:***
***≤7 days:***
***<2 kg:*** 150 mg/kg/24 hr ÷ Q12 hr
***≥ 2 kg:*** 225 mg/kg/24 hr ÷ Q8 hr
***>7 days:***
***<1.2 kg:*** 150 mg/kg/24 hr ÷ Q12 hr
***1.2–2 kg:*** 225 mg/kg/24 hr ÷ Q8 hr
***>2 kg:*** 300 mg/kg/24 hr ÷ Q6–8 hr
***Infant and child (IM/IV):*** 200–300 mg/kg/24 hr ÷ Q4–6 hr; **max. dose:** 24 g/24 hr
***Cystic fibrosis (IM/IV):*** 300–600 mg/kg/24 hr ÷ Q4–6 hr; **max. dose:** 24 g/24 hr
***Adult (IM/IV):*** 1–4 g/dose Q4–6 hr; **max. dose:** 24 g/24 h

May cause decreased platelet aggregation, bleeding diathesis, hypernatremia, hematuria, hypokalemia, hypocalcemia, allergy, rash, and increased AST. Like other penicillins, CSF penetration occurs only with inflamed meninges. **Do not** mix with aminoglycoside in same solution. May cause false-positive tests for urine protein and serum Coombs' test.

**Use with caution** with cephalosporin hypersensitivity and CHF (high sodium content). Half-life is prolonged with impaired hepatic and/or renal function **(adjust dose in renal failure; see Chapter 31).**

## TICARCILLIN AND CLAVULANATE

Timentin

***Antibiotic, penicillin (extended spectrum with beta-lactamase inhibitor)***

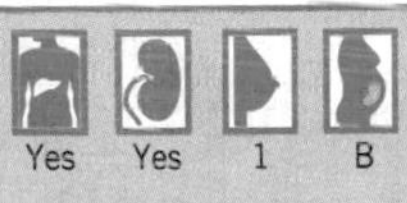


**Injection:** 3.1 g (3 g ticarcillin and 0.1 g clavulanate); contains 4.51 mEq $Na^+$ and 0.15 mEq $K^+$ per 1 g drug
**Premixed injection:** 3.1 g (3 g ticarcillin and 0.1 g clavulanate) in 100 mL; contains 18.7 mEq $Na^+$ and 0.5 mEq $K^+$ per 100 mL

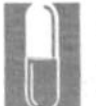

**All doses based on ticarcillin component.**
***Neonate:*** See *Ticarcillin.*
***Term neonate and infant <3 mo:*** 200–300 mg/kg/24 hr IV ÷ Q4–6 hr
***Infant ≥ 3 mo and child:***
***Mild/moderate infections:*** 200 mg/kg/24 hr IV ÷ Q6 hr
***Severe infections:*** 300 mg/kg/24 hr IV ÷ Q4-6 hr
**Max. dose:** 18–24 mg/24 hr
***Cystic fibrosis:*** See *Ticarcillin.*
***Adult:*** 3 g/dose IV Q4-6 hr IV
***UTI:*** 3 g/dose IV Q6–8 hr
**Max. dose:** 18–24 g/24 hr

*Continued*

For explanation of icons, see p. 698.

TICARCILLIN AND CLAVULANATE *continued*

Activity similar to ticarcillin except that beta-lactamase inhibitor broadens spectrum to include *S. aureus* and *H. influenzae*. See *Ticarcillin* for side effects. Like other penicillins, CSF penetration occurs only with inflamed meninges. May cause false-positive tests for urine protein and serum Coombs' test.

**Adjust dosage in renal impairment (see Chapter 31).**

## TOBRAMYCIN

Nebcin, Tobrex, AKTob, TOBI, and others

***Antibiotic, aminoglycoside***

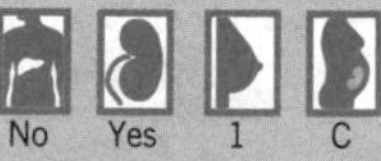


**Injection:** 10, 40 mg/mL; may contain phenol and bisulfites
**Powder for injection:** 1.2 g; preservative free
**Ophthalmic ointment (Tobrex, AKTob):** 0.3% (3.5 g)
**In combination with dexamethasone (TobraDex):** 0.3% tobramycin with 0.1% dexamethasone (3.5 g); contains 0.5% chlorbutanol
**Ophthalmic solution (Tobrex):** 0.3% (5 mL)
**In combination with dexamethasone:** 0.3% tobramycin with 0.1% dexamethasone (2.5, 5, 10 mL); contains 0.01% benzalkonium chloride and EDTA
**Nebulizer solution:** 300 mg/5 mL (TOBI, preservative free) (56s), 170 mg/3.4 mL (mixed in 0.45% NS, preservative free, use with eFlow nebulizer)

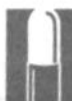

***Neonate, IM/IV (see following table):***

**TOBRAMYCIN**

| Post-conceptional Age (wk) | Postnatal Age (days) | Dose (mg/kg/dose) | Interval (hr) |
|---|---|---|---|
| ≤29* | 0–7 | 5 | 48 |
| | 8–28 | 4 | 36 |
| | >28 | 4 | 24 |
| 30–33 | 0–7 | 4.5 | 36 |
| | >7 | 4 | 24 |
| 34–37 | 0–7 | 4 | 24 |
| | >7 | 4 | 18–24 |
| ≥38 | 0–7 | 4 | 24 |
| | >7 | 4 | 12–18 |

*Or significant asphyxia, PDA, indomethicin use, poor cardiac output, reduced renal function.

***Child:*** 7.5 mg/kg/24 hr ÷ Q8 hr IV/IM
***Cystic fibrosis:*** 7.5–10.5 mg/kg/24 hr ÷ Q8 hr IV
***Adult:*** 3–6 mg/kg/24 hr ÷ Q8 hr IV/IM

*Continued*

TOBRAMYCIN *continued*

***Ophthalmic:***

***Tobramycin:***

***Child and adult:*** Apply thin ribbon of ointment into conjunctival sac(s) BID-TID; or 1–2 drops of solution to affected eye(s) Q4 hr

***Tobramycin with dexamethasone:***

***≥2 yr and adult:*** Apply ½ inch ribbon of ointment into conjunctival sac(s) TID-QID; or 1–2 drops of solution to affected eye(s) Q2 hr × 24–48 hr, then 1–2 drops Q4–6 hr

***Inhalation:***

***Cystic fibrosis prophylaxis therapy:***

***≥6 yr and adult:***

***TOBI:*** 300 mg Q12 hr administered in repeated cycles of 28 days on drug followed by 28 days off drug.

***Use with eFlow nebulizer:*** 170 mg Q12 hr administered in repeated cycles of 28 days on drug followed by 28 days off drug.

---

**Use with caution** in combination with neurotoxic, ototoxic, or nephrotoxic drugs; anesthetics or neuromuscular blocking agents; pre-existing renal, vestibular or auditory impairment; and in patients with neuromuscular disorders. May cause ototoxicity, nephrotoxicity, and neuromuscular blockade. Serious allergic reactions including anaphylaxis and dermatologic reactions including exfoliative dermatitis, toxic epidermal necrolysis, erythema multiforme, and Stevens-Johnson syndrome have been reported rarely. **Ototoxic effects synergistic with furosemide.**

Higher doses are recommended in patients with cystic fibrosis, neutropenia, or burns. **Adjust dose in renal failure (see Chapter 31).** Monitor peak and trough levels.

Therapeutic peak levels:

*6–10 mg/L in general*

*8–10 mg/L in pulmonary infections, neutropenia, osteomylitis, severe sepsis*

Therapeutic trough levels: <2 mg/L. Recommended serum sampling time at steady-state: trough within 30 min prior to the third consecutive dose and peak 30–60 min after the administration of the third consecutive dose.

**INHALATIONAL USE:** Transient voice alteration, bronchospasm, dyspnea, pharyngitis, and increased cough may occur. Transient tinnitus has been reported. For use with other medications in cystic fibrosis, use the following order of administration: bronchodilator first, chest physiotherapy, other inhaled medications (if indicated), and tobramycin last.

## TOLNAFTATE

Tinactin, Aftate, and many others

***Antifungal agent***

No No ? C

**Topical aerosol liquid [OTC]:** 1% (60, 120 mL); may contain 36% alcohol
**Aerosol powder [OTC]:** 1% (100, 105, 150 g); contains 14% alcohol and talc
**Cream [OTC]:** 1% (15, 21, 30 g)
**Gel [OTC]:** 1% (15 g)
**Topical powder [OTC]:** 1% (45, 90 g)
**Topical solution [OTC]:** 1% (10 mL)

---

***Child (≥ 2 yr) and adult:***

***Topical:*** apply 1–3 drops of solution or small amount of gel, liquid, cream or powder to affected areas BID–TID for 2–4 wk.

*Continued*

For explanation of icons, see p. 698.

TOLNAFTATE *continued*

May cause mild irritation and sensitivity. Contact dermatitis has been reported. **Avoid** eye contact. **Do not use** for nail or scalp infections. Discontinue use if sensitization develops.

## TOPIRAMATE

Topamax

***Anticonvulsant***

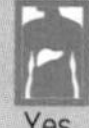
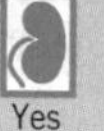
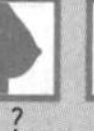
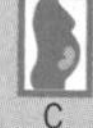

Yes Yes ? C

**Caps, sprinkle:** 15, 25 mg
**Tabs:** 25, 50, 100, 200 mg
**Oral suspension:** 6 mg/mL 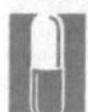

***Adjunctive therapy for partial onset seizures, primary generalized tonic clonic seizures, or Lennox-Gastaut syndrome (see remarks):***

***Child 2–16 yr:*** Start with 1–3 mg/kg/dose (**max. dose:** 25 mg/dose) PO QHS × 7 days; then increase by 1–3 mg/kg/24-hr increments at 1- to 2-wk intervals (divided daily dose BID) to response. Usual maintenance dose is 5–9 mg/kg/24 hr PO ÷ BID.

***≥17 yr and adult:*** Start with 25–50 mg PO QHS × 7 days; then increase by 25–50 mg/24-hr increments at 1-wk intervals until adequate response. Doses > 50 mg should be divided BID. Usual maintenance dose: 200–400 mg/24 hr. Doses above 1600 mg/24 hr have not been studied.

***Monotherapy for partial onset seizures or primary generalized tonic clonic seizures:***

***Child ≥ 10 yr and adult:*** Start with 25 mg PO BID × 7 days, then increase by 50 mg/24-hr increments at 1-wk intervals up to a **max. dose** of 100 mg PO BID at wk 4. If needed, dose may be further increased at weekly intervals by 100 mg/24 hr up to a recommended **max. dose** of 200 mg PO BID.

In primary generalized tonic clonic seizures, use a slower initial titration rate by reaching the assigned dose by the end of 8 wk; 6 mg/kg/24 hr for children 2–16 yr and 200 mg BID for adults. **Use with caution** in renal and hepatic dysfunction (decreased clearance) and sulfa hypersensitivity. **Reduce dose by 50% when creatinine clearance is < 70 mL/min.** Common side effects (incidence lower in children) include ataxia, cognitive dysfunction, dizziness, nystagmus, paresthesia, sedation, visual disturbances, nausea, dyspepsia, and kidney stones. Secondary angle closure glaucoma characterized by ocular pain, acute myopia and increased intraocular pressure has been reported and may lead to blindness if left untreated. Patients should be instructed to seek immediate medical attention if they experience blurred vision or periorbital pain. Oligohidrosis and hyperthermia have been reported primarily in children and should be monitored especially during hot weather and with use of drugs that predispose patients to heat-related disorders (e.g., carbonic anhydrase inhibitors and anticholinergics). Hyperchloremic, non-anion gap metabolic acidosis has also been reported. Suicidal behavior or ideation have been reported.

Drug is metabolized by and inhibits the CYP 450 2C19 isoenzyme. Phenytoin, valproic acid, and carbamazepine may decrease topiramate levels. Topiramate may decrease valproic acid, digoxin, and ethinyl estradiol (to decrease oral contraceptive efficacy), but may increase phenytoin levels. Alcohol and CNS depressants may increase CNS side effects. Carbonic anhydrase inhibitors (e.g., acetazolamide) may increase risk of metabolic acidosis, nephrolithiasis, or paresthesia.

*Continued*

TOPIRAMATE *continued*

Doses may be administered with or without food. Capsule may be opened and sprinkled on small amount of food (e.g., 1 teaspoonful of applesauce) and swallowed whole (**do not chew**). Maintain adequate hydration to prevent kidney stone formation.

## TRAZODONE

Many generics; previously available as Desyrel

***Antidepressant, triazolopyridine-derivative***

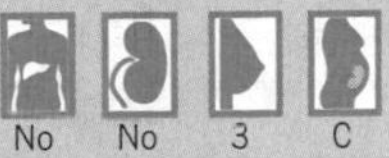


**Tabs:** 50, 100, 150, 300 mg

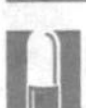

***Depression (titrate to lowest effective dose):***
***Child (6–18 yr):*** Start at 1.5–2 mg/kg/24 hr PO ÷ BID–TID; if needed, gradually increase dose Q3–4 days up to a **max.** of 6 mg/kg/24 hr ÷ TID
***Adult:*** Start at 150 mg/24 hr PO ÷ TID; if needed, increase by 50 mg/24 hr Q3–4 days up a **max.** of 600 mg/24 hr for hospitalized patients (400 mg/24 hr for ambulatory patients).

**Use with caution** in pre-existing cardiac disease, initial recovery phase of MI, in patients receiving antihypertensive medications,and electroconvulsive therapy. Common side effects include dizziness, drowsiness, dry mouth and diarrhea. Seizures, tardive dyskinesia, EPS, arrhythmias, priapism, blurred vision, neuromuscular weakness, anemia, orthostatic hypotension and rash have been reported. Monitor for clinical worsening of depression and suicidal ideation/behavior following the initiation of therapy or after dose changes.

Trazodone is CYP 450 3A4 isoenzyme substrate (may interact with inhibitors and inducers) and may increase digoxin levels and increase CNS effects of alcohol, barbiturates, and other CNS depressants. **Max.** antidepressant effect is seen at 2–6 wk.

## TRETINOIN

Retin-A, Retin-A Micro, Avita, Renova, and many others

***Retinoic acid derivative, topical acne product***

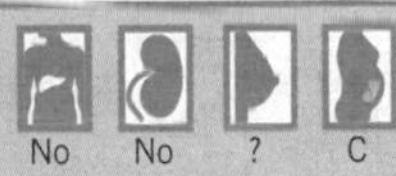


**Cream:** 0.02% (40 g), 0.025% (20, 45 g), 0.05% (20, 40, 45, 60 g), 0.1% (20, 45 g)
**Topical gel:** 0.01% (15, 45 g), 0.025% (15, 20, 45 g), 0.04% (20, 40 g); may contain 90% alcohol and may contain propylene glycol
**Topical gel (Retin-A Micro):** 0.04% (20, 45 g), 0.1% (20, 45 g); contains glycerin, propylene glycol, benzyl alcohol

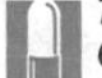

***Topical:***
***Child > 12 yr and adult:*** Gently wash face with a mild soap, pat the skin dry, and wait 20 to 30 min before use. Initiate therapy with either 0.025% cream or 0.01% gel and apply a small pea-sized amount to the affected areas of the face QHS. See remarks.

*Continued*

For explanation of icons, see p. 698.

TRETINOIN *continued*

**Contraindicated** in sunburns. **Avoid** excessive sun exposure. If stinging or irritation occurs, decrease frequency of administration to QOD. **Avoid** contact with eyes, ears, nostrils, mouth or open wounds. Local adverse effects include irritation, erythema, excessive dryness, blistering, crusting, hyperpigmentation or hypopigmentation, and acne flare-ups. Concomitant use of other topical acne products may lead to significant skin irritation. Onset of therapeutic benefits may be experienced within 2–3 wk with optimal effects in 6 wk. The gel dosage form is flammable and should **not** be exposed to heat or temperatures > 120°F.

## TRIAMCINOLONE

Azmacort, Nasacort HFA, Nasacort AQ, Kenalog, Aristospan, and others

***Corticosteroid***

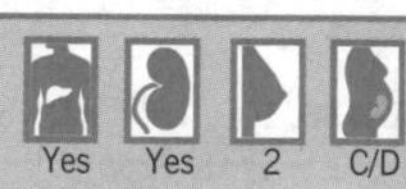


**Nasal spray:**

Nasacort HFA: 55 mcg/actuation (100 actuations per 9.3 g); contains dehydrated alcohol 0.7%

Nasacort AQ: 55 mcg/actuation (30 actuations per 6.5 g, 120 actuations per 16.5 g); contains benzalkonium chloride and EDTA

**Oral inhaler (Azmacort):** 75 mcg/actuation (240 actuations per 20 g)
**Oral syrup:** 4 mg/5 mL (120 mL)
**Cream (Kenalog and others):** 0.025%, 0.1% (15, 80, 454 g), 0.5% (15 g)
**Ointment (Kenalog and others):** 0.025%, 0.1% (15, 80, 454 g), 0.5% (15 g)
**Lotion (Kenalog and others):** 0.025%, 0.1% (60 mL)
**Topical aerosol (Kenalog):** 0.2 mg/2 second spray (23, 63 g); contains 10.3% alcohol
**Dental paste (Kenalog in Orabase and others):** 0.1% (5 g)
See Chapter 30 for potency rankings and sizes of topical preparations.
**Injection as acetonide:** 10 mg/mL (Kenalog-10) (5 mL), 40 mg/mL (Kenalog-40) (1, 5, 10 mL); contains benzyl alcohol
**Injection as hexacetonide:** 5 mg/mL (Aristospan Intralesional) (5 mL), 20 mg/mL (Aristospan Intra-articular) (1, 5 mL); contains benzyl alcohol

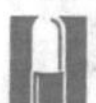

***Oral inhalation (titrate to lowest effective dose after symptoms are controlled):***

***Child 6–12 yr:*** 1–2 puffs TID–QID or 2–4 puffs BID; **max. dose:** 12 puffs/24 hr

***≥12 yr and adult:*** 2 puffs TID–QID or 4 puffs BID; **max. dose:** 16 puffs/24 hr

NIH-National Heart Lung and Blood Institute recommendations (divide daily doses BID–QID): See Chapter 24.

***Intranasal (titrate to lowest effective dose after symptoms are controlled):***

***Nasacort AQ:***

***Child 6–11 yr:*** Start with 1 spray in each nostril QD. If no benefit in 1 wk, dose may be increased to 2 sprays in each nostril QD.

***≥12 yr and adult:*** 2 sprays in each nostril QD (starting and **max. dose**).

***Nasacort HFA:***

***Child 6–11 yr:*** Start with 2 sprays in each nostril QD. Once desired effect is achieved, titrate dose to the mimimum effective dose.

***≥12 yr and adult:*** 2 sprays in each nostril QD. After 4–7 days, if needed, may increase to 4 sprays/nostril/24 hr ÷ QD–QID

*Continued*

TRIAMCINOLONE *continued*

***Topical:*** Apply to affected areas BID–TID
***Systemic use:*** Use ⅙ of cortisone dose. See Chapter 30.
***Intralesional, ≥12 yr and adult (Kenalog-10):*** 1 mg/site at intervals of 1 wk or more. May give separate doses in sites >1 cm apart, **not to exceed** 30 mg.

Rinse mouth thoroughly with water after each use of the oral inhalation dosage form. Nasal preparations may cause epistaxis, cough, fever, nausea, throat irritation, dyspepsia, and fungal infections (rarely). Topical preparations may cause dermal atrophy, telangiectasias and hypopigmentation. Topical steroids should be **used with caution** on the face and in intertriginous areas. See Chapter 8.

Dosage adjustment for hepatic failure with systemic use may be necessary. **Use with caution** in thyroid dysfunction, respiratory TB, occular herpes simplex, peptic ulcer disease, osteoporosis, hypertension, CHF, myasthenia gravis, ulcerative colitis, and renal dysfunction. Pregnancy category changes to "D" if used in the first trimester.

Shake oral inhalation and intranasal dosage forms before each use. **Avoid** SQ and IV administration with injectable dosage forms. Injectable forms contain benzyl alcohol.

## TRIAMTERENE
Dyrenium
***Diuretic, potassium sparing***

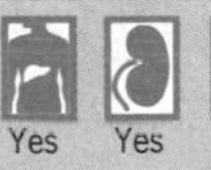
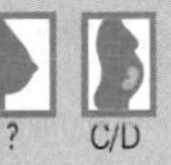

Yes Yes ? C/D

**Caps:** 50, 100 mg; contains benzyl alchohol and povidone

***Child:*** 1–2 mg/kg/24 hr ÷ BID PO. May increase up to a **max.** of 3–4 mg/kg/24 hr up to 300 mg/24 hr.
***Adult:*** 50–100 mg/24 hr ÷ QD–BID PO; **max. dose:** 300 mg/24 hr.

**Do not use** if GFR < 10 mL/hr. **Adjust dose in renal impairment (see Chapter 31).** Monitor serum electrolytes. May cause hyperkalemia, hyponatremia, hypomagnesemia and metabolic acidosis. Interstitial nephritis, thrombocytopenia and anaphylaxis have been reported.

Concurrent use of ACE inhibitors may increase serum potassium. **Use with caution** when administering medications with high potassium load (e.g., some penicillins), and in patients with hepatic impairment or on high potassium diets. Cimetidine may increase effects. This drug is also available as a combination product with hydrochlorothiazide. Administer doses with food to minimize GI upset. Pregnancy category changes to "D" if used in pregnancy-induced hypertension.

## TRILISATE

See *Choline Magnesium Trisalicylate*

For explanation of icons, see p. 698.

## TRIMETHOBENZAMIDE HCL

Tigan and others

***Antiemetic***

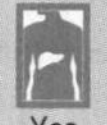 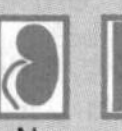 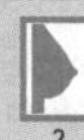 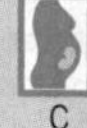

Yes No ? C

**Caps:** 300 mg

**Injection:** 100 mg/mL (2, 20 mL); may contain phenol or parabens

***Child (PO):*** 15–20 mg/kg/24 hr ÷ TID–QID.

***Alternative dosing:***

***<13.6 kg:*** 100 mg TID–QID

***13.6–40 kg:*** 100–200 mg/dose TID–QID

***>40 kg:*** 300 mg/dose TID–QID

***Adult:***

***PO:*** 300 mg/dose TID–QID

***IM:*** 200 mg/dose TID–QID

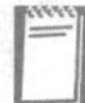

**Do not use** in premature or newborn infants. **Avoid** use in patients with hepatotoxicity, acute vomiting or allergic reaction. CNS disturbances are common in children (extrapyramidal symptoms, drowsiness, confusion, dizziness). Hypotension, especially with IM use, may occur. IM **not recommended** in children.

## TRIMETHOPRIM AND SULFAMETHOXAZOLE

See *Sulfamethoxazole and Trimethoprim*

## URSODIOL

Actigall, Urso 250, Urso Forte, and others

***Gallstone solubilizing agent, cholelitholytic agent***

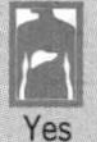 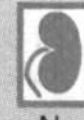 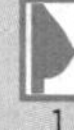 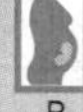 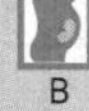

Yes No 1 B

**Oral suspension:** 20, 25, 50, 60 mg/mL

**Caps (Actigall and others):** 300 mg

**Tabs:**

**Urso 250:** 250 mg

**Urso Forte:** 500 mg

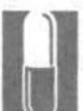

***Biliary atresia:***

***Infant (limited data):*** 10–15 mg/kg/24 hr QD PO

***TPN-induced cholestasis:***

***Infant and child (limited data, Gastroenterology 1996;111[3]:716–719):*** 30 mg/kg/24 hr ÷ TID PO

***Gallstone dissolution:***

***Adult:*** 8–10 mg/kg/24 hr ÷ BID–TID PO

***Cystic fibrosis (to improve fatty acid metabolism in liver disease):***

***Child:*** 15–30 mg/kg/24 hr ÷ QD–TID PO

**Contraindicated** in calcified cholesterol stones, radiopaque stones, bile pigment stones, or stones > 20 mm in diameter. **Use with caution** in patients with nonvisualizing gallbladder and chronic liver disease. May cause GI disturbance, rash, arthralgias, anxiety, headache, and elevated liver enzymes. Aluminum-containing antacids, cholestyramine, and oral contraceptives decrease ursodiol effectiveness. Dissolution of stones may take several mo. Stone recurrence occurs in 30%–50% of patients within 5 yr.

## VALACYCLOVIR
Valtrex
***Antiviral agent***

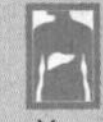 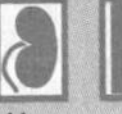 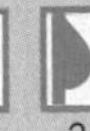 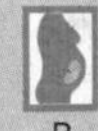 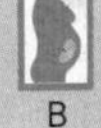
Yes Yes 2 B

**Tabs:** 500, 1000 mg
**Oral suspension:** 50 mg/mL

***Child:*** Recommended dosages based on steady-state pharmacokinetic data in immunocompromised children. Efficacy data is incomplete.

***To mimic an IV acyclovir regimen of 250 mg/m²/dose or 10 mg/kg/dose TID:***
***30 mg/kg/dose PO TID OR alternatively by weight:***
- ***4–12 kg:*** 250 mg PO TID
- ***13–21 kg:*** 500 mg PO TID
- ***22–29 kg:*** 750 mg PO TID
- ***≥30 kg:*** 1000 mg PO TID

***To mimic a PO acyclovir regimen of 20 mg/kg/dose 4 or 5 times a day:***
***20 mg/kg/dose PO TID OR alternatively by weight:***
- ***6–19 kg:*** 250 mg PO TID
- ***20–31 kg:*** 500 mg PO TID
- ***≥32 kg:*** 750 mg PO TID

***Herpes zoster (see remarks):***
***Adult (immunocompetent)*:** 1 g/dose PO TID × 7 days within 48–72 hr of onset of rash.

***Genital herpes:***
***Adolescent and adult:***
- ***Initial episodes:*** 1 g/dose PO BID × 10 days.
- ***Recurrent episodes:*** 500 mg/dose PO BID × 3 days.
- ***Suppressive therapy:*** 500–1000 mg/dose PO QD × 1 yr; then reassess for recurrences. Patients with < 9 recurrences per yr may be dosed at 500 mg/dose PO QD × 1 yr.

***Herpes labialis (cold sores).***
***Adolescent and adult:*** 2 g/dose PO Q12 hr × 1 day.

This pro-drug is metabolized to acyclovir and L-valine with better oral absorption than acyclovir. **Use with caution in hepatic or renal insufficiency (adjust dose; see Chapter 31)**. Thrombotic thrombocytopenic purpura/hemolytic uremic syndrome (TTP/HUS) has been reported in patients with advanced HIV infection and in bone marrow and renal transplant recipients. Probenecid or cimetidine can reduce the rate of conversion to acyclovir. Nausea, vomiting, and headache are common. See *Acyclovir* for additional drug interactions and adverse effects.

For initial episodes of genital herpes, therapy is most effective when initiated within 48 hr of symptom onset. Therapy should be initiated immediately after the onset of symptoms in recurrent episodes (no efficacy data when initiating therapy > 24 hr after onset of symptoms). Data are not available for use as suppressive therapy for periods > 1 yr.

Valacyclovir **CANNOT** be substituted for acyclovir on a one-to-one basis. Doses may be administered with or without food.

For explanation of icons, see p. 698.

## VALGANCICLOVIR

Valcyte

***Antiviral agent***

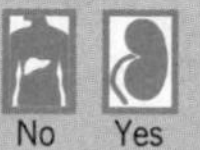 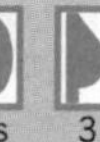 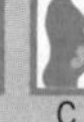 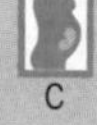

No Yes 3 C

**Tabs:** 450 mg
**Oral suspension:** 60 mg/mL

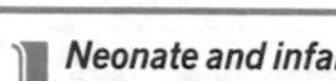

***Neonate and infant:***

***Symptomatic congenital CMV (from pharmacokinetic (PK) data in 8 infants 4–90 days old, mean: 20 days; and 24 neonates 8–34 days old):*** 15–16 mg/kg/dose PO BID. Additional PK, safety, and efficacy studies are required.

***Child:***

***CMV prophylaxis in liver transplantation (limited data based on a retrospective review in 10 patients, mean age 4.9 ± 5.6 yr):*** 15–18 mg/kg/dose PO QD × 100 days following transplantation resulted in 1 case of asymptomatic CMV infection detected by CMV antigenemia at day 7 of therapy. This patient then received a higher dose of 15 mg/kg/dose BID until 3 consecutive negative CMV antigenemia were achieved. The dose was switched back to a prophylactic regimen at day 46 posttransplant.

***Adolescent and adult:***

***CMV retinitis:***

***Induction therapy:*** 900 mg PO BID × 21 days with food

***Maintenance therapy:*** 900 mg PO QD with food

***CMV prophylaxis in heart, kidney, and kidney-pancreas transplantation:*** 900 mg PO QD starting within 10 days of transplantation until 100 days posttransplantation.

This pro-drug is metabolized to ganciclovir with better oral absorption than ganciclovir. **Contraindicated** with hypersensitivity to valganciclovir/ganciclovir; ANC < 500 $mm^3$; platelets < 25,000 $mm^3$; hemoglobin < 8 g/dL; and patients on hemodialysis. **Use with caution in renal insufficiency (adjust dose; see Chapter 31)**, bone marrow suppression, or receiving myelosupressive drugs or irradiation. May cause headache, insomnia, peripheral neuropathy, diarrhea, vomiting, neutropenia, anemia and thrombocytopenia. Use effective contraception during and for at least 90 days after therapy. See *Ganciclovir* for drug interactions and additional adverse effects.

Valganciclovir **CANNOT** be substituted for ganciclovir on a one-to-one basis. All doses are administered with food. **Avoid** direct contact with broken or crushed tablets with the skin or mucous membranes.

## VALPROIC ACID

Depakene, Depacon, and various generics

[Depakote: *See* Divalproex Sodium]

***Anticonvulsant***

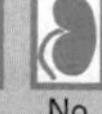 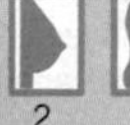 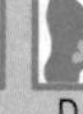

Yes No 2 D

**Caps:** 250 mg
**Syrup:** 250 mg/5 mL (473 mL); may contain parabens
**Injection (Depacon):** 100 mg/mL (5 mL)

*Continued*

VALPROIC ACID *continued*

***Oral:***
***Initial:*** 10–15 mg/kg/24 hr ÷ QD–TID
***Increment:*** 5–10 mg/kg/24 hr at weekly intervals to **max. dose** of 60 mg/kg/24 hr.
***Maintenance:*** 30–60 mg/kg/24 hr ÷ BID–TID. Due to drug interactions, higher doses may be required in children on other anticonvulsants.

***Intravenous (use only when PO is not possible):***
Use same PO daily dose ÷ Q6 hr. Convert back to PO as soon as possible.

***Rectal (use syrup, diluted 1:1 with water, given PR as a retention enema):***
***Load:*** 20 mg/kg/dose
***Maintenance:*** 10–15 mg/kg/dose Q8 hr

***Migraine prophylaxis:***
***Child (limited data):*** 15–30 mg/kg/24 hr PO ÷ BID
***Adult:*** Start with 500 mg/24 hr ÷ PO BID. Dose may be increased to a **max.** of 1000 mg/24 hr ÷ PO BID. If using divalproex sodium extended-release tablets, administer daily dose QD.

**Contraindicated** in hepatic disease. May cause GI, liver, blood, and CNS toxicity; weight gain; transient alopecia; pancreatitis (potentially life-threatening); nausea; sedation; vomiting; headache; thrombocytopenia; platelet dysfunction; rash (especially with lamotrigine); and hyperammonemia. Hepatic failure has occurred especially in children < 2 yr (especially those receiving multiple anticonvulsants, with congenital metabolic disorders, with severe seizure disorders with mental retardation, and with organic brain disease). Idiosyncratic life-threatening pancreatitis has been reported in children and adults. Hyperammonemic encephalopathy has been reported in patients with urea cycle disorders. Suicidal behavior or ideation have been reported.

Valproic acid is a substrate for CYP 450 2C19 isoenzyme and an inhibitor of CYP 450 2C9, 2D6 and 3A3/4 (weak). It increases amitriptyline/nortriptyline, phenytoin, diazepam and phenobarbital levels. Concomitant phenytoin, phenobarbital, topiramate, meropenem and carbamazepine may decrease valproic acid levels. Amitriptyline or nortriptyline may increase valproic acid levels. May interfere with urine ketone and thyroid tests.

**Do not give** syrup with carbonated beverages. Use of IV route has not been evaluated for > 14 days of continuous use. Infuse IV over 1 hr up to a **max. rate** of 20 mg/min. Depakote and Depakote ER are **NOT** bioequivalent; see package insert for dose conversion.

Therapeutic levels: 50–100 mg/L. Recommendations for serum sampling at steady-state: Obtain trough level within 30 min prior to the next scheduled dose after 2–3 days of continuous dosing. Levels of 50–60 mg/L and as high as 85 mg/L have been recommended for bipolar disorders. Monitor CBC and LFTs prior to and during therapy.

## VANCOMYCIN

Vancocin and others
***Antibiotic***

No Yes ? C/B

**Injection:** 0.5, 1, 5, 10 g
**Caps:** 125, 250 mg
**Oral solution:** 1 g (reconstitute to 250 mg/5 mL), 10 g (reconstitute to 500 mg/6 mL)

*Continued*

For explanation of icons, see p. 698.

VANCOMYCIN *continued*

***Neonate, IV (see following table):***

| | **Postnatal Age** | |
|---|---|---|
| **Weight (kg)** | **<7 Days** | **≥7 Days** |
| <1.2 | 15 mg/kg/dose Q24 hr | 15 mg/kg/dose Q24 hr |
| 1.2–2 | 10–15 mg/kg/dose Q12–18 hr | 10–15 mg/kg/dose Q8–12 hr |
| >2 | 10–15 mg/kg/dose Q8–12 hr | 15–20 mg/kg/dose Q8 hr |

***Infant and child, IV:***
- ***CNS and serious infections; and non-obese oncology patient without renal impairment:*** 60 mg/kg/24 hr ÷ Q6 hr
- ***Other infections:*** 40 mg/kg/24 hr ÷ Q6–8 hr
- **Max. dose:** 1 g/dose

***Adult:*** 2 g/24 hr ÷ Q6–12 hr IV; **max. dose:** 4 g/24 hr

***C. difficile colitis:***
- ***Child:*** 40–50 mg/kg/24 hr ÷ Q6 hr PO × 7–10 days
  - **Max dose:** 500 mg/24 hr; higher **max.** of 2 g/24 hr has also been used.
- ***Adult:*** 125 mg/dose PO Q6 hr × 7–10 days; dosages as high as 2 g/24 hr ÷ Q6–8 hr have also been used.

***Endocarditis prophylaxis for GU or GI (excluding esophageal) procedures (complete all antibiotic dose infusion(s) within 30 min of starting procedure):***
- ***Moderate-risk patients allergic to ampicillin or amoxicillin:***
  - ***Child:*** 20 mg/kg/dose IV over 1–2 hr × 1
  - ***Adult:*** 1 g/dose IV over 1–2 hr × 1
- ***High-risk patients allergic to ampicillin or amoxicillin:***
  - ***Child and adult:*** Same dose as moderate-risk patients plus gentamicin 1.5 mg/kg/dose (**max. dose:** 120 mg/dose) IV/IM ×1

Ototoxicity and nephrotoxicity may occur and may be exacerbated with concurrent aminoglycoside use. **Adjust dose in renal failure (see Chapter 31).** Low concentrations of the drug may appear in CSF with inflamed meninges.

Nausea, vomiting and drug-induced erythroderma are common. "Red man syndrome" associated with rapid IV infusion may occur. Infuse over 60 min (may infuse over 120 min if 60 min infusion is not tolerated). **Note:** Diphenhydramine is used to reverse red man syndrome. Allergic reactions have been reported.

Measuring serum levels is primarily indicated for enhancing efficacy. Toxicity relationship with serum levels has not been clearly established; earlier impure version of the drug ("Mississippi Mud") may have been more toxic. Although the monitoring of serum levels is controversial, there is a trend toward measuring trough levels in most patients. Therapeutic levels: trough: 5–15 mg/L with the additional suggestions: MRSA pneumonia 15–20 mg/L; CNS infections: 20 mg/L; endocarditis: 10–20 mg/L; and bacteremia: 10–15 mg/L. Peak level measurement (20–50 mg/L) has also been recommended for patients with burns, clinically nonresponsive in 72 hr of therapy, persistent positive cultures and CNS infections (≥ 30 mg/L).

*Continued*

VANCOMYCIN *continued*

*Recommended serum sampling time at steady-state:* Trough within 30 min prior to the third consecutive dose and peak 60 min after the administration of the third consecutive dose.

Metronidazole (PO) is the drug of choice for *C. difficile* colitis; vancomycin should be **avoided** due to the emergence of vancomycin-resistant enterococcus. Pregnancy category "B" is assigned with the oral route of administration.

## VARICELLA-ZOSTER IMMUNE GLOBULIN (HUMAN)

VariZig, VZIG

***Hyperimmune globulin, varicella-zoster***

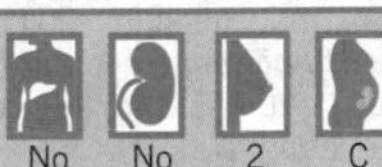


**Injection:** 125 U; contains 60–200 mg human immunoglobulin G, 0.1 M glycine, 0.04 M sodium chloride, and 0.01% polysorbate 80.
Product is available via an FDA-approved Expanded Access Protocol; see www.fffenterprises.com or call FFF Enterprises at 1-800-843-7477 for additional information.

***IM (preferred route) or IV (see remarks):***

***≤10 kg:*** 125 U
***10.1–20 kg:*** 250 U
***20.1–30 kg:*** 375 U
***30.1–40 kg:*** 500 U
***>40 kg:*** 625 U
**Max. dose:** 625 U/dose

**Contraindicated** in severe thrombocytopenia due to IM Injection, immunoglobulin A-deficiency (anaphylactic reactions may occur), and known immunity to varicella zoster virus. See Chapter 16 for indications. Dose should be given within 48 hr of exposure and no later than 96 hr post exposure. Local discomfort, redness and swelling at the injection site, and headache may occur.

Hyperviscosity of the blood may increase risk for thrombotic events. IM route is preferred over IV in patients with pre-existing respiratory conditions. Interferes with immune response to live virus vaccines such as measles, mumps and rubella; defer administration of live vaccines 5 mo or longer after VZIG dose. See latest AAP *Red Book* for additional information.

IM route is the preferred route by diluting each vial with 1.25 mL of diluent for a 100 U/mL concentration. **Avoid** IM injection into the gluteal region due to risk for sciatic nerve damage and **do not exceed** age-specific **single max. IM injection volume.** For IV administration, dilute each vial with 2.5 mL of diluent for a 50 U/mL concentration. IV doses are administered over 3–5 min.

## VASOPRESSIN

Pitressin and various generics, 8-Arginine Vasopressin

***Antidiuretic hormone analog***

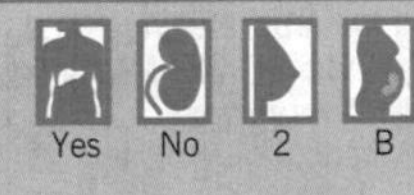


**Injection:** 20 U/mL (aqueous) (0.5, 1, 10 mL); contains 0.5% chlorobutanol

*Continued*

For explanation of icons, see p. 698.

VASOPRESSIN *continued*

***Diabetes insipidus:*** Titrate dose to effect.
***SC/IM:***
***Child:*** 2.5–10 U BID–QID
***Adult:*** 5–10 U BID–QID
***Continuous infusion (adult and child):*** Start at 0.5 milliunit/kg/hr (0.0005 U/kg/hr). Double dosage every 30 min PRN up to **max. dose** of 10 milliunit/kg/hr (0.01 U/kg/hr).

***Growth hormone and corticotropin provocative tests:***
***Child:*** 0.3 U/kg IM; **max. dose:** 10 U
***Adult:*** 10 U IM

***GI hemorrhage (IV):***
***Child:*** Start at 0.002–0.005 U/kg/min. Increase dose as needed to **max. dose** of 0.01 U/kg/min.
***Adult:*** Start at 0.2–0.4 U/min. Increase dose as needed to **max. dose** of 0.9 U/min.

***Cardiac arrest, ventricular fibrillation and pulseless ventricular tachycardia:***
***Child (use following 2 doses of epinephrine; limited data):*** 0.4 U/kg IV × 1
***Adult:*** 40 U IV × 1

**Use with caution** in seizures, migraine, asthma, and renal, cardiac, or vascular diseases. Side effects include tremor, sweating, vertigo, abdominal discomfort, nausea, vomiting, urticaria, anaphylaxis, hypertension and bradycardia. May cause vasoconstriction, water intoxication and bronchoconstriction. Drug interactions: lithium, demeclocycline, heparin and alcohol reduce activity; carbamazepine, tricyclic antidepressants, fludrocortisone and chlorpropamide increase activity.

**Do not** abruptly discontinue IV infusion (taper dose). Patients with variceal hemorrhage and hepatic insufficiency may respond to lower dosages. Monitor fluid intake and output, urine specific gravity, urine and serum osmolality and sodium.

## VECURONIUM BROMIDE

Norcuron and various generics
***Nondepolarizing neuromuscular blocking agent***

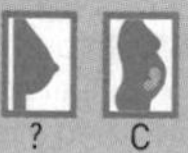


**Injection:** 10, 20 mg; diluent for reconstitution may contain benzyl alcohol

***Neonate:***
***Initial:*** 0.1 mg/kg/dose IV
***Maintenance:*** 0.03–0.15 mg/kg/dose IV Q1–2 hr PRN

***Infant (>7 wk–1 yr) (see remarks):***
***Initial:*** 0.08–0.1 mg/kg/dose IV
***Maintenance:*** 0.05–0.1 mg/kg/dose IV Q1 hr PRN

***>1 yr–adult (see remarks):***
***Initial:*** 0.08–0.1 mg/kg/dose IV
***Maintenance:*** 0.05–0.1 mg/kg/dose IV Q1 hr PRN; may administer via continuous infusion at 0.05–0.07 mg/kg/hr IV.

**Use with caution** in patients with renal or hepatic impairment, and neuromuscular disease. Dose reduction may be necessary in hepatic insufficiency. Infants (7 wk to 1 yr) are more sensitive to the drug and may have a longer recovery time. Children (1–10 yr) may require higher doses and more frequent supplementation than adults. Enflurane, isoflurane, aminoglycosides, beta-blockers, calcium channel blockers, clindamycin, furosemide, magnesium salts,

*Continued*

VECURONIUM BROMIDE *continued*

quinidine, procainamide, and cyclosporine may increase the potency and duration of neuromuscular blockade. Calcium, caffeine, carbamazepine, phenytoin, steroids (chronic use), acetylcholinesterases, and azathioprine may decrease effects. May cause arrhythmias, rash, and bronchospasm.

**Neostigmine, pyridostigmine or edrophonium are antidotes.** Onset of action within 1–3 min. Duration is 30–40 min. **See Chapter 1 for rapid sequence intubation.**

## VERAPAMIL

Isoptin, Isoptin SR, Calan, Calan SR, Verelan, Verelan PM, Covera-HS, and others

***Calcium channel blocker***

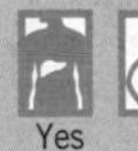
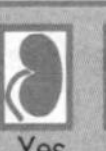
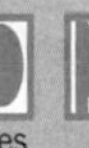
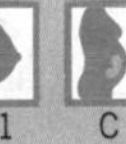

Yes Yes 1 C

**Tabs:** 40, 80, 120 mg
**Extended/sustained-release tabs:** 120, 180, 240 mg
**Extended/sustained-release caps:** 100, 120, 180, 200, 240, 300, 360 mg
**Injection:** 2.5 mg/mL (2, 4 mL)
**Oral suspension:** 50 mg/mL

***IV for dysrhythmias:*** Give over 2–3 min. May repeat once after 30 min.
***1–16 yr, for PSVT:*** 0.1–0.3 mg/kg/dose × 1; may repeat dose in 30 min; **max. dose:** 5 mg first dose, 10 mg second dose.
***Adult, for SVT:*** 5–10 mg (0.075–0.15 mg/kg) × 1; may administer second dose of 10 mg 15–30 min later.

***PO for hypertension:***
***Child:*** 4–8 mg/kg/24 hr ÷ TID
***Adult:*** 240–480 mg/24 hr ÷ TID–QID or divide QD–BID for sustained-release preparations.

**Contraindications** include hypersensitivity, cardiogenic shock, severe CHF, sick sinus syndrome, or AV block. **Use with caution** in hepatic and renal **(reduce dose in renal insufficiency; see Chapter 31)** impairment. **Due to negative inotropic effects, verapamil should not be used to treat SVT in an emergency setting in infants. Avoid IV use** in neonates and young infants due to apnea, bradycardia, and hypotension. Monitor ECG. **Have calcium and isoproterenol available to reverse myocardial depression.** May decrease neuromuscular transmission in patients with Duchenne's muscular dystrophy, and worsen myasthenia gravis.

Drug is a substrate of CYP 450 1A2, and 3A3/4; and an inhibitor of CYP 3A4 and P-gp transporter. Barbiturates, sulfinpyrazone, phenytoin, vitamin D and rifampin may decrease serum levels/effects of verapamil; quinidine and grapefruit juice may increase serum levels/effects. Verapamil may increase effects of beta-blockers (severe myocardial depression), carbamazepine, cyclosporine, digoxin, ethanol, fentanyl, lithium, nondepolarizing muscle relaxants, and prazosin.

## VITAMIN A

Aquasol A, Palmitate-A 5000, and many generics

***Vitamin, fat soluble***

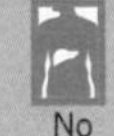
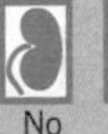
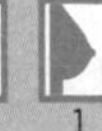
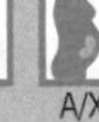

No No 1 A/X

**Caps:** 10,000 IU [OTC], 15,000 IU [OTC], 25,000 IU
**Tabs (Palmitate-A 5000):** 5,000 IU [OTC]
**Injection (Aquasol A):** 50,000 IU/mL (2 mL); contains polysorbate 80

*Continued*

For explanation of icons, see p. 698.

VITAMIN A *continued*

***U.S. RDA:*** See Chapter 21.
***Supplementation in measles (6 mo to 2 yr; see remarks):***
***6 mo–1 yr:*** 100,000 IU/dose QD PO × 2 days. Repeat 1 dose at 4 wk.
***1–2 yr:*** 200,000 IU/dose QD PO × 2 days. Repeat 1 dose at 4 wk.
***Malabsorption syndrome prophylaxis:***
***Child >8 yr and adult:*** 10,000–50,000 IU/dose QD PO of water miscible product.

**High doses above the U.S. RDA are teratogenic (category X).** The use of vitamin A in measles is recommended in children 6 mo to 2 yr of age who are either hospitalized or who have any of the following risk factors: immunodeficiency, ophthalmologic evidence of vitamin A deficiency, impaired GI absorption, moderate to severe malnutrition, and recent immigration from areas with high measles mortality. May cause GI disturbance, rash, headache, increased ICP (pseudotumor cerebri), papilledema and irritability. Large doses may increase the effects of warfarin. Mineral oil, cholestyramine and neomycin will reduce vitamin A absorption. See Chapter 21 for multivitamin preparations.

## VITAMIN $B_1$

See *Thiamine*

## VITAMIN $B_2$

See *Riboflavin*

## VITAMIN $B_3$

See *Niacin*

## VITAMIN $B_6$

See *Pyridoxine*

## VITAMIN $B_{12}$

See *Cyanocobalamin*

## VITAMIN C

See *Ascorbic Acid*

## VITAMIN D$_2$

See *Ergocalciferol*

## VITAMIN E/ALPHA-TOCOPHEROL

Aquasol E, Aquavit-E, Nutr-E-sol, and others

***Vitamin, fat soluble***

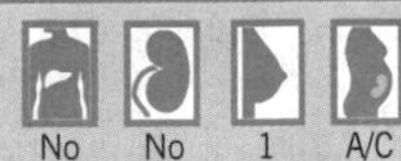


**Tabs [OTC]:** 100, 200, 400, 500, 800 IU
**Caps [OTC]:** 100, 200, 400, 1000 IU
**Drops (Aquasol E, Aquavit-E) [OTC]:** 50 IU/mL (12, 30 mL)
**Liquid (Nutr-E-sol) [OTC]:** 400 IU/15 mL (473 mL)

***U.S. RDA:*** See Chapter 21.
***Vitamin E deficiency, PO:*** Follow levels.
Use water miscible form with malabsorption.
***Neonate:*** 25–50 IU/24 hr
***Child:*** 1 IU/kg/24 hr
***Adult:*** 60–75 IU/24 hr
***Cystic fibrosis (use water miscible form):*** 5–10 IU/kg/24 hr PO QD; **max. dose:** 400 IU/24 hr.

Adverse reactions include GI distress, rash, headache, gonadal dysfunction, decreased serum thyroxine and triiodothyronine, and blurred vision. Necrotizing enterocolitis has been associated with large doses (> 200 units/24 hr). May increase hypoprothrombinemic response of oral anticoagulants (e.g., warfarin), especially in doses > 400 IU/24 hr.

One unit of vitamin E = 1 mg of DL-alpha-tocopherol acetate. In malabsorption, water miscible preparations are better absorbed. Therapeutic levels: 6–14 mg/L.

Pregnancy category changes to "C" if used in doses above the RDA. See Chapter 21 for multivitamin preparations.

## VITAMIN K

See *Phytonadione*

## VORICONAZOLE

VFEND

***Antifungal, triazole***

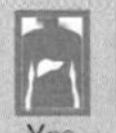

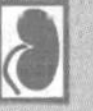

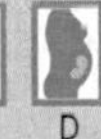


**Tabs:** 50, 200 mg; contains povidone
**Oral suspension:** 40 mg/mL (75 mL); contains sodium benzoate
**Injection:** 200 mg; contains 3200 mg sulfobutyl ether beta-cyclodextrin (SBECD)

*Continued*



For explanation of icons, see p. 698.

VORICONAZOLE *continued*

***IV (pediatric dosing not well established; see remarks):***
***Loading dose:*** 6 mg/kg/dose Q12 hr × 2 doses
***Maintenance dose:*** 4 mg/kg/dose Q12 hr; may be increased to 5 mg/kg/dose Q12 hr if needed or reduced to 3 mg/kg/dose Q12 hr if patient unable to tolerate.

***PO, > 12 yr (see remarks):***
***Invasive aspergillosis/Fusarium/Scedosporium/and other serious infections:***
***<40 kg:***
***Loading dose:*** 200 mg PO Q12 hr × 2 doses
***Maintenance dose:*** 100 mg PO Q12 hr; dose may be increased to 150 mg PO Q12 hr if response is inadequate.
***≥40 kg:***
***Loading dose:*** 400 mg PO Q12 hr × 2 doses
***Maintenance dose:*** 200 mg PO Q12 hr; dose may be increased to 300 mg PO Q12 hr if response is inadequate.
***Esophageal candidiasis (treat for a minimum 14 days and until 7 days after resolution of symptoms):***
***<40 kg:*** 100 mg PO Q12 hr
***≥40 kg:*** 200 mg PO Q12 hr

**Contraindicated** with concomitant administration with CYP 450 3A4 substrates that can lead to prolonged QTc interval (e.g., cisapride, pimozide, and quinidine); concomitant administration with rifampin, carbamazepine, barbiturates, ritonavir, efavirenz, and rifabutin (decreases voriconazole levels); concomitant administration with sirolimus, efavirenz, rifabutin, and ergot alkaloids (voriconazole increases levels of these drugs). Drug is a substrate and inhibitor for CYP 450 2C9, 2C19 (major substrate), and 3A4 isoenzymes. **Use with caution** in severe hepatic disease and galactose intolerance

Currently approved for use in invasive aspergillosis, candidal esophagitis, and *Fusarium* and *Scedosporium apiospermum* infections. Common side effects include GI disturbances, fever, headache, hepatic abnormalities, photosensitivity (**avoid** direct sunlight), rash (6%), and visual disturbances (30%). Serious but rare side effects include anaphylaxis, liver or renal failure, and Stevens-Johnson syndrome.

**Adjust dose in hepatic impairment** by decreasing only the maintenance dose by 50% for patients with a Child-Pugh Class A or B. **Do not use** IV dosage form for patients with GFR < 50 mL/min because of accumulation of the cyclodextrin excipient; switch to oral therapy if possible. Patients receiving concurrent phenytoin should increase their voriconazole maintenance doses (IV: 5 mg/kg/dose Q12 hr; PO: double the usual dose).

Administer IV over 1–2 hr with a **max. rate** of 3 mg/kg/hr at a concentration ≤ 5 mg/mL. Administer oral doses 1 hr before and after meals.

## WARFARIN
Coumadin and others
***Anticoagulant***

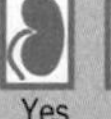
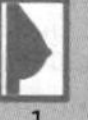
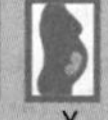

Yes Yes 1 X

**Tabs:** 1, 2, 2.5, 3, 4, 5, 6, 7.5, 10 mg
**Injection:** 5 mg

*Continued*

WARFARIN *continued*

***Infant and child (see remarks):*** To achieve an INR between 2 and 3.

***Loading dose on day 1:***
Baseline INR 1–1.3: 0.2 mg/kg/dose PO; **max. dose:** 10 mg/dose
Liver dysfunction or having undergone Fontan procedure: 0.1 mg/kg/dose PO; **max. dose:** 5 mg/dose

***Loading dose on days 2–4:***
If INR 1.1–1.3: Repeat day 1 loading dose
If INR 1.4–1.9: 50% of day 1 loading dose
If INR 2–3: 50% of day 1 loading dose
If INR 3.1–3.5: 25% of day 1 loading dose
If INR > 3.5: Hold doses until INR < 3.5 and restart according to the following maintenance dose guidelines.

***Maintenance dose:***
If INR 1.1–1.4: Increase previous dose by 20%
If INR 1.5–1.9: Increase previous dose by 10%
If INR 2–3: No change
If INR 3.1–3.5: Decrease previous dose by 10%
If INR > 3.5: Hold doses until INR < 3.5 and restart at 20% less than the last dose.

***Usual maintenance dose:*** ~0.1 mg/kg/24 hr PO QD; range: 0.05–0.34 mg/kg/24 hr. See remarks.

***Adult (see remarks):*** 5–10 mg PO QD × 2–5 days. Adjust dose to achieve the desired INR or PT. Maintenance dose range: 2–10 mg/24 hr PO QD.

**Contraindicated** in severe liver or kidney disease, uncontrolled bleeding, GI ulcers, and malignant hypertension. Acts on vitamin K–dependent coagulation factors II, VII, IX and X. Side effects include: fever, skin lesions, skin necrosis (especially in protein C deficiency), anorexia, nausea, vomiting, diarrhea, hemorrhage and hemoptysis.

Warfarin is a substrate for CYP 450 1A2, 2C8, 2C9, 2C18, 2C19 and 3A3/4. Chloramphenicol, chloral hydrate, cimetidine, delavirdine, fluconazole, fluoxetine, metronidazole, indomethacin, large doses of vitamins A or E, nonsteroidal anti-inflammatory agents, omeprazole, oxandrolone, quinidine, salicylates, SSRIs (e.g., fluoxetine, paroxetine, sertraline), sulfonamides, and zafirlukast may increase warfarin's effect. Ascorbic acid, barbiturates, carbamazepine, cholestyramine, dicloxacillin, griseofulvin, oral contraceptives, rifampin, spironolactone, sucralfate and vitamin K (including foods with high content) may decrease warfarin's effect.

Younger children generally require higher doses to achieve desired effect. A cohort study of 319 children found that infants < 1 yr required an average daily dose of 0.33 mg/kg and teenagers 11–18 yr required 0.09 mg/kg to maintain a target INR of 2–3. Children receiving Fontan cardiac surgery may require smaller doses than children with either congenital heart disease (without Fontan) or no congenital heart disease. (See *Chest* 2004;126:645S–687S and *Blood* 1999;94[9]:3007–3014 for additional information.)

Lower initial doses should be considered for patients with pharmacogenetic variations in CYP 2C9 (e.g., *2 and *3 alleles) and VKORC1 (e.g., 1639G>A allele) enzymes, elderly and/or debilitated patients, and patients with a potential to exhibit greater than expected PT/INR response to warfarin.

The INR (international ratio) is the recommended test to monitor warfarin anticoagulant effect. Monitor INR after 5–7 days of new dosage. The particular INR desired is based upon the indication and have been extrapolated from adults. An INR of 2–3 has been recommended for prophylaxis and treatment of DVT, pulmonary emboli, and bioprosthetic heart valves. An INR of 2.5–3.5 has been recommended for mechanical prosthetic heart valves and the prevention of recurrent systemic

*Continued*

For explanation of icons, see p. 698.

WARFARIN *continued*

emboli. If PT is monitored, it should be 1.5–2 times the control. Patients at high risk for bleeding may benefit from more frequent INR monitoring.

Onset of action occurs within 36–72 hr and peak effects occur within 5–7 days. IV dosing is equivalent to PO doses and is used in situations where oral dosing is not possible. **The antidote is vitamin K and fresh frozen plasma.**

## ZAFIRLUKAST

Accolate

***Anti-asthmatic, leukotriene receptor antagonist***

Yes No 3 B

**Tabs:** 10, 20 mg

***Asthma:***

***Child 5–11 yr:*** 10 mg PO BID

***Child ≥ 12 yr and adult:*** 20 mg PO BID

**Use with caution in hepatic insufficiency; 50%–60% reduction in clearance occurs in alcoholic cirrhosis**. May cause headache, dizziness, nausea, diarrhea, abdominal pain, vomiting, generalized pain, asthenia, myalgia, fever, LFT elevation, and dyspepsia. Eosinophilia, vasculitic rash, worsening pulmonary symptoms, cardiac complications, and/or neuropathy have been reported primarily in patients with oral steroid dose reduction. Hepatitis, hyperbilirubinemia, hepatic failure, and hypersensitivity reactions (e.g., urticaria, angioedema, and rashes) have also been reported.

Drug is a substrate for CYP 450 2C9 and inhibits CYP 450 2C9 and 3A4 isoenzymes. Erythromycin, terfenadine and theophylline decrease zafirlukast levels; aspirin increases levels. Zafirlukast may increase the effects of warfarin. Administer doses on an empty stomach, at least 1 hr prior or 2 hr after eating.

## ZIDOVUDINE

Retrovir, AZT

***Antiviral agent, nucleoside analogue reverse transcriptase inhibitor***

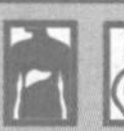
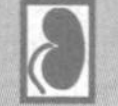
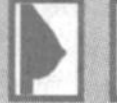
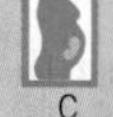

Yes Yes 3 C

**Caps:** 100 mg
**Tabs:** 300 mg
**Liquid:** 50 mg/5 mL (240 mL); contains 0.2% sodium benzoate
**Injection:** 10 mg/mL (20 mL)
**In combination with lamivudine (3TC) as Combivir:**
Tabs: 300 mg zidovudine + 150 mg lamivudine
**In combination with abacavir and lamivudine (3TC) as Trizivir:**
Tabs: 300 mg zidovudine + 300 mg abacavir + 150 mg lamivudine

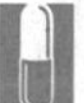

***HIV:*** See www.aidsinfo.nih.gov/guidelines.

***Prevention of vertical transmission:***

***14–34 wk of pregnancy:***

***Until labor:*** 600 mg/24 hr PO ÷ BID–TID

***During labor:*** 2 mg/kg/dose IV over 1 hr followed by 1 mg/kg/hr IV infusion until umbilical cord clamped.

*Continued*

ZIDOVUDINE *continued*

***Neonate and infant < 6 wk:*** 2 mg/kg/dose Q6 hr PO or 1.5 mg/kg/dose Q6 hr IV over 60 min. Begin within 12 hr of birth and continue until 6 wk of age.

***Premature infant:***

***<30 wk of gestation:*** 2 mg/kg/dose PO Q12 hr or 1.5 mg/kg/dose IV Q12 hr for first 4 wk of life; then increase dosing interval to Q8 hr thereafter.

***≥30 wk of gestation:*** 2 mg/kg/dose PO Q12 hr or 1.5 mg/kg/dose IV Q12 hr for first 2 wk of life; then increase dosing interval to Q8 hr thereafter. Dosage interval may be further reduced to Q6 hr when the child reaches full term (40 wk postconceptional age [PCA]).

***Needle stick prophylaxis:*** 200 mg/dose PO TID or 300 mg/dose PO BID × 28 days. Use in combination with lamivudine 150 mg/dose PO BID, and indinavir 800 mg/dose PO TID × 28 days.

See www.aidsinfo.nih.gov/guidelines for additional remarks.

**Use with caution** in patients with impaired renal or hepatic function. Dosage reduction is recommended in severe renal impairment and may be necessary in hepatic dysfunction. Drug penetrates well into the CNS. Most common side effects include: anemia, granulocytopenia, nausea and headache (dosage reduction, erythropoietin, filgrastim/GCSF or discontinuance may be required depending on event). Seizures, confusion, rash, myositis, myopathy (use > 1 yr), hepatitis and elevated liver enzymes have been reported. Macrocytosis is noted after 4 wk of therapy and can be used as an indicator of compliance. Lactic acidosis and severe hepatomegaly with steatosis, including fatal cases, have been reported.

**Do not use** in combination with stavudine because of poor antiretroviral effect. Effects of interacting drugs include: increased toxicity (acyclovir, trimethoprim-sulfamethoxazole); increased hematological toxicity (ganciclovir, interferon-alpha, marrow suppressive drugs); and granulocytopenia (drugs which affect glucuronidation). Methadone, atovaquone, cimetidine, valproic acid, probenecid and fluconazole may increase levels of zidovudine. Whereas, rifampin, rifabutin and clarithromycin may decrease levels.

**Do not administer IM**. IV form is incompatible with blood product infusions and should be infused over 1 hr (intermittent IV dosing). Despite manufacturer recommendations of administering oral doses 30 min prior to or 1 hr after meals, doses may be administered with food.

## ZINC SALTS

Galzin, Orazinc, Zincate, and others

***Trace mineral***

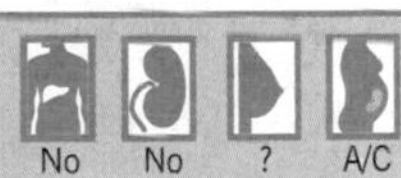


**Tabs as sulfate (Orazinc and others) [OTC], 23% elemental:** 66, 110, 200 mg
**Caps as sulfate (Orazinc, Zincate, and others) [OTC], 23% elemental:** 220 mg
**Tabs as gluconate, 14.3% elemental [OTC]:** 10, 15, 50 mg
**Caps as acetate** (Galzin), 25, 50 mg elemental per capsule
**Liquid as acetate:** 5 mg elemental Zn/mL
**Liquid as sulfate:** 10 mg elemental Zn/mL
**Injection as sulfate:** 1 mg, 5 mg elemental Zn/mL; may contain benzyl alcohol
**Injection as chloride:** 1 mg elemental Zn/mL (10, 50 mL)

*Continued*

For explanation of icons, see p. 698.

ZINC SALTS *continued*

***Zinc deficiency (see remarks):***
***Infant and child:*** 0.5–1 mg elemental Zn/kg/24 hr PO ÷ QD–TID.
***Adult:*** 25–50 mg elemental Zn/dose (100–220 mg Zn sulfate/dose) PO TID
***U.S. RDA:*** See Chapter 21.
For supplementation in parenteral nutrition, see Chapter 21.

Nausea, vomiting, GI disturbances, leukopenia, and diaphoresis may occur. Gastric ulcers, hypotension, and tachycardia may occur at high doses. Patients with excessive losses (burns) or impaired absorption require higher doses. Therapeutic levels: 70–130 mcg/dL.

May decrease the absorption of penicillamine, tetracycline and fluoroquinolones (e.g., ciprofloxacin). Drugs that increase gastric pH (e.g., $H_2$ antagonists and proton pump inhibitors) can reduce the absorption of zinc. Excessive zinc administration can cause copper deficiency.

Approximately 20%–30% of oral dose is absorbed. Oral doses may be administered with food if GI upset occurs. Pregnancy category is "A" for zinc acetate.

## ZONISAMIDE

Zonegran

***Anticonvulsant***

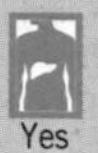
Yes
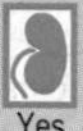
Yes
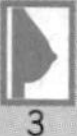
3
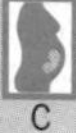
C

**Caps:** 25, 50, 100 mg

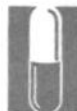

***Infant and child (data is incomplete):***
***Suggested dosing from a review of Japanese open-label studies for partial and generalized seizures:*** Start with 1–2 mg/kg/24 hr PO ÷ BID. Increase dosage by 0.5–1 mg/kg/24 hr Q2 wk to the usual dosage range of 5–8 mg/kg/24 hr PO ÷ BID.
***Recommended higher alternative dosing:*** Start with 2–4 mg/kg/24 hr PO ÷ BID–TID. Gradually increase dosage at 1- to 2-wk intervals to 4–8 mg/kg/24 hr; **max. dose:** 12 mg/kg/24 hr.
***Infantile spasms (regimen that was effective in a small study from Japan; additional studies are needed):*** Start with 2–4 mg/kg/24 hr PO ÷ BID. Then increase by 2–5 mg/kg/24 hr every 2–4 days until seizures disappear, up to a **max.** of 20 mg/kg/24 hr.

***>16 yr–adult:***
***Adjunctive therapy for partial seizures:*** 100 mg PO QD × 2 wk. Dose may be increased to 200 mg PO QD × 2 wk. Additional dosage increments of 100 mg/24 hr can be made at 2-wk intervals to allow attainment of steady-state levels. Effective doses have ranged from 100–600 mg/24 hr ÷ QD–BID; no additional benefit has been shown for doses > 400 mg/24 hr.

Since zonisamide is a sulfonamide, it is **contraindicated** in patients allergic to sulfonamides (may result in Stevens-Johnson syndrome or TEN). Common side effects of drowsiness, ataxia, anorexia, gastrointestinal discomfort, headache, rash and puritis usually occur early in therapy and can be minimized with slow dose titration. Urolithiasis has been reported. Children are at increased risk for hyperthermia and oligohydrosis especially in warm or hot weather. Suicidal behavior or ideation have been reported.

Although not fully delineated, therapeutic serum levels of 20–30 mg/L have been suggested as higher rates of adverse reactions have been seen at levels > 30 mg/L.

*Continued*

ZONISAMIDE *continued*

Zonisamide is a CYP 450 3A4 substrate. Phenytoin, carbamazepine, and phenobarbital can decrease levels of zonisamide.

**Use with caution** in renal or hepatic impairment; slower dose titration and more frequent monitoring is recommended. **Do not use** if GFR is < 50 mL/min. **Avoid** abrupt discontinuation or radical dose reductions. Swallow capsules whole and **do not** crush or chew.

## VII. BIBLIOGRAPHY


1. Package inserts of medications.
2. Drugs and Lactation Database (LactMed). United States National Library of Medicine, Toxicology Data Network. Available at http://toxnet.nlm.nih.gov/cgi-bin/sis/htmlgen?LACT.
3. Briggs GG et al: A Reference Guide to Fetal and Neonatal Risk: Drugs in Pregnancy and Lactation, 7th ed. Baltimore, Md, Lippincott Williams & Wilkins, 2005.
4. Pickering LK, ed. Red Book: 2006 Report of the Committee on Infectious Diseases, 27th ed. Elk Grove Village, Ill, American Academy of Pediatrics, 2006.
5. AIDSinfo: Information on HIV/AIDS Treatment, Prevention, and Research. U.S. Department of Health and Human Services. Available at www.hivatis.org.
6. Young TE, Mangum OB: Neofax: A Manual of Drugs Used in Neonatal Care, 20th ed. Montvale, NJ, Thomson Healthcare, USA, 2007.
7. Field JM et al, eds: Handbook of Emergency Cardiovascular Care for Healthcare Providers: Guidelines CPR ECC 2005. Dallas, Tex, American Heart Association, 2005.
8. McEvoy GK, Snow EK, eds: AHFS Drug Information. Stat!Ref electronic version. Bethesda, Md, American Society of Health-System Pharmacists. Available at www.ahfsdruginformation.com.
9. Facts and Comparisons: CliniSphere 2.0, electronic drug information service, Facts and Comparisons. St. Louis, Mo, Wolters Kluwer Health. Available at www.factsandcomparisons.com.
10. Micromedex Healthcare Series [Internet database]. Greenwood Village, Colo, Thomson Healthcare. Updated periodically.
11. Takemoto CK et al: Pediatric Dosage Handbook, 14th ed. Hudson, Ohio, Lexi-Comp, 2007.
12. National Institutes of Health: National Heart, Lung and Blood Institute—Expert Panel. Clinical Practice Guidelines: Guidelines for the Diagnosis and Management of Asthma. Available at www.nhlbi.nih.gov/guidelines/asthma/asthgdln.htm.
13. National High Blood Pressure Education Program Working Group on High Blood Pressure in Children and Adolescents: The Fourth Report on the Diagnosis, Evaluation, and Treatment of High Blood Pressure in Children and Adolescents. Pediatrics 2004;114:555–576.
14. Flynn JT, Daniels SR: Pharmacologic treatment of hypertension in children and adolescents. J Pediatr 2006;149:746–754.
15. Flynn JT, Pesko DA: Calcium channel blockers: Pharmacology and place in therapy of pediatric hypertension. Pediatr Nephrol 2000;15:302–316.
16. Monagle P et al: Antithrombotic therapy in children. Seventh ACCP Conference on Antithrombotic and Thrombolytic Therapy. Chest 2004;126:645S–687S.


For explanation of icons, see p. 698.

17. Yin T, Miyata T: Warfarin dose and the pharmacogenomics of CYP2C9 and VKORC1—rationale and perspectives. Thromb Res 2007;120:1–10.
18. American Thoracic Society: Targeted tuberculin testing and treatment of latent tuberculosis infection. Am J Respir Crit Care Med 2000;161:1376–1395.
19. Food and Drug Administration Safety Information and Adverse Event Reporting Program. Available at www.fda.gov/medwatch.

# Formulary Adjunct

*Jason W. Custer, MD*

## I. SYSTEMIC CORTICOSTEROIDS

### A. ENDOCRINE[1]

1. **Physiologic replacement:**
   a. Hydrocortisone: PO: 12–18 mg/m²/24 hr ÷ q8hr.
   b. Prednisolone: PO: 2.5–3.5 mg/m²/24 hr ÷ q12hr.

**Note** *See the body surface area nomogram (Fig. 30-1).*



2. **Stress dosing: For patients with adrenal insufficiency. Consider for patients on glucocorticoid therapy >2 weeks or patients in shock.**
   a. Ambulatory illnesses: Three times the physiologic replacement dose.
   b. Severe stress, including surgery: Hydrocortisone sodium succinate (Solu-Cortef): IV: 25–100 mg/m²/24 hr (give as continuous infusion). If IV access not available, administer 25 mg/m²/dose IM q6hr.
3. **Adrenal insufficiency:**
   a. Chronic: Provide physiologic replacement (see section I.A.1).
   b. Acute:
      (1) Fluids: Start hydration with 20 mL/kg $D_5$NS, then 60 mL/kg $D_5$NS administered over 24 hr.
      (2) Steroids: Hydrocortisone sodium succinate (Solu-Cortef), 50 mg/m² IV bolus, then begin continuous infusion over 24 hr as per "stress dosing" protocol.
4. **Congenital adrenal hyperplasia:**
   a. Non-salt losing: Provide physiologic replacement (see section I.A.1).
   b. Salt losing: Need to replace both mineralocorticoid and glucocorticoid.
      (1) Mineralocorticoid replacement: Fludrocortisone acetate (Florinef): PO: Usually 0.1 mg/m²/24 hr, with a range of 0.05–0.15 mg/24 hr. Dose adjusted for blood pressure and plasma renin activity.[1,2]
      (2) Glucocorticoid replacement (see section I.A.1) or stress dosing (see section I.A.2) as clinically indicated. Dose adjusted based on serum levels of steroid precursors.

### B. PULMONARY

1. **Airway edema:**
   a. Peri-extubation: Dexamethasone: PO/IV/IM: 0.5–2 mg/kg/24 hr ÷ q6hr. Begin 24 hr before extubation, and continue for 4–6 doses after extubation.
   b. Croup: Dexamethasone, 0.6 mg/kg/dose PO/IM/IV.[3,4] Recent studies suggest benefit of 0.6 mg/kg even in mild croup.[5] Inhaled budesonide, 2 mg q12hr (maximum: 4 doses).[6]

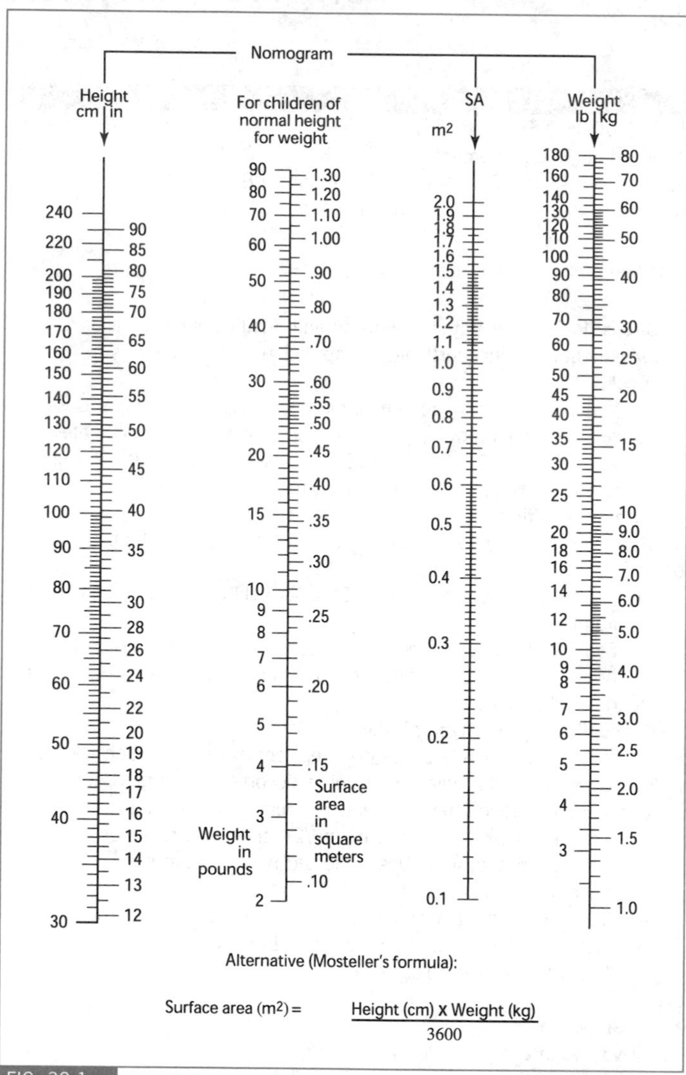


FIG. 30-1

Body surface area nomogram and equation. *(From Briars GL, Bailey BJ: Surface area estimation: Pocket calculator V nomogram. Arch Dis Child 1994;70:246–247.)*

2. **Acute asthma:**
a. Prednisone/prednisolone:
(1) PO: 2 mg/kg/24 hr ÷ q12–24 hr × 3 to 7 days.
(2) Maximum dose: 80 mg/24 hr.
b. Methylprednisolone:
(1) IV/IM: Load (optional) 2 mg/kg/dose × 1 dose.
(2) Maintenance: 2 mg/kg/24 hr ÷ q6–8hr.

### C. MISCELLANEOUS

1. **Antiemetic (chemotherapy induced): Dexamethasone.**
a. IV: Initial: 10 mg/m$^2$/dose (maximum dose: 20 mg).
b. Subsequent: 5 mg/m$^2$/dose q6hr.
2. **Cerebral edema: Dexamethasone.**
a. PO/IM/IV: Loading dose: 1–2 mg/kg/dose × 1 dose.
b. Maintenance: 1–1.5 mg/kg/24 hr ÷ q4–6hr (maximum dose: 16 mg/24 hr).
3. **Spinal cord injury: Methylprednisolone.**
a. 30 mg/kg bolus dose over 15 min, followed 45 min later by a continuous infusion of 5.4 mg/kg/hr × 23 hr.[7,8] Should be administered within 8 hr of injury for efficacy.
b. Methylprednisolone does not appear to be of benefit in acute head injury.
4. **Bacterial meningitis:**[9]
a. Indications:
(1) Dexamethasone recommended for children >6 weeks of age with *Haemophilus influenzae* type b meningitis.
(2) Dexamethasone could be considered for children >6 weeks of age with pneumococcal meningitis; still controversial.
b. Dose: Dexamethasone: 0.15 mg/kg/dose IV q6hr × 48 hr. Ideally given with or just before first parenteral antibiotic dose. Initiation >4 hr after parenteral antibiotics unlikely to be effective. Do not delay antibiotic therapy because of steroid administration.
5. **Idiopathic thrombocytic purpura:**[10]
a. Indications: Clinical bleeding.
b. Dose: Pulse steroid therapy with dexamethasone, 20–25 mg/m$^2$ IV × 4 days.[9]
6. **Transfusion reactions: Methylprednisolone:** IV: 0.5–1 mg/kg before initiation of blood product transfusion in patients with known transfusion reaction.[11]

### D. DOSE EQUIVALENCE OF COMMONLY USED STEROIDS (Table 30-1)

## II. INHALED CORTICOSTEROIDS FOR AIRWAY INFLAMMATION (Table 30-2)

TABLE 30-1

**DOSE EQUIVALENCE OF COMMONLY USED STEROIDS***

| Drug | Glucocorticoid Effect Equivalent to 100 mg Cortisol PO | Mineralocorticoid (mg): Sodium Retention Effect Equivalent to 0.1 mg Florinef[†] |
|---|---|---|
| Cortisone | 125 | 20 |
| Cortisol (hydrocortisone) | 100 | 20 |
| Prednisone | 20 | 50 |
| Prednisolone | 15 | 50 |
| Methylprednisolone | 15–20 | No effect |
| Triamcinolone | 10–20 | No effect |
| 9α-Fluorocortisol | 6.5 | 0.1 |
| Dexamethasone | 1.5–3.75 | No effect |

*The doses give approximately equivalent clinical effects. When using this table, select equipotent doses based on glucocorticoid or mineralocorticoid effects, because this is different for each drug.
[†]Total physiologic replacement for salt retention is usually 0.1 mg Florinef, regardless of size.

Modified from Kappy MS et al (eds): The Diagnosis and Treatment of Endocrine Disorders in Childhood and Adolescence, 4th ed. Springfield, Ill, Charles C Thomas, 1994, 769.

TABLE 30-2

**ESTIMATED COMPARATIVE DAILY DOSAGES FOR INHALED CORTICOSTEROIDS**

| | Low Dose (µg/day) | | Medium Dose (µg/day) | | High Dose (µg/day) | |
|---|---|---|---|---|---|---|
| Drug | Adult | Child | Adult | Child | Adult | Child |
| Beclomethasone 40 or 80 µg/puff | 80–240 | 80–160 | 240–640 | 160–320 | >640 | >320 |
| Budesonide DPI 200 µg/inhalation | 200–600 | 200–400 | 600–1200 | 400–800 | >1200 | >800 |
| Flunisolide 250 µg/puff | 500–1000 | 500–750 | 1000–2000 | 1000–1250 | >2000 | >1250 |
| Fluticasone MDI: 44, 110, 220 µg/puff | 88–264 | 88–176 | 264–660 | 176–440 | >660 | >440 |
| Triamcinolone Acetonide 100 µg/puff | 400–1000 | 400–800 | 1000–2000 | 800–1200 | >2000 | >1200 |

*Note:* The most important determinant of appropriate dosing is clinician's judgment of patient's response to therapy. Clinician must monitor patient's response on several clinical parameters and adjust dose accordingly. Stepwise approach to therapy emphasizes that once control of asthma is achieved, the dose of medication should be carefully titrated to minimum dose required to maintain control, thus reducing the potential for adverse effect. Reference point for range of doses in children is data on the safety of inhaled corticosteroids in children; in general, suggest that dose ranges are equivalent to those of beclomethasone dipropionate 200–400 µg/day (*low dose*), 400–800 µg/day (*medium dose*), and >800 µg/day (*high dose*). Metered-dose inhaler (MDI) dosages are expressed as the *activator dose* (amount of drug leaving activator and delivered to the patient), which is the labeling required in the United States. Dry-powder inhaler (DPI) doses are expressed as the amount of drug in the inhaler after activation. See formulary for brand names and side effects.

From Expert Panel Report II. Guidelines for the Diagnosis and Management of Asthma—Update on Selected Topics 2002. National Institutes of Health Pub. No. 02-5075. Bethesda, Md, National Asthma Education and Prevention Program, 2002.

## III. TOPICAL CORTICOSTEROIDS

### A. POTENCY

Table 30-3 provides a listing of topical steroids from the most potent (group I) to the least potent (group VII). Use intermediate- and low-potency steroids (groups IV–VII) for pediatric patients. Topical steroid use is contraindicated in the treatment of varicella.

### B. CAUTIONS

1. **Occlusive dressings (including waterproof diapers) increase systemic absorption of topical steroids; should not be used with high-potency preparations.**
2. **Topical steroids should be used with caution in intertriginous areas and on the face.**

### C. APPLICATION

Apply once or twice daily. Penetration of the skin is greatest with ointments, with decreasing effectiveness in gels, creams, and lotions. Prolonged use may result in cutaneous and systemic side effects.

### D. COVERAGE

A gram of topical cream or ointment should cover a 10 × 10-cm area. A 30- to 60-g tube will cover the entire body of an adult once.



## IV. INSULIN (Table 30-4)

For the management of diabetic ketoacidosis, see Chapter 10.

## V. PANCREATIC ENZYME SUPPLEMENTS (Table 30-5)

## VI. COMMON INDUCERS AND INHIBITORS OF THE CYTOCHROME P450 SYSTEM (Table 30-6)

## VII. OPHTHALMIC DRUGS (Table 30-7)

## VIII. PSYCHIATRIC DRUG FORMULARY (Table 30-8)

## IX. CHEMOTHERAPEUTIC AGENTS (Table 30-9)

## X. OXIDIZING AGENTS AND GLUCOSE-6-PHOSPHATE DEHYDROGENASE (G6PD) DEFICIENCY (Box 30-1)

*Text continued on p. 1051*

TABLE 30-3

**TOPICAL STEROID POTENCY RANKING (I—MOST POTENT, VII—LEAST POTENT)**

| Brand | Generic Name | Size |
|---|---|---|
| I | | |
| Temovate cr, ot 0.05% | Clobetasol propionate | 15, 30, 45 g |
| Diprolene ot, cr 0.05% | Betamethasone dipropionate | 15, 50 g |
| Psorcon ot 0.05% | Diflorasone diacetate | 15, 30, 60 g |
| Ultravate cr, ot 0.05% | Halobetasol dipropionate | 15, 45 g |
| II | | |
| Cyclocort ot 0.1% | Amcinonide | 15, 30, 60 g |
| Diprosone ot 0.05% | Betamethasone dipropionate | 15, 50 g |
| Elocon ot 0.1% | Mometasone furoate | 15, 45 g |
| Florone ot 0.05% | Diflorasone diacetate | 15, 30, 60 g |
| Halog cr, ot, sl 0.1% | Halcinonide | cr, ot: 15, 30, 60, 240 g<br>sl: 20, 60 mL |
| Lidex cr, gl, ot, sl 0.05% | Fluocinonide | 15, 30, 60, 120 g<br>sl: 20, 60 mL |
| Maxiflor ot 0.05% | Diflorasone diacetate | 15, 30, 60 g |
| Maxivate cr, ot 0.05% | Betamethasone dipropionate | 15, 45 g |
| Topicort cr, ot 0.25% | Desoximetasone | 15, 60 g |
| Topicort gl 0.05% | Desoximetasone | 15, 60 g |
| III | | |
| Aristocort A ot 0.1% | Triamcinolone acetonide | 15, 60 g |
| Cyclocort cr, lt 0.1% | Amcinonide | cr: 15, 30, 60 g<br>lt: 20, 60 mL |
| Diprosone cr 0.05% | Betamethasone dipropionate | 15, 45 g |
| Florone cr 0.05% | Diflorasone diacetate | 15, 30, 60 g |
| Lidex-E cr 0.05% | Fluocinonide | 15, 30, 60, 120 g |
| Maxiflor cr 0.05% | Diflorasone diacetate | 15, 30, 60 g |
| Maxivate lt 0.05% | Betamethasone dipropionate | 60 mL |
| Valisone ot 0.1% | Betamethasone valerate | 14, 45 g |
| IV | | |
| Aristocort ot 0.1% | Triamcinolone acetonide | 15, 60 g |
| Cordran ot 0.05% | Flurandrenolide | 15, 30, 60, 225 g |
| Elocon cr, lt 0.1% | Mometasone furoate | cr: 15, 45 g<br>lt: 30, 60 mL |
| Kenalog cr, ot 0.1% | Triamcinolone acetonide | 15, 60, 80, 240 g |
| Kenalog aerosol 0.2% | Triamcinolone acetonide | 63 mL |
| Dermatop cr, ot 0.1% | Prednicarbate | 15, 60 g |
| Synalar ot 0.025% | Fluocinolone acetonide | 20, 60 g |
| Topicort LP cr 0.05% | Desoximetasone | 15, 60 g |

*Note:* There are other topical steroid preparations containing dexamethasone, flumethasone, prednisolone, and methylprednisolone.

Cr, cream; gl, gel; lt, lotion; ot, ointment; sl, solution.

From Ferndale Laboratories, Ferndale, Michigan.

*Continued*

TABLE 30-3
TOPICAL STEROID POTENCY RANKING
(I—MOST POTENT, VII—LEAST POTENT)—cont'd

| Brand | Generic Name | Size |
|---|---|---|
| **V** | | |
| Cordran cr 0.05% | Flurandrenolide | 15, 30, 60 g |
| Kenalog lt 0.1% | Triamcinolone acetonide | 15, 60 mL |
| Kenalog ot 0.025% | Triamcinolone acetonide | 15, 60, 80, 240 g |
| Locoid cr, ot 0.1% | Hydrocortisone butyrate | 15, 45 g |
| Synalar cr 0.025% | Fluocinolone acetonide | 15, 60 g |
| Tridesilon ot 0.05% | Desonide | 15, 60 g |
| Valisone cr, lt 0.1% | Betamethasone valerate | cr: 15, 45, 110, 430 g<br>lt: 20, 60 mL |
| Westcort cr, ot 0.2% | Hydrocortisone valerate | ot: 15, 45, 60 g<br>cr: 15, 45, 60, 120 g |
| **VI** | | |
| Aclovate cr, ot 0.05% | Alclometasone dipropionate | 15, 45 g |
| Aristocort cr 0.1% | Triamcinolone acetonide | 15, 60 g |
| Kenalog cr, lt 0.025% | Triamcinolone acetonide | cr: 15, 60, 80<br>lt: 60 mL |
| Locoid sl 0.1% | Hydrocortisone butyrate | 20, 60 mL |
| Locorten cr 0.03% | Flumetasone pivalate | 15, 60 g |
| Synalar cr, sl 0.01% | Fluocinolone acetonide | cr: 15, 45, 60 g<br>sl: 20, 60 mL |
| Tridesilon cr 0.05% | Desonide | 15, 60 g |
| **VII** | | |
| Hytone cr, ot, lt 1% | Hydrocortisone | cr, ot: 30 g<br>lt: 120 mL |
| Hytone cr, ot, lt 2.5% | Hydrocortisone | cr, ot: 30 g<br>lt: 60 mL |

TABLE 30-4

CURRENTLY AVAILABLE INSULIN PRODUCTS

| Insulin* | Onset | Peak | Effective Duration |
|---|---|---|---|
| **Rapid acting** | 5–15 min | 30–90 min | 5 hr |
| Lispro (Humalog) | | | |
| Aspart (NovoLog) | | | |
| Glulisine (Apidra) | | | |
| **Short acting** | 30–60 min | 2–3 hr | 5–8 hr |
| Regular U100 | | | |
| Regular U500 (concentrated) | | | |
| Buffered regular (Velosulin) | | | |
| **Intermediate acting** | 2–4 hr | 4–10 hr | 10–16 hr |
| Isophane insulin (NPH, Humulin N/Novolin N) | | | |
| **Long acting** | | | |
| Glargine (Lantus) | 2–4 hr† | No peak | 20–24 hr |
| Detemir (Levemir) | Slow | 6–8 hr | 6–24 hr (dose-related) |
| **Premixed** | | | |
| 70% NPH/30% regular (Humulin 70/30) | 30–60 min | Dual | 10–16 hr |
| 50% NPH/50% regular (Humulin 50/50) | 30–60 min | Dual | 10–16 hr |
| 75% NPL/25% lispro (Humalog Mix 75/25) | 5–15 min | Dual | 10–16 hr |
| 70% NPA/30% aspart (NovoLog Mix 70/30) | 5–15 min | Dual | 10–16 hr |

*Assuming 0.1–0.2 U/kg per injection. Onset and duration vary significantly by injection site.

†Time to steady state.

L, lente; NPA, insulin aspart protamine (neutral protamine aspart); NPH, neutral protamine Hagedom; NPL, insulin lispro protamine (neutral protamine lispro).

Adapted with permission from American Diabetes Association: Practical Insulin: A Handbook for Prescribing Providers, 2nd ed. American Diabetes Association, 2007.

TABLE 30-5
**PANCRELIPASE***

| Product | Dosage Form[†] | Lipase (USP) Units | Amylase (USP) Units | Protease (USP) Units |
|---|---|---|---|---|
| Cotazym | C | 8000 | 30,000 | 30,000 |
| Cotazym-S | C, EC | 5000 | 20,000 | 20,000 |
| Creon | | | | |
| 5 | C, EC, DR, MS | 5000 | 16,600 | 18,750 |
| 10 | C, EC, DR, MS | 10,000 | 33,200 | 37,500 |
| 20 | C, EC, DR, MS | 20,000 | 66,400 | 75,000 |
| Pancrease | C, DR | 4500 | 20,000 | 25,000 |
| Pancrease MT | | | | |
| 4 | C, EC, MT | 4000 | 12,000 | 12,000 |
| 10 | C, EC, MT | 10,000 | 30,000 | 30,000 |
| 16 | C, EC, MT | 16,000 | 48,000 | 48,000 |
| 20 | C, EC, MT | 20,000 | 56,000 | 44,000 |
| Pancrecarb MS | | | | |
| 4 | C, EC, DR, MS | 4000 | 25,000 | 25,000 |
| 8 | C, EC, DR, MS | 8000 | 40,000 | 45,000 |
| 16 | C, EC, DR, MS | 16,000 | 52,000 | 52,000 |
| Ultrase | C, EC, MS | 4500 | 20,000 | 25,000 |
| Ultrase MT | | | | |
| 12 | C, EC, MT | 12,000 | 39,000 | 39,000 |
| 18 | C, EC, MT | 18,000 | 58,500 | 58,500 |
| 20 | C, EC, MT | 20,000 | 65,000 | 65,000 |
| Viokase | P (¼ tsp = 0.7 g) | 16,800/0.7 g | 70,000/0.7 g | 70,000/0.7 g |
| | T | 8000 | 30,000 | 30,000 |
| Zymase | C | 12,000 | 24,000 | 24,000 |

*See Formulary for side effects associated with administration. Avoid generics; they have been associated with treatment failure.

†Dosage forms: Capsule (C), delayed release (DR), enteric-coated (EC), microsphere (MS), minitab (MT), powder (P), tablet (T).

Modified from Taketomo CK et al: American Pharmaceutical Association Pediatric Dosage Handbook. Hudson, Ohio, Lexi-Comp, 1998, and Solvay Pharmaceuticals, Inc. 1994: Fact and Comparisons: September 1998, Scandipharm Product Information, July 1994 and May 1995.

TABLE 30-6

## INDUCERS AND INHIBITORS OF THE CYTOCHROME P450 SYSTEM

| Isoenzyme | Substrates (Drugs Metabolized by Isoenzyme) | Inhibitors | Inducers |
|---|---|---|---|
| CYP1A2 | Caffeine, tacrine, theophylline, lidocaine, R-warfarin | Cimetidine, ciprofloxacin, erythromycin, tacrine | Omeprazole, smoking, phenobarbital |
| CYP2B6 | Cocaine, ifosfamide, cyclophosphamide | Chloramphenicol | Phenobarbital |
| CYP2C9/10 | S-warfarin, phenytoin, tolbutamide, diclofenac, piroxicam | Amiodarone, fluconazole, lovastatin | Rifampin, phenobarbital |
| CYP2C19 | Diazepam, omeprazole, mephenytoin | Fluvoxamine, fluoxetine, omeprazole, felbamate | Rifampin, phenobarbital |
| CYP2D6 | Codeine, haloperidol, dextromethorphan, tricyclic antidepressants, phenothiazines, metoprolol, propranolol (4-OH), venlafaxine, risperidone, encainide, paroxetine, sertraline | Quinidine, fluoxetine, sertraline, amiodarone, propoxyphene | None known |
| CYP2E1 | Acetaminophen, alcohol | Disulfiram | Isoniazid, alcohol |
| CYP3A3/4 | Nifedipine, verapamil, cyclosporine, carbamazepine, terfenadine, cisapride, astemizole, tacrolimus, midazolam, alfentanil, diazepam, loratadine, ifosfamide, cyclophosphamide, ritonavir, indinavir | Erythromycin, cimetidine, clarithromycin, fluvoxamine, fluoxetine, ketoconazole, itraconazole, grapefruit juice, metronidazole, ritonavir, indinavir, mibefradil | Rifampin, phenytoin, phenobarbital, carbamazepine |

*Note:* The cytochrome P450 enzyme system is composed of different isoenzymes. Each isoenzyme metabolizes a unique group of drugs or substrates. When an ***inhibitor*** of a particular isoenzyme is introduced, the serum concentration of any drug or ***substrate*** metabolized by that particular isoenzyme will ***increase***. When an ***inducer*** of a particular isoenzyme is introduced, the serum concentration of drugs or ***substrates*** metabolized by that particular isoenzyme will ***decrease***.
CYP, cytochrome P450.

Modified from Hansten PD, Horn JR: Hansten and Horn's Drug Interaction Analysis and Management. Vancouver, BC, Canada, Applied Therapeutics, 1997.

TABLE 30-7

OPHTHALMIC DRUGS

| Brand Name | Ingredient | Indication | Dose |
|---|---|---|---|
| **Alocril** (≥3 yr)<br>Sol: 5 mL | Nedocromil sodium 2% (mast cell stabilizer), benzalkonium chloride | Allergic conjunctivitis | 1–2 gtt several times a day; remove contact lenses during therapy |
| **Alomide** (>2 yr)<br>Sol: 10 mL | Lodoxamide tromethamine 0.1% (mast cell stabilizer) | Vernal conjunctivitis and keratitis, keratoconjunctivitis | 1–2 gtt qid up to 3 mo |
| **Bleph-10** (>2 mo)<br>Sol: 2.5 mL, 5 mL, 15 mL<br>Oint: 3.5 g | Sulfacetamide sodium 10%<br>Sol: benzalkonium chloride;<br>Oint: phenylmercuric acetate | Conjunctivitis<br>Ophthalmic solution used as adjunct in trachoma | 1–2 gtt q2–3hr or small amount of oint q3–4hr for 7–10 days<br>Trachoma: 2 gtt q2hr w/ systemic therapy |
| **Corticosporin**<br>Oph susp: 7.5 mL<br><br>Oph oint: 3.5 g | Susp (per mL): polymyxin B sulfate (10,000 U), neomycin sulfate (0.35%), hydrocortisone (1%)<br>Oint (per g): polymyxin B sulfate (10,000 U), neomycin sulfate (0.35%), bacitracin zinc (400 U), hydrocortisone (1%) | Ocular inflammation associated with infection<br>**Contraindicated in fungal, viral, or mycobacterial infection**<br>Use with caution in glaucoma, or in corneal or scleral thinning | 1–2 gtt or small amount of oint tid–qid |
| **Garamycin**<br>Oph Sol 5 mL<br>Oph oint: 35 g | Gentamicin sulfate | Conjunctivitis | Severe infections: 2 gtt q1hr.<br>Mild-moderate infections: 1–2 gtt q4hr, or oint: bid–tid |
| **Ilotycin**<br>Oint: 1/8 oz | Erythromycin (5 mg/g) | Conjunctivitis<br>Prophylaxis of ophthalmia neonatorum | Small amount of oint ≥ qd<br>0.5–1 cm to each conjunctival sac |

From Prescribing Reference for Pediatricians. Spring–Summer 2001. Prescribing Reference, Inc., Haymarket Media Group, New York.

*Continued*

TABLE 30-7

OPHTHALMIC DRUGS—cont'd

| Brand Name | Ingredient | Indication | Dose |
|---|---|---|---|
| **Neosporin**<br>Oint: 3.75 g<br><br><br><br><br>Sol: 10 mL | Oint (per g): polymyxin B sulfate (10,000 U), bacitracin zinc (400 U), neomycin sulfate (3.5 mg)<br>Sol (per mL): polymyxin B sulfate (10,000 U), neomycin sulfate (1.75 mg), gramicidin (0.025 mg), 0.5% alcohol | Conjunctivitis | 1–2 gtt or small amount of oint bid–qid for 7–10 days<br>For acute infections, 1–2 gtt 2–4 × q1hr initially |
| **Ocuflox** (>1 yr)<br>Sol: 5 mL, 10 mL | Ofloxacin 0.3%, benzalkonium chloride | Conjunctivitis<br>Corneal ulcer | 1–2 gtt q2–4hr × 2 days, then qid × 5 days<br>1–2 gtt q30min while awake; at 4 hr and 6 hr during sleep × 2 days; then 1–2 gtt q1hr while awake × 5–7 days, then qid until treatment completion |
| **Poly-Pred**<br>Susp: 5 mL, 10 mL | Susp (per mL): prednisolone acetate (0.5%), neomycin sulfate (0.35%), polymyxin B sulfate (10,000 U) | Ocular inflammation associated with infection<br>**Contraindicated in fungal, viral, or mycobacterial infections**<br>Use with caution in glaucoma, or in corneal or scleral thinning | 1–2 gtt q3–4hr |
| **Polysporin**<br>Oint: 3.75 g | Oint (per g): polymyxin B sulfate (10,000 U), bacitracin zinc (500 U) | Conjunctivitis | 1–2 gtt q3–4hr; do not use >7 days |

TABLE 30-7
OPHTHALMIC DRUGS—cont'd

| Brand Name | Ingredient | Indication | Dose |
|---|---|---|---|
| **Polytrim** (>2 mo)<br>Sol: 10 mL | Trimethoprim sulfate (1 mg), polymyxin B sulfate (10,000 U/mL), benzalkonium chloride | Conjunctivitis | 1 gtt q3hr × 7–10 days |
| **Tobrex**<br>Sol: 5 mL<br>Oint: 3.5 g | Sol: tobramycin 0.3%, benzalkonium chloride<br>Oint: tobramycin 0.3%, chlorobutanol | Conjunctivitis | Severe infections: 2 gtt q1hr or 1/2″ of ointment q3–4hr<br>Mild-moderate infections: 1–2 gtt q4hr or 1/2″ of ointment bid–tid |
| **Vira-A** (>2 yr)<br>Oint: 3.5 g | Vidarabine 3% | Acute keratoconjunctivitis, recurrent epithelial keratitis caused by HSV 1 and 2 | 1/2″ in lower conjunctival sac 5 times daily (q3hr); continue for 7 more days (bid) after re-epithelialization |
| **Viroptic** (>6 yr)<br>Sol: 7.5 mL | Trifluridine 1%, contains thimerosal | Primary keratoconjunctivitis, recurrent epithelial keratitis caused by HSV 1 and 2 | 1 gtt q2hr while awake (maximum 9 gtt/day)<br>1 gtt q4hr × 7 days after re-epithelialization (maximum 21 days) |

TABLE 30-8

PSYCHIATRIC DRUG FORMULARY*

| Agent | Suggested Dose | Side Effects/Comments |
|---|---|---|
| **ANTIPSYCHOTICS** | | |
| Clozapine (Clozaril) | Starting dose: 6.25 mg/day<br>Titrate upward by 6.25 mg/wk in divided doses<br>Max dose: Prepubescent: 300 mg/day; adolescent: 400 mg/day | Obtain baseline EEG. Repeat EEG prn for sudden behavioral deterioration.<br>Monitor CBC. Because of potentially lethal hematologic changes, use is reserved for patients resistant to treatment. |
| Haloperidol (Haldol) | See Formulary | Obtain baseline ECG, HR, BP, LFTs. Check q3mo and with dose changes.<br>In general, anticholinergic effects include orthostatic hypotension, sedation, weight gain, dystonic reactions, tardive dyskinesia, akathisia, neuroleptic malignant syndrome. |
| Olanzapine (Zyprexa) | Prepubescent: 2.5 mg qd<br>Adolescent: 5 mg qd<br>Increase q3–4 days to maximum of 20 mg/day | See comments for haloperidol. |
| Risperidone (Risperdal) | Prepubescent: 2.5 mg qd<br>Adolescent: 0.5 mg/day qd–bid<br>Adult: 1 mg bid<br>Increase q wk 1 mg bid prn<br>Max dose: 3 mg bid | Renal/hepatic dosing.<br>See comments for haloperidol.<br>Hyperprolactinemia, amenorrhea, galactorrhea. |

*Note:* See formulary for stimulants (methylphenidate and amphetamine preparations), non-psychostimulants (clonidine), mood stabilizers (lithium, divalproex sodium, and carbamazepine), and tricyclic antidepressants (nortriptyline and imipramine).

BP, blood pressure; CBC, complete blood count; CNS, central nervous system; EEG, electroencephalogram; GI, gastrointestinal; HR, heart rate; LFT, liver function test; MAOIs, monoamine oxidase inhibitors.

From Physician's Desk Reference, 54th ed. Montvale, NJ, Medical Economics, 2000; Riddle MA et al: Anxiolytics, adrenergic agents and naltrexone. J Am Acad Child Adolesc Psychiatry 1999;38:546–556; Findling RL et al: The antipsychotics: A pediatric perspective. Pediatr Clin North Am 1998;45:1205–1232; Shoaf TL et al: Childhood depression: Diagnosis and treatment strategies in general pediatrics. Pediatr Ann 2001;30(3):130–171; Emslie GJ et al: Updates in the pharmacologic treatment of childhood depression. In Dunner DL, Rosenbaum JF (eds): The Psychiatric Clinics of North America Annual of Drug Therapy. Philadelphia, WB Saunders, 2000, 235–256; and Velosa JF, Riddle MA: Pharmacologic treatment of anxiety disorders in children and adolescents. Child Adolesc Psychiatr Clin North Am 2000;9:119–133.

*Continued*

TABLE 30-8
PSYCHIATRIC DRUG FORMULARY—cont'd

| Agent | Suggested Dose | Side Effects/Comments |
|---|---|---|
| **ANTIPSYCHOTICS—cont'd** | | |
| Quetiapine (Seroquel) | Prepubescent: 12.5–750 mg/day<br>Adolescent: 25–750 mg/day<br>Adult: 150–750 mg/day | See comments for haloperidol.<br>Baseline and semiannual ophthalmologic exam recommended; cataracts occurred in drug studies in canines. |
| Ziprasidone (Geodon) | 120 mg/day | Dyspepsia, constipation, nausea, abdominal pain, prolonged QTc.<br>Low incidence of extrapyramidal side effects. |
| **ANTIDEPRESSANTS/ANXIOLYTICS** | | |
| **Selective Serotonin Reuptake Inhibitors (SSRIs)** | | |
| Fluoxetine (Prozac) | Starting dose <12 yr: 5–10 mg/day<br>Maintenance: 10–30 mg/day<br>Starting dose ≥12 yr: 10 mg/day<br>Maintenance: 20–40 mg/day<br>Max dose: 60 mg/day | Do not use if MAOIs have been used in previous 14 days. Can cause GI upset, CNS side effects (headaches, nervousness, sedation), activate bipolar switchbacks. |
| Fluvoxamine (Luvox) | Starting dose <12 yr: 25 mg qhs<br>Maintenance: 100–200 mg/day<br>Starting dose ≥12 yr: 25–50 mg qhs<br>Maintenance: 150–300 mg/day | Contraindications: MAOIs, cisapride, terfenadine, astemizole.<br>Smoking increases levels. |
| Paroxetine (Paxil) | Starting dose <12 yr: 5–10 mg/day<br>Maintenance: 10–20 mg/day<br>Starting dose ≥12 yr: 10–20 mg/day<br>Maintenance: 20–40 mg/day | Purpura, hyponatremia, cytochrome P450 system (multiple drug interactions).<br>Also see comments for fluoxetine. |
| Sertraline (Zoloft) | Starting dose <12 yr: 25 mg/day<br>Maintenance: 100–150 mg/day<br>Starting dose ≥12 yr: 25–50 mg/day<br>Maintenance: 150–200 mg/day | See comments for fluoxetine. |
| Citalopram (Celexa) | <12 yr: 10–20 mg/day<br>≥12 yr: 10–40 mg/day | See comments for fluoxetine.<br>Multiple drug interactions. |

Continued

TABLE 30-8

PSYCHIATRIC DRUG FORMULARY—cont'd

| Agent | Suggested Dose | Side Effects/Comments |
|---|---|---|
| **ANTIDEPRESSANTS/ANXIOLYTICS—cont'd** | | |
| **Other Antidepressants/Anxiolytics** | | |
| Venlafaxine (Effexor) | Starting dose prepubescent: 37.5 mg/day<br>Maintenance: 75–150 mg/day<br>Starting dose adolescent: 37.5–75 mg/day<br>Maintenance: 150–300 mg/day | **Serotonin norepinephrine reuptake inhibitor.**<br>Nausea, dizziness, somnolence, constipation, xerostomia. |
| Nefazodone (Serzone) | Start 50 mg bid. Titrate to effectiveness by 50 mg q3 days<br>Max dose: Children: 300 mg/day; >12 yr: 600 mg/day | **5-HT blocker.**<br>Nausea, dizziness, priapism, agitiation, dry mouth, vision changes.<br>Contraindications: MAOIs, astemizole, cisapride, terfenadine. |
| Bupropion sustained release (Wellbutrin SR) | ≥18 yr: 100 mg bid × 3 days. If tolerated, increase by 100 mg tid (minimum q6hr)<br>Max daily dose: 450 mg/day<br>Max single dose: 150 mg/dose | CNS stimulation, weight change, dry mouth, headache, GI effects, insomnia.<br>Contraindications: Seizures, eating disorders, MAOIs. |
| Mirtazapine (Remeron) | ≥18 yr: Initially 15 mg qhs; increase q1–2wk | Obtain baseline CBC, LFTs; monitor periodically.<br>Side effects: Increased appetite, weight gain, dizziness, nausea, dry mouth, constipation, CNS effects (somnolence), hypotension/hypertension, elevated triglycerides, cholesterol. |
| Buspirone (BuSpar) | Prepubescent: 2.5–5 mg/day; increase by 2.5 mg/day q3–4 days<br>Max dose: 20 mg/day<br>Adolescent: 5–10 mg/day; increase by 5 mg/day q3–4 days<br>Max dose: 60 mg/day | **Anxiolytic.**<br>Tachycardia, headache, insomnia, confusion, dizziness, GI effects. |

TABLE 30-9

CHARACTERISTICS OF CHEMOTHERAPEUTIC AGENTS

| Drug Name (*Drug Class*) | Toxicity |
|---|---|
| **Asparaginase** (L-Asp, PEG-Asp, Elspar) *(Enzyme)* | DLT:* Pancreatitis, seizures, hypersensitivity reactions (both acute and delayed; less with PEG-modified), encephalopathy<br>Other: Nausea, pancreatitis, hyperglycemia, azotemia, fever, coagulopathy, sagittal sinus thrombosis and other venous thromboses, hyperammonemia<br>Long-term: Stroke |
| **Bleomycin** (Blenoxane) *(DNA strand breaker)* | DLT:† Anaphylaxis, pneumonitis<br>Other: Pain, fever, chills, mucositis, skin reactions<br>Long-term: Pulmonary fibrosis |
| **Busulfan** (Myleran) *(Alkylator)* | DLT: Myelosuppression, mucositis, seizures, hepatic veno-occlusive disease<br>Other: Hyperpigmentation, hypotension<br>Long-term: Infertility, endocardial fibrosis, secondary malignancy |
| **Carboplatin** (CBDCA, Paraplatin) *(DNA cross-linker)* | DLT:† Thrombocytopenia, nephrotoxicity<br>Other: Severe emesis, ototoxicity, peripheral neuropathy, optic neuritis (rare)<br>Long-term: Renal insufficiency, hearing loss |
| **Carmustine** (bis-chloronitrosourea, BCNU, BiCNU) *(Alkylator)* | DLT: Myelosuppression (prolonged cumulative)<br>Other: Vesicant; brownish discoloration of skin, hepatic and renal toxicity, severe emesis<br>Long-term: Pulmonary fibrosis, infertility, secondary malignancy |
| **Cisplatin** (*cis* platinum, CDDP, Platinol) *(DNA cross-linker)* | DLT:† Tubular and glomerular nephrotoxicity (related to cumulative dose), peripheral neuropathy<br>Other: Severe emesis, myelosuppression, ototoxicity, SIADH (rare), papilledema and retrobulbar neuritis (rare)<br>Long-term: Renal insufficiency, hearing loss, peripheral neuropathy |
| **Cladribine** (2-CdA, Leustatin) *(Nucleotide analogue)* | Myelosuppression, nausea and vomiting, headache, fever, chills, fatigue |
| **Cyclophosphamide** (CTX, Cytoxan) *(Alkylator prodrug)* | DLT: Leukopenia, cardiomyopathy<br>Other: Hemorrhagic cystitis (improved by mesna), emesis, direct ADH effect<br>Long-term: Infertility, cardiomyopathy, secondary malignancy, leukoencephalopathy |
| **Cytarabine** (Ara-C) *(Nucleotide analogue)* | DLT:† Myelosuppression, cerebellar toxicity<br>Other: Nausea and vomiting, anorexia, diarrhea, metallic taste, severe GI ulceration, conjunctivitis, lethargy, ataxia, nystagmus, slurred speech, respiratory distress rapidly progressing to pulmonary edema, influenza-like syndrome, fever |

*The dose-limiting toxicity (DLT) is the toxicity most likely to require adjustment or withholding of drug.

†Dose must be adjusted in renal insufficiency.

ADH, antidiuretic hormone; AML, acute myeloid leukemia; AST, aspartate transaminase; MAOI, monoamine oxidase inhibitors; SIADH, syndrome of inappropriate antidiuretic hormone.

*Continued*

TABLE 30-9

CHARACTERISTICS OF CHEMOTHERAPEUTIC AGENTS—cont'd

| Drug Name (*Drug Class*) | Toxicity |
|---|---|
| **Dacarbazine** (DIC, DTIC, imidazole carboxamide, DTIC-Dome) *(Alkylator)* | DLT: Myelosuppression<br>Other: Severe emesis, transaminitis, facial paresthesias (rare), rash<br>Long-term: Infertility |
| **Dactinomycin** (actinomycin D) *(Antibiotic)* | DLT: Myelosuppression, severe diarrhea<br>Other: Vesicant; nausea, acne, erythema, radiation recall, hepatic veno-occlusive disease<br>Long-term: Secondary malignancy |
| **Daunorubicin** (daunomycin) *(Anthracycline)* | DLT:[‡] Leukopenia, arrhythmia, congestive heart failure (related to cumulative dose)<br>Other: Stomatitis, emesis, vesicant, red urine, radiation recall<br>Long-term: Cardiomyopathy |
| **Doxorubicin** (Adriamycin) *(Anthracycline)* | Refer to daunorubicin |
| **Etoposide** (VP-16, VePesid) *(Topoisomerase inhibitor)* | DLT: Leukopenia, anaphylaxis (rare), transient cortical blindness<br>Other: Hyperbilirubinemia, transaminitis, peripheral neuropathy (rare), hypotension<br>Long-term: Secondary malignancy (AML) |
| **Fludarabine** (Fludara) *(Nucleotide analogue)* | Myelosuppression[†], anorexia, increased AST, somnolence, fatigue<br>Long-term: Peripheral neuropathy, immune suppression |
| **Fluorouracil** (5-FU, Adrucil) *(Nucleotide analogue)* | DLT: Myelosuppression (reversible with uridine), mucositis, severe diarrhea<br>Other: Hand-foot syndrome, tear duct stenosis, hyperpigmentation, loss of nails, cerebellar syndrome (rare), anaphylaxis |
| **Hydroxyurea** (Hydrea) *(Ribonucleotide reductase inhibitor)* | DLT: Leukopenia, pulmonary edema (rare)<br>Other: Megaloblastic erythropoiesis, hyperpigmentation, azotemia, transaminitis, radiation recall |
| **Idarubicin** (idamycin) *(Anthracycline)* | DLT: Arrhythmia, cardiomyopathy (cumulative)<br>Other: Vesicant; diarrhea, mucositis, enterocolitis<br>Long-term: Cardiomyopathy |
| **Ifosfamide** (isophosphamide, Ifex) *(Alkylator prodrug)* | DLT:[†] Myelosuppression, encephalopathy (rarely progressing to death), renal tubular damage<br>Other: Emesis, hemorrhagic cystitis (improved with mesna), direct ADH effect<br>Long-term: Secondary malignancy, infertility |
| **Lomustine** (CCNU) *(Alkylating agent)* | Myelosuppression, nausea and vomiting, disorientation, fatigue<br>Long-term: Secondary malignancy (leukemia) |

[‡]Dose must be adjusted in hyperbilirubinemia.

*Continued*

TABLE 30-9

CHARACTERISTICS OF CHEMOTHERAPEUTIC AGENTS—cont'd

| Drug Name (*Drug Class*) | Toxicity |
|---|---|
| **Mechlorethamine** (nitrogen mustard, $HN_2$ [mustine], Mustargen) (*Alkylator*) | DLT: Leukopenia, thrombocytopenia<br>Other: Severe emesis; vesicant (antidote: sodium thiosulfate); peptic ulcer (rare)<br>Long-term: Secondary malignancy, infertility |
| **Melphalan** (L-PAM, Alkeran) (*Alkylator*) | DLT: Prolonged leukopenia (6–8 wk), mucositis, diarrhea<br>Other: Pruritus, emesis<br>Long-term: Pulmonary fibrosis, secondary malignancy, infertility, cataracts |
| **Mercaptopurine** (6-MP) (*Nucleotide analogue*) | DLT: Hepatic necrosis and encephalopathy (especially doses >2.5 mg/kg/day)<br>Other: Vesicant; headache, diarrhea, nausea<br>Long-term: Cirrhosis |
| **Methotrexate** (MTX, amethopterin, Folex, Mexate) (*Folate antagonist*) | DLT:[§] Stomatitis, diarrhea, renal dysfunction, encephalopathy, cortical blindness, ventriculitis (intrathecal)<br>Other: Photosensitivity, erythema, excessive lacrimation, transaminitis<br>Long-term: Leukoencephalopathy, cirrhosis, pulmonary fibrosis, aseptic necrosis of bone, osteoporosis |
| **Mitoxantrone** (DHAD, DHAQ, dihydroxyanthracenedione dihydrochloride, Novantrone) (*DNA intercalator*) | DLT: Myelosuppression, cumulative cardiomyopathy<br>Other: Stomatitis, blue-green urine and serum<br>Long-term: Cardiomyopathy |
| **Paclitaxel** (Taxol) (*Tubulin inhibitor*) | DLT: Neutropenia, anaphylaxis, ventricular tachycardia and myocardial infarction (rare)<br>Other: Mucositis, peripheral neuropathy, bradycardia, hypertriglyceridemia<br>Long-term: Too soon to know |
| **Procarbazine** (Matulane) (*Alkylator*) | DLT: Encephalopathy; pancytopenia, especially thrombocytopenia<br>Other: Emesis, paresthesias, dizziness, ataxia, hypotension; adverse effects with tyramine-rich foods, ethanol, MAOIs, meperidine, and many other drugs<br>Long-term: Secondary malignancy, infertility |
| **Teniposide** (VM-26) (*Topoisomerase inhibitor*) | DLT: Leukopenia, anaphylaxis (rare)<br>Other: Hyperbilirubinemia, transaminitis<br>Long-term: Secondary malignancy (AML) |
| **Thioguanine** (6-TG, 6-thioguanine) (*Nucleotide analogue*) | DLT: Myelosuppression, bronchospasm and shock with rapid IV infusion, stomatitis, diarrhea<br>Other: Hyperbilirubinemia, transaminitis, decreased vibratory sensation, ataxia, dermatitis |

[§]Dose must be adjusted in renal insufficiency and in patients with third spacing.

Continued

TABLE 30-9

| CHARACTERISTICS OF CHEMOTHERAPEUTIC AGENTS—cont'd | |
|---|---|
| Drug Name (*Drug Class*) | Toxicity |
| **Thiotepa**<br>*(Alkylating agent)* | DLT: Cognitive impairment, leukopenia<br>Other: Increased AST, headache, dizziness, rash, desquamation<br>Long-term: Secondary malignancy (leukemia), impaired fertility, lower extremity weakness |
| **Topotecan** (Hycamptin)<br>*(Topoisomerase inhibitor)* | DLT: Leukopenia, peripheral neuropathy (rare), Horner syndrome<br>Other: Nausea, diarrhea, transaminitis, headache<br>Long-term: Too soon to know |
| **Vinblastine** (VBL, vincaleukoblastine, Velban)<br>*(Microtubule inhibitor)* | DLT:[‡] Leukopenia<br>Other: Vesicant (improved by hyaluronidase and applied heat); constipation, bone pain (especially in the jaw), peripheral and autonomic neuropathy, SIADH (rare) |
| **Vincristine** (VCR, Oncovin)<br>*(Microtubule inhibitor)* | DLT:[‡] Peripheral and autonomic neuropathy, encephalopathy<br>Other: Vesicant; bone pain, constipation, SIADH (rare) |
| CHEMOTHERAPY ADJUNCTS | |
| **Amifostine** | Indication: Reduces the toxicity of radiation and alkylating agents<br>Side effects: Hypotension (62%), severe nausea and vomiting, flushing, chills, dizziness, somnolence, hiccups, sneezing, hypocalcemia in susceptible patients (<1%), rigors (<1%), short-term reversible loss of consciousness (rare), mild skin rash |
| **Dexrazoxane** | Indication: Protective agent for doxorubicin-induced cardiotoxicity<br>Side effects: Myelosuppression |
| **Leucovorin** | Indication: Reduces methotrexate toxicity<br>Side effects: Allergic sensitization (rare) |
| **Mesna** | Indication: Reduces risk of hemorrhagic cystitis<br>Side effects: Headache, limb pain, abdominal pain, diarrhea, rash |

BOX 30-1

**OXIDIZING AGENTS AND G6PD DEFICIENCY**

| | |
|---|---|
| p-Aminosalicylic acid | Naphthalene* |
| Acetaminophen (Phenacetin)* | Nitrofurantoin (Furadantin) |
| Acetylsalicylic acid | Primaquine |
| Aniline dyes | Probenecid |
| Antipyrine | Sulfasalazine (Azulfidine) |
| Ascorbic acid† | Sulfacetamide (Sulamyd) |
| Chloramphenicol‡ | Sulfanilamide |
| Dapsone (diaminodiphenylsulfone) | Sulfisoxazole (Gantrisin)* |
| Fava beans | Sulfoxone* |
| Furazolidone (Furoxone) | Trisulfapyrimidine (Sultrin) |
| Henna | Vitamin K, water-soluble analogues only |
| Methylene blue* | |

*Note:* These drugs and chemicals may cause hemolysis of "reacting" (primaquine-sensitive) red blood cells (e.g., in patients with glucose-6-phosphate dehydrogenase [G6PD] deficiency).
*Only slightly hemolytic to G6PD A patients in very large doses.
†Hemolytic in G6PD Mediterranean but not in G6PD A or Canton.
‡In massive doses.



## REFERENCES


1. Kappy MS et al (eds): Diagnosis and Treatment of Endocrine Disorders in Childhood and Adolescence, 4th ed. Springfield, Ill, Charles C Thomas, 1994.
2. Migeon CJ, Wisniewski AB: Congenital adrenal hyperplasia owing to 21-hydroxylase deficiency: Growth, development, and therapeutic considerations. Endocrinol Metab Clin North Am 2001;30(1):193–206.
3. Geelhoed GC et al: Efficacy of a small dose of oral dexamethasone for outpatient croup: A double blind placebo controlled trial. BMJ 1996;313:140–142.
4. Rittichier KK, Ledwith CA: Outpatient treatment of moderate croup with dexamethasone: Intramuscular versus oral dosing. Pediatrics 2000;106:1344–1348.
5. Bjornson CL et al: A randomized trial of a single dose of oral dexamethasone for mild croup. NEJM 2004;351(13):1306–1313.
6. Roberts GW: Repeated dose inhaled budesonide versus placebo in the treatment of croup. J Pediatr Child Health 1999;35(2):170–174.
7. Bracken MB et al: A randomized controlled trial of methylprednisolone or naloxone in the treatment of acute spinal cord injury: Results of the Second National Acute Spinal Cord Injury Study. NEJM 1990;322(20):1405–1411.
8. Bracken MB: Pharmacological treatment of acute spinal cord injury: Current status and future projects. J Emerg Med 1993;11:43–48.
9. Pickering LK (ed): 2006 Red Book: Report of the Committee on Infectious Diseases, 27th ed. Elk Grove Village, Ill, American Academy of Pediatrics, 2006.
10. Adams DM et al: High dose oral dexamethasone therapy for chronic childhood idiopathic thrombocytopenic purpura. J Pediatr 1996;128:281–283.
11. Taketomo CK et al: American Pharmaceutical Association Pediatric Dosage Handbook. Hudson, Ohio, Lexi-Comp, 1998.

# Drugs in Renal Failure

*Rachel E. Rau, MD*

31

## I. DOSE ADJUSTMENT METHODS

### A. MAINTENANCE DOSE

In patients with renal insufficiency, the dose may be adjusted using the following methods:

1. **Interval extension (I):** Lengthen the intervals between individual doses, keeping the dose size normal. For this method, the suggested interval is shown.
2. **Dose reduction (D):** Reduce the amount of individual doses, keeping the interval between the doses normal. This method is particularly recommended for drugs in which a relatively constant blood level is desired. For this method, the percentage of the usual dose is shown.
3. **Interval extension and dose reduction (DI):** Lengthen the interval and reduce the dose.
4. **Interval extension or dose reduction (D, I):** In some instances, either the dose or the interval can be changed.

**Note** *These dose adjustments are for beyond the neonatal period. These dose modifications are only approximations. Each patient must be monitored closely for signs of drug toxicity, and serum levels must be measured when available. Drug dose and interval should be adjusted accordingly.*

### B. DIALYSIS

Quantitative effects of hemodialysis (He) and peritoneal dialysis (P) on drug removal are shown. *Y* indicates the need for a supplemental dose with dialysis. *N* indicates no need for adjustment. The designation *No* does not preclude the use of dialysis or hemoperfusion for drug overdose. *?* indicates no data available.

## II. ANTIMICROBIALS REQUIRING ADJUSTMENT IN RENAL FAILURE (Table 31-1)

## III. NONANTIMICROBIALS REQUIRING ADJUSTMENT IN RENAL FAILURE (Table 31-2)

*Text continued on p. 1076*

TABLE 31-1

ANTIMICROBIALS REQUIRING ADJUSTMENT IN RENAL FAILURE[1]

| | Pharmacokinetics | | | Adjustments in Renal Failure | | | | |
|---|---|---|---|---|---|---|---|---|
| Drug | Route of Excretion* | Normal $t_{1/2}$ (hr) | Normal Dose Interval | Method | CrCl (mL/min) | Dose | Interval | Supplemental Dose for Dialysis |
| Acyclovir (IV) | Renal | 2–3.5 | q8hr | DI | 25–50 | Nl | q12hr | Y (He) |
| | | | | | 10–25 | Nl | q24hr | N (P) |
| | | | | | <10 | 50% ↓ | q24hr | |
| Amantadine[†] | Renal | 10–28 | q12–24hr | DI | 30–50 | 50% ↓ | q24hr | N (He) |
| | | | | | 15–29 | 50% ↓ | q48–72hr | N (P) |
| | | | | | <15 | Nl daily dose | q7 days | |
| Amikacin | Renal | 1.5–3 | q8–12hr | I | Loading dose 5–7.5 mg/kg; subsequent doses are best determined by measurement of serum levels and assessment of renal insufficiency. | | | Y (He) Y (P) |
| Amoxicillin[‡] | Renal | 0.7–2 | q8–12hr | I | 10–30 | Nl | q12hr | Y (He) |
| | | | | | <10 | Nl | q24hr | N (P) |
| Amoxicillin/ clavulanate[‡] | Renal | 1 | q8–12hr | I | 10–30 | Nl | q12hr | Y (He) |
| | | | | | <10 | Nl | q24hr | N (P) |
| Amphotericin B | Renal (40% over 7 days) | Initial 15–48 hr Terminal 15 days | q24hr | D, I | Dosage adjustments are unnecessary with preexisting renal impairment; if decreased renal function is due to amphotericin B, daily dose can be decreased by 50% or dose given every other day. Therapy may be held until serum creatinine begins to decline. Can give 1–4 mg/L of peritoneal dialysis fluid ± low-dose IV therapy. | | | N (He) N (P) |
| Amphotericin B lipid complex (Abelcet) | Renal (1%) | 173 | q24hr | I | Renal toxicity is dose dependent. No firm guidelines for dose adjustments. | | | N (He) N (P) |

| | | | | | | | | |
|---|---|---|---|---|---|---|---|---|
| Amphotericin B, liposomal (AmBisome) | Renal (≤10%) | 100–153 | q24hr | I | No guidelines established. | | | N (He)<br>N (P) |
| Ampicillin[†] | Renal | 1–1.8 | q6–12hr | I | 10–30<br><10 | NI<br>NI | q6–12hr<br>q12hr | Y (He)<br>N (P) |
| Ampicillin/ sulbactam | Renal | 1–1.8 | q4–8hr | I | 15–29<br><15 | NI<br>NI | q12hr<br>q24hr | Y (He)<br>N (P) |
| Aztreonam | Renal (hepatic) | 1.3–2.2 | q6–12hr | D | 10–30<br><10 | 50% ↓<br>75% ↓ | NI<br>NI | Y (He)<br>N (P) |
| Cefaclor | Renal | 0.5–1 | q8–12hr | D | <10 | 50% ↓ | NI | Y (He)<br>Y (P) |
| Cefadroxil | Renal | 1–2 | q12–24hr | I | 10–25<br><10 | NI<br>NI | q24hr<br>q36hr | Y (He)<br>N (P) |
| Cefazolin | Renal | 1.5–2.5 | q8hr | I | 10–30<br><10 | NI<br>NI | q12hr<br>q24hr | Y (He)<br>N (P) |
| Cefdinir | Renal | 1.1–2.3 | q12–24hr | DI | <30 | 7 mg/kg/dose (children)<br>300 mg (adults) | q24hr<br>q24hr | Y (He)<br>N (P) |
| Cefepime[†] | Renal | 1.8–2.2 | q8–12hr | I | >50<br>10–50<br><10 | NI<br>NI<br>NI | q12hr<br>q16–24hr<br>q24–48hr | Y (He)<br>N (P) |
| Cefixime | Renal (hepatic) | 3–4 | q12–24hr | D | 21–60<br><20 | 25% ↓<br>50% ↓ | NI<br>NI | Y (He)<br>N (P) |

*Route in parentheses indicates secondary route of excretion.
[†]In adults; guidelines not established in children.
[‡]Should not use 875-mg tablet in patients with CrCl <30 mL/min.
CrCl, creatinine clearance; GFR, glomerular filtration rate; He, hemodialysis; Induct, induction; $K^+$, potassium; Maint, maintenance; $Na^+$, sodium; NI, normal; P, peritoneal dialysis; $t_{1/2}$, half-life.

*Continued*

TABLE 31-1

ANTIMICROBIALS REQUIRING ADJUSTMENT IN RENAL FAILURE—cont'd

| | Pharmacokinetics | | | Adjustments in Renal Failure | | | | |
|---|---|---|---|---|---|---|---|---|
| Drug | Route of Excretion* | Normal $t_{1/2}$ (hr) | Normal Dose Interval | Method | CrCl (mL/min) | Dose | Interval | Supplemental Dose for Dialysis |
| Cefotaxime | Renal | 1–1.5 | q6–12hr | D | <20 | 50% ↓ | NI | Y (He)<br>N (P) |
| Cefotetan | Renal (hepatic) | 3.5 | q12hr | I | 10–30<br><10 | NI<br>NI | q24hr<br>q48hr | Y (He)<br>N (P) |
| Cefoxitin | Renal | 0.75–1.5 | q4–8hr | I | 30–50<br>10–30<br><10 | NI<br>NI<br>NI | q8–12hr<br>q12–24hr<br>q24–48hr | Y (He)<br>N (P) |
| Cefpodoxime proxetil | Renal | 2.2 | q12hr | I | <30 | NI | q24hr | Y (He)[§]<br>N (P) |
| Cefprozil | Renal | 1.3 | q12–24hr | D | <30 | 50% ↓ | NI | Y (He)<br>N (P) |
| Ceftazidime | Renal | 1–2 | q8–12hr | I | 30–50<br>10–30<br><10 | NI<br>NI<br>NI | q12hr<br>q24hr<br>q24–48hr | Y (He)<br>Y (P) |
| Ceftibuten | Renal | 1.5–2.5 | q24hr | D | 30–49<br>5–29 | 50% ↓<br>75% ↓ | NI<br>NI | Y (He)<br>N (P) |
| Ceftizoxime | Renal | 1.6 | q6–12hr | I | 50–80<br>10–50<br><10 | NI<br>NI<br>NI | q8–12hr<br>q36–48hr<br>q48–72hr | Y (He)<br>N (P) |
| Cefuroxime (IV) | Renal | 1–2 | q8–12hr | I | 10–20<br><10 | NI<br>NI | q12hr<br>q24hr | Y (He)<br>N (P) |

| | | | | | | | | |
|---|---|---|---|---|---|---|---|---|
| Cephalexin | Renal | 0.5–2.5 | q6hr | I | 10–40 | NI | q8–12hr | Y (He) |
| | | | | | <10 | NI | q12–24hr | N (P) |
| Cephradine | Renal | 0.7–2 | q6–12hr | D, I | 10–50 | 50% ↓ | NI | Y (He) |
| | | | | | <10 | 75% ↓ | NI | N (P) |
| | | | | | *OR* | | | |
| | | | | | 25–50 | NI | q12hr | |
| | | | | | 10–25 | NI | q24hr | |
| | | | | | <10 | NI | q36hr | |
| Ciprofloxacin† | Renal (hepatic) | 3–5 | q8–12hr | D, I | <30 (IV) | 200–400 mg† | q18–24hr | Y (He) |
| | | | | | 30–50 (PO) | 250–500 mg† | q12hr | Y (P) |
| | | | | | <30 (PO) | 250–500 mg† | q18hr | |
| Clarithromycin | Renal/hepatic | 3–9 | q12hr | DI | <30 | 50% ↓ | q12–24hr | No data<br>Dose after He |
| Ertapenem† | Renal | 2.5–4 | q12–24hr | D | ≤30 | 50% ↓ | NI | Y (He) |
| Erythromycin | Hepatic (renal) | 1.5–2 | q6–12hr | D | <10 | 25%–50% ↓ | NI | N (He)<br>N (P) |
| Ethambutol | Renal (hepatic) | 2.5–3.6 | q24hr | I | 10–50 | NI | q24–36hr | Y (He) |
| | | | | | <10 | NI or reduced | q48hr | N (P) |
| Famciclovir† | Renal (hepatic) | 2–3 | 500 mg q8hr | DI | <u>*Herpes zoster treatment*</u>‡ | | | Y (He) |
| | | | | | 40–59 | 500 mg | q12hr | ? (P) |
| | | | | | 20–39 | 500 mg | q24hr | |
| | | | | | <20 | 250 mg | q24hr | |

‡For patients on hemodialysis, administer 3 times per week.

*Continued*

TABLE 31-1

ANTIMICROBIALS REQUIRING ADJUSTMENT IN RENAL FAILURE—cont'd

| | Pharmacokinetics | | | Adjustments in Renal Failure | | | | |
|---|---|---|---|---|---|---|---|---|
| Drug | Route of Excretion* | Normal $t_{1/2}$ (hr) | Normal Dose Interval | Method | CrCl (mL/min) | Dose | Interval | Supplemental Dose for Dialysis |
| Famciclovir—cont'd | | | | | *Recurrent genital herpes treatment*[†] | | | |
| | | | | | 40–59 | 500 mg | q12hr × 1 day | |
| | | | | | 20–39 | 500 mg | Single dose | |
| | | | | | <20 | 250 mg | Single dose | |
| | | | | | *Recurrent genital herpes suppression*[†] | | | |
| | | | | | 40–59 | 250 mg | q12hr | |
| | | | | | 20–39 | 125 mg | q12hr | |
| | | | | | <20 | 125 mg | q24hr | |
| | | | | | *Recurrent orolabial or genital herpes in HIV-infected patients*[†] | | | |
| | | | | | 40–59 | 500 mg | q12hr | |
| | | | | | 20–39 | 500 mg | q12hr | |
| | | | | | <20 | 250 mg | q24hr | |
| Fluconazole[†] | Renal | 15.2–30 | q24hr | D | ≤50 | 50% ↓ | NI | Y (He)<br>N (P) |
| Flucytosine | Renal | 2.5–7.4 | q6hr | I | 20–40 | NI | q12hr | Y (He) |
| | | | | | 10–20 | NI | q24hr | Y (P) |
| | | | | | <10 | NI | q24–48hr | |
| Foscamet | Renal | 2–4.5 | Induct: q8hr<br>Maint: q24hr | D | See package insert for adjustments for induction and maintenance. | | | Y (He)<br>N (P) |

| Ganciclovir | Renal | 2.5–3.6 | Induct: | DI | *Induction IV* | | | Y (He)§ |
|---|---|---|---|---|---|---|---|---|
| | | | q12hr IV | | 50–69 | 2.5 mg/kg | q12hr | N (P) |
| | | | Maint: | | 25–49 | 2.5 mg/kg | q24hr | |
| | | | q24hr IV | | 10–24 | 1.25 mg/kg | q24hr | |
| | | | OR | | <10 | 1.25 mg/kg | 3 times/wk after He | |
| | | | q8hr PO | | | | | |
| | | | | | *Maintenance IV* | | | |
| | | | | | 50–69 | 2.5 mg/kg | q24hr | |
| | | | | | 25–49 | 1.25 mg/kg | q24hr | |
| | | | | | 10–24 | 0.625 mg/kg | q24hr | |
| | | | | | <10 | 0.625 mg/kg | 3 times/wk after He | |
| | | | | | *Maintenance PO*† | | | |
| | | | | | 50–69 | 1500 mg | q24hr | |
| | | | | | | *OR* 500 mg | q8hr | |
| | | | | | 25–49 | 1000 mg | q24hr | |
| | | | | | | *OR* 500 mg | q12hr | |
| | | | | | 10–24 | 500 mg | q24hr | |
| | | | | | <10 | 500 mg | 3 times/wk after He | |

*Continued*

TABLE 31-1
ANTIMICROBIALS REQUIRING ADJUSTMENT IN RENAL FAILURE—cont'd

| | Pharmacokinetics | | | Adjustments in Renal Failure | | | | |
|---|---|---|---|---|---|---|---|---|
| Drug | Route of Excretion* | Normal $t_{1/2}$ (hr) | Normal Dose Interval | Method | CrCl (mL/min) | Dose | Interval | Supplemental Dose for Dialysis |
| Gentamicin[‖] | Renal | 0.5–5 | q8–24hr | I | 40–60 | NI | q12hr | Y (He) |
| | | | | | 20–40 | NI | q24hr | Y (P)[¶] |
| | | | | | <20 | NI | Monitor levels | |
| Imipenem/ cilastatin | Renal | 1–1.4 | q6–8hr | DI | 41–70 mL/ min/ 1.73 m² | 50% ↓ in max daily dose | q6hr | Y (He) N (P) |
| | | | | | 21–40 mL/ min/ 1.73 m² | 63% ↓ in max daily dose | q8hr | |
| | | | | | 6–20 mL/min/ 1.73 m² | 75% ↓ in max daily dose | q12hr | |
| | | | | | ≤5 mL/min/ 1.73 m² | Should not receive imipenem unless on He. | | |
| Isoniazid | Hepatic (renal) | 2–5 (slow)[#] 0.5–1.5 (fast) | q24hr | D | <10 | 50% ↓ | NI | Y (He) N (P) |
| Kanamycin | Renal | 1.8–5 | q8hr | DI | GFR > 50 mL/min | 10%–40% ↓ | q12hr | Y (He) Y (P)e |
| | | | | | GFR 10–50 mL/min | 30%–70% ↓ | q12–18hr | |
| | | | | | GFR < 10 mL/min | 70%–80% ↓ | q24–48hr | |

| | | | | | | | | |
|---|---|---|---|---|---|---|---|---|
| Lamivudine[†,**] | Renal | 1.4–7 | q12hr | DI | 30–49 | NI | q24hr | Y (He) |
| | | | | | 15–29 | First dose 100%, then 66% | q24hr | N (P) |
| | | | | | 5–14 | First dose 100%, then 33% | q24hr | |
| | | | | | <5 | First dose 33%, then 17% | q24hr | |
| Levofloxacin[†] | Renal (hepatic) | 6–8 | q12–24hr | DI | *500 mg q24hr regimen* | | | N (He) |
| | | | | | 20–49 | First dose 500 mg, then 250 mg | q24hr | N (P) |
| | | | | | 10–19 | First dose 250–500 mg, then 250 mg | q48hr | |
| | | | | | *750 mg q24hr regimen* | | | |
| | | | | | 20–49 | 750 mg | q48hr | |
| | | | | | 10–19 | 500 mg | q48hr | |
| | | | | | *250 mg q24hr regimen* | | | |
| | | | | | 10–19 | 250 mg | q48hr | |
| Loracarbef | Renal | 0.78–1 | q12hr | D, I | 10–49 | 50% ↓ | NI | Y (P) |
| | | | | | *OR* | NI | q24hr | N (P) |
| | | | | | <10 | NI | q3–5 days | |

[||]Subsequent doses best determined by measurement of serum levels and assessment of renal insufficiency.
[¶]May add to peritoneal dialysate to obtain adequate serum levels.
[#]Rate of acetylation of isoniazid.
**GFR ≥5 mL/min: Give full dose as first dose; GFR <5 mL/min: Give 33% of full dose as first dose.

*Continued*

TABLE 31-1

ANTIMICROBIALS REQUIRING ADJUSTMENT IN RENAL FAILURE—cont'd

| | Pharmacokinetics | | | Adjustments in Renal Failure | | | | |
|---|---|---|---|---|---|---|---|---|
| Drug | Route of Excretion* | Normal $t_{1/2}$ (hr) | Normal Dose Interval | Method | CrCl (mL/min) | Dose | Interval | Supplemental Dose for Dialysis |
| Meropenem | Renal | 1–1.5 | q8hr | DI | 26–50 | NI | q12hr | Y (He) |
| | | | | | 10–25 | 50% ↓ | q12hr | N (P) |
| | | | | | <10 | 50% ↓ | q24hr | |
| Metronidazole | Hepatic (renal) | 6–12 | q6–8hr | D | <10 | 50% ↓ | NI | Y (He) N (P) |
| Norfloxacin | Hepatic (renal) | 2–4 | q12hr | I | 10–50 | NI | q12–24hr | N (He) |
| | | | | | <10 | NI | q24hr | N (P) |
| Oseltamivir[†] | Renal | 1–10 | q12–24hr | I | *Treatment of influenza* | | | ? |
| | | | | | 10–30 | 75 mg | q24hr | |
| | | | | | <10 | No recommended dosage regimen. | No recommended dosage regimen. | |
| | | | | | *Prophylaxis of influenza* | | | |
| | | | | | 10–30 | 75 mg | q48hr | |
| | | | | | <10 | No recommended dosage regimen. | No recommended dosage regimen. | |
| Oxacillin | Renal hepatic) | 0.3–1.8 | q4–12hr | D | <10 | Use lower range of usual dose. | NI | N (He) N (P) |

| | | | | | | | | |
|---|---|---|---|---|---|---|---|---|
| Penicillin G–aqueous K⁺ and Na⁺ (IV) | Renal (hepatic) | 0.5–1.2 | q4–6hr | I | 10–30<br><10 | NI<br>NI | q8–12hr<br>q12–18hr | Y (He)<br>N (P) |
| Penicillin V K⁺ (PO) | Renal (hepatic) | 30–40 min | q6hr | I | <10 | NI | q8hr | Y (He)<br>N (P) |
| Pentamidine | Renal | 6.4–9.4 | q24hr | I | 10–30<br><10 | NI<br>NI | q36hr<br>q48hr | N (He)<br>N (P) |
| Piperacillin | Renal (hepatic) | 0.39–1 | q4–6hr | I | 20–40<br><20 | NI<br>NI | q8hr<br>q12hr | Y (He)<br>N (P) |
| Piperacillin/tazobactam | Renal | Piperacillin: 0.39–1<br>Tazobactam: 0.7–1.6 | q6–8hr | DI | 20–40<br><20 | 30% ↓<br>30% ↓ | q6hr<br>q8hr | Y (He)<br>N (P) |
| Rifabutin[†] | Renal (hepatic) | 16–69 | q12–24hr | D | <30 | 50% ↓ | NI | N (He)<br>N (P) |
| Rifampin | Hepatic (renal) | 3–4 | q12–24hr | D | 10–50<br><10 | NI–50% ↓<br>50% ↓ | NI<br>NI | N (He)<br>N (P) |
| Streptomycin sulfate | Renal | 2–4.7 | q24hr | DI | 50–80<br>10–50<br><10 | 7.5 mg/kg<br>7.5 mg/kg<br>7.5 mg/kg | q24hr<br>q24–72hr<br>q72–96hr | Y (He)<br>N (P) |
| Sulfamethoxazole/trimethoprim (cotrimoxazole) | Sulfamethoxazole: Hepatic (renal)<br>Trimethoprim: Renal (hepatic) | Sulfamethoxazole: 9–12<br>Trimethoprim: 6–11 | q12hr | D | 15–30<br><15 | 50% ↓<br>Not recommended. | NI<br>Not recommended. | Y (He)<br>N (P) |

*Continued*

TABLE 31-1

ANTIMICROBIALS REQUIRING ADJUSTMENT IN RENAL FAILURE—cont'd

| | Pharmacokinetics | | | Adjustments in Renal Failure | | | | |
|---|---|---|---|---|---|---|---|---|
| Drug | Route of Excretion* | Normal $t_{1/2}$ (hr) | Normal Dose Interval | Method | CrCl (mL/min) | Dose | Interval | Supplemental Dose for Dialysis |
| Sulfisoxazole | Renal | 4–8 | q6hr | I | 10–50 | NI | q8–12hr | Y (He) |
| | | | | | <10 | NI | q12–24hr | Y (P) |
| Tetracycline | Renal (hepatic) | 6–12 | q6hr | I | 50–80 | NI | q8–12hr | N (He) |
| | | | | | 10–50 | NI | q12–24hr | N (P) |
| | | | | | <10 | NI | q24hr | |
| Ticarcillin[††] | Renal | 0.9–1.3 | q4–6hr IV | I | 10–30 | NI | q8hr | Y (He) |
| | | | q6–8hr IM | | <10 | NI | q12hr | N (P) |
| Ticarcillin/ clavulanate[††] | Renal | Ticarcillin: 0.9–1.3 | q4–6hr | I | 10–30 | NI | q8hr | Y (He) |
| | | Clavulanate: 1–1.5 | | | <10 | NI | q12hr | N (P) |
| | | | | | <10 *AND* hepatic impairment | NI | q24hr | |
| Tobramycin[‖] | Renal | 0.5–5 | q6–8hr | I | Any degree of renal insufficiency | 2.5 mg/kg; subsequent doses determined by levels | Determined by levels | Y (He) Y (P)[¶] |
| Valacyclovir[†] | 88% as acyclovir in urine | Valacyclovir: ~30 min | q12–24hr | DI | <u>*Herpes zoster (adults)*</u> | | | Y (He) |
| | | Acyclovir: 2–3 | | | 30–49 | 1 g | q12hr | N (P) |
| | | | | | 10–29 | 1 g | q24hr | |
| | | | | | <10 | 500 mg | q24hr | |

| | | | | |
|---|---|---|---|---|
| | | *Genital herpes (adol/adults): Initial episode* | | |
| | | 10–29 | 1 g | q24hr |
| | | <10 | 500 mg | q24hr |
| | | *Genital herpes (adol/adults): Recurrent episode* | | |
| | | <10 | 500 mg | q24hr |
| | | *Genital herpes (adol/adults): Suppressive* | | |
| | | <10 | 500 mg | q24hr (for usual dose of 1 g q24hr) |
| | | | *OR* | |
| | | | 500 mg | q48hr (for usual dose of 500 mg q24hr) |
| | | *Herpes labialis (adol/adults)* | | |
| | | 30–49 | 1 g | q12hr × 2 doses |
| | | 10–29 | 500 mg | q12hr × 2 doses |
| | | <10 | 500 mg | Single dose |

[††]May inactivate aminoglycosides in patients with renal impairment.

*Continued*

TABLE 31-1

ANTIMICROBIALS REQUIRING ADJUSTMENT IN RENAL FAILURE—cont'd

| | Pharmacokinetics | | | Adjustments in Renal Failure | | | | |
|---|---|---|---|---|---|---|---|---|
| Drug | Route of Excretion* | Normal $t_{1/2}$ (hr) | Normal Dose Interval | Method | CrCl (mL/min) | Dose | Interval | Supplemental Dose for Dialysis |
| Valganciclovir (see ganciclovir) | | | | | | | | |
| Vancomycin[||] | Renal | 2.2–8 | q6–12hr | I | >90 | NI | q6hr | Y/N (He)[††] |
| | | | | | 70–89 | NI | q8hr | N (P) |
| | | | | | 46–69 | NI | q12hr | |
| | | | | | 30–45 | NI | q18hr | |
| | | | | | 15–29 | NI | q24hr | |
| | | | | | <15 | 10–20 mg/kg | Subsequent doses best determined by levels. | |

[‡‡]If using high-flux hemodialysis (polysulfone polyamide and polyacrylonitrile), give supplemental dose after dialysis.

TABLE 31-2

NONANTIMICROBIALS REQUIRING ADJUSTMENT IN RENAL FAILURE[1]

| | Pharmacokinetics | | | Adjustments in Renal Failure | | | | Supplemental Dose for Dialysis |
|---|---|---|---|---|---|---|---|---|
| Drug | Route of Excretion* | Normal $t_{1/2}$ (hr) | Normal Dose Interval | Method | CrCl (mL/min) | Dose | Interval | |
| Acetaminophen | Hepatic | 2–4 | q4hr | I | 10–50 | NI | q6hr | N (He) |
| | | | | | <10 | NI | q8hr | N (P) |
| Acetazolamide | Renal | 2.4–5.8 | q6–24hr | I | 10–50 | NI | q12hr | ? |
| | | | | | <10 | Avoid use. | | |
| Allopurinol | Renal | 1–3 | q6–12hr | D | 10–50 | 50% ↓ | NI | ? |
| | | | | | <10 | 70% ↓ | NI | |
| Aminocaproic acid | Renal | 1–2 | q4–6hr | D | Oliguria/ESRD | 75% ↓ | NI | ? |
| Aspirin[†] | Hepatic (renal) | 3–10 | q4hr | I | 10–50 | NI | q4–6hr | Y (He) |
| | | | | | <10 | Avoid use. | | N (P) |
| Atenolol | Renal (GI) | 3.5–7 | q24hr | D, I | 15–35 | 1 mg/kg *OR* 50 mg | q24hr | Y (He) N (P) |
| | | | | | <15 | 1 mg/kg *OR* 50 mg | q48hr | |
| Azathioprine[‡] | Hepatic (renal) | 0.7–3 | q24hr | D, I | 10–50 | NI | q36hr | Y (He) |
| | | | | | | *OR* 25% ↓ | NI | ? (P) |
| | | | | | | NI | q48hr | |
| | | | | | <10 | *OR* 50% ↓ | NI | |

*Route in parentheses indicates secondary route of excretion.

[†]With large doses, the $t_{1/2}$ is prolonged up to 30 hr.

[‡]Azathioprine rapidly converted to mercaptopurine ($t_{1/2}$ = 0.5–4 hr).

Continued

TABLE 31-2

**NONANTIMICROBIALS REQUIRING ADJUSTMENT IN RENAL FAILURE—cont'd**

| | Pharmacokinetics | | | Adjustments in Renal Failure | | | | Supplemental Dose for Dialysis |
|---|---|---|---|---|---|---|---|---|
| Drug | Route of Excretion* | Normal $t_{1/2}$ (hr) | Normal Dose Interval | Method | CrCl (mL/min) | Dose | Interval | |
| Bismuth subsalicylate | Hepatic (renal) | Salicylate: 2–5<br>Bismuth: 21–72 days | q3–4hr | D | Avoid use in patients with renal failure. | | | NA |
| Calcium supplements | GI | Variable | Variable | | <25 | May require dosage adjustment depending on calcium level. | | |
| Captopril | Renal (hepatic) | 0.98–12.4 | q6–24hr | D | 10–50<br><10 | 25% ↓<br>50% ↓ | NI<br>NI | Y (He)<br>N (P) |
| Carbamazepine | Hepatic (renal) | Initial: 25–65<br>Subsequent: 8–17 | q6–24hr | D | <10 | 25% ↓ (monitor serum levels) | NI | N (He)<br>N (P) |
| Cetirizine | Renal (hepatic) | 6.2–9 | q12–24hr | D | *<u>≤6 yr with renal impairment</u>*<br>Use not recommended.<br>*<u>6–11 yr</u>*<br>Any degree of Insufficiency<br>*<u>≥12 yr</u>*<br>11–31<br><11 | <br><br><br><2.5 mg<br><br><br>5 mg<br>Use not recommended. | <br><br><br>q24hr<br><br><br>q24hr<br>Use not recommended. | N (He)<br>? (P) |
| Chloral hydrate | Renal | 8–11 | q6–8hr | NA | <50 | Avoid use. | | NA |

| | | | | | | | | |
|---|---|---|---|---|---|---|---|---|
| Chloroquine | Renal (hepatic) | 3–5 days | q6hr–7 days | D | <10 | 50% ↓ | NI | N (He)<br>N (P) |
| Chlorothiazide | Renal | 0.75–2 | q12–24hr | NA | <50 | May be ineffective. Use not recommended. | | NA |
| Cimetidine | Renal (hepatic) | 1.4–2 | q6–12hr | D, I | >40 | NI | q6hr | N (He) |
| | | | | | 20–40 | NI | q8hr | N (P) |
| | | | | | | *OR* 25% ↓ | NI | |
| | | | | | <20 | NI | q12hr | |
| | | | | | | *OR* 50% ↓ | NI | |
| Codeine | Hepatic (renal) | 2.5–3.5 | q4–6hr | D | 10–50 | 25% ↓ | NI | ? |
| | | | | | <10 | 50% ↓ | NI | |
| Desloratadine | Renal (GI) | 27 | q24hr | I | Any degree of renal impairment | NI | q48hr | N (He)<br>N (P) |
| Digoxin[§] | Renal | 18–48 | q12–24hr | D, I | _*Digitalizing dose*_ | | | N (He) |
| | | | | | ESRD | 50% ↓ | NA | N (P) |
| | | | | | _*Maintenance dose*_ | | | |
| | | | | | 10–50 | 25%–75% ↓ | NI | |
| | | | | | | *OR* NI | q36hr | |
| | | | | | <10 | 75%–90% ↓ | NI | |
| | | | | | | *OR* NI | q48hr | |
| Diphen-hydramine | Hepatic | 2–8 | q6–8hr | I | 10–50 | NI | q6–12hr | N (He) |
| | | | | | <10 | NI | q12–18hr | N (P) |

[§]Decrease loading dose by 50% in end-stage renal disease because of decreased volume of distribution.
CrCl, creatinine clearance; GFR, glomerular filtration rate; He, hemodialysis; MDH, 10-monohydroxy metabolite; NA, not applicable; maint, maintenance dose; P, peritoneal dialysis.

*Continued*

TABLE 31-2

NONANTIMICROBIALS REQUIRING ADJUSTMENT IN RENAL FAILURE—cont'd

| | Pharmacokinetics | | | Adjustments in Renal Failure | | | | Supplemental |
|---|---|---|---|---|---|---|---|---|
| Drug | Route of Excretion* | Normal $t_{1/2}$ (hr) | Normal Dose Interval | Method | CrCl (mL/min) | Dose | Interval | Dose for Dialysis |
| Disopyramide[‖] | Renal (GI) | 3.15–10 | q6hr | I | 30–40 | NI | q8hr | N (He) |
| | | | | | 15–30 | NI | q12hr | N (P) |
| | | | | | <15 | NI | q24hr | |
| EDTA calcium chloride[‖] | Renal | 1.5 (IM) | q4hr IM | D, I | *Serum creatinine: IV dose* | | | ? |
| | | 0.3 (IV) | q12hr IV | | ≤2 mg/dL | 1 g/m² | q24hr × 5 days | |
| | | | | | 2–3mg/dL | 500 mg/m² | q24hr × 5 days | |
| | | | | | 3–4mg/dL | 500 mg/m² | q48hr × 3 doses | |
| | | | | | >4 mg/dL | 500 mg/m² | Once weekly | |
| Enalapril (IV: Enalaprilat) | Renal (hepatic) | 1.3–6.3 (PO) | q6–24hr | D | 10–50 | 0%–25% ↓ | NI | Y (He) |
| | | | | | <10 | 50% ↓ | NI | N (P) |
| | | 5.1–38 (IV) | | | Use not recommended in infants and children ≤16 yr with GFR <30 mL/min/1.73m². | | | |
| Enoxaparin[‖,¶] | Renal | 4.5–7 | q12hr | I | <30 | NI | q24hr | ? |
| Famotidine | Renal | 0.8–5 | q8–12hr | D, I | 10–50 | 50% ↓ | NI | N (He) |
| | | | | | | *OR* NI | q24hr | N (P) |
| | | | | | <10 | NI | q36–48hr | |
| Felbamate | Renal | 20–30 | q6–8hr | D | Any degree of renal impairment | 50% ↓ | NI | ? |
| Fentanyl | Renal (hepatic) | 2–4 | q30min–1hr | D | 10–50 | 25% ↓ | NI | NA |
| | | | | | <10 | 50% ↓ | NI | |

| | | | | | | | | |
|---|---|---|---|---|---|---|---|---|
| Fexofenadine | GI (renal) | 14–18 | q12hr | I | Any degree of renal impairment | NI | q24hr | ? |
| Flecainide | Renal/hepatic | 8–27 | q8–12hr | D | <20 | 25%–50% | NI | N (He)<br>N (P) |
| Furosemide | Renal (hepatic) | 0.5 | q6–24hr PO<br>q6–12hr IV | | Avoid use in oliguric states. | | | N (He)<br>N (P) |
| Gabapentin[‖] | Renal (hepatic) | 4.7–9 | q8hr | DI | 30–59<br>15–29<br><15 | 200–700 mg<br>200–700 mg<br>100–300 mg | q12hr<br>q24hr<br>q24hr | Y (He)<br>N (P) |
| Hydralazine[#] | Hepatic (renal) | 2–8 | q4–6hr (IV) | I | 10–50<br><10 | NI<br>NI | q8hr<br>q8–16hr (fast acetylator)<br>q12–24hr (slow acetylator) | N (He)<br>N (P) |
| Insulin (regular)** | Hepatic (renal) | 1.5 | Variable | D | 10–50<br><10 | 25% ↓<br>50%-75% ↓ | NI<br>NI | N (He)<br>N (P) |
| Levetiracetam[‖] | Renal | 5–8 | q12hr | D | *Adults*<br>50–80<br>30–50<br><30<br>ESRD on dialysis | <br>500–1000 mg<br>250–750 mg<br>250–500 mg<br>500–1000 mg | <br>NI<br>NI<br>NI<br>q24hr | Y (He)<br>N (P) |

[‖]Guidelines in adults; guidelines not established in children.
[¶]Monitor antifactor Xa closely.
[#]Dose interval varies for rapid and slow acetylators with normal and impaired renal function.
**Renal failure may cause hyposensitivity or hypersensitivity to insulin; adjust to clinical response and blood glucose.

*Continued*

TABLE 31-2

NONANTIMICROBIALS REQUIRING ADJUSTMENT IN RENAL FAILURE—cont'd

| | Pharmacokinetics | | | Adjustments in Renal Failure | | | | Supplemental |
|---|---|---|---|---|---|---|---|---|
| Drug | Route of Excretion* | Normal $t_{1/2}$ (hr) | Normal Dose Interval | Method | CrCl (mL/min) | Dose | Interval | Dose for Dialysis |
| Lisinopril | Renal | 11–13 | q24hr | D | 10–30<br><10<br>Use not recommended for children with CrCl <30 mL/min/1.73m². | 50% ↓<br>75% ↓ | NI<br>NI | Y (He)<br>N (P) |
| Lithium | Renal | 18–24 | q6–8hr | D | 10–50<br><10 | 25%–50% ↓<br>50%–75% ↓ | NI<br>NI | Y (He)<br>N (P) |
| Loratadine | Renal/hepatic | Loratadine: 8.4<br>Metabolite: 28 | q24hr | I | <30 | NI | q48hr | N (He)<br>N (P) |
| Meperidine | Renal (hepatic)<br>Normeperidine: Renal | 2.3–4 | q3–4hr | D | 10–50<br><10 | 25% ↓<br>50% ↓ | NI<br>NI | ? |
| Methadone | Hepatic (renal) | 4–87 | q3–6hr | D | <10 | 25%–50% ↓ | NI | N (He)<br>N (P) |
| Methyldopa | Hepatic (renal) | 1–3 | q6–12hr PO<br>q6–8hr IV | I | >50<br>10–50<br><10 | NI<br>NI<br>NI | q8hr<br>q8–12hr<br>q12–24hr | Y (He)<br>N (P) |
| Metoclopramide | Renal | 2.5–6 | q6hr PO<br>q6–8hr IV | D | 40–50<br>10–40<br><10 | 25% ↓<br>50% ↓<br>50%–75% ↓ | NI<br>NI<br>NI | N (He)<br>? (P) |
| Midazolam | Hepatic (renal) | 2.2–6.8 | Variable | D | <10 | 50% ↓ | NI | NA |

| | | | | | | | | |
|---|---|---|---|---|---|---|---|---|
| Milrinone | Renal | 1.5–3.8 | Continuous infusion | D | 50 mL/min/1.73 $m^2$<br>40 mL/min/1.73 $m^2$<br>30 mL/min/1.73 $m^2$<br>20 mL/min/1.73 $m^2$<br>10 mL/min/1.73 $m^2$<br>5 mL/min/1.73$m^2$ | 0.43 mcg/kg/min<br>0.38 mcg/kg/min<br>0.33 mcg/kg/min<br>0.28 mcg/kg/min<br>0.23 mcg/kg/min<br>0.2 mcg/kg/min | NA<br>NA<br>NA<br>NA<br>NA<br>NA | NA |
| Morphine | Hepatic (renal) | 1–6.2 | Variable | D | 10–50<br><10 | 25% ↓<br>50% ↓ | NI<br>NI | N (He)<br>? (P) |
| Neostigmine | Hepatic (renal) | 0.5–2.1 | Variable | D | 10–50<br><10 | 50% ↓<br>75% ↓ | NI<br>NI | ? |
| Oxcarbazepine | Renal | Oxcarbazepine: 2<br>MHD: 9 | q12hr | D | <30 | 50% ↓ in initial dose and slower titration | NI | ? |
| Pancuronium bromide | Renal (hepatic) | 1.8 | q30–60min OR continuous infusion | D | 10–50<br><10 | 50% ↓<br>Avoid use. | NI | ? |
| Phenazopyridine | Renal (hepatic) | ? | q8hr for 2 days | I | 50–80<br><50 | NI<br>Avoid use. | q8–16hr | NA |
| Phenobarbital | Hepatic (renal, 30%) | 37–120 | q8–12hr | I | <10 | NI | q12–16hr | Y (He)<br>Y (P) |

*Continued*

TABLE 31-2

NONANTIMICROBIALS REQUIRING ADJUSTMENT IN RENAL FAILURE—cont'd

| | Pharmacokinetics | | | Adjustments in Renal Failure | | | | Supplemental Dose for Dialysis |
|---|---|---|---|---|---|---|---|---|
| Drug | Route of Excretion* | Normal $t_{1/2}$ (hr) | Normal Dose Interval | Method | CrCl (mL/min) | Dose | Interval | |
| Primidone | Hepatic (renal, 20%) | Primidone: 10–12<br>Metabolite: 16 | q6–12hr | I | >50 | NI | q8hr | Y (He) |
| | | | | | 10–50 | NI | q8–12hr | ? (P) |
| | | | | | <10 | NI | q12–24hr | |
| Procainamide | Hepatic (renal) | Procainamide: 1.7–4.7<br>NAPA: 6–8 | q3–6hr PO<br>q4–6hr IM | I | *Oral* | | | Y (He) |
| | | | | | 10–50 | NI | q6–12hr | N (P) |
| | | | | | <10 | NI | q8–24hr | |
| | | | | | *IV (adult) maintenance* | | | |
| | | | | | 10–50 | 33% ↓ | NI | |
| | | | | | <10 | 67% ↓ | NI | |
| | | | | | *IV (adult) loading dose* | | | |
| | | | | | Severe renal impairment | 12 mg/kg | NA | |
| Propylthiouracil | Hepatic (renal) | 1.5–5 | q8–12hr | D | GFR 10–50 | 25% ↓ | NI | ? |
| | | | | | GFR < 10 | 50% ↓ | NI | |

| | | | | | | | | |
|---|---|---|---|---|---|---|---|---|
| Quinidine | Renal | 2.5–8 | q4–12hr | D | <10 | 25% ↓ | NI | Y (He)<br>N (P) |
| Ranitidine | Renal (hepatic) | 1.8–2.5 | q12hr PO<br>q6–8hr IV/IM | D | 10–50<br><10 | 50% ↓<br>75% ↓ | NI<br>NI | N (He)[††]<br>N (P) |
| Spironolactone | Renal (hepatic) | Spironolactone: 1.3–1.4<br>Canrenone: 13–24 | q6–24hr | I | 10–50<br><10 | NI<br>Avoid use. | q12–24hr | NA |
| Terbutaline (IV/PO) | Renal (hepatic) | 2.9–14 | Variable | D | GFR: 10–50 mL/min<br>GFR < 10 mL/min | 50% ↓<br>Avoid use. | NI | ? |
| Thiopental | Hepatic (renal) | 3–11.5 | One-time dose | D | <10 | 25% ↓ | NI | NA |
| Triamterene | Hepatic (renal) | 1.6–2.5 | q12–24hr | I | 10–50<br><10 | NI<br>Avoid use. | q12hr[‡‡] | NA |
| Verapamil | Renal (hepatic) | 2–8 | Variable | D | <10 | 25%–50% ↓ | NI | N (He)<br>N (P) |

[††]Adjust dose schedule to administer dose at the end of dialysis.

## REFERENCES


1. Taketomo C, et al: Pediatric Dosage Handbook, 14th ed. Hudson, Ohio, Lexi-Comp, 2007–2008.
2. American Society of Health-System Pharmacists: American Hospital Formulary Service. Bethesda, Md, The Society, 1998.
3. Johnson C, Simmons W: Dialysis of drugs. Pharm Practice News 1988;(Dec):30–33.
4. Micromedex Healthcare Series (electronic version). Thomson Micromedex, Greenwood Village, Colo. Available at http://www.thomsonhc.com. Accessed October 25, 2007.
5. Aronoff G et al: Drug prescribing in renal failure: Dosing guidelines for adults, 4th ed. Philadelphia, American College of Physicians, 1999.

# Index

Note: Page numbers followed by f indicate figures, page numbers followed by t indicate tables, and page numbers followed by b indicate boxed material. Entries in *italics* indicate color plates.

## A

**B**

## E

**J**

## O

**S**

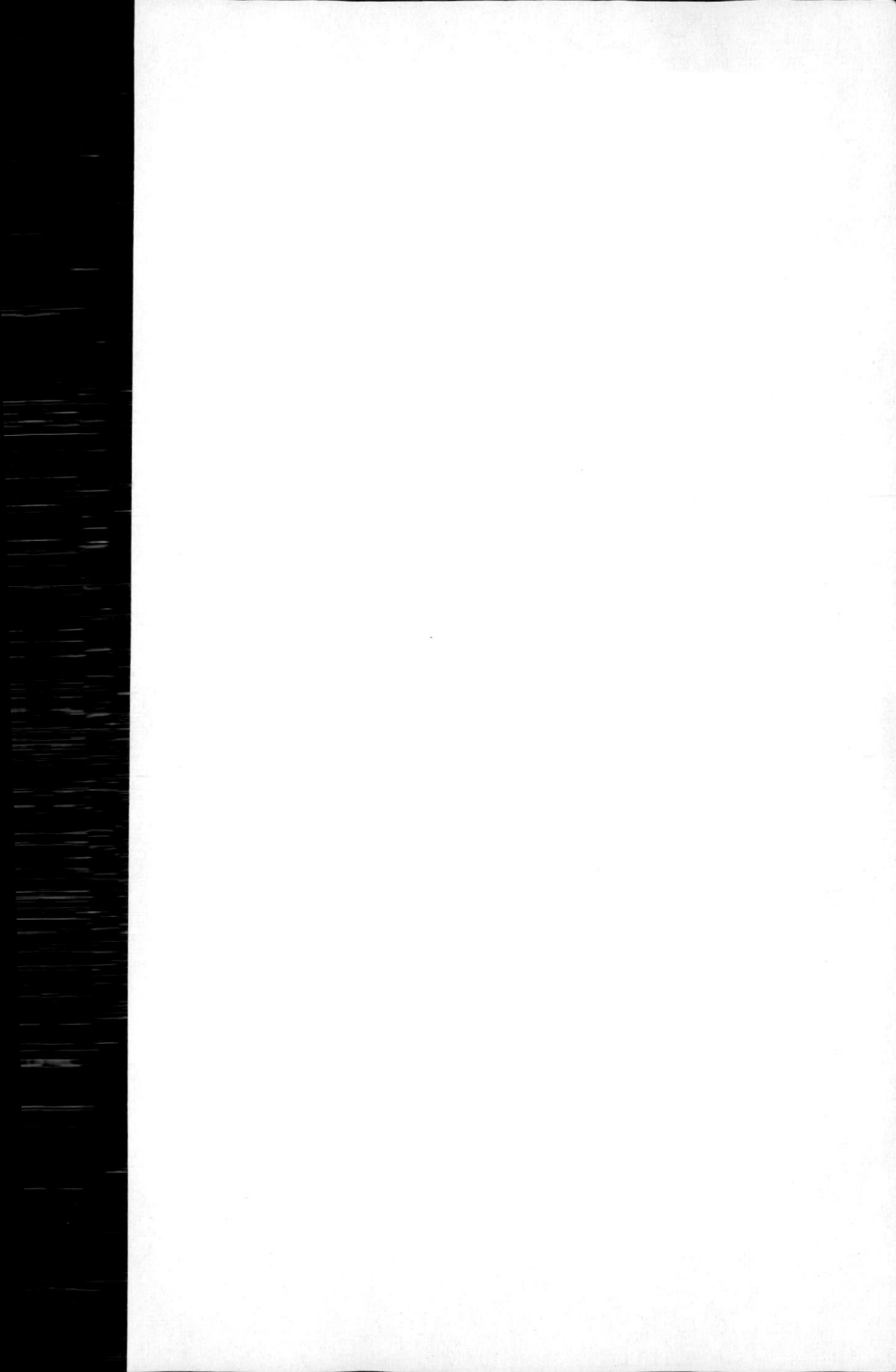

CUSTER, JASON W.
THE HARRIET LANE
HANDBOOK - 18th EDITION

## CLASSIFYING ASTHMA SEVERITY AND INITIATING TREATMENT IN CHILDREN 5–11 YEARS OF AGE

Assessing severity and initiating therapy in children who are not currently taking long-term control medication

| Components of severity | | Classification of asthma severity (5–11 years of age) | | | |
|---|---|---|---|---|---|
| | | | Persistent | | |
| | | **Intermittent** | **Mild** | **Moderate** | **Severe** |
| **Impairment** | Symptoms | ≤2 days/week | >2 days/week but not daily | Daily | Throughout the day |
| | Nighttime awakenings | ≤2×/month | 3–4×/month | >1×/week but not nightly | Often 7×/week |
| | Short-acting $beta_2$-agonist use for symptom control (not prevention of EIB) | ≤2 days/week | >2 days/week but not daily | Daily | Several times per day |
| | Interference with normal activity | None | Minor limitation | Some limitation | Extremely limited |
| | Lung function | • Normal $FEV_1$ between exacerbations<br>• $FEV_1$ >80% predicted<br>• $FEV_1$/FVC >85% | • $FEV_1$ = >80% predicted<br>• $FEV_1$/FVC >80% | • $FEV_1$ = 60%–80% predicted<br>• $FEV_1$/FVC = 75%–80% | • $FEV_1$ <60% predicted<br>• $FEV_1$/FVC <75% |
| **Risk** | Exacerbations requiring oral systemic corticosteroids | 0–1/year (see note) | ≥2/year (see note) → | | |
| | | ← Consider severity and interval since last exacerbation. Frequency and severity may fluctuate over time for patients in any severity category. → | | | |
| | | Relative annual risk of exacerbations may be related to $FEV_1$. | | | |
| **Recommended step for initiating therapy** | | Step 1 | Step 2 | Step 3, medium-dose ICS option | Step 3, medium-dose ICS option, or step 4 |
| | | | | and consider short course of oral systemic corticosteroids | |
| **(See next page for treatment steps.)** | | In 2–6 weeks, evaluate level of asthma control that is achieved, and adjust therapy accordingly. | | | |

Key: EIB, exercise-induced bronchospasm; $FEV_1$, forced expiratory volume in 1 second; FVC, forced vital capacity; ICS, inhaled corticosteroids

**Notes**

- The stepwise approach is meant to assist, not replace, the clinical decision making required to meet individual patient needs.
- Level of severity is determined by both impairment and risk. Assess impairment domain by patient's/caregiver's recall of previous 2–4 weeks and spirometry. Assign severity to the most severe category in which any feature occurs.
- At present, there are inadequate data to correspond frequencies of exacerbations with different levels of asthma severity. In general, more frequent and intense exacerbations (e.g., requiring urgent, unscheduled care, hospitalization, or ICU admission) indicate greater underlying disease severity. For treatment purposes, patients who had ≥2 exacerbations requiring oral systemic corticosteroids in the past year may be considered the same as patients who have persistent asthma, even in the absence of impairment levels consistent with persistent asthma.

*From NAEPP—Expert Panel Report 3: Guidelines for the diagnosis and management of asthma, August 2007. Available at www.nhlbi.nih.gov/guidelines/asthma/asthgdln.htm.*

## STEPWISE APPROACH FOR MANAGING ASTHMA IN CHILDREN 5–11 YEARS OF AGE

| Intermittent asthma | Persistent asthma: Daily medication. Consult with asthma specialist if step 4 care or higher is required. Consider consultation at step 3. | | | | | |
|---|---|---|---|---|---|---|
| **Step 1** | **Step 2** | **Step 3** | **Step 4** | **Step 5** | **Step 6** | Step up if needed (first, check adherence, inhaler technique, environmental control, and comorbid conditions) ↑ |
| *Preferred:* SABA PRN | *Preferred:* Low-dose ICS<br>*Alternative:* Cromolyn, LTRA, Nedocromil, or Theophylline | *Preferred:* EITHER: Low-dose ICS + either LABA, LTRA, or Theophylline<br>OR<br>Medium-dose ICS | *Preferred:* Medium-dose ICS + LABA<br>*Alternative:* Medium-dose ICS + either LTRA or Theophylline | *Preferred:* High-dose ICS + LABA<br>*Alternative:* High-dose ICS + either LTRA or Theophylline | *Preferred:* High-dose ICS + LABA + oral systemic corticosteroid<br>*Alternative:* High-dose ICS + either LTRA or Theophylline + oral systemic corticosteroid | *Assess control*<br>Step down if possible (and asthma is well controlled at least 3 months) ↓ |

Each step: Patient education, environmental control, and management of comorbidities.
Steps 2–4: Consider subcutaneous allergen immunotherapy for patients who have allergic asthma (see notes).

Quick-relief medication for all patients

- SABA as needed for symptoms. Intensity of treatment depends on severity of symptoms: up to 3 treatments at 20-minute intervals as needed. Short course of oral systemic corticosteroids may be needed.
- Caution: Increasing use of SABA or use >2 days a week for symptom relief (not prevention of EIB) generally indicates inadequate control and the need to step up treatment.

Key: **Alphabetical order is used when more than one treatment option is listed within either preferred or alternative therapy.** ICS, inhaled corticosteroid; LABA, long-acting inhaled beta$_2$-agonist; LTRA, leukotriene receptor antagonist; SABA, short-acting inhaled beta$_2$-agonist

Notes:

- The stepwise approach is meant to assist, not replace, the clinical decision making required to meet individual patient needs.
- If alternative treatment is used and response is inadequate, discontinue it and use the preferred treatment before stepping up.
- Theophylline is a less desirable alternative due to the need to monitor serum concentration levels.
- Step 1 and step 2 medications are based on Evidence A. Step 3 ICS + adjunctive therapy and ICS are based on Evidence B for efficacy of each treatment and extrapolation from comparator trials in older children and adults—comparator trials are not available for this age group; steps 4–6 are based on expert opinion and extrapolation from studies in older children and adults.
- Immunotherapy for steps 2–4 is based on Evidence B for house-dust mites, animal danders, and pollens; evidence is weak or lacking for molds and cockroaches. Evidence is strongest for immunotherapy with single allergens. The role of allergy in asthma is greater in children than in adults. Clinicians who administer immunotherapy should be prepared and equipped to identify and treat anaphylaxis that may occur.

*From NAEPP—Expert Panel Report 3: Guidelines for the diagnosis and management of asthma, August 2007. Available at www.nhlbi.nih.gov/guidelines/asthma/asthgdln.htm.*

## CLASSIFYING ASTHMA SEVERITY AND INITIATING TREATMENT IN YOUTHS ≥12 YEARS OF AGE

Assessing severity and initiating treatment for patients who are not currently taking long-term control medications

| Components of severity | | Classification of asthma severity ≥12 years of age | | | |
|---|---|---|---|---|---|
| | | | Persistent | | |
| | | Intermittent | Mild | Moderate | Severe |
| Impairment<br><br>Normal $FEV_1$/FVC:<br>8–19 yr 85%<br>20–39 yr 80%<br>40–59 yr 75%<br>60–80 yr 70% | Symptoms | ≤2 days/week | >2 days/week but not daily | Daily | Throughout the day |
| | Nighttime awakenings | ≤2×/month | 3–4×/month | >1×/week but not nightly | Often 7×/week |
| | Short-acting beta$_2$-agonist use for symptom control (not prevention of EIB) | ≤2 days/week | >2 days/week but not daily, and not more than 1 time on any day | Daily | Several times per day |
| | Interference with normal activity | None | Minor limitation | Some limitation | Extremely limited |
| | Lung function | • Normal $FEV_1$ between exacerbations<br>• $FEV_1$ >80% predicted<br>• $FEV_1$/FVC normal | • $FEV_1$ >80% predicted<br>• $FEV_1$/FVC normal | • $FEV_1$ >60% but <80% predicted<br>• $FEV_1$/FVC reduced 5% | • $FEV_1$ <60% predicted<br>• $FEV_1$/FVC reduced >5% |
| Risk | Exacerbations requiring oral systemic corticosteroids | 0–1/year (see note) | ≥2/year (see note) → | | |
| | | ← Consider severity and interval since last exacerbation. Frequency and severity may fluctuate over time for patients in any severity category. → | | | |
| | | Relative annual risk of exacerbations may be related to $FEV_1$ | | | |
| Recommended step for initiating treatment | | Step 1 | Step 2 | Step 3 and consider short course of oral systemic corticosteroids | Step 4 or 5 and consider short course of oral systemic corticosteroids |
| (See next page for treatment steps.) | | In 2–6 weeks, evaluate level of asthma control that is achieved and adjust therapy accordingly. | | | |

Key: $FEV_1$, forced expiratory volume in 1 second; FVC, forced vital capacity; ICU, intensive care unit

**Notes**

- The stepwise approach is meant to assist, not replace, the clinical decision making required to meet individual patient needs.
- Level of severity is determined by both impairment and risk. Assess impairment domain by patient's/caregiver's recall of previous 2–4 weeks and spirometry. Assign severity to the most severe category in which any feature occurs.
- At present, there are inadequate data to correspond frequencies of exacerbations with different levels of asthma severity. In general, more frequent and intense exacerbations (e.g., requiring urgent, unscheduled care, hospitalization, or ICU admission) indicate greater underlying disease severity. For treatment purposes, patients who had ≥2 exacerbations requiring oral systemic corticosteroids in the past year may be considered the same as patients who have persistent asthma, even in the absence of impairment levels consistent with persistent asthma.

*From NAEPP—Expert Panel Report 3: Guidelines for the diagnosis and management of asthma, August 2007. Available at www.nhlbi.nih.gov/guidelines/asthma/asthgdln.htm.*

## STEPWISE APPROACH FOR MANAGING ASTHMA IN YOUTH ≥12 YEARS OF AGE AND ADULTS

| Intermittent asthma | Persistent asthma: Daily medication<br>Consult with asthma specialist if step 4 care or higher is required.<br>Consider consultation at step 3. | | | | |
|---|---|---|---|---|---|
| **Step 1** | **Step 2** | **Step 3** | **Step 4** | **Step 5** | **Step 6** |
| *Preferred:*<br>SABA PRN | *Preferred:*<br>Low-dose ICS<br>*Alternative:*<br>Cromolyn, LTRA, Nedocromil, or Theophylline | *Preferred:*<br>Low-dose ICS + either LABA, OR Medium-dose ICS<br>*Alternative:*<br>Low-dose ICS + either LTRA, Theophylline, or Zileuton | *Preferred:*<br>Medium-dose ICS + LABA<br>*Alternative:*<br>Medium-dose ICS + either LTRA, Theophylline, or Zileuton | *Preferred:*<br>High-dose ICS + LABA<br>AND<br>Consider Omalizumab for patients who have allergies | *Preferred:*<br>High-dose ICS + LABA + oral corticosteroid<br>AND<br>Consider Omalizumab for patients who have allergies |

↑ Step up if needed

(first, check adherence, environmental control, and comorbid conditions)

*Assess control*

Step down if possible

(and asthma is well controlled at least 3 months) ↓

Each step: Patient education, environmental control, and management of comorbidities.

Steps 2–4: Consider subcutaneous allergen immunotherapy for patients who have allergic asthma (see notes).

Quick-relief medication for all patients

- SABA as needed for symptoms. Intensity of treatment depends on severity of symptoms: up to 3 treatments at 20-minute intervals as needed. Short course of oral systemic corticosteroids may be needed.
- Use of SABA >2 days a week for symptom relief (not prevention of EIB) generally indicates inadequate control and the need to step up treatment.

Key: **Alphabetical order is used when more than one treatment option is listed within either preferred or alternative therapy**. EIB, exercise-induced bronchospasm; ICS, inhaled corticosteroid; LABA, long-acting inhaled beta$_2$-agonist; LTRA, leukotriene receptor antagonist; SABA, short-acting inhaled beta$_2$-agonist

Notes:

- The stepwise approach is meant to assist, not replace, the clinical decision making required to meet individual patient needs.
- If alternative treatment is used and response is inadequate, discontinue it and use the preferred treatment before stepping up.
- Zileuton is a less desirable alternative due to limited studies as adjunctive therapy and the need to monitor liver function. Theophylline requires monitoring of serum concentration levels.
- In step 6, before oral systemic corticosteroids are introduced, a trial of high-dose ICS + LABA + either LTRA, theophylline, or zileuton may be considered, although this approach has not been studied in clinical trials.
- Step 1, 2, and 3 preferred therapies are based on Evidence A; step 3 alternative therapy is based on Evidence A for LTRA, Evidence B for theophylline, and Evidence D for zileuton. Step 4 preferred therapy is based on Evidence B, and alternative therapy is based on Evidence B for LTRA and theophylline and Evidence D for zileuton. Step 5 preferred therapy is based on Evidence B. Step 6 preferred therapy is based on Expert Panel Report 2 (1997) and Evidence B for omalizumab.
- Immunotherapy for steps 2–4 is based on Evidence B for house-dust mites, animal danders, and pollens; evidence is weak or lacking for molds and cockroaches. Evidence is strongest for immunotherapy with single allergens. The role of allergy in asthma is greater in children than in adults.
- Clinicians who administer immunotherapy or omalizumab should be prepared and equipped to identify and treat anaphylaxis that may occur.

*From NAEPP—Expert Panel Report 3: Guidelines for the diagnosis and management of asthma, August 2007. Available at www.nhlbi.nih.gov/guidelines/asthma/asthgdln.htm.*

PEDIATRIC BASIC LIFE SUPPORT ALGORITHM

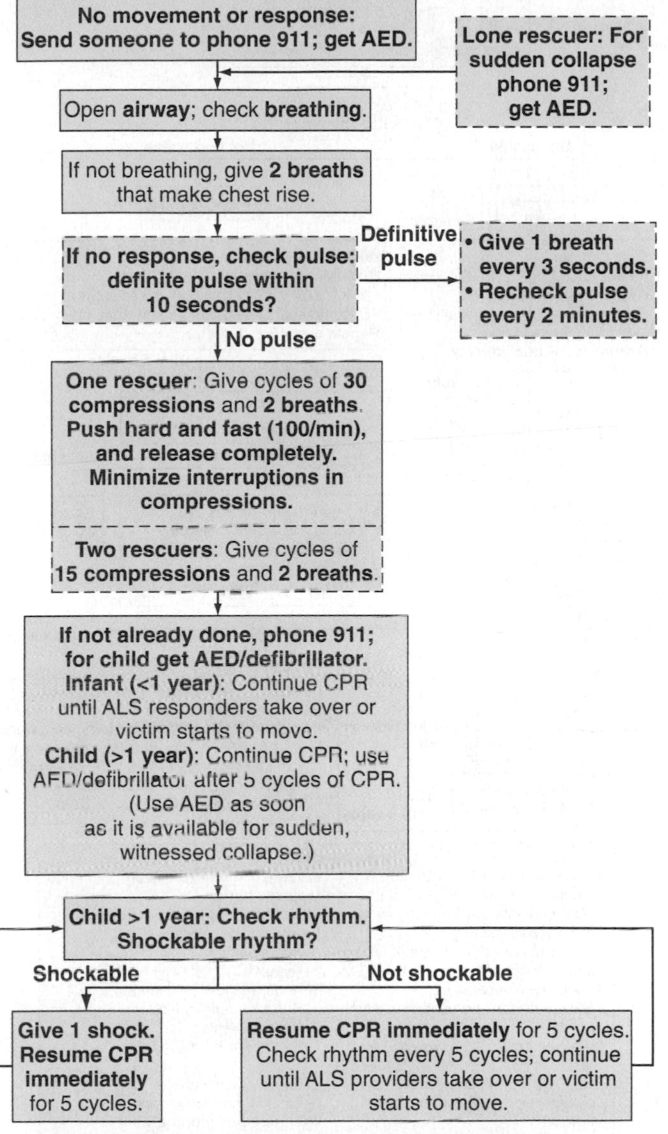


From 2005 American Heart Association Guidelines for Cardiopulmonary Resuscitation and Emergency Cardiovascular Care. Part 11: Pediatric Basic Life Support. Circulation 2005;112:156–166.

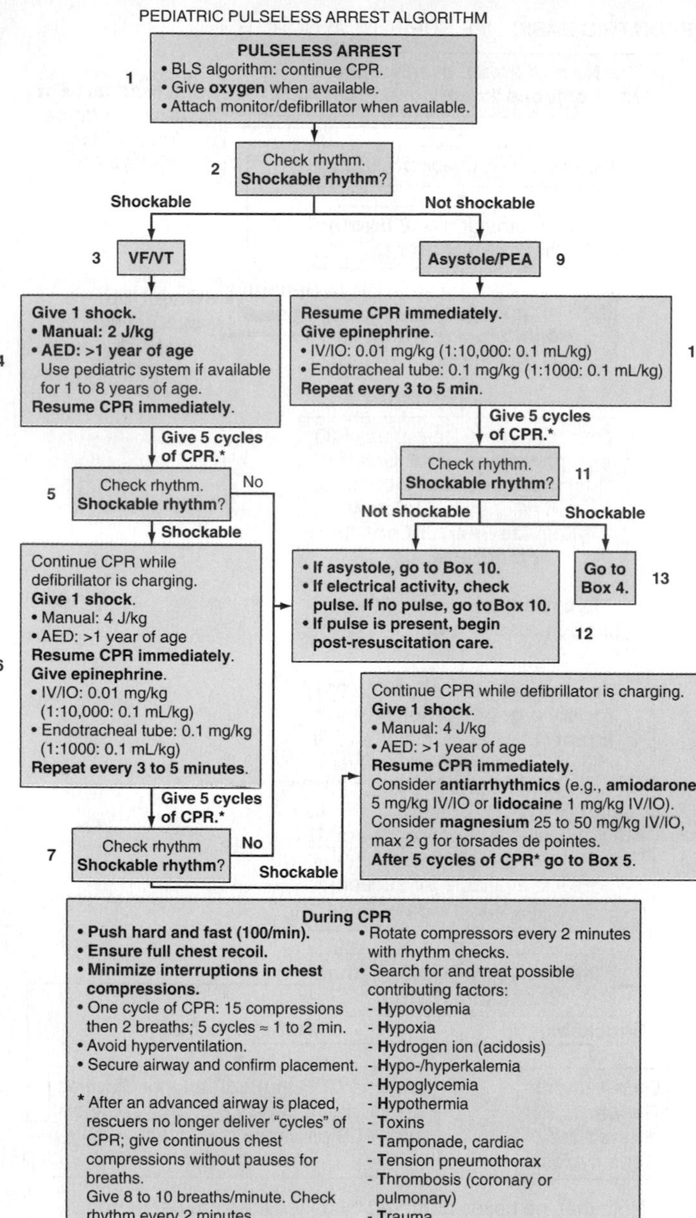


From 2005 American Heart Association Guidelines for Cardiopulmonary Resuscitation and Emergency Cardiovascular Care. Part 12: Pediatric Advanced Life Support. Circulation 2005;112:167–187.

PEDIATRIC BRADYCARDIA ALGORITHM

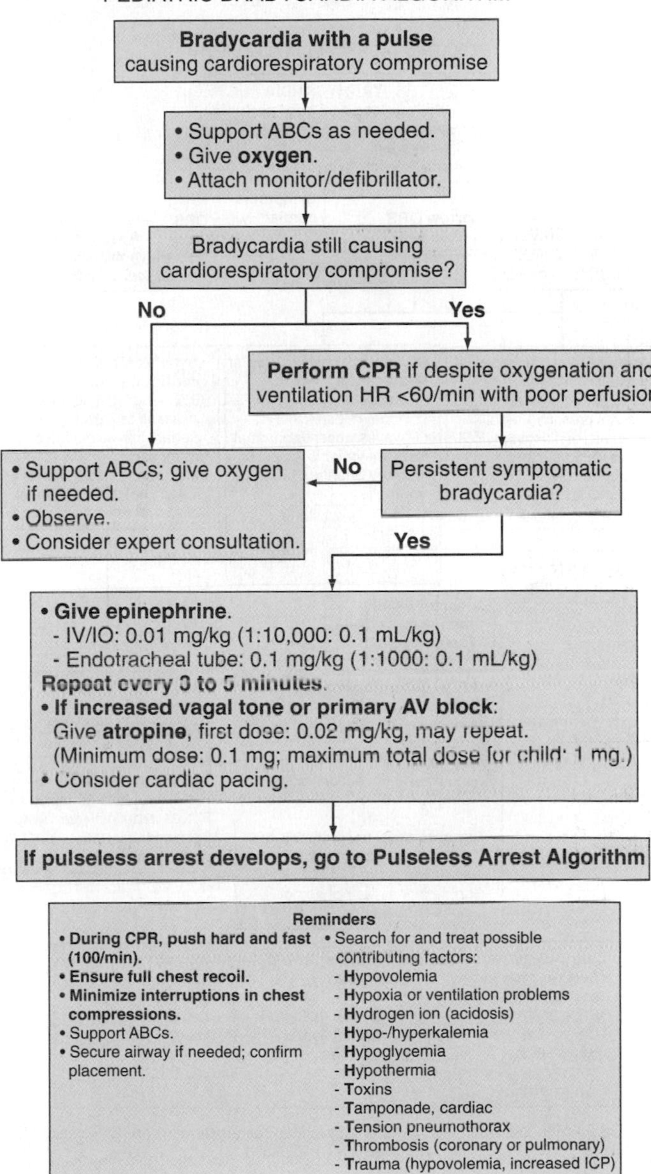

**Bradycardia with a pulse**
causing cardiorespiratory compromise
• Support ABCs as needed.
• Give **oxygen**.
• Attach monitor/defibrillator.
Bradycardia still causing cardiorespiratory compromise?
No
Yes
**Perform CPR** if despite oxygenation and ventilation HR <60/min with poor perfusion.
• Support ABCs; give oxygen if needed.
• Observe.
• Consider expert consultation.
No
Persistent symptomatic bradycardia?
Yes
• **Give epinephrine.**
- IV/IO: 0.01 mg/kg (1:10,000: 0.1 mL/kg)
- Endotracheal tube: 0.1 mg/kg (1:1000: 0.1 mL/kg)
**Repeat every 3 to 5 minutes.**
• **If increased vagal tone or primary AV block**:
Give **atropine**, first dose: 0.02 mg/kg, may repeat.
(Minimum dose: 0.1 mg; maximum total dose for child: 1 mg.)
• Consider cardiac pacing.
**If pulseless arrest develops, go to Pulseless Arrest Algorithm**
**Reminders**
• **During CPR, push hard and fast (100/min).**
• **Ensure full chest recoil.**
• **Minimize interruptions in chest compressions.**
• Support ABCs.
• Secure airway if needed; confirm placement.
• Search for and treat possible contributing factors:
- **H**ypovolemia
- **H**ypoxia or ventilation problems
- **H**ydrogen ion (acidosis)
- **H**ypo-/hyperkalemia
- **H**ypoglycemia
- **H**ypothermia
- **T**oxins
- **T**amponade, cardiac
- **T**ension pneumothorax
- **T**hrombosis (coronary or pulmonary)
- **T**rauma (hypovolemia, increased ICP)

From 2005 American Heart Association Guidelines for Cardiopulmonary Resuscitation and Emergency Cardiovascular Care. Part 12: Pediatric Advanced Life Support. Circulation 2005;112:167–187.

PEDIATRIC TACHYCARDIA ALGORITHM

**TACHYCARDIA**
**With pulses and poor perfusion**
- Assess and support ABCs as needed
- Give **oxygen**
- Attach monitor/defibrillator

↓ **Symptoms persist**

**Evaluate QRS duration**

**Narrow QRS (≤0.08 sec)** → **Evaluate rhythm with 12-lead ECG or monitor**

**Wide QRS (>0.08 sec)** → **Possible ventricular tachycardia**

From "Evaluate rhythm with 12-lead ECG or monitor":

**Probable Sinus Tachycardia**
- Compatible history consistent with known cause
- P waves present/normal
- Variables R-R; constant P-R
- Infants: rate usually <220 bpm
- Children: rate usually <180 bpm

↓ **Search for and treat cause**

**Probable Supraventricular Tachycardia**
- Compatible history (vague, nonspecific)
- P waves absent/abnormal
- HR not variable
- History of abrupt rate changes
- Infants: rate usually ≥220 bpm
- Children: rate usually ≥180 bpm

**Consider vagal maneuvers (no delays)** →

↓

- **If IV access readily available:**
  **Give adenosine** 0.1 mg/kg (maximum first dose 6 mg) by rapid bolus
  May double first dose and give once (maximum second dose 12 mg)

  **or**
- **Synchronized cardioversion:**
  0.5 to 1 J/kg: if not effective, increase to 2 J/kg
  Sedate if possible but do not delay cardioversion

→ Expert consultation advised

From "Possible ventricular tachycardia":

- **Synchronized cardioversion:**
  0.5 to 1 J/kg; if not effective, increase to 2 J/kg
  Sedate if possible but don't delay cardioversion
- May attempt **adenosine** if it does not delay electrical cardioversion

↓

**Expert consultation advised**
- **Amiodarone** 5 mg/kg IV over 20 to 60 minutes

  **or**
- **Procainamide** 15 mg/kg IV over 30 to 60 minutes

Do not routinely administer amiodarone and procainamide together

***During Evaluation***
- Secure, verify airway and vascular access when possible
- Consider expert consultation
- Prepare for cardioversion

***Treat Possible Contributing Factors:***
- **H**ypovolemia
- **H**ypoxia
- **H**ydrogen ion (acidosis)
- **H**ypo-/hyperkalemia
- **H**ypoglycemia
- **H**ypothermia
- **T**oxins
- **T**amponade, cardiac
- **T**ension pneumothorax
- **T**hrombosis (coronary or pulmonary)
- **T**rauma (hypovolemia)

From 2005 American Heart Association Guidelines for Cardiopulmonary Resuscitation and Emergency Cardiovascular Care. Part 12: Pediatric Advanced Life Support. Circulation 2005;112:167–187.